Core Curriculum for
Neonatal Intensive Care Nursing

Core Curriculum for
Neonatal Intensive Care Nursing

Fourth Edition

Edited by

M. Terese Verklan, PhD, CCNS, RNC
Associate Professor, Neonatal Clinical Nurse Specialist
University of Texas Health Science Center at Houston
Houston, Texas

Marlene Walden, PhD, RN, NNP-BC, CCNS
Professor, Clinical Nursing
Director, Neonatal Nurse Practitioner Program
The University of Texas

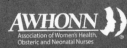
AWHONN
Association of Women's Health,
Obstetric and Neonatal Nurses

AMERICAN
ASSOCIATION
of CRITICAL-CARE
NURSES

SAUNDERS

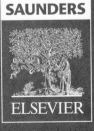

ELSEVIER

National
Association of
Neonatal
Nurses

BP45

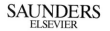

SAUNDERS
ELSEVIER

11830 Westline Industrial Drive
St. Louis, Missouri 63146

CORE CURRICULUM FOR NEONATAL INTENSIVE CARE NURSING   ISBN: 978-1-4377-0260-6
Copyright © 2010, 2004, 1999, 1993 by Saunders, an imprint of Elsevier Inc.

Notice

Knowledge and best practice in this field are constantly changing. As new research and experience broaden our knowledge, changes in practice, treatment and drug therapy may become necessary or appropriate. Readers are advised to check the most current information provided (i) on procedures featured or (ii) by the manufacturer of each product to be administered, to verify the recommended dose or formula, the method and duration of administration, and contraindications. It is the responsibility of the practitioner, relying on their own experience and knowledge of the patient, to make diagnoses, to determine dosages and the best treatment for each individual patient, and to take all appropriate safety precautions. To the fullest extent of the law, neither the publisher nor the editors assume any liability for any injury and/or damage to persons or property arising out of or related to any use of the material contained in this book.

Library of Congress Cataloging-in-Publication Data

Core curriculum for neonatal intensive care nursing / edited by M. Terese Verklan, Marlene Walden.—4th ed.
    p. ; cm.
    Includes bibliographical references and index.
    ISBN 978-1-4377-0260-6 (pbk. : alk. paper)   1. Neonatal intensive care—Outlines, syllabi, etc.   I. Verklan, M. Terese.   II. Walden, Marlene, 1956-
    [DNLM: 1. Neonatal Nursing—methods—Outlines.   2. Intensive Care, Neonatal—methods—Outlines.   WY 18.2 C7968 2010]
    RJ253.5.C67 2010
    618.92'01—dc22

                                                    2009000759

Managing Editor: Michele D. Hayden
Senior Developmental Editor: Laurie K. Gower
Publishing Services Manager: Deborah L. Vogel
Project Manager: Pat Costigan
Book Designer: Amy Buxton

Printed in the United States of America

Last digit is the print number: 9 8 7 6 5 4 3 2 1

Working together to grow
libraries in developing countries

www.elsevier.com | www.bookaid.org | www.sabre.org

ELSEVIER   BOOK AID International   Sabre Foundation

10/2/09

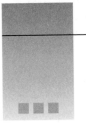

Foreword

Continuing the unique partnership that began in 1996, the Association of Women's Health, Obstetric and Neonatal Nurses; the National Association of Neonatal Nurses; and the American Association of Critical-Care Nurses have collaborated once again on this fourth edition of the *Core Curriculum for Neonatal Intensive Care Nursing*.

We applaud the efforts of editors Terese Verklan and Marlene Walden, as well as the many clinician experts who contributed and reviewed neonatal nursing content. We appreciate and recognize the commitment to professional collegiality and dedication to providing high-quality nursing care for critically ill infants and their families that made this book possible.

Kim L. Armour, CNP, APN, RDMS, MSN
President, Association of Women's Health, Obstetric and Neonatal Nurses

Peggy Gordin, MS, RN, NEA-BC, FAAN
President, National Association of Neonatal Nurses

Caryl Goodyear-Bruch, RN, PhD, CCRN
President, American Association of Critical-Care Nurses

To Mom and Dad, Cindy, Paul, and Theresa George—thank you for showing me I have no boundaries.
MTV

To my loving parents, Bobby and Wanda; my brother, Michael; and my sister, Sharlene. Also to my professional colleagues who teach me so much; but most important, to the babies and families who have taught me the art of neonatal nursing.
MW

Contributors

Debra C. Armentrout, RNC, NNP, PhD
Assistant Professor, Pediatrics
University of Texas Health Science Center
Houston, Texas

Debbie Fraser Askin, MN, RNC
Associate Professor, Faculty of Nursing
University of Manitoba
Neonatal Nurse Practitioner
St. Boniface General Hospital
Winnipeg, Manitoba, Canada

Teresa Bailey, RNC, MSN, APN
Neonatal Nurse Practitioner
Pediatrix Medical Group
Austin, Texas

Kathleen Benjamin, BSN, MSN, NNP-BC
Neonatal Nurse Practitioner
The Children's Hospital
Aurora, Colorado

Carol Botwinski, BS, MS, EdD, ARNP,
NNP-BC
Assistant Professor, Nursing
University of Tampa
Tampa, Florida

S. Louise Bowen, RNC, MSN, ARNP, CMTE,
CNA, BC
Director, Transport Services
All Children's Hospital
St. Petersburg, Florida

Holly A. Boyd, RN, MSN, NNP-BC
Neonatal Nurse Practitioner
Texas Children's Hospital
Houston, Texas

Wanda Todd Bradshaw, RNC, MSN, NNP,
PNP, CCRN
Assistant Clinical Professor, School of Nursing
Duke University
Durham, North Carolina

M. Colleen Brand, MSN, NNP-BC
Neonatal Nurse Practitioner
Texas Children's Hospital
Houston, Texas

Anne B. Broussard, DNS, CNM, CNE,
FACCE
Coordinator, BSN Program
Iberia General Hospital and Medical Center/
LEQSF Regents Professor in Nursing
Professor, College of Nursing and Allied
Health Professions
The University of Louisiana at Lafayette
Lafayette, Louisiana

Carol Turnage Carrier, MSN, RN, CNS
Neonatal Clinical Nurse Specialist
Texas Children's Hospital
Houston, Texas

Dianne S. Charsha, RNC, MSN, CRNP
Associate Chief Nursing Officer
Cooper University Hospital
Camden, New Jersey

William Diehl-Jones, BSc, MSc, PhD, BScN,
RN
Associate Professor, Faculty of Nursing
and Department of Biological Sciences
University of Manitoba
Scientist, Manitoba Institute for Child Health
Winnipeg, Manitoba, Canada

Georgia R. Ditzenberger, NNP-BC, PhD
Assistant Professor, School of Medicine and
Public Health
Department of Pediatrics, Division of
Neonatology
University of Wisconsin
Director Neonatal Advanced Practice Nursing
and Research
Meriter Hospital, Inc.
Madison, Wisconsin

Christine Domonoske, BS, PharmD
Neonatal Clinical Pharmacist
Memorial Hermann Texas Medical Center
Children's Memorial Hermann
Houston, Texas

Susan Arana Furdon, MS, RNC, NNP
Neonatal Clinical Nurse Specialist
Neonatal Nurse Practitioner
Albany Medical Center
Albany, New York

Martha Goodwin, BSN, MSN, NNP
Neonatal Nurse Practitioner Coordinator
Children's Mercy Hospital
Faculty, Neonatal Nurse Practitioner Program
University of Missouri—Kansas City
Kansas City, Missouri

Brenda Hueske Halbardier, BSN, MSN, NNP
Assistant Professor, Pediatrics
University of Texas Health Science Center
    Medical School
Houston, Texas

**Gina M. Heiss-Harris, RNC, DNP, NNP-BC,
    CCRN**
Neonatal Nurse Practitioner
Pediatrix Medical Group
Austin, Texas

Pat Hummel, MA, APN, NNP, PNP
Neonatal Nurse Practitioner
Pediatric Nurse Practitioner
Loyola University Medical Center
Maywood, Illinois

**Helen M. Hurst, DNP, RNC, MSN,
    APRN-CNM**
Instructor, College of Nursing and Allied
    Health Professions
University of Louisiana at Lafayette
Lafayette, Louisiana

**Carole Kenner, DNS, BSN, MSN, RNC,
    FAAN**
Dean/Professor, College of Nursing
University of Oklahoma
Oklahoma City, Oklahoma

Nanette Landry, BSN, MS, CNM
Certified Nurse Midwife
Aurora Nurse-Midwives
Aurora, Colorado

Linda Lane-Ehret, RNC, MSN, NNP
Neonatal Nurse Practitioner
The Children's Hospital
Denver, Colorado

Judy Wright Lott, DSN, RNC, NNP
Dean and Professor, Louise Herrington
    School of Nursing
Baylor University
Dallas, Texas

Carolyn Houska Lund, RN, MS, FAAN
Neonatal Clinical Nurse Specialist
ECMO Coordinator
Children's Hospital Oakland
Oakland, California

Lynn Lynam, ADN, BSN, MSN, PhD
Clinical Research Scientist, Maternal
    Infant Care
GE Healthcare
Laurel, Maryland

Barbara E. Pappas, RNC, MSN, NNP
Neonatal Nurse Practitioner
Blank Children's Hospital
Des Moines, Iowa

Kathleen Pitts, RN, MSN, MPH, CPNP, NNP
Neonatal Nurse Practitioner
Baylor College of Medicine
Houston, Texas

Sharyl L. Sadowski, AB, BSN, MSN, RNC
Neonatal Nurse Practitioner
Outreach Educator
University of Illinois at Chicago Perinatal
    Center
Chicago, Illinois

**Julieanne Schiefelbein, MAppSc, MA (Ed),
    CNM, RNC, NNP, PNP**
Neonatal Nurse Practitioner
Pediatric Nurse Practitioner
Primary Children's Medical Center
Salt Lake City, Utah

Bonita Shviraga, BSN, MS, CNM
Certified Nurse Midwife
The Medical Center of Aurora
Aurora Nurse-Midwives
Aurora, Colorado

Joan Renaud Smith, ADN, BSN, MSN, RNC, NNP
Neonatal Nurse Practitioner
St. Louis Children's Hospital
St. Louis, Missouri

Leann Sterk, MS, NNP, CNS
Neonatal Nurse Practitioner
Clinical Nurse Specialist
Rapid City Regional Hospital
Rapid City, South Dakota

Laura Stokowski, RNC, MS
Staff Nurse
Inova Fairfax Hospital for Children
Falls Church, Virginia

Tanya Sudia-Robinson, PhD, RN
Professor, College of Nursing
Mercer University
Macon, Georgia

Diane M. Szlachetka, RNC, MSN, APRN
Neonatal Nurse Practitioner
Baystate Medical Center
Springfield, Massachusetts

Karen A. Thomas, PhD, RN
Professor, School of Nursing
University of Washington
Seattle, Washington

M. Terese Verklan, PhD, CCNS, RNC
Associate Professor, Neonatal Clinical Nurse Specialist
University of Texas Health Science Center at Houston
Houston, Texas

Marlene Walden, PhD, RN, NNP-BC, CCNS
Professor, Clinical Nursing
Director, Neonatal Nurse Practitioner Program
The University of Texas
Austin, Texas

Brenda Walker, MSN, RNC
Neonatal Clinical Nurse Specialist
Iowa Health Des Moines—Methodist, Lutheran, Blank
Des Moines, Iowa

Catherine L. Witt, MS, NNP-BC
Neonatal Nurse Practitioner
NNP Services of Colorado
Denver, Colorado

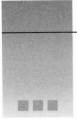

Reviewers

Leslie Altimier, RN, MSN
Director, Women's and Children's Services
Mercy Hospital Anderson
Cincinnati, Ohio

Gail A. Bagwell, RN, MSN
Clinical Nurse Specialist—Perinatal Outreach
Nationwide Children's Hospital
Columbus, Ohio

Beverly B. Bowers, PhD, RN, CNS
Assistant Dean, Faculty Development and
    Professional Continuing Education
Assistant Professor, College of Nursing
The University of Oklahoma
Oklahoma City, Oklahoma

Joyce M. Butler, MSN, RNC, CNNP
Clinical Instructor/CNNP Coordinator
University of Mississippi Medical Center
Jackson, Mississippi

Terri A. Cavaliere, MS, RNC, NNP
Neonatal Nurse Practitioner, North Shore
    University Hospital
Manhasset, New York
Clinical Assistant Professor, School of Nursing
State University of New York at Stony Brook
Stony Brook, New York

Jody Farrell, MSN, PNP
Clinical Coordinator
University of California, San Francisco
    Children's Medical Center
San Francisco, California

Mary M. Kaminski, RNC, MS, CNNP
Clinical Instructor, College of Nursing
The Ohio State University
Neonatal Nurse Practitioner
Nationwide Children's Hospital
Columbus, Ohio

Andrea C. Morris, MSN, RNC, CCRN
Neonatal Clinical Nurse Specialist
Citrus Valley Medical Center
West Covina, California

Barbara Pascoe, RN, BA, MA
Director, Maternity and Pediatrics
Concord Hospital
Concord, New Hampshire

Beth Shields, PharmD
Clinical Pharmacy Specialist in Pediatrics
Special Operations Supervisor in Pediatrics
Rush University Medical Center
Chicago, Illinois

Janet L. Thigpen, RNC, MN, CNNP
Neonatal Nurse Practitioner, School of
    Medicine
Emory University
Atlanta, Georgia

Robin L. Watson, RN, MN, CCRN
Clinical Nurse Specialist, Neonatal/Pediatrics
Harbor–UCLA Medical Center
Torrance, California

Preface

The provision of intensive care to the high-risk neonate challenges every neonatal care provider. Research and refinements in technology have made "high-tech" modalities such as ECMO, nitric oxide, and hypothermia available to many more hospitals. The art and science of neonatal nursing is never stochastic. We learn from scientists, researchers, multidisciplinary colleagues, and of course, our infants and their families. At a minimum, we are expected to enhance our application of clinical knowledge by utilizing an evidence-based approach to improve patient outcomes. The role of the nurse is frequently to bring together all of the pieces of the puzzle to ensure comprehensive, clinically excellent, and compassionate care to sick newborns and their families.

The fourth edition of *Core Curriculum for Neonatal Intensive Care Nursing* is intended as a clinical resource. It is divided into sections and designed in an outline format so that it may be used as an easy reference. The first section, *Antepartum, Intrapartum, and Transition to Extrauterine Life,* addresses clinical issues related to factors that affect the fetus and the neonate's ability to successfully adapt to postnatal life. Information is also presented as to how we can assist in the recognition of the high-risk fetus/neonate and plan interventions that support the physiologic demands of the neonate during transition. *Cornerstones of Clinical Practice* presents concepts common to the delivery of quality care to all high-risk newborns and families. A new chapter has been added that addresses the late preterm infant specifically since recent research has indicated this group of neonates has a high risk of morbidity and mortality when they are treated the same way as a healthy term neonate. The third section, *Pathophysiology: Management and Treatment of Common Disorders,* provides a systems approach to the assessment and management of the disease processes high-risk neonates commonly present with. The last section, *Professional Practice,* focuses on the caregiver to strengthen competency with respect to research utilization, in addition to providing an overview of universal ethical and legal issues that may be encountered in the practice of neonatal nursing.

This text is the collaborative effort of the three major nursing specialty associations: the Association of Women's Health, Obstetric and Neonatal Nurses (AWHONN); the American Association of Critical-Care Nurses (AACN); and the National Association of Neonatal Nurses (NANN). The book brings together experts in the care of the high-risk neonate, all having the common goal of providing a comprehensive resource for the management and care of sick newborns. We are honored to be the editors of such an outstanding collaborative effort.

M. Terese Verklan
Marlene Walden

Contents

SECTION ONE
ANTEPARTUM, INTRAPARTUM, AND TRANSITION TO EXTRAUTERINE LIFE

1 Uncomplicated Antepartum, Intrapartum, and Postpartum Care, 1
BONITA SHVIRAGA AND NANETTE LANDRY
Terminology, 1
Normal Maternal Physiologic Changes by Systems, 1
Antepartum Care, 6
Normal Labor and Birth, 11
Puerperium: "Fourth Trimester", 17

2 Antepartum-Intrapartum Complications, 20
ANNE B. BROUSSARD AND HELEN M. HURST
Anatomy and Physiology, 20
Conditions Related to the Antepartum Period, 24
Conditions Related to the Intrapartum Period, 28
Obstetric Analgesia and Anesthesia, 35

3 Perinatal Substance Abuse, 41
KATHLEEN PITTS
Introduction, 41
Drugs of Abuse, 42
Stimulants, 46
Cannabinoids, 49
Narcotics and Opioids, 50
Sedatives/Hypnotics, 52
Inhalants, 53
Other (Antidepressants), 53
General Management Recommendations, 58
Nursing Interventions, 59
Drug Screening, 63
Breastfeeding, 64
Problems Associated with Maternal Drug Use, 65
Ethical and Legal Considerations, 67

4 Adaptation to Extrauterine Life, 72
M. TERESE VERKLAN
Anatomy and Physiology, 72
Routine Care Considerations in the Transition Nursery, 77
Recognition of the Sick Newborn Infant, 82
Parent Teaching, 88

5 Neonatal Deliver Room Resuscitation, 91

BARBARA ELIZABETH PAPPAS AND BRENDA WALKER
Definitions, 91
Anatomy and Physiology, 92
Risk Factors, 93
Anticipation and Preparation for Resuscitation, 94
Equipment for Neonatal Resuscitation, 95
Apgar Scoring, 95
Decision-Making Process, 97
Unusual Situations, 103
Complications of Resuscitation, 107
Postresuscitation Care, 107

SECTION TWO
CORNERSTONES OF CLINICAL PRACTICE

6 Thermoregulation, 110

M. COLLEEN BRAND AND HOLLY BOYD
Identifying Infants at Risk, 110
Physiology of Thermoregulation, 111
Mechanisms of Heat Transfer, 113
Strategies for Managing Thermoregulation, 114

7 Physical Assessment, 120

SUSAN ARANA FURDON AND KATHLEEN BENJAMIN
Perinatal History, 120
Gestational-Age Instruments, 123
Classification of Growth and Maturity, 127
Physical Examination, 132

8 Fluid and Electrolyte Management, 156

BRENDA HUESKE HALBARDIER
Fluid Balance, 156
Disorders of Fluid Balance, 159
Electrolyte Balance and Disorders, 161
Acid-Base Balance and Disorders, 168

9 Glucose Management, 172

DEBRA ARMENTROUT
Glucose Homeostasis, 172
Hypoglycemia, 173
Infant of Diabetic Mother, 177
Hyperglycemia, 178
Transient or Permanent Neonatal Diabetes, 179

10 Nutritional Management, 182

GEORGIA R. DITZENBERGER
Anatomy and Physiology of the Premature Infant's Gastrointestinal Tract, 182
Nutritional Requirements, 186
Parenteral Nutrition (PN), 190
Enteral Feedings: Human Milk and Commercial Formulas for Term, Special-Needs, and
    Premature Infants, 194
Enteral Feeding Methods, 199
Nursing Interventions to Facilitate Tolerance of Enteral Feedings, 202
Nutritional Assessment and Standards for Adequate Growth, 203

11 Developmental Support, 208
CAROL TURNAGE CARRIER
Barriers to Infant Development in the NICU Setting, 208
Developmental Care Standards, 209

12 Pharmacology, 233
CHRISTINE D. DOMONOSKE
Principles of Pharmacology, 233
Pharmacodynamics, 234
Pharmacokinetics, 236
Medication Categories, 243
Central Nervous System (CNS) Medications, 246
Nursing Implications for Medication Administration in the Neonate, 250

13 Laboratory Concepts and Test Interpretation, 252
DIANE M. SZLACHETKA
Laboratory Tests in the NICU, 252
Purpose of Laboratory Testing, 255
Process of Laboratory Collection, 255
Concepts of Laboratory Test Interpretation, 258
Principles of Test Utilization, 259
Iatrogenic Sequelae of Laboratory Testing—Preventive Strategies, 260
Decision—Questions to Ask Prior to Obtaining a Laboratory Test, 262
Laboratory Interpretation—Decision Tree, 264

14 Radiologic Evaluation, 270
LINDA LANE
Basic Concepts, 270
Terminology, 270
X-Ray Views Commonly Used in the Newborn Infant, 271
Radiographic Densities, 272
Risks Associated with Radiographic Examination in the Neonate, 272
Approach to Interpreting an X-Ray, 272
Respiratory System, 274
Pulmonary Parenchymal Disease, 275
Pulmonary Air Leaks, 279
Miscellaneous Causes of Respiratory Distress, 280
Thoracic Surgical Problems, 281
Cardiovascular System, 284
Gastrointestinal System, 287
Skeletal System, 293
Indwelling Lines and Tubes, 294
Diagnostic Imaging, 296

15 Common Invasive Procedures, 299
GINA M. HEISS-HARRIS AND TERESA BAILEY
Airway Procedures, 299
Circulatory Access Procedures, 307
Blood Sampling Procedures, 320
Miscellaneous Procedures, 324

16 Pain Assessment and Management, 333
MARLENE WALDEN
Definition of Pain, 333
Neonatal Intensive Care Unit Procedures That Cause Pain, 333

Physiology of Acute Pain in Preterm Neonates, 334
Standards of Practice, 336
Pain Assessment, 336
Pain Assessment Instruments, 338
Nursing Care of the Infant in Pain, 340
Pain Management at End of Life, 344
Parents' Role in Pain Assessment and Management, 345

17 Families in Crisis, 347
CAROLE KENNER
Crisis and the Birth of the Sick or Premature Infant, 347
Specific Population of Parents: Adolescents, 349
The Family in Crisis, 349
Summary of Parental Needs to Be Met by NICU Staff, 359

18 Patient Safety, 361
JOAN RENAUD SMITH

19 Discharge Planning and Transition to Home Care, 383
PAT HUMMEL
Introduction, 383
General Principles, 383
Health Care Trends, 384
Discharge Criteria Must Be Established and Individualized to the Infant and Family, 385
Parental Needs and Role in the Discharge and Transition to Home Process, 386
Discharge Planning and Transition to Home, 387
Neonatal Teaching Needs, 392
Family and Infant Care Postdischarge, 393

20 Genetics: From Bench to Bedside, 399
JULIEANNE SCHIEFELBEIN
Basic Genetics, 399
Chromosomal Defects, 402
Prenatal Diagnosis, 402
Postnatal Testing, 406
Human Genome Project, 406
Genetic Counseling, 407
Newborn Care, 408

21 Intrafacility and Interfacility Neonatal Transport, 415
S. LOUISE BOWEN
Historical Aspects, 415
Philosophy of Neonatal Transport, 416
Intrafacility Neonatal Transport, 416
Interfacility Neonatal Transport, 417
Selection of Transport Vehicles, 418
Transport Personnel, 419
Transport Equipment, 421
Neonatal Transport Process, 422
Documentation, 427
Safety, 428
Disaster Preparation, 429
Air Transport Considerations, 430
Legal and Ethical Considerations, 430
Total Quality Management, 431

22 Care of the Extremely Low Birth Weight Infant, 434

DIANNE SUSAN CHARSHA

Prenatal Considerations, 434

Delivery Room Management, 435

Admission to the NICU, 436

Parameters of Clinical Assessment and Nursing Management, 437

23 Care of the Late Preterm Infant, 447

BARBARA ELIZABETH PAPPAS AND BRENDA WALKER

SECTION THREE
PATHOPHYSIOLOGY: MANAGEMENT AND TREATMENT OF COMMON DISORDERS

24 Respiratory Distress, 453

DEBBIE FRASER ASKIN

Lung Development, 453

Physiology of Respiration, 455

Respiratory Disorders, 455

Pulmonary Air Leaks (Pneumomediastinum, Pneumothorax, Pneumopericardium, Pulmonary Interstitial Emphysema), 475

Pulmonary Hypoplasia, 477

Pulmonary Hemorrhage, 477

Other Causes of Respiratory Distress, 478

25 Apnea, 484

MARTHA GOODWIN

Definitions of Apnea, 484

Types of Apnea, 484

Pathogenesis of Apnea in the Premature Infant, 485

Causes of Apnea, 487

Evaluation for Apnea, 488

Management Techniques, 489

Home Monitoring, 491

26 Assisted Ventilation, 494

DEBBIE FRASER ASKIN AND WILLIAM DIEHL-JONES

Physiology, 494

Treatment Modalities, 499

Nursing Care of the Patient Requiring Respiratory Support or Conventional Mechanical Ventilation, 502

High-Frequency Ventilation, 505

Nursing Care During Therapy, 511

Medications Used During Ventilation Therapy, 513

Weaning from Conventional Ventilation, 516

Interpretation of Blood Gas Values, 517

27 Extracorporeal Membrane Oxygenation, 521

CAROLYN HOUSKA LUND

ECMO: A Historical Perspective, 521

Criteria for Use of ECMO, 522

Venoarterial Perfusion, 522

Venovenous Perfusion, 523

Circuit Components and Additional Devices, 524

Physiology of Extracorporeal Circulation, 526
Care of the Infant During ECMO, 527
Post-ECMO Care, 531
Parental Support, 531
Follow-up and Outcome, 531

28 **Cardiovascular Disorders, 534**
SHARYL L. SADOWSKI
Cardiovascular Embryology and Anatomy, 535
Congenital Heart Defects, 542
Risk Assessment and Approach to Diagnosis of Cardiac Disease, 544
Defects with Increased Pulmonary Blood Flow, 553
Obstructive Defects with Pulmonary Venous Congestion, 560
Obstructive Defects with Decreased Pulmonary Blood Flow, 562
Mixed Defects, 567
Congestive Heart Failure, 573
Postoperative Cardiac Management, 576
Postoperative Disturbances, 578

29 **Gastrointestinal Disorders, 589**
WANDA T. BRADSHAW
Gastrointestinal Embryonic Development, 589
Functions of the Gastrointestinal Tract, 590
Assessment of the Gastrointestinal System, 590
Abdominal Wall Defects, 595
Obstructions of the Gastrointestinal Tract, 599
Necrotizing Enterocolitis, 612
Short Bowel Syndrome, 615
Biliary Atresia, 617
Cholestasis, 618
Gastroesophageal Reflux, 620
Multisystem Disorders with Gastrointestinal Involvement, 623

30 **Endocrine Disorders, 638**
LAURA STOKOWSKI
The Endocrine System, 638
Pituitary Gland Disorders, 640
Thyroid Gland Disorders, 641
Adrenal Gland Disorders, 649
Disorders of Sexual Development, 655
Pancreatic Disorders, 662

31 **Hematologic Disorders, 666**
WILLIAM DIEHL-JONES AND DEBBIE FRASER ASKIN
Development of Blood Cells, 666
Coagulation, 671
Anemia, 672
Hemorrhagic Disease of the Newborn, 678
Disseminated Intravascular Coagulation, 679
Thrombocytopenia, 681
Polycythemia, 684
Inherited Bleeding Disorders, 685
Transfusion Therapies, 686
Recombinant Hematopoietic Growth Factors, 690
Evaluation by Complete Blood Cell Count, 691

32 Immunology and Infectious Disease, 694
JUDY WRIGHT LOTT
Immune System, 695
Transmission of Infectious Organisms in the Neonate, 698
Diagnosis and Therapy, 699
History, Sites, and Types of Neonatal Infection, 706
Infection with Specific Pathogens, 708
Infection Control, 720

33 Renal and Genitourinary Disorders, 724
CAROL BOTWINSKI
Embryology, 724
Renal Anatomy, 725
Renal Hemodynamics, 726
Renal Physiology, 726
Acute Renal Failure, 728
Hypertension, 731
Potter Syndrome (Oligohydramnios Syndrome), 733
Autosomal Recessive Polycystic Kidney Disease, 735
Multicystic Dysplastic Kidney Disease, 735
Hydronephrosis, 736
Renal Vein Thrombosis, 738
Urinary Tract Infections, 739
Patent Urachus, 740
Hypospadias, 741
Exstrophy of the Bladder, 742
Undescended Testicles (Cryptorchidism), 744
Circumcision, 745

34 Neurologic Disorders, 748
LYNN LYNAM AND M. TERESE VERKLAN
Anatomy of the Neurologic System, 748
Physiology of the Neurologic System, 751
Neurologic Assessment, 752
Neurologic Disorders, 753
Intracranial Hemorrhages, 766
Seizures, 771
Hypoxic–Ischemic Encephalopathy, 774
Periventricular Leukomalacia, 778
Meningitis, 779

35 Congenital Anomalies, 782
LEANN STERK
Specific Disorders, 786
Nonchromosomal Abnormalities, 794
Deformation Abnormalities, 805
Congenital Metabolic Problems, 806
Disorders of Metabolism, 807

36 Neonatal Dermatology, 813
CATHERINE L. WITT
Anatomy and Physiology of the Skin, 813
Care of the Newborn Infant's Skin, 815
Assessment of the Newborn Infant's Skin, 816
Common Skin Lesions, 817

37 Ophthalmologic and Auditory Disorders, 832

DEBBIE FRASER ASKIN AND WILLIAM DIEHL-JONES

Anatomy of the Eye, 832
Patient Assessment, 834
Pathologic Conditions and Management, 834
Anatomy of the Ear, 844
Innervation, 846
Patient Assessment, 847

SECTION FOUR
PROFESSIONAL PRACTICE

38 Foundations of Neonatal Research, 850

KAREN A. THOMAS

Research and Generation of Nursing Knowledge, 850
Research Process and Components of a Research Study, 851
Quantitative Research, 853
Qualitative Research, 854
Areas of Exploration in Neonatal Nursing, 854
Nurses as Consumers of Research, 854
Ethics in Research and Nurses as Advocates, 856

39 Ethical Issues, 860

TANYA SUDIA-ROBINSON

Examining Ethical Issues in the NICU, 860
Principles of Biomedical Ethics, 860
Other Approaches to Ethical Issues, 862
Case Analysis Model, 863
The Nurse's Role in Ethical Issues, 863
Consulting the Hospital Ethics Committee, 864

40 Legal Issues, 865

M. TERESE VERKLAN

Nursing Process, 865
Standard of Care, 866
Malpractice, 869
Liability, 869
Advance Practice, 873
Documentation, 874
Informed Consent, 877
Professional Liability Insurance, 878

Appendix A, 882

Index, 885

1 Uncomplicated Antepartum, Intrapartum, and Postpartum Care

BONITA SHVIRAGA and NANETTE LANDRY

OBJECTIVES

1. Identify normal physiologic changes of each system in pregnancy.
2. Describe parameters to assess gestational age and establish pregnancy dating.
3. Discuss genetic screening options for pregnancy.
4. Identify medications that may cause congenital malformations.
5. Outline components of prenatal care, including history, physical, laboratory, and diagnostic testing.
6. Explain tests of fetal lung maturity.
7. Identify six methods of antepartum fetal surveillance.
8. Discuss the normal stages of labor and delivery.
9. Describe low-risk labor management, including fetal monitoring guidelines.
10. Discuss normal immediate postpartum recovery and related postpartum nursing assessments and management.

■
■■ Antepartum, intrapartum, and postpartum care are not usually included within the practice parameters of the neonatal nurse. Yet an understanding of the normal processes of pregnancy, birth, and postpartum recovery provides a framework for beginning to understand factors that affect the developing fetus and the high-risk neonate. This chapter discusses uncomplicated antepartum, intrapartum, and postpartum nursing care. In addition, an overview of the normal physiologic changes that can be expected in a healthy mother is included.

TERMINOLOGY

A. **Calculation of gestation:** 280 days, 40 postmenstrual weeks, or 10 lunar months counted from the first day of the last menstrual period. (Actual duration of gestation from conception to estimated date of confinement is 38 weeks, assuming a 28-day cycle.)
B. **Trimesters:** division of gestation into three segments of approximately equal duration.
   1. First trimester: 0 to 12 weeks.
   2. Second trimester: 13 to 27 weeks.
   3. Third trimester: 28 to 40 weeks.
C. **Preterm, term, and postterm pregnancy:** *term*, 37 to 42 weeks; *preterm*, <37 completed weeks; and *postterm*, >42 weeks.

NORMAL MATERNAL PHYSIOLOGIC CHANGES BY SYSTEMS

A. **Alimentary tract and perinatal nutrition.**
   1. The recommended caloric intake for the average woman of childbearing age is 2200 kcal/day. During pregnancy there is an increased caloric need of 300 kcal/day to support the

growing fetus and increased maternal metabolic rate, resulting in a caloric requirement of 2500 kcal/day during pregnancy (Pillitteri, 2007). Pregnant teenagers need an additional 100 to 200 kcal/day. Total recommended weight gain for women with normal body mass index (BMI) is 25 to 35 pounds, and for underweight women a gain of up to 40 pounds may be recommended (Johnson et al., 2007). Limiting weight gain to 15 pounds is recommended for obese women (Johnson et al., 2007).

2. Routine supplementation of folic acid 0.4 mg is recommended for women of childbearing age to prevent neural tube defect (Blackburn, 2007; Perry, 2006).

3. Approximately 50% of pregnancies are affected by morning sickness during the first trimester. Increased incidence of nausea and vomiting is associated with increased levels of human chorionic gonadotropin (hCG) and progesterone (Pillitteri, 2007). Decreased glucose levels and increased estrogen levels may also increase nausea (Pillitteri, 2007).

4. The stomach loses tone and has decreased motility and delayed emptying time because of the effects of progesterone (Blackburn, 2007).

5. Relaxation of the pyloric sphincter and upward displacement of the diaphragm in combination with increased intraabdominal pressure from the enlarging uterus can result in gastroesophageal reflux and heartburn (Blackburn, 2007).

6. The small bowel has reduced motility and hypertrophy of the duodenal villi to increase absorption of nutrients (Blackburn, 2007). In the colon, constipation is a problem because of mechanical obstruction from the uterus, reduced motility, and increased water absorption. As pregnancy progresses, the appendix and cecum are displaced toward the right costal margin, causing the physical findings in appendicitis to be altered in pregnant women (Blackburn, 2007).

7. The gallbladder has decreased muscle tone and motility after 14 weeks as a result of the effects of progesterone (Blackburn, 2007). The gallbladder empties much more slowly and high residual volumes increase until 20 weeks and remain high until term. High levels of estrogen may decrease water absorption by the gallbladder's mucosa, leading to dilute bile with resulting inability to sequester cholesterol. This increase in cholesterol may lead to gallstone formation during the second and third trimesters of pregnancy (Blackburn, 2007). Decreased gallbladder tone may also lead to increased retention of bile salts, resulting in pruritus and cholestasis gravidarum (Blackburn, 2007). Cholestasis gravidarum has been associated with increased risk of stillbirth and preterm deliveries (Kroumpouzos, 2007).

8. The liver is displaced upward by the enlarging uterus; however, hepatic size and hepatic blood flow remain essentially unchanged in pregnancy (Blackburn, 2007). Estrogen may cause altered production of plasma proteins, bilirubin, serum enzymes, and serum lipids (Blackburn, 2007). Alterations in liver lab values such as reduced serum albumin, elevated alkaline phosphatase, and elevated serum cholesterol may mimic liver disease (Blackburn, 2007). Serum levels of bilirubin, aspartate aminotransferase (AST), and alanine aminotransferase (ALT) are unchanged in normal pregnancy and may be used as an indicator of hepatic compromise during pregnancy (Blackburn, 2007). During labor, alkaline phosphatase levels may increase further, and AST, ALT, and lactic dehydrogenase levels may increase as a result of stress of labor (Blackburn, 2007).

B. **Respiratory system.**
   1. The increased vascularity and vascular congestion of the upper respiratory tract resulting from increased levels of estrogen results in hypersecretion of mucus from the nasopharynx resulting in nasal stuffiness, sinus congestion, and epistaxis (nosebleed) during pregnancy (Lowdermilk and Perry, 2006).
   2. Maternal oxygen requirements increase during pregnancy as a result of increased maternal metabolic rate, fetal oxygen requirements, and increased tissue mass (Lowdermilk and Perry, 2006).
   3. The chest wall profile changes. Increased levels of estrogen and relaxin cause relaxation of intercostal ligaments with resulting increased chest expansion and chest circumference and an increase in the subcostal margin angle (Blackburn, 2007; Cunningham et al., 2005). The diaphragm is elevated by 4 cm in the third trimester (Lowdermilk and Perry, 2006).

4. Respiratory changes during pregnancy include a 30% to 40% increase in tidal volume, 20% to 30% decrease in expiratory reserve volume, 20% decrease in residual volume, and a 20% decrease in functional residual capacity (Blackburn, 2007). Forced expiratory volume does not change in pregnancy and is a reliable indicator of asthma status in pregnant women (Blackburn, 2007). Progesterone, estradiol, and prostaglandins increase the sensitivity of the respiratory center to carbon dioxide (Blackburn, 2007; Lowdermilk and Perry, 2006). Maternal $Paco_2$ levels decrease to 32 mm Hg and oxygen levels rise to 106 mm Hg early in pregnancy to allow fetal placental exchange (Pillitteri, 2007). Respiratory rate may be slightly increased by 1 to 2/minute (Pillitteri, 2007). As a result of these cumulative respiratory changes, pregnant women may experience physiologic dyspnea. Although pulmonary function is not impaired, respiratory diseases may be more serious during pregnancy (Cunningham et al., 2005).

C. **Skin.**
   1. Because of elevated levels of estrogen, spider angiomas (vascular red elevations with tiny vessels branching out from a central body) are frequently seen on the neck, face, throat, and arms. Palmar erythema, diffuse or blotchy spots on the palms, is common in two thirds of white women and one third of black women (Cunningham et al., 2005).
   2. Striae gravidarum, or "stretch marks," occur in women with a genetic predisposition to stretching of the skin or connective tissue. Stretching due to the increased activity of adrenocorticosteroids, estrogens, and relaxin may cause separation and rupture of areas of connective tissue of the skin leading to pink or red streaks on the abdomen, thighs, and breast (Blackburn, 2007; Lowdermilk and Perry, 2006; Pillitteri, 2007). After pregnancy, striae do not completely resolve; however, they turn a silvery-white color (Pillitteri, 2007). Studies have not found evidence to support the use of topical agents to prevent striae (Blackburn, 2007).
   3. Increased pigmentation is due to increased levels of estrogen, progesterone, and melanocyte-stimulating hormone. This is most marked on the nipples, areolas, perineum, and the midline of the lower portion of the abdomen (commonly called the linea nigra) (Blackburn, 2007).
   4. Sun-sensitive hyperpigmentation of the face, called chloasma or melasma and also referred to as the "mask of pregnancy," results in a dark, blotchy appearance of the face, forehead, and upper lip and occurs in 45% to 70% of women, with an increased incidence in women with dark hair and dark complexions (Blackburn, 2007). There is a genetic predisposition to melasma (Blackburn, 2007).
   5. During gestation a greater percentage of the hair remains in the anagen (growth) phase, which decreases normal hair loss. Hair loss commonly occurs between 2 and 4 months after delivery and is due to an increase in the telogen (resting) phase of hair growth. The hair returns to a normal growth phase within 1 to 5 months (Papoutsis and Kroumpouzos, 2007).
   6. Changes in secretory glands occur during pregnancy. Sebaceous gland activity changes are variable, with resulting changes in acne unpredictable (Papoutsis and Kroumpouzos, 2007). Eccrine sweat gland activity increases as a result of increased thyroid activity, body weight, and metabolic activity and may result in miliaria and dyshidrotic eczema (Blackburn, 2007).
   7. Changes in the nails are uncommon but may occur beginning in the first trimester. These changes include brittleness, distal separation of the nail bed, subungual hyperkeratosis, whitish discoloration (leukonychia), and transverse grooving (Blackburn, 2007; Papoutsis and Kroumpouzos, 2007). The cause is unknown (Blackburn, 2007).

D. **Urinary system.**
   1. Structural renal changes begin during the first trimester and are a result of estrogen, progesterone, and prostaglandin E_2 secretion; pressure from the enlarging uterus; and increase in blood volume (Blackburn, 2007; Lowdermilk and Perry, 2006). The kidneys enlarge, the ureters dilate, hyperplasia of the smooth muscle walls of the ureters occurs, and the ureters elongate (Lowdermilk and Perry, 2006). Hydronephrosis occurs in 80% of pregnant women (Blackburn, 2007). Bladder capacity also increases to 1000 ml (Pillitteri, 2007). The consequences of these changes include the following:

    a. An increase in asymptomatic bacteriuria that may lead to cystitis and pyelonephritis.

    b. Difficulty in diagnosing obstruction on x-ray examination and interference with studies of glomerular filtration, renal blood flow, and tubular function. Accuracy of 24-hour urine collection results may also be affected (Blackburn, 2007).

    c. Vesicoureteral reflux, which may occur especially during the third trimester, as a result of decreased bladder tone (Blackburn, 2007).

  2. Urodynamic and hemodynamic changes also occur in the renal system during pregnancy.

    a. Mean 24-hour urine output increases from 1475 to 1919 ml, and the mean number of daily voids increases as well (Blackburn, 2007).

    b. The renal plasma flow increases by 75%, with a 25% decrease in the third trimester (Gordon, 2007). The increased renal plasma flow is accompanied by an increase in glomerular filtration rate of 50%, which leads to an increase in creatinine clearance and a decrease in nitrogen levels, as reflected by decreased blood urea nitrogen (BUN) and serum creatinine levels (Pillitteri, 2007).

    c. An increased filtration of sodium is balanced by an increased reabsorption of sodium by the renal tubules.

    d. The lower renal threshold for glucose excretion negates using urine glucose measurements in the management of diabetes mellitus.

    e. Proteinuria of trace to 1+ may occur as a result of an increased load of amino acids (Blackburn, 2007). Although this level of proteinuria may not indicate pathology, the pregnant woman with proteinuria and hypertension should be evaluated for preeclampsia (Lowdermilk and Perry, 2006).

E. Cardiovascular system.

  1. There is an increase in maternal blood volume by 1500 ml or 30% to 50% from the end of the first trimester, peaking at 28 to 32 weeks (Lowdermilk and Perry, 2006). If plasma volume increases faster than red blood cell (RBC) production, a hemodilutional pseudoanemia may result (Pillitteri, 2007).

  2. There is an increase in maternal heart rate, increasing by 10 to 20 beats above the nonpregnant state by the third trimester. Stroke volume increases during the first and second trimesters and then decreases during the third trimester. Pregnancies with multiples have a greater increase in maternal cardiac output (Blackburn, 2007).

  3. Because the heart is displaced leftward and upward by the enlarging uterus, the cardiac silhouette increases on x-ray films.

  4. Altered cardiac sounds in pregnancy include splitting of the first heart sound, an audible S_3 heart sound, systolic flow murmurs (90% of pregnant women), and transient diastolic murmurs (20% of pregnant women) (Blackburn, 2007; Cunningham et al., 2005).

  5. Blood pressure remains at the prepregnancy level in the first trimester and drops during the second trimester at approximately 24 weeks of gestation by 5 to 10 mm Hg systolic and 10 to 15 mm Hg diastolic. It returns to normal prepregnancy levels at the end of pregnancy (Blackburn, 2007).

  6. In late pregnancy, pressure obstruction of the inferior vena cava may occur in the supine position. The resulting 25% fall in cardiac output is called supine hypotension (Blackburn, 2007).

  7. Blood stagnates in the lower extremities because of compression of the pelvic veins and the inferior vena cava, contributing to dependent edema, varicosities of the legs and vulva, and hemorrhoid formation (Cunningham et al., 2005).

F. Breasts.

  1. Early changes in the breasts (beginning by 4 weeks of gestation) include tingling, heaviness, tenderness, and enlargement in response to increased levels of estrogen (Lowdermilk and Perry, 2006). These symptoms usually subside at the end of the first trimester.

  2. The areolas enlarge and darken. Sebaceous glands on the areolae, Montgomery's tubercles, increase activity in preparation for lactation and therefore become more prominent (Blackburn, 2007; Papoutsis and Kroumpouzos, 2007).

  3. Estrogen, progesterone, human placental lactogen (hPL), hCG, prolactin, and luteal and placental hormones cause hyperplasia of the breast tissue and development of lactiferous ducts and lobular alveolar tissue during the second and third trimesters (Lowdermilk and Perry, 2006; Pillitteri, 2007). Physical examination may reveal palpable milk ducts and excretion of colostrum from the nipples.

4. Colostrum, which is a high-protein precursor of breast milk, may be expressed as early as 16 weeks of pregnancy (Pillitteri, 2007).

5. The breast is capable of lactogenesis after 16 weeks. Compared to milk produced after a term delivery, the milk produced after delivery of a preterm infant (i.e., <34 weeks) has higher protein content, higher antiinfective properties, including secretory IgA and lactoferrin, and higher oligosaccharides, fat, sodium, chloride, and iron (Blackburn, 2007).

G. Skeletal changes.

1. Compensating for the anteriorly positioned growing uterus, the lower portion of the back curves. This lordosis shifts the center of gravity backward over the lower extremities and causes low back pain, a common complaint in pregnancy (Gordon, 2007).

2. Sacroiliac and pubic symphysis joints loosen during pregnancy because of the hormone relaxin (Gordon, 2007).

3. Alteration in the center of gravity, loosening of the joints, and an unsteady gait increase the risk of falls in pregnancy.

4. Numbness, tingling, weakness, and aching in the upper extremities are a result of marked lordosis. Symptoms are the result of anterior flexion of the neck in the cervicodorsal region, producing traction on the brachial plexus and ulnar and median nerves (Lowdermilk and Perry, 2006).

5. Although serum calcium levels decrease during pregnancy, serum ionized calcium levels are unchanged. The National Institutes of Health (NIH) consensus panel recommends 1200 to 1500 mg calcium during pregnancy and lactation (Gordon, 2007).

6. Bone turnover is low in the first trimester and then increases in the third trimester when peak fetal calcium transfer occurs; however, osteoporosis is not associated with pregnancy bone turnover (Gordon, 2007).

H. Hematologic changes.

1. Plasma volume is increased 15% by the end of the first trimester, undergoes a rapid expansion during the second trimester, peaks at 32 to 34 weeks, and then plateaus near term. Plasma volume at or near term is 40% to 45% (~1500 ml) above prepregnant levels (Cunningham et al., 2005).

2. The white blood cell (WBC) count rises progressively during pregnancy and labor. It then returns to normal pregnancy levels, ranging from 5,000 to 12,000 cells/microliter (mcl) and increases up to 25,000 cells/mcl in labor and the early postpartum period (Blackburn, 2007).

3. The RBC count rises up to 33% during the first trimester with an average increase of 30% to 35% throughout pregnancy (Blackburn, 2007). The increase in plasma volume changes the ratio of RBCs to plasma, causing a drop in hematocrit. This "physiologic anemia of pregnancy" reaches the lowest levels at 30 to 34 weeks; then as the hematocrit begins to rise, a closer to normal ratio of RBCs to plasma results in a higher hematocrit near term (Gordon, 2007).

4. Iron requirements are increased by 800 mg in pregnancy, with total fetal requirements of 350 to 400 mg of iron (Pillitteri, 2007). Fetal iron requirements are greatest during the third trimester (Gordon, 2007). Serum ferritin levels fall until 30 to 32 weeks, with the greatest decrease between 12 and 25 weeks (Blackburn, 2007).

5. Pregnancy has been called a "hypercoagulable state." The platelet count decreases slightly, but remains within the normal range (Blackburn, 2007). Fibrinogen is increased by 50% to 80%, and factors VII through X increase (Blackburn, 2007; Pillitteri, 2007). Bleeding and clotting times remain normal (Gordon, 2007). The incidence of thromboembolism increases five- to six-fold (Gordon, 2007) and is greatest during the postpartum period (Pettker and Lockwood, 2007).

6. Pregnancy is known to result in altered immunologic function so that the "foreign fetus" is accommodated. Therefore a decrease in cellular immunity may account for improvement of certain autoimmune diseases in pregnancy and an increased susceptibility to

infection (Gordon, 2007). The humoral immunity system characterized by antibody-mediated immunity remains intact (Gordon, 2007).

I. **Endocrine and Metabolic Changes**

1. **Thyroid:** The thyroid enlarges during pregnancy; however, there is little transplacental transfer of the hormones triiodothyronine (T_3) and thyroxine (T_4). Thyroid-binding globulin (TBG) increases during the first trimester owing to the effects estrogen has on the liver. TBG plateaus at approximately 10 to 15 weeks and results in increases in total T_4 and total T_3 levels (Blackburn, 2007; Mestman, 2007). hCG has thyrotropic activity and can activate thyroid-stimulating hormone (TSH) receptors and also increase secretion of T_4 (Blackburn, 2007). Serum portions of T_3 and T_4 are normal unless a maternal iodine deficiency is present (Mestman, 2007). Increased hCG levels are associated with decreased TSH levels in early pregnancy. There is a transient decrease in TSH during the first trimester, with a return to normal levels by the second trimester (Blackburn, 2007). Fetal thyroid function appears to be independent of maternal thyroid function.

2. **Carbohydrate metabolism** (Cunningham et al., 2005):
   a. Characterized by mild fasting hypoglycemia, postprandial hyperglycemia, and hyperinsulinemia.
   b. The basal metabolic rate is increased by 25%.
   c. Peripheral resistance to insulin is referred to as the "diabetogenic effect of pregnancy." Its purpose is to ensure sustained postprandial supply of glucose for the fetus. By term there is a 50% to 70% reduction in the action of insulin. The hormones responsible for this effect are hPL, progesterone, and estrogen. HPL may increase lipolysis, leading to increased free fatty acids, which increases tissue resistance to insulin.
   d. Glucose is actively transported to the fetus; however, insulin and glycogen do not cross the placenta. During pregnancy, hyperglycemic states rapidly change to fasting states, resulting in hypoglycemia. In this fasting state, there is an increase in levels of fatty acids, triglycerides, and cholesterol. This switch in fuels from glucose to lipids is referred to as accelerated starvation, and ketonuria rapidly occurs.

ANTEPARTUM CARE

A. **Initial antepartum visit.**
   1. A thorough obstetric history is obtained:
      a. Gravidity (G), indicating the number of pregnancies, and parity (P), indicating the number of births. The obstetric history is often written as "G_ P _ _ _ _". A four-number parity is often used, which includes the number of elective and spontaneous abortions and the number of living children.
         (1) *G* indicates the number of times the woman has been pregnant, including this pregnancy.
         (2) *P* represents the number of term deliveries, number of preterm deliveries, total number of abortions (elective and spontaneous before 20 weeks, including ectopic pregnancies), and number of living children.
         (3) For example, G5P1121 indicates this is a woman's fifth pregnancy, she has had one term delivery, one preterm delivery, and two abortions and has one living child.
      b. Information regarding course of pregnancy and delivery: Weeks of completed gestation for each pregnancy, weight of newborn at birth, any maternal or neonatal complications, duration of labor in hours, type of delivery (vaginal, forceps, vacuum, or operative), reason for any cesarean delivery as well as any information known about uterine scar and postoperative course.
      c. Medical history: including infections (hepatitis, HIV, HSV, rubella, varicella, sexually transmitted infections, and tuberculosis), psychosocial assessment, substance use, and family history.
      d. Genetic history: ethnicity; maternal age (>35 years); paternal age (>50 years); family history of genetic disorders, such as Down syndrome, Fragile X; neural tube defect; mental retardation; and cystic fibrosis. Ethnic predispositions to certain genetic disorders are:

■ TABLE 1-1
■ ■ **Prenatal Screening Tests***

Test	Reason for Screening Test
Blood type, Rh status, antibody screen	Identifies fetuses at risk of isoimmune disease
Hemoglobin or hematocrit	Baseline laboratory studies: rule out anemia
Rubella antibody screen	Identifies women susceptible to acquiring rubella during pregnancy; susceptible women should be immunized *after* delivery
Tuberculin skin testing	Identifies infected women for treatment
Hepatitis B surface antigen	Identifies women whose offspring can be treated at birth to prevent hepatitis B infection
Serologic test for syphilis (VDRL or rapid plasmin reagin)	Treatment reduces fetal/neonatal morbidity; mandated by law in most states
Human immunodeficiency virus	Identifies women for treatment and perinatal therapy to decrease transmission to the fetus
Urinalysis	
Glucose, ketones, protein	Screen for diabetes, pregnancy-induced hypertension, and renal disease
RBCs, WBCs, bacteria	Possible urinary tract infection
Diabetes screen (24 to 28 weeks)	Fasting and glucose tolerance tests to rule out gestational diabetes
Papanicolaou smear	Identifies cervicitis and precancerous and cancerous lesions
Neisseria gonorrhoeae and *Chlamydia*[†] cultures	Identify treatable sexually transmitted diseases, most of which can cause fetal or neonatal morbidity
Triple screen (maternal serum for AFP, human chorionic gonadotropin, estriol)	Tests done at 16 to 20 weeks at mother's discretion after counseling; AFP screens for neural tube defects, Down syndrome; combination of three tests very sensitive in identifying Down syndrome

AFP, Alpha-fetoprotein; *VDRL*, Venereal Disease Research Laboratory.
*Laboratory tests may vary from one center to another. Certain tests may be ordered if the patient is at specific risk (i.e., hemoglobinopathy screen to rule out sickle cell disease in a black patient whose status is unknown or with a family history). Ultrasonography is considered by some to be a screening tool for congenital anomalies. Cystic fibrosis testing is recommended for all couples planning a pregnancy, particularly for those ethnic groups at highest risk (e.g., Caucasians and Ashkenazi Jews).
[†]Some centers also screen for *Mycoplasma hominis* and group B streptococcus colonization.
Adapted from Clinic Protocol for Department of Obstetrics and Gynecology, University of Colorado Health Sciences Center; O'Neill, P., Davies, J., LeBel, A., and Hobbins, J.: Maternal factors affecting the newborn. In P.J. Threen, J. Deacon, J.A. Hernandez, and D.M. Hall (Eds.): *Assessment and care of the well newborn* (2nd ed.). St. Louis, 2005, Saunders.

      (1) African Americans: sickle cell anemia
      (2) Ashkenazi Jews: Tay-Sachs, Canavan, familial dysautonomia
      (3) Cajuns: Tay-Sachs
      (4) French Canadians: Tay-Sachs
      (5) Mediterranean descent: β-thalassemia and sickle cell disease
      (6) Southeast Asians: α-thalassemia
    e. History of pregnancy loss or neonatal death (Blackburn, 2007).
    f. Exposure to teratogens (Blackburn, 2007).
    g. History of current pregnancy.
  2. Perform a complete physical examination, including a complete pelvic examination.
  3. Initial laboratory work (Table 1-1), including genetic screening blood work such as screens for ethnically linked disorders.

Assessment of Gestational Age

A. Last menstrual period (LMP): Estimating gestational age by counting from the LMP is a reliable method.

1. A menstrual history should include frequency and duration of menstrual periods, heaviness of menstrual flow, menarche, and hormonal contraceptive use.
2. The estimated date of confinement (EDC) or due date may be determined by Nägele's rule: EDC = First day of LMP − 3 months + 7 days + 1 year.

B. **Pelvic examination and fundal height.**
1. Determination of the size of the uterus during an early examination (before 12 to 14 weeks) is relatively accurate if the mother is of normal height and not grossly obese.
2. Fundal height measurements (in centimeters) are made from 20 weeks on to assess growth and approximate gestational age ± 2 cm. The uterus is generally at the umbilicus at 20 weeks.

C. **Quickening is the first feeling of fetal movement.**
1. Primigravida: has quickening by 18 to 20 weeks.
2. Multigravida: has quickening by 16 to 18 weeks.

D. **Fetal heart tones:** Can be detected by an electronic Doppler device as early as 9 weeks and commonly by 12 weeks, and may be auscultated with a fetoscope by 19 to 20 weeks.

E. **Ultrasonography.**
1. Crown–rump measurement during the first trimester (6 to 12 weeks) most accurately reflects gestational age plus or minus 5 to 6 days with 90% accuracy (Platt, 2005). Gestational sac measurements prior to 6 weeks of gestation are not as accurate and should be followed up with subsequent ultrasound when the fetus is visible (Platt, 2005).
2. Fetal heart motion can be detected by real-time ultrasonography as early as 6 weeks' gestation by vaginal ultrasonography (Richards, 2007).
3. Biparietal diameter is the most frequently used method of establishing gestational age; it is most accurate between 12 and 20 weeks (Platt, 2005). The BPD has an accuracy of ±7 days between 14 and 21 weeks with a 95% confidence interval (Richards, 2007).
4. Abdominal circumference can be used to assess gestational age and intrauterine growth restriction. Use of abdominal circumference to assess gestational age is best done before 14 weeks (Platt, 2005).
5. Fetal femur length may also be used to determine gestational age in the second trimester and is accurate ±7 days (Platt, 2005).
6. Although placental grading is not used to date pregnancies, the amount of calcium deposits in the placenta increases as gestation progresses (Pillitteri, 2007). It may be helpful to look at placental grading when considering other ultrasound parameters to determine gestational age: Grade 0, 12 to 24 weeks; Grade 1, 30 to 32 weeks; Grade 2, 36 weeks; Grade 3, 37 to 38 weeks.
7. Reliability of ultrasound dating after 26 weeks is low and reliability of single parameters is poor (Platt, 2005). Beyond 30 weeks of gestation, accuracy of ultrasound measurements is ±2 to 3 weeks (Richards, 2007). Assessment of multiple parameters along with serial ultrasounds may be done to determine gestational age.

Genetic Screening

A. **All patients who present for care at ≤20 weeks should be offered noninvasive and invasive genetic screening regardless of age (American College of Obstetricians and Gynecologists [ACOG], 2007).**

B. **Noninvasive screening for chromosomal abnormalities (ACOG, 2007).**
1. First-trimester integrated screening at 10 to 14 weeks includes ultrasound measurement of fetal nuchal translucency and/or biochemical markers. Biochemical markers include α-fetoprotein (AFP), β-hCG, unconjugated estriol, inhibin A, and pregnancy-associated plasma protein A (PAPP-A).
2. Serum integrated biochemical marker screening in first and second trimester where nuchal translucency measurement is not an option. Single report in second trimester.
3. Nuchal translucency is a more reliable screen for multiples because interpretation of biochemical markers is difficult in multiple gestations (Simpson and Otaño, 2007).
4. All patients should be offered screening for cystic fibrosis, and if carrier status is detected then the partner should be screened and, if indicated, counseled (ACOG, 2005).

5. Second-trimester ultrasound at 18 to 20 weeks for review of systems.
6. Second-trimester biochemical marker screening at 15 to 20 weeks: screens for open neural tube defects (NTDs), Down syndrome, Trisomy 13, and Trisomy 18. For other potential genetic problems, screens with up to four markers—AFP, estriol, hCG, and inhibin A—with increased detection of chromosomal abnormalities with additional markers.

C. **Invasive screening.**
   1. Chorionic villus sampling (CVS) at 9 to 11 weeks: transabdominal or transvaginal aspiration of trophoblastic tissue with a catheter under ultrasound guidance (Simpson and Otaño, 2007). Risk of pregnancy loss is similar to amniocentesis. If CVS is performed for an increased risk of NTD, cystic hygroma, or other suspected anomaly, then the risk is increased (Simpson and Otaño, 2007).
   2. Amniocentesis at 18 to 20 weeks: aspiration of approximately 20 ml of amniotic fluid with a spinal needle inserted through the maternal abdomen into the uterine cavity under ultrasound guidance. Direct chromosomal analysis of fluid and AFP measurement is performed. Risk of procedural pregnancy loss: 1 in 400 (Simpson and Otaño, 2007).

Antepartum Visits

A. **Frequency:** Obstetric visits are recommended every 4 weeks until 28 weeks, then every 2 to 3 weeks until 36 weeks, and then weekly. If no ultrasound has been done or is not planned, additional visits may be necessary by 18 to 20 weeks to establish the presence of heart tones with a fetoscope and the presence of quickening (Johnson et al., 2007).

B. **Routine assessments:** Weight, blood pressure, fundal height, fetal presentation, fetal heart tones, fetal movement, abnormal bleeding or discharge, signs of preterm labor, signs of preeclampsia, psychosocial state.

C. **Lab and diagnostic assessments.**
   1. 24- to 28-week visit: a 1-hour oral glucose challenge test.
      a. 50-g oral glucose challenge test for gestational diabetes is performed. A level greater than 135 mg/dl is abnormal. A 3-hour oral glucose tolerance test is performed on all patients with an abnormal oral glucose challenge test screen result. The diagnosis of gestational diabetes is made if two values are elevated (plasma values: fasting, 95 mg/dl; at 1 hour, 180 mg/dl; at 2 hours, 155 mg/dl; and at 3 hours, 140 mg/dl) (Expert Committee on the Diagnosis and Classification of Diabetes Mellitus, 2000).
      b. Obtain repeat hemoglobin and hematocrit determinations to recheck for anemia. Repeat at 36 weeks if anemia is detected.
   2. 28-week visit: obtain a repeat antibody titer for Rh-negative mothers; administer Rh immunoglobulin, 300 mg, if no anti-D antibody has been detected.
   3. Ultrasonography may be indicated to evaluate fetal growth, amniotic fluid volume, Doppler flow, or placental assessment.
   4. 36-week visit: repeat HIV, syphilis, gonorrhea, and chlamydia culture if indicated.
   5. 35- to 37-week visit: obtain a vaginal/rectal group B streptococcus (GBS) culture. The culture result is reliable for 5 weeks (Centers for Disease Control and Prevention [CDC], 2002).

Antepartum Fetal Surveillance

A. **Fetal Movement Counts or Fetal Kick Counts (Druzin et al., 2007).**
   1. Fetal movement periods last approximately 40 minutes, and quiet periods last approximately 20 minutes.
   2. Decrease in fetal movements precedes fetal death; therefore, fetal movement counts are a cost-effective method to monitor fetal well-being.

B. **Nonstress test (NST).** This is the most widely used screening method for fetal well-being and is indicated for patients at risk of placental insufficiency and may be started as early as 30 to 32 weeks' gestation.

1. Some indications for NST include postterm pregnancy, diabetes mellitus, hypertension, previous stillbirths, intrauterine growth restriction, decreased fetal movements, and Rh disease.
2. Testing is repeated once or twice weekly. A *reactive* NST result is two fetal heart rate (FHR) accelerations, defined as a 15-beat rise from baseline that lasts for at least 15 seconds with return to baseline during a 20-minute period. A *nonreactive* test result is no FHR accelerations after 40 minutes (Druzin et al., 2007).
3. A reactive test result is reassuring, with risk of fetal death approximately 5 in 1000. A nonreactive result is an indication for further testing.

C. **Contraction stress test (CST).**
   1. CST evaluates the reserve function of the placenta. Indications for use are the same as for use of the NST. The CST is most often used after a nonreactive NST result (Druzin et al., 2007).
   2. Done by evaluating three spontaneous contractions in a 10-minute period, or attaining three contractions in a 10-minute period through nipple stimulation (endogenous oxytocin) or intravenous oxytocin challenge test (exogenous). The contractions should be of moderate intensity and last 40 to 60 seconds in the 10-minute period.
   3. CST simulates a labor pattern and allows the fetus to be stressed as in normal labor. The CST looks for FHR decelerations in relation to the onset of uterine contractions.
      a. A positive CST result is defined as late decelerations of the FHR that are present with the majority of contractions in a 10-minute window. Delivery should be considered with a positive CST result.
      b. Findings may also be considered suspicious or equivocal, unsatisfactory, or as showing hyperstimulation. These cases require retesting in the next 24 hours for adequate interpretation of fetal well-being (Druzin et al., 2007).

D. **Biophysical profile.**
   1. The biophysical profile uses real-time ultrasonography to evaluate five parameters, each receiving either 0 or 2 points; the maximum score is 10 points, with management based on the assigned score.
   2. Modified biophysical profile: NST/amniotic fluid index (AFI) (Druzin et al., 2007).
      a. NST is an indicator of present fetal condition.
      b. Amniotic fluid index (AFI) is a marker of longer-term fetal status.

E. **Amniotic fluid index.**
   1. Decreased amniotic fluid volume (oligohydramnios) is associated with uteroplacental insufficiency. It may also be indicative of fetal genitourinary or lung anomalies. Increased incidence of perinatal mortality with oligohydramnios (Tarsa and Moore, 2005).
   2. Polyhydramnios may be associated with chromosomal disorders, maternal diabetes, and anatomic anomalies such as tracheoesophageal fistula (Gilbert, 2007).
   3. Measurement of amniotic fluid:
      a. Single vertical pocket measurement of 2 cm considered adequate.
      b. The four-quadrant measure is the AFI, and it varies by gestational age. AFI of <5 at term is used as cutoff for oligohydramnios (Tarsa and Moore, 2005).

Laboratory Assessments for Documenting Fetal Lung Maturity

1. Lecithin/sphingomyelin (L/S) ratio equal to or greater than 2.0 indicates fetal lung maturity and occurs when fetal lung surfactant is present in amniotic fluid (at approximately 35 weeks). Positive predictive value is 95% (Ghidini and Locatelli, 2005).
2. Phosphatidylglycerol (PG), a minor component of surfactant, is also present in amniotic fluid at approximately 35 weeks and increases rapidly at 37 weeks. PG is reported as present or absent with a positive predictive value of 95% to 100% (Ghidini and Locatelli, 2005). Measurement of PG is a more reliable test of lung maturity in mothers with diabetes than is measurement of the L/S ratio.
3. Fetal lung maturity assay measures surfactant/albumin ratio in amniotic fluid. It is less expensive, is easier to perform, and has fewer false-negative results than the L/S ratio

or PG measurement. Positive predictive value is 96% to 100% (Ghidini and Locatelli, 2005).

4. Lamellar body counts (LB) are a storage form of surfactant (Druzin et al., 2007). Test is inexpensive and may be performed in 15 minutes with <1 ml of amniotic fluid. Results have a 97% to 98% positive predictive value (Ghidini and Locatelli, 2005).

Maternal Infections

A. **TORCH infections** (Thureen et al., 2005) (Table 1-2).
   1. Acronym rarely used as diagnostic grouping but frequently used clinically to refer to five infectious diseases: *t*oxoplasmosis, *o*thers (e.g., parvovirus, congenital syphilis), *r*ubella, *c*ytomegalovirus infection, and *h*erpes simplex. They all cross the placenta and may adversely affect the fetus.
B. **Sexually transmitted infections** (Thureen et al., 2005) (Table 1-3).
C. **Other communicable diseases** (Thureen et al., 2005) (Table 1-4).
D. **Chorioamnionitis** (Thureen et al., 2005).
   1. An infection of the chorion, amnion, and amniotic fluid that may cause perinatal morbidity and mortality usually associated with prolonged labor and ruptured membranes but can also be found in women with intact membranes.
   2. Usually an ascending infection, commonly caused by *Escherichia coli*, group B streptococcus, anaerobic streptococci, and bacteroids.
E. **Infection with group B streptococcus.**
   1. Approximately 10% to 30% of women are colonized with group B streptococcus (GBS; formerly *Streptococcus agalactiae*) (Dinsmoor, 2005). Colonization can be transient, chronic, or intermittent.
   2. GBS may cause severe invasive disease in neonates. The majority of neonatal GBS infections occur during the first week of life and present as sepsis or pneumonia (CDC, 2002). There has been a 70% decline in neonatal GBS infection since intrapartum prophylaxis was instituted in the 1990s (CDC, 2002). The infection rate is 5.1 in 1000 infants born to colonized mothers without risk factors and increases to 41 in 1000 infants if there is premature labor and delivery, prolonged rupture of membranes, or intrapartum fever (Dinsmoor, 2005).
   3. All women should be screened at 35 to 37 weeks of gestation for rectal-genital group B streptococcus. Cultures are considered reliable for 5 weeks. Any woman with positive culture results should be given antibiotic prophylaxis during labor (CDC, 2002).

NORMAL LABOR AND BIRTH

A. **Stages and phases of labor:** There are three stages of labor.
   1. First stage: onset of contractions to complete dilatation has three phases.
      a. Latent phase: onset of labor to time when the slope of cervical dilatation changes.
      b. Active phase: approximately 4 cm to complete cervical dilatation. Maximum slope is from 5 to 9 cm and is time when labor progresses rapidly.
      c. Transition: portion of active phase from 8 to 10 cm with intense contraction and beginning of descent.
   2. Second stage: complete dilatation to delivery of infant. Maximum fetal descent coincides with transition and second stage.
   3. Third stage: Time from delivery of infant to delivery of placenta.

Intrapartum Labor Management

A. **Admission.**
   1. History, review of prenatal records, contractions, membrane status, bleeding, fetal movement, and nutritional status.
   2. Physical examination: vital signs, fetal heart tones, contraction pattern, abdominal examination (Leopold maneuvers, estimated fetal weight, scars), extremities, vaginal

Text continued on p. 17

TABLE 1-2

■ **TORCH Infections**

Infection/Incubation	Transmission	Detection	Maternal Effects	Neonatal Effects	Incidence and Prevention
Cytomegalovirus Incubation: unknown	Intimate contact with infected secretions (breast milk, cervical mucus, semen, saliva, and urine) Transplacentally Organ transplantation	IgM titer	Clinically "silent"; only 1% to 5% acquire symptoms: low-grade fever, malaise, arthralgia, hepatomegaly	Infection is most likely to occur with maternal primary infection; 90% of infected infants are free of symptoms at birth, but 5% to 15% of these may have long-term sequelae, 5% with severe involvement at birth: IUGR, microcephaly, periventricular calcification, deafness, blindness, chorioretinitis, mental retardation, hepatosplenomegaly	Primarily occurs in 1% to 2% of pregnant women; 90% of adult population in United States are seropositive. Rigorous personal hygiene throughout pregnancy to prevent infection if not infected
Herpes simplex virus Incubation: 2 to 10 days	Intimate mucocutaneous exposure Passage through an infected birth canal Ascending infection, especially with rupture of membranes Transplacentally (rare) if initial infection occurs during pregnancy	Suspect with vesicles on cervix, vagina, or external genital area; painful lesions Presumptive diagnosis by fluorescent antibody or Papanicolaou smear on vesicular fluid Confirm diagnosis by vesicle culture	Painful genital lesions Primary infection commonly associated with fever, malaise, myalgias Numbness, tingling, burning, itching, and pain with lesions Lymphadenopathy Urinary retention	Rare transplacental transmissions have resulted in miscarriages Mortality rate of 5% to 60% if neonatal exposure is with active primary infection Neurologic or ophthalmic sequelae Disseminated infection in 70% of cases, with jaundice, respiratory distress, and CNS involvement	Estimated 300,000 new cases per year 1:3000 to 20,000 live births with perinatal transmission Up to 80% of women delivering infected infants have no history of genital herpes; cesarean delivery if known active infection Avoid genital contact when male has penile lesions; use condoms

Infection/Incubation	Mode of Transmission	Signs and Symptoms	Fetal/Neonatal Effects	Comments
Rubella Incubation: 14 to 21 days	Nasopharyngeal secretions Transplacentally	Pink maculopapular rash on face, neck, arms, and legs lasting 3 days Lymph node enlargement, fever, malaise, headache History of exposure 3 weeks earlier	Fetal infection rate greatest before 11 weeks and after 35 weeks, but severe sequelae occur with first-trimester infection; includes deafness (60% to 70%), eye defects (10% to 30%), CNS anomalies (10% to 25%), congenital heart disease (10% to 20%)	Since introduction of vaccine in late 1960s, rubella is rare Occurs more commonly in springtime Vaccine is contraindicated during pregnancy; vaccinate susceptible women postpartum
Toxoplasmosis (protozoa, *Toxoplasma gondii*) Incubation: 2 to 3 weeks	Eating raw meat containing *T. gondii* Ingesting *T. gondii* cysts secreted in feces of infected cats Transplacentally Impossible to transmit to others because the infecting organisms are tissue bound and are not secreted	Serologic antibody testing ELISA 90% of infected women have no symptoms Posterior cervical lymphadenopathy Malaise Premature labor and delivery	Severity varies with gestational age (usually, earlier infection results in more severe effects) Neurologic, ophthalmologic, and co-sequelae are variable IUGR Hydrocephalus Microcephaly	Incidence varies throughout the world (1 to 4 infants per 1000 live births) 20% to 30% of U.S. women have been exposed Incidence of congenital toxoplasmosis infection in the United States is 1:1000 to 8000 Reduce contact with cats during pregnancy

Serologic antibody titer testing (IgG-specific rubella antibody) Virus isolation from throat (Rubella testing)

CNS, Central nervous system; *ELISA,* enzyme-linked immunosorbent assay; *IgG,* immunoglobulin G; *IgM,* immunoglobulin M; *IUGR,* intrauterine growth restriction; *TORCH,* toxoplasmosis, *o*ther infections (e.g., congenital syphilis), *r*ubella, *c*ytomegalovirus infection, and *h*erpes simplex.

From Thureen, P.J., Davies, J.K., Lebel, A., and Hobbins, J.C.: Maternal factors affecting the newborn. In P.J. Thureen, J. Deacon, J.A. Hernandez, and D.M. Hall (Eds.): *Assessment and care of the well newborn* (2nd ed.). St. Louis, 2005, Saunders.

■ TABLE 1-3
■ ■ **Sexually Transmitted Infections**

Infection/Agent/Incubation	Detection	Maternal Effects	Neonatal Effects	Incidence
Acquired immunodeficiency syndrome Human immunodeficiency virus Incubation: variable, months to years	ELISA for screening Western blot or indirect immunofluorescence assay p24 antigen for acute infection before seroconversion		30% chance of transmission from infected mother Syndrome develops in up to 65% of infected infants within a few months after birth	1991: estimated 200,000 cases in the United States; 0.15% of all women who delivered were infected
Chlamydiosis Bacterium: *Chlamydia trachomatis* Incubation: variable but more than 1 week	Culture of endocervical and urethral specimens ELISA or fluorescent antibody	Most cases asymptomatic Mucopurulent cervicitis on swab specimen is less sensitive and specific Occasionally premature rupture of membranes, preterm labor, IUGR, infertility, chorioamnionitis	30% to 40% of exposed infants have conjunctivitis Frequently associated with other sexually transmitted infections	Most common sexually transmitted infection 3% to 18% have pneumonia Estimated 4 million cases occur annually in the United States, with prevalence rates in female patients of 8% to 20% 70% of infections may be asymptomatic
Gonorrhea Bacteria: *Neisseria gonorrhoeae*, gram-negative diplococcus Incubation: 10 days	Endocervical, oral, or rectal cultures Genital or blood cultures Gram stain of lesions	60% to 80% of those infected are free of symptoms Occasionally pelvic peritonitis, premature rupture of membranes, postpartum endometritis, chorioamnionitis, increased infertility, ectopic pregnancy	Purulent conjunctivitis Sepsis or meningitis	More than 1 million cases are reported in the United States each year Incidence in pregnancy ranges from 1% to 10%, depending on the population

Organism/Incubation				
Human papillomavirus Incubation: unknown (3 months to years)	Single or multiple irregular painless papules in the genital or perianal area Colposcopy used as adjunct in equivocal situations Cervical cytologic testing	Significant number of lesions enlarge during pregnancy Usually multicentric in pregnancy Viral lesions probably more frequent in pregnant women because of increased hormone levels Increasing incidence noted in STI clinics and private offices Peak occurrence at ages 15 to 35 Associated with other STIs	Potential transmission of laryngeal papillomas Very rare (<1:1000 to 1500 pregnancies in which mothers have genital condyloma)	Estimated 40 to 60 million people infected worldwide
Syphilis Spirochete: *Treponema pallidum* Incubation: 3 weeks on average	VDRL test Rapid plasma reagin test Fluorescent treponemal antibody absorption test	Primary chancre: painless ulcerative lesion Secondary syphilis: fever and malaise, red macules on palms or soles of feet Generalized lymphadenopathy Early latent (positive serologic finding <1 year's duration) syphilis Latent (cardiovascular) syphilis Neurosyphilis	Vary depending on gestation Stillbirth IUGR Nonimmune hydrops Premature labor	100,000 cases are reported in the United States each year; 80% of these women are of reproductive age 3850 cases of congenital syphilis in 1992 70% to 100% fetal transmission rate in primary maternal disease
Trichomoniasis Protozoa: *Trichomonas vaginalis* Incubation: 4 to 20 days	"Wet prep" saline examination Papanicolaou smear Dysuria Urinalysis	Malodorous, discolored vaginal discharge	Infant contact through infected vagina Usually asymptomatic	Not reported to CDC but estimated in as many as 20% of pregnancies Estimates of 10% to 15% of all cases of vaginitis

CDC, Centers for Disease Control and Prevention; *ELISA*, enzyme-linked immunosorbent assay; *IUGR*, intrauterine growth retardation; *STD*, sexually transmitted disease; *VDRL*, Venereal Disease Research Laboratory.

From Thureen, P.J., Davies, J.K., Lebel, A., and Hobbins, J.C.: Maternal factors affecting the newborn. In P.J. Thureen, J. Deacon, J.A. Hernandez, and D.M. Hall (Eds.): *Assessment and care of the well newborn* (2nd ed.). St. Louis, 2005, Saunders.

■ TABLE 1-4
■ ■ Other Communicable Diseases

Infection/Agent/Incubation	Mode of Transmission	Maternal Effects	Neonatal Effects	Incidence and Prevention
Influenza virus Incubation: 24 to 72 hours	Respiratory secretions	Usually brief but incapacitating disease Death occurs from secondary bacterial pneumonia	Any risk of malformation has been confined to first trimester Most studies fail to support teratogenicity	Killed virus vaccine Vaccine during pregnancy is indicated if mother is at medical risk because of other diseases
Mumps Paramyxovirus Incubation: 16 to 18 days	Respiratory secretions	Spontaneous abortion rate is increased twofold	Teratogenicity is unknown	Avoid pregnancy for 3 months after vaccination
Parvovirus B19 (fifth disease) DNA virus Incubation: 4 to 14 days	Respiratory secretions	Erythema Elevated temperature Arthralgia	Spontaneous abortions	Risk for women with primary infection during the first 20 weeks of pregnancy is 15% to 17% 200,000 to 300,000 cases in the United States each year
Hepatitis B	Sexually Perinatally Transplacentally Blood, stool, and saliva transmission	Fever, jaundice, malaise, hepatosplenomegaly Premature labor	Increased stillbirth rate Infected infants usually symptom-free at birth	One third of infants born to HBsAg-positive mothers will have HBsAg/HBeAg positivity and anti-HBe negativity
Varicella (chickenpox) Varicella-zoster virus Incubation: 11 to 21 days	Probably by aerosolized respiratory droplets Portal of entry is the respiratory tract Transplacentally	Severe in adults Risk of premature labor as a result of high temperature Risk of varicella pneumonia appears to be increased during pregnancy	2% of infants with maternal infection in the first trimester have cutaneous scarring, eye abnormalities, and retardation At risk if maternal rash onset 5 days before to 2 days after delivery; severe disseminated neonatal disease may develop, and one third die	90% of women are immune In the United States occurs in less than 0.1% of pregnancies

DNA, Deoxyribonucleic acid; HBsAg, hepatitis B surface antigen; HBeAg, hepatitis B "e" antigen.
From Thureen, P.J., Davies, J.K., Lebel, A., and Hobbins, J.C.: Maternal factors affecting the newborn. In P.J. Thureen, J. Deacon, J.A. Hernandez, and D.M. Hall (Eds.): Assessment and care of the well newborn (2nd ed.). St. Louis, 2005, Saunders.

examination (dilatation, effacement, station), pelvis, speculum examination if history warrants to assess for ruptured membranes (Nitrazine, ferning, pooling, Valsalva).

B. **Management of low-risk patient.** The patient should be identified as being low or high risk on the basis of available data. ACOG recommends that low-risk patients have auscultation of FHR every 30 minutes in the first stage and every 15 minutes in the second stage, and high-risk patients every 15 minutes in the first stage and every 5 minutes in the second stage (Garite, 2007).

1. A nonreassuring FHR detected by auscultation is indication for electronic fetal monitoring: bradycardia, tachycardia, or FHR decelerations.

2. Electronic fetal monitoring—recommendation to use National Institute of Child Health and Human Development terminology (National Institute of Child Health and Human Development Research Planning Workshop, 1997):

   a. FHR baseline evaluated over a 10-minute segment.
     (1) Normal baseline is 110 to 160 beats per minute (bpm).
     (2) Bradycardia is <110 bpm.
     (3) Tachycardia is >160 bpm.

   b. Fetal heart rate patterns associated with increased incidence of fetal compromise:
     (1) Severe bradycardia: rate <80 bpm for more than 3 minutes
     (2) Repetitive late decelereations: a symmetric fall in the FHR, beginning at or after the peak of the uterine contraction and returning to baseline only after the contraction has ended
     (3) Undulating baseline: a pattern of rapid change between tachycardia (rate >160 bpm) and bradycardia (rate <100 bpm)
     (4) Any nonreassuring pattern associated with explained poor or absent baseline variability: a flat or nearly flat baseline
     (5) Absence of accelerations

   c. Uterine activity may be measured by external palpation, external tocodynamometer, or intrauterine pressure catheter to assess frequency, duration, and intensity of contractions.

C. **Second-stage management.**

1. Fetal descent/pushing
   a. ACOG (2003) recommends adherence to a 2-hour time limit for primipara and 1 hour for multipara (3 hours for primipara and 2 hours for multipara with epidurals). Research has shown no significant relationship between second-stage duration and perinatal mortality, 5-minute Apgar scores <7, neonatal seizures, or admission to NICU (Varney et al., 2004). Current recommendations state that critical factor is time of duration of active pushing rather than overall duration (Roberts and Hanson, 2007); therefore, passive descent and to evaluation of fetal descent relative to time spent actively pushing is advised.

D. **Third stage—time from the birth of the baby to the delivery of the placenta.**

1. Normal duration from 0 to 30 minutes.

PUERPERIUM: "FOURTH TRIMESTER"

The period from delivery through the sixth week is known as the "fourth trimester." Under the Newborns' and Mothers' Health Protection Act of 1996, minimum federal standards mandate health plans to provide coverage for 48 hours after a normal vaginal birth and 96 hours after a cesarean birth unless the attending health provider and mother agree on early discharge (Crum, 2006b).

A. **Uterine involution.**

1. Involution begins immediately after delivery. The fundus is generally firm at the level of the umbilicus and generally decreases by one finger breadth daily. It is not palpable abdominally by 2 weeks.

B. **Breasts/breastfeeding.**

1. During the first 2 to 3 postpartum days, high-protein colostrum secretion provides the infant with nutrition. It also has high concentrations of immunoglobulin A, lactoferrin, and oligosaccharide to protect the infant against infection (Blackburn, 2007).

2. On the second or third postpartum day, milk secretion begins and breast engorgement may occur. Engorgement generally resolves spontaneously within 24 to 36 hours. In non-breastfeeding mothers, lactation ceases within 1 week.

3. Mature milk is established by the end of the first or second week. Milk production is based on supply–demand, and suckling provides a sensory nerve stimulus to secrete prolactin and oxytocin to increase milk production (Blackburn, 2007). If needed, various regimens exist to increase milk supply, including the use of Brewer's yeast and metoclopramide (Reglan).

4. Establishment of breastfeeding is facilitated by early initiation of breastfeeding, rooming-in, breastfeeding on demand, not using pacifiers, and not providing formula supplementation unless medically indicated. Postpartum breastfeeding support contributes to successful initiation and continuation of breastfeeding.

C. Immunizations.

1. Rubella vaccination should be administered in the immediate postpartum period to all women who are not immune (Crum, 2006a). $Rh_o(D)$ immune globulin (RhoGAM) suppresses the immune response; therefore, if the woman needs $Rh_o(D)$ immune globulin and a rubella vaccine, the rubella vaccine can be delayed until the postpartum week 6 visit or, if given with $Rh_o(D)$ immune globulin, she should be retested for rubella immunity 3 months after administration (Crum, 2006b).

2. $Rh_o(D)$ immune globulin (300 mcg given intramuscularly) is administered to the Rh-negative mother with an Rh-positive newborn within 72 hours of delivery to prevent sensitization from fetal–maternal transfusion of Rh-positive fetal erythrocytes (Crum, 2006b).

3. Tdap (Tetanus, diphtheria, and pertussis): Women who have not previously received a dose of Tdap, including breastfeeding women, should receive Tdap after delivery, before leaving the hospital or birthing center if 2 years or more have elapsed since the last Td (tetanus diphtheria) immunization (CDC, 2007). Tdap can be administered with other vaccines.

D. Emotional changes.

1. Postpartum blues may occur from birth to 14 days postpartum. Mild, transient symptoms of emotional lability may be caused by hormonal changes, sleep deprivation, role adjustment, and physiologic changes. Symptoms may be more intense if there are neonatal problems.

2. Postpartum depression may occur from birth throughout 6 months postpartum and evaluation includes diagnostic criteria for depression. There are various screening tools such as the Beck or Edinburgh Postpartum Depression scales. A rare severe form of postpartum depression is postpartum psychosis, which may encompass suicidal thoughts or delusional behaviors.

3. Postpartum thyroiditis may cause symptoms of fatigue and depression. Women with postpartum depression should be evaluated for thyroiditis.

REFERENCES

American College of Obstetricians and Gynecologists: Dystocia and augmentation of labor. *Practice Bulletin No. 49.* Washington, DC, 2003, American College of Obstetricians and Gynecologists.

American College of Obstetricians and Gynecologists: ACOG Committee opinion. Update on carrier screening for cystic fibrosis. *Report No. 325.* Washington, DC, 2005, American College of Obstetricians and Gynecologists.

American College of Obstetricians and Gynecologists: ACOG practice bulletin: Screening for fetal chromosomal abnormalities. *Practice Bulletin No. 77.* Washington, DC, 2007, American College of Obstetricians and Gynecologists.

Blackburn, S.T.: *Maternal, fetal, and neonatal physiology: A clinical perspective* (3rd ed.). St. Louis, 2007, Saunders.

Centers for Disease Control and Prevention: *Recommended adult immunization schedule, United States. October 2006-2007.* Retrieved February 3, 2008, from http://www.cdc.gov/vaccines/recs/schedules/downloads/adult/07-08/adult-schedule-11x17.pdf, 2007.

Centers for Disease Control and Prevention: *Prevention of perinatal group B streptococcal disease. Revised guidelines from CDC. MMWR Recommendation and Reports,* August 16, 2002 / 51(RR11);1-22. Retrieved February 2, 2008, from http://www.cdc.

gov/mmwr/preview/mmwrhtml/rr5111a1.htm, 2002.

Crum, K.: Maternal physiologic changes. In D.L. Lowdermilk and S.E. Perry (Eds.): *Maternity nursing* (7th ed.). St. Louis, 2006a, Mosby, pp. 454-465.

Crum, K.: Nursing care during the fourth trimester. In D.L. Lowdermilk and S.E. Perry (Eds.): *Maternity nursing* (7th ed.). St. Louis, 2006b, Mosby, pp. 466-495.

Cunningham, F.G., Leveno, K.J., Bloom, S.L., et al.: *Williams' obstetrics* (22nd ed.). New York, 2005, McGraw-Hill.

Dinsmoor, M.: Group B streptococcus. In J.R. Queenan, J.C. Hobbins, and C.Y. Spong (Eds.): *Protocols for high-risk pregnancies* (4th ed.). Malden, MA, 2005, Blackwell, pp. 329-333.

Druzin, M., Smith, J., Jr., Gabbe, S., and Reed, K.: Antepartum fetal evaluation. In S.G. Gabbe, J.R. Niebyl, and J.L. Simpson (Eds.): *Obstetrics: Normal and problem pregnancies* (5th ed.). Philadelphia, 2007, Churchill Livingstone, pp. 267-300.

Expert Committee on the Diagnosis and Classification of Diabetes Mellitus: Report of the expert committee on the diagnosis and classification of diabetes mellitus. *Diabetes Care*, 23(Suppl 1):S4-S19, 2000.

Garite, T.: Intrapartum fetal evaluation. In S.G. Gabbe, J.R. Niebyl, and J.L. Simpson (Eds.): *Obstetrics: Normal and problem pregnancies* (5th ed.). Philadelphia, 2007, Churchill Livingstone, pp. 364-395.

Ghidini, A. and Locatelli, A.: Indices of maturity. In J.R. Queenan, J.C. Hobbins, and C.Y. Spong (Eds.): *Protocols for high-risk pregnancies* (4th ed.). Malden, MA, 2005, Blackwell, pp. 89-95.

Gilbert, W.: Amniotic fluid disorders. In S.G. Gabbe, J. R. Niebyl, and J.L. Simpson (Eds.): *Obstetrics: Normal and problem pregnancies* (5th ed.). Philadelphia, 2007, Churchill Livingstone, pp. 834-845.

Gordon, M.: Maternal physiology. In S.G. Gabbe, J.R. Niebyl, and J.L. Simpson (Eds.): *Obstetrics: Normal and problem pregnancies* (5th ed.). Philadelphia, 2007, Churchill Livingstone, pp. 55-84.

Johnson, T., Gregory, K., and Niebyl, J.: Preconception and prenatal care: Part of the continuum. In S.G. Gabbe, J.R. Niebyl, and J.L. Simpson (Eds.): *Obstetrics: Normal and problem pregnancies* (5th ed.). Philadelphia, 2007, Churchill Livingstone, pp. 111-137.

Kroumpouzos, G.: Intrahepatic cholestasis of pregnancy. In S.G. Gabbe, J.R. Niebyl, and J.L. Simpson (Eds.): *Obstetrics: Normal and problem pregnancies* (5th ed.). Philadelphia, 2007, Churchill Livingstone, pp. 1112-1113.

Lowdermilk, D.L. and Perry, S.E.: *Maternity nursing* (7th ed.). St. Louis, 2006, Mosby.

Mestman, J.H.: Thyroid and parathyroid diseases in pregnancy. In S.G. Gabbe, J.R. Niebyl, and J.L.

Simpson (Eds.): *Obstetrics: Normal and problem pregnancies* (5th ed.). Philadelphia, 2007, Churchill Livingstone, pp. 1011-1037.

National Institute of Child Health and Human Development Research Planning Workshop: Electronic fetal heart rate monitoring: Research guidelines for interpretation. *Journal of Obstetric, Gynecologic, and Neonatal Nursing*, 26(6):635-640, 1997.

Papoutsis, J. and Kroumpouzos, G.: Dermatologic disorders of pregnancy. In S.G. Gabbe, J.R. Niebyl, and J.L. Simpson (Eds.): *Obstetrics: Normal and problem pregnancies* (5th ed.). Philadelphia, 2007, Churchill Livingstone, pp. 1178-1192.

Perry, S.: Genetics, conception, and fetal development. In D.L. Lowdermilk and S.E. Perry (Eds.): *Maternity nursing* (7th ed.). St. Louis, 2006, Mosby, pp. 175-207.

Pettker, C. and Lockwood, C.: Thromboembolic disorder. In S.G. Gabbe, J.R. Niebyl, and J.L. Simpson (Eds.): *Obstetrics: Normal and problem pregnancies* (5th ed.). Philadelphia, 2007, Churchill Livingstone, pp. 1064-1079.

Pillitteri, A.: *Maternal and child health nursing: Care of the childbearing and childrearing family* (5th ed.). Philadelphia, 2007, Lippincott Williams & Wilkins.

Platt, L.: Assessment of gestational age. In J.R. Queenan, J.C. Hobbins, and C.Y. Spong (Eds.): *Protocols for high-risk pregnancies* (4th ed.). Malden, MA, 2005, Blackwell, pp. 64-74.

Richards, D.S.: Ultrasound for pregnancy dating, growth, and the diagnosis of fetal malformations. In S.G. Gabbe, J.R. Niebyl, and J.L. Simpson (Eds.): *Obstetrics: Normal and problem pregnancies* (5th ed.). Philadelphia, 2007, Churchill Livingstone, pp. 215-244.

Roberts, J. and Hanson, L.: Best practices in second stage labor care: Maternal bearing down and positioning. *Journal of Midwifery and Women's Health*, 52:238-245, 2007.

Simpson, J. and Otaño, L.: Prenatal genetic diagnosis. In S.G. Gabbe, J.R. Niebyl, and J.L. Simpson (Eds.): *Obstetrics: Normal and problem pregnancies* (5th ed.). Philadelphia, 2007, Churchill Livingstone, pp. 152-183.

Tarsa, M. and Moore, T.: Oligohydramnios. In J.R. Queenan, J.C. Hobbins, and C.Y. Spong (Eds.): *Protocols for high-risk pregnancies* (4th ed.). Malden, MA, 2005, Blackwell, pp. 428-433.

Thureen, P., Davies, J., LeBel, A., et al.: Maternal factors affecting the newborn. In P.J. Thureen, J. Deacon, J. Hernandez, and D. Hall (Eds.): *Assessment and care of the well newborn* (2nd ed.). St. Louis, 2005, Saunders, pp. 3-26.

Varney, H., Kriebs, J., and Gegor, C.: *Varney's midwifery* (4th ed.). Boston, 2004, Jones & Bartlett.

2 Antepartum-Intrapartum Complications

ANNE B. BROUSSARD and HELEN M. HURST

OBJECTIVES
1. List maternal risk factors that may exist before pregnancy.
2. Discuss the effects of hypertension and diabetes on the maternal-placental-fetal complex.
3. Categorize intrapartum conditions that may result in complications for the newborn infant.
4. Assess the fetus/neonate for effects of tocolytic drugs.
5. Describe the effect on the fetus/neonate of these intrapartum crises: abruptio placentae, placenta previa, cord prolapse, and shoulder dystocia.
6. List neonatal complications associated with breech delivery.
7. Examine the effect of obstetric analgesia/anesthesia and cesarean birth on the newborn infant.

An understanding of maternal complications enhances the ability of the nurse to anticipate and recognize neonatal complications and intervene appropriately. The purpose of this chapter is to provide a comprehensive view of possible neonatal complications resulting from maternal risk factors. These risk factors may exist before the pregnancy or develop during the antepartum and intrapartum periods (Table 2-1).

ANATOMY AND PHYSIOLOGY

A. **The fetus.** The fetus is a part of the maternal-placental-fetal complex.
B. **Conditions and substances that affect the pregnant woman.** These have the potential to affect placental functions of respiration, nutrition, excretion, and hormone production. Decreased placental function can in turn adversely affect the fetus.
C. **The placenta.** The traditional concept of the placenta as a barrier to noxious substances has long been superseded by the concept of the placenta as a sieve that permits transport of desirable and undesirable substances to the fetus. The placental membrane separating maternal and fetal circulations consists of several tissue layers; it thins to three layers after 20 weeks (Davidson et al., 2008).
D. **Placental transport mechanisms.** These mechanisms, including passive and facilitated diffusion, are affected by a number of factors (Baschat, 2006; Burton et al., 2007; Ross et al., 2007).
   1. Placental area.
      a. To supply the increased growth needs of the fetus, the placenta normally increases in size as the pregnancy advances.
      b. A placenta that is not keeping pace with fetal growth or that has decreased functional area as a result of infarct or separation does not allow optimal transport of materials between the fetus and the mother.
      c. The outcome of decreased functional placental area can include a decrease in fetal growth, fetal or neonatal distress, and even fetal or neonatal death.
   2. Concentration gradient.
      a. Passive and facilitated diffusion of unbound substances dissolved in maternal and fetal plasma occurs in the direction of lesser concentration.

■ TABLE 2-1
■ ■ **Prenatal High-Risk Factors**

Factor	Maternal Implications	Fetal/Neonatal Implications
SOCIAL-PERSONAL		
Low income level and/or low educational level	Poor antenatal care Poor nutrition ↑ Risk preeclampsia	Low birth weight IUGR
Poor diet	Inadequate nutrition ↑ Risk anemia ↑ Risk preeclampsia	Fetal malnutrition Prematurity Small for gestational age
Living at high altitude	Hemoglobin	Prematurity IUGR ↑ Hemoglobin (polycythemia)
Multiparity more than 3	↑ Risk antepartum/postpartum hemorrhage	Anemia Fetal death
Weight less than 45.5 kg (100 lb)	Poor nutrition Cephalopelvic disproportion Prolonged labor	IUGR Hypoxia associated with difficult labor and birth
Weight more than 91 kg (200 lb)	↑ Risk hypertension ↑ Risk cephalopelvic disproportion ↑ Risk diabetes	↓ Fetal nutrition ↑ Risk macrosomia
Age less than 16 years	Poor nutrition Poor antenatal care ↑ Risk preeclampsia ↑ Risk cephalopelvic disproportion	Low birth weight ↑ Fetal death
Age more than 35 years	↑ Risk preeclampsia ↑ Risk cesarean birth	↑ Risk congenital anomalies ↑ Chromosomal aberrations
Smoking 1 pack per day or more	↑ Risk hypertension ↑ Risk cancer	Placental perfusion ↓ O_2 and nutrients available Low birth weight IUGR Preterm birth
Use of addictive drugs	↑ Risk poor nutrition ↑ Risk infection with intravenous drugs ↑ Risk HIV, hepatitis C ↑ Risk abruptio placentae	↑ Risk congenital anomalies ↑ Risk low birth weight Neonatal withdrawal Lower serum bilirubin
Excessive alcohol consumption	↑ Risk poor nutrition Possible hepatic effects with long-term consumption	↑ Risk fetal alcohol syndrome
PREEXISTING MEDICAL DISORDERS		
Diabetes mellitus	↑ Risk preeclampsia, hypertension Episodes of hypoglycemia and hyperglycemia ↑ Risk cesarean birth	Low birth weight Macrosomia Neonatal hypoglycemia ↑ Risk congenital anomalies ↑ Risk respiratory distress syndrome
Cardiac disease	Cardiac decompensation Further strain on mother's body ↑ Maternal death rate	↑ Risk fetal death ↑ Perinatal death
Anemia Less than 11 g/dl hemoglobin Less than 32% hematocrit	Iron-deficiency anemia Low energy level ↓ Oxygen-carrying capacity	Fetal death Prematurity Low birth weight

■ TABLE 2-1
■ ■ Prenatal High-Risk Factors—cont'd

Factor	Maternal Implications	Fetal/Neonatal Implications
Hypertension	↑ Vasospasm ↑ Risk irritability of central nervous system → Convulsions ↑ Risk cerebrovascular accident ↑ Risk renal damage	↓ Placental perfusion → Low birth weight Preterm birth
Thyroid disorder Hypothyroidism	↑ Infertility ↑ Basal metabolic rate, goiter, myxedema	↑ Spontaneous abortion ↑ Risk congenital goiter
Hyperthyroidism	↑ Risk postpartum hemorrhage ↑ Risk preeclampsia Danger of thyroid storm	Mental retardation → cretinism ↑ Incidence congenital anomalies ↑ Incidence preterm birth ↑ Tendency to thyrotoxicosis
Renal disease (moderate to severe)	↑ Risk renal failure	↑ Risk IUGR ↑ Risk preterm birth
Exposure to diethylstilbestrol	↑ Infertility, spontaneous abortion ↑ Cervical incompetence ↑ Risk breech presentation	↑ Spontaneous abortion ↑ Risk preterm birth

OBSTETRIC CONSIDERATIONS
PREVIOUS PREGNANCY

Stillborn	↑ Emotional/psychologic distress	↑ Risk IUGR ↑ Risk preterm birth
Habitual abortion	↑ Emotional/psychologic distress ↑ Possibility diagnostic study	↑ Risk abortion
Cesarean birth	↑ Possibility repeat cesarean birth	↑ Risk preterm birth ↑ Risk respiratory distress
Rh or blood group sensitization	↑ Financial expenditure for testing	Hydrops fetalis Icterus gravis Neonatal anemia Kernicterus Hypoglycemia
Large baby	↑ Risk cesarean birth ↑ Risk gestational diabetes ↑ Risk instrument-assisted birth	Birth injury Hypoglycemia

CURRENT PREGNANCY

Rubella (first trimester)		Congenital heart disease Cataracts Nerve deafness Bone lesions Prolonged virus shedding
Rubella (second trimester)		Hepatitis Thrombocytopenia IUGR Encephalopathy
Cytomegalovirus		
Herpesvirus type 2	Severe discomfort Concern about possibility of cesarean birth, fetal infection	Neonatal herpesvirus type 2 Hepatitis with jaundice Neurologic abnormalities
Syphilis	↑ Incidence abortion	↑ Fetal death Congenital syphilis
Urinary tract infection	↑ Risk preterm labor Uterine irritability	↑ Risk preterm birth

■ TABLE 2-1
■ ■ **Prenatal High-Risk Factors—cont'd**

Factor	Maternal Implications	Fetal/Neonatal Implications
Abruptio placentae and placenta previa	↑ Risk hemorrhage Bed rest Extended hospitalization	Fetal/neonatal anemia Intrauterine hemorrhage ↑ Fetal death
Preeclampsia/eclampsia (pregnancy-induced hypertension)	See "Hypertension"	↓ Placental perfusion → Low birth weight
Multiple gestation	↑ Risk postpartum hemorrhage	↑ Risk preterm birth ↑ Risk fetal death
Elevated hematocrit	↑ Viscosity of blood	Fetal death rate 5 times normal rate
More than 41%		
Spontaneous premature rupture of membranes	↑ Uterine infection	↑ Risk preterm birth ↑ Fetal death

From Davidson, M.R., London, M.L., and Ladewig, P.A.: *Olds' Maternal-newborn nursing & women's health across the lifespan* (8th ed.). Boston, 2008, Pearson Prentice Hall, pp. 343-344.

    b. The greater the concentration gradient, the faster will be the rate of diffusion.

    c. Concentration gradients are maintained when dissolved substances are removed from the plasma by metabolism, cellular uptake, or excretion. For example, the excretion of CO_2 from the maternal lungs maintains the concentration gradient for CO_2, permitting fetal plasma CO_2 to cross from fetal plasma to maternal plasma. Inefficient maternal excretion of CO_2 may lead to maternal respiratory acidosis and fetal acidosis.

  3. Diffusing distance.

    a. The greater the distance between maternal and fetal blood in the placenta, the slower will be the diffusion rate of substances.

    b. Any edema that develops in the placental villi increases the distance between the fetal capillaries within the villi and the maternal arterial blood in the intervillous spaces, thus slowing the diffusion rate of substances between the maternal and fetal circulations.

    c. Edema of villi may occur in:

      (1) Maternal diabetes.

      (2) Transplacental infections.

      (3) Erythroblastosis fetalis.

      (4) Twin-to-twin transfusion syndrome (donor twin).

      (5) Fetal congestive heart failure.

    d. Thinning of the placental membrane in the second half of pregnancy decreases diffusing distance, thus increasing the functional efficiency of the placenta. However, this change also facilitates the passage of drugs in pregnancy and the intrapartum period.

  4. Uteroplacental blood flow.

    a. At term, uterine blood flow is 750 ml per minute or more, representing 10% to 15% of the maternal cardiac output.

    b. Decreased blood flow to the uterus or within the intervillous spaces will decrease the transport of substances to and from the fetus.

    c. Causes of decreased uteroplacental blood flow include:

      (1) Maternal vasoconstriction in hypertension, cocaine abuse, diabetic vasculopathy, and smoking.

      (2) Maternal vasodilatation caused by vasodilators, antihypertensives, and regional anesthetics with sympathetic blockade actions.

      (3) Decreased maternal cardiac output in supine hypotension.

(4) Decreased maternal blood flow in intervillous spaces resulting from edema of the placental villi.

(5) Hypertonic uterine contractions.

(6) Severe maternal physical stress.

(7) Degenerative placental changes near term.

5. Fetal factors.

    a. Fetal tachycardia, often seen with fetal hypoxia, is analogous to an adult's "blowing off CO_2"; the increased heart rate increases the delivery of CO_2 to the placenta for diffusion to the maternal circulation.

    b. Conversely, fetal bradycardia resulting from hypoxia or anoxia leads to an increased CO_2 level.

    c. Umbilical cord compression leads to CO_2 accumulation and acidosis.

    d. Fetal pH during labor is usually 0.1 to 0.15 unit less than the maternal pH; this difference increases the transport of acidophilic substances from the mother to the fetus and reduces albumin binding of drugs, resulting in more free drug in the fetal bloodstream.

CONDITIONS RELATED TO THE ANTEPARTUM PERIOD

Preeclampsia and Eclampsia

Hypertension in pregnancy, including acute gestational hypertension, preeclampsia, and chronic hypertension, is a major cause of maternal-fetal morbidity and death in the United States (Walfisch and Hallak, 2006). The main pathophysiologic events in preeclampsia are vasospasm, hematologic changes, and endothelial damage, leading to tissue hypoxia and multiple organ involvement (Sibai, 2007).

A. Incidence: Incidence is 5% to 10% of all pregnancies (Sibai, 2007; Walfisch and Hallak, 2006).

B. Etiology/predisposing factors.

1. The exact cause of preeclampsia and eclampsia has not been determined, although current theories involve an immunologic basis, genetic predisposition, dietary deficiencies or excesses, abnormal trophoblast invasion, alterations in coagulation, damage to vascular endothelium, and lack of cardiovascular adaptation (Sibai, 2007).

2. Preeclampsia and eclampsia are associated with primigravidas, younger and older women, family history of preeclampsia or previous personal history of severe preeclampsia, obesity, diabetes, chronic hypertensive or renal disease, thrombophilias, multifetal gestation, or large fetus. Other predisposing factors include placental abruption, fetal death, and intrauterine growth restriction (IUGR) in previous pregnancies (Sibai, 2007; Walfisch and Hallak, 2006).

C. Clinical presentation.

1. A blood pressure (BP) of 140/90 mm Hg or above after week 20 of pregnancy. Severe preeclampsia is characterized by a BP of 160/110 or above.

2. Proteinuria due to decreased renal perfusion resulting in the development of glomerular capillary endotheliosis.

3. Edema due to salt retention and decreased plasma colloid osmotic pressure, evidenced by sudden and excessive weight gain, may or may not be present (35% of normotensive patients develop edema). However, following 12 hours of bedrest, generalized edema of the body and face is abnormal (Walfisch and Hallak, 2006).

4. Other signs and symptoms: headache, hyperreflexia with clonus, visual and retinal changes, irritability, nausea and vomiting, epigastric pain, dyspnea, and oliguria.

D. Potential complications.

1. Maternal.

    a. Eclampsia (grand mal seizure).

    b. Cardiopulmonary failure and pulmonary edema.

    c. Hepatic rupture.

    d. Cerebrovascular accident.

    e. Renal cortical necrosis.

      f. Disseminated intravascular coagulation.

      g. HELLP syndrome (i.e., *h*emolysis, *e*levated *l*iver function test results, and *l*ow *p*latelet count).

      h. Retinal detachment.

  2. Placental/fetal.

      a. Premature placental aging, placental infarction, and decrease in amniotic fluid.

      b. Abruptio placentae in 0.5% to 10% of cases, depending upon the severity of the disease (Walfisch and Hallak, 2006).

      c. IUGR resulting from decreased placental blood flow.

      d. Fetal distress.

      e. Preterm birth.

E. Assessment and management.

  1. Severe preeclampsia (Sibai, 2007; Walfisch and Hallak, 2006).

      a. Primary goals of management include prevention of seizures (via limitation of stimuli and drug therapy), prevention of complications (via frequent systems assessments and lab studies), and birth of a live infant.

      b. Seizure precautions.

      c. Placental-fetal function tests: continuous electronic fetal monitoring; fetal movement; ultrasonography to determine fetal age and detect IUGR; serial nonstress tests, contraction stress tests, biophysical profile, and/or umbilical artery Doppler studies; and amniocentesis to determine fetal lung maturity.

      d. Medications.

         (1) Use of intravenous (IV) magnesium sulfate as a central nervous system (CNS) depressant to prevent seizures. A transient decrease in BP often occurs. Monitor fetal heart for decreased variability. Therapy is continued for at least 24 hours postpartum.

         (2) Use of antihypertensives is indicated when systolic BPs are greater than 180 or diastolic BPs are greater than 110:

            (a) Hydralazine (Apresoline). Monitor fetus for signs of hypoxia (tachycardia, bradycardia, or late decelerations), which can occur with a sudden decrease in maternal BP.

            (b) Labetalol hydrochloride. Used to increase uteroplacental perfusion. Monitor fetus for transient bradycardia.

         (3) Use of corticosteroids to increase fetal lung maturity when birth can be delayed for 48 hours and the woman is at less than 34 weeks of gestation.

      e. Delivery by induction or cesarean section if fetus is mature or if worsening maternal condition warrants.

  2. Eclampsia (Sibai, 2007; Walfisch and Hallak, 2006).

      a. Immediate notification of physician or midwife.

      b. Bolus administration of IV magnesium sulfate.

      c. Safety measures for woman during and after seizures.

      d. Support of respirations with airway, oxygen, and suctioning.

      e. Monitor fetal heart for transient bradycardia, rebound tachycardia, decreased variability, and late decelerations (Ghulmiyyah and Sibai, 2007).

      f. Continuous maternal assessment, including assessment for abruptio placentae.

      g. Laboratory work: complete blood count (CBC), clot observation, serum creatinine, liver function tests, fibrinogen, arterial blood gases, and electrolytes.

      h. Delivery by induction or cesarean section according to the status of the maternal-placental-fetal complex.

  3. Assessment of newborn infant for the following:

      a. IUGR.

      b. Preterm gestational age.

      c. Hypoxia and acidosis.

      d. Possible adverse drug effects on neonate:

         (1) Signs of hypermagnesemia when maternal administration of high doses of magnesium sulfate occurs near the time of birth: respiratory depression and neuromus-

cular depression, as evidenced by weakness, lethargy, hypotonia, flaccidity, and poor suck (Wilson et al., 2007).

(2) Hypotension, bradycardia, hypoglycemia, respiratory depression, and transient tachypnea, with maternal administration of labetalol (Murray and McKinney, 2006).

Diabetes Mellitus

The woman with insulin-dependent diabetes who becomes pregnant, and the pregnant woman in whom gestational diabetes mellitus (GDM) or type 1 diabetes develops, are at risk during the antepartum period because of altered carbohydrate metabolism. The fetus/neonate is therefore also at risk. Strict control of maternal blood glucose concentration and anticipatory management of the newborn infant are important elements of perinatal care.

A. **Incidence:** Of all pregnancies, 3% to 5% are complicated by diabetes mellitus and 1% to 6% by GDM (Ang et al., 2006).

B. **Etiology and predisposing factors in gestational diabetes.**
   1. In the second half of pregnancy, secretion of estrogen, progesterone, and human placental lactogen increases cellular resistance to insulin. The pancreas of the woman who is predisposed to diabetes cannot meet the increased demand for insulin, which leads to hyperglycemia.
   2. Risk factors for GDM include maternal obesity; a family history of diabetes; age greater than 25 years; member of an ethnic group at risk for diabetes (Native North American, Hispanic, African American, Pacific Islanders, and South or East Asian Americans) (Jones, 2008); and a history of having had an infant who was large for gestational age (LGA), who had a congenital anomaly, whose gestation resulted in hydramnios, or who was stillborn.

C. **Clinical presentation and screening for gestational diabetes.**
   1. Women at high risk for GDM should be screened at the first prenatal visit in addition to the routine testing at 26 to 28 weeks, because GDM may be asymptomatic or evidenced only by subtle changes (Landon et al., 2007).
   2. Women with average risk for GDM should be screened with a 1-hour glucose tolerance test, and an abnormally high value requires further testing (Landon et al., 2007).
   3. The American College of Obstetricians and Gynecologists (ACOG) indicates that if a woman is considered to be low risk for GDM, glucose screening may not be required (ACOG, 2001).

D. **Potential complications.**
   1. Maternal.
      a. Hypoglycemic reactions in the first trimester.
      b. Ketoacidosis in the second and third trimesters.
      c. Progression of vasculopathy, nephropathy, and retinopathy with preexisting diabetes.
      d. Hydramnios.
      e. Pregnancy-induced hypertension.
      f. Anemia.
      g. Infections such as monilial vaginitis and urinary tract infections.
   2. Fetal/neonatal: Outcomes can be improved via careful attention to prepregnancy and pregnancy glycemic control (Landon et al., 2007).
      a. Macrosomia (weight greater than 4000 g) with possible traumatic vaginal birth such as with shoulder dystocia. IUGR when the mother has vascular disease (Davidson et al., 2008).
      b. Fetal death.
      c. Respiratory distress syndrome.
      d. Hypoglycemia, hypocalcemia, and hypomagnesemia.
      e. Polycythemia, hyperviscosity, and hyperbilirubinemia.
      f. Cardiomyopathy with congestive heart failure.
      g. Congenital malformation as a consequence of poorly controlled preexisting diabetes: renal anomalies such as Potter syndrome, polycystic kidneys, and double ureters;

neural tube defects; skeletal defects such as caudal regression syndrome and spina bifida; cardiac anomalies such as patent ductus arteriosus, transposition of the great vessels, endocardial cushion defects, and ventricular septal defect; and gastrointestinal defects such as tracheoesophageal fistula, bowel atresia, and imperforate anus. Currently, 30% to 50% of perinatal mortality results from congenital malformations in pregnancies in which the mother has diabetes.

E. **Assessment and management.**
   1. In preexisting diabetes (Landon et al., 2007):
      a. Preconception counseling is provided, with optimal control of blood glucose levels. Insulin is considered the therapy of choice because oral antidiabetic agents can cause fetal and newborn hypoglycemia and teratogenic effects (Ang et al., 2006; Ricci, 2007). The woman should begin taking 0.4 mg of folic acid daily, and continue through the first trimester, to reduce the risk for neural tube defects.
      b. Glycosylated hemoglobin tests may be performed before conception and during the pregnancy to assess glucose control during the previous 1 to 2 months. Levels beyond the normal range are associated with increased congenital anomalies.
      c. Home blood glucose monitoring, diet, and either insulin pump therapy or several daily injections of insulin are prescribed to maintain tight control of the blood glucose concentration (60 to 120 mg/dl). Tight control is associated with decreased risk of macrosomia, respiratory distress syndrome, congenital anomalies, and perinatal death, as well as maternal urinary tract infection and preterm labor.
      d. Women are evaluated early in pregnancy for evidence of diabetic retinopathy and nephropathy.
      e. At 16 weeks of gestation, the woman should be offered maternal serum alpha-fetoprotein (MSAFP) testing, accompanied by a comprehensive ultrasound at 18 to 20 weeks to assess for the presence of neural tube defects or other anomalies. An alternative choice of testing may be the triple screen (MSAFP, maternal serum unconjugated estriol, and hCG) or the quad test, which includes inhibin A in addition to the three elements of the triple screen (Jones, 2008). Serial ultrasounds may be performed to evaluate fetal growth. Fetal echocardiography is also recommended, as well as Doppler umbilical artery velocimetry.
      f. Weekly prenatal visits are made after 28 weeks, with fetal assessment by means of nonstress tests, biophysical profiles, and daily fetal movement counting.
      g. Before any decision is made about induction of labor, amniocentesis is performed to determine the lecithin/sphingomyelin (L/S) ratio and the presence of phosphatidylglycerol. Delivery is accomplished before term if maternal or fetal complications develop.
      h. Insulin is given intravenously during labor if blood glucose values are above 140 mg/dl. Glucose levels are monitored every hour to ensure optimum titration of insulin in order to decrease the risk of neonatal rebound hypoglycemia.
   2. In gestational diabetes (Landon et al., 2007):
      a. A 2000- to 2500-calorie diet with no simple carbohydrates is recommended;
      b. Fasting and 2-hour postprandial glucose levels are checked weekly; and
      c. Nonstress testing begins at 40 weeks in the well-controlled mother.
   3. In the neonate:
      a. Assess for gestational age and size (LGA or IUGR).
      b. Assess for
         (1) Respiratory distress;
         (2) Hypoglycemia, hypocalcemia, and hypomagnesemia;
         (3) Polycythemia and hyperviscosity;
         (4) Complications resulting from decreased blood flow, erythrocyte hemolysis, and thrombosis;
         (5) Congenital malformations; and
         (6) Birth injuries: fractured clavicles, intracranial bleeding, facial nerve paralysis, brachial palsy, and skull fractures.

CONDITIONS RELATED TO THE INTRAPARTUM PERIOD
Preterm Labor

Preterm labor is defined as labor occurring at greater than 20 and less than 37 completed weeks of gestation. If preterm labor is recognized in time, measures can be taken to attempt to stop the contractions. The prognosis for the fetus improves with each week of pregnancy gained.

A. **Incidence:** In 2004, 12.5% of live births in the United States were preterm (March of Dimes, Preterm birth overview).

B. **Etiology/predisposing factors.**
   1. The exact cause of preterm labor is unknown, although chorioamnionitis and other infections such as periodontitis and bacterial vaginosis have been implicated (Meis, 2007).
   2. A number of maternal factors have been associated with an increased incidence of preterm labor: maternal age (<16 or >40), socioeconomic effects (lower socioeconomic status or educational level, African American race, poor nutrition, inadequate prenatal care), medical/obstetric history (use of assisted reproductive technologies, anemia, preexisting or gestational hypertension or diabetes, preterm labor or birth, one or more midtrimester pregnancy losses, short interpregnancy interval, uterine anomalies and cervical insufficiency, systemic and genitourinary tract infections, polyhydramnios, immunologic factors, abruptio placentae, and placenta previa), and lifestyle factors (use of alcohol, cigarettes, and illicit drugs such as cocaine and domestic violence or other stressors) (Iams and Romero, 2007; Ricci, 2007).
   3. Fetal factors contributing to the development of preterm labor may include congenital anomalies and complications from multifetal gestation (Iams and Romero, 2007).
   4. Risk scoring systems, designed to screen women during pregnancy, have a predictive value of only 17% to 34% (Svigos et al., 2006). Many women who give birth before term do not have any known risk factors.

C. **Clinical presentation.**
   1. Painless or painful uterine contractions.
   2. Low, dull, intermittent, or constant backache.
   3. Intermittent or constant menstrual-like cramping.
   4. Intermittent pelvic pressure that may extend along the inner thigh.
   5. Abdominal cramps, which may be accompanied by diarrhea.
   6. Increased vaginal discharge, which may be mucoid, watery, or slightly bloody.
   7. Spontaneous premature rupture of membranes.
   8. A generalized feeling that something is wrong.
   9. Progressive cervical effacement and dilatation unless intervention is performed.

D. **Potential complications.**
   1. Maternal.
      a. No particular physical complications other than adverse reactions from tocolytic agents.
      b. Emotional stress and financial issues.
   2. Fetal/neonatal.
      a. Preterm birth with an increase in neonatal morbidity and death.
      b. Adverse reactions to tocolytic agents.

E. **Assessment and management.**
   1. Screening of pregnant women at the first and subsequent prenatal visits for preterm labor risk factors.
   2. Teaching all pregnant women the symptoms of preterm labor and the actions to take if they occur (lie down on the left side and drink several glasses of fluid; report to the physician or midwife if contractions are still occurring after 1 hour).
   3. Helping high-risk women modify their risk factors and take measures to prevent preterm labor (e.g., stop smoking, improve nutrition and hydration, treat infections, decrease work hours and stress, increase rest, and avoid nipple preparation or sexual activity that may initiate signs of preterm labor).

4. Although regular cervical examinations and ultrasonographic evaluation of the cervix are being performed by some providers, these methods are still being evaluated for specificity and sensitivity as predictors of preterm birth (Svigos et al., 2006).

5. Use of home contraction monitoring systems has not been proven effective in identifying women who will deliver preterm (Iams and Romero, 2007).

6. Treatment decisions may be based on the results of a fetal fibronectin test performed on vaginal secretions. The test is valued for its negative predictive value in symptomatic women—a negative result means that preterm labor will most likely not begin within 2 weeks of sampling, preventing unnecessary and potentially harmful pharmacologic treatment (Iams and Romero, 2007; Svigos et al., 2006).

7. Although episodes of preterm labor are widely treated with hospitalization, hydration with IV fluid, bed rest in the left lateral position, and pelvic rest, there is little evidence that these interventions are effective (Davidson et al., 2008). Corticosteroid therapy is recommended for women at risk for preterm birth to reduce the incidence of neonatal morbidity and death from respiratory distress syndrome.

8. When appropriate and not contraindicated, use of one of the following medications may prolong pregnancy 24 hours or more, allowing enough time for concurrent corticosteroid therapy to benefit the fetus and/or for transfer of the mother to a hospital with a level III nursery (Iams and Romero, 2007; Meis, 2007).

    a. Ritodrine (Yutopar), given intravenously, inhibits uterine contractility. Potential fetal/neonatal side effects include tachycardia, fetal hyperglycemia and neonatal hypoglycemia and hypocalcemia, cardiac failure, neonatal hyperbilirubinemia, hypotension, and paralytic ileus (Ricci, 2007).

    b. Magnesium sulfate, given intravenously for uterine relaxation. Signs of hypermagnesemia in the neonate when maternal administration of high doses of magnesium sulfate occurs near the time of birth: respiratory depression and neuromuscular depression, as evidenced by weakness, lethargy, hypotonia, flaccidity, and poor suck (Wilson et al., 2007).

    c. Terbutaline (Brethine), given subcutaneously. Potential fetal/neonatal side effects are the same as for ritodrine but are generally fewer and less serious.

    d. Indomethacin (Indocin) given prior to 32 weeks, either rectally or orally. Contraindications to its use include fetal renal anomalies, oligohydramnios, IUGR, chorioamnionitis, ductal dependent cardiac defects, and twin-to-twin transfusion syndrome. Fetal side effects include oligohydramnios, constriction of the ductus arteriosus, and neonatal pulmonary hypertension.

    e. Nifedipine (Procardia), a calcium channel blocker, is given orally and is being used more frequently as a tocolytic because of its relative lack of maternal-fetal side effects. It is contraindicated in cardiac disease, hypertension, and intrauterine infection.

9. For women with preterm rupture of the membranes and/or preterm labor, prophylactic antibiotic therapy is initiated to prevent neonatal group B streptococcal infection.

10. If the measures noted above are not successful, and the cervix continues to efface and dilate, the following measures are important:

    a. To allow the amniotic fluid to cushion the fetal skull, no rupture of the membranes is performed.

    b. The head is delivered in a slow, controlled fashion. There is no justification for elective cesarean delivery of all preterm infants.

    c. Cesarean delivery is often suggested for the preterm fetus with a breech presentation because of the risk of cord prolapse and the potential risk of difficult birth of the head.

Abruptio Placentae

In abruptio placentae, the placenta separates suddenly, prematurely, and in varying degrees from the uterine wall during pregnancy or labor. It is a common cause of bleeding in the second half of pregnancy.

A. Incidence: Placental abruption occurs in 1 of 100 pregnancies (March of Dimes, Placental conditions).

B. Etiology/predisposing factors.
1. Although the cause of abruptio placentae has not been definitively established, there is a high correlation with hypertensive disorders during pregnancy, cocaine and crack use, trauma, and placental abnormalities (circumvallate). Additional predisposing factors include uterine fibroids or malformations, polyhydramnios and multifetal pregnancy, increased parity, history of previous abruption, chorioamnionitis, preterm premature rupture of membranes, and maternal cigarette smoking and poor nutrition (Francois and Foley, 2007). Short cord is also considered a risk factor.

C. Clinical presentation.
1. The abruption is classified as grade 1, 2, or 3 according to clinical findings and degree of coagulopathy (Francois and Foley, 2007).
2. Maternal signs and symptoms.
   a. Mild labor pains with persistent cramping to sharp, continuous abdominal pain.
   b. Board-like and tender abdomen.
   c. Dark or bright red vaginal bleeding (unless the bleeding is concealed behind the placenta), ranging from spotting to frank hemorrhage. In 20% to 30% of patients with abruption, there is no visible evidence of bleeding (Konje and Taylor, 2006).
   d. Uterine hyperactivity.
   e. Enlargement of the uterus as blood accumulates, with increasing abdominal girth.
3. Fetal distress.
   a. Loss of fetal heart tones or movement.
   b. Tachycardia.
   c. Late or variable decelerations.
   d. Decreased fetal heart rate variability.
   e. Sinusoidal fetal heart rate pattern.

D. Potential complications.
1. Maternal (Francois and Foley, 2007; Konje and Taylor, 2006).
   a. Anemia.
   b. Hypovolemic shock, sometimes resulting in anterior pituitary necrosis (Sheehan syndrome).
   c. Couvelaire uterus (blood forced between the muscle fibers of the uterus).
   d. Disseminated intravascular coagulation.
   e. Acute renal failure.
   f. Postpartum hemorrhage.
   g. Fetomaternal hemorrhage.
   h. Death.
2. Fetal/neonatal.
   a. Anemia.
   b. Preterm birth.
   c. Hypoxia and asphyxia with intrauterine fetal demise.
   d. Hypovolemia.
   e. Long-term neurobehavioral problems.
   f. 20% to 30% incidence of fetal death; sudden infant death syndrome.
   g. IUGR.

E. Assessment and management.
1. Any episode of bleeding during pregnancy in an Rh-negative woman requires a Kleihauer-Betke test and the administration of Rh immunoglobulin (Konje and Taylor, 2006).
2. Management decisions are based on the severity of the abruption, complications, gestational age, and maternal-fetal status.
3. Management if fetus is stable and maternal hematologic status can be maintained:
   a. Ultrasonography to locate placenta and determine degree of placental separation and location of hematoma.
   b. Bed rest in left lateral position, close assessment of abdomen for rigidity and pain, and close assessment of vaginal bleeding.

    c. Monitoring of maternal vital signs and continuous monitoring of fetal heart for brady-cardia, late decelerations, and prolonged decelerations.

    d. Placement of large-bore IV cannula for possible administration of fluids and blood products.

    e. CBC, coagulation studies, and type and cross-match for blood.

    f. Possible collection of urine for drug screening.

    g. Possible induction of labor and/or vaginal birth.

    h. Notify the neonatal intensive care unit (NICU) and the neonatologist/pediatrician.

4. Preparation for cesarean birth if fetal distress or severe hemorrhage occurs:

    a. Inform and support parents and ensure that surgical consent is obtained.

    b. Laboratory tests as above.

    c. Prepare the abdomen and insert an indwelling urinary catheter.

Placenta Previa

Placenta previa is a placenta that is implanted in the lower part of the uterus near the cervix (marginal) or in varying degrees (partial or total) over the cervix. Cervical dilation at or near term is accompanied by bleeding from the placenta. Placenta previa is a common cause of bleeding in the second half of pregnancy, when the lower uterine segment stretches and thins.

A. Incidence: The incidence is 1 per 200 births in the United States (March of Dimes, Placental conditions, 2008).

B. Etiology/predisposing factors (Francois and Foley, 2007).

  1. The precise cause of placenta previa is unknown, but it occurs most frequently in multiparous and older women.

  2. Other associated and predisposing factors include previous placenta previa, prior cesarean birth, living in higher altitudes, cigarette smoking, multifetal gestation, and prior curettage.

C. Clinical presentation (Konje and Taylor, 2006).

  1. Bright red, painless vaginal bleeding. Although the first bleeding episode may be slight in amount, more blood is usually lost in subsequent episodes. Ten percent of women with a placenta previa will also have a placental abruption.

  2. Uterine contractions occur in 25% of cases, but otherwise the uterus is usually soft and nontender.

  3. If an ultrasound is performed at less than 20 weeks of gestation, a low-lying placenta may be noted. However, at this gestational age, the lower uterine segment is not yet fully developed and this is not diagnostic of a placenta previa.

  4. Failure of presenting part of fetus to become engaged. Fetus may lie transversely or be in a breech position.

D. Potential complications.

  1. Maternal.

    a. Anemia.

    b. Hypovolemic shock.

    c. Endometritis.

    d. Decreased contractile strength of the lower uterine segment, which can lead to postpartum hemorrhage and need for hysterectomy.

    e. Abnormal placental implantation (placenta accreta, percreta, and increta).

    f. Air embolism.

  2. Fetal/neonatal.

    a. Hypoxia and asphyxia.

    b. IUGR.

    c. Fetal hemorrhage, anemia, and death.

    d. Prematurity.

    e. Infection.

E. Assessment and management.

  1. Treatment and delivery decisions are based on amount of bleeding, gestational age, cervical status, grade of previa, and condition and presentation of fetus (Konje and Taylor,

2006). Any episode of bleeding during pregnancy in an Rh-negative woman requires a Kleihauer-Betke test and the administration of Rh immunoglobulin.

2. Marginal or partial placenta previa with minimal bleeding is managed conservatively:
   a. Ultrasonography to confirm diagnosis and to rule out IUGR.
   b. No vaginal examinations.
   c. Bed rest and activity level at home or in the hospital determined by clinical presentation.
   d. Avoidance of intercourse and orgasm, which can cause uterine contractions.
   e. Amniocentesis for fetal lung maturity if there is any question about term status.
   f. If the fetus is mature, vaginal birth can be accomplished if the placenta is anterior and bleeding continues to be minimal (with an anterior placenta, bleeding may be decreased as a result of compression of the placenta between the fetal head and the symphysis pubis) (Konje and Taylor, 2006).

3. Partial or total placenta previa with greater amounts of bleeding is handled as noted above, except that vaginal birth may not be possible. In addition:
   a. Frequent assessment of vaginal bleeding, with pad counts and/or weighing of pads.
   b. Frequent assessment of maternal vital signs and fetal heart tones, and palpation of abdomen.
   c. Laboratory work: CBC, type, and cross-match for possible blood transfusion.
   d. With significant bleeding, placement of IV lines with 16-gauge catheters for blood administration.
   e. Method of delivery.
      (1) Vaginal delivery may be performed if bleeding remains minimal and the placenta is anterior.
      (2) If bleeding is significant, cesarean delivery is performed.

Umbilical Cord Prolapse

Umbilical cord prolapse is an event that is life threatening to the fetus and requires immediate and effective management by the nurse. It occurs when the cord falls below the presenting part or is compressed between the presenting part and the pelvis or cervix.

A. **Incidence:** Varies from 1 in 265 to 600 births (Steer and Danielian, 2006; Watts, 2008).

B. **Etiology/predisposing factors.**
   1. The fetal presenting part does not fill the pelvic inlet well, and the cord slips past it, often when the membranes rupture.
   2. Predisposing factors include amniotomy with a high presenting part, premature rupture of membranes, abnormally long cord, malpresentation (transverse lie and breech presentation), premature or small-for-gestational-age fetus, multifetal pregnancy, polyhydramnios, cephalopelvic disproportion that prevents fetal engagement, lack of engagement before the onset of labor (as is common with multiparous women), and abnormal placentation (Watts, 2008).

C. **Clinical presentation.**
   1. Cord is protruding from vagina or is palpable on vaginal examination.
   2. In an occult prolapse, cord is not visible or palpable but is located between the presenting part and the pelvis or cervix.
   3. More commonly occurs with a high station of presenting part, and membranes are often ruptured.
   4. Fetal heart changes can include increase in fetal heart rate, uniform accelerations, bradycardia, and variable decelerations.

D. **Potential complications.**
   1. Maternal.
      a. Trauma to the birth canal from rapid forceps delivery.
      b. General anesthesia resulting in uterine atony with subsequent postpartum bleeding.
      c. Blood loss from cesarean birth.
   2. Fetal/neonatal.
      a. Perinatal mortality increases as increased time elapses between cord prolapse and birth.

     b. Fetal anoxia leading to long-range neurologic complications.

     c. Neonatal infection.

E. Assessment and management.

  1. Assessments on admission to labor and delivery.

     a. Presenting part and its station.

     b. Dilation of cervix.

     c. Status of membranes.

     d. Estimation of fetal weight and fetal heart rate.

  2. Assessment for presence of polyhydramnios or lack of engagement of presenting part. Ambulation during labor and artificial rupture of membranes may be contraindicated.

  3. Assessment after artificial or spontaneous rupture of membranes.

     a. Monitor fetal heart for changes as indicated above.

     b. Perform vaginal examination to detect prolapse if indicated.

  4. If prolapse has occurred:

     a. Keep the examining hand in vagina to push the presenting part away from the cord until birth of fetus. The provider may also attempt to replace the prolapsed cord into the uterus (Steer and Danielian, 2006).

     b. An alternative measure is to insert an indwelling catheter to fill the mother's bladder with sterile saline solution in order to elevate the fetal presenting part so that it is off the cord (Steer and Danielian, 2006).

     c. Help woman into knee-chest or steep Trendelenburg position, with hips elevated and head down (Steer and Danielian, 2006).

     d. Monitor fetal heart rate continuously and palpate cord lightly for continued pulsation. Administer oxygen to the woman as indicated for fetal distress.

     e. Tocolytic agents such as terbutaline may be used.

     f. If the cervix is fully dilated and the fetal station is below the ischial spines, vaginal birth may be expedited. Emergency cesarean delivery may be preferable, especially if the cervix is not fully dilated and the fetus exhibits a nonreassuring heart rate pattern.

Shoulder Dystocia

Shoulder dystocia is an acute emergency in which the physician or midwife is unable to deliver the shoulders of the infant by the usual maneuvers after birth of the head.

A. Incidence: Incidence is 0.2% to 3% of all births (Gherman, 2006).

B. Etiology/predisposing factors.

  1. The fetal shoulders are too broad to be delivered between the symphysis pubis and the sacrum.

  2. Factors associated with shoulder dystocia include maternal obesity, fetus more than 4000 g, history of previous shoulder dystocia, poorly controlled maternal diabetes, contracted pelvic outlet, multiparity, and postdate pregnancy. However, up to 50% to 60% of cases occur with fetuses less than 4000 g (Gherman, 2006).

C. Clinical presentation.

  1. Slow active phase of labor.

  2. Second stage longer than 2 hours, with slow descent of head.

  3. After birth of the head, it recoils against the perineum and restitution does not occur ("turtling"). The usual traction from below is not successful in delivering the neonate.

D. Complications.

  1. Maternal.

     a. Vaginal, cervical, or perineal lacerations.

     b. Ruptured uterus.

     c. Postpartum hemorrhage or infection.

     d. Bladder trauma.

  2. Fetal/neonatal.

     a. Birth injuries such as brachial palsy, Erb palsy, facial nerve palsy, or fractured clavicle or humerus.

     b. Anoxia, perinatal depression, hypoxic-ischemic encephalopathy.

     c. Intrapartum or neonatal death.

E. Assessment and management (Gherman, 2006).

  1. Anticipate shoulder dystocia if descent of the head is slow and estimated weight is large. Make sure the woman's bladder is empty before birth occurs.

  2. If shoulder dystocia occurs, the physician or midwife will:

     a. Use the McRoberts maneuver (an exaggerated lithotomy position).

     b. Have the nurse apply firm suprapubic pressure to attempt to release the anterior shoulder.

     c. Perform or extend the episiotomy. However, this intervention alone will not resolve the problem, because the etiology is not soft-tissue dystocia.

     d. If the above are not effective, perform other maneuvers to expedite birth:

       (1) Turn the woman onto her side or pull the hips off the bed to free the sacrum.

       (2) Turn the woman on all fours to widen the pelvic outlet if this can be easily accomplished (the Gaskin maneuver).

       (3) Manually rotate shoulders from the anteroposterior to the oblique diameter in the pelvis.

       (4) Use the Wood corkscrew maneuver, in which both hands are inserted internally to rotate the posterior shoulder to the anterior position for delivery under the pubic bone, with the maneuver repeated for the other shoulder.

       (5) Extract posterior shoulder and arm.

       (6) The Zavanelli maneuver can be performed to push the fetal head back into the vagina so that a cesarean birth can be done, but it is rarely used.

Breech Presentation

A. Incidence: Incidence is 14% at 29 to 32 weeks, 2.2% to 3.7% at term, and overall 3% to 4% of all labors (Penn, 2006). Incidence increases in multiple gestation and in preterm birth.

B. Etiology/predisposing factors.

  1. Maternal.

     a. Polyhydramnios or oligohydramnios.

     b. Uterine anomalies.

     c. Contracted pelvis.

     d. Use of anticonvulsant medications or alcohol abuse.

  2. Placental/fetal.

     a. Placenta previa or cornual placenta.

     b. Multifetal gestation.

     c. IUGR or fetal anomalies, especially those related to CNS problems.

     d. Short cord.

     e. Preterm fetus.

C. Clinical presentation.

  1. Woman feels fetus kicking in the lower abdomen.

  2. Fetal heart sounds are heard loudest above the umbilicus.

  3. Use of Leopold maneuvers indicates head is in the fundal area and the breech is in the pelvis.

  4. On vaginal examination, it is found that the presenting part is soft, no fontanelles are felt, and the genitalia may be identified.

D. Assessment and management.

  1. A procedure that may help the fetus turn from breech to cephalic presentation is postural exercise, in which the woman assumes either the knee-chest or an elevated-hip posture several times a day until the fetus turns (Penn, 2006).

  2. The physician may attempt external cephalic version after 37 weeks with or without the use of a uterine relaxant and if the fetus remains in a cephalic presentation, vaginal birth. However, in many cases the fetus reverts to breech (Penn, 2006).

  3. Assessments on admission to labor and delivery:

    a. Perform Leopold maneuvers and vaginal examination to determine presentation.

    b. Report clinical findings immediately to the physician or midwife.

4. Ultrasonography may be ordered to confirm breech presentation, determine degree of flexion of fetal head, evaluate size of fetal head, estimate fetal weight, diagnose fetal anomalies, and locate placenta.

5. A trial of labor for vaginal birth for the term breech may be attempted.

    a. The fetal position must be a frank or complete breech with the head flexed, and the pelvis must be adequate.

    b. The estimated fetal weight must be approximately 2000 to 3800 g (Lanni and Seeds, 2007), and no other indications for cesarean birth must exist.

    c. The nurse should perform, at the time of rupture of the membranes, a vaginal examination to check for prolapsed cord and should monitor the fetal heart tones closely.

    d. Meconium in the amniotic fluid is not necessarily a sign of fetal hypoxia when the fetus is in a breech position. However, meconium aspiration at the time of birth may be a serious complication.

    e. The woman may receive an episiotomy, and Piper forceps may be used to assist in delivery of the neonate's head. The nurse may be asked to apply suprapubic pressure to keep the neonate's head flexed while the physician or midwife performs certain maneuvers during the birth.

6. Many physicians will perform cesarean delivery when the fetus is breech in these situations: estimated fetal weight less than 1500 g or more than 4000 g, small pelvis, arrest of progress, nonreassuring fetal heart rate, lack of expertise in performing breech delivery, preterm fetus, hyperextension of head, and footling breech (Lanni and Seeds, 2007).

7. Assessment of the neonate may reveal:

    a. Edema of the external genitalia.

    b. A continuation of the frank breech position for a period of time after the birth.

E. Complications.

1. In numerous studies, poorer neonatal outcomes that are attributed to vaginal breech birth were affected by fetal anomalies and preterm birth rather than mode of birth (Lanni and Seeds, 2007; Penn, 2006).

2. Fetal/neonatal complications resulting from vaginal birth (Penn, 2006).

    a. Prolapsed cord.

    b. Asphyxia from slow birth of fetal head or from compression of umbilical cord between pelvis and head during birth.

    c. Aspiration of amniotic fluid with potential for meconium aspiration syndrome.

    d. Genital damage in the male infant.

    e. CNS injuries such as intracranial hemorrhage, brachial plexus injury, and severed spinal cord, especially if fetal head is hyperextended.

OBSTETRIC ANALGESIA AND ANESTHESIA

Most anesthesiologists, obstetricians, and midwives would agree that there is no method of pharmacologic pain relief that is completely safe for all laboring women. In addition, side effects or adverse reactions in the woman affect the fetus to some degree. For this reason, nonpharmacologic methods of pain management (e.g., labor support, freedom of movement, hypnosis, acupressure and acupuncture, application of heat or cold, listening to music, breathing techniques, massage, hydrotherapy, and transcutaneous electrical nerve stimulation [TENS]) should be as routinely provided as pharmacologic methods and may provide sufficient pain relief for many women.

Obstetric Analgesia

Obstetric analgesia is given by either the intramuscular (IM) or the IV route and in as small a dose as possible. The most commonly used analgesics are butorphanol (Stadol) and nalbuphine (Nubain).

A. Potential side effects or complications.
1. Maternal.
    a. Respiratory depression.
    b. Nausea and vomiting.
    c. Orthostatic hypotension.
    d. Drowsiness and dizziness.
2. Fetal/neonatal.
    a. Decreased fetal activity and variability, sinusoidal pattern, and late decelerations if mother experiences hypotension.
    b. Neonatal respiratory depression and respiratory acidosis.
    c. Thermoregulation problems related to lethargy and/or hypotonia.
B. Assessment and management.
1. Avoid administration of analgesics close to birth if possible.
2. Administer IV analgesics slowly; give during a uterine contraction to minimize amount of drug the fetus receives.
3. Observe the woman for side effects and monitor the fetus continuously with electronic fetal monitor or intermittent auscultation.
4. With maternal hypotension, turn the woman onto her left side, increase IV infusion of fluids, and closely monitor fetal heart tones and maternal BP.
5. Have naloxone (Narcan), oxygen, and ventilatory equipment available for use with the newborn infant if respiratory depression occurs.
6. Document use of analgesic and transmit this information to the nursery nurse.
7. In the nursery, observe the neonate for side effects of maternal analgesia.

Obstetric Anesthesia

Several types of anesthesia are used with women in labor and delivery. General anesthesia is used primarily for emergency cesarean and complicated vaginal births when it is not possible to have immediate and effective regional anesthesia. Regional anesthesia includes continuous lumbar epidural, spinal, and pudendal block. Local anesthesia involves perineal infiltration prior to episiotomy, birth, and/or perineal repair.
A. Potential complications with general anesthesia.
1. Maternal.
    a. Vomiting and aspiration of gastric contents, with acid pneumonitis (Mendelson syndrome) as a consequence.
    b. Respiratory depression.
    c. Cardiac irritability and arrest.
    d. Hypotension or hypertension.
    e. Tachycardia.
    f. Laryngospasm.
    g. Postpartum uterine atony.
2. Fetal/neonatal.
    a. Decreased fetal cardiac variability and movements.
    b. Neonatal respiratory depression and hypotonicity.
    c. Fetal depression in proportion to the amount of anesthesia.
B. Assessment and management with general anesthesia.
1. The woman must have nothing by mouth while in labor if there is a strong possibility that she will receive general anesthesia.
2. Note the time of her last meal.
3. Physician may order 30 ml of clear antacid to be administered before general anesthesia to increase the pH of the stomach contents in case of aspiration.
4. Endotracheal tube and cricoid pressure are techniques used by the anesthesiologist to prevent aspiration.
5. Place a wedge under the right hip to cause displacement of the uterus from the aorta and vena cava and to prevent supine hypotensive syndrome during surgery.

6. Monitor the woman's cardiorespiratory status during and after surgery, and uterine bleeding postoperatively.
7. Monitor the newborn infant after surgery for complications.

C. Potential complications with regional anesthetics.
   1. Maternal.
      a. With spinal and epidural anesthesia:
         (1) Hypotension due to sympathetic blockade.
         (2) Allergic reaction to the injected anesthetic.
         (3) Toxic reaction to overdose or intravascular injection, with seizure activity.
         (4) Respiratory paralysis from inadvertent high spinal anesthesia.
         (5) Headaches after spinal anesthesia.
         (6) Failure of anesthetic to be effective.
         (7) Urinary retention during labor and in the postpartum period.
         (8) Slowing of labor, with need to use oxytocin and forceps if anesthetic is given too early.
         (9) Formation of a hematoma that compresses the spinal cord, with potential for permanent damage.
         (10) Paralysis (rare).
      b. With epidural anesthesia:
         (1) Shearing off of epidural catheter.
         (2) Trauma to spinal cord or nerve roots.
         (3) Some evidence of increased malposition and instrumental delivery (Hawkins et al., 2007).
         (4) Back pain and postdural puncture headache.
         (5) "Epidural shakes" and "epidural fever" (involuntary shivering that leads to an elevated temperature). Fever may also be caused by a decrease in hyperventilation and dissipation of heat (Murray and McKinney, 2006).
      c. With pudendal block (Hawkins et al., 2007; Murray and McKinney, 2006).
         (1) Sciatic nerve trauma.
         (2) Perforated rectum.
         (3) Anesthetic toxicity.
         (4) Broad-ligament hematoma.
   2. Fetal/neonatal.
      a. Toxic reaction from overdose or intravascular injection.
      b. Fetal compromise with prolonged maternal hypotension, as evidenced by late decelerations, bradycardia, and either increased or decreased variability.
      c. Hyperthermia with epidural anesthesia (Murray and McKinney, 2006).

D. Assessment and management with regional anesthetics.
   1. Note history of allergies to local anesthetics.
   2. Prehydrate with 500 to 1000 ml IV fluid before spinal or epidural anesthesia to minimize hypotensive effects from sympathetic blockade.
   3. Position and reassure woman during administration of anesthetic. To prevent supine hypotension, a small roll may be placed under the right hip.
   4. Monitor woman's BP after administration of spinal or epidural anesthetic; monitor fetal heart after any type of regional anesthesia.
   5. Monitor bladder distention and catheterize if necessary.
   6. Complications and their management.
      a. Hypotension.
         (1) Signs and symptoms.
            (a) Decreased baseline BP.
            (b) Dizziness or affected vision.
            (c) Nausea and vomiting.
         (2) Management.
            (a) Increase IV fluids.
            (b) Displace uterus from aorta and vena cava.

        (c) Administer oxygen and IV ephedrine as ordered.

        (d) Monitor the fetus for hypoxia and the fetus/newborn for side effects of ephedrine (tachycardia, jitteriness, and increased muscular activity).

  b. High spinal.

    (1) Signs and symptoms.

      (a) Breast numbness, indicating a rising level of anesthesia.

      (b) Sensation of inability to breathe.

      (c) Respiratory arrest.

    (2) Management.

      (a) Notify anesthesia immediately.

      (b) Maintain airway and ventilation.

      (c) Monitor fetal heart tones.

  c. Toxic reaction.

    (1) Signs and symptoms.

      (a) Metallic taste.

      (b) Ringing in ears.

      (c) Slurring of speech.

      (d) Numbness of tongue and mouth.

      (e) Seizures.

      (f) Cardiovascular and respiratory depression.

    (2) Management.

      (a) Cardiorespiratory support.

      (b) Drugs to control seizures.

      (c) Monitor the newborn infant for seizures, bradycardia, apnea, and hypotonia.

  d. Allergic reaction.

    (1) Signs and symptoms.

      (a) Bronchospasm.

      (b) Laryngeal edema.

      (c) Urticaria.

    (2) Management: use of IV antihistamine such as diphenhydramine (Benadryl).

Cesarean Delivery

A. Incidence: The cesarean birth rate in the United States was 29.1% in 2004. The primary cesarean section rate was 18.1% and the vaginal birth after cesarean section (VBAC) rate was 1.1% (March of Dimes, Delivery method overview). Possible reasons for the increasing cesarean rate include the use of continuous electronic fetal monitoring, increased number of labor inductions with failure of induction, decline in vaginal breech birth and VBACs, decreased operative vaginal deliveries, repeat cesareans, increased multifetal pregnancies, changes in obstetric training, medical-legal issues, parental-societal expectations of the outcome of the pregnancy, and some evidence that women may be requesting elective cesarean (Dickinson, 2006; Landon, 2007).

B. Indications.

  1. Maternal.

    a. Cephalopelvic disproportion.

    b. Failure to progress in labor or failed induction.

    c. Previous classic (vertical) uterine cesarean incision.

    d. Cardiac disease.

    e. Active herpes.

  2. Placental.

    a. Abruptio placentae.

    b. Placenta previa.

    c. Placental insufficiency.

  3. Fetal.

    a. Distress.

    b. Breech or other malpresentation.

    c. Multifetal gestation.

    d. Congenital anomalies such as myelomeningocele and anterior abdominal wall defects.

C. Potential complications.

  1. Maternal.

    a. Infection.

    b. Anemia.

    c. Hemorrhage.

    d. Morbidity and death from anesthesia.

    e. Inadvertent operative injuries.

    f. Pulmonary embolus and atelectasis.

    g. Thrombophlebitis.

  2. Fetal/neonatal.

    a. Asphyxia.

    b. Iatrogenic preterm birth.

    c. Respiratory distress syndrome caused by retained fluid in the lungs.

    d. Persistent pulmonary hypertension (Murray and McKinney, 2006).

    e. Anemia from blood loss caused by incision of placenta and lack of full placental transfusion.

D. Assessment and management.

  1. Perform usual interventions to prepare the woman for operative delivery.

  2. Notify infant's physician per policy.

  3. Give an antacid if ordered.

  4. Remove fetal scalp electrode before surgery.

  5. Place wedge under woman's right hip to displace the uterus to the left to avoid supine hypotension and fetal hypoxia.

  6. Follow Neonatal Resuscitation Program (NRP) protocols for neonatal care following birth.

REFERENCES

American College of Obstetricians and Gynecologists: *ACOG Practice Bulletin No. 30:* Gestational diabetes. Washington, DC, September 2001, ACOG.

Ang, C., Howe, D., and Lumsden, M.: Diabetes. In D. James, P. Steer, C. Weiner, and B. Gonik (Eds.): *High risk pregnancy: Management options* (3rd ed.). Philadelphia, 2006, Saunders, pp. 986-1004.

Baschat, A.A.: Fetal growth disorders. In D. James, P. Steer, C. Weiner, and B. Gonik (Eds.): *High risk pregnancy: Management options* (3rd ed.). Philadelphia, 2006, Saunders, pp. 240-271.

Burton, G.J., Sibley, C.P., and Jauniaux, E.R.M.: Placental anatomy and physiology. In S.G. Gabbe, J.R. Niebyl, and J.L. Simpson (Eds.): *Obstetrics: Normal and problem pregnancies* (5th ed.). Philadelphia, 2007, Churchill Livingstone, pp. 3-25.

Davidson, M.R., London, M.L., and Ladewig, P.A.: *Olds' maternal-newborn nursing & women's health across the lifespan* (8th ed.). Upper Saddle River, NJ, 2008, Pearson Education.

Dickinson, J.E.: Cesarean section. In D. James, P. Steer, C. Weiner, and B. Gonik (Eds.): *High risk pregnancy: Management options* (3rd ed.). Philadelphia, 2006, Saunders, pp. 1543-1556.

Francois, K.E. and Foley, M.R.: Antepartum and postpartum hemorrhage. In S.G. Gabbe, J.R. Niebyl, and J.L. Simpson (Eds.): *Obstetrics: Normal and problem pregnancies* (5th ed.). Philadelphia, 2007, Churchill Livingstone, pp. 456-485.

Gherman, R.B.: Shoulder dystocia. In D. James, P. Steer, C. Weiner, and B. Gonik (Eds.): *High risk pregnancy: Management options* (3rd ed.). Philadelphia, 2006, Saunders, pp. 1443-1449.

Ghulmiyyah, L.M. and Sibai, B.M.: Gestational hypertension-preeclampsia and eclampsia. In J.T. Queenan, C.Y. Spong, and C.J. Lockwood (Eds.): *Management of high-risk pregnancy* (5th ed.). Malden, MA, 2007, Blackwell, pp. 271-279.

Hawkins, J.L., Goetzl, L., and Chestnut, D.H.: Obstetric anesthesia. In S.G. Gabbe, J.R. Niebyl, and J.L. Simpson (Eds.): *Obstetrics: Normal and problem pregnancies* (5th ed.). Philadelphia, 2007, Churchill Livingstone, pp. 396-427.

Iams, J.D. and Romero, R.: Preterm birth. In S.G. Gabbe, J.R. Niebyl, and J.L. Simpson (Eds.): *Obstetrics: Normal and problem pregnancies* (5th ed.). Philadelphia, 2007, Churchill Livingstone, pp. 668-712.

Jones, S.: Genetics, embryology, and preconceptual/prenatal assessment and screening. In S. Orshan (Ed.): *Maternity, newborn, and women's health nursing: Comprehensive care across the lifespan.* Philadelphia, 2008, Lippincott Williams & Wilkins, pp. 355-428.

Konje, J.C. and Taylor, D.J.: Bleeding in late pregnancy. In D. James, P. Steer, C. Weiner, and B. Gonik (Eds.): *High risk pregnancy: Management options* (3rd ed.). Philadelphia, 2006, Saunders, pp. 1259-1275.

Landon, M.B.: Cesarean delivery. In S.G. Gabbe, J.R. Niebyl, and J.L. Simpson (Eds.): *Obstetrics: Normal and problem pregnancies* (5th ed.). Philadelphia, 2007, Churchill Livingstone, pp. 486-520.

Landon, M.B., Catalano, P.M., and Gabbe, S.G.: Diabetes mellitus complicating pregnancy. In S.G. Gabbe, J.R. Niebyl, and J.L. Simpson (Eds.), *Obstetrics: Normal and problem pregnancies* (5th ed.). Philadelphia, 2007, Churchill Livingstone, pp. 976-1010.

Lanni, S.M. and Seeds, J.W.: Malpresentations. In S.G. Gabbe, J.R. Niebyl, & J.L. Simpson (Eds.): *Obstetrics: Normal and problem pregnancies* (5th ed). Philadelphia, 2007, Churchill Livingstone, pp. 428-455.

March of Dimes: *Delivery method overview*. Retrieved January 23, 2008, from http://marchofdimes.com/peristats/tlanding.aspx?reg=99&lev=0&top=8&slev=1&dv=qf

March of Dimes: *Placental conditions*. Retrieved February 11, 2008, from http://www.marchofdimes.com/professionals/14332_1154.asp

March of Dimes: *Preterm birth overview*. Retrieved January 23, 2008, from http://marchofdimes.com/peristats/tlanding.aspx?reg=99&lev=0&top=3&slev=1&dv=qf

Meis, P.J.: Prevention of preterm birth. In J.T. Queenan, C.Y. Spong, and C.J. Lockwood (Eds.): *Management of high-risk pregnancy* (5th ed.). Malden, MA, 2007, Blackwell, pp. 326-332.

Murray, S.S. and McKinney, E.S.: *Foundations of maternal-newborn nursing* (4th ed.). St. Louis, 2006, Saunders.

Penn, Z.: Breech presentation. In D. James, P. Steer, C. Weiner, and B. Gonik (Eds.): *High risk pregnancy: Management options* (3rd ed). Philadelphia, 2006, Saunders, pp. 1334-1358.

Ricci, S.S.: *Essentials of maternity, newborn, and women's health nursing*. Philadelphia, 2007, Lippincott Williams, & Wilkins.

Ross, M.G., Ervin, M.G., and Novak, D.: Fetal physiology. In S.G. Gabbe, J.R. Niebyl, & J.L. Simpson (Eds.), *Obstetrics: Normal and problem pregnancies* (5th ed.). Philadelphia, 2007, Churchill Livingstone, pp. 26-54.

Sibai, B.M.: Hypertension. In S.G. Gabbe, J.R. Niebyl, and J.L. Simpson (Eds.): *Obstetrics: Normal and problem pregnancies* (5th ed.). Philadelphia, 2007, Churchill Livingstone, pp. 863-912.

Steer, P.J. and Danielian, P.: Fetal distress in labor. In D. James, P. Steer, C. Weiner, and B. Gonik (Eds.): *High risk pregnancy: Management options* (3rd ed.). Philadelphia, 2006, Saunders, pp. 1450-1472.

Svigos, J., Robinson, J., and Vigneswaran, R.: Threatened and actual preterm labor including mode of delivery. In D. James, P. Steer, C. Weiner, and B. Gonik (Eds.): *High risk pregnancy: Management options* (3rd ed.). Philadelphia, 2006, Saunders, pp. 1304-1320.

Walfisch, A. and Hallak, M.: Hypertension. In D. James, P. Steer, C. Weiner, and B. Gonik (Eds.): *High risk pregnancy: Management options* (3rd ed.). Philadelphia, 2006, Saunders, pp. 772-797.

Watts, N.: High-risk labor and childbirth. In S. Orshan (Ed.): *Maternity, newborn, and women's health nursing: Comprehensive care across the lifespan*. Philadelphia, 2008, Lippincott Williams & Wilkins, pp. 629-670.

Wilson, B.A, Shannon, M.T., Shields, K.M., Stang, C.L., et al.: *Nurse's drug guide 2007*. Upper Saddle River, NJ, 2007, Prentice Hall.

3 Perinatal Substance Abuse

■■■

KATHLEEN PITTS

OBJECTIVES

1. Describe three behavioral or psychologic signs of an infant exposed to cocaine in utero.
2. Describe the effects of cocaine, alcohol, and tobacco abuse on lactation.
3. Describe five physical characteristics of an infant with a diagnosis of fetal alcohol syndrome (FAS).
4. List four nonpharmacologic nursing interventions appropriate for withdrawing infants.
5. List three psychologic characteristics of women who abuse substances and/or alcohol.
6. Discuss four suggested nursing interventions to use when working with mothers who abuse substances and/or alcohol.
7. List the five areas used to categorize symptoms of an infant with neonatal abstinence syndrome (NAS).

INTRODUCTION

Prevalence

1. Epidemiologic evidence from the United States indicates that males are more likely than females to have opportunities to initiate illegal drug use, but females are generally just as likely as males to initiate illegal drug use once the opportunity is presented (Van Etten and Anthony, 2001). In addition, using controlled drugs, women are just as likely to become drug dependent once they initiate extramedical drug use.
2. "In the United States illicit drug use is the ninth leading contributing cause of death" (Ebrahim and Gfroerer, 2003). The use and abuse of licit and illicit drugs in society have increased alarmingly during the past 25 to 30 years. Patterns of alcohol and substance abuse have also changed and polydrug use has become more prevalent.
   a. Perinatal exposure is associated with high morbidity and mortality rates, and as a consequence, substance and alcohol abuse in pregnancy is a problem with devastating social, medical, and economic implications.
   b. The National Survey on Drug Use and Health (NSDUH) reported that approximately 40.9% of women aged 12 or older reported using an illicit drug at *some point in their lives*, 11.8% of females aged 12 and older reported *past year* use of an illicit drug and 6.2% reported *past month* use of an illicit drug (Substance Abuse and Mental Health Services Administration [SAMHSA], January 26, 2007).
   c. There is great variability of drug and alcohol use in young pregnant women depending on ethnicity, country, and region of country. Continued efforts to screen and intervene are encouraged so that effective services for both mother and infant can be developed (Crome and Kumar, 2007).
3. Half of women who use illicit drugs are of childbearing age (15 to 44 years).
   a. Data collected from the National Hospital Discharge Survey in the United States, between 1979 and 1990, identified a 576% increase in the number of drug-using parturient women.
   b. 5.5% of pregnant women continue to use illicit drugs, and prenatal episodes of substance and alcohol use are not declining significantly.
   c. From 1996 to 1998, 1 of 14 U.S. women of childbearing age reported using illicit drugs in the past month and only one quarter of them had abstained from illicit use during the third trimester (Ebrahim and Gfroerer, 2003).

    d. When urine and meconium analysis is used, a three- to six-fold increase over maternal self-report is reported (urine, 13% to 18%; meconium, 31%) (Nordstrom-Klee et al., 2002).

  4. Racial Trends

    a. Estimates for lifetime history of illegal drug use indicate that use is highest among white women (51.2%), followed by African American women (36.0%), Hispanic women (26.2%), and women of other race/ethnicity groups (20.2%; prevalence estimates for illegal drug use and for recently active use of marijuana and cocaine were highest among women aged 15 to 24) (National Institute of Drug Abuse [NIDA], 2007).

The following chapter presents the illicit drugs used in pregnancy and the adverse effects they have on the pregnancy, fetus, and neonate. Management recommendations and nursing interventions for both prenatal and postnatal care of mother and neonate are outlined. Finally, a brief overview of the general and psychologic profile of the substance-using mother, gender-specific treatment and aftercare needs, and ethical and legal issues is presented.

DRUGS OF ABUSE

Categories of drugs presented in the first section include those in Box 3-1.

Tobacco and Nicotine

A. Incidence of smoking in pregnancy.

  1. Ranges from 15% to 20%.

  2. More than half of pregnant women (54%) who admitted to using illicit drugs in 1996 through 1998 also used tobacco and alcohol (Bennett, 1999; Ebrahim and Gfroerer, 2003).

  3. Rate of tobacco use is second to alcohol use.

  4. Adolescents (12 to 17 years of age) who smoke cigarettes are 12 times as likely to use illicit drugs and 23 times as likely to consume heavy amounts of alcohol.

  5. Whites smoke more heavily than blacks or Hispanics (2002-2005) (SAMHSA, February 9, 2007).

  6. Pregnant women (17.3%) and recent mothers (23.8%) were less likely to be current cigarette smokers (smoked in past month) than women who were not recent mothers (30.6%) (SAMHSA, February 9, 2007).

  7. Pregnant women who were current cigarette smokers were more likely to report smoking cigarettes during their first trimester (22.9%) than second trimester (14.3%) or third trimester of pregnancy (15.3%) (SAMHSA, February 9, 2007).

  8. Younger pregnant women were more likely than their older counterparts to smoke cigarettes during their pregnancy: 24.3% of pregnant women aged 15 to 17 and 27.1% of pregnant women aged 18 to 25 compared with 10.6% of pregnant women aged 26 to 44 smoked cigarettes during their pregnancy in the past month of the survey (SAMHSA, February 9, 2007).

■ BOX 3-1
■ **CATEGORIES OF DRUGS**

■ Cannabinoids	■ Narcotics/opioids
■ Designer/club drugs	■ Sedatives/hypnotics
■ Ethyl alcohol	■ Stimulants
■ Hallucinogens	■ Tobacco/nicotine
■ Inhalants	■ Other (antidepressants)

9. Environmental tobacco smoke (ETS):
   a. Reduces birth weight (BW) in nonsmoking mothers (Dejmek et al., 2002).
   b. Can further compromise high-risk infants by increasing long-term respiratory problems.
B. **Pharmacology.**
   1. Tobacco is a central nervous system (CNS) stimulant.
   2. The active constituents of cigarette smoke are nicotine, tar, carbon monoxide, and cyanide (approximately 4000 compounds found in cigarette smoke).
   3. Nicotine is water and lipid soluble and crosses the placenta.
   4. Carbon monoxide combines with hemoglobin to form carboxyhemoglobin. It is this form that impairs oxygenation for both the mother and fetus, yielding profound fetal hypoxia. Other effects are placental vasoconstriction and vasospasm.
   5. There is a dose-related response between the number of cigarettes smoked and neonatal effects.
C. **Effects on pregnancy** (Mahoney and Larig, 2001).
   1. Spontaneous abortion.
   2. Placenta previa.
   3. Abruptio placentae.
   4. Preterm labor.
   5. Premature rupture of membranes (PROM).
   6. Cesarean section.
D. **Effects on the fetus and newborn infant.**
   1. Increase in intrauterine growth restriction (IUGR)
      a. Decrease in BW (it declines as tobacco exposure increases, but is not a linear relation) (England et al., 2002; Secker-Walker and Vacek, 2003).
      b. Decrease in head circumference.
      c. Decrease in length.
      d. Reduced abdominal circumference and femur length (Jaddoe et al., 2007)
   2. Small increased risk of congenital malformations, including CNS malformations, hypospadias, inguinal hernia, eye and ear malformations, polycystic kidneys, aortopulmonary septum defects, gastroschisis, and skull deformities (Haustein, 1999).
   3. Neurobehavioral effects, suggesting that children exposed to prenatal nicotine do less well on tests of cognitive, psychomotor, and language skills and in general academic achievement (Ernst et al., 2001; Huizink and Mulder, 2006).
   4. Sudden infant death syndrome (SIDS) increased (Martinez et al., 2006)
      a. with the number of cigarettes smoked (dose-dependent relationship observed);
      b. in households with exposure to tobacco smoke before or after birth; and
      c. in those families in which only paternal smoking occurred.
   5. Increased cost of hospitalization. "The smoking attributable neonatal cost in the U.S. represent almost $367 million in 1996 dollars; these costs range from less than a million in smaller states to over $35 million in California alone. All of these costs are preventable" (Adams et al., 2002).
   6. Perinatal mortality was seen with an increase of 150% in women who smoke (Andres and Day, 2000).
E. **Nursing considerations.**
   1. Regular documentation of all growth parameters.
   2. Education regarding risk factors associated with SIDS. Recommend and encourage:
      a. Infants should be placed for sleep in a supine position for every sleep. Side sleeping is not as safe as supine sleeping and is not advised (American Academy of Pediatrics [AAP] Task Force on Sudden Infant Death Syndrome, 2005).
      b. Head to remain uncovered during sleep.
      c. Smoke-free environment for the infant.
      d. Avoidance by smokers of sharing bed with the infant.
      e. Provide the mother opportunity to complete infant cardiopulmonary resuscitation (CPR).
      f. Encourage all efforts for smoking cessation.

Alcohol

A. Incidence of alcohol use in pregnancy.

 1. In 2002, 3% of pregnant women aged 15 to 44 used illicit drugs in the past month, 3% reported binge alcohol use, and 17% reported smoking cigarettes in the past month. Among pregnant women aged 15 to 44, 9.8% reported drinking alcohol during the past month, 4.1% reported binge alcohol use, and less than 1% reported heavy alcohol use (Office of Applied Studies, 2002).

B. Pharmacology.

 1. Alcohol is an anxiolytic analgesic with a depressant effect on the CNS.
 2. Alcohol is absorbed rapidly from the stomach (20%) and the intestines (80%). It is metabolized by the liver (95%) and eliminated by the kidneys and lungs (both total 5%). Fetal ethanol concentration is eliminated only by maternal hepatic biotransformation.
 3. Ethanol reaches the fetus through diffusion across the placental membranes and impairs normal placental function by altering the transfer of essential nutrients to the fetus. Ethanol is metabolized into acetaldehyde and then to acetate. Acetaldehyde is more toxic than ethanol.
 4. Alcohol is a teratogen. Effects in infants are directly related to dose levels, chronicity of alcohol use, gestational stage (timing of use), and duration of exposure (Martinez et al., 2006).

C. Dosage of alcohol.

 1. No safe level of alcohol consumption has been established for pregnant women. The AAP Committee on Substance Abuse and Committee on Children with Disabilities (2000) statement reads, "Because there is no safe amount of alcohol consumption during pregnancy, abstinence from alcohol for women who are pregnant or who are planning a pregnancy is recommended."
 2. Risk to the fetus appears greatest with
    a. 3 oz of absolute alcohol per day (equivalent to six standard drinks).
    b. Binge drinking (equivalent to 5 oz or more at one sitting).
 3. With lower levels of alcohol consumption, the degree and severity of effect on an infant are variable.
 4. Short- and long-term outcome is associated with both chronicity and quantity. The most affected children are born to women in the chronic stages of alcoholism. Long-term outcomes have shown significant negative input in learning and memory skills at a 10-year follow-up (Richardson et al., 2002).

D. Effects on pregnancy.

 1. Increase in spontaneous abortion (twofold to fourfold in moderate and heavy drinkers).
 2. Increased risk of abruptio placentae.
 3. Breech presentation: 70% of FAS newborns are delivered breech.
 4. Decrease in abnormalities and growth restriction, which can be prevented when drinking ceases during any period of the pregnancy.
 5. Increase in extreme preterm delivery (Sokol et al., 2007).

E. Effects on the fetus and neonate.

 1. FAS is the leading cause of mental retardation, and the only preventable cause.
 2. Incidence:
    a. One of the *Healthy People 2010* objectives (objective 16-18) targets a reduction in the occurrence of FAS. The CDC and five states (Alaska, Arizona, Colorado, New York, and Wisconsin) have collaboratively developed the Fetal Alcohol Syndrome Surveillance Network (FASSNet). The goal of the project is to monitor occurrence of FAS and to evaluate prevention, education, and intervention methods (Centers for Disease Control and Prevention, 2002).
    b. In the United States during the 1980s and 1990s, FAS was estimated to be 0.5 to 2 per 1000 live births (0.08 per 1000 live births reported in other countries) (May and Gossage, 2001; Riley et al., 2003).

    c. The incidence of fetal alcohol effects (FAE) is 4 per 1000 live births. The combined rate of FAS, FAE, alcohol-related neurodevelopmental disorder (ARND), and alcohol-related birth defects (ARBD) may be as high as 9.1 per 1000 live births (Jones and Bass, 2003). Prevalence rate is 2.5 to 5.6 per 1000 live births among Native Americans/Alaskan Natives from two states (National Institute on Alcohol Abuse and Alcoholism, 2000, 2002).

    d. FAS occurs in all socioeconomic groups, with a higher incidence in low socioeconomic groups.

    e. First-born children appear less likely to have FAS than subsequent offspring, and there is significant risk (increase of 406 times) of a sibling having FAS with a documented case in the family.

    f. Maternal risk factors associated with FAS, FAE, ARBD, or ARND include:

        (1) Advanced maternal age.

        (2) Low socioeconomic status.

        (3) Frequent binge drinking.

        (4) Family and friends with problems with alcohol.

        (5) Poor social and psychologic indicators.

  3. Five diagnostic categories are used to describe effects of alcohol exposure:

    a. FAS with a confirmed history of maternal alcohol intake.

    b. FAS with phenotypic features but no confirmed history of maternal alcohol intake.

    c. Partial FAS—confirmed history of maternal alcohol intake, some facial abnormalities, and one of the following: CNS abnormalities, growth restriction, or behavioral or cognitive disabilities.

    d. ARBD—some adverse birth outcomes related to prenatal alcohol exposure. Congenital anomalies may include

        (1) Cardiac: atrial or ventricular septal defects, tetralogy of Fallot;

        (2) Skeletal;

        (3) Renal: aplastic or dysplastic kidneys, hydronephrosis;

        (4) Ocular: strabismus, optic nerve hypoplasia, increased tortuosity of the retinal vessels, impaired vision (Stromland and Pinazo-Duran, 2002); and

        (5) Auditory: conductive or neurosensory hearing loss.

    e. ARND—CNS abnormalities related to prenatal alcohol exposure. CNS neurodevelopmental abnormalities can be one of the following:

        (1) Decreased cranial size at birth.

        (2) Structural brain abnormalities (e.g., microcephaly, agenesis of corpus callosum, cerebellar hypoplasia).

        (3) Neurologic signs: as age appropriate (e.g., impaired fine motor skills, neurosensory hearing loss, poor eye-hand coordination) (Hannigan and Armant, 2000).

        (4) Evidence of behavioral or cognitive abnormalities that are inconsistent with developmental level and unexplained by hereditary or environmental factors alone.

F. Neonatal withdrawal from alcohol.

  1. Withdrawal symptoms from alcohol are relatively mild in comparison with infant narcotic withdrawal.

  2. Onset is between birth and 12 hours after birth.

  3. Symptoms include the following:

    a. Hypertonia.

    b. Tremors.

    c. Opisthotonos.

    d. Weak suck and poor feeding pattern.

  4. Infants sleep little, cry more, and often engage in exaggerated mouthing behavior.

G. Nursing considerations.

  1. Careful and thorough assessment.

  2. Documentation of growth parameters (to include head circumference, length, and birth weight).

  3. Careful examination of facial features over a period of time.

4. Regular neurologic assessment for symptoms of neonatal withdrawal patterns.
5. Genetics consultation is indicated should FAS be suspected.
6. Family counseling and assessment of parenting skills.

STIMULANTS

This class of drugs include amphetamines, caffeine, cocaine, dextroamphetamines, methamphetamines (MDMA [ecstasy], crystal meth), and methylphenidates (Ritalin).

Cocaine

A. **Incidence of cocaine use in pregnancy.**
1. The National Institute on Drug Abuse conducted the National Pregnancy and Health Survey in 1992 to 1993 surveying 4 million women who gave birth. The statistics showed that 221,000 women used illegal drugs during their pregnancy and 45,000 reported using cocaine.
2. The Maternal Lifestyle Study, which included 8627 mother-infant pairs from May 1993 to May 1995, showed that of the women ages 18 to 25 years (49%), 26 to 35 years (44%), and 36 to 49 years (8%), 13% admitted to having used cocaine, and 59% of these used cocaine during their pregnancy (Klitsch, 2002).
3. Substance abuse admissions decreased from 17% (1995) to 14% (2005) for cocaine as primary drug of choice.
4. Smoking and inhalation are the first and second most frequent routes of administration. Smoking has decreased but inhalation has increased (14% to 22%; 1995-2005).
5. There has been an increase in admissions for whites, decrease in blacks, and little to no change in Hispanics for either smoking or inhalation (SAMHSA, February 9, 2007).
B. **Pharmacology.**
1. Cocaine is a CNS stimulant taken for its mood-altering properties.
2. It is one of the most powerful addictive substances of abuse.
3. It may be taken orally, sublingually, intranasally, or intravenously or inhaled ("crack").
4. Cocaine is derived from the leaves of the South and Central American plant *Erythroxylon coca.*
5. Crack cocaine is made by mixing cocaine powder with ammonia, water, and baking soda. The resulting mixture cracks when heated and releases the cocaine vapor, which is inhaled. Smoking crack offers a peak effect within 60 to 90 seconds, a high lasting only 5 to 10 minutes, and is the most popular form.
6. Cocaine is fat soluble and has a relatively low molecular weight, making passage through the blood-brain barrier and across the placenta very easy.
7. Cocaine is metabolized and made water soluble by plasma and liver cholinesterases for excretion in the urine. Metabolism is slower in the fetus and newborn infant, with metabolites persisting in the infant's urine for 4 to 14 days (metabolites in an adult can be detected up to 72 hours in urine).
8. Cocaine inhibits the reuptake of both norepinephrine and dopamine. "The resulting excess of these neurotransmitters at the postsynaptic receptor sites results in a prolonged stimulation" (Ostrea et al., 2005). The stimulation is what gives the euphoric "high." The hypothalamus is affected by the diminished reuptake of norepinephrine, causing a lack of appetite.
9. Peripheral vasoconstriction, tachycardia, hypertension, and hyperthermia are adverse effects that can lead to acute myocardial infarction, cerebrovascular accident, pulmonary edema, and renal and bowel infarction if heavy use continues.
10. Cocaine is rarely used alone; it is associated with polydrug use and should be a red flag for all health care providers.
C. **Effects on pregnancy.**
1. Use is associated with little to no prenatal care, which contributes to the poor pregnancy outcomes. Women are fearful about the legal ramifications to themselves and their children

(present or future) if they present in a clinic to a professional. Medical complications related to maternal cocaine use include the following:

    a. Anorexia (decreased uptake of norepinephrine acts through the hypothalamus to decrease appetite).

    b. Anemia.

    c. Cardiac disease.

  2. Sexually transmitted diseases or infections may be present.

    a. Gonorrhea.

    b. Syphilis.

    c. Hepatitis B.

    d. Hepatitis C (4% to 7% per pregnancy) (Yeung et al., 2001) increases fourfold to fivefold with hepatitis B virus coinfection.

    e. Human immunodeficiency virus (HIV) infection.

Two major side effects of cocaine use—vasoconstriction and hypertension—are responsible for most of the adverse complications listed in Box 3-2.

D. Effects on the fetus and neonate (Ostrea et al., 2005).

  1. Congenital malformations are not increased. However, there is multiorgan dysfunction in the neonate:

    a. Central nervous system: abnormal sleep patterns, electroencephalogram, and cry; seizures/tremors; cerebral infarction.

    b. Sensory organs: abnormal brainstem auditory-evoked response, increase in auditory startle response.

    c. Cardiovascular: atrial/ventricular arrhythmia, hypertension, decreased cardiac output.

    d. Respiratory: apnea, abnormal breathing patterns (periodic).

    e. Renal: ectopia.

    f. Gastrointestinal: increased incidence of early-onset necrotizing enterocolitis and intestinal perforation not related to NEC.

    g. Eye: vascular, disruptive lesions; retinal hemorrhage.

E. Neonatal withdrawal from cocaine.

  1. Signs of CNS irritability after birth are considered to be an effect of cocaine rather than withdrawal. Infants may be restless, irritable, tremulous, and hypertonic.

  2. Following an initial hyperirritability period, infant may exhibit drowsiness and/or lethargy.

  3. Changes in behavioral state displayed may include

    a. difficulty responding to the human voice and face;

    b. difficulty maintaining alert states, alternating between periods of sleep and agitation;

    c. depressed interactive behaviors and poor responses to environmental stimuli;

    d. poor response to comforting by caregivers;

    e. startle that is easily elicited;

    f. rapid change in state; and

    g. getting distressed easily (exhibited by rapid respirations, frantic gaze aversion, color changes, and/or disorganized motor activity).

  4. Neuromotor deficits may include hypertonic or hypotonic muscle tone, abnormal movements, and abnormal suck-swallow pattern (causing poor feeding).

■ BOX 3-2
■ **OBSTETRIC EFFECTS OF COCAINE**

■ Abruptio placentae	■ Precipitous delivery
■ Fetal hypoxia and stillbirth	■ Pregnancy-induced hypertension
■ Meconium staining	■ Preterm labor
■ Spontaneous abortion	

F. Limited follow-up studies.
 1. Controversial research findings suggest that a high-risk environment may play a greater role in cognitive and behavioral deficits than prenatal exposure (Keller and Snyder-Keller, 2000). Maternal psychologic function has been found to have influenced the overall functional outcome of the child (Accornero et al., 2002).
 2. Improvement in state control abilities seen at 1 month.
 3. Hypertonia may persist for up to 2 years. Infants with cocaine-related hypertonia exhibit lower cognitive scores.
 4. Weight and length normalize at 1 year of age, but head circumference remains smaller throughout the first 2 years of life.
 5. Significant effects on cognitive development are seen at 2 years; however, the child is twice as likely to have significant delay. No significant motor delay is seen (Singer et al., 2002).
 6. No significant adverse effects are seen according to the level of cocaine exposure on the Mental Development Index (MDI), Psychomotor Development Index (PDI), or Infant Behavior Record of the Bayley Scales of Infant Development (Frank et al., 2001, 2002).

G. Nursing considerations.
 1. Hospital costs for cocaine-exposed infants have been estimated to be $5200 more than for nonexposed infants.
 2. Symptom management usually does not require pharmacologic intervention.
 3. Address the needs of prematurity more than substance exposure.
 4. Keep environmental stimuli to a minimum.
 5. Provide swaddling and frequent small feeds as needed.
 6. Arrange for supportive care for the mother prior to discharge.

Amphetamines (3,4-Methylenedioxymethamphetamine [MDMA])

A. Incidence
 1. It has been reported that between 1992 and 1998 incidence increased; however, since that time the prevalence has stabilized.
 2. Persons aged 18 to 25 were more likely than those aged 26 or older to be past-year users of LSD, phencyclidine (PCP), and "ecstasy" (NIDA, 2007).
 3. Methamphetamine use in the past year among the civilian, noninstitutionalized population aged 12 or older declined overall between 2002 and 2005.
 4. In 2005, an estimated 1.3 million persons aged 12 or older (0.5%) had used methamphetamine in the past year; an estimated 556,000 of these were female and 741,000 male.
 5. The number of recent methamphetamine initiates (i.e., persons who used methamphetamine for the first time in the 12 months before the survey) remained relatively stable between 2002 and 2004 but decreased between 2004 and 2005 (318,000 and 192,000 persons, respectively).
 6. Data from 2002 to 2005 indicate that persons in the West (1.2%) were more likely to have used methamphetamine in the past year than persons in the Midwest (0.5%), South (0.5%), and Northeast (0.1%); these findings were consistent for both females and males (NSDUH, January 26, 2007).
 7. The prevalence of past-year prescription psychotherapeutic drug misuse among women aged 15 to 44 was generally lower among those who were currently pregnant than those who were not. When disaggregated according to age, the pattern of lower rates of nonmedical use among women who were pregnant held for those aged 18 to 25 and for those aged 26 or older for any prescription drug, pain relievers, and tranquilizers. Among women aged 15 to 17, however, rates of misuse of any prescription drug, pain relievers, stimulants, methamphetamine, and sedatives tended to be higher among those who were pregnant than those who were not, but these differences did not reach statistical significance (Office of Applied Studies, 2002).
 8. MDMA is inexpensive and easy to access.
 9. MDMA appeals to a younger age-group of users.

B. **Pharmacology.**
 1. Amphetamines are a group of drugs that act as CNS stimulants. Sympathomimetic drugs usually are used for appetite suppression, weight loss, depression, hyperkinesis, and treatment of narcolepsy.
 2. Consists of amphetamine, dextroamphetamine, methamphetamine, MDMA ("ecstasy," Adam, bean, E, M, roll, X, XTC, and lovers' speed), crystal methamphetamine (batu, crank, crystal, glass, hiropon, ice, meth, shabu, shards, speed, Tina, ventano, vidrio, and white cross), and methylphenidate (Ritalin).
 3. Amphetamines can be inhaled, injected, smoked, or taken orally.
 4. They are neurotoxic.
 5. They cause vasoconstriction and hypertension.
 6. Intense physical and psychologic exhilaration is produced. Duration is 2 to 14 hours, depending on the dose. Effects are similar to those of cocaine.
 7. MDMA was reclassified as a Schedule I drug in 1985 and is now a banned substance. (MDMA is an amphetamine that has hallucinogenic properties similar to mescaline's.)
 8. Crystal methamphetamine is a colorless, odorless form of d-methamphetamine, also a powerful stimulant. It is often compared with crack cocaine because it produces similar physiologic effects. It may be inhaled or injected, with the effect lasting up to 12 hours (U.S. Department of Justice, 2002).
C. **Effects on pregnancy** (Martinez et al., 2006).
 1. Prematurity, abruptio placentae, hypertension, cardiac arrhythmias, myocardial infarction, clefting, and fetal growth restriction deficits.
 2. When teratogenicity has been produced in human studies, only a small increase was documented in the following: CNS and cardiac anomalies/defects (26 per 1000 live births), cleft palate, limb reduction and/or musculoskeletal anomalies (38 per 1000 live births), and congenital defects have been found.
D. **Effects on the fetus and neonate.**
 1. IUGR (low birth weight, length, and head circumference).
 2. Animal studies have shown varying results that indicate some teratogenicity (CNS and cardiac defects) (Ostrea et al., 2005).
 3. High incidence of retroplacental hemorrhage.
E. **Neonatal withdrawal from amphetamines.**
 1. Characterized by abnormal sleep patterns, poor feeding, tremors, abnormal weight gains, and state disorganization.
 2. Diaphoresis, episodes of agitation alternating with lassitude, miosis, and vomiting can occur shortly after birth.
 3. Frantic fist sucking, high-pitched cry, loose stools, fever, yawning, hyperreflexia, and excoriation when both cocaine and amphetamines were used.
F. **Nursing considerations.**
 1. Provide supportive care to the mother. Refer to social services to assist with underlying psychologic morbid issues.
 2. Promote and facilitate frequent and positive visits with infant.

CANNABINOIDS

Marijuana

A. **Incidence of marijuana use.**
 1. The most commonly used illicit drug and usually used in conjunction with other drugs or alcohol, with an estimated overall incidence of 4.8% to 5.4% for the U.S. population.
 2. The 2006 National Survey on Drug Use and Health Findings Report (NSDUH) indicates that there were 2.1 million persons aged 12 or older who had used marijuana for the first time within the past 12 months. This estimate is similar to estimates from past NSDUH surveys dating back to 2002 (SAMHSA, July 19, 2007).
B. **Pharmacology.**
 1. Marijuana has both depressant and mild hallucinogenic effects on the CNS.

2. It is usually smoked in a cigarette or pipe; alternatively, it can be cooked in biscuits or cakes.
3. It comes from the dried leaves and flowering tops of the plant *Cannabis sativa*.
4. Hashish is more potent and is prepared by drying and compressing the resin of flowering tops and leaves of the female cannabis plant.
5. The psychoactive ingredient is tetrahydrocannabinol (THC), which has a high affinity for lipids and accumulates in the fatty tissues throughout the body.
6. Placental transfer is highest in the first trimester of pregnancy.
7. Smoking marijuana increases the blood carbon monoxide level and may result in hypoxia.
8. The THC content in marijuana has changed from the 1960s by 15-fold. Therefore, the risks and consequences of this strength cannot be equated to studies performed in the past.

C. Effects on pregnancy.
1. Harm associated with the same adverse effects as those who use tobacco.
2. Effects are limited, inconsistent, and conflicting. Controversial issues relate to
   a. length of gestation (shortened) and
   b. duration of labor and outcome (preterm delivery).

D. Effects on the fetus and neonate.
1. Limited studies have been conducted, with controversial findings:
   a. Congenital anomalies.
   b. IUGR as a result of increase in carboxyhemoglobin.
   c. Some evidence of neonatal withdrawal (tremulousness, alterations of sleep patterns, prolonged startle, high-pitched cry), but usually does not persist beyond 1 month.
   d. Significant association between SIDS and paternal marijuana use in all periods (Klonoff-Cohen and Lam-Kruglick, 2001).

NARCOTICS AND OPIOIDS

This class includes (a) natural opioids: morphine and opium; (b) semisynthetic opioids: heroin and methadone; and (c) synthetic opioids: propoxyphene (Darvon), hydromorphone hydrochloride (Dilaudid), and oxycodone (OxyContin).

A. Incidence of opiate use in pregnancy.
1. In 2000 heroin was ranked second to cocaine as the most serious drug problem by 20% of the Pulse Check sources (Pulse Check is a grouping of cities that are part of the Committee of Epidemiologic Workshop Group sponsored by NIDA investigating different aspects of substance use and trends).
2. Heroin use increased from 22% in 1999 to 26% in 2000 as a serious drug problem.
3. There are no current national prevalence data that give accurate statistics on heroin drug use by pregnant women in the United States. However, it has been estimated that each year between 100,000 and 375,000 women use illicit drugs during pregnancy.
4. Among pregnant women ages 15 to 44 years, 3.3% reported using illicit drugs in the month prior to the interview (based on the combined 1999 and 2000 NHSDA samples). This rate is significantly lower than the rate among nonpregnant women ages 15 to 44 years (7.7%). Among pregnant women ages 15 to 17 years, the rate of use was 12.9%, nearly equal to the rate for nonpregnant women of the same age (13.5%).
5. In California in 1992, 1.1% of urine samples from pregnant women were positive for cocaine and 1.4% positive for opiates. Black women had the highest rates: 7.8% for cocaine and 2.5% for opiates. NIDA has reported that as of December 1999, data from 20 cities in the United States have shown a trend in which marijuana and heroin abuse had increased (NIDA, 2003).
6. There were no gender differences in injection use in the past year. Males and females were similar in the proportion who injected the drug in the past year (42.0% and 40.7%, respectively) (SAMHSA, July 19, 2007).

7. The proportion of primary heroin admissions who injected the drug declined from 69% in 1995 to 63% in 2005, whereas the proportion of primary heroin admissions who inhaled the drug increased from 27% in 1995 to 33% in 2005.
8. There is a varying degree of NAS in infants (48% to 94%) when women use opiates during pregnancy (Osborn et al., 2005).
9. There has been an increase in oxycodone use and emergency department visits in the United States (89% between 1993 and 1999; increase in 68% in 2000) (U.S. Department of Justice, 2001).

B. **Pharmacology.**
   1. Opiates are CNS depressants.
   2. They are derived from the opium poppy, *Papaver somniferum.*
   3. Heroin is a semisynthetic opiate that may be sniffed, smoked, or injected.
   4. Heroin is quick acting and produces a sense of euphoria within 10 seconds after injection.
   5. Heroin is much stronger than morphine and readily crosses the placental barrier.
   6. Methadone, a synthetic opiate, is usually taken orally but can be injected. Methadone also crosses the placental barrier.
   7. Methadone is absorbed slowly and has a long duration of action, making it suitable for treatment of heroin addicts.
   8. Methadone in pregnancy is preferred to heroin because
      a. the drug level delivered to the fetus is more stable and reduces the risk of fetal withdrawal, and
      b. there is less risk of infection from the use of contaminated needles.
   9. Opiates interfere with the normal menstrual cycle, thereby reducing fertility. Many addicted women do not realize they are pregnant until between the 5th and 7th months.
   10. Oxycodone is manufactured by modifying thebaine, an alkaloid found in opium. It is an opiate agonist, used for moderate to high pain relief and is highly addictive (trade names are Percocet, Percodan, Tylox, and OxyContin.)

C. **Effects on pregnancy.**
   1. Pregnant addicts may present with a number of medical complications related to their drug use:
      a. Anorexia.
      b. Anemia.
      c. Cardiac disease.
      d. Thrombosis.
      e. Abscesses.
   2. Sexually transmitted diseases or infections may also be present:
      a. Gonorrhea.
      b. Syphilis.
      c. Hepatitis B and C.
      d. HIV.
   3. Women may be polydrug abusers.
   4. Many of the effects of opiate use in pregnancy are correlated directly to the amount of prenatal care received and the maternal lifestyle, rather than to the drug itself.
   5. Morbidity and mortality rates are lower in infants born to methadone-dependent women who have adequate prenatal care.
   6. Spontaneous abortions are common.
   7. Obstetric complications include those listed in Box 3-3.

D. **Effects on the fetus and neonate.**
   1. Hypoxia due to an unstable intrauterine environment and reduction in placental blood flow.
   2. Lower Apgar scores.
   3. NAS. Concern about the administration of naloxone, a narcotic antagonist for respiratory depression, has been raised. Rapid withdrawal and seizures may result, and urgent treatment for withdrawal may be needed.

■ BOX 3-3
■ **OBSTETRIC COMPLICATIONS OF METHADONE**

■ Toxemia	■ Precipitous delivery
■ Abruptio placentae	■ Breech delivery
■ Premature labor	■ Fetal distress
■ Shorter-than-average labor	■ Stillbirth

4. Meconium aspiration and aspiration pneumonia.
5. IUGR.
6. Lower incidence of respiratory distress syndrome.
7. Lower degrees of physiologic jaundice.
8. Congenital infections.
9. Increased incidence of SIDS.
10. Low birth weight.
11. Microcephaly.
12. Increased chromosomal aberrations (heroin-only-exposed infants).

E. **Results of follow-up studies.**
   1. Inconsistent. There may be alterations in physical growth and in neurologic, behavioral, and cognitive functioning in early infancy and childhood (Hans and Jeremy, 2001).

F. **Comparison of methadone with heroin.**
   1. With adequate prenatal care in a low-dose methadone program, perinatal outcome is improved in terms of prematurity, fetal loss, and medical complications (Burns et al., 2007; Dashe et al., 2002).
   2. Both groups of infants present with low birth weight; however, methadone infants are generally larger.
   3. Infants exposed to both methadone and heroin may exhibit signs of NAS. However, NAS usually occurs later in infants exposed to methadone because it is stored in the fetal lung, liver, and spleen and metabolized after birth. Very little heroin is stored by the fetus (Weiner and Finnegan, 2006).

SEDATIVES/HYPNOTICS

This class of drugs includes barbiturates (Seconal, Nembutal, Amytal, Tuinal, phenobarbital) and benzodiazepines (Ativan, Halcion, Librium, Rohypnol, Valium, and Xanax). Street names include downers, forget-me pill, ludes, roofenol, roofies, rophies, ruffies, sopers, trenks, 714s, yellow jackets, reds, blues, rainbow.

A. **Incidence of sedative and hypnotic use.**
   1. Not generally the primary drug of abuse. Used to induce sleep or to decrease anxiety related to alcohol withdrawal or to accentuate the effects of alcohol or other drugs.
   2. Popular to use and desired due to no outward signs of use; no odor detected.

B. **Pharmacology.**
   1. Benzodiazepines largely replaced short-acting barbiturates in the 1960s. They are used in combination with alcohol for a sedative effect or to take the edge off withdrawal from cocaine.
   2. They act on the CNS but without significant CNS depression. Also, they alter the balance of the neurotransmitter, gamma-aminobutyric acid (GABA), in the limbic system of the brain-regulating emotional state.
   3. Onset is 30 to 45 minutes and can last for 3 to 5 hours. Its half-life in adults is 20 to 60 hours and can be 4 times longer in neonates (mean plasma half-life in the neonate is about 31 hours).
   4. They are highly addictive.

C. **Effects on pregnancy and on the fetus and neonate.**
   1. They are readily transmitted across the placenta; concentration in fetal blood is similar to maternal circulation owing to high lipid solubility.
   2. Substantial accumulation may occur in adipose tissue; a high concentration also is present in the brain, lungs, and heart.
   3. Side effects may include abortion, malformations, IUGR, functional deficits, carcinogenesis, and mutagenesis (Iqbal et al., 2002).
   4. Fetuses exposed to long-acting benzodiazepines on a long-term basis showed neonatal hypotonicity, failure to feed, and/or withdrawal syndrome (Perault et al., 2000).
   5. There is inconsistent research showing risk of congenital malformations.
   6. Regular use of benzodiazepines in mothers showed infants who had side effects similar to FAS.

INHALANTS

Examples of inhalants include benzene, Freon, gasoline, lighter fluid, nitrous oxide, shoe polish, toluene, and typewriter correction fluid.

A. **Pharmacology.**
   1. Two main categories:
      a. Volatile solvents and aerosols (solvents: glue [toluene], typewriter correction fluid, and gasoline; aerosols: spray paint and cooking sprays).
      b. Nitrites (amyl nitrites [poppers, snappers], butyl nitrite, isopropyl nitrite [rush, locker room], and nitrous oxide [laughing gas, whippets]).
   2. CNS depressants that cause alcohol-like intoxication symptoms.
   3. Short-acting heart stimulant and vasodilator. Nitrites decrease blood pressure, increase heart rate, and reduce oxygen flow to the brain.
   4. Effects take place immediately (30 to 60 seconds) and can last 15 minutes to several hours.
   5. Readily cross the placenta.

B. **Effects on pregnancy.**
   1. Long-term use results in
      a. accidents (owing to memory loss, heightened sense of power, judgment problems).
      b. tissue damage (permanent damage to brain, bone marrow, liver, kidneys, and other major organs).
      c. sudden "sniffing" death (related to cardiac failure).
      d. suffocation (when plastic bags are used to inhale solvent vapors).
   2. Excessive use may cause glaucoma, blood cell damage (can trigger methemoglobinemia), acquired immunodeficiency syndrome (AIDS), and rupture of lungs (if high-pressure tank is used).

C. **Effects on the fetus and neonate.**
   1. Fetal dysmorphogenesis syndrome (similar to FAS) has been associated with these exposures.
   2. High concentrations of toluene exposure have been reported to include the following deficits: small for gestational age (SGA), microcephalic, short palpebral fissures, deep-set eyes, small face, low-set ears, micrognathia, spatulate fingertips, small fingernails, developmental delay, language impairment, hyperactivity, and cerebellar dysfunction (Jones and Balster, 1997).

OTHER (ANTIDEPRESSANTS)

A. **Pharmacology.**
   1. Three categories (in terms of the neurotransmitters affected):
      a. Selective serotonin reuptake inhibitors (SSRIs)—SSRIs (e.g., Zoloft, Lexapro, Prozac, Paxil, Celexa) are the most commonly prescribed antidepressants. SSRIs increase the amount of serotonin by hindering the process involved in eliminating serotonin (which

is called reuptake). After serotonin is released from a nerve cell, the reuptake process removes any serotonin that is not used. Because the reabsorption of serotonin is blocked, the level of serotonin is increased.

    b. Tricyclic antidepressants (TCAs)—TCAs (e.g., Elavil, Nortriptyline) increase serotonin, norepinephrine, and dopamine by also blocking the reuptake process (the removal of these neurotransmitters). Because of more adverse side effects, TCAs are prescribed less often than SSRIs.

    c. Monoamine oxidase inhibitors (MAOIs)—MAOIs (e.g., Nardil, Marplan) inhibit the action of an enzyme called monoamine oxidase, which breaks down certain neurotransmitters. As a result, the amounts of serotonin and norepinephrine are increased. MAOIs are less prescribed than SSRIs and TCAs because of possible severe side effects and drug interactions.

    d. Wellbutrin is a dopamine and norepinephrine reuptake inhibitor (DNRI), which increases both dopamine and norepinephrine by blocking the removal of these two neurotransmitters.

  2. All antidepressants cross the placenta to some degree.

B. Effects on the fetus and neonate.

  1. SSRIs were found to increase preterm labor, respiratory problems, prematurity, low Apgar scores, neonatal convulsions, hypoglycemia, some congenital malformations (Lennestal and Kallen, 2007; Maschi et al., 2008; Wogelius et al., 2006). Association is seen with anencephaly, omphalocele, and craniosynostosis (Alwan et al., 2007).

  2. First-trimester use of paroxetine (Seroxat, Paxil) (levels greater than 25 mg/day) found to increase major congenital and cardiac malformations (Bar-Oz et al., 2007; Berard et al., 2007).

  3. Third-trimester use of SSRIs and TCAs had an increased risk for respiratory distress syndrome, endocrine and metabolic disturbances, hypoglycemia, temperature regulation disorders, and convulsions (Davis et al., 2007).

Neonatal Abstinence Syndrome (Ostrea et al., 2005)

Neonatal abstinence is described as a generalized disorder (multisystem) characterized by 21 signs most commonly seen in withdrawing infants (Finnegan, 1990) (see Table 3-1).

  1. More than two thirds of neonates born to opiate-dependent women will exhibit signs of NAS.

  2. Onset varies from shortly after birth to 2 weeks of age.

  3. Majority of signs appear within 72 hours of birth (see Table 3-2).

  4. Duration ranges from 8 to 16 weeks or longer.

  5. Presentation of NAS is variable. It can be mild and transient, intermittent, or delayed in onset or waver between acute and subacute withdrawal.

  6. Chronic drug users have more severe withdrawal.

  7. The closer to delivery the drug is taken, the greater the delay of onset and the more severe the signs (Weiner and Finnegan, 2006).

The degree or severity of NAS is influenced by the following factors: (1) type of drug used, (2) half-life of drug, (3) time of last drug exposure prior to birth, (4) dose taken (if known), (5) quality of labor, (6) type of anesthesia and/or analgesia used, (7) maturity and status of neonate, (8) gestational age, and (9) nutritional status of mother and infant.

Methods for Scoring Neonatal Abstinence Syndrome

There are three methods used to score or rate NAS:

  1. Finnegan's Neonatal Abstinence Score (Modified Finnegan Score).

  2. Neonatal Drug Withdrawal Scoring System (Lipsitz Tool) (Lipsitz, 1975).

  3. Neonatal Withdrawal Inventory (Zahorodny, 1998).

Modified Finnegan Scoring Tool (original 32 items) has 21 items scored every 4 hours. Individual NAS symptoms are weighted (numerical score 1 to 5) according to the presence and severity

■ TABLE 3-1
■ ■ **Neonatal Signs of Withdrawal**

System	Sign
Neurologic	Hypertonia
	Tremors
	Hyperreflexia
	Irritability and restlessness
	High-pitched cry
	Sleep disturbances
	Seizures
Autonomic	Yawning
	Nasal stuffiness
	Sweating
	Sneezing
	Low-grade fever
	Skin mottling
Gastrointestinal	Diarrhea
	Vomiting
	Poor feeding
	Regurgitation
	Dysmature swallowing
	Excessive sucking
Respiratory	Tachypnea
Miscellaneous	Skin excoriation

■ TABLE 3-2
■ ■ **Onset of Drug Withdrawal Symptoms after Delivery**

Drug	Onset of Withdrawal Symptoms after Delivery
Alcohol	3 to 12 hours after delivery
Narcotics (heroin, methadone)	48 to 72 hours; may be as late as 4 weeks
Barbiturates	4 to 7 days on average (1 to 14 days possible)
Cocaine	48 to 72 hours

Source: American Academy of Pediatrics Committee on Drugs: Neonatal drug withdrawal. *Pediatrics, 101*(6):1079-1088, 1998.

of the symptom exhibited. Scores >8 or greater are recommended to receive pharmacologic treatment.

Neonatal Drug Withdrawal Scoring System is an 11-item scale, each symptom scored 0 to 3 according to the severity of symptoms. Pharmacologic treatment is recommended for a score of 4 or greater (Lipsitz, 1975).

Neonatal Withdrawal Inventory is a 27-item scale originally tested using an actigraph to objectively measure movement (Zahorodny et al., 1998).

Other key points:

1. The NAS scoring system used should be based on the individual institution/neonatology service guidelines.
2. Good studies yielding evidence for the selection of the best pharmacologic treatment for neonates is lacking (Osborn et al., 2005).

3. There has been little advancement in NAS management or research since the 1970s. Finnegan is held as the gold standard as well as the theoretical background on which studies are based (Marcellus, 2007).

Neonatal Abstinence Scoring System (Finnegan Score)

1. The Neonatal Abstinence Scoring System assists in the detection of the onset of withdrawal symptoms and charts the progression and response to therapeutic intervention (see Table 3-3).
2. The scoring system can be used to assess withdrawal from both opioid and nonopioid CNS depressants (Weiner and Finnegan, 2006).
3. Assess all high-risk infants 2 hours after birth and then every 4 hours.
4. If, at any point, the score is 8 or greater, the scoring should be initiated every 2 hours and should be continued for a minimum of 24 hours.
5. If pharmacotherapy is not required, the infant is scored for the first 96 hours of life.
6. If the infant scores 8 or higher on three consecutive scoring times, the infant should be evaluated for pharmacotherapy.
7. NAS symptoms often mimic common neonatal metabolic conditions (such as hypoglycemia, hypocalcemia, sepsis, and meningitis). A complete blood cell count and measurement of calcium and glucose levels are recommended before therapy is initiated.

Pharmacologic Treatment of Neonatal Abstinence Syndrome

1. Approximately 50% to 60% of infants exposed in utero to opiates will require pharmacologic intervention (Weiner and Finnegan, 2006).

■ TABLE 3-3
■ ■ **Neonatal Abstinence Scoring System**

Signs	Score			
	0	**1**	**2**	**3**
Tremors (muscle activity of limbs)	Normal	Minimally ↑ when hungry or disturbed	Moderately or markedly ↑ when undisturbed, subside when fed or held snugly	Marked even when undisturbed, going on to seizure-like movements
Irritability (excessive crying)	None	Slightly ↑	Moderate to severe when disturbed or hungry	Marked even when undisturbed
Reflexes	Normal	Increased	Markedly increased	
Stools	Normal	Explosive, but normal frequency	Explosive, more than 8/day	
Muscle tone	Normal	Increased	Rigidity	
Skin abrasions	No	Redness of knees and elbows		Breaking of skin
Respiratory rate/minute	<55	55 to 75	76 to 95	
Repetitive sneezing	No	Yes		
Repetitive yawning	No	Yes		
Vomiting	No	Yes		
Fever	No	Yes		

Scoring: Identification of newborn with narcotic withdrawal when score >17 (78% probability).
Source: Lipsitz, P.J.: A proposed narcotic withdrawal score for use with newborn infants: A pragmatic evaluation of its efficacy. *Clinical Pediatrics, 14*(6):592-594, 1975.

2. Begin pharmacologic treatment only when withdrawal is not controlled by supportive measures.
3. Pharmacologic agents used to treat NAS are provided in Table 3-4.
4. Opiates are used for NAS due to opiate exposure and sedatives for nonopiate or polydrug exposure (Osborn et al., 2005). Opiates used for NAS due to opiate withdrawal have included tincture of opium, paregoric (contains anhydrous morphine with antispasmodics, camphor, 45% ethanol, and benzoic acid), morphine, and methadone. Sedatives used for opiate withdrawal have included clonidine (an alpha$_2$ presynaptic blocker), chlorpromazine, phenobarbitone, and diazepam (AAP Committee on Infectious Diseases, 1998).

■ TABLE 3-4
■ ■ **Drugs Used to Reduce Opioid Withdrawal in Neonates**

Name	Dosing	Recommendations
Tincture of opium	0.1 ml/kg or 2 drops/kg with feedings every 4 hours After 3 to 5 days' stabilization, taper by decreasing dose without altering frequency	Preferred over paregoric; 25-fold dilution contains the same concentration of morphine as in paregoric
Paregoric	0.1 ml/kg or 2 drops/kg with feedings every 4 hours; may be increased by 2 drops/kg every 3 to 4 hours until stabilized After 3 to 5 days' stabilization, taper by decreasing dose without altering frequency	Infants have greater physiologic sucking and weight gain Use of paregoric declined because of potential toxic effects of ingredients
Morphine	Parenteral: 0.1 mg/kg Oral: 4 mg/ml	Oral route provides less analgesic than parenteral Respiratory depressant; can be life threatening
Methadone	0.05 to 0.1 mg/kg every 6 hours with increases of 0.05 mg/kg until stable After controlling, dose every 12 to 24 hours Discontinue after weaning to 0.05 mg/kg/day	Treat NAS from opioid withdrawal
Clonidine	Oral: 0.5 to 1.0 mg/kg single dose Maintenance: 3 to 5 mg/kg/day in divided doses every 4 to 6 hours	May have immediate reversal of symptoms Treatment shorter than phenobarbital Oral liquid not available
Chlorpromazine	IM/PO: 0.55 mg/kg every 6 hours	CNS and GI signs produced by withdrawal are controlled Multiple side effects
Phenobarbital	Loading dose: 16 mg/kg per 24 hours Maintenance: 2 to 8 mg/kg per 24 hours When stabilized, decrease by 10% to 25% per day Blood levels 24 to 48 hours after loading dose: 20 to 30 mg/ml	Good choice for nonnarcotic-related withdrawal signs Does not relieve GI symptoms
Diazepam	1 to 2 mg every 8 hours	Multiple side effects

CNS, central nervous system; *GI*, gastrointestinal; *IM*, intramuscular; *NAS*, Neonatal abstinence syndrome; *PO*, by mouth.
Source: Naegle, M.A. and D'Avanzo, M.A.: Addictions and substance abuse: *Strategies for advanced practice nursing*. Upper Saddle River, NJ, 2001, Prentice Hall, p. 244. Adapted from American Academy of Pediatrics Committee on Drugs: Neonatal drug withdrawal. *Pediatrics, 101*(6):1079-1088, 1998.

5. Oral morphine is the opiate of choice. The second-line drugs are paregoric and tincture of opium (used less because of their high alcohol content).
6. Opiates do not make the infant drowsy or interfere with infant feeding. They are effective for controlling a variety of gastrointestinal disturbances.
7. Once withdrawal is controlled, pharmacologic treatment can be gradually weaned.
8. *Control* is defined as meeting the following conditions:
   a. Scores of 8 or less.
   b. Infant is easily consoled.
   c. Infant maintains a rhythmic sleep and feeding cycle.
   d. Steady weight gain.

Iatrogenic Neonatal Abstinence Syndrome

1. Opiates are used extensively in the care of critically ill neonates and infants as analgesics and sedatives to assist in ventilation.
2. Abrupt cessation of these drugs may result in signs of withdrawal (NAS) following prolonged use.
3. It is recommended to wean from opiates with the assistance of the same neonatal abstinence scoring system.

Nonpharmacologic Treatment of Neonatal Abstinence Syndrome

1. Swaddling, settling, massage, relaxation baths, pacifiers, and waterbeds (Crocetti et al., 2007; D'Apolito, 1999; King Edward Memorial Hospital, 2006).

GENERAL MANAGEMENT RECOMMENDATIONS

A. **Document maternal drug use:** Review history, drug of choice, and pattern during prenatal period.
B. **Obtain toxicology screening** for all infants when there is a moderate to strong suspicion of use. For urine, obtain the earliest urine possible. Consent may be needed in some states. Follow the Health Insurance Portability and Accountability Act (HIPAA) guidelines set by your institution.
C. **Consider HIV testing** pending the mother's consent and your hospital's policy. If no prenatal care, HIV testing may be part of admission maternal serology panel.
D. **If a careful physical examination reveals abnormalities, investigate further:** Any malformations, growth restriction, or microcephaly noted is cause for additional screening for congenital infections and possible referral to genetics or dysmorphologist on staff.
E. **Obtain additional tests:** Follow unit protocol to obtain cranial and renal ultrasound, electroencephalogram, visual evoked response, ophthalmologic examination, and brainstem auditory-evoked response prior to discharge.
F. **Observe carefully and monitor consistently** for signs of feeding intolerance and difficulty. Observe mother during feeding and offer helpful suggestions.
G. **Evaluate for signs of withdrawal** (see Table 3-3).
H. **Counsel and educate the mother regarding breastfeeding:** Provide lactation specialist referral in-house and support group contact numbers.
I. **Initiate a careful and comprehensive plan of care for discharge:** Attention to maintaining continuity of care after discharge for both mother and infant is imperative (Payot and Berner, 2000).
J. **Consult with social services and other health care providers:** Make referrals to appropriate agencies or for foster care, if needed (this includes all cases of FAS/FAE). The mother must be clearly informed of all medical, social, and legal circumstances regarding her and the infant. Consider using a translation service (or designated person in the hospital—not a family member) if there is any doubt about language competency. This process needs to be well documented in the medical chart.

NURSING INTERVENTIONS

A. The infant: Each infant presents with a variable prenatal history, delivery scenario, and response to the environment. Table 3-5 provides strategies that the nurse and parent can use to help ease the prenatal exposure to drug sequelae in the neonatal nursery, newborn nursery, and at home.

B. Mother-nurse interactions.

1. Nurses must confront their own feelings regarding these issues. Many nurses still harbor punitive and negative attitudes toward these mothers, rather than positive and supportive ones.

2. Addiction is a chronic disease requiring ongoing health care intervention. All patients should be treated in a professional manner. Nurses need to be knowledgeable about substance exposure and addiction theories to be effective change agents with mothers and the family.

3. Develop a therapeutic relationship with the mother by establishing trust. Proceed slowly and take cues from the mother at a comfortable pace for her.

4. Provide consistency in caregivers, preferably with a primary nurse or team. Provide support to the mother by being present during dialogs, rounds, and consults with neonatologists and other health care providers. Help her interpret what she heard in terms understandable to her.

5. Provide clear information and specific guidelines for expected behavior of both the mother and the infant. Provide the mother with realistic expectations of the infant's behavior and progress. Be sensitive to the fact that repeated explanation of skills or information already presented in the past may be required.

6. Present truthful information and education in a nonjudgmental manner while allowing opportunity for the mother's concerns, fears, and questions to be addressed.

■ TABLE 3-5
■ ■ **Strategies for Caring for Infants Prenatally Exposed to Drugs**

Infant Behavior	Behavior Description	Strategies
Vomiting or poor feeding	Infants frequently display gastrointestinal difficulties throughout their first year of life. Vomiting is frequent during the first 6 to 9 months, as are intermittent constipation and diarrhea. These difficulties tend to increase irritability and discomfort. If allowed, some infants sleep up to 20 hours per day during the first 6 months of life and miss feedings. They are therefore at risk for inadequate nutrition and failure to thrive.	■ If necessary, wake infant for feeding. ■ Give small quantities of food. ■ Allow infant to rest frequently during feeding. ■ Have infant upright for feeding. After feeding, place infant in side-lying or prone position to prevent aspiration of milk. ■ If infant vomits, clean skin immediately to prevent irritation from stomach acid.
Uncoordinated sucking and swallowing	A variety of abnormal oral-motor behaviors have been observed, including a preemie-like suck pattern, poorly coordinated suck-swallow patterns, inability to stabilize tongue in midline, and (occasionally) tongue thrusting and tongue tremors. These abnormal patterns increase feeding time. Consequently, a great deal of infant energy is required, and stress and frustration may occur in the mother and infant.	■ Hold infant in sitting position with arms forward in slight trunk flexion (curve) during feeding. ■ Keep infant's chin tucked downward. Infants prenatally exposed to drugs often push head back, which causes an abnormal swallow pattern. ■ If sucking is difficult for infant, support infant's chin or chin and cheeks with your hand. ■ Play soft, rhythmic music to help infant relax and to facilitate rhythmic sucking.

■ TABLE 3-5

■ ■ **Strategies for Caring for Infants Prenatally Exposed to Drugs—cont'd**

Infant Behavior	Behavior Description	Strategies
Weak pull-to-sit development	Infants often are slow in learning the pull-to-sit movement; frequently, it is accomplished with head lag or excessive effort after 6 months of age. (Infants normally pull to sit with no head lag by 4 months.) Some of those prenatally exposed to drugs who are able to pull to sit with no head lag may compensate by pulling their arms back into a strong W position. Usually pull to sit is accomplished with arms forward and some trunk flexion. The skill is a developmental milestone that indicates abdominal and neck muscle strength; it later affects the quality and endurance of balance, sitting, walking, and protective reflexes.	■ Move the infant from the supine to sitting position, supporting the head so that it does not lag. ■ While moving the infant into the sitting position, support the shoulders close to the infant's body with head forward (neck flexion). With the infant semireclined (45-degree angle), encourage it to assist with pull to sit. Give additional head support if needed to prevent head lag and to bring the infant's arms forward into the midline position. ■ Place the infant in a supported sitting position and move it slowly backward within the range of head control. Then slowly rock or move the infant back and forth to strengthen the neck and abdominal muscles.
Irritability and difficulty sleeping	Exposure to drugs in utero can cause the infant's state to vary from highly irritable to very passive. Most of these infants, however, are highly irritable and often have difficulty sleeping. Irritable infants can reach a frantic-cry state, which needs to be avoided. If the infant is passive, interaction needs to take place during quiet alert, not hyperalert, states. Caregivers need to monitor their interactions by being alert to infant behavioral and psychologic cues that indicate stress and adjust interactions appropriately. Caregivers will be affected by infant irritability, resulting in frustration and feelings of inadequacy in the mothering role and in infant-caregiver attachment. The caregiver needs to be made aware of behavior typical in infants prenatally exposed to drugs. Subsequently, the quality of their relationship will improve, negative judgments about infant will be reduced, and the likelihood of child abuse will decrease.	■ Reduce noise in the environment. ■ Turn down the lights. ■ Swaddle the infant in a cotton blanket in flexed position with its arms close to the body. ■ Hold the swaddled infant close. ■ Put the infant in a bunting-type wrapper and carry close to the body. ■ Rock the infant slowly and rhythmically, either horizontally or with the head supported vertically, whichever soothes. ■ Place in a front-pack carrier. ■ Walk with the infant. ■ Give child pacifier. ■ Provide hydrotherapy (warm bath). ■ Respond to stress cues by stopping the activity with the infant. This response will give the infant a timeout. ■ Provide a firm, calm touch to the midchest, back, or soles of the infant's feet. ■ Play a soft music or sing or hum quietly. ■ Provide background noise (e.g., a hair dryer or vacuum cleaner), often called white noise, which may calm the infant. ■ If all else fails, place the infant in a quiet, darkened room with no outside stimulation. (Caregivers report this works with both premature and full-term infants exposed prenatally to drugs.)

■ TABLE 3-5
■ ■ **Strategies for Caring for Infants Prenatally Exposed to Drugs—cont'd**

Infant Behavior	Behavior Description	Strategies
Tremors, trembling, and extraneous movement	Tremors of the hands, arms, legs, chin, and tongue are commonly observed in infants prenatally exposed to drugs, although usually more pronounced and intense in younger infants. Tremors and tremulousness of movements have been observed in infants older than 1 year, but the intensity is diminished. In younger infants, tremors are primarily observed when infants are at rest. As they get older, fewer and less intense at-rest tremors occur, and intention tremors emerge. They tend to increase as the infant tires. Intention tremors occur when the infant is actively attempting a specific motor movement, for example, reaching for a toy. Intervention is often successful with intention tremors of arms and hands. Signs of stress often occur after persisting with an activity that elicits intention tremors because physical movements are difficult, and more energy and time are required to accomplish a task. Fine-motor development is at risk. Some infants prenatally exposed to drugs exhibit constant extraneous movements that make it difficult for them to soothe themselves. These extraneous movements slow acquisition of organized intentional motor control and visual-motor skills.	■ Swaddling and holding the infant close may be helpful for early at-rest tremors and extraneous movement. ■ Hold the infant semireclined (almost sitting) with arms and shoulders forward to reduce the effort exerted by the infant to maintain the arm at midline while reaching for, holding, or manipulating toys. ■ Touch the tremulous area firmly and calmly. Touch the chest firmly and calmly.
Stiffness and rigidity	Stiffness and rigidity, or increased extensor tone, are often seen in infants prenatally exposed to drugs. The increased muscle tone, which causes these infants to frequently roll over at a few weeks of age, interferes with normal motor development, ability to cuddle, and pull to sit, and it delays the control of arms at midline. Increased extensor tone in infants tends to diminish slowly. By 1 year of age, some degree of increased tone usually remains and diminishes the quality and smoothness of gross-motor patterns as well as balance and protective reactions. These infants often arch their backs when held in a variety of positions, or when being fed. Arching occurs up to 12 months of age. More energy is used to accomplish fine- and gross-motor tasks; thus, some level of frustration is created.	■ Bathe the infant in warm water. ■ Try gentle, calming massage. ■ Swaddle in flexion with shoulders and arms close to body. ■ Place the infant in baby hammock to help ease rigidity, to maintain the infant in slight spinal flexion, and to inhibit abnormal extension pattern. ■ Do not leave the infant supine if the position maintains or increases stiffness, for example, head pushing back with scapular retraction (shoulder blades pinching together), or arms pushing into the *W* position. Instead, put infant in cloth, sling-style seat, as this position inhibits abnormal extension pattern. ■ Discourage the use of baby walkers, as they are known to further increase extensor tone.

■ TABLE 3-5
■ ■ **Strategies for Caring for Infants Prenatally Exposed to Drugs—cont'd**

Infant Behavior	Behavior Description	Strategies
Arms in *W* position	A large majority of infants prenatally exposed to drugs exhibit scapular retraction and/or resistance or weakness when attempting to bring arms to midline. When supine, arms are typically widespread and in a *W* position, or one arm is in a unilateral *W* position. As these infants develop, difficulty continues in bringing arms to midline or sustaining a midline position. Younger infants compensate by locking their hands together, but when they release them, their arms snap backward into a *W* position, much like a rubber-band effect. When infants are older, they can use their arms against increased extensor tone and thus use large amounts of active energy to maintain control. Fine-motor performance is compromised, and development of bimanual skills is difficult. Maintaining hands at midline is an important developmental step in acquiring fine-motor skills.	■ Swaddle the infant with arms in the midline position. ■ Carry or hold the infant in a semireclining position with shoulders forward so that the infant will experience arms at midline without excessive effort. ■ Place the infant in a cloth, sling-style infant seat. ■ Use reverse figure-eight strap to sustain arms in the forward position while the infant is in cloth, sling-style seat or in a prone or sitting position. The infant can have a successful experience without struggling for control. ■ Use a Forth infant feeder chair to position the child and assist in keeping arms at midline. This strategy can be used for infants who cannot tolerate the reverse figure-eight strap.

Source: Lewis, K.D., Bennett, B., and Schmeder, N.H.: The care of infants menaced by cocaine abuse. *MCN American Journal of Maternal Child Nursing, 14*(5):324-329, 1989.

7. Assist mothers to attach emotionally to their infants by encouraging and facilitating touch. Allow the mother to assist with caregiving skills and personalize her achievements.

8. Provide positive reinforcement and immediate feedback for all caretaking activities and interactions.

9. Parent education should be culturally sensitive, goal directed, and tailored to the mother's education level. Provide clear steps of the caretaking tasks and clinical milestones that both the mother and infant must meet before discharge.

10. Explain the infant's behavior in simple terms. Engage in discussion about the infant's oversensitivity to the environment and to excessive handling (stimulation).

11. Explain and remind mother that the infant's behavior is not a rejection of her.

12. Teach mothers how to intervene early with crying infants by explaining that the infants are not yet able to quiet themselves. Dealing with stressful parenting situations are areas in which these women have difficulty in their daily lives. It is often this type of stress that has been, or can be, a trigger for continued substance use. Serving as a role model by talking and demonstrating ways to problem-solve and reduce the stress may serve the mother well in future situations. They are not unlike other mothers who may need to share the issues that are causing them problems. Be open to allowing them to vent their frustrations, then redirect their focus on the infant's progress or setbacks and needs today.

13. Provide and introduce kangaroo care (skin to skin) time if the mother desires.

14. Recognize that substance-using mothers and exposed infants require increased flexibility and intense commitment of energy, time, and patience.

DRUG SCREENING

A. Policy.

1. The AAP considers the practice of performing drug screening unethical for the primary reason of detecting illegal use. It set forth a policy statement for neonatal drug withdrawal that includes guidelines for screening (AAP Committee on Drugs, 2001, www.aap.org/policy/re9746.html). Maternal characteristics that suggest screening include those in Box 3-4.

2. Drug screening during pregnancy must be accompanied with a reporting process that includes provision of rehabilitation and supportive services and long-term involvement of court or social services without criminal prosecution (e.g., use of family drug courts) (Martinez et al., 2006).

B. Method.

1. Accuracy of drug screening is dependent on
   a. Laboratory used,
   b. Test used,
   c. Minimum drug in sample considered positive (see Table 3-6),
   d. Reliability of the testing procedure, and
   e. Drug-use pattern of person being tested (one-time dose, moderate use, etc.).

2. Thin-layer chromatography (TLC) is the most popular, inexpensive method that hospitals use despite high false-negative rates and poor sensitivity in the detection of low quantities of marijuana, PCP, LSD, MDA, MDMA, mescaline, or fentanyl.

3. Enzyme immunoassay (EIA) (other types of this method, e.g., enzyme multiplied immunoassay test [EMIT]; radioimmunoassay [RIA]; fluorescent polarization immunoassay), [FPIA]; high-performance TLC [HPTLC]), and gas chromatography/mass spectrometry (GC/MS), available in larger hospitals, offer a 5- to 10-drug panel analysis.

4. All positive tests are confirmed by Western blot or another analysis run.

■ BOX 3-4
■ **MATERNAL CHARACTERISTICS FOR DRUG SCREENING**

■ No prenatal care
■ Previous unexplained fetal demise
■ Abruptio placentae
■ Hypertensive episodes

■ Severe mood swings
■ Myocardial infarction or cerebrovascular accident
■ Repeated spontaneous abortions

■ TABLE 3-6
■ ■ **Basic Urine Drug Screen for Illicit Drug Use**

Class	Screening Cutoff	Confirmation Cutoff
Amphetamines	1000 ng/ml	Amphetamines, 500 ng/ml Methamphetamines, 500 ng/ml
Cannabinoids	50 ng/ml	THC-COOH, 15 ng/ml
Cocaine	300 ng/ml	Benzoylecgonine, 150 ng/ml
Opiates	300 ng/ml	Codeine, 300 ng/ml Morphine, 300 ng/ml
Phencyclidine	25 ng/ml	Phencyclidine, 25 ng/ml

Source: Naegle, M.A. and D'Avanzo, M.A.: *Addictions and substance abuse: Strategies for advanced practice nursing.* Upper Saddle River, NJ, 2001, Prentice Hall, p. 118.

C. **Urine.**
   1. Most common method used (inexpensive, rapid, and available in any hospital laboratory).
   2. Can be collected noninvasively, stored, and frozen easily for a long time.
   3. Limitation is that it can only detect "recent" use (5 days after marijuana use, 3 days after cocaine use, 2 days after heroin use, and 12 hours after alcohol use).
   4. Cannot measure quantity or frequency of drug use.
D. **Blood.**
   1. Requires invasive collection.
   2. Elimination half-life dependent on actual drug compound.
E. **Meconium.**
   1. Meconium accumulates throughout the pregnancy and therefore provides higher sensitivity (detects three times more drug users than urine) (Bar-Oz et al., 2003).
   2. May detect second-trimester drug exposure.
   3. Limited availability in hospitals and more expensive.
   4. Easy to obtain (collected noninvasively) and abundant quantity. Can provide an approximate 20-week historical snapshot of exposure (must be collected in the first 2 days of life).
   5. Ethical and clinical considerations still in question for widespread implementation (Marcellus, 2007).
F. **Neonatal hair and nails.**
   1. Detects long-term drug use and can stay positive for up to 3 months after birth (Bar-Oz et al., 2003; Garcia-Bournissen et al., 2007).
   2. Three times more sensitive than urine screen.
   3. Curly black hair has higher affinity for binding drug metabolites than brown hair.
   4. Parents may be reluctant to provide sample of hair.

BREASTFEEDING

Alcohol, caffeine, nicotine, and marijuana can all have a large effect on the production, volume, composition, and ejection of breast milk in addition to direct effects on infants (Martinez et al., 2006; Ostrea et al., 2005).

A. **Nicotine and smoking.**
   1. Elimination half-life of nicotine in milk ($t_{1/2} = 97 \pm 20$ minutes) slightly exceeds the half-life of nicotine in serum ($t_{1/2} = 81 \pm 9$ minutes). Actual nicotine detected in milk is 1.5 to 3 times that found in maternal plasma (AAP Committee on Drugs, 2001).
   2. No clear long-term effects of breastfeeding while smoking have been established.
   3. Evidence demonstrates a less detrimental effect of respiratory illnesses in infants whose mothers smoked and breastfed than for those mothers who smoked and bottle-fed (AAP Committee on Drugs, 2001).
   4. If mothers continue to smoke, recommend not smoking during nursing or directly in the infant's presence. Smoke immediately after breastfeeding or during an infant's long nap.
   5. Mothers should be encouraged to decrease the number of cigarettes and to consider smoking cessation programs.
B. **Alcohol.**
   1. Use of alcohol during lactation should be discouraged.
   2. Moderate to heavy drinking has been shown to interfere with oxytocin release, causing inhibition of the letdown reflex.
   3. Alcohol crosses into the breast milk and leads to changes in the infant's sleep-wake patterning and gross motor development. Infants fall asleep sooner, but sleep for shorter periods and spend less time in active sleep (Mennella and Garcia-Gomez, 2001).
C. **Cocaine and amphetamines.**
   1. Breastfeeding is contraindicated with active use.
   2. Cocaine remains in the system for up to 60 hours after maternal ingestion.
   3. Adverse effects seen may include cocaine intoxication, poor sleeping patterns, irritability, vomiting, diarrhea, tremulousness, and seizures.

D. **Marijuana.**
   1. Breastfeeding is not recommended.
   2. Impairment of deoxyribonucleic acid (DNA) and ribonucleic acid (RNA) formation and of use of essential proteins has been reported.
   3. No long-term effect has been shown in research to date.
E. **Heroin.**
   1. Heroin-dependent women should not breastfeed.
   2. Adverse side effects include tremors, restlessness, vomiting, and poor feeding and sleep patterns.
F. **Methadone.**
   1. In 2001 the AAP eliminated the dose restriction for methadone and stated that methadone is compatible with breastfeeding.
   2. There is no clear indication of how much methadone is present in breast milk; transfer is considered minimal.
   3. Women who are taking methadone and are breastfeeding should be educated about the effects of methadone and the use of illicit drugs.
   4. Breastfeeding by a woman using methadone should not be stopped abruptly; the infant should be weaned gradually to prevent withdrawal.
G. **Sedatives/hypnotics.**
   1. Long-term use of diazepam by women has been reported to cause sedation and lethargy in those neonates who are breastfed. Effects may result in feeding difficulties or weight loss.
   2. Recommend to discontinue breastfeeding in those infants that present with signs of weight loss or lethargy.
H. **Hepatitis B virus.**
   1. Breastfeeding is not a contraindication.
   2. Hepatitis B virus (HBV) has been detected in breast milk of women who have tested positive for hepatitis B surface antigen (Gardner et al., 1998). An infant should receive hepatitis B immunoglobulin and vaccine as indicated by AAP and hospital guidelines.
I. **Hepatitis C virus.**
   1. Research does not show breastfeeding as an important risk to hepatitis C virus (HCV) transmission when nipples are not traumatized (bleeding) and HCV is not active (Yeung et al., 2001).
   2. Benefits and risks of breastfeeding should be explained to the mother to allow her to make an informed decision (AAP Committee on Infectious Diseases, 1998).
J. **Human immunodeficiency virus.**
   1. It is recommended that women who are HIV seropositive be counseled not to breastfeed. The HIV antigen has been isolated in breast milk. "The probability of HIV-1 infection per liter of breast milk ingested by an infant is similar in magnitude to the probability of heterosexual transmission of HIV-1 through unprotected sex acts in adults" (Richardson et al., 2003).
   2. Women who are HIV seronegative but at high risk for seroconversion should be given information concerning the transmission of HIV through breast milk and methods to reduce the risk of becoming infected.

PROBLEMS ASSOCIATED WITH MATERNAL DRUG USE

A. **Characteristics of women with a substance-use disorder (Box 3-5).**
B. **Psychologic profile of women with a substance-use disorder (Box 3-6).**
C. **Maternal–infant relationships.**
   1. The attachment process between mother and infant is based on reciprocity. Maternal characteristics found to negatively affect the development of this relationship include the following:
      a. "More disengaged from their infants."
      b. "Display a higher degree of emotional instability" (inability to attach or securely attach to the infant).

■ BOX 3-5
■ **CHARACTERISTICS OF WOMEN WITH A SUBSTANCE USE DISORDER**

- Dysfunctional family of origin
- Lack of a positive relationship with their own parents
- Little to no positive parenting role models in their lives
- One or more parent with a history of substance abuse
- History of trauma as a child (physical, emotional, and/or sexual abuse)
- Lack of education (less than 16 years of formal education)
- Unemployed and poor vocational skills
- Maintain chaotic lifestyles
- Homeless or living in an unstable or dangerous environment
- Poor or lack of prenatal care (fear of legal reprisal)
- Reliance of public assistance for health care during hospitalization
- Lack network of social support (estranged from family members)
- Single, divorced, or separated
- Patterns of abuse by their spouses or significant others (domestic violence)
- Biological father of infant or partner often a substance abuser; enables woman to maintain addiction and not involved in parenting
- Limited knowledge about child development and child-care skills

■ BOX 3-6
■ **PSYCHOLOGIC PROFILE OF WOMEN WITH A SUBSTANCE USE DISORDER**

- Inability to ask for help
- Lack the ability to establish positive personal relationships
- Comorbidity (depression, anxiety, codependency, PTSD, etc.)
- Low self-esteem (high sense of guilt, shame, and unworthiness, poor ego development, and insecure)
- Lack coping mechanisms and skills
- Impulsive: lack ability to be future-oriented

    c. "Unpredictable and unavailable in caregiving."
    d. "Display a lack of enjoyment and communication in interactions with infant."
    e. Possess "less sensitivity to identify cues that their infant displays." (Johnson, 2001)
  2. Factors in the infant that contribute to impaired maternal-infant interaction include the following:
    a. Extreme irritability, with arching and writhing behavior.
    b. Difficulty or resistance to being comforted.
    c. Rarely reaches alert state.
    d. Low threshold for stimulation, easily disturbed, and unable to transition well from state to state.
    e. Erratic sleep patterns, spending less time in active sleep.
    f. Difficult to feed and poor weight gain.
D. Continuity of care and follow-up.
  1. Develop a discharge plan that focuses on an interdisciplinary approach. Include short- and long-term follow-up. Areas that require attention include abuse and neglect, attachment, and development—not just the immediate postnatal time period.
  2. Lack of continuity of care is often due to limited treatment and home visitation programs that accept both mothers and infants. Be aware of what resources are available in the com-

munity. This is an important first step toward advocating for the infant and ensuring future success of recovery for the mother.

3. Referrals should be made early to a local drug rehabilitation program and other appropriate community resources (e.g., the Women, Infants, and Children program [WIC], lactation phone support, nearby or hospital-based clinic, Planned Parenthood, and women's shelters and centers).

E. **Treatment, rehabilitation, and recovery.**
1. "There are no simple predictors of women's substance abuse treatment outcomes" (Comfort et al., 2003).
2. Abstinence is found to be related to length of stay in a treatment program.
3. Treatment success may involve multiple treatment program attempts and completion as well as variety of types of treatment (outpatient vs. residential).
4. Recovery is considered a long-term process.
5. Definition of successful recovery is controversial.

F. **Gender-specific treatment needs.**
1. Treatment programs that allow women to bring infants or children with them are essential.
2. Drug treatment should include a program that
   a. Offers a multifaceted and integrative approach to recovery;
   b. Incorporates gender-based theories (women's psychosocial development) (Angove and Fothergill, 2003);
   c. Integrates parenting and child-rearing guidance and skill mastery;
   d. Directs and identifies children's behavior appropriately;
   e. Enhances the self-esteem of women and relationship building;
   f. Offers supportive psychotherapy (group and individual);
   g. Provides anger control, conflict management, and stress-reduction skills;
   h. Offers a supportive environment that provides multiple role models; and
   i. Supports a full range of ancillary services (child care services, social services, medical support, vocational, educational, and aftercare).

G. **Nursing considerations.**
1. Prenatal care, drug treatment programs, and coordinated aftercare can make a significant difference in improving pregnancy and childhood outcomes. Key points to be aware of when working with mothers with a substance abuse disorder and their infants are as follows:
   a. Polydrug use is more common than use of a single substance or alcohol alone (D'Apolito and Hepworth, 2001; Greene and Goodman, 2003).
   b. Research and statistics on incidence and outcomes of the substance-exposed infant remain conflicting and controversial.
   c. Outcomes of the substance-exposed infant are based on a multifactorial perspective (genetic, biologic, environmental, and social areas).
   d. Short-term deficits may not be representative of long-term outcomes.
   e. The overall adverse drug effects infants present with are often subtle. The four areas targeted in all prenatal exposed infants are affect, attention, arousal, and action— termed the "four A's" of infancy (Lester and Tronick, 1994).
   f. Evidence-based research must be included at all levels of the neonatal intensive care unit (NICU) and each nurse plays a vital part in furthering research development with ideas and problem-solving strategies.
   g. Opportunities for changing the addicted woman's behavior and her view of health care providers can be influenced by the care she and her infant receive while hospitalized.

ETHICAL AND LEGAL CONSIDERATIONS

A. **Ethical principles.** When interacting with women and substance use/abuse, consider the following:
1. Justice: what is the equitable allocation of health, social resources, and treatment for women who use/abuse alcohol and substances?

2. Beneficence: is one providing advocacy for what is best for the mother and child? That which is doing good can also include preventing harm that threatens someone.
3. Nonmaleficence: not doing harm. (Although nonmaleficence and beneficence are closely related, it is still important that the requirement to avoid harm is much stronger than the requirement to do good.)
4. Autonomy: the freedom to live your life. This becomes maternal autonomy versus fetal rights when the woman is pregnant. To be autonomous, one needs
   a. Liberty of action: no one is stopping you;
   b. Freedom of choice: you have alternatives available; and
   c. Effective deliberation: you are able to make a rational decision (Tiedje, 1998).
B. **Legal implications.**
   1. Legal statutes vary depending on country and state of residence. "In March 2001, the Supreme Court determined that nonconsensual drug screening of pregnant women by clinicians in a public hospital violated the woman's Fourth Amendment rights to be secure against unreasonable search and seizure" (Marshall et al., 2003).
   2. No state has passed a law criminalizing pregnancy and drug use, but an estimated 250 women in more than 30 states have been prosecuted on the theory of "fetal abuse."
   3. Most countries have mandatory laws obligating health care providers to report existing or suspected child abuse and neglect. Thus, notification to the authorities may be necessary after delivery if health care providers are concerned about safety of the infant and/or the parents' ability to care for the infant.
C. **Criminal model vs. the harm-reduction model.**
   1. Experts in the field of perinatal substance abuse believe that substance abuse is an illness and do not support prosecution of mothers (Catlin, 1997; Lowinson et al., 1997).
   2. Fear of prosecution may deter women from seeking prenatal care and treatment for their drug problems. Lack of prenatal care and poverty are two of the major preventable factors that contribute to adverse pregnancy outcomes among pregnant drug users (Garcia, 1997; Wilkinson and Pickett, 2007). The harm-reduction model balances what is best for each individual with protection of the public good (Tiedje, 1998).
   3. The rights and needs of the mother and those of the fetus require a view of being inter-related. In this manner, solutions may be developed to support both.
   4. Drug courts are an alternative to incarceration of women with a substance use disorder. There are 940 drug courts operating in 49 states, with 441 courts in the planning stages. The judges in these courts require abstinence, altered behavior through a combination of graduated sanctions, mandated drug testing, case management, and supervised treatment and aftercare programs.

REFERENCES

Accornero, V.H., Morrow, C.F., Bandstra, E.S., et al.: Behavioral outcome of preschoolers exposed prenatally to cocaine: Role of maternal behavioral health. *Journal of Pediatric Psychology, 27*(3):259-269, 2002.

Adams, E.K., Miller, V.P., Ernst, C., et al.: Neonatal health care costs related to smoking during pregnancy. *Journal of the American Medical Association, 287*(2):195-202, 2002.

Alwan, S., Reefhuis, J., Rasmussen, S.A., et al.: Use of selective serotonin-reuptake inhibitors in pregnancy and the risk of birth defects. *New England Journal of Medicine, 356*(26):2684-2692, 2007.

American Academy of Pediatrics Committee on Drugs: The transfer of drugs and other chemicals into human milk. *Pediatrics, 108*(3):776-789, 2001.

American Academy of Pediatrics Committee on Infectious Diseases: Hepatitis C virus infection. *Pediatrics, 101*(3 Part 1):481-485, 1998.

American Academy of Pediatrics Committee on Substance Abuse and Committee on Children with Disabilities: Fetal alcohol syndrome and alcohol-related neurodevelopmental disorders. *Pediatrics, 106*(2):358-361, 2000.

American Academy of Pediatrics Task Force on Sudden Infant Death Syndrome: The changing concept of sudden infant death syndrome: Diagnostic coding shifts, controversies regarding the sleeping environment, and new variables to consider in reducing risk. *Pediatrics, 116*(5):1245-1255, 2005.

Andres, R.L. and Day, M.: Perinatal complications associated with maternal tobacco use. *Seminars in Neonatology, 5*(3):231-241, 2000.

Angove, R. and Fothergill, A.: Women and alcohol: Misrepresented and misunderstood. *Journal of Psychiatric and Mental Health Nursing, 10*(2):213-219, 2003.

Bar-Oz, B., Einarson, T., Einarson, A.: Paroxetine and congenital malformations: Meta-analysis and consideration of potential confounding factors. *Clinical Therapeutics, 29*(5):918-926, 2007.

Bar-Oz, B., Klein, J., Karaskov, T., and Koren, G.: Comparison of meconium and neonatal hair analysis for detection of gestational exposure to drugs of abuse. *Archives of Disease in Childhood: Fetal and Neonatal Edition, 88*(2):F98-F100, 2003.

Bennett, A.D.: Perinatal substance abuse and the drug-exposed neonate. *Advanced Nurse Practitioner, 7*(5):32-36, 1999.

Berard, A., Ramos, E., Rey, E., et al.: First trimester exposure to paroxetine and risk of cardiac malformations in infants: The importance of dosage. *Birth Defects Research Part B: Developmental and Reporductive Toxicology, 80*(1):18-27, 2007.

Burns, L., Mattick, R.P., Lim, K., et al.: Methadone in pregnancy: Treatment retention and neonatal outcomes. *Addiction, 102*(2):264-270, 2007.

Catlin, A.J.: Commentary on Deborah L. Burns' article. Positive toxicology screening in newborns: Ethical issues in the decision to legally intervene. *Pediatric Nursing, 23*(1):76-78, 1997.

Centers for Disease Control and Prevention: Fetal alcohol syndrome—Alaska, Arizona, Colorado and New York, 1995-1997. *Morbidity and Mortality Weekly Report MMWR, 51*(20):433-435, 2002.

Comfort, M., Sockloff, A., Loverro, J., and Kaltenbach, K.: Multiple predictors of substance-abusing women's treatment and life outcomes: A prospective longitudinal study. *Addictive Behaviors, 28*(2):199-224, 2003.

Crocetti, M.T., Amin, D.D., and Jansson, L.M: Variability in the evaluation and management of opiate-exposed newborns in Maryland. *Clinical Pediatrics, 46*(7):632-635, 2007.

Crome, I.B. and Kumar, M.T.: Epidemiology of drug and alcohol use in young women. *Seminars in Fetal and Neonatal Medicine, 12*(2):98-105, 2007.

D'Apolito, K.: Comparison of a rocking bed and standard bed for decreasing withdrawal symptoms in drug-exposed infants. *MCN The American Journal of Maternal Child Nursing, 24*(3):138-144, 1999.

D'Apolito, K. and Hepworth, J.: Prominence of withdrawal symptoms in polydrug-exposed infants. *Journal of Perinatal and Neonatal Nursing, 14*(4):46-60, 2001.

Dashe, J.S., Sheffield, J.S., Olscher, D.A., et al.: Relationship between maternal methadone dosage and neonatal withdrawal. *Obstetrics and Gynecology, 100*(6): 1244-1249, 2002.

Davis, R.L, Rubanowice, D., McPhillips, H., et al: Risks of congenital malformations and perinatal events among infants exposed to antidepressant medication during pregnancy. *Pharmacoepidemiology and Drug Safety, 16*(10):1086-1094, 2007.

Dejmek, J., Solansky, I., Podrazilova, K., and Sram, R.J.: The exposure of nonsmoking and smoking mothers to environmental tobacco smoke during different gestational phases and fetal growth. *Acta Paediatrica, 91*(3):323-328, 2002.

Ebrahim, S.H. and Gfroerer, J.: Pregnancy-related substance use in the United States during 1996-1998. *Obstetrics and Gynecology, 101*(2):374-379, 2003.

England, I.J., Kendrick, J.S., Gargiullo, P.M., et al.: Measures of maternal tobacco exposure and infant birth weight at term. *European Journal of Pediatrics, 161*(8):445-448, 2002.

Ernst, M., Moolchan, E.T. and Robinson, M.L.: Behavioral and neural consequences of prenatal exposure to nicotine. *Journal of American Academy of Child & Adolescent Psychiatry, 40*(6):630-641, 2001.

Finnegan, L.P.: Neonatal abstinence syndrome. In N. Nelson (Ed.): *Current therapy in neonatal-perinatal medicine* (2nd ed.). Ontario, 1990, BC Decker, pp. 3-25.

Frank, D.A., Augustyn, M., Knight, W.G., et al.: Growth, development and behavior in early childhood following prenatal cocaine exposure: A systematic review. *Journal of the American Medical Association, 285*(12):1613-1625, 2001.

Frank, D.A., Jacobs, R.R., Beeghly, M., et al.: Level of prenatal cocaine exposure and scores on the Bayley Scales of Infant Development: Modifying effects of caregiver, early intervention, and birth weight. *Pediatrics, 110*(6):1143-1152, 2002.

Garcia, S.: Ethical and legal issues associated with substances abuse by pregnant and parenting women. *Journal of Psychoactive Drugs, 29*(1):101-111, 1997.

Garcia-Bournissen, F., Rokach, B., Karaskov, T., et al.: Cocaine detection in maternal and neonatal hair: Implications to fetal toxicology. *Therapeutic Drug Monitoring, 29*(1):71-76, 2007.

Garcia-Bournissen, F., Rokach, B., Karaskov, T., et al.: Methamphetamine detection in maternal and neonatal hair: Implications for fetal safety. *Archives of Disease in Childhood: Fetal & Neonatal Edition, 92*(5):F351-355, 2007.

Gardner, S.L., Snell, B.J., and Lawrence, R.A.: Breast feeding the neonate with special needs. In G.B. Merenstein and S.L. Gardner (Eds.): *Handbook of neonatal intensive care* (6th ed.). St. Louis, 2006, Mosby, pp. 224-246, 1998.

Greene, C. and Goodman, M.H.: Neonatal abstinence syndrome: Strategies for care of the drug-exposed infant. *Neonatal Network, 22*(4):15-25, 2003.

Hannigan, J.H. and Armant, D.R.: Alcohol in pregnancy and neonatal outcome. *Seminars in Neonatology, 5*(3):243-254, 2000.

Hans, S.I. and Jeremy, R.J.: Postneonatal mental and motor development of infants exposed in utero to opioid drugs. *Infant Mental Health Journal, 22*(3):300-315, 2001.

Haustein, K.O: Cigarette smoking, nicotine and pregnancy. *Human Experiments in Toxicology, 18*(4):202-205, 1999.

Huizink, A.C. and Mulder, E.J.: Maternal smoking, drinking or cannabis use during pregnancy and neurobehavioral and cognitive functioning in human offspring. *Neuroscience & Biobehavioral Reviews, 30*(1): 24-41, 2006.

Iqbal, M.M., Sobhan, T., and Ryals, T.: Effects of commonly used benzodiazepines in the fetus, the neonate and the nursing infant. *Psychiatric Service, 53*(1):39-49, 2002.

Jaddoe, V.W., Verburg, B.O., de Ridder M.A., et al.: Maternal smoking and fetal growth characteristics in different periods of pregnancy: The generation R study. *American Journal of Epidemiology*, 165(10):1207-1215, 2007.

Johnson, M.O.: Mother-infant interaction and maternal substance use/abuse: An integrative review of research literature in the 1990s. *The Online Journal of Knowledge Synthesis for Nursing*, February 16(8):2, 2001.

Jones, H.E. and Balster, R.L.: Neurobehavioral consequences of intermittent prenatal exposure to high concentrations of toluene. *Neurotoxicology and Teratology*, 19(4):305-313, 1997.

Jones, M.W. and Bass, W.T.: Fetal alcohol syndrome. *Neonatal Network*, 22(3):63-70, 2003.

Keller, R.W., Jr., and Snyder-Keller, A.: Prenatal cocaine exposure. *Annals of the New York Academy of Sciences*, 909:217-232, 2000.

King Edward Memorial Hospital: NCCU Clinical Guidelines, section 17: *Neonatal abstinence syndrome*. Perth: King Edward Memorial Hospital, 2006, p. 2. Retrieved December 27, 2007, from http://speciosum.curtin.edu.au/nas/NAS_Guideline.pdf

Klitsch, M.: Prenatal cocaine and opiate use are linked to a wide variety of health hazards. *Perspectives on Sexual and Reproductive Health*, 34(4), 2002. Retrieved December 29, 2007, from www.guttmacher.org/pubs/journals/3421802.htm

Klonoff-Cohen, H. and Lam-Kruglick, P.: Maternal and paternal recreational drug and sudden infant death syndrome. *Archives of Pediatrics & Adolescent Medicine*, 155(7):765-770, 2001.

Lennestal, R. and Kallen, B.: Delivery outcome in relation to maternal use of some recently introduced antidepressants. *Journal of Clinical Psychopharmacology*, 27(6):603-613, 2007.

Lester, B.M. and Tronick, E.: The effect of prenatal cocaine exposure and child outcome: Lessons from the past. *Infant Mental Health Journal*, 15(2):107-120, 1994.

Lipsitz, P.J.: A proposed narcotic withdrawal score for use with newborn infants. A pragmatic evaluation of its efficacy. *Clinical Pediatrics*, 14:592-594, 1975.

Lowinson, J.H., Ruiz, P., Millman, R.B., and Langrod, J.G. (Eds.): *Substance abuse: A comprehensive textbook* (3rd ed.). Baltimore, 1997, Williams & Wilkins.

Mahoney, D. and Larig, S.: Substance-related problems and childbearing. In M.A. Naegle and C.E. D'Avanzo (Eds.): *Addictions and substance abuse: Strategies for advanced practice nursing*. Upper Saddle River, NJ, 2001, Prentice Hall Health, pp. 221-270.

Marcellus, L.: Is meconium screening appropriate for universal use? Science and ethics say no. *Advances in Neonatal Care*, 7(4):207-214, 2007.

Marcellus, L.: Neonatal abstinence syndrome: Reconstructing the evidence. *Neonatal Network*, 26(1):33-39, 2007.

Marshall, M.F., Menikoff, J., and Paltrow, L.M.: Perinatal substance abuse and human subjects research: Are privacy protections adequate? *Mental Retardation and Developmental Disabilities Research Reviews*, 9(1):54-59, 2003.

Martinez, A., Partridge, J.C., and Taeusch, H.W.: Perinatal substance abuse. In: H.W. Taeusch, R.A.

Ballard, and C.A. Gleason (Eds.): *Avery's diseases of the newborn*. Philadelphia, 2006, Saunders, pp. 106-126.

Maschi, S., Clavenna, A., and Campi, R.: Neonatal outcome following pregnancy exposure to antidepressants: A prospective controlled cohort study. *International Journal of Obstetrics & Gynaecology*, 115(2):283-289, 2008.

May, P.A. and Gossage, J.P.: Estimating the prevalence of fetal alcohol syndrome: A summary. *Alcohol Research and Health*, 25(3):159-167, 2001.

Mennella, J.A. and Garcia-Gomez, P.L.: Sleep disturbances after acute exposure to alcohol in mothers' milk. *Alcohol*, 25(3):153-158, 2001.

National Institute on Alcohol Abuse and Alcoholism: *Alcohol alert no. 50*. Rockville, MD, 2000, U.S. Department of Health and Human Services. Retrieved December 27, 2007, from www.niaaa.nih.gov/publications/aa50.htm

National Institute on Alcohol Abuse and Alcoholism: *Alcohol alert no. 55*. Rockville, MD, 2002, U.S. Department of Health and Human Services. Retrieved December 27, 2007, from www.niaaa.gov/publications/aa55.htm

National Institute of Drug Abuse: *Info Facts: MDMA (Ecstasy)*. National Institutes of Health, Department of Health and Human Services. Retrieved December 27, 2007, from http://www.nida.nih.gov/Infofacts/ecstasy.html

Nordstrom-Klee, B., Delaney-Black, V., Covington, C., et al.: Growth from birth onwards of children prenatally exposed to drugs: A literature review. *Neurotoxicology and Teratology*, 24(4):481-488, 2002.

Office of Applied Studies, Substance Abuse and Mental Health Administration (SAMHSA): *National household survey on drug abuse (NHSDA)*, 2002. Retrieved December 27, 2007, from http://www.oas.samhsa.gov/NSDUH/2k6NSDUH/2k6results.cfm#2.6

Osborn, D.A., Jeffrey, H.E., and Cole, M.J: Opiate treatment for opiate withdrawal in newborn infants. *Cochrane Database of Systematic Reviews*, 1:1-23, 2005.

Ostrea, E.M., Jr., Posecion, E.W.C., and Villanueva, M.E.U.T.: The infant of the drug-dependent mother. In M.G. MacDonald, M.D. Mullett, and M.M.K. Seshia (Eds.): *Avery's neonatology: Pathophysiology and management of the newborn*. Philadelphia, 2005, Lippincott, pp. 1572-1616.

Payot, A. and Berner, M.: Hospital stay and short-term follow-up of children of drug-abusing mothers born in an urban community hospital—A retrospective review. *European Journal of Pediatrics*, 159(9):679-683, 2000.

Perault, M.C., Favreliere, S., Minet, P., and Remblier, C.: Benzodiazepines and pregnancy. *Therapie*, 55(5):587-595, 2000.

Richardson, B.A., John-Stewart, G.C., Hughes, J.P., et al.: Breast milk infectivity on human immunodeficiency virus type 1 infected mothers. *Journal of Infectious Diseases*, 187(5):736-740, 2003.

Richardson, G.A., Ryan, C., Willford, J., et al.: Prenatal alcohol and marijuana exposure: Effects on neuropsychological outcomes at 10 years. *Neurotoxicology and Teratology*, 24(3):309-320, 2002.

Riley, E.P., Guerri, C., Calhoun, F., et al.: Prenatal alcohol exposure: Advancing knowledge through international collaborations. *Alcoholism: Clinical and Experimental Research, 27*(1):118-135, 2003.

Secker-Walker, R.H. and Vacek, P.M.: Relationships between cigarette smoking during pregnancy, gestational age, maternal weight gain, and infant birthweight. *Addictive Behaviors, 28*(1):55-66, 2003.

Singer, L.T., Arendt, R., Minnes, S., et al.: Cognitive and motor outcomes of cocaine-exposed infants. *Journal of the American Medical Association, 287*(15):1952-1960, 2002.

Sokol, R.J., Janisse, J.J., and Louis, J.M.: Extreme prematurity: An alcohol-related birth effect. *Alcoholism: Clinical & Experimental Research, 31*(6):1031-1037, 2007.

Stromland, K. and Pinazo-Duran, S.K.: Ophthalmic involvement in the fetal alcohol syndrome: Clinical and animal model studies. *Alcohol and Alcoholism, 37*(1):2-8, 2002.

Substance Abuse and Mental Health Services Administration: *Methamphetamine use. The National Survey on Drug Use and Health (NSDUH).* January 26, 2007. Retrieved December 27, 2007, from http://www.oas. samhsa.gov/2k7/meth/meth.htm

Substance Abuse and Mental Health Services Administration: *Cigarette use among pregnant women and recent mothers. The National Survey on Drug Use and Health (NSDUH).* February 9, 2007. Retrieved December 29, 2007, from http://www.oas.samhsa.gov/2k7/ pregCigs/pregCigs.pdf

Substance Abuse and Mental Health Services Administration: *Demographic and geographic variations in injection drug use. The National Survey on Drug Use and Health (NSDUH).* July 19, 2007. Retrieved January 24, 2008, from http://www.oas.samhsa.gov/2k7/idu/ idu.pdf

Tiedje, L.B.: Ethical and legal issues in the care of substance-using women. *Journal of Obstetric, Gynecologic and Neonatal Nursing, 27*(1):92-98, 1998.

U.S. Department of Health and Human Services, National Institutes of Health, National Institute on Drug Abuse (NIDA), Division of Epidemiology, Services and Prevention Research: *Drug use among racial/ethnic minorities* (NIH Publication No. 03-3888), Washington, D.C., 2003, Author.

U.S. Department of Justice: *Crystal methamphetamine, Information Bulletin,* August. Johnstown, PA, 2002, National Drug Intelligence Center. Retrieved December 29, 2007, from http://www.usdoj.gov/ndic/ pubs1/1837/index.htm

U.S. Department of Justice: *OxyContin diversion and abuse, Information Bulletin,* August. Johnstown, PA, 2001, National Drug Intelligence Center. Retrieved December 29, 2007, from http://www.usdoj.gov/ ndic/pubs/651/651t.htm

Van Etten, M.L., and Anthony, J.C.: Male-female differences in transitions from first drug opportunity to first use: Searching for subgroup variation by age, race, region, and urban status. *Journal of Women's Health and Gender Based Medicine, 10*(8):797-804, 2001.

Weiner, S.M. and Finnegan, L.P.: Drug withdrawal in the neonate. In G.B. Merenstein and S.L. Gardner (Eds.): *Handbook of neonatal intensive care* (6th ed.). St. Louis, 2006, Mosby, pp. 3-22.

Wilkinson, R.G. and Pickett, K.E.: The problems of relative deprivation: Why some societies do better than others. *Social Science and Medicine, 65*(7):1965-1978, 2007.

Wogelius, P., Norgaard, M., Gislum, M.: Maternal use of selective serotonin reuptake inhibitors and risk of congenital malformations. *Epidemiology, 17*(6):701-704, 2006.

Yeung, L.T., King, S.M., and Roberts, E.A.: Mother-to-infant transmission of hepatitis C virus. *Hepatology, 34*(2):223-229, 2001.

Zahorodny, W., Rom, C., Whitney, W., et al.: The neonatal withdrawal inventory: A simplified score of newborn withdrawal. *Journal of Developmental and Behavioral Pediatrics, 19*(2):89-93, 1998.

4 Adaptation to Extrauterine Life

■■■

M. TERESE VERKLAN

OBJECTIVES
1. Identify primary features of fetal circulation.
2. Identify physiologic changes that occur during transition to extrauterine life.
3. Identify routine care considerations for a newborn infant during the transition period.
4. Identify signs and symptoms of common problems in the transition period.
5. Define the methods and intervention times for parental teaching.

■
■■ The transition period is considered to be the first 6 to 10 hours of life, but more than a period of time, it is a process of physiologic change in the newborn infant that begins in utero as the child prepares for the transition from intrauterine placental support to extrauterine self-maintenance. The fetus prepares for transition during the course of gestation in such ways as storing glycogen, producing catecholamines, and depositing brown fat. The neonate's ability to accomplish the transition to extrauterine life will depend on gestational age and the quality of placental support during gestation as well as any physical defects or anomalies that may affect major organ systems.

ANATOMY AND PHYSIOLOGY

Characteristics of Placental/Fetal Circulation

A. Placenta.
 1. Blood oxygenation and elimination of waste products of metabolism. Transfer of O_2 and CO_2 across the placenta is by simple diffusion.
 2. High rate of metabolism. The placenta uses one-third of all the oxygen and glucose supplied to it by the maternal circulation for its own metabolic needs.
 3. Low-resistance circuit. The placenta receives approximately 50% of fetal cardiac output.
 4. Characteristics of uterine venous blood as it enters the intervillous space: Pco_2 of 38 mm Hg, Po_2 of 40 to 50 mm Hg, and pH of 7.36.
B. Fetal shunts/blood flow (Fig. 4-1) (Moore and Persaud, 2008).
 1. Umbilical vein (Po_2 32 to 35 mm Hg). It carries oxygenated blood from the placenta to the fetus.
 2. Ductus venosus. Forty to sixty percent of the umbilical venous blood bypasses the liver through the ductus venosus to the inferior vena cava (IVC). It is a low-resistance channel that allows a significant portion of relatively well-oxygenated blood to enter the heart directly; the other half passes through the liver and enters the IVC via the hepatic veins. This mixing of blood slightly lowers the Po_2.
 3. IVC blood and the blood from the coronary sinuses (Po_2 = 25 to 28 mm Hg). This blood is largely deflected across the right atrium, through the foramen ovale, and into the left atrium. In contrast, most of the blood from the superior vena cava (SVC), also returning to the right atrium, is deflected to the right ventricle (see item 6, below). The crista dividens (lower edge of the septum secundum) separates the flow of blood from the IVC into two streams, with 50% to 60% of the blood from the IVC being diverted across the foramen ovale into the left atrium (Blackburn, 2007) and the remainder of blood from the

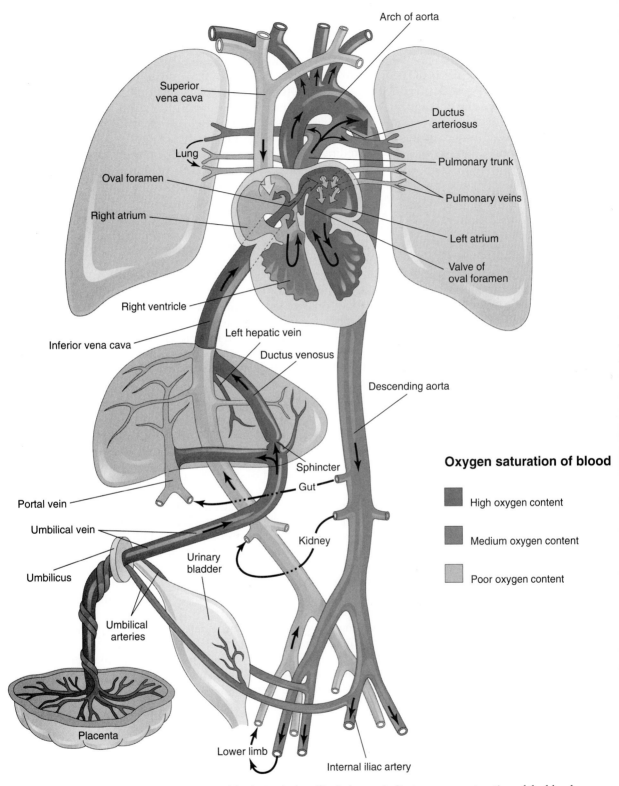

Oxygen saturation of blood

- High oxygen content
- Medium oxygen content
- Poor oxygen content

FIGURE 4-1 ■ Simplified scheme of fetal circulation. Shaded areas indicate oxygen saturation of the blood; arrows show course of fetal circulation. Organs are not drawn to scale. (From Moore, K.L. and Persaud, T.V.N.: *The developing human: Clinically oriented embryology* [8th ed.]. Philadelphia, 2008, Saunders.)

IVC remaining in the right atrium and mixing poorly oxygenated blood from the superior vena cava and coronary sinus.

4. Left atrium. Blood is received from the right atrium via the foramen ovale and mixes with a small amount of blood returning from the lungs via the pulmonary veins.

5. Left ventricular blood (Po$_2$ = 25 to 28 mm Hg). Virtually all this blood is from the IVC by way of the right atrium–foramen ovale–left atrium pathway. Left ventricular blood is pumped out through the aorta to the brain from the upper part of the aortic arch. Approximately 90% of the blood from the ascending aorta feeds the coronary, carotid, and subclavian arteries and thus the brain and upper extremities.

6. The SVC. Unoxygenated blood returning from the brain and upper extremities is received by the SVC. Ninety-seven percent enters the right atrium and flows to the right ventricle through the tricuspid valve; only 3% flows to the left atrium via the foramen ovale.

7. Right atrium. Some mixing occurs here between the unoxygenated SVC blood and the oxygenated IVC blood not shunted directly into the left atrium via the foramen ovale.

8. Right ventricle. The dominant ventricle (Po$_2$ = 19 to 22 mm Hg) ejects about 66% of the total cardiac output. Most of the blood is shunted across the ductus arteriosus, away from the lungs, and into the descending aorta to supply the kidneys and intestines. It then divides into two arteries, which subsequently return back to the placenta.

9. Ductus arteriosus. Equal in size to the aorta, it connects the pulmonary artery to the descending aorta. The blood flows right to left (pulmonary artery to aorta) across the ductus arteriosus because of high pulmonary vascular resistance and low placental resistance. Patency is maintained by the low oxygen tension in utero and by the vasodilating effect of prostaglandin E$_2$.

10. Low pulmonary blood flow (only 10% to 12% of the right ventricular output). This results from high pulmonary vascular resistance (Blackburn, 2007).

11. Descending aorta. It supplies the kidneys and intestines, divides into two arteries, and returns blood to the placenta for oxygenation.

Fetal Lung Characteristics

A. **Decreased blood flow.** In part, the decrease is caused by compression of the pulmonary capillaries by the fetal lung fluid.

B. **Pulmonary arteries.** The small pulmonary arteries of the fetus have a thick, muscular medial layer; they are very reactive and are actively constricted by the low Po$_2$ normally present during fetal life. Pulmonary vascular resistance increases throughout fetal life.

C. **Lung fluid secretion.** Fetal lungs actively secrete fluid; secretion of fluid is decreased near term. At term the lung contains 30 ml of plasma ultrafiltrate per kilogram of body weight. This is comparable to a postnatal thoracic gas volume of 25 ml/kg. An adequate fluid volume is necessary for lung development. Fluid moves into and out of the lungs through the trachea.

D. **Fetal breathing.** In utero fetal breathing movements have been detected as early as 11 weeks of gestation. They contribute to lung development.

E. **Surfactant.** Surfactant is secreted into the amniotic fluid by the fetal lung before 20 weeks of gestation. The absolute quantity of surfactant increases throughout gestation in both the lung and amniotic fluid and can support extrauterine respiration at approximately week 34 of gestation.

Fetal Metabolism and Hematology

A. **Glucose.** Fetal blood glucose concentrations are 70% to 80% of maternal blood glucose concentrations. Glucose is exchanged via the placenta by facilitated diffusion.

B. **Glycogen.** Large glycogen stores (2 to 10 times that of an adult) provide large energy reserves to sustain the newborn infant through the transition period.

C. **Hemoglobin.** Fetal hemoglobin has an increased affinity for oxygen. Fetal hemoglobin is progressively replaced by adult hemoglobin from weeks 32 to 36 of gestation and is approximately 80% of the total hemoglobin at term.

Labor

A. **Placenta.** Maternal placental perfusion ceases with uterine contractions.

B. **Stress hormones**. High concentrations of stress hormones (predominantly norepinephrine) are released as a direct effect of the resultant hypoxia on the adrenal medulla.

Cardiopulmonary Adaptation at Birth

A. **Cardiovascular adaptation (Fig. 4-2) (Moore and Persaud, 2008).**
1. Umbilical cord is clamped.
    a. Placenta is separated from the circulation, and the umbilical arteries and veins constrict.
    b. As the low-resistance placental circuit is removed, there is a resultant increase in systemic blood pressure; the systemic vascular resistance then exceeds the pulmonary vascular resistance.
2. The three major fetal shunts (ductus venosus, foramen ovale, and ductus arteriosus) functionally close during transition (Alvaro and Rigatto, 2005).
    a. Ductus arteriosus. The lungs now provide more efficient oxygenation of the blood, and the arterial oxygen tension rises. This rise in Po_2 is a potent stimulus to constriction of the ductus arteriosus. Increased pulmonary blood flow increases the metabolism of circulating prostaglandins, and the loss of prostaglandins contributed by the placenta enhances the constrictive effects of oxygen on the ductus.
    b. Foramen ovale. The fall in pulmonary vascular resistance results in a drop in right ventricular and right atrial pressure, and the increased systemic vascular resistance results in an increase in left atrial and left ventricular pressures, causing the foramen ovale to close against the atrial septum.
        (1) The foramen ovale becomes sealed by the deposit of fibrin and cell products during the first month of life.
        (2) Until the foramen ovale is anatomically sealed, anything that produces a significant increase in right atrial pressure can reopen the foramen ovale and allow a right-to-left shunt.
    c. Ductus venosus. Absent umbilical venous return leads to closure of the ductus venosus. It functionally closes within 2 to 3 days and becomes the ligamentum venosum.
3. Postnatal circulation (see Fig. 4-2) (Moore and Persaud, 2008).
    a. Systemic venous blood enters the right atrium from the SVC and the IVC.
    b. Poorly oxygenated blood enters the right ventricle and passes through the pulmonary artery into the pulmonary circulation for oxygenation.
    c. The oxygenated blood returns to the left atrium through the pulmonary veins.
    d. This blood passes through the left ventricle and into the aorta to supply the systemic circulation with oxygenated blood.

B. **Pulmonary adaptation (Blackburn, 2007).**
1. The lungs as the organ of gas exchange. Intermittent breathing begins in utero long before delivery and, after birth, is a continuation of movements and reflexes that have been well established.
2. Stimuli for initiating respiration. The mild hypercapnia, hypoxia, and acidosis that result from normal labor are due partially to the intermittent cessation of maternal-placental perfusion with contractions. The decreased pH stimulates the respiratory center directly; the low Po_2 and high Pco_2 stimulate the respiratory center by means of central and peripheral chemoreceptors (Hansen and Corbet, 2005). Other stimuli include cold, light, noise, and touch.
3. Entry of air into lungs with the first breath.
    a. Aeration of the lungs drives fluid into the interstitium; it is then absorbed through the lymphatic and pulmonary circulation. The rate at which this process occurs is variable, and fine crackling rales may be audible throughout the lungs until this process is completed.

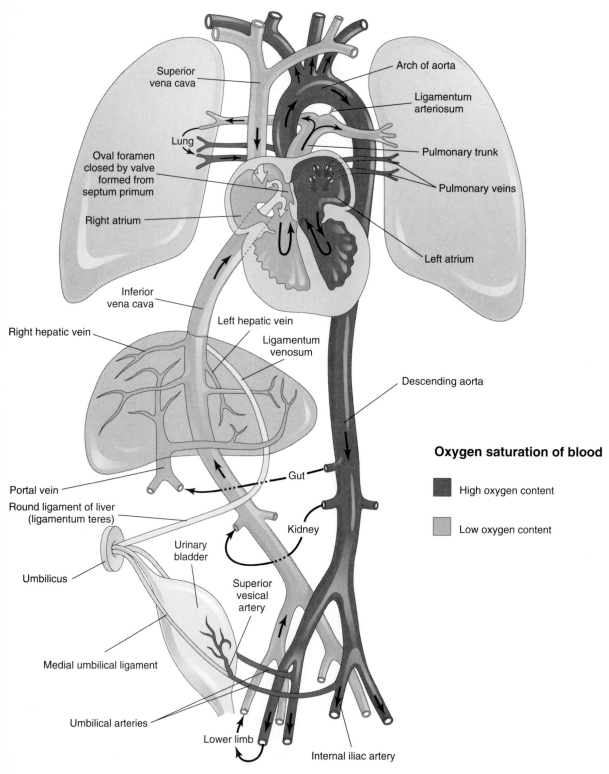

FIGURE 4-2 ■ Simplified representation of circulation after birth. Adult derivatives of fetal vessels and structures that become nonfunctional at birth are also shown. Arrows indicate course of neonatal circulation. Organs are not drawn to scale. (From Moore, K.L. and Persaud, T.V.N.: *The developing human: Clinically oriented embryology* [8th ed.]. Philadelphia, 2008, Saunders.)

   b. The pulmonary vessels respond to the increase in Po_2 with vasodilation. Pulmonary vascular resistance progressively decreases until adult levels are reached by 6 to 8 weeks of age (Blackburn, 2007).

4. Inspiration of air and expansion of lungs. After the thoracic squeeze (during labor and vaginal delivery, this empties the lungs of approximately one third of the fetal lung fluid), the subsequent recoil of the chest wall causes inspiration of air and expansion of the lungs. Negative intrathoracic pressures generated with the first breath may be as high as 20 to 70 cm H_2O because of the mechanical advantage created by the high resting level of the diaphragm in the nonaerated lung (Niermeyer and Clarke, 2006). Subsequent breaths in the normal newborn infant require 15 to 20 cm H_2O pressure.

5. Respiratory augmentation. Head's paradoxic reflex is a vagally mediated hyperinflation triggered by distention of stretch receptors in the large airways.

6. Work of inspiration. This is predominately related to overcoming the surface tension of the walls of the terminal lung units at the gas-tissue interface. On expiration, the ability to retain air depends on surfactant.
   a. Surfactant is a complete lipoprotein produced by type II alveolar pneumocytes; surfactant release increases in response to increased catecholamine levels at birth.
   b. Surfactant has the ability to lower the surface tension at an air-liquid interface.
   c. As the surfactant lowers the surface tension in the alveolus at end-expiration, it stabilizes the alveoli and prevents collapse.

7. There is an increase in the functional residual capacity with each breath. Less inspiratory pressure is thus required for subsequent breaths.

8. Lung compliance. Improves in the hours after delivery as a result of circulating catecholamines. The increased levels of catecholamines (especially of epinephrine) also clear the lungs by decreasing the secretion of the lungs' fluids and increasing their absorption through the lymphatic system.

ROUTINE CARE CONSIDERATIONS IN THE TRANSITION NURSERY*

A. Assessment/observation. Within 2 hours of birth, the neonate's health status should be evaluated and the neonate assessed for risks that may complicate transition to extrauterine life (American Academy of Pediatrics [AAP] and American College of Obstetricians and Gynecologists [ACOG], 2007).
   1. Body measurements. Head circumference, length, and weight are recorded.
   2. Vital sign assessment. Vital signs recorded on admission will include heart rate, respiratory rate, and axillary temperature. Universal blood pressure screening in the well newborn infant is not warranted (American Academy of Pediatrics Policy Statement [AAP], 1993).
   3. Gestational age assessment. Weight, head circumference, and length are graphed against the assessed gestational age and record (refer to Chapter 7).
   4. Clinical changes. During the first hours of life, vital signs stabilize and the newborn proceeds through sleep-wake cycles associated with readiness to feed behaviors (Verklan, 2002). The time sequence of changes is altered in infants with low Apgar scores, immaturity, maternal medications, and intrinsic disease (refer to Chapter 5).
   5. Head-to-toe physical examination (refer to Chapter 7). The following findings seen during transition are within normal limits as the infant progresses through the physiologic changes described under cardiopulmonary adaptation, above.
      a. Skin.
         (1) Acrocyanosis. Vasoconstricted peripheral vessels result in a mottled appearance; peripheral pulses are decreased initially. (These findings are sequelae of catecholamine release, mild acidosis, and cold stress.)
         (2) Petechiae of the face and facial bruising. A vertex presentation, a rapid second stage of labor, or a tight nuchal cord may result in these skin changes. (With severe facial bruising, central color may be assessed by looking at the mucous membranes in the mouth.)

---

*Gardner and Johnson, 2006; Sansoucie and Cavaliere, 2007.

   b. Head.
      (1) The neonate's head is large relative to the body. During a vaginal delivery, considerable molding of the skull bones may take place to facilitate passage through the birth canal. Molding resolves during the first hours and days.
      (2) Caput succedaneum (edema of the presenting part of the scalp, caused by pressure that restricts the return of venous and lymph flow during vaginal delivery), may be present.
   c. Respirations/breath sounds.
      (1) Initially, coarse rales and moist tubular breath sounds. These breath sounds may continue until clearing of lung fluid is complete.
      (2) Prolonged expiratory phase.
      (3) Respiratory rate of 30 to 60 breaths per minute.
      (4) Grunting and retracting (intercostal and substernal). These findings may be present during the first hours of life as lung fluid is cleared.
   d. Heart sounds.
      (1) Second heart sound may be loud during the first 2 hours; splitting of the second heart sound is usually detectable at 2 to 4 hours of age and increases during the next 12 hours (pulmonic ahead of aortic component).
      (2) Soft grade 2/6 systolic murmur may be present; represents a left-to-right shunt across the ductus arteriosus before its closure.
   e. Heart.
      (1) Normal heart rate 120 to 160 beats per minute (bpm); increased initially, with a mean peak of 180 bpm, and then decreased or irregular.
      (2) Consistently high or low heart rate suggests a pathologic condition.
   f. Intestines.
      (1) Blood flow is reduced initially.
      (2) As the bowel begins to fill with air, normal motility and bowel sounds are present within 15 minutes.
      (3) The normal term neonate passes meconium within the first 24 hours after birth. If a term neonate has not passed meconium by 48 hours after birth, the lower gastrointestinal tract may be obstructed (AAP and ACOG, 2007.)
   g. Urinary function.
      (1) Urine is normally passed within the first 24 hours after birth.
      (2) Failure to void within the first 24 hours may indicate genitourinary obstruction or abnormality (AAP and ACOG, 2007).
   h. Extremities. Findings may include deformities resulting from the intrauterine position.
B. **Thermoregulation considerations in the nursery (Blake and Murray, 2006).** The admission assessment and observation should be done in a controlled environment, such as a radiant warmer or incubator, that both provides warmth and prevents heat loss so that the infant maintains a normal temperature without increasing oxygen consumption, using glucose stores, or exceeding brown fat stores in the process of nonshivering thermogenesis (mediated by norepinephrine released by cold stress). Normal axillary ranges are 36.5 to 37.5° C (97.7 to 99.5° F for the term neonate and 36.3 to 36.9° C (97.3 to 98.6° F) for the preterm neonate. Hypothermia and hyperthermia occur when the infant's attempts to maintain a normal temperature fail, which has serious metabolic consequences for the newborn infant (refer to Chapter 6).
   1. Monitor temperature. Check axillary temperature every 30 minutes to 1 hour during transition while the infant is under a radiant warmer. Avoid hyperthermia (skin temperature greater than 37° C or axillary temperature greater than 37.5° C). NOTE: Monitoring the axillary temperature allows time for successful intervention before a fall in core temperature indicates failure of the body's heat-regulation mechanism.
   2. First bath. Delay bath until body temperature has stabilized and is within normal limits. Check temperature 30 minutes after the bath and 1 hour after transfer to open crib.
   3. Temperature. Check temperature at least every 4 hours until the infant's condition is stable, and then every 8 hours until discharge. Temperatures may need to be monitored every 30 minutes until stable.

4. Environmental temperature (incubator or warmer). Record environmental temperature with temperature checks of the infant to monitor its environmental requirements. NOTE: These requirements can be checked against the normal ranges of neutral thermal environmental temperature needs as a tool in evaluating an infant's condition.

C. **Transition nursery medications (AAP and ACOG, 2007).**

1. Eye care. Administered to both eyes before 1 hour of age in all neonates, regardless of type of delivery.
   a. Recommendation. Apply a 1- to 2-cm ribbon of sterile ophthalmic ointment containing 0.5% erythromycin, or 1% tetracycline, or an ophthalmic solution of 2.5% povidone-iodine for prophylaxis of ophthalmia neonatorum due to *Neisseria gonorrhoeae*. Prophylaxis for *Chlamydia trachomatis* requires erythromycin or tetracycline.
   b. Procedure. Instill medication into conjunctival sac within 1 hour of birth; however, this may be delayed until after the first breastfeeding. The medication should not be flushed from the eye after application. A new tube is used for each infant.

2. Vitamin K_1 (phytonadione). Administer vitamin K within 1 hour of birth.
   a. Recommendation. Every neonate should receive a single parenteral 0.5- to 1-mg dose of natural vitamin K (phytonadione) (AAP and ACOG, 2007). Administer 0.5 mg if the infant weighs less than 1.5 kg and 1 mg if infant weighs more than 1.5 kg.
   b. Risk of deficiency. Maternal dietary inadequacy of vitamin K, hepatic immaturity, reduced liver stores, and absence of intestinal flora predispose the child to deficiency of vitamin K; gut bacteria are a substantial source. Vitamin K is needed to promote the hepatic biosynthesis of vitamin K–dependent clotting factors, including prothrombin (factor II), proconvertin (factor VII), plasma thromboplastin component (factor IX), and Stuart factor (factor X). Deficiency results in hemorrhagic disease of the newborn (HDN).
      (1) Classic HDN. The disease occurs at 1 to 7 days of life. The infant is healthy at birth but develops cutaneous or gastrointestinal (GI) bleeding. Other sites of bleeding include nasal bleeding or bleeding after circumcision. Classic HDN can be prevented with vitamin K prophylaxis.
      (2) Early HDN. Maternal exposure to drugs, including warfarin, anticonvulsants, and antituberculosis drugs, may affect coagulation. Severe or life-threatening hemorrhage may occur during delivery or in the first day of life. Intracranial hemorrhage is a common complication. Early HDN is the only type that cannot be prevented by vitamin K prophylaxis.
      (3) Late HDN. The late form of HDN may occur between 1 and 3 months of life. Acute intracranial hemorrhage is the most common initial finding and is often fatal or neurologically devastating. Other findings include gastrointestinal or mucous membrane bleeding. Late HDN can be prevented by vitamin K prophylaxis.

3. Hepatitis vaccine and hepatitis B immunoglobulin (HBIG).
   a. Rate of hepatitis B virus (HBV) infection. If the mother is HBsAg and HBeAg positive, the baby has a 90% risk of HBV infection in the first 12 months if treatment is not received. There is a 20% risk of HBV infection if the mother is positive for HBsAg only (Lott, 2007).
   b. Chronicity. In the absence of treatment, the neonate will likely become a carrier, and eventually develop primary hepatocellular carcinoma (Lott, 2007).
   c. Maternal HbsAg-positive treatment recommendations:
      (1) Child is bathed as soon as temperature is stable.
      (2) Hepatitis B vaccine (Engerix-B, 10 mcg, or Recombivax-HB, 5 mcg) and HBIG, 0.5 ml IM (prepared from plasma to contain a high titer of antibody against HBsAg), should be administered before 12 hours of age (AAP, 2003); may be given concurrently at different sites; 85% to 95% effective in preventing both HBV infection and the chronic carrier state.
      (3) Remaining doses of hepatitis B vaccine are given at 1 and 6 months of age.

    d. Maternal HBsAg-negative treatment recommendations:

       (1) Hepatitis B vaccine should be administered to all infants, including those born to HBsAg-negative mothers.

       (2) Hepatitis B vaccine (Engerix-B, 10 mcg, or Recombivax-HB, 5 mcg) is administered prior to discharge from the hospital. The second dose is administered at 1 to 2 months of age and the third dose at 6 to 18 months of age.

    e. Unknown maternal HBsAg status at delivery. Follow schedule for maternal HBsAg positive. Additional HBIG administration will depend on the results of maternal serologic screening done within 12 hours after delivery.

    f. Premature infants with birth weight less than 2 kg born to HBsAg-negative mothers should receive the vaccine just before hospital discharge if the infant weighs more than 2 kg or the dose is delayed until 2 months of age when other routine immunizations are given. All premature infants born to HBsAg-positive mothers should receive immunoprophylaxis (HBIG) and vaccine beginning as soon as possible after birth, followed by appropriate postvaccination testing (AAP Committee on Infectious Diseases, 2000).

D. Glucose needs/first feeding (McGowan et al., 2006).

  1. The stress of delivery causes increased conversion of fats and glycogen to glucose for the increased energy needs of temperature maintenance, skeletal muscles, and breathing and crying. Breakdown products of this conversion are glucose, free fatty acids, and glycerol.

  2. Hepatic glycogen is mobilized immediately after birth in response to the increased catecholamines to provide a continuing source of glucose to the brain in the absence of placental supply; in a healthy term infant, up to 90% of the hepatic glycogen stores may be consumed by 3 hours of life.

  3. Blood glucose concentration at birth is about 85% of the maternal level. The last maternal meal, the duration of labor, the mode of delivery, the type and amount of IV fluids administered to the mother, and medications given to the mother all influence the actual concentration of glucose. The glucose level then falls for 1 to 2 hours, followed by an increase and stabilization at mean levels of approximately 70 mg/dl by the age of 3 hours in healthy, nonstressed infants (Stanley and Pallotto, 2005).

  4. A screening blood glucose test (on capillary whole blood) should be performed in infants with risk factors at 30 minutes to 1 hour of age. A glucose level less than 40 mg/dl at any time in any newborn infant is an indication for evaluation and treatment. The goal is to maintain the glucose value at greater than 40 mg/dl in the first day and greater than 40 to 50 mg/dl thereafter. NOTE: The whole-blood glucose level on the screening test is usually 10% to 15% lower than the corresponding serum or plasma level because the erythrocytes will continue to metabolize the glucose in the sample. Risk factors include the following:

    a. Asphyxia, cold stress, increased work of breathing, and sepsis, which lead to an increased metabolic response and increased use of glucose.

    b. Reduced stores of glucose in premature and small-for-gestational-age infants.

    c. Hyperinsulinemia in infants of mothers with diabetes or gestational diabetes and in large-for-gestational-age infants, resulting in rapid removal of glucose from the circulation.

    d. Any symptoms of a low blood glucose level. An infant may have jitteriness, irritability, seizures, hypothermia, temperature instability, lethargy, poor feeding, emesis, apnea, pallor, cyanosis, and weak or high-pitched cry (see also Common Problems and Clinical Presentation, item F: Metabolic Problems, on p. 86). NOTE: Capillary samples from an unwarmed heel may lead to a falsely low glucose value because of stasis of blood and ongoing transfer of glucose to the cells.

  5. Early, frequent feedings should be given on demand; frequency is not to exceed 4 hours between feedings (maximum of 3 hours between feedings for infants weighing <2.5 kg). Allow the infant to begin feeding when he or she is demanding nutrition and when evaluation findings are within normal limits; nursing or formula feeding can be used (type of formula is by family's or physician's choice).

   a. Evaluation before feeding.
      (1) Physical examination. Bowel tones are normal, and abdomen is soft and nontender. Sucking reflex is normal, with no excessive mucus. Passage of an orogastric tube is indicated before feeding if questions exist regarding esophageal patency. Anus and nares are patent. The respiratory rate is less than 60 breaths per minute and the pattern of breathing is normal.
      (2) Contraindications to nippling the feeding or to breastfeeding (consider gavage feeding for these infants).
         (a) Choanal atresia.
         (b) Respiratory rate greater than 60 breaths per minute without other signs of respiratory distress.
         (c) Weak suck.
         (d) Absent coordination of suck and swallow.
      (3) Contraindications to any enteral feedings.
         (a) Cyanosis.
         (b) Severe birth asphyxia.
         (c) Shock.
         (d) Increased work of breathing and oxygen requirement.
         (e) Suspicion of gastrointestinal obstruction.
   b. Sterile-water "test" feeding. It is difficult to evaluate an infant's ability to suck and swallow with sterile water because most infants do not like the taste and on occasion will refuse to suck or swallow; therefore, it is advisable to forgo "sips of water" in favor of a thorough evaluation before feeding.
   c. Dextrose 5%. Use of dextrose 5% is not indicated as a "test" feeding because studies show that it is more irritating to lungs after aspiration than is formula. Moreover, it is not indicated after a feeding.
   d. Guidelines for feeding in transition nursery for transient asymptomatic hypoglycemia:
      (1) May breastfeed or be offered formula (by nipple or gavage) if there are no contraindications to enteral feedings (see Contraindications, item a (3), on p. 81), and the infant is active and vigorous.
      (2) Check glucose level 1 hour after feeding is given.
   e. Indications for IV glucose infusion (see Initial Stabilization of the Sick Newborn Infant, on p. 87):
      (1) Hypoglycemia is persistent and symptomatic.
      (2) Enteral feedings are contraindicated.
      (3) Oral feedings do not maintain normal glucose levels.
      (4) Initial glucose screening level is less than 40 mg/dl.

E. **Ongoing teaching in the transition nursery.**
   1. Discuss with family the infant's ability to see and hear, with a preference for black-white contrast initially, and the sound of a higher-pitched voice.
   2. Demonstrate or point out infant's response to stimuli (tactile, visual, auditory): self-consolability, body movements, gaze, head turning.
   3. Discuss physical findings.
      a. Transient: head molding, acrocyanosis, birth trauma, positional deformities.
      b. Permanent: congenital anomalies, birthmarks.
   4. A stable infant may stay with the family from birth through recovery to postpartum period with appropriate observation and teaching provided by all staff members in contact with the family unit.

F. **Transfer of infant from the transition nursery when the following are stable.**
   1. Temperature, heart rate, respiratory rate.
   2. Glucose level.
   3. Normal physical assessment findings, or abnormal findings that do not require continuous observation or immediate intervention or treatment.

RECOGNITION OF THE SICK NEWBORN INFANT

Review of Perinatal History (Fanaroff et al., 2001)

A. **Ultrasonographic-biophysical profile:** estimated date of confinement, evidence of congenital anomalies, twins, breech, preterm, and intrauterine growth restriction.

B. **Medications or history of substance abuse:** alcohol, nicotine, cocaine, opiates, marijuana, amphetamines, tocolytics, anticonvulsants, anticoagulants, and analgesics/anesthetics.

C. **Maternal illnesses:** pregnancy-induced hypertension, diabetes, intrapartum fever/infection (e.g., with group B streptococcus, genital herpes simplex virus, human immunodeficiency virus, and varicella), HBsAg positive, thyroid disease, inherited disorders, and cardiac disease.

D. **Perinatal fetal distress, delivery complications:** abnormal fetal heart rate pattern, meconium staining of the amniotic fluid, rapid delivery, difficult delivery, rupture of membranes more than 18 hours before delivery.

E. **Cesarean delivery and indications**: breech presentation, fetal distress, placenta previa, abruptio placentae, cephalopelvic disproportion, failure to progress in labor.

Physical Assessment

A. **Skin.**
　1. Cyanotic.
　2. Pale.
　3. Mottled.
　4. Cool to touch.
　5. Poor perfusion.

B. **Respiratory system.**
　1. Poor color.
　2. Tachypnea.
　3. Decreased air entry.
　4. Increased work of breathing: grunting, flaring, and retracting.
　5. Apnea.
　6. Unequal breath sounds.
　7. Oxygen requirement.

C. **Cardiovascular system.**
　1. Abnormal heart sounds such as murmur.
　2. Weak, absent, or unequal pulses.
　3. Hepatosplenomegaly.

D. **Central nervous system.**
　1. Hypertonic or hypotonic.
　2. Jitteriness, tremors.
　3. Lethargy.
　4. Bulging fontanelle (record baseline head circumference).
　5. Seizures.
　6. Irritability, high-pitched cry.

E. **Morphologic features.**
　1. Congenital anomalies (e.g., abdominal wall defects, imperforate anus).
　2. Severe birth trauma.
　3. Absent or decreased limb movement.
　4. Asymmetry.

F. **GI tract.**
　1. Abdominal distention (measure baseline abdominal girth).
　2. Increased gastric contents on aspiration.
　3. Inability to pass an orogastric tube.
　4. Excessive mucus.
　5. Emesis soon after birth or after first feeding.

Diagnostic Tools (Bradshaw et al., 2006)

A. **Pulse oximetry (peripheral monitoring of oxygen saturation).**
  1. Oxygen saturation (Sao_2) of blood is that percentage of the total hemoglobin concentration that is chemically combined with oxygen.
  2. A baseline Pao_2 value should be obtained to confirm the infant's oxygen level.
  3. For hyperoxic study, administer 100% oxygen to differentiate between pulmonary and cardiac disease. (In infants with pulmonary disease, saturation will improve, whereas in infants with cyanotic heart disease, little or no change will occur. Use caution to avoid exposing the ductus arteriosus to high oxygen levels in ductal-dependent cardiac lesions.)
B. **Arterial blood gas determinations.** If oxygen requirement persists, pulse oximetry saturations in room air are decreased and cyanosis is present.
C. **Chest x-ray examination.** Anteroposterior and lateral views are needed if respiratory distress is present or cardiac disease is suspected.
D. **Transillumination.** Use a high-intensity light placed over the side of the chest in question if pneumothorax or pneumomediastinum is suspected.
E. **Whole-blood glucose screening test or serum glucose determination if indicated by history or assessment results** (see Routine Care Considerations in the Transition Nursery, item D: Glucose Needs/First Feeding, on p. 80).
F. **Hematocrit determination.**
  1. History of blood loss.
  2. Plethoric or pale infant.
  3. Twins (to rule out twin-to-twin transfusion).
  4. Heel-stick (capillary) samples tend to have higher results of approximately 10%.
  5. Hematocrit variations. Highest hematocrit is at 2 to 4 hours of age and then progressively falls as a result of the beginning of red blood cell breakdown and the cessation of erythropoiesis in response to a comparatively oxygen-enriched environment.
G. **Complete blood cell count with differential examination of the white blood cells.**
  1. As part of a sepsis diagnostic evaluation.
  2. To screen for normal and abnormal hematologic indices.
H. **Blood culture as part of a diagnostic evaluation for sepsis.**
I. **Urine sample collection.**
  1. Urinalysis.
  2. Screening test for drugs of abuse.
J. **Lumbar puncture:** Performed at the discretion of the physician as part of a diagnostic evaluation for sepsis.
K. **Ultrasonography, computed tomography, and magnetic resonance imaging.**
  1. Cranial evaluation for abnormal central nervous system (CNS) findings.
  2. Abdominal examination if history of two-vessel cord to rule out renal anomalies.
L. **Echocardiography and electrocardiography:** As part of a diagnostic study for a congenital cardiac defect.
M. **Passage of orogastric tube.**
  1. To check patency of esophagus in infants with excessive pooling of mucus in the oropharynx.
  2. To decompress a distended abdomen.
  3. To measure and assess gastric contents (>25 ml and/or significant bile in the stomach indicates obstruction).

Common Problems and Clinical Presentation

A. **Birth trauma** (refer to Chapter 2).
B. **Birth asphyxia** (Rehan and Phibbs, 2005; Vannucci, 2002).
  1. Birth asphyxia is defined as interference with gas exchange resulting in compromised oxygen delivery, accumulation of CO_2, and a switch to anaerobic metabolism.
  2. Fetal distress is indicated by an abnormal fetal heart rate pattern, meconium staining of the amniotic fluid, scalp pH less than 7.20, and Apgar scores less than 5 at 1 minute of age and less than 7 at 5 minutes of age.

3. Pathophysiologic sequelae include:
   a. Decreasing Po_2. The tissue hypoxia that ensues leads to anaerobic metabolism with release of lactic acid into the circulation.
   b. Respiratory acidosis from elevated levels of carbon dioxide.
   c. Metabolic acidosis.
      (1) Results in high pulmonary vascular resistance.
      (2) Leads to decreased surfactant release.
   d. Hypoxic-ischemic damage to less vital organs such as kidney and gut after redistribution of blood to vital organs.
   e. The myocardium depends on its stored reserves of glycogen for energy as its supply of oxygen falls. Eventually this reserve is consumed and the myocardium is simultaneously exposed to progressively lower Po_2 and pH levels. The combined effects lead to reduced myocardial function with decreased blood flow to vital organs (Rehan and Phibbs, 2005).
4. All newborn infants have some degree of respiratory acidosis and hypoxia during labor and vaginal delivery; a healthy term infant has increased tolerance and reserves. The asphyxiated newborn infant has more prolonged hypoxia and respiratory acidosis and may have additional metabolic acidosis, hypothermia, and hypoglycemia.
5. Clinical findings.
   a. Mild to moderate perinatal asphyxia.
      (1) Extended awake, alert state (45 minutes to 1 hour).
      (2) Dilated pupils.
      (3) Normal muscle tone.
      (4) Active suck.
      (5) Regular or slightly increased respiratory rate.
      (6) Normal or slightly increased heart rate.
   b. Moderate to severe perinatal asphyxia.
      (1) Hypothermia.
      (2) Hypoglycemia.
      (3) Pupils constricted.
      (4) Respiratory distress manifested by grunting, flaring, retracting, tachypnea, and oxygen requirement.
      (5) Seizures (subtle and multifocal clonic; 12 to 24 hours of age).
      (6) Acute tubular necrosis following reduced blood flow to the kidneys.
      (7) Hypotonia initially, lethargy.
      (8) Bradycardia.
   c. Severe perinatal asphyxia, which requires constant monitoring in a level II (intermediate care) or level III (intensive care) nursery.
      (1) Pale skin, poor perfusion.
      (2) Cerebral edema.
      (3) Seizures.
      (4) Apnea.
      (5) Intracranial hemorrhage.
C. **Pulmonary problems (Hagedorn et al., 2006).**
   1. Air Leak: 2% to 10% of healthy term neonates develop spontaneous air leak, and 16% to 36% of neonates who require ventilatory support, including CPAP.
      a. Tachypnea, unequal breath sounds, shift of heart tones, and distant heart tones.
      b. Transillumination of chest is positive for free air.
   2. Retained lung fluid, respiratory distress syndrome (because of prematurity or birth asphyxia), and pneumonia.
      a. Decreased air entry with respiratory distress syndrome and pneumonia.
      b. Increased work of breathing: grunting, flaring, and retracting.
      c. Tachypnea, apnea.
      d. Decreased saturations (Sao_2), cyanosis, continued oxygen requirement.
   3. Aspiration syndromes (meconium, blood).
      a. Coarse rales.

      b. Tachypnea.

      c. Barrel chest.

  4. Upper airway obstruction (e.g., choanal atresia or micrognathia).

  5. Extrapulmonary (e.g., phrenic nerve injury with resultant diaphragmatic paralysis or eventration of the diaphragm).

D. Cardiovascular problems (Knight and Washington, 2006).

  1. Congenital heart disease.

      a. Acyanotic lesions.

          (1) Patent ductus arteriosus with a left-to-right shunt.

          (2) Ventricular septal defect.

          (3) Atrial septal defect.

          (4) Endocardial cushion defect or atrioventricular canal defects.

      b. Obstructive lesions.

          (1) Aortic stenosis.

          (2) Coarctation of the aorta.

          (3) Pulmonary valve stenosis or atresia.

          (4) Hypoplastic left heart syndrome.

      c. Admixture of lesions.

          (1) Normal or increased pulmonary blood flow.

             (a) Complete transposition of the great vessels.

             (b) Truncus arteriosus.

             (c) Anomalous venous connections of the pulmonary veins.

          (2) Decreased pulmonary blood flow.

             (a) Tetralogy of Fallot.

             (b) Tricuspid valve atresia.

  2. Persistent fetal shunts.

      a. Patent ductus arteriosus with right-to-left shunt.

      b. Persistent pulmonary hypertension.

  3. Clinical findings.

      a. Cyanosis with or without increased work of breathing, decreased oxygen saturations. NOTE: Absence of any signs of abnormal respiratory function in the presence of cyanosis suggests congenital heart disease.

      b. Unequal or absent pulses, bounding pulses, decreased blood pressure in the lower extremities, and decreased perfusion.

      c. Increased precordial activity, shift of point of maximal impulse (PMI) of heart tones to right, murmur.

      d. Congestive heart failure, indicated by tachypnea, moist breath sounds, tachycardia, peripheral edema, cardiomegaly, and hepatomegaly.

E. Hemodynamics.

  1. Acute hypovolemic shock.

      a. Internal hemorrhage resulting from birth trauma; intracranial hemorrhage.

      b. External hemorrhage resulting from placenta previa or abruptio placentae; cord accident; fetal-maternal or twin-to-twin transfusion.

      c. Respiratory distress, pallor, poor perfusion, hypotension, weak or absent pulses, anemia.

  2. Polycythemia.

      a. Plethoric, cyanotic, or excessively flushed with crying.

      b. Hypoglycemia.

      c. CNS symptoms, including jitteriness, hypotonia, lethargy, and seizures.

  3. Anemia.

      a. Acute or chronic blood loss.

      b. Hemolysis from sepsis or ABO/Rh blood group incompatibilities.

      c. Reduced red blood cell production, manifested by severe asphyxia, sepsis, and aplastic anemia.

      d. Pale skin, murmur, tachypnea, normal arterial blood pressure, signs of congestive heart failure, including hepatosplenomegaly and increased vascular markings on x-ray film.

F. **Metabolic problems.**
  1. Hypoglycemia (McGowan et al., 2006).
      a. Observed in infants who are large or small for gestational age, infants of diabetic mothers, premature infants, and stressed infants such as those with sepsis, cold stress, or respiratory distress.
      b. Clinical findings:
          (1) Jitteriness, irritability.
          (2) Seizures.
          (3) Hypothermia, temperature instability.
          (4) Lethargy.
          (5) Poor feeding, emesis.
          (6) Apnea.
          (7) Cardiorespiratory distress, cyanosis, oxygen requirement.
          (8) Pallor.
          (9) Tachycardia.
          (10) Weak or high-pitched cry.
  2. Adverse effects of maternal medications; maternal use of illicit drugs.
      a. Magnesium sulfate. Infants present with respiratory depression, decreased muscle tone, and decreased serum calcium concentration.
      b. Tocolytics. Infants may present with hypoglycemia.
      c. Narcotics. Infants present with apnea, respiratory depression, and periodic breathing.
      d. Cocaine. Infants may present with apnea, poor muscle tone initially and then irritability and agitation, tremors, and feeding difficulties.
      e. Marijuana or methadone. Infants present with hyperthermia, agitation, and diarrhea.
      f. Alcohol. Infants have fetal alcohol syndrome with dysmorphic and behavioral abnormalities.
G. **Infection (see also Chapter 32).**
  1. Generalized bacterial or viral disease; acquired in utero or nosocomial.
  2. Clinical findings. NOTE: Nearly 90% of neonates with early-onset group B streptococcus have signs of infection within 12 hours of birth (median age is 8 hours) (Edwards et al., 2006).
      a. Temperature instability.
      b. Tachypnea, apnea.
      c. Respiratory distress, cyanosis.
      d. Tachycardia.
      e. Cool, mottled skin; weak pulses; capillary refill lasting longer than 2 seconds; and and hypotension.
      f. Disseminated intravascular coagulation.
      g. Hepatosplenomegaly.
      h. Unexplained jaundice.
      i. Purpura, petechiae.
      j. Hypoglycemia or hyperglycemia.
      k. Poor feeding, emesis, and abdominal distention.
      l. Lethargy, poor muscle tone.
  3. In utero viral infection. Infant may be small for gestational age with microcephaly.
H. **Congenital anomalies (frequently obvious on gross examination).**
  1. Diaphragmatic hernia.
      a. Immediate onset, at birth, of significant respiratory distress.
      b. Shift in heart tones, decreased or unequal breath sounds, bowel tones heard in chest, scaphoid abdomen, and cyanosis.
  2. Esophageal atresia with or without tracheoesophageal fistula.
      a. Excessive amniotic fluid.
      b. Increased pooling of secretions in the oropharynx, respiratory distress, unable to place orogastric tube.

3. Abdominal wall defects: omphalocele and gastroschisis.
4. Limb anomalies: amniotic banding, talipes equinovarus, polydactyly, and syndactyly.
5. Neural tube defects.
6. Intestinal obstructions.
7. Chromosomal abnormalities such as trisomy 21 or trisomy 18.
8. Urogenital abnormalities: exstrophy of bladder, hypospadias, epispadias, and ambiguous genitalia.

Initial Stabilization of the Sick Newborn Infant

A. Short-term observation in transition nursery to monitor trends before the infant's transfer to a neonatal intensive care unit (NICU).
1. The infant may be capable of resolving the problem on his or her own if given time (e.g., correction of mild acidosis from asphyxia, clearing of lung fluid, stabilization of blood glucose concentration, and stabilization of blood pressure).
2. Monitor and record trends (i.e., improved respiratory rate toward normal, improved perfusion, and normal glucose screens).

B. Avoid excessive handling.
1. Organize care and interventions to avoid frequent, unnecessary stimulation of an already stressed infant.
2. Use pulse oximeter or cardiorespiratory monitor to reduce hands-on determination of vital signs.
3. Reduce background stimulation such as loud noises or bright lights.
4. Use nonnutritive sucking to lower activity levels and reduce energy needs.
   a. Infant may be more comfortable in a prone position.
   b. Crying can be stressful and is similar to a Valsalva maneuver, with prolonged exhalation, obstructed venous return, quick inspiratory gasp, and right-to-left shunting at the foramen ovale.
   c. Crying depletes energy reserves and increases oxygen consumption.

C. Provide a neutral thermal environment (refer to Chapter 6).
1. Observe infant for apnea and hypotension during warming.
2. Avoid hyperthermia.

D. Supply glucose.
1. Oral administration of glucose for a blood glucose level of less than 40 mg/dl in an otherwise healthy asymptomatic neonate; early, frequent feedings by nipple, gavage, or nursing.
   a. Give at least 0.5 to 1 ounce of formula by nipple or gavage if there are no contraindications to enteral feedings and the infant is free of symptoms (see Routine Care Considerations in the Transition Nursery, on p. 77). If condition is stable, infant may be allowed to nurse 5 to 10 minutes on each breast.
   b. Begin maintenance formula at 50 to 70 kcal/kg/day or breastfeed on demand every 2 to 3 hours.
   c. Check blood glucose 30 minutes to 1 hour after feeding.
   d. Consider giving a formula designed for premature infants when treating hypoglycemia orally.
      (1) These formulas provide 50% of carbohydrate in the form of glucose polymers that are easily absorbed; salivary amylase retains its activity in the infant's stomach because of increased gastric pH and is effective in the digestion of glucose polymers (Blackburn, 2007).
      (2) Approximately 50% of the fats are provided as medium-chain triglycerides (MCTs). As MCTs are absorbed from the stomach, they may also increase the level of plasma ketones, which can be used as an alternative substrate to glucose for brain metabolism (Blackburn, 2007).
      (3) The process of absorbing fat (fatty acid oxidation and ketogenesis) spares glucose for brain energy needs; free fatty acids and ketones promote glucose production by providing essential gluconeogenic cofactors.

(4) Healthy newborn infants respond to a protein meal by preferentially increasing glucagon, which elicits a glycemic response.

2. Intravenous administration of glucose for hypoglycemia (see Routine Care Considerations in the Transition Nursery, item D: Glucose Needs/First Feeding on p. 80) is as follows:

   a. Provide bolus (2 ml/kg) of 10% dextrose in water ($D_{10}W$), followed by an infusion of 4 to 6 mg/kg/minute; $D_{10}W = 100$ mg/ml.

   b. Monitor therapy with frequent glucose checks and titrate the infusion rate and concentration to meet the infant's needs. NOTE: Do not administer an IV bolus of glucose greater than $D_{10}W$ because of reactive hypoglycemia and hypertonicity of the solution. Always follow a glucose bolus with a continuous infusion of glucose.

E. **Supply oxygen:** Assess needs with a pulse oximeter or with arterial blood gas determinations and close observation.

   1. Extended oxygen use in the transition nursery requires notification of the physician and transfer to a level II or III setting.

   2. Provide warmed, humidified oxygen by oxygen hood, continuous positive airway pressure by nasal prongs, or assisted ventilation by endotracheal tube according to the infant's needs (refer to Chapter 26).

   3. Monitor oxygen provided with an oxygen analyzer. Record blow-by oxygen in liters per minute and as distance from the infant's face.

F. **Supply volume expanders, including blood and normal saline solution.**

   1. For hypotension and blood loss.

   2. Requires IV line placement and transfer to level II or III nursery for continued management and observation, including cardiorespiratory monitoring and blood pressure checks to adjust therapy as necessary.

G. **Naloxone hydrochloride (Narcan).**

   1. Administer drug for severe respiratory depression with a normal heart rate and color in the delivery room and history of maternal narcotic administration within the past 4 hours.

   2. Do not use naloxone if the mother has a history of opioid dependency: may precipitate acute withdrawal symptoms.

H. **Antibiotics.**

   1. As indicated by history, current status of the infant, and initial results of sepsis evaluation.

   2. Administer via peripheral IV or heparin-lock IV line.

PARENT TEACHING

Before Delivery

A. **History.** Review obstetric history; anticipate needs of the infant at delivery.

B. **Complications.** If there are expected complications (preterm delivery, congenital anomalies) and time permits, discuss the anticipated plan of care with the family.

   1. Discuss plans for managing the infant, including plans for transfer to a level II or III nursery and any special equipment that may be used (oxygen hood, incubator, ventilator, monitors).

   2. Allow the parents to tour the NICU if possible.

C. **Parental support.** Encourage parents to express their feelings, fears, and misgivings; involve support people.

At Delivery

A. **After drying the neonate, place on the mother's chest or abdomen when possible with uncomplicated deliveries.** A warm blanket should be placed over the baby's back. Use the family's birth plan as much as possible.

B. **After delivery room assessment, return the infant to the family if the infant's condition is stable.**

C. Answer questions regarding acrocyanosis, Apgar scores, and morphologic findings.

D. Allow parents time to visit, breastfeed, and see extended family.

During Transition

A. "Introduce" the newborn to the family by noting unique features (dimples, long eyelashes, hair color).

B. Encourage the support person to touch and talk to the infant.

C. Discuss physical findings such as caput succedaneum, head molding, positional deformities, and birthmarks.

D. Discuss the infant's sensory capabilities, including seeing, hearing, and smell.

E. Listen to the parents. Allow them to express their reactions as they compare their "dream" infant with the real infant they now have (too tiny, not the right sex, deformed, or premature).

F. After completion of admission procedures, the infant is returned to the family for feeding and visiting.

G. Allow the family to participate in the infant's care, such as giving the first bath or first feeding.

Postpartum Period (Early Discharge)

A. **Parental involvement.** Involve the parents in evaluation of their learning needs; begin teaching as soon as delivery occurs.

B. **Short hospital stays and family instruction.** With shorter hospital stays, there is less time available for teaching and an increased importance of teaching. This may be the only information many families receive on care of a newborn infant.

  1. Classes; videotaped lectures.
      a. Cardiopulmonary resuscitation; safety.
      b. Breastfeeding.
      c. Developmental milestones.
  2. Follow-up visits by the nurse to the home and phone calls from postpartum nurses. Encourage families to call the nursery if they have questions about their newborn's care.
  3. Follow-up visit with the primary care provider within 48 to 72 hours. Encourage the family to select a primary care provider and assist in making an appointment for the first visit.
  4. Return visit for newborn screening if needed.

Transfer to Level II or III Setting

A. Provide prenatal teaching—if possible, with visits to NICU.

B. Provide information booklets, with location, phone numbers, visiting regulations, parent-to-parent groups, and necessary support personnel.

C. **Bring the mother to the infant's bedside if the infant is unable to return to the mother after delivery.** Allow family members to be near the infant as much as possible and encourage them to see past the equipment to the infant and his or her special needs (gentle touch, stroking, soft voice, a familiar person).

D. **When the infant is stable, allow family members to visit in the privacy of their postpartum room or a parent room if condition warrants; for example, an infant with a heparin lock for antibiotics can be taken to the mother's room to nurse.**

E. **Provide a picture and footprints of the infant for the family.** This is especially important if transfer to a level II or III nursery will be to another facility.

F. **Facilitate the family in keeping in contact with the transfer facility, and be available to explain information given to the family.**

REFERENCES

Alvaro, R.E. and Rigatto, H.: Cardiorespiratory adjustments at birth. In M.G. Macdonald, M.M.K. Seshia, and M.D. Mullett (Eds.): *Avery's neonatology: Pathophysiology and management of the newborn* (6th ed.). Philadelphia, 2005, Lippincott Williams and Wilkins, pp. 284-303.

American Academy of Pediatrics: *Report of the committee on infectious disease* (26th ed.). Elk Grove Village, IL, 2003, American Academy of Pediatrics.

American Academy of Pediatrics and American College of Obstetricians and Gynecologists: *Guidelines for perinatal care* (6th ed.). Elk Grove Village, IL, and Washington, DC, 2007, American Academy of Pediatrics and American College of Obstetricians and Gynecologists.

American Academy of Pediatrics Committee on Infectious Diseases: Update on timing of hepatitis B vaccine for premature infants and for children with lapsed immunizations. *Pediatrics,* 94(3):403-404, 2000.

American Academy of Pediatrics Policy Statement: Routine evaluation of blood pressure, hematocrit, and glucose in newborns (RE9322). *Pediatrics,* 92(3): 474-476, 1993.

Blackburn, S.T.: *Maternal, fetal, and neonatal physiology: A clinical perspective* (3rd ed.). St. Louis, 2007, Saunders.

Blake, W.W. and Murray, J.A.: Heat balance. In G.B. Merenstein and S.L. Gardner (Eds.): *Handbook of neonatal intensive care* (6th ed.). St. Louis, 2006, Mosby, pp. 122-138.

Bradshaw, W.T., Turner, B.S., and Pierce, J.R.: Physiologic monitoring. In G.B. Merenstein and S.L. Gardner (Eds.): *Handbook of neonatal intensive care* (6th ed.). St. Louis, 2006, Mosby, pp. 139-156.

Edwards, M.S., Nizet, V., and Baker, C.J.: Group B streptococcal infections. In J.S. Remington, J.O. Klein, C.B. Wilson, and C.J. Baker (Eds.): *Infectious diseases of the fetus and newborn infant* (6th ed.). Philadelphia, 2006, Saunders, pp. 403-464.

Fanaroff, A.A., Kiwi, R., and Shah, D.M.: Antenatal and intrapartum care of the high-risk neonate. In M.H. Klaus and A.A. Fanaroff (Eds.): *Care of the high-risk neonate* (5th ed.). Philadelphia, 2001, Saunders, pp. 1-44.

Gardner, S.L. and Johnson, J.L.: Initial nursery care. In G.B. Merenstein and S.L. Gardner (Eds.): *Handbook of neonatal intensive care* (6th ed.). St. Louis, 2006, Mosby, pp. 79-121.

Hagedorn, M.I.E., Gardner, S.L., Dickey, L.A., and Abham, S.H.: Respiratory diseases. In G.B. Merenstein and S.L. Gardner (Eds.): *Handbook of neonatal intensive care* (6th ed.). St. Louis, 2006, Mosby, pp. 595-698.

Hansen, T.N. and Corbet, A.: Control of breathing. In H.W. Taeusch, R.A. Ballard, and C.A. Gleason (Eds.): *Avery's diseases of the newborn* (8th ed.). Philadelphia, 2005, Saunders, pp. 616-633.

Knight, S.E. and Washington, R.L.: Cardiovascular diseases and surgical interventions. In G.B. Merenstein and S.L. Gardner (Eds.): *Handbook of neonatal intensive care* (6th ed.). St. Louis, 2006, Mosby, pp. 699-735.

Lott, J.W.: Immune system. In C. Kenner and J.W. Lott (Eds.): *Comprehensive neonatal care: An interdisciplinary approach* (4th ed.). St. Louis, 2007, Saunders, pp. 203-220.

McGowan, J.E., Price-Douglas, W., and Hay, W.W.: Glucose homeostasis. In G.B. Merenstein and S.L. Gardner (Eds.): *Handbook of neonatal intensive care* (6th ed.). St Louis, 2006, Mosby, pp. 368-390.

Moore, K.L. and Persaud, T.V.N.: *The developing human: Clinically oriented embryology* (8th ed.). Philadelphia, 2008, Saunders, pp. 366-374.

Niermeyer, S. and Clarke, S.B.: Delivery room care. In G.B. Merenstein and S.L. Gardner (Eds.): *Handbook of neonatal intensive care* (6th ed.). St. Louis, 2006, Mosby, pp. 54-78.

Rehan, V.K. and Phibbs, R.H.: Delivery room management. In M.G. Macdonald, M.M.K. Seshia, and M.D. Mullett (Eds.): *Avery's neonatology: Pathophysiology and management of the newborn* (6th ed.). Philadelphia, 2005, Lippincott Williams and Wilkins, pp. 304-326.

Sansoucie, D.A. and Cavaliere, T.A.: Assessment of the newborn and infant. In C. Kenner and J.W. Lott (Eds.): *Comprehensive neonatal care. An interdisciplinary approach* (4th ed.). St. Louis, 2007, Saunders, pp. 677-718.

Stanley, C.A. and Pallotto, E.K.: Disorders of carbohydrate metabolism. In H.W. Taeusch, R.A. Ballard, and C.A. Gleason (Eds.): *Avery's diseases of the newborn* (8th ed.). Philadelphia, 2005, Saunders, pp. 1410-1422.

Vannucci, R.C.: Perinatal asphyxia. In A.A. Fanaroff and R.J. Martin (Eds.): *Neonatal-perinatal medicine: Diseases of the fetus and infant* (7th ed.). St. Louis, 2002, Mosby, pp. 867-879.

Verklan, M.T.: Physiologic variability during transition to extrauterine life. *Critical Care Nursing Quarterly,* 24(4):41-56, 2002.

5 Neonatal Delivery Room Resuscitation

BARBARA ELIZABETH PAPPAS and BRENDA WALKER

OBJECTIVES

1. Describe three anatomically unique features of the neonate that require special consideration during resuscitation.
2. Compare three physiologic characteristics of the neonate that make neonatal resuscitation different from adult resuscitation.
3. List three antepartum and intrapartum factors that indicate the neonate may be at risk for developing asphyxia.
4. Identify the equipment needed for neonatal resuscitation.
5. Review the components of neonatal resuscitation as outlined by the Neonatal Resuscitation Program (NRP) of the American Heart Association/American Academy of Pediatrics.
6. Recognize three neonatal disease states, congenital malformations, or special situations that may alter the resuscitation process.
7. Describe three potential complications of neonatal resuscitation.
8. Discuss the postresuscitative needs of the neonate.
9. Verbalize three risk factors that may leave the neonate at risk for cardiopulmonary arrest after the initial period of stabilization.
10. Recall two controversial therapies relating to neonatal resuscitation.
11. Discuss ethical considerations surrounding resuscitation of periviable or marginally viable neonates or those with unpredictable life expectancy.

Few neonates require resuscitation at birth. Although approximately 10% of all newborn infants require some assistance at birth, less than 1% require full resuscitative measures (International Liaison Committee on Resuscitation, May 2006). Most neonates only require basic stabilization, including thermal and airway management. Neonates requiring more advanced resuscitation often have respiratory insufficiency or depression.

Neonates at risk for resuscitation benefit from prompt, organized, and efficient interventions tailored to their needs and response. High-functioning resuscitation teams are optimal. Such teams require appropriate education and training in neonatal resuscitation. Formalized education, hands-on experience with equipment, periodic review, and mock codes are all beneficial in promoting the resuscitation skills necessary for a smooth and coordinated resuscitation.

The risk for cardiopulmonary arrest does not stop once the neonate leaves the delivery environment. Physical and physiological vulnerabilities continue to place the neonate at risk. Efforts should be made to minimize the neonate's risk. Prevention is key and although studies regarding neonatal rapid response teams are not available, rapid response teams should be considered as an avenue to reduce the need for resuscitation in the neonatal period.

DEFINITIONS

Newly born: time of the infant's life from birth to the first hours after birth.
Neonate: refers to the first 28 days of the infant's life.
Infant: neonatal period extending through the first 12 months of life.

ANATOMY AND PHYSIOLOGY

A. **Physiologic and anatomic characteristics.** Normal characteristics specific to the neonate differ from the adult, leaving the neonate at significant risk for compromise. A thorough understanding of the uniqueness of the neonate often allows anticipation and intervention before the neonate is compromised to the point of cardiac failure. Unique characteristics specific to the neonate include the following:

1. Large head in proportion to body size. At risk for
   a. Insensible water loss (IWL),
   b. Heat loss: no insulating fat layer, and
   c. Minimal insulation and moisture retention from hair.
2. Large surface area/body size ratio. At risk for
   a. IWL and
   b. Heat loss.
3. Decreased muscle mass. At risk for
   a. Increased potential for heat loss through external gradient,
   b. Decreased ability to flex body to conserve heat, causing increased surface area in premature or ill neonate, and
   c. Decreased ability to generate heat.
4. Decreased subcutaneous fat (premature birth, intrauterine growth restriction). At risk for
   a. Decreased heat production (from brown fat metabolism) and
   b. Increased heat loss (from lack of insulation and decreased flexion).
5. Thinner epidermal layer.
   a. Increased IWL; the more premature the greater the loss.
   b. Decreased support of internal gradient to maintain heat.
   c. Increased risk for breakdown and injury can contribute to increased IWL.
6. Immature systems.
   a. Central nervous system: impaired ability to regulate vasomotor stability, resulting in impaired perfusion and poor autoregulation of blood pressure and temperature regulation.
   b. Neuromuscular system: decreased ability to shiver and generate heat.
   c. Liver: ability to metabolize drugs and mobilize glucose stores is decreased.
   d. Kidneys: risk for decreased perfusion with compromise, ability to excrete drugs and fluids is impaired.
   e. Gastrointestinal tract: gastric distention and respiratory compromise related to decreased gastrointestinal motility and forced air entry with bag-and-mask ventilation.
   f. Metabolism: decreased stores, decreased ability to convert stored glucose, inefficient energy production from stored glucose, and increased utilization of glucose results in hypoglycemia.
   g. Respiratory system: decreased absorption of lung fluid if cesarean section without trial of labor, decreased surface area for gas exchange, decreased availability of surfactant, and increased risk for aspiration from gastric distention.
   h. Immune system: increased predisposition to infection, immature immune response despite adequate cell counts.
7. Glottis positioned anteriorly in the hypopharynx.
   a. Intubation may be difficult.
   b. The neonate is predisposed to airway compromise from positioning.
8. Short neck.
   a. Lack of clarity in identifying landmarks contributes to difficulty in intubation.
   b. Tendency for hyperextension and flexion of neck.
9. Preferential nasal breathing.
   a. Preferential nose breather; patency is essential to airway maintenance.
   b. Anatomic patency must be confirmed.
   c. Increased airway resistance with edema from nasal suctioning.

10. Venous access.
    a. Small and superficial veins: access is difficult, vessels fragile.
    b. Vasoconstriction associated with acidosis, hypothermia, hypoglycemia, and shock.
    c. Umbilical access. Normal cord includes two arteries and one vein. Inadvertent cannulization of the portal vein with umbilical vein catheterization can lead to liver damage with chemical resuscitation.
11. Unknown physical variations make resuscitation and stabilization challenging.
    a. Lack of adequate perinatal information (i.e., ultrasound, genetic testing).
    b. Gross physical assessment only.

RISK FACTORS

Risk factors are warning signs that alert the perinatal team to the possibility of a crisis and the need for anticipatory preparation of neonatal resuscitation.

A. **Antepartum:** conditions during pregnancy that predispose mother and fetus to stress and can interfere with successful transition of the fetus to extrauterine life.
   1. Maternal age less than 16 years or more than 35 years.
   2. Maternal diabetes.
   3. Hemorrhage, anemia.
   4. Maternal substance abuse.
   5. Maternal drug therapy such as magnesium sulfate, adrenergic blocking agents, over-the-counter or herbal medications.
   6. No or late entry to prenatal care.
   7. Polyhydramnios or oligohydramnios.
   8. Maternal cardiac, renal, pulmonary, thyroid, endocrine, gastrointestinal, or neurologic disease.
   9. Premature rupture of membranes.
   10. Anatomic abnormalities of the uterus.
   11. Isoimmunization, Rh, or ABO (blood group) incompatibilities.
   12. Hypertension (pregnancy-induced hypertension, chronic).
   13. Multiple gestation.
   14. Postterm gestation.
   15. Discrepancy in size and dates.
   16. Previous pregnancy complication or fetal loss.
   17. Diminished or absent fetal activity.

B. **Intrapartum period:** conditions that predispose the fetus to difficult transition to extrauterine life or signs that the fetus is not tolerating the stresses of labor. Unsuccessful transition may ensue.
   1. Abnormal fetal positioning or presentation (e.g., breech position).
   2. Cesarean delivery.
   3. Fetal heart rate abnormalities (e.g., bradycardia, tachycardia).
   4. Nonreassuring fetal heart rate pattern.
   5. Maternal or fetal intrapartum blood loss (e.g., abruptio placenta, placental previa).
   6. Maternal sedation, anesthesia, or analgesia (e.g., narcotics in the previous 4 hours).
   7. Maternal fever or infection (e.g., chorioamnionitis).
   8. Prolonged labor (>24 hours or second stage >2 hours).
   9. Premature labor.
   10. Precipitous delivery.
   11. Prolonged rupture of membranes (>18 hours).
   12. Prolapse of the umbilical cord.
   13. Fetal malformations.
   14. Meconium-stained amniotic fluid.
   15. Uterine hyperstimulation.
   16. Instrument-assisted delivery (e.g., vacuum or forceps).
   17. Macrosomia.

C. **Newly born period:** signs or conditions in the delivery room or during the transitional period that indicate the neonate is having difficulty making all the physiologic changes needed for successful adaptation from intrauterine to extrauterine life.
1. Congenital malformations (e.g., cardiac, respiratory, gastrointestinal, neurologic, genitourinary).
2. Cardiac arrhythmia or murmur (e.g., tachycardia or bradycardia).
3. Extreme color change (e.g., cyanosis, plethora, pallor, mottling).
4. Prolonged or delayed capillary refill time.
5. Respiratory distress (e.g., apnea, tachypnea, grunting, altered breath sounds, excessive secretions).
6. Temperature instability.
7. Hypertonia/hypotonia.
8. Hypotension.
9. Seizures.
10. Hypoglycemia.
11. Prematurity.
12. Postmaturity.
13. Anemia or polycythemia.
14. Feeding difficulty or intolerance.
15. Seemingly well, then clinically deteriorates.

ANTICIPATION OF AND PREPARATION FOR RESUSCITATION

Anticipation and preparation for resuscitation requires an evidence-based multidisciplinary approach. Internationally, the Neonatal Resuscitation Program is recognized as the gold standard for neonatal resuscitation. Program content is based on the American Academy of Pediatrics and American Heart Association's Guidelines for Cardiopulmonary Resuscitation and Emergency Cardiovascular Care of Pediatric and Neonatal Patients: Neonatal Resuscitation Guidelines. The Guidelines are based on the International Liaison Committee on Resuscitation (ILCOR) consensus on science statement regarding treatment recommendations for neonatal resuscitation. All units and facilities caring for newborn infants and neonates must be adequately staffed, prepared, and equipped to deliver resuscitative care when anticipated or unexpected resuscitation needs arise.

A. **Education and competency development.**
1. Completion of educational program on neonatal resuscitation (e.g., NRP) does not equate to competency or confidence.
2. Development and implementation of regular mock code system for education and quality improvement.
3. Annual competency evaluation and review is also recommended.
4. Establish a quality improvement process for reviewing neonatal codes (e.g., effectiveness of call system, response times, and drug doses).

B. **General preparation.**
1. Promote development of effective teams. Effective teams demonstrate clear communication and strong leadership and management.
2. Consider the development and utilization of a rapid response team.
3. Evaluate and update equipment frequently.
4. Arrange for periodic evaluation and maintenance of electrical equipment by the biomedical engineering department on a regularly scheduled basis.
5. Schedule periodic evaluation and maintenance of all respiratory equipment.
6. Formulate supply replacement procedures. Evaluate and replace supplies as quickly as possible after use (use equipment checklist).
7. Test alerting system for rapid, consistent response of personnel.

C. **Delivery room preparation.**
1. Anticipate the needs of the neonate by evaluation of gestational age, risk factors (e.g., meconium, infection), and immediate status at birth (e.g., crying, tone).
   a. Formulate a plan before anticipated need if possible (e.g., endotracheal tube size, drug doses, concentrations, and handling equipment).

    b. Promote effective communication between personnel, departments, and institutions that encourages identification and notification of high-risk situations and preparedness.

  2. Prewarm room to minimize thermal losses in the newly born infant. Use a polyethylene wrap or plastic bag for neonate <32 weeks or <1500 g.

  3. Assemble equipment in an organized, easily available system. Check function of equipment routinely and before use.

  4. Ensure safety of team members and utilization of standard precautions.

  5. Preheat warmer, hat, blankets, and nest (blanket rolls or bendable positioning device). Approximately 15 to 30 minutes (heat output set on high) is required to thoroughly warm the mattress on a radiant warmer bed. Assemble alternative heat sources to bedside as needed (i.e., warming pad).

  6. Identify and assemble available team members and designate roles.

  7. Position resuscitation algorithms and charts easily within view of the resuscitative area.

  8. Promote family-centered care through active family communication and involvement in decision making.

D. Personnel roles.

  1. Personnel roles should be defined by institutional policies and job descriptions in addition to state laws, license regulations, and scope of practice definitions.

  2. Preparedness for resuscitation should exist at every delivery. Every delivery should be attended by at least one person skilled in neonatal resuscitation who is immediately available and solely responsible for initiating resuscitation and stabilization of the neonate. Additional qualified personnel should be available for more complex situations.

  3. A family-centered approach should include a designated support and communication liaison to the family. Family support should not be left unassigned. Family presence during resuscitation has not been shown to be detrimental to the outcome of the neonate.

E. Non–delivery room preparation. As with delivery room resuscitation, being prepared for unforeseen events throughout the entire infant's hospitalization can facilitate success in a time of crisis. Unlike delivery room events, non–delivery room resuscitation is often unpredictable and risks ill preparedness. The following events may precipitate respiratory or circulatory compromise:

  1. Apnea.

  2. Choking or aspiration (i.e., feedings).

  3. Unwitnessed cardiac arrest.

  4. Seizure.

  5. Hypoxia or airway obstruction.

  6. Infection.

  7. Postoperative period.

  8. Air leak syndromes.

  9. Severe anemia (i.e., subgaleal hemorrhage, abruption).

  10. Shock.

EQUIPMENT FOR NEONATAL RESUSCITATION

Not every item on the equipment list (Box 5-1) will be used, but it is important to have appropriate sizes and supply quantities to support a prolonged effort. Ensuring that equipment is functional and up to date is vital to a successful resuscitation. It is important that staff members be familiar with the equipment they will be using and practice with it frequently.

APGAR SCORING

The Apgar score (Table 5-1) is a descriptive tool for documenting the status of the newborn post delivery. Generally scored during or after resuscitation and stabilization at 1 and 5 minutes, it describes the infant's physiologic condition in five categories: color, heart rate, reflex irritability, muscle tone, and respiratory effort. When the 5-minute score is less than 7, the Apgar score should be determined every 5 minutes until 20 minutes of age. The scores are not used for decision

■ BOX 5-1
■ **NEONATAL RESUSCITATION EQUIPMENT LIST**

Thermoregulation Equipment
- Radiant warmer with firm mattress and/or other heat source
- Warmed linens
- Recloseable, food-grade polyethylene bag/wrap

Suction Equipment
- Bulb syringe
- Mechanical suction with tubing
- Suction catheters: 5F or 6F, 8F, 10F, 12F, and 14F
- 8F feeding tube with 20-ml syringe
- Meconium aspiration device

Bag-and-Mask Equipment
- Oxygen source with flow meter (flow rate up to 10 ml/min) and tubing
- Positive pressure ventilation device capable of delivering 90% to 100% oxygen
- Face mask (preterm and term) with cushioned rim

Airway
- Laryngoscope with straight blades 00 (optional), 0 and 1 size
- Extra batteries and bulb for laryngoscope
- Endotracheal tubes: 2.5, 3, 3.5, and 4 mm
- Stylet (optional)
- Carbon dioxide detector
- Scissors
- Tape or securing device for endotracheal tube (latex-free preferred)
- Pectin-based skin preparation (approved for neonate)
- Oral airways: size 000, 00, and 0, or 30-, 40-, and 50-mm lengths
- Laryngeal mask airway, size 1 (optional)

Medications
- Epinephrine 1:10,000 (0.1-0.3 ml/kg)
- Isotonic crystalloid (normal saline or Ringer's lactate)
- Sodium bicarbonate 4.2% (0.5 mEq/ml)
- Naloxone hydrochloride (0.4 mg/ml)
- Surfactant (optional)
- Dextrose 10%
- Normal saline for flushes
- Umbilical vessel catheterization supplies (refer to umbilical catheter procedure, Chapter 15)
- Syringes (1, 3, 5, 10, and 20 ml) and syringe labels
- Needleless puncture device or needles (25, 21, and 18 gauge)

Miscellaneous
- Blood gas syringes or supplies for blood gas evaluation
- Cardiac monitor or pulse oximeter (optional)
- Stethoscope—neonatal size
- Clock with second hand (timer optional)
- Standard precaution supplies: gloves and personal protection equipment
- Pulse oximeter with probe
- Transport incubator to maintain temperature for transfer to nursery

Premature Neonate Supplies
- Compressed air source (tank or wall) with oxygen blender
- Polyethylene wrap or plastic bag
- Chemically activated warming pad

■ TABLE 5-1
■ ■ **Apgar Score**   **Gestational Age:** _____ **Weeks**

Sign	0	1	2	1 Minute	5 Minutes	10 Minutes	15 Minutes	20 Minutes
Color	Blue or pale	Acrocyanotic	Completely pink					
Heart rate	Absent	<100/minute	>100/minute					
Reflex irritability	No response	Grimace	Cry or active withdrawal					
Muscle tone	Limp	Some flexion	Active motion					
Respiration	Absent	Weak cry: Hypoventilation	Good: Crying					
			Total					

		Resuscitation			
Comments:		1 Minute	5 Minutes	10 Minutes	15 Minutes	20 Minutes
	Oxygen					
	PPV/NCPAP					
	ETT					
	Chest compressions					
	Epinephrine					

ETT, Endotracheal tube; *NCPAP*, nasal continuous positive airway pressure; *PPV*, positive pressure ventilation.

making during resuscitation. The scores are influenced by interventions, gestational age, maternal medications, and cardiorespiratory and neurologic conditions (e.g., malformations, hypoglycemia). An expanded Apgar score has been proposed by the American Academy of Pediatrics and American College of Obstetricians and Gynecologists to record the correlation of infant's status with resuscitative interventions. Narrative documentation detailing interventions (e.g., ventilation, medications, and oxygen) should accompany the scoring.

DECISION-MAKING PROCESS

A. **Decision making** during resuscitation requires quick and frequent assessment, intervention, and evaluation. The initial steps to resuscitation should be preceded by four questions that facilitate fact finding and assist in preparation and decision making.
   1. Ask the following questions:
      a. What is the gestational age?
      b. Is the amniotic fluid clear?
      c. Is the neonate breathing or crying?
      d. Is the neonate's muscle tone appropriate for gestational age?
B. **Initial steps.** At most deliveries, the following five steps are the only interventions necessary. Initial steps should be initiated within a few seconds and completed as quickly as possible unless meconium is present and the neonate is not vigorous.
   1. Prevent hypothermia and hyperthermia, which may increase metabolic requirements and contribute to respiratory distress, metabolic acidosis, and hypoglycemia.
      a. Place and keep the neonate in a preheated environment (radiant heat source or incubator). Stable neonates should be placed on maternal chest if possible. Supplement environmental support with warmed linens.

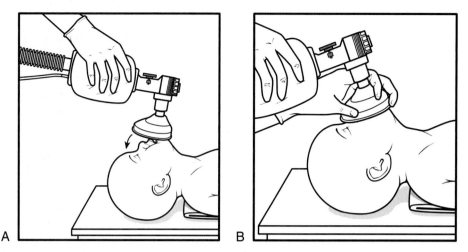

A   B

FIGURE 5-1 ■ Correct head position for airway management. (From Kattwinkel, J. [Ed.]: *Textbook of neonatal resuscitation* [5th ed.]. Elk Grove Village, IL, 2006, American Academy of Pediatrics/American Heart Association.)

    b. Avoidance of drafts, for example, sidewalls up on radiant warmer; limit door open and closing; and keep bed away from ventilation drafts.

  2. Open the airway.

    a. Position infant on the back or side if infant has an open spinal defect, with the neck slightly extended.

      (1) Care should be taken to avoid hyperextension or flexion of the neck (Fig. 5-1).

      (2) A shoulder pad may help maintain the correct airway position, especially for neonates with a large occiput.

      (3) When supine, the infant's head should be in the "sniffing" position.

    b. Clear airway.

      (1) Use the least invasive method possible. May wipe nose and mouth with towel, suction with bulb syringe, or suction catheter to mechanical suction. The suction pressure should be approximately 100 mm Hg.

      (2) Vigorous or prolonged deep suctioning can result in trauma, bradycardia, or apnea induced by stimulation of the posterior pharynx and vagus nerve.

      (3) When meconium-stained fluid is present and the neonate is not vigorous (heart rate less than 100, depressed respirations, and decreased muscle tone), suction the trachea with 12F or 14F suction catheter or endotracheal tube attached to suction device prior to additional stimulation. Repeat intubation and suctioning until clear of meconium or heart rate indicates continued deterioration.

      (4) A vigorous neonate born through meconium-stained fluid should have mouth and nose cleared with bulb syringe or large-bore suction catheter. Clinical judgment must be used.

  3. Continued thermal and airway support.

    a. Maintain dry, warm environment.

      (1) Dry thoroughly.

      (2) Remove wet linen immediately after drying infant and replace with dry linen.

      (3) Provide additional heat source as necessary. Do not use warm water gloves or microwaved heat source (e.g., blankets, saline bag).

    b. Reposition airway.

  4. Evaluate respirations.

    a. If apneic, gently slap or flick the soles of the infant's feet.

    b. Gently rub the back, trunk, and extremities.

    c. Attempts to stimulate should be brief, no more than two attempts. If respirations do not begin, proceed to bag-and-mask ventilation (unless diaphragmatic hernia is suspected, in which case intubate the trachea and ventilate the infant through the endo-tracheal tube with the resuscitation bag).

5. Begin supplemental oxygen at any time if central cyanosis is present, heart rate is greater than 100 beats per minute (bpm), and respirations are adequate.
   a. Use 100% oxygen with a flow of at least 5 l/minute. Deliver oxygen by mask, cupped hand holding tubing over infant's face, flow-inflating bag and mask, or T-piece resuscitator. The closer the oxygen source to the face, the higher will be the oxygen concentration delivered.
   b. When using a flow-inflating bag and mask, allow some oxygen to escape the mask to prevent a buildup of pressure within the bag-and-mask system.
   c. Continue oxygen delivery until infant pinks and then slowly withdraw the oxygen per pulse oximeter and neonate status, ensuring adequate delivery for the infant to remain pink.
   d. Pulse oximetry should be available for all neonates. Oximetry levels may take more than 10 minutes to rise to 90% or more in the full-term, stable neonate. Occasional dips in oxygen saturation to a high 80% range may be considered normal in the first few days of life when unaccompanied by other changes in status.
6. Evaluate frequently and simultaneously the following:
   a. Airway: assess for alignment, secretions, and inadvertent extubation.
   b. Respiratory effort: rate, breath sounds, work of breathing (grunting, flaring, retracting, depth), symmetry of chest movement.
   c. Heart rate: count for 6 seconds and multiply by 10. Obtain heart rate by
      (1) palpation at the base of the umbilical cord stump and
      (2) auscultation of the apical heartbeat with a stethoscope.
   d. Color.
      (1) Infant should have pink lips and a pink trunk.
      (2) Peripheral cyanosis of hands and feet is usually normal.
      (3) Central cyanosis of tongue and gums is abnormal and requires supplemental oxygen.

C. **Positive-pressure ventilation.**
   1. Bag-and-mask ventilation.
      a. Initiate when
         (1) apnea or gasping respirations,
         (2) heart rate is less than 100 bpm,
         (3) color remains cyanotic despite supplemental oxygen, or
         (4) need for continued ventilation is determined by frequent assessment of the infant's response to interventions.
      b. Equipment.
         (1) Resuscitation devices—resuscitation bags should not be larger than 750 ml and should be connected to oxygen source; blended oxygen preferred for neonates <32 weeks.
            (a) Self-inflating bags must have a reservoir to deliver high concentrations of oxygen, should have a pressure gauge and a pressure-release valve; cannot deliver free-flow oxygen or continuous positive airway pressure (CPAP).
            (b) Flow-inflating (anesthesia) bags must have a gas source, pressure gauge, and flow control valve; deliver free-flow oxygen of 21% to 100% if positive end-expiratory pressure (PEEP) valve is present; and usually lack pressure-release valve.
            (c) T-piece resuscitator—requires compressed gas source and allows manual setting of inspiratory pressure and PEEP.
         (2) Mask of proper size should be used to obtain adequate seal. Appropriate sizing should have the mask covering the chin, mouth, and nose but not the eyes.
         (3) Equipment should always be present and ready for use, preset and checked before each use.
      c. Procedure.
         (1) Assemble, set, and test the equipment.

(2) Position and open airway as in "Initial Steps," item B, Open the Airway under Neonatal Resuscitation, p. 98.

(3) Apply mask and ensure proper seal. Be careful not to apply too much pressure to the neonate's face or neck.

(4) Observe for gentile chest rise and fall. Rate of ventilation is 40 to 60 breaths per minute. Volume of lung is small, approximately 5 to 8 ml/kg. Adequate ventilation is gentle but sufficient pressure to improve heart rate, color, and muscle tone. Pressure of 30 cm H_2O or more may be needed for diseased lungs.

(5) Effective ventilation and signs of improvement include increasing heart rate, improving color, spontaneous breathing, and improving muscle tone.

(6) After 30 seconds of ventilation, pause to check 6-second heart rate. Continue ventilation and for signs of improvement every 30 seconds until the neonate begins spontaneous breathing and the heart rate is greater than 100 bpm.

(7) If manual ventilation is ineffective or if there is a need for prolonged ventilation, endotracheal intubation should be performed.

d. Exceptions.

(1) Meconium-stained fluid and nonvigorous neonate as in "Initial Steps," item B, Open the Airway, p. 98.

(2) Blocked airway or impaired lung function (e.g., airway malformations, lung disease, congenital heart disease, diaphragmatic hernia, and pneumothorax)—perform intubation, i.e., insert orogastric tube with diaphragmatic hernia.

e. Orogastric tube placement.

(1) Ventilation for more than several minutes (with or without compressions) can cause air to accumulate in the stomach.

(2) Ensure the tube is placed through the mouth rather than the nose to maximize ventilation through the nose.

(3) Aspirate contents, secure in place, and leave open to air.

2. Ventilation via endotracheal tube.

a. Indications.

(1) The neonate does not respond to manual ventilation, as evidenced by inadequate chest rise, lack of spontaneous respirations, continued heart rate less than 100, diminished muscle tone, diminished breath sounds, or persistent central cyanosis.

(2) Suspected mechanical blockage or impaired lung function (e.g., diaphragmatic hernia).

(3) Prolonged ventilation is required.

(4) Tracheal suctioning is required.

(5) Extreme prematurity.

(6) Surfactant administration.

(7) Chemical resuscitation.

(8) Administration of chest compression to facilitate coordination of compressions and ventilation, maximize efficiency of ventilation.

b. Equipment (Box 5-1).

c. Laryngeal mask airway.

(1) Airway device useful when positive pressure ventilation (PPV) ineffective or endotracheal intubation not feasible or unsuccessful (e.g., airway congenital anomalies)

(2) Soft, inflatable mask inserted into mouth and guided along hard palate until mask covers larynx.

(3) Limitations—cannot be used to suction meconium from airway, leaks with high pressures, may be ineffective with chest compression, unable to deliver endotracheal medications.

d. Endotracheal intubation (see Chapter 15).

(1) Should be a clean procedure.

(2) Perform intubation.

(3) Confirm placement of endotracheal tube.

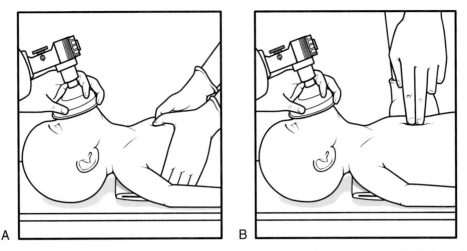

A   B

FIGURE 5-2 ■ ■ Two techniques for providing chest compressions. (From Kattwinkel, J. [Ed.]: *Textbook of neonatal resuscitation* [5th ed.]. Elk Grove Village, IL, 2006, American Academy of Pediatrics/American Heart Association.)

     (4) Secure tube.

     (5) Observe for dislocation of endotracheal tube or unplanned extubation (e.g., central cyanosis, bradycardia, decreased chest movement, breath sounds absent or diminished, CO_2 detector does not indicate presence of CO_2, distended abdomen, air noises audible over stomach, or no mist or fogging in tube).

D. Chest compressions.

  1. Chest compressions should be initiated when the heart rate is less than 60 bpm after 30 seconds of ventilation with 100% oxygen.

  2. Should always be accompanied by ventilation with 100% oxygen available; requires second person.

  3. Use one of the following two methods (Fig. 5-2):

    a. Thumb technique (Preferred).

     (1) Place both thumbs side by side or on small neonate one over the other. Location is the lower third of the infant's sternum above the xiphoid process.

     (2) Flex thumbs at first joint and apply pressure vertically.

     (3) Encircle the infant's torso with hands and provide support for the back. If hands are too small, ensure that the infant is on a firm surface.

    b. Two-finger technique.

     (1) Place the tips of the middle finger and either the index finger or the ring finger of one hand over the lower third of the infant's sternum.

     (2) Place the other hand under the infant's back to provide support.

     (3) Compressions should squeeze the heart between the spinal column and the sternum.

       (a) Force of compression should be straight down to minimize rib or lung damage.

       (b) Depress the sternum approximately one third of the anterior–posterior diameter of the chest and release to allow heart to refill.

       (c) Fingers or thumbs should remain in contact with the chest at all times, both during compression and release. Lack of contact with chest wall increases the risk for complications and wastes time relocating landmarks for compression area.

     (4) Compression/ventilation ratio of 3:1.

       (a) Provide three compressions, pause for a single ventilation. This will equal 90 compressions to 30 ventilations, or 120 events per minute.

       (b) Optimally the neonate's trachea should be intubated during compressions.

(c) Reevaluate respiratory effort and heart rate every 30 seconds during compressions and ventilations.

(5) Indications for discontinuing chest compressions.

(a) Heart rate greater than 60 bpm.

(b) After 10 minutes of asystole or 20 minutes of complete and adequate resuscitative measures.

E. Chemical resuscitation. Most neonatal resuscitations do not require medications or volume expanders. When medications are required, an umbilical catheter may be the fastest and most direct route. Intravenous administration of resuscitation medications is preferable whenever available. A peripheral intravenous (IV) line may also be used to administer medications or volume expanders (see Chapter 15). If unable to place umbilical catheter or IV line, intraosseous access may be an acceptable alternative.

1. Indications.

   a. Stimulate the heart.

   b. Increase tissue perfusion.

   c. Correct metabolic acidosis.

   d. Replace volume.

   e. Reverse respiratory depression related to maternal narcotics.

2. Medications and solutions.

   a. Epinephrine, a cardiac stimulant, increases the heart rate and strength of contractions; causes peripheral vasoconstriction; and increases blood flow through coronary arteries and the brain.

   (1) Indications for use:

   (a) Heart rate is less than 60 bpm despite 30 seconds of effective assisted ventilation and another 30 seconds of coordinated chest compression and ventilation.

   (b) Heart rate is undetectable while ventilations and compressions are initiated.

   (2) Response: the heart rate should increase by more than 60 beats per minute within 30 seconds of administration. If this does not happen, dosing may be repeated every 3 to 5 minutes, given intravenously if possible.

   b. Volume expanders are fluids that increase the neonate's circulating blood volume to correct hypovolemia and facilitate tissue perfusion. Normal saline, Ringer's lactate, and O Rh-negative blood may be used, normal saline being the preferred fluid.

   (1) Indicated when there is suspected shock and the neonate is not responding to resuscitation.

   (a) Weak or absent peripheral pulses.

   (b) Low blood pressure.

   (c) Persistent bradycardia or tachycardia.

   (d) Pallor, mottling, or cyanosis despite good oxygenation.

   (e) Poor perfusion.

   (f) Diminished or limp muscle tone.

   (g) Continued respiratory depression or apnea.

   (2) Dose: 10 ml/kg given over 5 to 10 minutes intravenously.

   (3) Response: increase in blood pressure, improvement of skin perfusion, and increase in the intensity of pulses should occur within minutes. Procedure may be repeated if necessary.

   c. Sodium bicarbonate, a base buffer, raises the pH of the blood.

   (1) Use during resuscitation is controversial.

   (2) Adequate ventilation required to remove by-product of carbon dioxide.

   (3) Indications for use:

   (a) Documented or suspected metabolic acidosis.

   (b) Evidence of prolonged asphyxia.

   (4) Dose: For a concentration of 4.2% solution (0.5 mEq/ml), the dose is 2 mEq/kg (4 ml/kg) given intravenously only.

   (a) Sodium bicarbonate can be very damaging to lung tissue and should not be given per endotracheal tube. It is also caustic and hypertonic and must be administered in a large vein.

   (5) Response: The pH should change, and tone and respirations improve.

    d. Naloxone hydrochloride, a short-acting narcotic antagonist, displaces narcotics from receptor sites and reverses the physiologic depressant effects of the narcotic.
        (1) Indications for use.
            (a) Continued respiratory depression after positive pressure ventilation has restored a normal heart rate and color *and*
            (b) a history of maternal narcotic administration within the 4 hours before delivery.
        (2) Not the first intervention for respiratory depression. Use should follow ventilatory support and other initial steps of resuscitation.
        (3) Administration to neonate of narcotic-addicted mother may cause severe withdrawal (i.e., seizures and/or cardiorespiratory arrest).
        (4) Dose: Concentration is 1 mg/ml, the dose is 0.1 mg/kg given rapidly intravenously.
        (5) Response: Respiratory depression should decrease within seconds or minutes (depending on route) after administration. Duration of action is widely variable (1 to 4 hours). Monitor closely for return of respiratory depression. May be repeated several times if needed.

UNUSUAL SITUATIONS

A. Respiratory
  1. Choanal atresia/upper-airway obstruction.
    a. Definitions and characteristics.
        (1) Bony or soft tissue obstruction of the posterior nares; may be bilateral or unilateral.
        (2) Respiratory distress may be present immediately after birth because of blockage of the primary airway, the nose.
        (3) May present with cyanosis when quiet or at rest, pinks with crying.
        (4) Inability to pass small-gauge suction catheter or nasogastric tube may be an indicator of choanal atresia.
    b. Management.
        (1) Stimulate neonate to cry, thereby using the secondary airway (mouth) for ventilation.
        (2) Insert an oral airway or endotracheal tube as an oral airway into the posterior pharynx.
        (3) Infants with more complicated craniofacial malformations may require endotracheal intubation.
  2. Robin sequence.
    a. Definitions and characteristics:
        (1) Small mandible causing displacement of the tongue posteriorly into the pharynx, causing partial or complete obstruction.
        (2) Presents with apnea, stridor, and cyanosis.
    b. Management:
        (1) Maintain patent airway by turning the neonate onto the stomach (prone), which should cause the tongue to fall forward and open the airway.
        (2) If this is not effective, insert an oral airway; or a large catheter (12F) or small endotracheal (2.5 mm) nasally to the posterior pharynx. A laryngeal mask airway may be effective but is not recommended for removal of meconium.
        (3) Position prone.
  3. Pulmonary hypoplasia.
    a. Definitions and characteristics.
        (1) Underdeveloped lungs resulting from insufficient space within the thoracic cavity for normal development.
        (2) Associated with Potter syndrome, dysplastic renal conditions, chronic oligohydramnios, and diaphragmatic hernia.
    b. Clinical presentation: deterioration may be acute.
        (1) Inability to ventilate lungs adequately exhibited by poor chest movement, decreased breath sounds, and cyanosis.

(2) Very high pressures required to expand small, stiff lungs.

(3) High risk of pulmonary air leak.

(4) Low and/or descending Apgar scores.

(5) Poor perfusion.

(6) Diminished muscle tone.

(7) Respiratory and/or metabolic acidosis.

  c. Management.

(1) Intubate.

(2) Ventilate with 100% oxygen and as much pressure as necessary to expand the lungs (i.e., adequate chest rise and fall).

(3) Transilluminate and auscultate chest frequently, assessing for pulmonary air leaks. Be prepared for emergency evacuation of air leak.

4. Congenital diaphragmatic hernia.

  a. Definitions and characteristics (see Chapter 29).

(1) Herniation of the abdominal contents into the chest cavity early in gestational development.

(2) Pulmonary hypoplasia arises secondary to compression from abdominal organs and limited capacity for growth in the thoracic cavity.

(3) Most commonly occurs on the left.

(4) May present with a scaphoid abdomen.

(5) Severity of symptoms is associated with the amount of lung compression and pulmonary hypoplasia. May present with rapid respiratory distress and descending Apgar scores at the time of delivery or with respiratory distress later during transition.

(6) Breath sounds absent or decreased on the side of defect.

(7) Bowel sounds audible in the chest.

(8) Heart sounds may be audible on the right side if left-sided defect.

(9) Prenatal diagnosis possible through ultrasound. Polyhydramnios often present.

  b. Management.

(1) Consider immediate endotracheal intubation and ventilation to minimize overdistention of the stomach resulting from bag-and-mask ventilation.

(2) Provide gastric decompression per oral or nasogastric tube.

(3) Systemic hypotension and respiratory or metabolic acidosis commonly occur. Aggressive management necessary to minimize pulmonary hypertension.

(4) Extracorporeal membrane oxygenation (ECMO) and nitric oxide may be used for infants not responding to conventional therapies.

5. Esophageal atresia/tracheoesophageal fistula.

  a. Definitions and characteristics.

(1) Failure of the trachea to differentiate and separate appropriately from the esophagus during gestational development (see Chapter 29).

(2) Excessive coughing, drooling, choking, gasping, or cyanosis. May cause airway obstruction, aspiration, and respiratory distress.

(3) Failure to pass oral or nasogastric tube.

  b. Management.

(1) Oral or nasogastric decompression of esophageal pouch to decrease risk of aspiration.

(2) Position prone or side lying to facilitate secretion drainage.

6. Hydrops fetalis.

  a. Definition and characteristics.

(1) Generalized subcutaneous edema usually accompanied by ascites and pleural or pericardial effusion (see Chapter 29).

  b. Management.

(1) Maintain airway through positioning and endotracheal intubation.

(2) Thoracentesis or paracentesis may be required to improve ventilation and oxygenation.

(3) Volume expansion may be necessary due to extravascular fluid shift.

B. Abdominal wall defects.
1. Definition and characteristics.
   a. Gastroschisis: herniation of stomach, liver, or intestines through a defect next to the umbilical cord, usually to the right of the cord.
   b. Omphalocele: midline herniation of the bowel into the umbilical cord.
   c. Exstrophy of the bladder: externalization and aversion of the bladder, urethra, or ureteral orifices through a defect in the lower portion of the abdominal wall.
2. Clinical risks.
   a. Fluid and heat loss through the exposed viscera (exposure increases the surface area).
   b. Potential for visceral damage from drying or trauma.
   c. Increased risk of infection.
3. Management.
   a. Handle the defect gently and use a sterile technique.
   b. Position the infant to allow adequate visceral perfusion.
      (1) Gastroschisis and omphalocele: Position the infant supine with lateral support to keep the defect in the midline position, promoting optimal blood flow in the superior mesenteric artery. If the defect lies even slightly to the side, the superior mesenteric artery may kink and perfusion may be compromised.
      (2) Avoid prone position. Position the infant on the side, preferably the right side, to prevent kinking of the superior mesenteric artery where it exits the abdomen.
      (3) Place the infant in a sterile bowel bag from the axillary region down. Place sterile gauze moistened with sterile saline in the bag to cover contact with the defect.
   c. Ensure a neutral thermal environment.
   d. Observe for hypovolemia. Provide adequate fluid support and maintenance. Fluid losses will be higher than normal.
   e. Place an orogastric tube to intermittent suction to prevent gastric and intestinal inflation, which would complicate repair.
   f. Consider the use of latex precautions.
C. Neural tube defects.
1. Most common types and characteristics.
   a. Anencephaly: most severe form, in which the neural tube fails to close and the brain is exposed. Death most common in the newborn period.
   b. Encephalocele: defect in closure of the neural tube at the proximal end, with outpouching of brain tissue through or at the base of the skull.
   c. Myelomeningocele: defect in closure of the neural tube at the distal end, with exposure of the neural tube. Occurs at any level of the spinal column.
2. Acute clinical problems.
   a. Heat and fluid losses through an open defect.
   b. Increased risk of infection and potential leakage of cerebral spinal fluid (CSF).
   c. Potential for damage of exposed nervous system tissue as a result of trauma.
   d. Difficulty in handling the infant because of exposed tissue.
   e. Ethical and legal questions of viability or organ donation from infants with anencephaly.
3. Management.
   a. Initiate latex precautions immediately to minimize the risk of development of latex allergies.
   b. Cover the defect with sterile, saline solution–soaked sponges and a plastic barrier to prevent heat and fluid losses. Place a protective barrier between the defect and the anus if myelomeningocele to prevent contamination.
   c. Observe for leakage of CSF.
   d. Maintain neonate in a neutral thermal environment.
   e. Keep neonate on the side or prone.
   f. Assisted ventilation may be given, with the neonate in a side-lying or prone position as necessary.
   g. Manage all defects regardless of degree in the same manner, no matter how severe. Discuss viability issues after resuscitation and stabilization.

D. Congenital heart disease (includes structural defects and conduction disorders).
  1. Definition and characteristics.
     a. Cardiac anomalies causing respiratory or cardiac decompensation.
     b. Persistent cyanosis despite adequate ventilation with 90% to 100% oxygen.
     c. Presentation may range from peaceful tachypnea or respiratory distress without increase in work of breathing to severe shock and cardiorespiratory arrest.
     d. Murmur may be present.
     e. Conduction disorders not always associated with structural anomalies.
  2. Management.
     a. Cardiorespiratory support as symptoms indicate.
     b. Hyperoxia test in 100% oxygen. If arterial oxygen does not increase, it may be indicative of cardiac disease.
E. Multiple gestation.
  1. Definitions and characteristics.
     a. May be small for gestational age or intrauterine growth restricted.
     b. Compression deformations may be present.
     c. Distress may be related to placental abnormalities, compromise of cord blood flow, or mechanical complications during delivery.
  2. Management.
     a. Delivery of multiples may be unexpected.
     b. Separate resuscitation team for each neonate.
     c. Twin-to-twin transfusion may require volume resuscitation of donor twin.
     d. Premature delivery common.
     e. Systematic and planned approach for mobilizing extra resuscitative teams is necessary to ensure appropriate resuscitation of unexpected multiples.
     f. Ensure adequate supplies and equipment are available, in addition to back-up supplies, to manage multiple prolonged resuscitative efforts.
F. Premature.
  1. Definitions and characteristics.
     a. Multisystem immaturity.
     b. Fragile skin, especially with very low birth weight (VLBW).
     c. Susceptible to trauma from resuscitative intervention.
     d. Susceptible to infection.
     e. Increased thermal instability.
  2. Management.
     a. Have additional trained personnel available for full resuscitation.
     b. Thermal stability
        (1) Increase the temperature of the delivery room.
        (2) Use additional heat sources to maintain a thermal-neutral environment.
        (3) Preheat radiant warmer.
        (4) Thermal wrapping with recloseable, food-grade polyethylene bag and portable warming pad for neonates less than 28 weeks or 1500 g. Monitor temperature closely.
        (5) Use a prewarmed transport unit during transfer.
     c. Respiratory support for neonates less than 32 weeks postmenstrual age.
        (1) Oxygen
           (a) Use a blender to titrate oxygen as necessary
           (b) If resuscitating with less than 100% oxygen, increase oxygen if no appreciable improvement within 90 seconds.
           (c) Use a pulse oximeter.
        (2) Ventilation
           (a) Avoid excessive pressures: peak inspiratory pressure and CPAP.
           (b) Consider CPAP if the heart rate >100 beats/min, spontaneous respirations with respiratory distress, and decreased pulse oximetry.
           (c) Elective endotracheal intubation.

      (3) Administration of surfactant. Presentation in the delivery room may range from mild respiratory distress to severe shock and cardiorespiratory arrest.

  d. Neuroprotection

      (1) Be as gentle as possible with the tiny neonate (i.e., drying, ventilating, and cardiopulmonary resuscitation).

      (2) Maintain head in midline positioning as much as possible.

      (3) Avoid iatrogenic hyperthermia.

      (4) Keep head of bed flat or elevated 15 to 30 degrees.

      (5) Infuse fluids slowly and cautiously.

      (6) Avoid delivering excess positive pressure or CPAP.

      (7) Use pulse oximeter and blood gases to adjust ventilation and oxygen concentration gradually and appropriately.

  e. Infection control

      (1) Implement strategies to reduce nosocomial infection (i.e., ventilator-associated pneumonia, catheter-related bloodstream infections).

      (2) Use sterile supplies (i.e., sterile water) when possible for very low birth weight infants.

      (3) Minimize use of tape and adhesives.

  f. Provide developmental care to promote physiologic stability.

  g. If at all possible, the family and the primary care physician, along with the neonatal team, should explore viability issues and expected outcome before the birth.

COMPLICATIONS OF RESUSCITATION

A. Trauma.

  1. Skin: bruises and abrasions from chest compressions, handling, and tape application and removal.

  2. Mucosa: laryngoscopy and intubation can cause trauma to and bleeding of the gums, lips, pharynx, and trachea.

  3. Internal organ damage from chest compressions.

B. Pulmonary air leaks.

  1. Pneumothorax.

  2. Pneumomediastinum.

  3. Pneumopericardium.

C. Complications related to the use of umbilical vessel catheters.

  1. Vessel perforation.

  2. Accidental blood loss.

  3. Thrombus and emboli.

  4. Intermittent vascular spasm.

  5. Organ and vessel endothelial damage from the infusion of hypertonic solutions.

  6. Organ ischemia from the blockage of major vessels by the catheter tip.

  7. Sepsis.

D. Intracranial hemorrhage.

  1. Subarachnoid.

  2. Periventricular.

  3. Intraventricular.

  4. Extracranial hemorrhage (i.e., subgaleal hemorrhage).

POSTRESUSCITATION CARE

The goal of postresuscitation care is to evaluate the infant's condition for complications, avoid intensifying conditions that may impair outcome (i.e., hypothermia, hypoglycemia), and help diagnose and treat underlying disease.

A. Assess oxygenation, ventilation, and acid-base balance.

  1. Check blood gas concentrations (capillary, arterial, and venous).

  2. Correlate findings with the neonate's clinical condition.

   3. Correlate findings with transcutaneous and/or pulse oximetry–monitoring devices.
   4. Adjust the neonate's respiratory and oxygen support as needed. Assess for increased or return of respiratory distress.
B. **Monitor glucose concentrations to ensure normoglycemia.**
   1. Serial screening of blood glucose.
   2. Treat hypoglycemia and adjust maintenance dextrose infusion if IV fluids are required. Bolus infusions ($D_{10}W$, 2 ml/kg) may be required to elevate serum glucose in addition to maintenance infusion.
   3. Feeding may not be recommended depending on infant's status.
C. **Volume and electrolyte support.**
   1. Assess perfusion and evaluate for anemia, polycythemia, and hypovolemia.
   2. Calculate the fluid volume received during resuscitation and estimate volume deficiencies.
   3. Determine the amount needed (in milliliters per kilogram per day).
   4. Adjust IV rate as needed. Include all fluids in fluid calculations.
   5. Monitor the urine output. Keep an accurate account of the intake.
D. **Chest and abdominal x-ray examination for pneumothorax, pneumomediastinum, pneumo-pericardium, and pneumoperitoneum.**
   1. Assess endotracheal tube position.
   2. Assess the position of umbilical catheters.
   3. Evaluate for lung and cardiac disease.
   4. Rule out fractures and anomalies.
E. **Monitor vital signs.**
   1. Provide a neutral thermal environment to prevent the sequelae of hypothermia or hyperthermia.
   2. Continue the assessment of perfusion and capillary refill in seconds.
   3. Monitor the blood pressure, preferably arterial.
   4. Continuous cardiorespiratory monitoring is recommended. Assess the heart rate and respiratory rate as needed.
   5. Monitor for seizure activity.
F. **Screen for infection.**
   1. Evaluate maternal history: titers, cultures, pretreatment, and risk factors.
   2. Obtain a complete blood cell count, differential cell count, platelet count, and C-reactive protein.
   3. Obtain blood, tracheal, and viral cultures and for sensitivity testing as indicated.
   4. If the index of suspicion is high and the neonate's condition is stable, lumbar puncture may be performed for cerebral spinal fluid analysis.
G. **Support family.**
   1. Provide a family-centered approach to care. Actively collaborate with family regarding decision making.
   2. Report the neonate's condition to mother and significant others.
   3. Make appropriate referrals to ancillary support services.
H. **Documentation.**
   1. Accurate charting including descriptive and often minute-by-minute documentation reveals the events, interventions, and infant responses to the resuscitative efforts.
   2. Include pertinent perinatal factors, physical findings, procedures and care performed, infant response, and team communication.
   3. Vital signs, medications, laboratory findings, and other factual data should also be included.
   4. Developmental support and the infant's behavioral response to care should be integrated into resuscitation and stabilization documentation.
I. **Safety**
   1. Ensure the neonate is accurately identified.
   2. Nurse-to-nurse communication should include a thorough history of resuscitation and stabilization.
   3. Reconcile medications if the neonate is transferred to another unit or another hospital.

J. Ethics.
   1. Collaboration with the family is essential with all decision making.
   2. Noninitiation or discontinuation of resuscitation may be appropriate in the delivery room when extreme prematurity or severe congenital anomalies are involved (i.e., confirmed trisomy 13 or 18, gestational age <23 weeks or birth weight <400 g; anencephaly).
   3. Information at or around the time of delivery is often incomplete. Resuscitative options may include initiation of therapy and reevaluation of treatment decision making after more information is available.
   4. Consult hospital ethics committee or legal counsel if needed.
K. Controversial therapies in resuscitation.
   1. Room air versus 100% oxygen in positive-pressure ventilation.
   2. Cerebral versus total body hypothermia for neonatal encephalopathy.

REFERENCES

American Academy of Pediatrics: 2005 American Heart Association (AHA) guidelines for cardiopulmonary resuscitation (CPR) and emergency cardiovascular care (ECC) of pediatric and neonatal patients: Neonatal resuscitation guidelines. *Pediatrics, 117*(5):e1029-e1038, 2006.

American Academy of Pediatrics and American College of Obstetricians and Gynecologists: *Guidelines for Perinatal Care* (6th ed.). Washington, DC, 2007, American Academy of Pediatrics and American College of Obstetricians and Gynecologists, p. 46.

American Academy of Pediatrics and American College of Obstetricians and Gynecologists: The Apgar score. *Pediatrics, 117*(4):1444-1448, 2006.

Kattwinkel, J. (Ed.): *Textbook of neonatal resuscitation* (5th ed.). Elk Grove Village, IL, 2006, American Academy of Pediatrics and American Heart Association.

Sayeed, S.A.: The marginally viable newborn: Legal challenges, conceptual inadequacies, and reasonableness. *Journal of Law, Medicine, & Ethics*, Fall:600-610, 2006.

6 Thermoregulation

M. COLLEEN BRAND and HOLLY A. BOYD

OBJECTIVES

1. Discuss the importance of thermoregulation in the care of newborn infants.
2. Identify newborns at increased risk for thermal instability.
3. Review symptoms of thermal stress in newborns.
4. Describe the physiologic processes involved in thermoregulation.
5. Compare mechanisms of heat transfer involved in newborn thermoregulation.
6. Apply strategies for managing the thermal environment.

Thermoregulation is a cornerstone in the care of newborn infants (Sherman et al., 2006). It is well known that keeping babies warm is key to the survival of sick newborns. In the 1950s, Silverman demonstrated that hypothermia increased morbidity and mortality (Silverman et al., 1958). The World Health Organization (WHO) recognizes thermoregulation of the newborn as a major threat to the health of newborns throughout the world ("Thermal Protection of the Newborn," 1997). Managing the thermal environment is crucial in caring for preterm infants and becomes increasingly important in care of the very low birthweight (VLBW) and the extremely low birthweight (ELBW) infant (Knobel and Holditch-Davis, 2007).

IDENTIFYING INFANTS AT RISK FOR THERMAL INSTABILITY

A. **Thermal instability.**
   The definition of thermal instability in the neonate is when body temperature is outside the expected normal range (Blake and Murray, 2006). Normal temperature ranges vary slightly depending on the resource, but in general the following ranges can be used.
   1. Axillary temperature 36.5° to 37.5° C (97.7° to 99.5° F) for term and 36.3° to 36.9° C (97.3° to 98.6° F) for preterm neonates (Blackburn, 2007; Blake and Murray, 2006; "Thermal Protection of the Newborn," 1997).
   2. Skin temperature 35.5° to 36.5° C (95.9° to 97.7° F) for term and 36.2° to 37.2° C (97.2° to 98.9° F) for preterm neonates (Blackburn, 2007).
B. **Temperature monitoring.**
   Accurate temperature measurements are important and a neonate's temperature can be measured by a variety of methods. The goal is measurement or estimation of core temperature. Rectal temperature should not be used routinely in neonates because of the risk of perforation and vagal stimulation (Blake and Murray, 2006; "Thermal Protection of the Newborn," 1997).
   1. Esophageal temperature monitoring is difficult to obtain and impractical for general temperature monitoring.
   2. Tympanic membrane thermometry is rapid and noninvasive, but accuracy in the unstable or very premature newborn population has not been established.
   3. Axillary temperatures are safe and easy to measure and correlate well with core temperature methods (Blake and Murray, 2006; "Thermal Protection of the Newborn," 1997). Disposable digital or electronic thermometers are used in most nurseries.
      a. The thermometer should be held in the midaxillary space for the time specified by the manufacturer.

   b. Ill neonates need axillary temperature measurements every 1 to 4 hours.
   c. Full-term, healthy neonates may be assessed every 4 to 8 hours.
   d. Continuous skin temperature monitoring is required for neonates using a servo-controlled mode in an incubator or radiant warming bed and may detect peripheral vasoconstriction as an early indication of cold stress (Blackburn, 2007).
      (1) Attach skin thermistors with insulated probe covers.
      (2) The neonate should not lie on the probe.
      (3) Avoid placing thermistors in areas of brown adipose tissue (BAT) such as the axilla.
      (4) Document incubator or radiant warming bed temperature simultaneously with all body temperature assessments.
      (5) Direct sunlight, phototherapy, or heat lamps increase the risk of hyperthermia.
      (6) A dislodged temperature probe may lead to hyperthermia. Current incubators and radiant warmers are equipped with safety alarms to alert staff to dislodged probes.
      (7) Never use a radiant warmer in the manual mode because of the risk of hyperthermia.
C. **Infants at risk for thermal instability.**
   1. Many infants are at risk for hypothermia because of large surface area, limited brown fat stores, decreased subcutaneous fat, limited glycogen stores, high transepidermal water loss and lack of muscle tone or activity (Blackburn, 2007; Knobel and Holditch-Davis, 2007; Mance, 2008). These risk factors are frequently found in infants with the following conditions.
      a. Prematurity.
      b. Small for gestational age.
      c. Central nervous system (CNS), endocrine, or cardiorespiratory abnormalities.
      d. Hypoglycemia, electrolyte imbalances, infection, or nutritional problems.
      e. Open skin defects (e.g., abdominal wall defects, neural tube defects).
      f. Exposure to neuromuscular blocking agents, analgesics, and/or anesthetics.
   2. Infants are at risk for hyperthermia because of their limited ability to dissipate heat (Baumgart, 2008; Blackburn, 2007).
      a. Iatrogenic overheating.
      b. Hypermetabolism (e.g., sepsis, cardiac problems, drug withdrawal).
      c. Infection.
      d. Dehydration.
      e. Medication effects (e.g., prostaglandin administration, immunizations).
      f. CNS injury or malformation (e.g., intraventricular hemorrhage, birth trauma, meningitis, spinal neurenteric cysts).
      g. Maternal fever (hyperthermia at delivery).
      h. Maternal epidural anesthesia.
      i. Use of excessive clothing or blankets.
D. **Symptoms of thermal stress in newborns, including hypothermia and hyperthermia, are presented in Box 6-1.**

PHYSIOLOGY OF THERMOREGULATION

A. **Like all mammals, infants are homeothermic, which means they have a physiologic response to changes in ambient temperature in an attempt to maintain a normal core temperature.** Despite this, the ability to maintain a normal temperature is limited. This is particularly true in premature and low birthweight newborns. The term *poikilothermic* is sometimes used to describe the response of premature infants to cold stress, meaning they are unable to maintain their core temperature above that of the environment (Baumgart, 2008).
B. **Thermoregulation is a balance of heat loss, heat gain, and heat production** (Blake and Murray, 2006). This gain or loss through heat transfer is dependent on the presence of a temperature gradient. Heat is transferred from higher to lower temperatures. The more premature, lower birth weight, and/or critically ill an infant is, the more likely it is that

■ BOX 6-1
■ **SYMPTOMS OF THERMAL STRESS IN NEWBORNS**

Hypothermia
- Apnea
- Bradycardia
- Central cyanosis
- Coagulation defects (i.e., pulmonary hemorrhage)
- Hypoglycemia
- Hypotonia
- Hypoxia
- Feeding Intolerance (abdominal distension, emesis, increased residuals)
- Increased metabolic rate
- Irritability
- Lethargy
- Metabolic acidosis
- Peripheral vasoconstriction (pallor, decreased capillary refill time)
- Poor weight gain (chronic hypothermia)
- Pulmonary vasoconstriction (persistent pulmonary hypertension of the newborn)
- Respiratory distress (decreased surfactant synthesis and activity)
- Shivering (mature neonates in presence of severe hypothermia)
- Weak cry or suck

Hyperthermia
- Apnea
- Central nervous system depression
- Dehydration (Increased insensible water loss)
- Flushed/red skin
- Hypernatremia
- Irritability
- Lethargy
- Poor feeding
- Seizures
- Sweating (term neonates)
- Tachycardia
- Tachypnea
- Warm to touch
- Weak or absent cry

Baumgart, S.: Iatrogenic hyperthermia and hypothermia in the neonate. *Clinics in Perinatology, 35*(1):183-197, 2008; Blackburn, S.: *Maternal, fetal, and neonatal physiology: A clinical perspective* (3rd ed.). St. Louis, 2007, Saunders, pp. 700-723; Mance, M.J.: Keeping infants warm: Challenges of hypothermia. *Advances in Neonatal Care, 8*(1):6-12, 2008.

thermoregulation will be a problem. It is important that caregivers understand the principles of thermoregulation and intervene to maintain a neutral thermal environment for the infant.

1. Physical methods of heat production or conservation (Blackburn, 2007; Blake and Murray, 2006).
    a. Shivering is the mainstay of heat production in adults; neonates rarely shiver and then, only after prolonged cold stress.
    b. Increased muscular activity from restlessness, hyperactivity, or crying may be seen in healthy term neonates.
    c. Posture may increase or decrease surface area.
2. Nonshivering thermogenesis is the newborn's main method for generating heat (Baumgart, 2008; Blackburn, 2007; Blake and Murray, 2006).
    a. It indicates heat production through the metabolism of BAT.

  b. BAT metabolism is stimulated by thermal receptors in the skin that are most prominent over the trigeminal area of the face.
  - (1) These thermal receptors stimulate the hypothalamus, which controls heat production.

  c. Thermogenin, a protein found in BAT mitochondria, regulates BAT metabolism.
  - (1) The major function is anaerobic heat production, which requires both oxygen and glucose.

  d. Metabolism of BAT releases nonesterified fatty acids that compete with bilirubin for albumin-binding sites.

  e. Properties of BAT (Baumgart, 2008; Blackburn, 2007).
  - (1) Located in the mediastinum, around the great vessels, kidneys, adrenal glands, axilla, nape of the neck, and between the scapulas.
  - (2) A heavy concentration of blood vessels gives BAT its characteristic brown color and serves to conduct heat into the circulation.
  - (3) Production begins at 26 to 28 weeks of gestation.
  - (4) Stores increase until 3 to 5 weeks postnatal age.
  - (5) A reduced quantity is available in preterm infants.
  - (6) Cannot be replenished once used.

3. Subcutaneous fat provides insulation (Blackburn, 2007).
  a. Heat transfer from neonatal organs to the skin surface is increased because of the neonate's decreased subcutaneous (SQ) fat.
  b. SQ fat accounts for only 16% of the body fat in neonates, compared with approximately 30% in adults.
  c. The more premature or SGA the infant, the less SQ fat is available.

4. Increased surface-area-to-weight ratio allows for heat transfer to the environment (Blackburn, 2007).
  a. Term neonates have 3 times the surface-area-to-weight ratio as adults.
  b. Preterm neonates have 5 times the surface-area-to-weight ratio as adults and this ratio is even higher in ELBW infants.
  c. Full-term neonates can decrease heat loss from exposed body surfaces by assuming a flexed position.
  d. Preterm neonates have a limited ability to maintain body flexion.
  e. Critically ill or sedated neonates often lie in an extended position unless positioned by caregivers.

5. Transepidermal water loss (TEWL) increases heat loss through evaporation. The more immature the infant, the greater the degree of TEWL (Blake and Murray, 2006).

6. Norepinephrine is released in response to cold stress (Blackburn, 2007).
  a. Peripheral vasoconstriction is triggered in an attempt to decrease heat loss.
  b. Nonshivering thermogenesis is stimulated, which leads to
  - (1) Consumption of BAT,
  - (2) Depletion of glycogen stores, and
  - (3) Increased oxygen consumption.
  - (4) Lactic acid production results in metabolic acidosis, which leads to
    - (a) Pulmonary vasoconstriction and
    - (b) Decreased blood flow to vital organs (shock).

MECHANISMS OF HEAT TRANSFER

A. Heat transfer occurs between the neonate and the environment through four mechanisms (Blake and Murray, 2006; Mance, 2008).
  1. Conduction: heat transfer via direct contact.
  a. Heat loss occurs when neonates come in contact with any cold surface, such as a mattress, x-ray plate, or scale.
  b. Heat gain occurs when neonates come in contact with surfaces warmer than the body, such as a chemical warming mattress or warm blankets.

    c. The heat transfer rate varies with the temperature gradient and the amount of skin contacting the surface.

    d. Conduction of heat occurs more rapidly from the skin to a metal object than from the skin to a cloth surface.

  2. Convection: heat transfer via air currents.

    a. This is the mode of heat transfer that provides heat gain in incubators.

    b. Heat transfer increases with

      (1) An increased temperature gradient between skin and air,

      (2) Increased air flow, and

      (3) An increase in the skin surface area that is exposed to the air.

  3. Radiation: heat transfer of radiant energy without direct contact through absorption and emission of infrared rays.

    a. This is the mode of heat transfer used by radiant warming beds.

    b. Transfer depends on

      (1) The temperature gradient,

      (2) Surface absorptive properties, and

      (3) The distance and angle between the skin surface area and the heat source.

    c. Transfer is independent of

      (1) Ambient temperature,

      (2) Airflow, and

      (3) Other heat loss mechanisms.

        (a) Accounts for a major source of incubator heat loss if the incubator walls are cooler than the body. Conversely, a greenhouse effect can occur if an incubator is placed in sunlight, because of the transmission of heat from the sun through the incubator walls.

  4. Evaporation: heat loss by conversion of liquid into vapor.

    a. Rate of heat transfer depends on air speed and relative humidity.

    b. Evaporation of amniotic fluid accounts for 25% of neonatal heat loss at delivery. Heat loss occurs at a rate of 0.5° F (0.3° C)/minute, resulting in 3° to 4° C (5° F) decrease in temperature over 10 minutes (Blackburn, 2007; Dahm and James, 1972).

    c. High total body water content, immature skin, and relatively large body surface-area-to-weight ratio in preterm neonates increase evaporative heat loss. This is more significant in VLBW and ELBW infants.

    d. Increased activity, tachypnea (through respiratory insensible water loss), and radiant warming beds augment loss.

    e. Halogen phototherapy increases evaporative heat loss through increased TEWL (Grunhagen et al., 2002).

STRATEGIES FOR MANAGING THERMOREGULATION

A. Hypothermia is the predominant thermoregulatory problem of newborns. It is exaggerated in premature infants and becomes significantly more critical as the gestational age and birth weight decrease. Management is dependent on being proactive and using measures to reduce heat loss before hypothermia occurs, then providing a neutral thermal environment (NTE) to maintain normothermia. Once hypothermia or hyperthermia occurs, it is imperative to take appropriate measures to correct the problem.

  1. NTE is the ideal environmental temperature in which body temperature is maintained within a normal range while the metabolic rate, and thus oxygen and glucose consumption, is minimal (Baumgart, 2008; Blackburn, 2007; Hey, 1969; Mance, 2008). The NTE table (Table 6-1) offers a starting point of temperature ranges based on age and weight but should then be adjusted according to the needs of individual infants. Premature infants weighing <800 g are not represented in this table and should have a starting incubator temperature of 36.5° C (97.7° F) (Blake and Murray, 2006).

  2. Strategies to decrease heat loss.

    a. Reduce conductive heat loss.

      (1) Use warm blankets at delivery.

■ TABLE 6-1
■ ■ **Neutral Thermal Environmental Temperatures**

Age and Weight	Range of Temperature (° C)	Age and Weight	Range of Temperature (° C)
0 to 6 hours		72 to 96 hours	
<1200 g	34 to 35.4	<1200 g	34 to 35
1200 to 1500 g	33.9 to 34.4	1200 to 1500 g	33 to 34
1501 to 2500 g	32.8 to 33.8	1501 to 2500 g	31.1 to 33.2
>2500 g	32 to 33.8	>2500 g	29.8 to 32.8
6 to 12 hours		4 to 12 days	
<1200 g	34 to 35.4	<1500 g	33 to 34
1200 to 1500 g	33.5 to 34.4	1501 to 2500 g	31 to 33.2
1501 to 2500 g	32.2 to 33.8	>2500 g	
>2500 g	31.4 to 33.8	4 to 5 days	29.5 to 32.6
12 to 24 hours		5 to 6 days	29.4 to 32.3
<1200 g	34 to 35.4	6 to 8 days	29 to 32.2
1200 to 1500 g	33.3 to 34.3	8 to 10 days	29 to 31.8
1501 to 2500 g	31.8 to 33.8	10 to 12 days	29 to 31.4
>2500 g	31 to 33.7	12 to 14 days	
24 to 36 hours		<1500 g	32.6 to 34
<1200 g	34 to 35	1501 to 2500 g	31 to 33.2
1200 to 1500 g	33.1 to 34.2	>2500 g	29 to 30.8
1501 to 2500 g	31.6 to 33.6	2 to 3 weeks	
>2500 g	30.7 to 33.5	<1500 g	32.2 to 34
36 to 48 hours		1501 to 2500 g	30.5 to 33
<1200 g	34 to 35	3 to 4 weeks	
1200 to 1500 g	33 to 34.1	<1500 g	31.6 to 33.6
1501 to 2500 g	31.4 to 33.5	1501 to 2500 g	30 to 32.7
>2500 g	30.5 to 33.3	4 to 5 weeks	
48 to 72 hours		<1500 g	31.2 to 33
<1200 g	34 to 35	1501 to 2500 g	29.5 to 32.2
1200 to 1500 g	33 to 34	5 to 6 weeks	
1501 to 2500 g	31.2 to 33.4	<1500 g	30.6 to 32.3
>2500 g	30.1 to 33.2	1501 to 2500 g	29 to 31.8

Adapted from Scopes, J.W. and Ahmed, I.: Range of critical temperatures in sick and premature babies. *Archives of Disease in Childhood, 41*:417, 1966. For their table, Scopes and Ahmed had the walls of the incubator 1° to 2° C warmer than the ambient air temperatures.
Generally speaking, the smaller infants in each weight group will require a temperature in the higher portion of the temperature range. Within each time range, the younger the infant, the higher the temperature required. All infants who weighed more than 2500 g were born at more than 36 weeks of gestation.
From Klaus, M.H. and Fanaroff, A.A.: *Care of the high-risk neonate* (5th ed.). Philadelphia, 2001, Saunders.

(2) Preheat surfaces for delivery room resuscitation.
(3) Warm cold scales or use warmed cover on scales.
(4) Cover x-ray plates with warmed linen.
(5) Warm incubator mattress, linens, clothing, and diapers prior to use.
(6) Avoid placing neonates directly on a warming surface to prevent burns.
(7) Warm the stethoscope and hands prior to examining the neonate or performing care.
(8) Use an appropriately warmed, chemically activated mattress in the delivery room, on transport, or during special procedures (Almeida et al., 2000; Blake and Murray, 2006).
(9) Encourage parental skin-to-skin (kangaroo) care (Baumgart, 2008; "Thermal Protection of the Newborn," 1997).

   b. Reduce convective heat loss.

     (1) Warm delivery room to >26° C (78.8° F) (Knobel et al., 2005).

     (2) Keep ambient temperature of nursery/neonatal intensive care unit (NICU) warm, 72° to 78° F (22° to 26° C) (American Academy of Pediatrics and American College of Obstetricians and Gynecologists, 2007).

     (3) Transport neonates in an enclosed incubator.

     (4) Work inside incubator via portholes.

     (5) Use plastic sleeves on portholes according to manufacturer guidelines.

     (6) Maintain flexed position with bunting or positioning aids.

     (7) Avoid drafts.

     (8) Use transparent plastic across radiant warming bed sides to decrease airflow across bed.

     (9) Use a knit cap made of some insulating material other than stockinette, which is ineffective for reducing convective heat loss. Consider using a knit cap

       (a) In the delivery room, once the head is thoroughly dry;

       (b) When the infant is being held; and

       (c) When the infant is being weaned from the incubator.

     (10) Warm all gas sources (e.g., oxygen).

   c. Reduce evaporative heat loss.

     (1) Thoroughly dry neonate at delivery.

     (2) Replace wet towels with warm, dry ones.

     (3) Delay initial bath until the temperature has stabilized ("Thermal Protection of the Newborn," 1997).

       (a) Provide an additional heat source during bath.

       (b) Bathe only in a draft-free area.

       (c) Bathe one body part, dry it, then proceed to another body part.

     (4) Humidify oxygen.

   d. Reduce heat loss by radiation.

     (1) Prewarm the radiant warmer or incubator

     (2) Prewarm ventilator circuits.

     (3) Do not place incubators/beds near cold outer walls.

     (4) Consider thermal window blinds and incubator covers (Fig. 6-1).

     (5) Use double-walled incubators.

     (6) Cover transport incubator with thermal shield (Fig. 6-2).

     (7) Use clothing inside incubator to decrease exposed surface area and provide thermal insulation.

3. Additional considerations for managing VLBW and ELBW infants:

   a. Use of a polyethylene bag or wrap helps prevent hypothermia by decreasing evaporative water loss and to a lesser degree conductive heat loss if used immediately after delivery. Polyethylene transmits energy wavelengths produced by radiant warmers (Knobel and Holditch-Davis, 2007; Knobel et al., 2005; LeBlanc, 1991; Lund et al., 2007; Mance, 2008; "Summary of Major Changes," 2005; Vohra et al., 1999, 2004). Polyethylene bags should be

     (1) Used in patients less than 28 weeks of gestation or less than 1500 g;

     (2) Applied immediately after birth and before drying, leaving the infant's head (and therefore access to the airway) open; head and face should be dried thoroughly and cap applied; and

     (3) Removed once the infant is placed in a warm environment in the nursery.

   b. Transfer from warming bed to incubator once admission procedures are completed.

   c. Consider use of a hybrid incubator (an incubator that converts from warming bed to incubator at the touch of a button.

   d. Humidification may be required to maintain an NTE for VLBW and ELBW infants (Blackburn, 2007; Hammarlund and Sedin, 1979; Harpin and Rutter, 1985; Knobel and Holditch-Davis, 2007; Lund et al., 2007; Mance, 2008).

     (1) Humidification reduces TEWL and therefore evaporative heat loss.

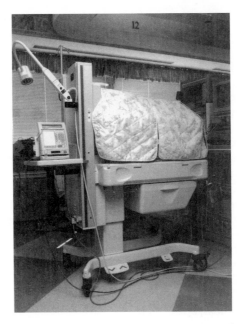

FIGURE 6-1 ■ Incubator with cover. Covering the incubator decreases radiant heat loss, a major factor in incubator use. (Courtesy Barbara Noerr, Palmyra, PA.)

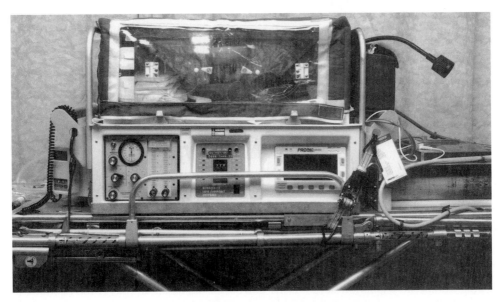

FIGURE 6-2 ■ Thermal cover on a neonatal transport incubator. The thermal cover decreases radiant heat loss. Prevention of radiant heat loss is important during external transports in cold climates. (Courtesy Barbara Noerr, Palmyra, PA.)

(2) This can be accomplished by humidifying incubators or adding humidity to a polyethylene tent under a radiant warming bed.

(3) Provide humidity at 70% to 90% for the first 7 days of life (Lund et al., 2007).

(4) Some recommendations have emerged that indicate humidity should be reduced to 50% during the second week of life as humidity may slow maturation of the skin (Agren et al., 2006).

(5) Plexiglas heat shields should not be used under the radiant warming bed as heat may build up because of a greenhouse effect (Blackburn, 2007).

    e. Occlusive barriers applied to the skin reduce TEWL and therefore evaporative heat loss, but must be removed like other adhesives and may cause skin breakdown (Lund et al., 2007).

    f. Emollients may be beneficial in decreasing evaporative heat loss, but study results remain mixed as to whether there is an increased risk of infection related to their use (Lund and Kuller, 2007).

4. Rewarming when hypothermia occurs should begin immediately (Blake and Murray, 2006).

    a. An external heat source should be provided.

    b. Any avenue of heat loss should be stopped.

    c. Rewarm slowly, about 0.5° C (0.9° F) per hour to avoid apnea, tachycardia, and overheating (Baumgart, 2008; Blake and Murray, 2006).

    d. The reason for hypothermia should be investigated.

5. Typically hyperthermia in the neonate is iatrogenic, and while hyperthermia occurs less often than hypothermia, it can be just as dangerous (Baumgart, 2008; Blake and Murray, 2006; "Thermal Protection of the Newborn," 1997).

    a. Evaluate for environmental cause, and if present,

      (1) Move away from heat source or if in an incubator lower the temperature,

      (2) Partially undress and uncover infant,

      (3) Remove positioning devices and allow extended posture to increase skin exposure and allow heat loss, and

      (4) Bathe using warm water (slightly cooler than skin temperature).

    b. Evaluate for dehydration and weight loss.

    c. Consider systemic infection as well as localized infection such as cellulitis, septic arthritis, osteomyelitis, omphalitis, and mastitis.

6. Weaning from a thermal controlled environment (incubator) is an essential stride in preparation for discharge to home. Potentially, weight gain will slow because of the increased energy expenditure shown to occur when an infant is weaned from an incubator (Dohlberg et al., 2004). Successful weaning is likely to occur when the following conditions are present (Blake and Murray, 2006):

    a. Weight is at least 1500 g.

    b. Has had at least five consecutive days of weight gain.

    c. Is tolerating feedings.

    d. Is free of major medical conditions.

    e. Proceed with weaning over at least a day.

    f. Fully dress and swaddle the neonate inside the incubator.

    g. Decrease the incubator temperature slowly.

    h. Assess the neonate's temperature frequently.

    i. Once weaned to an open crib, keep the neonate away from drafts and monitor body weight daily.

Summary

Managing the thermoregulation needs of the newborn is an essential role of the neonatal nurse. In addition, thermoregulation in the VLBW and ELBW infant presents a complex challenge because of their physical characteristics and immaturity and require specific knowledge and attention to detail.

REFERENCES

Agren, J., Sjors, G., and Sedin, G.: Ambient humidity influences the rate of skin barrier maturation in extremely preterm infants. *Journal of Pediatrics,* *148*(5):613-617, 2006.

Almeida, B., Chandley, J., and Rubin, L.: Improving admission temperature of very low birthweight newborn: An interventional trial. *Pediatric Research,* *47:* 282A, 2000.

American Academy of Pediatrics and American College of Obstetricians and Gynecologists: *Guidelines of perinatal care* (6th ed.). Elk Grove Village, IL, 2007, American Academy of Pediatrics and American College of Obstetricians and Gynecologists, p. 60.

Baumgart, S.: Iatrogenic hyperthermia and hypothermia in the neonate. *Clinics in Perinatology, 35*(1):183-197, 2008.

Blackburn, S.: *Maternal, fetal, and neonatal physiology: A clinical perspective* (3rd ed.). St. Louis, 2007, Saunders, pp. 700-723.

Blake, W. and Murray, J.: Heat balance. In G.B. Merenstein and S.L. Gardner (Eds.): *Handbook of neonatal intensive care.* St. Louis, 2006, Mosby, pp. 122-138.

Dahm, L.S. and James, L.S.: Newborn temperature and calculated heat loss in the delivery room. *Pediatrics, 49*:504-512, 1972.

Dohlberg, S., Mimouni, F.B., and Weintraub, V.: Energy expenditure in infants weaned from a convective incubator. *American Journal of Perinatology, 21*:253-256, 2004.

Grunhagen, D.J., De Boer, M.G.J., DeBeaufort, A.J., and Walther, F.J.: Transepidermal water loss during halogen spotlight phototherapy in preterm infants. *Pediatric Research, 51*(3):402-405, 2002.

Hammarlund, K. and Sedin, G.: Transepidermal water loss in newborn infants, III: Relation to gestational age. *Acta Paediatrica Scandinavica, 68*(6):795-801, 1979.

Harpin, V.A. and Rutter, N.: Humidification of incubators. *Archives of Disease in Childhood, 60*(3):219-224, 1985.

Hey, E.N.: The relation between environmental temperature and oxygen consumption in the new-born baby. *Journal of Physiology, 200*(3):589-603, 1969.

Knobel, R. and Holditch-Davis, D.: Thermoregulation and heat loss prevention after birth and during neonatal intensive care unit stabilization of extremely low-birthweight infants. *Journal of Obstetric, Gynecologic and Neonatal Nursing, 36*(3):280-287, 2007.

Knobel, R.B., Vohra, S., and Lehmann, C.U.: Heat loss prevention in the delivery room for preterm infants: A national survey of newborn intensive care units. *Journal of Perinatology, 25*(8):514-518, 2005.

LeBlanc, M.H.: Thermoregulation: Incubators, radiant warmers, artificial skins, and body hoods. *Clinics in Perinatology, 18*(3):403-422, 1991.

Lund, C. and Kuller, J.: Integumentary system. In C. Kenner and J.W. Lott (Eds.): *Comprehensive neonatal care: An interdisciplinary approach* (4th ed.). St. Louis, 2007, Saunders, pp. 65-91.

Lund, C.H., Kuller, J., Raines, D., Ecklund, S., Archambault, M.E., and O'Flaherty, P.: *Neonatal skin care: Evidence based guidelines* (2nd ed.). Washington, DC, 2007, Association of Women's Health, Obstetric and Neonatal Nurses.

Mance, M.J.: Keeping infants warm: Challenges of hypothermia. *Advances in Neonatal Care, 8*(1):6-12, 2008.

Sherman, T.I., Greenspan, J.S., St. Clair, N., Touch, S.M., and Shaffer, T.H.: Optimizing the neonatal thermal environment. *Neonatal Network, 25*(4):251-260, 2006.

Silverman, W.A., Fertig, J.W., and Berger, A.P.: The influence of the thermal environment upon the survival of newly born premature infants. *Pediatrics, 22*(5):876-886, 1958.

Summary of major changes to the 2005 AAP/AHA emergency cardiovascular care guidelines for neonatal resuscitation: Translating evidence-based guidelines to the NRP. *NRP Instructor Update, 15*, 2005. Retrieved from http://www.aap.org/nrp/pdf/nrp-summary.pdf **Accessed October 6, 2008.**

Thermal protection of the newborn: a practical guide, 1997. Retrieved August 22, 2008, from http://www.who.int/reproductive-health/publications/MSM_97_2_Thermal_protection_of_the_newborn/thermal_protection_newborn2.pdf

Vohra, S., Frent, G., Campbell, V., Abbott, M., and Whyte, R: Effect of polyethylene occlusive skin wrapping on heat loss in very low birth weight infants at delivery: A randomized trial. *Journal of Pediatrics, 134*(5):547-551, 1999.

Vohra, S., Roberts, R.S., Zhang, B., Janes, M., and Schmidt, B.: Heat loss prevention (HeLP) in the delivery room: A randomized controlled trial of polyethylene occlusive skin wrapping in very preterm infants. *Journal of Pediatrics, 145*(6):750-753, 2004.

7 Physical Assessment

SUSAN ARANA FURDON and KATHLEEN BENJAMIN

OBJECTIVES

1. Review key aspects of the perinatal history as it relates to physical assessment of the newborn.
2. Describe methods of determining gestational age (GA).
3. Relate growth pattern and maturity to classification of newborns by GA and weight.
4. Describe a systematic approach in the examination of the newborn infant.

■■ A comprehensive newborn physical examination requires a synthesis of perinatal and neo-natal risk factors with a systematic approach to the examination. An understanding of growth, maturity, and GA risk factors provides a framework for defining wellness or subsequent problems. The nurse is in a unique position of providing a detailed observation and description within the context of these factors.

PERINATAL HISTORY (SEE CHAPTERS 1, 2, 3, AND 4)

Elements of a perinatal history focus on the relationship of maternal medical condition and the overall growth and maturity of the infant. Communication from obstetric staff to pediatric staff of fetal anomalies and risk factors for abnormal growth or fetal well-being is essential.

A. **Family history.**
   1. Known inherited diseases/conditions: http://www.nlm.nih.gov/medlineplus/geneticdisorders.html.
      a. Cystic fibrosis, Down syndrome (translocation only), fragile X syndrome, cleft lip/palate, neural tube defects, dwarfism and osteogenesis imperfecta, muscular dystrophy.
      b. Hereditary anemia: sickle cell anemia, thalassemia.
      c. Genetic brain disorder: leukodystrophy, phenylketonuria, Tay-Sachs disease, Wilson disease.
   2. Chronic disorders or disabilities: diabetes, hypertension, mental retardation, cardiac lesions, renal disease, and seizures.
B. **Maternal medical history.**
   1. General health: age, body mass index, physical activity, diet, and exposure to potential teratogens.
   2. Chronic illness: diabetes, cardiac disease, hypertension, asthma, thyroid disorder, systemic lupus erythematosus, herpes simplex virus, and anxiety/depression disorder.
   3. Surgical procedures and hospitalizations.
   4. Medications before and during pregnancy.
C. **Obstetric history.**
   1. History of infertility: abnormal uterine structure, hormonal imbalance, and treatment.
   2. Previous pregnancies (gravida): number of live born, term versus preterm, spontaneous or elective abortions.
   3. Birth weight(s) of live born and neonatal problems identified.
   4. Previous fetal demise or neonatal death(s): age of infant and reason for death.
D. **Social history:** early identification of family stressors or support and barriers to teaching.
   1. Marital status and consanguinity.

2. Financial support, socioeconomic status, and education level.
3. Tobacco, alcohol, and illicit drug use.
4. History of depression.
5. Domestic violence.
6. Religious and cultural considerations.
7. Factors affecting teaching.
   a. Primary language.
   b. Sensory deficits.
E. **Pregnancy history.**
   1. Prenatal care: timing of first visit, compliance to follow-up.
   2. Estimated date of confinement.
      a. Last menstrual period.
      b. Ultrasound dating.
      c. Birth date calculator (wheel).
   3. Single vs. multiple gestation.
   4. Weight gain and nutritional status.
   5. Blood group incompatibility and risk for isoimmunization: maternal blood type and Rh status.
      a. antepartum administration of Rho(D) immunoglobulin prophylaxis for D negative blood group.
      b. positive antibody screen (examples: Cc, Ee, Kell, and Duffy).
      c. serial fetal surveillance for positive isoimmunization status: antibody titers, ultrasounds, amniocentesis, fetal transfusion.
   6. Maternal serum screening: triple or quad screen.
   7. GBS culture at 35 to 37 weeks of gestation.
   8. Congenital infection: rubella, syphilis, cytomegalovirus, hepatitis, human immunodeficiency virus, herpes simplex virus, human papillomavirus, chlamydia, gonorrhea, and parvovirus. Congenital West Nile Virus has also been reported (O'Leary et al., 2006).
   9. Maternal diabetes.
      a. gestational or type 1.
      b. classification.
      c. glucose control.
   10. Hypertensive disorders.
       a. gestational hypertension (formerly called pregnancy-induced hypertension [PIH]).
       b. preeclampsia/eclampsia.
       c. chronic hypertension.
       d. hemolysis, elevated liver enzymes, and low platelet count (HELLP syndrome).
   11. Abnormal fetal growth: fundal height, serial ultrasounds.
       a. Intrauterine growth restriction (IUGR) factors: multiple maternal, placental, uterine, and fetal factors limit intrauterine growth potential (Breeze & Lees, 2007; Lawrence, 2006).
          (1) Previous small-for-gestational-age (SGA) or IUGR baby.
          (2) Age greater than 35 or less than 16 years, single marital status, low socioeconomic status.
          (3) Malnutrition, low pregnancy weight gain, active Crohn disease, untreated celiac disease.
          (4) Unexplained history of miscarriage or stillbirth (fetal loss at greater than 20 weeks of gestation).
          (5) Multiple gestation.
          (6) Tobacco exposure.
             (a) Nicotine releases catecholamines, reduces prostacyclin synthesis.
             (b) Vasoconstriction and increased vascular resistance decreases placental delivery of nutrients and oxygen.
             (c) Associated with placental abruption and late fetal death.
             (d) IUGR rates 3 to 4.5 times that for nonsmokers.

(7) Hypertensive/vascular disorders causing placental insufficiency.
  (a) Chronic hypertension. Incidence 4 times greater, with severe versus mild hypertension.
  (b) Preeclampsia.
  (c) Advanced diabetes mellitus.
  (d) Placental or umbilical cord abnormalities or disruption.
(8) Chronic renal failure.
(9) Congenital infections: toxoplasmosis, rubella, cytomegalovirus, and herpes virus (TORCH); cytomegalovirus most common association.
(10) Congenital malformations and chromosomal abnormalities.
  b. Large-for-gestational-age (LGA) infant (Lawrence, 2007).
  (1) Maternal race.
  (2) Maternal diabetes.
  (3) Obesity.
  (4) Previous LGA infant.
12. Fetal anomaly: ultrasound, fetal echocardiography (ECHO), and amniocentesis.
13. Placental or vascular abnormality:
  a. abnormal cord insertion: accreta, velamentous.
  b. abnormal umbilical artery Doppler studies: reverse end-diastolic flow, increased middle cerebral flow velocity.
  c. twin-to-twin transfusion.
14. Amniotic fluid volume: polyhydramnios and oligohydramnios.
15. Recurrent urinary tract infections.
F. Labor and delivery.
  1. History of presenting problem.
    a. Labor: preterm labor, post dates.
    b. bleeding.
    c. acute abdominal pain.
    d. hypertension.
    e. trauma.
  2. Infection risks:
    a. Symptoms of chorioamnionitis: maternal or fetal tachycardia, maternal fever ≥100.4° F, uterine tenderness, elevated maternal white blood cell (WBC) count.
    b. Group B streptococcus (GBS) (Winn, 2007).
  3. Risk factors that increase neonatal early-onset GBS infection: preterm premature rupture of membranes (PPROM), prolonged rupture of membranes >18 hours.
  4. Intrapartum chemoprophylaxis for GBS colonization.
    a. Preterm labor with intact membranes is associated with occult intraamniotic infection (American Academy of Pediatrics and the American College of Obstetricians and Gynecologists [AAP/ACOG], 2007).
  5. Fetal lung maturity.
    a. Less than 5% risk of respiratory distress syndrome if mature fetal lung maturity test after 34 weeks of gestation.
    b. Antenatal corticosteroids administered for anticipated preterm delivery at <34 weeks of gestation are effective in decreasing neonatal morbidity and mortality (AAP/ACOG, 2007).
    c. Optimal benefit of glucocorticosteroid: 24 hours after administration for up to 7 days; may be beneficial at <24 hours of treatment (AAP, ACOG Perinatal Guidelines, 2007).
  6. Spontaneous vs. induced labor, indication for induction of labor
  7. Cord prolapse.
  8. Fetal distress and nonreassuring fetal heart tracing.
  9. Analgesic and anesthetic prior to and at delivery.
  10. Mode of delivery: vaginal, cesarean, assisted (forceps and vacuum); indication for cesarean.
  11. Presentation: vertex, breech, brow, chin, and arm.

12. Appearance of amniotic fluid.
    a. Clear: normal.
    b. Green: meconium stained.
    c. Yellow: old meconium, old blood, and sepsis.
    d. Cloudy: sepsis.
13. Shoulder dystocia (Benjamin, 2005).
    a. Multifactorial:
       (1) Maternal risk factors: uterine abnormalities, diabetes, maternal body proportions.
       (2) Infant risk factors: macrosomia, transverse lie, poor tone, 5-minute Apgar <5.
    b. Intrapartum events:
       (1) Mechanical forces of labor alone.
       (2) Vaginal breech delivery/operative vaginal delivery.
       (3) Prolonged duration of labor.
       (4) Precipitous delivery.
       (5) Prolonged head-to-body interval at delivery.
G. **Newborn resuscitation (see Chapter 5).**

GESTATIONAL-AGE INSTRUMENTS

The principal basis for use of GA instruments is that fetal maturity follows a predictable, organized course and that characteristics are common to a given GA (Sansoucie and Cavaliere, 2007).

A. **General considerations.**
   1. Use neonatal assessment tools from birth to 5 days, before physical characteristics change.
   2. Perform within 48 hours of birth for highest accuracy.
   3. Consider problems with accuracy of gestational-age assessments for periviable fetus at 22 to 26 weeks of gestation when making treatment or withdrawal of care decisions (Higgins et al., 2005).
B. **Most common tools.**
   1. Dubowitz: clinical assessment of GA (Dubowitz et al., 1970).
      a. Scores criteria: 10 neurologic and 11 external (physical).
      b. Combined total score correlated to weeks of gestation.
      c. Combined score has higher correlation (±2 weeks, 95% confidence) than either component separately.
      d. SGA infants: external signs underscored and neurologic signs overscored; combined score reliable.
   2. Ballard: newborn maturity rating.
      a. Simplified system based on Dubowitz's method, less time to use.
      b. Eliminates active tone scoring, passive tone more useful than active tone.
      c. Six neurologic and six physical criteria, scores totaled.
      d. GA maturity rating assigned using form chart.
   3. New Ballard Score (Ballard et al., 1991).
      a. Modified to assess GA of 20 to 44 weeks.
      b. Accurate within 2 weeks of gestation; sick or well infants.
      c. For 20 to 26 weeks of gestation: most accurate when scored within first 12 hours of life.
      d. Limitations.
         (1) Examination should be done twice by two different examiners for objectivity.
         (2) Infant must be in a quiet, alert state.
         (3) Scoring affected by
            (a) Breech and positional deformities,
            (b) Neurologic disorders and asphyxia, and
            (c) Infants affected by maternal medications.

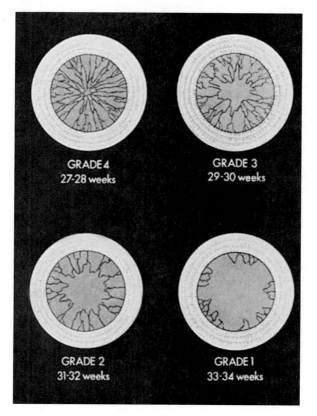

GRADE 4
27-28 weeks

GRADE 3
29-30 weeks

GRADE 2
31-32 weeks

GRADE 1
33-34 weeks

FIGURE 7-1 ■ Grading system for assessment of gestational age by examination of anterior vascular capsule of lens. (From Hittner, H.M., Hirsch, N.J., and Rudolph, A.J.: Assessment of gestational age by examination of the anterior vascular capsule of the lens. *Journal of Pediatrics, 91*[3]:455-458, 1977.)

    4. Embryonic vessels on the lens: from 27 to 34 weeks of gestation, examination of the anterior vascular capsule of the lens is helpful in determining GA by examining the level of remaining embryonic vessels on the lens (Fig. 7-1).

C. GA examination (Fig. 7-2): Use the chart for scoring each criterion.

    1. Technique for assessment of neurologic criteria.

      a. Posture.

        (1) Evaluates degree of arm and leg flexion and extension and leg abduction.

        (2) Flexion and hip adduction increases with increasing GA.

        (3) Early in gestation the infant's resting posture is hypotonic.

        (4) Observe infant's posture while supine and quiet.

      b. Square window.

        (1) Evaluates flexion when the wrist is at a right angle to the forearm.

        (2) Angle decreases with increasing GA because of the influence of maternal hormones at the end of pregnancy.

        (3) Findings do not change after birth.

        (4) Flex infant's hand on the forearm between examiner's thumb and index finger. Use sufficient pressure to get full flexion. Visually measure angle between hypothenar eminence and ventral aspect of forearm.

      c. Arm recoil.

        (1) Evaluates degree of arm flexion and the strength of recoil.

        (2) Place infant supine, flex arms for 5 seconds, then fully extend arms by pulling the hands downward, then release.

      d. Popliteal angle.

        (1) The angle decreases with increasing GA.

NEUROMUSCULAR MATURITY

	−1	0	1	2	3	4	5
Posture							
Square Window (wrist)	>90°	90°	60°	45°	30°	0°	
Arm Recoil		180°	140°−180°	110°−140°	90°−110°	<90°	
Popliteal Angle	180°	160°	140°	120°	100°	90°	<90°
Scarf Sign							
Heel to Ear							

SCORE

Neuro-
muscular _____
Physical _____
Total _____

PHYSICAL MATURITY

Skin	sticky friable transparent	gelatinous red, translucent	smooth pink, visible veins	superficial peeling &/or rash, few veins	cracking pale areas rare veins	parchment deep cracking no vessels	leathery cracked wrinkled
Lanugo	none	sparse	abundant	thinning	bald areas	mostly bald	
Plantar Surface	heel–toe 40-50 mm: −1 <40 mm: −2	>50 mm no crease	faint red marks	anterior transverse crease only	creases ant. 2/3	creases over entire sole	
Breast	imperceptible	barely perceptible	flat areola no bud	stippled areola 1-2 mm bud	raised areola 3-4 mm bud	full areola 5-10 mm bud	
Eye/Ear	lids fused loosely: −1 tightly: −2	lids open pinna flat stays folded	sl. curved pinna; soft; slow recoil	well-curved pinna; soft but ready recoil	formed & firm instant recoil	thick cartilage ear stiff	
Genitals male	scrotum flat, smooth	scrotum empty faint rugae	testes in upper canal rare rugae	testes descending few rugae	testes down good rugae	testes pendulous deep rugae	
Genitals female	clitoris prominent labia flat	prominent clitoris small labia minora	prominent clitoris enlarging minora	majora & minora equally prominent	majora large minora small	majora cover clitoris & minora	

MATURITY RATING

score	weeks
−10	20
−5	22
0	24
5	26
10	28
15	30
20	32
25	34
30	36
35	38
40	40
45	42
50	44

FIGURE 7-2 ■ New Ballard Score, expanded to include extremely premature infants. (From Ballard, J.L., Khoury, J.C., Wedig, K., et al.: New Ballard Score, expanded to include extremely premature infants. *Journal of Pediatrics, 119*[3]:417-423, 1991.)

    (2) Position infant supine, pelvis flat on surface; hold thigh in knee-chest position with left index finger and thumb. Place right index finger behind infant's ankle and extend leg with gentle pressure.

    (3) Measure the angle between the lower leg and thigh, posterior to the knee.

  e. Scarf sign.

    (1) Position infant supine; take hand and pull across chest and around neck as far posterior as possible toward the opposite shoulder. Assist maneuver by lifting elbow across body.

    (2) Observe the position of the elbow to the midline of the infant's body.

      f. Heel to ear.

        (1) Position infant supine, pelvis flat on the bed. Draw foot to head as near as it will extend without force.

        (2) Observe distance between the foot and head and the degree of knee extension. Knee is left free and may draw down alongside abdomen.

  2. Physical examination criteria: observe and grade according to Figure 7-2.

    a. Skin.

      (1) With increasing GA, transparency decreases and more texture develops, vessels become obscured.

      (2) As gestation progresses beyond 38 weeks, subcutaneous tissue decreases, causing wrinkling and desquamation.

    b. Lanugo.

      (1) Fine, downy hair that covers the body of the fetus from 20 to 28 weeks.

      (2) At 28 weeks it begins to disappear around the face and anterior aspect of the trunk.

      (3) At term a few patches may be present over the shoulders.

    c. Plantar creases.

      (1) Creases first appear on the anterior portion of the foot, between 28 and 30 weeks of gestation, and extend toward the heel as gestation progresses.

      (2) An infant with IUGR and early loss of vernix caseosa may have more plantar creases than expected for size.

      (3) After 12 hours, the skin begins to dry and plantar creases are no longer a valid indicator of GA.

    d. Breast development.

      (1) Nipple size and amount of breast tissue are examined.

      (2) A 1- to 2-mm nodule of breast tissue is palpable by about 36 weeks and grows to approximately 10 mm by 40 weeks of gestation.

    e. Eyes and ears.

      (1) Evaluated for fused eyelids.

      (2) At 26 to 30 weeks of gestation, fused eyelids open.

      (3) Assess ear formation and amount of pinna cartilage.

      (4) Inward curving of the upper pinna usually begins by 34 weeks of gestation and by 40 weeks extends to the lobe.

      (5) Before 34 weeks the pinna has little cartilage and will stay folded on itself.

      (6) By 36 weeks there is some cartilage, and the pinna will spring back from being folded.

    f. Genitalia.

      (1) Female infant: evaluate development of the labia minora and majora and prominence of the clitoris.

        (a) Early in gestation the clitoris is prominent, with small, widely separated labia.

        (b) By 40 weeks, fat deposits have increased in size in the labia majora, so that the labia majora completely cover the labia minora.

      (2) Male infant: evaluate presence of testes, degree of descent into scrotum, and development of rugae on the scrotum.

        (a) The testes begin to descend from the abdomen at 28 weeks.

        (b) At 37 weeks the testes can be palpated high in the scrotum.

        (c) At 40 weeks the testes are completely descended and the scrotum is covered with rugae.

        (d) As gestation progresses, the scrotum becomes more pendulous.

D. Clinical estimate of GA (AAP/ACOG, 2007; AAP, 2004).

  1. Determination of GA on all newborns is recommended.

  2. Use standard terminology.

    a. GA is the time between the last menstrual period and the day of delivery.

    b. Expressed in completed weeks of gestation.

  3. Assign GA after review of all history and examination findings.

  4. Document marked discrepancy between obstetric and physical data.

5. Classify.
   a. Preterm: infant born on or before the end of the 37th week of gestation.
      (1) Subcategory: "late preterm" defined as between 34 6/7 and 36 6/7 weeks of gestation (Engle, 2006).
      (2) Replaces the phrase *near term*, emphasizes the higher morbidity and mortality of premature infants.
         (a) Term: infant born from the first day of the 38th week to the last day of the 42nd week.
         (b) Postterm: infant delivered from the first day of the 43rd week.

CLASSIFICATION OF GROWTH AND MATURITY

The intrauterine growth pattern reflects fetal well-being. This pattern is influenced by maternal health or disease, placental function, medications, nutrition, and smoking. There are multiple reasons to classify growth and maturity of the newborn infant.

■ Assist in identification of the most commonly occurring problems in the newborn period.
■ Estimate dating if there is no prenatal care.
■ Examine discrepancy between weight and GA.
■ Standardize reports of health statistics.

A. **Measurement.**
   1. Comparison of newborn's measurements should be of population-based growth curves, representing the patient in gender, race, geographic region for altitude, and other environmental variances.
   2. For clinical purposes, use of 10th and 90th percentile range is reasonable (Fletcher, 1998).
B. **Obtain measurements.**
   1. Type.
      a. Normal-appearing infants: weight, length, head circumference, and abdominal circumference.
      b. Dysmorphic appearance: may require more extensive measurements.
   2. Birth weight.
      a. Obtain as soon as possible after delivery.
      b. Express in grams.
      c. Weigh unclothed infant when quiet: (weight can be falsely increased with significant motion) (Fletcher, 1998).
      d. Classifications (regardless of GA) (AAP/ACOG, 2007).
         (1) Low birth weight: <2500 g birth weight.
         (2) Very low birth weight: <1500 g birth weight.
         (3) Extremely low birth weight: <1000 g birth weight.
   3. Length: crown-to-heel measurement.
      a. Most variable measurement: requires full extension of normally flexed infant.
      b. Measure length with infant supine and leg extended, head to heel.
      c. Accuracy facilitated by use of measurement board.
      d. Use crown-to-rump measurement to establish proportionality when length falls below norms (referenced data in *Smith's Recognizable Patterns of Human Malformation* [Jones, 2005]).
         (1) Congenital dwarfism.
         (2) When lower-extremity anomalies make crown-to-heel measurement unreliable.
   4. Head circumference (HC): indication of normal brain growth.
      a. Measurement of largest occipitofrontal circumference.
      b. Apply paper measurement tape firmly around head above the eyebrow ridges, from most prominent frontal to occipital areas.
      c. Occipitofrontal circumference as measured may be erroneous: significant cranial molding, craniosynostosis, caput, and cephalohematoma need to be noted along with the measurement.
      d. Consider parent head size vs. intracranial pathology when head size is of concern.

C. Plot newborn's weight, length, and head circumference by GA on standardized growth charts.

1. Centers for Disease Control and Prevention (CDC) national reference for term infants: www.cdc.gov.growthcharts.
2. Commonly used charts: Colorado Intrauterine Growth Chart (Fig. 7-3) (Lowdermilk and Perry, 2007).
   a. Colorado growth charts developed in 1960s.
   b. Other limitations of Lubchenco data (Thomas et al., 2000).
      (1) Charts developed at mile-high elevation (Denver); 10th percentile is lower than data from centers at sea level.
      (2) Overestimates number of infants greater than 90th percentile and less than 10th percentile.

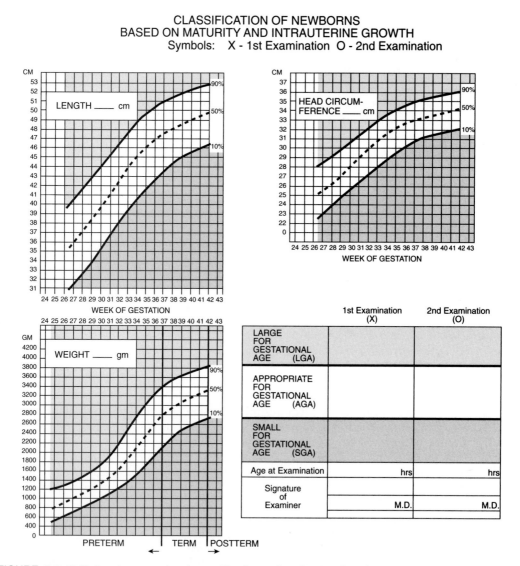

**CLASSIFICATION OF NEWBORNS
BASED ON MATURITY AND INTRAUTERINE GROWTH
Symbols: X - 1st Examination   O - 2nd Examination**

FIGURE 7-3 ■ Estimating gestational age: Newborn classification based on maturity and intrauterine growth. (In Lowdermilk, D.L. and Perry, S.E.: *Maternity & women's health care* [9th ed.]. St. Louis, 2007, Mosby; modified from Lubchenco, L., et al.: Intrauterine growth in length and head circumference as estimated from live births at gestational ages from 26 to 42 weeks. *Journal of Pediatrics*, 37:403, 1966; Battaglia, F. and Lubchenco, L.: A practical classification of newborn infants by weight and gestational age. *Journal of Pediatrics*, 71[2]:159-163, 1967.)

(3) Population sample only whites and primarily low socioeconomic groups.

(4) Leads to inaccurate classification of SGA and LGA that is gender and race specific.

3. Pediatrix Medical Group Inc. Growth Chart (Thomas et al., 2000) (Fig. 7-4).

   a. GA had largest influence on each growth parameter (head circumference, birth weight, length).

     (1) Infants of less than 30 weeks of GA: overall lower growth parameters with respect to the Lubchenco chart.

     (2) Infants of greater than 36 weeks of GA: larger and heavier.

   b. Gender and race differences found in 1996 to 1998 population data.

     (1) Females smaller than males.

     (2) Black infants smaller than Hispanic and white infants at each GA.

   c. Revised charts reflecting race, gender, GA, and multiple birth differences are needed.

4. Babson and Benda fetal-infant growth graph (Fenton, 2003).

   a. Allows evaluation of catch-up growth by extending intrauterine growth from 22 weeks to 10 weeks post-term.

   b. CDC growth charts could be used after 50 weeks.

   c. Original 1976 chart updated in 2003 with growth data from the National Institute of Child Health and Human Development Neonatal Research Network.

   d. Useful in neonatal intensive care units as it reflects preterm infants' postnatal weight and length delay in comparison to head growth.

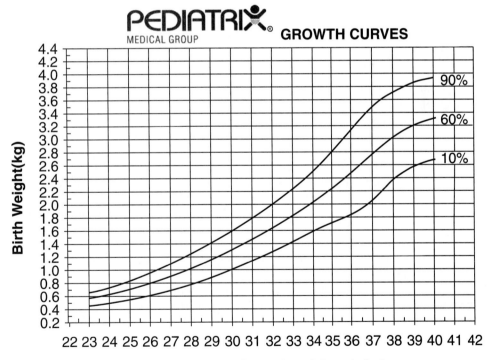

FIGURE 7-4 ■ These growth curves represent an estimate of intrauterine growth based on data from 80,011 neonates admitted to 114 neonatal intensive care units (birth weight above 250 g and gestational age of 22 to 42 weeks). Gender, race, and multiple births had a small but significant effect on each parameter (see the Clinical Research Center at Pediatrix U, www.pediatrixu.com/clinical_research_center.asp). These curves are a reference for the clinician to assess neonates' intrauterine and postnatal growth. The CDC national references (http://www.cdc.gov/growthcharts/) may also be used for term infants. © 2001 Pediatrix Medical Group, Inc. Reproduction of this material by any means without the express written permission of Pediatrix Medical Group, Inc., is prohibited. Please see www.pediatrix.com for updated information.

   e. Open access with credit given, available online at http://www.biomedcental.com/
   1471-2431/3/13.
D. Compare weight with GA to determine size classification (weight compared with established norm).
   1. SGA: birth weight less than 10th percentile.
   2. Appropriate for gestational age (AGA): birth weight within 10th and 90th percentiles.
   3. LGA: birth weight greater than 90th percentile.
E. Compare all growth parameters (head circumference, birth weight, and length) with GA.
   1. IUGR.
      a. Process of slowing of intrauterine growth rate.
      b. IUGR infants may or may not be SGA.
      c. Below expected norms for weight and length at birth based on GA, race, and gender.
   2. Classifications (Britton, 2001).
      a. Symmetric.
         (1) Proportional decreased growth.
         (2) Measurements for weight, length, and HC all within the same growth curve, all
            less than 10th percentile.
         (3) Etiology: decreased growth potential or reduced fetal cells (see Pregnancy
            History).
            (a) Intrauterine congenital infection.
            (b) Congenital malformation.
            (c) Chromosomal disorder.
      b. Asymmetric (head-sparing IUGR).
         (1) Disproportionate reduction in weight and length at birth compared with head
            circumference.
         (2) Weight below expected norms for GA, race, and gender.
         (3) Etiology: normal number of cells; reduced cell size.
            (a) Uteroplacental insufficiency.
            (b) Maternal malnutrition.
            (c) Extrinsic factors occurring late in pregnancy.
F. Determine neonatal mortality risk based on classification of newborns by standardized birth weight norms and GA.
   1. Morbidity and mortality statistics: standardized reporting of reproductive health
      statistics.
   2. Establishment of level of risk for short- and long-term complications.
      a. Higher morbidity and mortality if term infants at or below the 3rd percentile of weight
         for GA (McIntire et al., 1999).
      b. Preterm infants: no specific birth weight thresholds for morbidity and mortality.
   3. Mortality risk (Fig. 7-5).
   4. Morbidity risk by birth weight and GA (Fig. 7-6).
G. Identify infants at risk for respiratory disease, hypoglycemia, and thermal instability based on classification(s):
   1. Preterm: problems with immaturity of body systems: respiratory distress syndrome,
      necrotizing enterocolitis (NEC), and patent ductus arteriosus.
   2. Late preterm (Engle, 2006; McIntire and Leveno, 2008).
      a. Subgroup of later-gestation preterm infants with increased morbidity and mortality
         compared with term infants.
      b. GA ≥34 and <37 weeks.
      c. Potential problems: temperature instability, hypoglycemia, respiratory distress, apnea,
         bradycardia, feeding difficulty, and hyperbilirubinemia.
   3. Postterm: problems associated with placental insufficiency—asphyxia and meconium
      aspiration.
   4. IUGR.
      a. Typical appearance of infant (Southgate and Pittard, 2001).
         (1) Head disproportionately large for trunk.
         (2) Extremities appear wasted.

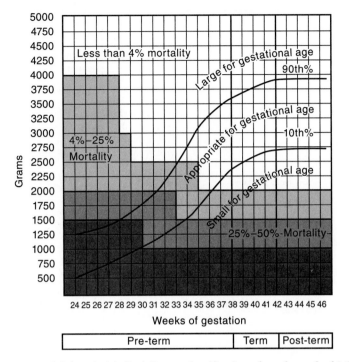

FIGURE 7-5 ■ University of Colorado Medical Center classification of newborns by birth weight and gestational age and by neonatal mortality risk. (From Battaglia, F. and Lubchenco, L.: A practical classification of newborn infants by weight and gestational age. *Journal of Pediatrics, 71*[2]:159-163, 1967.)

    (3) Facial appearance: "wizened old man."

    (4) Large anterior fontanelles with cranial sutures wide or overlapping.

    (5) Thin umbilical cord, diminished Wharton jelly.

    (6) Scaphoid abdomen.

    (7) Skin: loose, decreased subcutaneous fat, dry, flaky, little or no vernix caseosa.

  b. Potential problem list (Lawrence, 2006).

    (1) Hypoglycemia due to high metabolic rate and decreased glycogen stores (Doctor et al., 2001).

    (2) Hypothermia: high demand plus inadequate adipose tissue to maintain temperature.

    (3) Polycythemia: increased red blood cell production in utero caused by chronic hypoxia or endocrine/metabolic or chromosomal disorder.

    (4) Hypoxia: birth asphyxia and meconium aspiration.

    (5) Infection.

    (6) Problems related to etiology of growth restriction.

    (7) Long-term morbidity and mortality dependent on etiology.

5. LGA infant.

  a. Typical appearance.

    (1) Macrosomia.

    (2) Infant of diabetic mother (IDM).

      (a) Hairy ear (Clark, 2000).

      (b) Characteristic large body with head circumference within normal limits for GA (insulin does not cross the blood-brain barrier).

  b. Potential problem list (Lawrence, 2007).

    (1) Abnormal glucose metabolism after birth, hyperinsulinemia and hypoglycemia.

    (2) Birth trauma from difficult extraction (fractured clavicle, brachial plexus injury) or asphyxia.

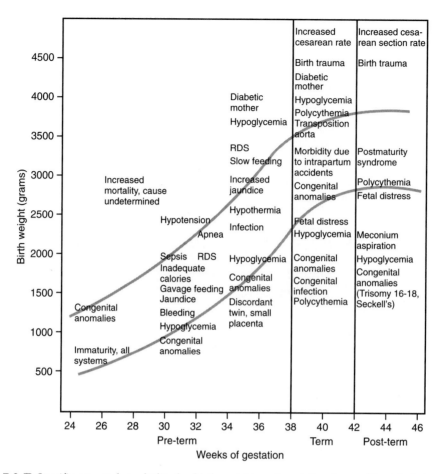

FIGURE 7-6 ■ Specific neonatal morbidity by birth weight and gestational age. (From Lubchenco, L.O.: *The high-risk infant*. Philadelphia, 1976, Saunders.)

(3) Complications from operative or assisted delivery: respiratory distress, adverse effects of anesthesia.

(4) Iatrogenic prematurity: overestimation of fetal GA.

(5) Association with other problems related to infant of diabetic mother: respiratory distress syndrome, hypoglycemia, hypocalcemia, polycythemia, hyperbilirubinemia, and congenital anomalies.

(6) Pulmonary hypertension.

(7) Poor feeding.

(8) Thermal instability as a result of central nervous system (CNS) trauma or infection.

(9) Beckwith-Wiedemann syndrome, LGA, macroglossia, hypoglycemia, umbilical hernia, undescended testes.

PHYSICAL EXAMINATION

A systematic approach to the physical examination of the newborn should be performed in the first 12 to 18 hours of life after successfully transitioning. This prevents pertinent omissions and provides a detailed description that can be utilized in communication of alterations in anatomic structure or changes in physiology or function. These observations ultimately must be made within the context of the patient's history and GA. Communication to the primary care provider is essential for further evaluation and prompt treatment.

A. **Assessment techniques.**
  1. Examine in well-lit room; direct light should not be in infant's face.
  2. Warm hands and equipment.
  3. Keep infant warm by using overhead heat source or uncovering small areas at a time to prevent hypothermia.
  4. Complete detailed observations prior to physical contact.
  5. Order of examination:
     a. Depends on the purpose of the examination and the current state of the infant (Fletcher, 1998).
     b. Generally: least invasive observations to most disturbing techniques.
     c. Observe skin throughout the examination.
     d. Evaluate neurobehavior within the context of the infant's behavioral state.
  6. Document physical examination in patient care record inclusive of description of abnormalities and vital signs.

B. **Timing of examinations (AAP/ACOG, 2007).**
  1. Recognize life-threatening symptoms and address those prior to a comprehensive examination.
  2. Modify elements of examination based on infant's state or illness.
  3. Initial examination in delivery room.
     a. Apgar scoring.
     b. Inspection for birth injury or major congenital malformation.
     c. Evaluation of pulmonary and cardiovascular adjustment to extrauterine life.
     d. Notification of primary care provider.
        (1) Apgar score <5.
        (2) Maternal fever.
        (3) Abnormal examination findings.
        (4) Evidence of and/or suspected substance abuse.
  4. Comprehensive newborn examination.
     a. Within 12 to 18 hours of life: evaluation of size, growth, and GA; transition to extrauterine life; and congenital anomalies.
     b. Discharge examination: focus on problem(s) during hospitalization, problems with feeding and weight gain, and ability of parent(s) to meet infant's needs.

C. **General appearance: initial impression.**
  1. State: indicator of well-being.
     a. Sleep states: deep sleep and light sleep.
     b. Awake states: quiet alert, actively alert, and crying.
  2. Color (Sniderman and Taeusch, 2005).
     a. Most reliable indicator of color: mucous membranes. Other areas include conjunctiva, nail beds, lips, buccal mucosa, earlobes, and soles of feet.
     b. Lighting and color of blankets can affect perception of color.
     c. Central cyanosis; always abnormal
        (1) Recognition influenced by hematocrit, temperature, and environmental factors.
        (2) Central cyanosis: superficial capillaries exceed 5 g/dl unsaturated hemoglobin (Roberton, 2000).
        (3) Variety of etiologies: cardiac, pulmonary, infection, metabolic, neurologic, and hematologic.
     d. Acrocyanosis.
        (1) Suggests instability of peripheral circulation.
        (2) Cyanosis limited to hands, feet, and circumoral area (lips).
        (3) May be a result of cold, stress, shock, and polycythemia.
        (4) Normal finding for 24 to 48 hours after birth.
     e. Pallor: pale, white appearance.
        (1) Reflects poor perfusion and circulatory failure or acidosis.
        (2) With bradycardia indicates anoxia or vasoconstriction found in shock, sepsis, or severe respiratory distress.
        (3) With tachycardia can indicate anemia.

     f. Plethora: ruddy or red appearance.
       (1) May indicate polycythemia.
     g. Jaundice: yellow pigmentation in skin or conjunctiva due to deposition of bilirubin.
       (1) Abnormal in the first 24 hours of life. Needs immediate investigation.
       (2) Cephalocaudal progression.
     h. Mottling: checkerboard red and white pattern.
       (1) May be normal in neonatal period, especially in preterm infants. Reflects vasomotor instability and unequal capillary blood to cutaneous tissue.
       (2) May be seen in cold stress, hypovolemia, and sepsis.
       (3) Cutis marmorata: exaggerated marbling greatest on extremities but also present on trunk (Fletcher, 1998).
     i. Harlequin sign: distinct midline demarcation.
       (1) Pale on one side and red on the opposite side.
       (2) Owing to immature autoregulation of blood flow.
  3. Respiratory effort.
     a. Rate.
       (1) Normal 40 to 60 respirations per minute.
       (2) Rate can vary with activity of infant.
     b. Quality: absence of "work of breathing."
       (1) Retractions: occur more often in premature as a result of highly compliant chest wall (Bates and Balistreri, 2002).
       (2) Nasal flaring: diameter of nares increased as mechanism to decrease airway resistance.
       (3) Expiratory grunting: increase in intrathoracic pressure to prevent volume loss during expiration as a result of alveolar collapse.
  4. Wheezing: due to increased airway resistance. High-pitched rhonchi heard more loudly on expiration.
  5. Stridor: partially obstructed airway.
  6. Nutritional status.
     a. Well nourished: increased subcutaneous fat, without loose skin.
     b. Growth restricted: thin and wasted appearance, no subcutaneous fat, loose skin.
  7. Tone.
     a. Based on GA expectations.
     b. Initial position reflects intrauterine position and may reflect limitation of movement or increased pressure on head, trunk, or extremities.
     c. Degree of flexion and amount of resistance demonstrated with examiner's extension of extremities.
     d. Decreased flexion (hypotonia) or increased flexion (hypertonia) should be evaluated further.
  8. Congenital defects.
     a. Determine if malformation (abnormal shape or structure) or deformation (fully formed but influenced by in utero environment).
     b. Describe anatomic structures fully: size, number, shape, position, color, texture, continuity, and alignment (Sniderman and Taeusch, 2005).
  9. Temperature (see Chapter 6).
D. **Skin (see Chapter 36).**
  1. General considerations.
     a. Findings differ with GA, especially with extremely low birth weight.
     b. Indicators of underlying illness: petechiae, pigmentation, rashes, and pustules.
     c. Congenital lesions may not be apparent at birth; influenced by maternal hormones.
     d. Differentiate between findings at birth vs. injury after birth (medical interventions).
     e. Use basic descriptors: color, quantity, size, shape, pattern of distribution, and texture (Lund and Kuller, 2007).
  2. Skin is soft, smooth, and opaque and should be warm to the touch; cold, clammy skin may indicate shock.

3. Inspect lesions, rashes, bruises, and birthmarks. Differentiate between benign findings and those suspicious of infection or hematologic or neurologic disturbance.
4. Palpate for texture (raised, flat) unless lesion is open.
5. Vernix caseosa.
   a. White or yellow material on the skin; discolored with postmaturity, hemolytic disease, and meconium staining.
   b. Sebaceous gland secretions and exfoliated skin cells.
   c. Presents during third trimester and decreases with increasing GA.
6. Lanugo: fine soft hair covering face, trunk.
   a. Amount and distribution are GA dependent.
   b. Covers entire body in preterm, disappears at 32 to 37 weeks from face and lower back.
   c. At term, present on upper back and limbs.
7. Erythema toxicum (newborn rash).
   a. Erythematous macules, each containing a central papule (yellow or white).
   b. Papules contain eosinophils in a fluid that is sterile.
   c. Persist for several days and then resolve spontaneously.
   d. Most often located on trunk, arms, and perineal areas.
   e. Never located on soles of feet or palms of hands.
8. Pustular melanosis.
   a. Benign, transient, nonerythematous pustules and vesicles.
   b. Single or clusters, rupture leaves scaly white lesion.
9. Ecchymosis: nonblanching blue or black area.
   a. Extravasation of blood into tissue.
   b. Related to trauma of blood vessels.
10. Petechiae.
    a. Tiny red or purple nonblanching pinpoint macules.
    b. Benign when found on presenting part; result from areas of compression during delivery.
    c. More diffuse distribution suggests general thrombocytopenia.
    d. Require further evaluation when progressive (Lund and Kuller, 2007).
11. Vascular nevi.
    a. Common cutaneous malformation(s) that can occur anywhere on body.
    b. May present at birth or may develop in early infancy.
    c. Types.
       (1) Nevus simplex or capillary hemangiomas (stork bite).
           (a) Macular patches with diffuse borders.
           (b) Found on forehead, nape of neck, glabella, and eyelids.
           (c) Blanch when pressure is applied.
           (d) Resolve spontaneously.
       (2) Nevus flammeus (port wine stain).
           (a) Flat, sharply defined lesion.
           (b) Most common on back of neck.
           (c) If present over the face following branches of trigeminal nerve (forehead and upper eyelid), may be associated with Sturge-Weber syndrome.
           (d) Will not blanch with pressure.
           (e) May fade with time but will not resolve.
12. Café au lait spots.
    a. Light tan or brown macules with well-defined borders.
    b. Deeper pigmentation than surrounding skin.
    c. Six or more may be pathologic.
13. Strawberry hemangioma(s).
    a. Red, raised, circumscribed, and compressible.
    b. Can occur anywhere on the body.
    c. Proliferate: increase in size and number.

  d. Most involute spontaneously.

  e. No treatment is required unless they affect vital function.

  f. Occur with increasing frequency with decreased GA.

 14. Epidermolysis bullosa.

  a. Blistering internally and externally.

  b. May be either autosomal dominant or recessive.

 15. Staphylococcal scalded skin syndrome.

  a. Skin response to *Staphylococcus aureus*.

  b. Scalded skin appearance.

 16. Sucking blisters: skin erosion on thumbs, index fingers, wrist, or forearm from intrauterine sucking.

E. Head.

 1. General considerations.

  a. Up to 90% of the congenital malformations present at birth are apparent on the head and neck (Jones, 2005).

  b. Review perinatal history, abnormal ultrasound findings, and mode of delivery.

  c. Many variations are transient or racial, sexual, or familial traits.

 2. Obtain head circumference (HC) measurements.

  a. Measurement reflects brain growth.

  b. Predictable measurement: follows norms for GA and weight.

  c. Usually HC falls on same percentile curve as length. Determine etiology of abnormal growth if length and HC differ by greater than one quartile (Sansoucie and Cavaliere, 2007).

  d. HC should be 2 cm larger than the chest circumference. Normal = 32 to 38 cm for full-term AGAs.

   (1) Microcephalic: poor brain growth, atrophy, or premature cranial synostosis.

   (2) Macrocephalic: familial (follows persistently higher but consistent growth curve) and pathologic (hydrocephalus: increase in cerebrospinal fluid results in increasing HC).

 3. Observe shape and symmetry; may reflect effect of birth process or in utero position or significant anatomic defect.

  a. Molding.

   (1) Occurs with vaginal delivery from a vertex position; adaptive mechanism to facilitate passage through birth canal.

   (2) Elongation of head with prominence of occiput and overriding sagittal suture line.

   (3) Resolution in first week of life.

   (4) Not uncommon for overriding sutures to persist longer than 1 week in the extremely low birth weight infant.

  b. Rounded head occurs with delivery by cesarean section without labor; flat head with increased occipital-frontal diameter occurs with breech delivery.

  c. Abnormal prominence, depressions, or flattening.

  d. Abnormal shape of skull.

   (1) Plagiocephaly: asymmetric appearance of head, flattened on one side.

   (2) Craniosynostosis: premature closing of one or more of cranial sutures.

   (3) Anencephaly: failed closure of neural tube without skull formation.

 4. Palpate sutures and fontanelles (Fig. 7-7).

  a. Sutures: check for mobility of sutures by placing thumb on opposite sides of suture and alternately pushing (gently).

   (1) Well approximated.

   (2) Overriding.

    (a) Molding.

    (b) Fused suture: premature synostosis.

   (3) Wide sutures.

    (a) May be wide in the absence of increased intracranial pressure.

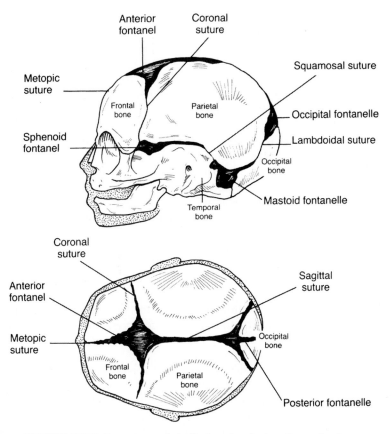

FIGURE 7-7 ■ Two views of skull, showing fontanelles and sutures.

(b) Widened lambdoid suture: indicates increased pressure.
(c) Sagittal and metopic sutures normally wider in black infants (Fletcher, 1998).
(4) Craniotabes: soft demineralized area typically found in parietal and occipital regions along the lambdoidal suture line.
   (a) Under gentle pressure, the area will collapse and then recoil.
   (b) Infant engaged in the vertex position for a prolonged period.
   (c) Pressure of skull against maternal pelvis results in delayed ossification or reabsorption of bone.
b. Anterior fontanelle.
   (1) Location: junction of sagittal and coronal sutures.
   (2) Shape: diamond.
   (3) Size: measures 4 to 6 cm at the largest diameter (bone to bone).
   (4) Normally closes at 18 months.
c. Posterior fontanelle.
   (1) Location: junction of lambdoidal and sagittal sutures.
   (2) Shape: triangular.
   (3) Size: usually fingertip.
   (4) Normally closes by 2 months of age.
d. Abnormal findings.
   (1) Third fontanelle: between anterior and posterior fontanelles along the sagittal suture (may be associated with congenital anomalies).
   (2) Size: large fontanelle, considerable racial variations; not pathognomonic for any condition (Fletcher, 1998).
   (3) Closed fontanelles with immobile, rigid sutures suggest premature synostosis.
   (4) Bruit over temporal, frontal, or occipital area associated with high-output cardiac failure and arteriovenous malformation.

(5) Abnormal tension.
    (a) Bulging, tense, full fontanelle: associated with increased intracranial pressure secondary to hydrocephalus, birth injury, bleeding, or infection.
    (b) Depressed fontanelle: associated with dehydration.

5. Palpate soft tissue findings on scalp, face, and neck (Furdon and Clark, 2001).
  a. Caput succedaneum: common finding in infants born in the vertex position as a result of compression of local blood vessels.
    (1) Maximal swelling present at birth.
    (2) Edema extends across suture lines and has poorly defined borders.
    (3) Edema can shift to dependent position.
    (4) ± Ecchymosis, petechiae, or purpura.
    (5) Disappears within 24 to 48 hours.
  b. Cephalohematoma: subperiosteal hemorrhage due to traumatic delivery.
    (1) Typically not present at birth, increases in size over the first day of life.
    (2) Unilateral; fixed, firm, and palpable mass.
    (3) Swelling does not cross suture lines.
    (4) Often no ecchymosis.
    (5) Poor tone, feeding, and decreased activity may be indication of underlying skull fracture.
    (6) Resolution may not occur for several months, often leaving a calcified "knot."
  c. Subgaleal hemorrhage: owing to forces that compress and drag the head through the pubic outlet.
    (1) Is a clinical emergency.
    (2) Ballotable scalp mass present at birth that is mobile, not fixed.
    (3) Swelling crosses suture lines and fontanelles, poorly defined margins.
    (4) Rapidly can increase in size and shape with significant acute blood loss, resulting in shock as the presenting symptom.
    (5) Bleeding, seen as swelling, can expand to orbital ridges, around the ears and dissect along tissue planes into the neck.
    (6) Least common of the birth injuries; however, has the greatest potential for complications.

6. Inspect the scalp.
  a. Intact skin.
  b. Normal hair pattern (direction of growth) and distribution (Furdon and Clark, 2003).
    (1) Color concordant racially with parents; genetic disorders can present with hypopigmentation of scalp hair.
    (2) Localized patches of hypopigmentation; e.g., white forelock: Waardenburg syndrome.
    (3) Areas of diffuse or localized absence or abundance of hair.
    (4) Hair texture: brittle, fragile, twisted, wooly, excessively kinky.
    (5) Anterior and posterior hair margins.
  c. Abnormal findings.
    (1) Lacerations or abrasions as the result of instruments at delivery or scalp electrode.
    (2) Vesicles: electrode site and behind the ears.
    (3) Cutis aplasia: localized absence of skin associated with trisomy 13.
    (4) Hair whorls: spiral hair growth pattern; multiple hair whorls or abnormal placement may represent abnormal brain growth or development.
    (5) Anterior hairline well onto the forehead.

7. Note position infant holds head at rest.
  a. Reflects fetal position.
  b. Usual position: anterior neck flexion.
  c. Observe for full range of motion.

F. Face.
1. Observe for symmetry and location of eyes, nose, and mouth.
  a. Divide the face into thirds for inspection: one third, forehead; one third, eyes and nose; and one third, mouth and chin.

      b. At rest and with crying or sucking.

      c. Asymmetry when infant crying: facial palsy.

2. Observe relationship and location of eyes, nose, and mouth.

  a. Eyes.

    (1) Spacing and size.

      (a) Space between inner and outer canthus of one eye approximates the width between the two inner canthi.

      (b) Hypertelorism (widened distance between orbits); hypotelorism (decreased distance between orbits) associated with various syndromes.

    (2) Number: anophthalmos (absent); cyclopia (one).

    (3) Conjunctiva and sclera.

      (a) Subconjunctival hemorrhage: result from pressure on fetal head during delivery.

      (b) Sclera color usually white.

      (c) Blue sclera: extreme prematurity, osteogenesis imperfecta, other chromosomal associations.

      (d) Yellow sclera: jaundiced.

    (4) Cornea, iris, and pupils.

      (a) Cornea relatively cloudy at birth:

        (i) Term infant: cloudiness resolves within a few days.

        (ii) Asymmetric or dense cloudiness: abnormal.

        (iii) Infantile cataracts: rubella, cytomegalovirus, familial association, and chromosomal defect.

      (b) Iris: dark blue until 3 to 6 months of age, then eye color may change.

        (i) Brushfield's spots: speckled appearance; occurs in 75% of infants with trisomy 21; also normal (Fletcher, 1998).

        (ii) Coloboma: cleft-shaped fissure (keyhole shape); can be sporadic or in association with trisomy 13 or choanal atresia, posterior coloboma, heart defect, choanal atresia, retardation, genital and ear abnormalities (CHARGE) sequence.

      (c) Pupils.

        (i) PERRL (pupils equal, round, and react to light).

        (ii) White color: abnormal.

      (d) Red reflex: reflection of ophthalmoscope's light on the retina.

      (e) Color range: red (light-skinned infant) to yellow (dark-skinned infant).

        (i) White: congenital cataracts.

        (ii) Absence: retinoblastoma, glaucoma, or hemorrhage.

    (5) Symmetry of eye movements.

      (a) Eyelids.

        (i) Should open to above midpoint of pupil when the eye is in a neutral position.

        (ii) Edema: related to birth process or chemical irritation with eye prophylaxis.

        (iii) Fused eyelids: extreme prematurity; generally not fused by 28 weeks of gestation; should not be used as an indicator of viability or nonviability.

        (iv) Ptosis: abnormal drooping of one or both eyelids.

      (b) Palpebral fissures.

        (i) Slant is primarily racially determined.

        (ii) Variations typical of several syndromes.

      (c) Epicanthal folds.

        (i) Vertical fold of skin at inner canthus of eye on either side of the nose.

        (ii) Common in trisomy 21.

        (iii) Manifestation of in utero compression (Potter facies).

      (d) Eyelashes, eyebrows.

        (i) Appear at 20 to 23 weeks.

        (ii) Abnormalities.

          a) Absent lashes or long lashes.

          b) High-arched eyebrows or synophrys (meeting of eyebrows in middle).

  b. Nose.

    (1) Shape and size.

      (a) Positional deformities often due to birth process; resolve without treatment.

      (b) Abnormal shape: may be associated with a congenital syndrome.

      (c) Abnormal: flat, broad nasal bridge.

    (2) Patency of nostrils.

      (a) Place a cold, metal object under each nostril and observe for fogging: presence of airflow.

      (b) Causes of nasal obstruction.

        (i) Choanal atresia or stenosis: membranous or bony obstruction; unilateral or bilateral.

        (ii) Iatrogenic: swollen mucosa from suction catheters.

        (iii) Inflammation and secretions.

  c. Mouth, tongue, and perioral region.

    (1) Mouth should be symmetric and positioned in the midline:

      (a) Microstomia: very small mouth; may be associated with trisomy 18.

      (b) Macrostomia: large mouth; often associated with mucopolysaccharidosis, Beckwith-Wiedemann syndrome, or hypothyroidism.

      (c) Suck and swallow develops at 32 to 34 weeks, and root and gag response at 36 weeks. They should be elicited during the examination.

    (2) Cleft upper lip: can vary from a niche in the lip to a complete separation extending up onto the floor of the nose.

    (3) Thin upper lip in association with flat philtrum: fetal alcohol syndrome.

    (4) Soft and hard palate should be visually inspected, then palpated (Merritt, 2005):

      (a) Presence of submucous or membranous clefts.

      (b) Narrow or high arch palate may indicate a decrease in neuromotor activity or sucking in utero.

    (5) Mucosal cysts.

      (a) Epithelial or Epstein's pearls: small, white epidermal cysts commonly found on the hard and soft palates and on gum margins and disappear after a few weeks.

      (b) Bohn nodule: equivalent to milia on the skin.

      (c) Gingival or alveolar cysts.

    (6) Dental eruptions and neonatal teeth.

      (a) If mobile or poor root formation: generally removed.

      (b) Consult with pediatric dentist; may be primary teeth.

    (7) Frenulum.

      (a) Small lingual frenulum normal ("tongue tied").

      (b) Short frenulum that limits tongue movement: abnormal; tip of tongue will form an inverted V shape.

    (8) Tongue.

      (a) Large tongue (macroglossia): generally part of syndrome (Beckwith-Wiedemann).

      (b) Large tongue can obstruct the airway.

      (c) Protruding tongue: trisomy 21 and Beckwith-Wiedemann.

    (9) Thrush: oral moniliasis: usually contracted from mothers with vaginal moniliasis at time of delivery.

      (a) Lacy white material present on surface of oral mucous membranes.

      (b) Does not wipe away with a cotton-tipped swab.

3. Observe other facial features.

  a. Nasolacrimal ducts.

    (1) Tears are rare until 2 to 4 months of age.

    (2) Obstruction: visible mass.

4. Inspect facial skin.
   a. Milia: 1-mm white or yellow papules without erythema; resolve spontaneously within first weeks of life.
   b. Miliaria: clear, thin vesicles 1 to 2 mm that develop in sweat glands; primarily seen on forehead, scalp, and creases.
   c. Lacerations, ecchymosis, abrasions from forceps.
   d. Petechiae over head and neck: typically from nuchal cord, rapid second stage of labor.
   e. Pits or sinus: facial cleft syndromes.
5. Observe for size of jaw and relationship to maxilla.
   a. Micrognathia: abnormally small jaw with normal-sized tongue.
      (1) May present serious airway problem.
      (2) Seen in Pierre Robin, Treacher Collins, and de Lange syndromes.
G. **Ears (Sansoucie and Cavaliere, 2007).**
   1. Note presence or absence of external ear.
   2. Determine position and rotation.
      a. Helix attaches to scalp at a point horizontal to the inner canthus of the eye.
      b. Normal: 30% of pinna above imaginary line drawn from the inner canthi of the eyes toward the occiput and tragus (cartilaginous projection in front of the external meatus of the ear).
      c. Cranial molding may distort landmarks; ears may appear low-set.
      d. Low-set ears may be associated with various syndromes and chromosomal abnormalities.
   3. Check for presence of ear canals; visualization of eardrums not typically necessary.
   4. Examine for abnormal findings.
      a. Microtia: disorganized or dysplastic ear.
         (1) Associated with atresia of auditory meatus and conductive hearing loss.
         (2) Variations.
            (a) Lop ear: helix folded downward because of inadequate development of the antihelix.
            (b) Cup ear: small cup-shaped ear.
      b. Preauricular pits and sinus.
         (1) Pinpoint openings at base of helix or front of tragus.
         (2) Increased risk of congenital deafness and renal abnormalities.
      c. Preauricular ear appendages (tags).
         (1) Single or multiple; vary in size.
         (2) Differentiate from accessory auricle or tragus.
         (3) Consistently seen in Goldenhar syndrome: syndrome with wide range of facial, ear, and vertebral defects (Jones, 2005).
         (4) Associated with urinary tract abnormalities (Kohelet and Arbel, 2000) and other brachial arch abnormalities: cleft lip, cleft palate, and hypoplasia of mandible.
H. **Neck and clavicles.**
   1. Inspect and palpate neck.
      a. Mass: note location.
         (1) Most common: cystic hygroma.
            (a) Multiloculated cyst arising from lymphatic channels typically located posterior to the sternocleidomastoid muscle and extending into the scapula and axillary and thoracic compartments.
            (b) Can distort the anatomy of the airway.
         (2) Thyroglossal duct cyst or branchial cleft cyst.
      b. Webbing.
         (1) Excessive skinfold extending from the mastoid process to the shoulders.
         (2) Associated with Turner and Noonan syndromes and trisomy 21.
      c. Torticollis: rotation limited due to constant position of head to one side.
   2. Gently palpate neck and clavicles.
      a. Crepitus: due to fractured bone ends rubbing together.

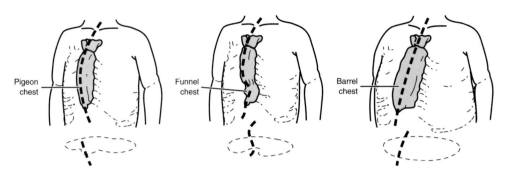

FIGURE 7-8 ■ Different chest shapes. (Adapted from Alexander, M.M. and Brown, M.S.: *Pediatric history taking and physical diagnosis for nurses* [2nd ed.]. St. Louis, 1979, Mosby.)

     (1) Swelling, discoloration, or tenderness associated with fractured clavicle.

     (2) Observe for asymmetric arm movement with the Moro reflex or signs of pain with manipulation.

I. **Chest and lungs.**

  1. Review influencing factors: GA, timing of examination, intrapartum and delivery history, maternal drugs, and cool environment.

  2. Inspect the shape and size of the chest (Fig. 7-8).

    a. Compare size relationship of the thorax and abdomen.

    b. Normal: round symmetric shape with the anterior-posterior diameter approximately the same as the transverse diameter.

    c. Large or barrel-shaped chest: associated with air trapping and hyperinflation.

    d. Pigeon chest or protrusion of sternum: associated with Marfan syndrome.

    e. Chest wall itself depressed or funnel shaped: pectus excavatum; no clinical significance.

    f. Short sternum: associated with trisomy 18.

    g. Rib margins apparent in premature infants: thinner layers of muscle and fat.

  3. Observe.

    a. Color: refer to C. General Appearance: Initial Impression, p. 133.

    b. Respiratory rate and pattern.

      (1) Should be evaluated at rest and before any manipulation.

      (2) Rate: normal—40 to 60 breaths per minute, easy, unlabored and typically abdominal or diaphragmatic.

      (3) Tachypnea: rate greater than 60 breaths per minute—lung pathology, cardiac disease, infection, overheating, fever, and pain.

      (4) Bradypnea or shallow respirations: CNS depression.

      (5) Periodic breathing: 5- to 20-second pauses without changes in color, tone, or heart rate.

      (6) Apnea: cessation of breathing for more than 20 seconds. May be accompanied by bradycardia, change in muscle tone, or color change; apnea of prematurity, infection, respiratory insufficiency, gastroesophageal reflux.

      (7) Slow, gasping respirations: respiratory failure and acidosis.

    c. Depth and ease of respirations.

      (1) Normal: irregular and varying depth.

      (2) Chest pulled inward as abdomen rises with inspiration as a result of normal diaphragmatic excursion.

      (3) Retractions: accessory muscles used.

        (a) Note depth (minimal, marked).

        (b) Subcostal, substernal: common after birth. Persistence may indicate respiratory problems.

        (c) Intercostal.

      (4) Nasal flaring retractions, tachypnea, and grunting—symptomatic of respiratory distress.

4. Auscultate breath sounds.
    a. Compare and contrast each side of chest.
    b. Presence of air entry: normal, fair, or poor.
    c. Asymmetric breath sounds: pneumothorax, cystic adenomatoid malformation, or congenital diaphragmatic hernia (CDH).
    d. Normal breath sounds: clear and equal, little differentiation between inspiration and expiration.
    e. Adventitious breath sounds.
        (1) Crackles: fine or coarse, lower pitched, fine crackles heard on inspiration, often present after birth due to clearing lung fluid.
        (2) Wheeze: high pitched usually heard on exhalation, reactive airway.
        (3) Rhonchi: low pitched, arise from partial obstruction by mucus or secretions.
        (4) Stridor: rough, harsh sound worse during inspiration, caused by reduced airway diameter (edema, mass, vascular ring).
        (5) Diminished breath sounds: atelectasis, effusion, decreased air entry, poor respiratory effort.
        (6) Peristaltic sounds: bowel sounds indicate CDH.
        (7) Friction rub: pleural effusion.
5. Inspect breasts and nipples.
    a. Size.
        (1) Based on GA.
        (2) Enlarged breasts: effects of maternal estrogen, transient.
        (3) Unilateral redness or firmness indicates sepsis.
    b. Location and symmetry: widespread nipples—distance between nipples more than 25% of full chest circumference; may indicate variety of conditions (Sansoucie and Cavaliere, 2007).
    c. Number: supernumerary nipples; small, raised, pigmented areas vertical with main nipple line 5 to 6 cm below normal nipple; familial.
    d. Discharge.
        (1) Witch's milk.
            (a) Milky discharge produced in response to maternal hormones.
            (b) Lasts for several weeks to months.
        (2) Purulent: mastitis due to staphylococcal infection.
J. **Heart and cardiovascular system.**
    1. General considerations: congenital heart defects are associated with other congenital malformations, chromosomal defects, maternal medication or substance use (phenytoin [Dilantin], alcohol), maternal health or illness (diabetes), viral illness, and familial association.
    2. Observe color.
    3. Heart rate: normal range 120 to 160 beats per minute (bpm) varies with infant behavioral state.
        a. Bradycardia: rate less than 100 bpm.
            (1) May be associated with apnea, cerebral defects, vagal response, congenital heart block.
            (2) Term infant in deep sleep can have heart rate of 80 to 90 bpm; should increase as infant awakens.
        b. Tachycardia: more than 160 bpm sustained.
            (1) May be associated with respiratory distress, anemia, congestive heart failure, hyperthermia, shock, and supraventricular tachycardia.
        c. Brief irregularities are common; identification of abnormality cannot be made by auscultation alone.
    4. Location of point of maximal intensity.
        a. Normal: lateral to midclavicular line at the 4th intercostal space.
        b. Shift in location can indicate tension pneumothorax.
        c. Right-side location: dextrocardia, CDH.
        d. Observe precordial activity.

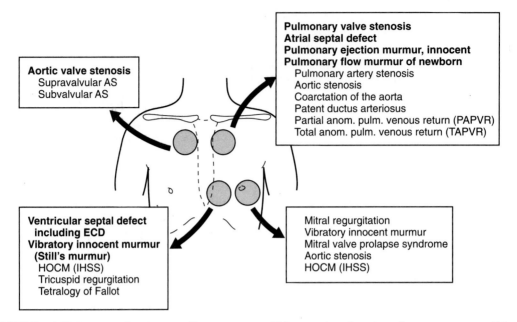

FIGURE 7-9 ■ Diagram showing systolic murmurs audible at various locations. Less common conditions are shown in lighter type. *AS,* Aortic stenosis; *ECD,* endocardial cushion defect; *HOCM,* hypertrophic obstructive cardiomyopathy; *IHSS,* idiopathic hypertrophic subaortic stenosis. (From Park, M.K.: *Pediatric cardiology for practitioners* [5th ed.]. St. Louis, 2008, Mosby.)

    (1) Within 6 hours of birth may be visible along left sternal border (Southgate and Pittard, 2001).
    (2) Visible for longer periods in premature infants.
    (3) Associated with congestive heart failure, heart disease, and fluid overload.
5. Auscultate heart sounds.
  a. First heart sound.
    (1) Accentuated at birth.
    (2) Increase in intensity: patent ductus arteriosus, ventricular septal defect, tetralogy of Fallot, anemia, hyperthermia, and arteriovenous fistula.
  b. Second heart sound.
    (1) Sound produced by closure of aortic and pulmonary valves.
    (2) No splitting of heart sound: pulmonary atresia, transposition of the great artery, or truncus arteriosus.
  c. Muffled heart sounds: may indicate pneumopericardium, pneumomediastinum, or CDH.
6. Auscultate murmur: turbulence in blood flow (Fig. 7-9).
  a. Can be innocent or pathologic (underlying cardiovascular disease).
  b. Timing of appearance.
    (1) First 48 hours of life: can be related to cardiovascular transition; should be followed up.
    (2) Audible after transition complete: ventricular septal defect, turbulence in pulmonary arteries secondary to obstruction; severe outflow tract obstruction.
  c. Location and radiation.
    (1) Describe as interspace, midclavicular, midsternal, or axillary.
    (2) Transmission: auscultate back or axilla.
  d. Timing within cycle.
    (1) Continuous: extends beyond second heart sound into diastole.
    (2) Systolic ejection murmur: occurs before the first heart sound; ends at or before second heart sound; flow across pulmonary valve.

e. Loudness or quality.
   (1) Grade 1: barely audible.
   (2) Grade 2: soft but easily audible.
   (3) Grade 3: moderately loud but no thrill.
   (4) Grade 4: loud with thrill.
   (5) Grade 5: loud; audible with stethoscope placed lightly on chest.
   (6) Grade 6: loud; audible with stethoscope placed near chest.
7. Palpate pulses: strength and equality (upper to lower and side to side).
   a. Brachial, radial, and palmar.
   b. Femoral, popliteal, posterior tibial, and dorsalis pedis.
   c. Grading scale (Vargo, 1996).

   0: Not palpable.
   +1: Very difficult to palpate; weak, thready, easily obliterated with pressure.
   +2: Difficult to palpate; may be obliterated with pressure.
   +3: Easy to palpate; not easy to obliterate with pressure; found in normal pulses.
   +4: Strong and bounding; not obliterated with pressure; associated with patent ductus arteriosus.

   d. Absent femoral: associated with coarctation of aorta.
8. Assess capillary refill or perfusion.
   a. Press and release skin over abdomen until area blanches.
   b. Count number of seconds until color returns to area.
   c. Normal: less than or equal to 3 seconds.
9. Blood pressure (Fig. 7-10).
   a. Depends on gestational age and chronologic age.
   b. Differential greater than 20 mm Hg between upper- and lower-extremity blood pressure indicates obstruction (coarctation of aorta).
   c. Blood pressure (BP) in lower extremities should be slightly higher than in the upper extremities.

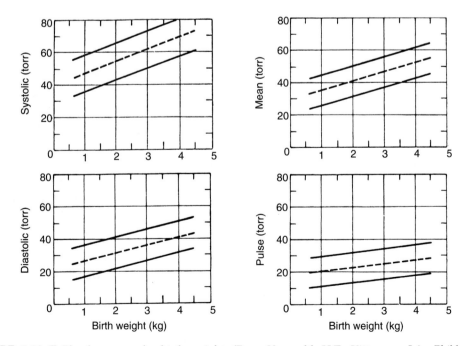

FIGURE 7-10 ■ Blood pressure by birth weight. (From Versmold, H.T., Kitterman, J.A., Phibbs, R.H., et al.: Aortic blood pressure during the first 12 hours of life in infants with birth weight 610 to 4200 grams. *Pediatrics, 67*[5]:607-613, 1981.)

K. Abdomen.

1. General considerations: review history for feeding intake, emesis, stooling, maternal medications affecting bowel function, maternal blood type, and intrauterine infection.
2. Observe abdomen: slightly rounded, soft, and symmetric.
    a. Scaphoid abdomen: abdominal contents in chest (diaphragmatic hernia). May appear slightly concave at birth, but will become distended as bowel fills with air.
    b. Decreased abdominal tone or muscles in abdominal wall, with visible bowel loops and margins of spleen and liver (prune belly syndrome) (Woods and Brandon, 2007).
    c. Distention: obstruction, infection, masses, or enlargement of an abdominal organ.
3. Observe for abdominal wall defect (Thigpen, 2007).
    a. Etiology: disruption in migration of abdominal contents from the umbilical cord and defect in the development of abdominal wall musculature.
    b. Omphalocele: abdominal contents usually covered with a membrane; umbilical cord inserts into sac; commonly associated with cardiac lesions, trisomy 13, trisomy 18, Beckwith-Wiedemann syndrome.
    c. Gastroschisis: abdominal wall defect resulting in protrusion of abdominal contents not covered with a membrane.
        (1) Typically located to the right of midline.
        (2) Abdominal contents often thickened, edematous, and matted as a result of exposure to amniotic fluid.
    d. Umbilical hernia: bulge at umbilicus related to weakness in abdominal muscle.
4. Palpate gently for enlargement in liver or presence of masses.
    a. Normal: liver edge 1 to 2 cm below right costal margin in midclavicular line.
    b. Begin palpation in right lower quadrant and progress upward so liver edge will not be missed.
    c. Enlarged liver: congenital heart disease, infection, hemolytic disease, and arteriovenous malformation.
    d. A normal spleen is rarely palpable; palpable spleen more than 1 cm below left costal margin is abnormal.
    e. Abdominal mass: most often of urinary tract origin.
5. Palpate kidneys and bladder.
    a. Place one hand under the flank and palpate gently from above with the fingertips of the other hand.
    b. Normal kidney in term infant is 4.5 to 5 cm from pole to pole.
    c. Further evaluation needed: absence of palpable kidney or enlarged kidneys.
    d. Bladder can be palpated 1 to 4 cm above pubic symphysis when urine present.
6. Auscultate for bowel sounds.
    a. Absent or hyperactive bowel sounds may indicate obstruction.
7. Inspect the umbilical cord (Thigpen, 2007).
    a. Important clues to fetal growth, development, and well-being.
    b. Normal: bluish white, moist, and gelatinous.
    c. Diameter of cord varies and is related to Wharton jelly.
        (1) Supportive covering protecting the cord vessels from compression or occlusion.
        (2) Increases with GA.
        (3) Thin cord may reflect placental insufficiency and intrauterine growth restriction.
    d. Total length of cord: normal 30 to 90 cm.
        (1) Length determined by intrauterine space and fetal activity.
        (2) Infants with limited fetal activity (Down syndrome, congenital neuromuscular disorders) have short cords.
    e. Presence of knots.
    f. Color: green or yellow (meconium); red (blood); depth of staining correlates with duration of exposure.
    g. Number of vessels.
        (1) Normally contains two arteries and one vein.
        (2) Single umbilical artery may be associated with renal anomalies.

    h. Urine draining from umbilicus: patent urachus (embryologic communication between bladder and umbilicus).

L. Genitalia and anus.

  1. General considerations.

    a. Review pertinent history.

      (1) GA; appearance changes with GA.

      (2) Oligohydramnios or polyhydramnios: possible renal/urinary or gastrointestinal/pulmonary anomaly.

      (3) Family history: associated genetic predisposition.

    b. Congenital defects are relatively rare but highly stressful to parents.

    c. Normal variations are more common than pathologic conditions.

    d. Genitourinary anomalies are highly associated with other system disorders (see Chapter 33).

    e. Breech deliveries can cause significant bruising and edema of genitalia and perineum.

    f. No circumcision should be done in infants with epispadias, hypospadias, or chordee.

  2. General inspection and palpation: position infant supine for examination.

    a. Gender identification: if not clearly distinguishable, do not assign sex until further evaluation. Inform parents of ambiguity and need for further testing.

    b. Anus: locate position in relation to genitalia and determine patency.

      (1) Anal opening: approximately midline.

      (2) Slightly more anterior to genitalia in females.

      (3) Check for anal wink in any infant suspected of neural tube defect; stroke anal opening lightly; observe positive constriction.

    c. Passage of meconium; ensures open communication only.

      (1) Fistulas: anteriorly or posteriorly placed; may be accompanied with bowel distention.

        (a) Rectovaginal fistula (female) or rectoperineal fistula (male).

      (2) Constant dribbling of loose stool: suspect neural tube defect.

    d. Inguinal area (Parker, 2007).

      (1) Assess for hernia(s) when inguinal mass observed.

      (2) Groin bulge: may be unilateral or bilateral; increase in size with crying or straining or spontaneously reduce.

      (3) Palpate from lower abdomen along the inguinal canal to the labia or scrotum.

      (4) Attempt to gently compress bowel back toward abdomen. Irreducible hernias are at high risk for incarceration and subsequent necrosis.

  3. Male.

    a. Penis: inspect size, appearance, and foreskin.

      (1) Normal.

        (a) Straight, may be erect.

        (b) Size proportionate to body, average term length 2.5 to 3.5 cm from pubic bone to glans tip (Goodwin and Caldamone, 2005).

        (c) Glans covered by prepuce (foreskin) in uncircumcised infant.

        (d) Physiologic phimosis: tight, nonretractable foreskin; does not retract until 2 to 3 years of age.

        (e) Prepuce: foreskin or fold of skin over the glans.

          (i)   Amount and distribution: hooded (appearance of distal foreskin).

          (ii) Small, white epithelial cysts on distal prepuce.

      (2) Abnormal.

        (a) Chordee: curving or bowing of penis; sometimes occurs in conjunction with hypospadias.

        (b) Micropenis: less than 2.5 cm in the term neonate.

    b. Determine position of urinary meatus.

      (1) Normal: midline at the glans tip.

      (2) Abnormal.

(a) Hypospadias (Stokowski, 2004):
   (i) Urethral opening located at the ventral surface of the penis; associated with chordee, meatal stenosis, inguinal hernia, and undescended testes.
   (ii) May be blind dimple or pit in the glans at expected location of meatus
(b) Epispadias: urethral opening located on the dorsal surface of the penis.

  c. Urine: observe strength, direction of stream, and color.
    (1) Normal.
      (a) Straight, forceful, and continuous stream.
      (b) Most newborns void within first 24 hours of birth.
      (c) Uric acid crystals (flaky, rust colored) are a normal variant.
    (2) Abnormal.
      (a) Altered stream direction may indicate urinary obstruction; urine from perineum or abdomen indicates urinary fistula.
      (b) Abnormal color: red (hemoglobin or myoglobin), brown (bilirubin), brown-yellow (concentrated).

  d. Scrotum and testes: inspect for size, symmetry, color, presence of rugae, and location of testes.
    (1) Normal.
      (a) Firm, smooth testes of equal size palpable in scrotal sac; undescended testes in inguinal canal normal for preterm infants.
      (b) Darker skin pigmentation.
    (2) Abnormal: scrotal swelling or discoloration, nonpalpable testes.
      (a) Cryptorchidism, extrascrotal testes position—needs further investigation with ultrasound and karyotyping.
      (b) Nonpalpable testes: if not detected in phenotypic male, evaluate for virilizing adrenal hyperplasia.
      (c) Bifid scrotum: deep midline cleft in the scrotum.
      (d) Hydrocele: unilateral or bilateral fluid collection in scrotal sac, + transillumination.
      (e) Testicular torsion: blue discoloration, palpable firm mass, tender or nontender, – transillumination. May be surgical emergency.

4. Female.
  a. Labia and clitoris: separate labia and exert gentle downward traction to evaluate structures.
    (1) Normal: smooth, wrinkling with weight loss, hyperpigmented from hormonal influence.
    (2) Edematous at birth due to maternal hormones.
    (3) Perineum is smooth, no dimpling; fingertip width.
    (4) Abnormal.
      (a) Labia bulge may indicate inguinal hernia or ectopic ovary.
      (b) Labioscrotal fusion, female virilization.
      (c) Clitoromegaly, pseudohermaphroditism.
      (d) Genitourinary (GU) anomalies: abnormal spacing between orifices.
      (e) Rugae: ambiguous genitalia.

  b. Vagina.
    (1) Normal: pink, patent.
      (a) White or blood-tinged discharge due to hormonal influence (pseudomenstruation); can persist 2 to 4 weeks.
      (b) Redundant hymen tissue and vaginal skin tags are common.
    (2) Abnormal.
      (a) Rectovaginal fistula: feces from vagina, indicates rectovaginal fistula.
      (b) Imperforate hymen: secretions pool in vagina; can be confused with enlarged Bartholin cysts.
      (c) Hydrometrocolpos: membrane covering vaginal opening causes uterine enlargement and pooling of vaginal secretions; seen as perineal or suprapubic mass.

    c. Urethral meatus.

        (1) Normal position: below clitoris; often obscured by hymen.

        (2) Abnormal: anterior displacement.

  5. Intersex conditions.

M. Back, spine, and extremities.

  1. General considerations.

    a. Influencing factors: GA, maternal hormones, in utero position, delivery mode/history, and timing of examination.

    b. Many abnormalities are deformations from compression and contracture in utero rather than congenital defects.

    c. Review for relevant history (Brand, 2007).

        (1) Elevated maternal alfa-fetoprotein (neural tube defects).

        (2) Maternal diabetes mellitus (sacral agenesis).

        (3) Maternal deficiency folic acid or zinc; use of anticonvulsant medication.

        (4) Decreased fetal movement (congenital neuromuscular disorders).

        (5) Postnatal *S. aureus* sepsis (risk for osteomyelitis).

        (6) Family history (hip dysplasia).

  2. Observe infant at rest: appropriate number of limbs and digits; size and symmetry of upper and lower extremities; movement, position of comfort, range of motion, and trauma.

  3. Palpate for joint or bone swelling, tenderness, or crepitus.

  4. Back: position infant prone.

    a. Inspect for symmetry of sides, scapula position and symmetry, spine alignment and integrity, and presence of dermal lesions over spine or masses.

    b. Inspect skin.

        (1) Mongolian spots.

            (a) Normal variant; macular gray-blue lesions from melanocyte concentration in dermis.

            (b) Most commonly in lumbosacral region but can be found on legs, back, and shoulders.

            (c) Occurs more often in black, Hispanic, Asian, and Native American infants.

            (d) Benign; fade during childhood.

        (2) Subtle cutaneous findings can indicate hidden spinal defects; observe for sacral pits or dimples, sacral tracts (pilonidal cysts), skin tag, abnormal hair distribution or hair tufts, unusual pigmentation, hemangiomas, or lipomas (Brand, 2007).

        (3) Asymmetry of gluteal fold: suggests underlying mass (lipoma) or tethered cord (Brand, 2007).

    c. Congenital spine defects.

        (1) Closed spinal dysraphism (Brand, 2007).

            (a) Spinal lipoma.

            (b) Dermoid tumor.

            (c) Tethered cord.

            (d) Split cord malformation.

            (e) Skin tags and appendages, human tail.

            (f) Dermal sinus tract

        (2) Neural tube defect.

            (a) Failure of posterior neural tube closure (see Chapters 34 and 35).

            (b) Defect can be open, with spine and nerves exposed or covered with skin or tissue.

        (3) Sacrococcygeal teratoma: tumor (mainly benign).

        (4) Scoliosis: lateral spine curvature; evaluate for associated GU tract anomalies.

  5. Extremities.

    a. Upper extremities.

        (1) Absent humerus, radius, or ulna: associated with syndromes.

        (2) Clavicle or humerus fractures: associated with birth injury or osteogenesis imperfecta.

        (3) Blisters on hands or forearms: in utero sucking.

(4) Brachial plexus injury: stretching or tearing of nerve roots by lateral traction on shoulder during birth (Volpe, 2008); or pressure from the maternal sacral promontory during fetal descent (Jennet et al., 2002).

(a) Erb palsy ("waiter's tip"): paralysis of arm with intact grasp; asymmetric Moro reflex.

(b) Klumpke paralysis: forearm paralysis with absent grasp.

(c) Total brachial plexus injury; because the neonate cannot move the shoulder, the arms remain extended and turned inward, with the flaccid hand suggesting a "waiter's tip" hand.

(5) Observe the shape of hands and digits.

(a) Syndactyly: webbing between adjacent digits of hands.

(b) Polydactyly: supernumerary digits.

(c) Clinodactyly: congenital deviation of digits.

(d) Brachydactyly: shortened digit from shortened finger joint; normal variant; associated with achondroplasia and trisomy 21.

(6) Simian crease: single palmar crease; normal variant, positive finding in less than 50% of trisomy 21 infants (Sansoucie and Cavaliere, 2007).

(7) Nails: yellowing from meconium or postmaturity; dysplasia with chromosomal defects.

b. Buttocks.

(1) Observe for blanching or cyanosis of extremities or buttocks while umbilical catheters in use; indicates circulation compromise and potential necrosis.

(2) Dimple on buttocks can indicate congenital anomaly of femur (Fletcher, 1998).

c. Hips.

(1) Positional hip abduction: persistent joint flexion or contraction with knee extension resulting from prolonged breech position in utero.

(2) Developmental dysplasia of the hip (Witt, 2003).

(a) Asymmetric creases of buttocks and thighs due to shortened adductor muscles.

(b) Uneven knee level (positive Galeazzi sign) when positioned prone with feet level and knees at a 90-degree angle.

(c) Ortolani maneuver: detects dislocated hips.

(d) Barlow maneuver: determines dislocatable hips (Fig. 7-11).

d. Lower extremities.

(1) Legs normally slightly bowed with everted feet.

(2) Genu recurvatum: knee hyperextension; related to in utero position.

(a) Usually found in breech position, females more often than males.

(b) Associated with Ehlers-Danlos, Marfan, Klinefelter, and Turner syndromes.

(c) Mild cases are benign; severe cases may require splinting/casting.

(3) Limb or digit amputation (amniotic band syndrome).

(a) Strands of amnion can wrap around any digit or more frequently, a limb.

(b) Causes constriction and amputation.

(4) Metatarsus adductus (Furdon and Reu Donlon, 2002).

(a) May be positional or structural.

(b) Convex shape to lateral border of foot (C shaped).

(c) Adduction at tarsal-metatarsal joint; wider space between first and second toes.

(5) Talipes equinovarus; clubfoot.

(a) May be positional or structural.

(b) Inversion deformity of heel (sole points medially), forefoot incurving and ankle in equinus posture (toes pointing down and heel pointing up).

(6) Talipes calcaneovalgus: related to intrauterine position; sole of foot is flattened against uterine wall.

(7) Rocker bottom feet: arch looks like rocker bottom.

N. Neurologic examination.

1. General considerations.

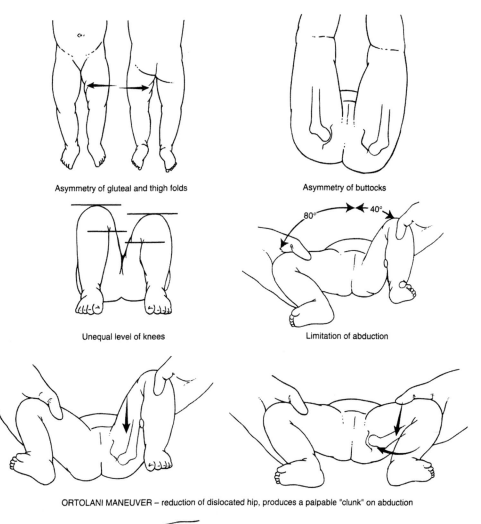

Asymmetry of gluteal and thigh folds

Asymmetry of buttocks

Unequal level of knees

Limitation of abduction

ORTOLANI MANEUVER – reduction of dislocated hip, produces a palpable "clunk" on abduction

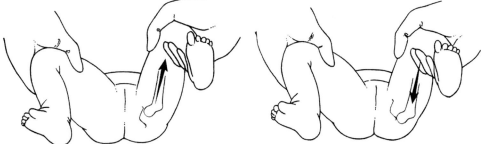

BARLOW MANEUVER – dislocation of unstable hip, produces a palpable "clunk" on adduction with gentle downward pressure

FIGURE 7-11 ■ Assessment of newborn infant for dislocated or unstable hip includes gluteal and thigh folds, buttocks, knees, abduction, Ortolani maneuver, and Barlow maneuver. (From Nichols, F.H. and Zwelling, E.: *Maternal-newborn nursing: Theory and practice.* Philadelphia, 1997, Saunders.)

    a. Repeat examination of abnormal findings; assess changes over time.
    b. Review history: familial, genetic, or neurologic diagnosis; birth trauma; difficult delivery; perinatal depression; maternal medication, alcohol, and/or drugs.
    c. GA is an important consideration; responses of preterm infant are immature.
    d. Timing and sequence of examination may alter the neurologic examination (Volpe, 2008).

       (1) Optimal timing for older newborns is about two thirds between feedings.

       (2) Clinical condition may necessitate exclusion of parts of examination.

2. Observe for skin lesions related to neurologic disorders (Jones, 2005).
   a. Neurofibromatosis: café au lait spots, greater than 1.5 cm in length or in numbers of six or greater.
   b. Sturge-Weber syndrome: nevus flammeus noted unilaterally, following the trigeminal nerve tract on the face and possibly involving the upper trunk.
   c. Tuberous sclerosis: areas of hypopigmented (white) macules on the skin.

3. Assess posture: assess infant in quiet awake, quiet active, or light sleep state(s); unswaddled; position supine with head midline.
   a. Term infant lies with arms adducted, hips abducted and partially flexed, moderate flexion of all extremities, and with loosely clenched fists.
   b. Preterm infant becomes more hypotonic with decreasing GA.
   c. Abnormal.
      (1) Persistent neck extension (opisthotonos).
      (2) Obligate thumb flexion (cortical thumb).
      (3) Elbow flexion with dorsum of hands on bed.
      (4) Frog-leg position at greater than 36 weeks of gestation.

4. Observe spontaneous movement.
   a. Term infant moves limbs smoothly.
   b. Preterm infant's movements may be jittery and jerky, with tremors.
   c. Environmental stimuli or discomfort produces mass movements.
   d. Coarse tremors and brief chin trembling are normal.
   e. Jittery: rhythmic movements of equal intensity.
      (1) Occurs more after startle or crying.
      (2) Distinguish between tonic and clonic seizures using gentle restraint: tremors will stop; seizures will continue.

5. Cry.
   a. Lusty, with normal pitch: normal term infant.
   b. Weak or monotonous cry: depressed, ill, or preterm infant.
   c. High-pitched cry: neurologic or metabolic abnormalities, drug withdrawal.

6. Tone.
   a. With decreasing GA, it may be more difficult to distinguish between random movement and true recoil.
   b. Note weak, absent, or unequal responses.
   c. Assess resistance to movement (passive tone).
      (1) Limb recoil, heel-to-ear, scarf sign.
      (2) Tendon reflex: only patellar reflex is reliable at birth; note sustained clonus.
   d. Assess resistance to gravity (active tone).
      (1) Traction response: pull-to-sit, ventral suspension; note degree of resistance.
      (2) Ventral and horizontal suspension.

7. Reflexes.
   a. Developmental reflexes (primitive reflexes): should be elicited in the normal term infant. Note any exaggerated or absent responses.
      (1) Sucking reflex: gently stimulate lips; infant opens mouth and begins to suck.
         (a) Evaluate the coordination and strength of the suck with a gloved finger.
         (b) Present at birth even in the premature infant, although it is not as strong as at term.
      (2) Rooting reflex: stroke cheek: infant turns head and opens mouth toward the stimulated side.
      (3) Palmar grasp: stroke the infant's palm with finger; infant will grasp the finger.
         (a) Attempts to remove the finger will elicit a tighter grasp.
         (b) Grasp should be equal bilaterally.
      (4) Tonic neck reflex (fencing position).
         (a) Position the infant supine. Turn the infant's head to one side.

      (b) The infant will extend the upper extremity on the side where the head is turned and flex the opposite upper extremity.

    (5) Moro reflex (startle reflex): "head drop" method preferred depending on the infant's condition (Sniderman and Taeusch, 2005). The high-risk neonate can be startled by making a loud noise close to the ear and noting the response.

      (a) Hold infant supine in a neutral position several inches off the bed.

      (b) Hold one hand behind the upper back and other supporting head. Infant's arms should cover the chest.

      (c) Head is held midline and dropped back 1 cm with supportive hand.

      (d) Infant will partially abduct shoulder, extend, and then smoothly adduct arms.

        (i)   Evaluate arm responses only.

        (ii) Repeat two or three times as needed for detailed observation.

        (iii) Asymmetric response may indicate brachial plexus injury.

    (6) Stepping reflex: Hold the infant upright, allowing the soles of the feet to touch a flat surface; infant will alternate stepping movements.

    (7) Babinski reflex.

      (a) Stimulate sole of foot; infant will either flex or extend toes.

      (b) Persistent absence of reflex can indicate CNS depression or spinal nerve dysfunction.

  b. Spinal reflexes.

    (1) Truncal incurvation reflex (Galant reflex).

      (a) Hold infant in ventral suspension.

      (b) Apply firm pressure along the side parallel to spine.

      (c) Infant should flex pelvis toward the stimulated side.

      (d) Indicates T2-S1 innervation.

    (2) Anocutaneous reflex (anal wink).

      (a) Stimulate perianal skin.

      (b) External sphincter constricts.

      (c) Indicates S4-5 innervation.

8. Cranial nerves.

  a. Olfactory (I).

    (1) Not usually assessed in newborns.

    (2) Can attempt in infants with strong scents such as clove or peppermint placed under nose; evaluate for sniffing, grimace, or startle reflex.

  b. Optic (II).

    (1) Evaluate visual acuity and fields by using tracking methods.

    (2) Watch for wandering or persistent nystagmus.

    (3) Check pupils for size and constriction in response to light.

  c. Oculomotor (II), trochlear (IV), and abducens (VI) nerves: supply pupils and extraocular muscles.

    (1) Observe pupil response to light.

    (2) Evaluate eye size and symmetry.

    (3) "Doll's-eyes" test (vestibular response): move infant's head from side to side, eyes should move away from the direction of rotation.

    (4) Fixed position or movement in same direction may indicate brainstem or oculomotor dysfunction.

  d. Trigeminal nerve (V): supplies sensory nerves of jaw and face.

    (1) Touch the cheek; infant will demonstrate rooting reflex.

    (2) Place a gloved finger in the infant's mouth to evaluate sucking and biting reflex.

  e. Facial nerve (VII): controls facial expression.

    (1) Observe for symmetric movement of the face.

    (2) Inability to wrinkle brow or close eyes with crying indicates injury.

  f. Auditory nerve (VIII): tested only grossly without proper auditory equipment (see 9, Sensory Function Responses).

  g. Glossopharyngeal nerve (IX): evaluate and inspect tongue movements and elicit gag reflex.

    h. Vagus nerve (X): supplies the soft plate, pharynx, and larynx.

        (1) Listen to cry: determine the presence or absence of stridor, hoarseness, or aphonia.

        (2) Evaluate infant's ability to swallow.

    i. Accessory nerve (XI): supplies neck muscles (sternocleidomastoid and trapezius).

        (1) Turn infant's head from midline to one side.

        (2) Infant should attempt to bring head back to midline.

    j. Hypoglossal nerve (XII): supplies tongue muscles. Evaluate suck, swallow, and gag reflexes.

9. Sensory function responses.

    a. Touch.

        (1) Painful stimulus to a foot elicits a withdrawal reflex.

        (2) Touch sole of the foot with a pin to provoke flexion of the limb and extension of the contralateral limb.

        (3) Absence of flexion in the stimulated leg is abnormal.

    b. Light: shining a penlight into the infant's eye results in eyelid closure.

    c. Sound.

        (1) Ring a bell sharply within a few inches of the infant's ear while the infant is lying supine.

        (2) Response is based on observable attentiveness to the sound.

        (3) A brainstem auditory evoked response is recommended in the newborn period for all infants.

REFERENCES

American Academy of Pediatrics and American College of Obstetricians and Gynecologists: *Guidelines for perinatal care* (6th ed.). Elk Village Grove, IL, 2007, American Academy of Pediatrics and American College of Obstetricians and Gynecologists.

American Academy of Pediatrics: Policy statement. Age terminology during the perinatal period. *Pediatrics,* 114(5):1362-1364, 2004.

Ballard, J.L., Khoury, J.C., Wedig, K., et al.: New Ballard Score, expanded to include extremely premature infants. *Journal of Pediatrics,* 119(3):417-423, 1991.

Bates, M.D. and Balistreri, W.F.: The neonatal gastrointestinal tract. Part 1: Development of the human digestive system. In A.A. Fanaroff and R.J. Martin (Eds.): *Neonatal-perinatal medicine: Diseases of the fetus and infant* (7th ed.). St. Louis, 2002, Mosby.

Benjamin, K.: Part I Injuries to the brachial plexus: Mechanism of injury and identification of risk factors. *Advances in Neonatal Care,* 5(4):181-189, 2005.

Bernstein, D.: Evaluation of the cardiovascular system: history and physical examination. In Behrman, R.E., Kliegman, R.M. (Eds.): *Nelson textbook of pediatrics* (17th ed). Philadelphia, 2004, Saunders.

Brand, M.C.: Part 3: Examination of the newborn with closed spinal dysraphism. *Advances in Neonatal Care,* 7(1):30-40, 2007.

Breeze, A.C.G. and Lees, C.C.: Prediction and perinatal outcomes of fetal growth restriction. *Seminars in Fetal and Neonatal Medicine,* 12:383-397, 2007.

Britton, B.A.: Intrauterine growth retardation: A review and update. *Central Lines,* 17(5):16-23, 2001.

Clark, D.A.: *Atlas of neonatology.* Philadelphia, 2000, Saunders.

Doctor, B.A., O'Riordan, M.A., Kirchner, H.L., et al.: Perinatal correlates and neonatal outcomes of small for gestational age infants born at term gestation. *American Journal of Obstetrics and Gynecology,* 185(3):652-659, 2001.

Donovan, E.F., Tyson, J.E., Ehrenkranz, R.A., et al.: Inaccuracy of Ballard scores before 28 weeks' gestation. National Institute of Child Health and Human Developmental Neonatal Research Network. *Journal of Pediatrics,* 135(2 Pt 1):147-152, 1999.

Dubowitz, L.M.S., Dubowitz, V., and Goldberg, C.: Clinical assessment of gestational age in the newborn infant. *Journal of Pediatrics,* 77(1):1-10, 1970.

Engle, W.A.A.: A recommendation for the definition of "late preterm" (near-term) and the birth weight-gestational age classification system. *Seminars in Perinatology,* 30:2-7, 2006.

Fenton, T.R.: A new growth chart for preterm babies: Babson and Benda's chart updated with recent data and a new format. *BMC Pediatrics,* 3:13, 2003.

Fletcher, M.A.: *Physical diagnosis in neonatology.* Philadelphia, 1998, Lippincott-Raven.

Furdon, S.A. and Clark, D.A: Differentiating scalp swelling in the newborn. *Advances in Neonatal Care,* 1:22, 2001.

Furdon, S.A. and Clark, D.A.: Scalp hair characteristics in the newborn infant. *Advances in Neonatal Care,* 3(6):286-296, 2003.

Furdon, S.A. and Reu Donlon, C.: Examination of the newborn foot: Positional and structural abnormalities. *Advances in Neonatal Care,* 2(5):248-258, 2002.

Goodwin, G. and Caldamone, A.: Ambiguous genitalia in the newborn. In H.W. Taeusch, R.A. Ballard and

C.A. Gleason (Eds.): *Avery's diseases of the newborn* (8th ed.). Philadelphia, 2005, Saunders, p. 1378.

Higgins, R.D., Delivoria-Papadopoulos, M., and Raju, T.N.K.: Executive summary of the workshop on the border of viability. *Pediatrics, 115*(5), 2005.

Jennet, R.J., Tarby, T.J., and Krauss, R.L.: Erb's palsy contrasted with Klumpe's and total palsy: Different mechanisms are involved. *American Journal of Obstetrics and Gynecology, 186*(6):112-116, 2002.

Jones, K.L.: Facial features as major feature. In K.L. Jones (Ed.): *Smith's recognizable patterns of human malformation* (5th ed.). Philadelphia, 2005, Saunders, p. 250.

Kohelet, D. and Arbel, E.: A prospective search for urinary tract abnormalities in infants with isolated preauricular tags. *Pediatrics, 105*(5):e61, 2000.

Lawrence, E.J.: Part 1. A mater of size: evaluating the growth-restricted neonate. *Advances in Neonatal Care, 6*(6):313-322, 2006.

Lawrence, E.J.: A matter of size: Part 2. Evaluating the large-for-gestational-age neonate. *Advances in Neonatal Care, 7*(4):187-197, 2007.

Lowdermilk, D.L. and Perry, S.E.: *Maternity & women's health care* (9th ed). St. Louis, 2007, Mosby.

Lund, C.H. and Kuller, J.M.: Integumentary system. In C. Kenner and J.W. Lott (Eds.): *Comprehensive neonatal care: An interdisciplinary approach* (4th ed.). St. Louis, 2007, Saunders, p. 65.

McIntire, D.D., Bloom, S.L., Casey, B.M., and Leveno, K.J.: Birth weight in relation to morbidity and mortality among newborn infants. *New England Journal of Medicine, 340*(16):1234-1238, 1999.

McIntire, D.D. and Leveno K.J.: Neonatal mortality and morbidity rates in late preterm births compared with births at term. *Obstetrics and Gynecology. 111*(1):35-41, 2008.

Merritt, L.: Part 2. Physical assessment of the infant with cleft lip and/or palate. *Advances in Neonatal Care, 5*(3): 125-134, 2005.

O'Leary, D.R, Kuhn, S., and Kniss, K.L., et al.: Birth outcomes following West Nile Virus infection of pregnant women in the United States: 2003-2004. *Pediatrics, 117*(3):e537-e545, 2006.

Parker, L.: Genitourinary system. In C. Kenner and J.W. Lott (Eds.): *Comprehensive neonatal care: An interdisci-*plinary approach (4th ed.). St. Louis, 2007, Saunders, p. 175.

Roberton, N.R.C.: Clinical examination. In S.K. Sinha and S.M. Donn (Eds.): *Manual of neonatal and respiratory care*. Armonk, NY, 2000, Futura, p. 45.

Sansoucie, D.A. and Cavaliere, T.A.: Newborn and infant assessment. In C. Kenner and J.W. Lott (Eds.): *Comprehensive neonatal care: An interdisciplinary approach* (4th ed.). St. Louis, 2007, Saunders, p. 677.

Sniderman, S. and Taeusch, H.W.: Initial evaluation: History and physical examination of the newborn. In H.W. Taeusch, R.A. Ballard and C.A. Gleason (Eds.): *Avery's diseases of the newborn* (8th ed.). Philadelphia, 2005, Saunders, p. 301.

Southgate, W.M. and Pittard, W.B.: Classification and physical examination of the newborn infant. In M.H. Klaus and A.A. Fanaroff (Eds.): *Care of the high-risk neonate* (5th ed.). Philadelphia, 2001, Saunders, p. 100.

Stokowski, A.A.: Hypospadias in the neonate. *Advances in Neonatal Care, 4*(4):206-215, 2004.

Thigpen, J.: Gastrointestinal system. In C. Kenner and J.W. Lott (Eds.): *Comprehensive neonatal care: An interdisciplinary approach* (4th ed.). St. Louis, 2007, Saunders, p. 92.

Thomas, P., Peabody, J., Turnier, V., and Clark, R.H.: A new look at intrauterine growth and the impact of race, altitude, and gender. *Pediatrics, 106*(2), 2000. Retrieved March 5, 2003, from www.pediatrics.org/cgi/content/full/106/2/e21.

Vargo, L.: Cardiovascular assessment of the newborn. In E. Tappero and M. Honeyfield (Eds.): *Physical assessment of the newborn* (2nd ed.). Petaluma, CA, 1996, NICU Ink, pp. 81, 87, 90.

Volpe, J.H.: *Neurology of the newborn* (5th ed.). Philadelphia, 2008, Saunders.

Winn, H.N.: Group B streptococcus infection in pregnancy. *Clinics in Perinatology, 34*:387-392, 2007.

Witt, C.: Detecting developmental dysplasia of the hip. *Advances in Neonatal Care, 3*(2):65-75, 2003.

Woods, A.G. and Brandon D.H.: Prune belly syndrome. A focused physical assessment. *Advances in Neonatal Care, 7*(3):132-143, 2007.

8 Fluid and Electrolyte Management

BRENDA HUESKE HALBARDIER

OBJECTIVES

1. Identify the influences on fluid and electrolyte homeostasis in the newborn infant.
2. Describe fluid and electrolyte management in the neonate.
3. Compare fluid and electrolyte management of the full-term infant and the prematurely born newborn.
4. Discuss acid-base balance in the neonatal period.

■■■ An essential part of the successful transition to extrauterine life is the achievement of fluid, electrolyte, and acid-base homeostasis and control. Because mature control of these processes may not occur for days to weeks after birth, premature and other stressed neonates can have transient disturbances of fluid, electrolyte, and acid-base balance.

FLUID BALANCE

Physiologic and Assessment Considerations

A. **Fluid homeostasis in the fetus and neonate.**
   1. Body water distribution. Water, the most abundant component of the body, is distributed in two main compartments: intracellular fluid (ICF) and extracellular fluid (ECF); the latter is composed of intravascular and interstitial spaces. As gestation progresses, the fetus undergoes changes in total body water (TBW) content and its distribution:
      a. Early in gestation, water makes up 95% of total body weight, with the majority in ECF compartments.
      b. By term, water makes up 75% of body weight and a greater proportion has shifted from ECF to ICF compartments. These changes are largely due to increases in body fat content.
   2. Fluid adjustments after birth.
      a. An acute increase in intravascular volume occurs after birth. Timing of cord clamping can influence the volume increase.
      b. A physiologic contraction of ECF volume occurs with diuresis in the first week of life, resulting in postnatal weight loss. This is reflected in a weight loss of 5% to 10% in term infants and up to 20% in preterm infants. This may be related to levels of circulating atrial natriuretic peptide (Modi et al., 2000).
B. **Regulation of fluid balance.**
   1. Renal mechanisms.
      a. Because water and electrolyte balance is regulated by the placenta, the role of the fetal kidneys is primarily to maintain amniotic fluid volume. Fetal nephrons are functional but immature until 34 weeks. Renal blood flow, renal tubular function, and glomerular filtration rate (GFR) are all immature in the fetus and in the extremely premature infant (Vogt et al., 2001).
      b. After birth, renal blood flow increases as renal vascular resistance falls. Improved renal function in the days after birth from increased GFR is more pronounced in the term than in the preterm infant.

    c. Both term and preterm infants can dilute urine; however, when faced with a rapid fluid load, the preterm infant may have a delayed response, resulting in fluid retention.

    d. Reabsorption of sodium, bicarbonate, and glucose is limited in the newborn infant.

    e. The use of antenatal steroids has been associated with decreased insensible water losses (IWLs), less frequent incidence of hypernatremia, and an earlier diuresis. The exact mechanism of action is not known (Omar et al., 1999).

  2. Hormonal mechanisms.

    a. Antidiuretic hormone (ADH) is released by the posterior pituitary in response to a variety of stimuli, including hypotension and hyperosmolality. ADH influences water balance by stimulating the kidneys to conserve water. In the absence of ADH, the distal tubules remain impermeable to water, which is excreted as urine.

    b. Because of decreased responsiveness to ADH, neonates cannot efficiently concentrate urine in response to fluid deprivation.

C. Fluid losses in the neonatal period.

  1. Renal losses: Urine output ranges from 1 to 4 ml/kg/hour. Highest flow rates occur during the physiologic reduction in ECF.

  2. IWLs: These are the nonmeasurable losses that occur through the skin and respiratory system. Factors influencing IWLs are summarized in Box 8-1.

    a. Transepidermal water loss (TEWL): TEWL occurs as body water diffuses through the immature epidermis and is lost to the atmosphere. Skin features such as poor keratinization, high water content, low subcutaneous fat, large surface area, and high degree of skin vascularity all predispose the premature infant to high evaporative losses.

      (1) TEWL increases with decreasing gestational age (Lund and Kuller, 2007).

      (2) TEWL is the major source of IWL in very premature infants.

      (3) TEWL is highest on the first day after birth, decreasing on subsequent days as the barrier function of the skin improves. This improvement slows with decreasing gestational age, taking several weeks for the development of a fully functional stratum corneum in the extremely premature infant (Lund and Kuller, 2007).

      (4) TEWL is closely related to ambient relative humidity. TEWL increases with decreasing ambient humidity.

      (5) TEWL does not appear to be influenced by antenatal steroids or gender (Jain et al., 2000).

      (6) Failure to account for TEWL increases the possibility of inaccurate estimates of fluid needs, with resultant fluid and electrolyte imbalances.

■ BOX 8-1
■ **ENVIRONMENTAL INFLUENCES ON INSENSIBLE WATER LOSS (IWL)**

Factors That May Increase IWL:	Factors That May Decrease IWL:
Extreme prematurity	Increasing gestation
Postnatal age less than 1 week	Increasing postnatal age
Low relative ambient humidity	High relative ambient humidity
Radiant warmer use	Double-walled incubator use
High ambient temperature	Neutral thermal environment
Hyperthermia	Heat shields/plastic blankets
Convection; drafts	Humidification of inspired gases
Ventilation with dry gases	Ointments or transparent dressings on skin
Tachypnea	Clothing
High minute ventilation	
Phototherapy	
Activity	

      b. Respiratory losses: roughly 0 to 10 ml/kg/day; related to the temperature and humidity of inspired gases and to minute ventilation.

   3. Stool losses: estimated to be 5 ml/kg/day in the first week of life, increasing to 10 ml/day thereafter.

   4. Other losses are possible. These include but may not be limited to gastric drainage, enterostomies, surgical wounds, and pleural fluid drainage.

D. Fluid therapy.

   1. Goal of fluid therapy: The goal is to permit physiologic, adaptive fluid and electrolyte changes to occur appropriately (Davis and Avner, 2002; Kerr et al., 2006).

   2. General principles guiding fluid volume decisions. No fixed fluid administration schedules are appropriate for all infants.

      a. During the first 3 to 5 days after birth, fluid intake should be at a level that allows a reasonable weight loss yet avoids intracellular dehydration. Provision of 60 to 100 ml/kg/day, depending on the degree of control over IWL, is a typical starting point. Extremely premature infants require more fluid relative to body weight because of a larger IWL. Fluids given to correct shock, hypoglycemia, or acidosis must be taken into account.

      b. Fluid intake is gradually increased on subsequent days to 150 to 175 ml/kg/day, although fluids may be restricted longer for infants with severe cardiorespiratory disorders, renal failure, and postasphyxial syndrome.

      c. Infants with ongoing fluid losses (chest tube drainage, gastric drainage, enterostomy drainage, diarrhea) may need replacement of these volumes with appropriate fluids.

      d. It is generally recommended to use birth weight, rather than current body weight, to calculate fluids on a per-kilogram basis until birth weight is reachieved.

   3. Fluid constituents.

      a. Dextrose 10% in water is most commonly used for initial fluid therapy. Decreasing dextrose concentrations may be prescribed initially for infants who weighed less than 1 kg at birth, because of the incidence of hyperglycemia in this population.

      b. Electrolytes are not usually added to maintenance intravenous (IV) fluids for the first 24 to 48 hours after birth. Serum electrolyte levels and urine output are used to determine when to add these electrolytes to IV fluids.

E. Assessment of fluid balance: Quantifying fluid requirements in extremely preterm infants is difficult. Fluid restriction places the infant at risk for dehydration, whereas fluid excess places the infant at risk for intravascular fluid overload (Davis and Avner, 2002). Close monitoring of hydration status is imperative, with some infants requiring assessment of their fluid balance as often as every 6 to 8 hours.

   1. Body weight: Weight changes with alterations in fluid balance only if there is a net change in TBW; internal shifts of body fluid may not be detected by weight alone. Because the procedure for weighing the ELBW infant is prone to errors and a significant source of stress for the infant, some neonatal intensive care units (NICUs) have abandoned weighing these infants in the first few days after birth. In-bed electronic scales may be used; however, weights obtained in this manner can be affected by the amount of equipment attached to the infant and how the neonate is handled during weighing.

   2. Urine volume: For greatest possible accuracy, urine output must be measured right after it occurs; urine collected onto diapers lying under radiant warmers may evaporate before the diapers are weighed for determination of output.

   3. Specific gravity of urine: an indirect measure of urine osmolality. Normal values (1.002 to 1.012) reflect a normal urine osmolality (100 to 300 mOsm/l). Specific gravity is an unreliable predictor of urine osmolality if glucose, blood, or protein is present.

   4. Assessment parameters:

      a. Physical assessment: quality of skin turgor, mucous membranes, presence of edema, appearance of eyes, and level of anterior fontanelle.

      b. Hemodynamic assessment: pulse quality, blood pressure, and perfusion (capillary refill time, temperature, and acid–base balance).

   5. Laboratory evaluation of hydration status: serum sodium level, osmolality, blood urea nitrogen (BUN), creatinine, and/or hematocrit.

DISORDERS OF FLUID BALANCE

Disorders of fluid balance in the newborn infant do not always fit neatly into categories such as "fluid depletion" or "fluid excess"; some involve elements of both. One such disorder is septic shock, in which low intravascular volume (a fluid deficit) can coexist with interstitial and cellular edema (a fluid surplus). For simplicity, an attempt is made here to group clinical conditions according to the primary effect on TBW (e.g., decreased, as in dehydration, or increased, as in congestive heart failure), even though there may be an overlap.

Fluid Depletion

A. **Pathophysiology:** Fluid can be lost from the body acutely or gradually. Sudden loss of body fluid can result in signs and symptoms of shock. If lost fluid is not restored, the body will attempt to compensate by retaining sodium and water. Gradual or chronic fluid loss, even though central blood pressure may be maintained, can result in serious metabolic disturbances.

B. **Causes and precipitating factors.**
1. Extreme prematurity (<28 weeks of gestation, <800 g). The large TEWL and rapid contraction of the ECF result in a sodium excess that cannot be excreted efficiently by the kidneys. If fluid intake is inadequate, hyperosmolar hypernatremic dehydration ensues.
2. Acute blood loss/hypovolemia: hemorrhagic losses at birth, postnatal internal hemorrhage, surgical blood loss, or the removal of large volumes for laboratory tests.
3. Diarrhea.
4. Diabetes insipidus (pure renal water loss from failure to secrete or respond to ADH). This condition is treated with intranasally administered arginine vasopressin (DDAVP).
5. Abdominal or pleural cavity exposure during surgery.
6. Unreplaced losses from gastric suction.
7. Medications that may cause diuresis: caffeine and theophylline.
8. Breastfeeding malnutrition: inadequate intake in a breastfed infant with a cycle of reduced milk production and decreasing demand, resulting in severe malnutrition, dehydration, and hypernatremia.

C. **Clinical presentation and assessment.**
1. Weight loss if net reduction in TBW.
2. Low urine output (<0.5 ml/kg/hour); possibly high specific gravity. Urine output may be normal or even high in the ELBW infant during postnatal diuresis.
3. Poor skin turgor (gently pinched skin is slow to retract) and dry skin and mucous membranes.
4. Hemodynamic changes: tachycardia or decreased pulses with peripheral vasoconstriction (pale, cool, mottled skin with prolonged capillary filling time), increased core-peripheral temperature differential, central blood pressure either normal or low.
5. In breastfeeding malnutrition, possible excessive sleepiness, disinterest in feeding, or irritability.

D. **Diagnostic studies.**
1. Serum sodium can be low, normal, or high, depending on the cause of dehydration/fluid loss.
2. With dehydration, BUN and creatinine levels may be elevated.
3. Hematocrit levels may be increased or decreased with blood loss.
4. Blood gas values may reveal metabolic acidosis in the infant with hypovolemia.

E. **Patient care management.**
1. Hypovolemic states (shock, hemorrhage) are managed acutely with volume replacement and vasoactive inotropic agents, as described elsewhere in this text.
2. The type of fluid given to replace other fluid deficits depends on the constituents of lost fluid (e.g., free water loss, electrolyte loss) and the infant's electrolyte levels. Determination of the fluid constitution can be guided by evaluating the electrolyte composition of the fluid being lost.
3. Management of severe dehydration involves replacing the free water deficit slowly over several days to avoid a rapid fall in serum osmolality.

F. Fluid management of hypernatremic hyperosmolar dehydration in the preterm infant.
1. Prevention of TEWL is more effective than replacing these losses. This is because the fluid lost is mostly solute free, whereas replacement fluids contain solutes that can aggravate hyperosmolality.
2. The single method or combination of methods most effective in reducing TEWL has yet to be proved. Each of the following strategies will decrease TEWL to some degree.
    a. Use of incubators rather than radiant warmers. TEWL is higher under radiant warmers because of the lower ambient relative humidity and increased air currents the neonate is exposed to when on a radiant warmer.
    b. Supplemental humidity. Devices to saturate the air immediately surrounding the infant can be used with both incubators and radiant warmers. Humidifier temperature, airflow setting, and seasonal ambient relative humidity variations can significantly affect the achievable humidity level.
    c. Heat shields or plastic film "blankets" increase ambient humidity by using the infant's own trapped evaporative losses.
    d. Semipermeable dressings (adhesive or nonadhesive) may help reduce TEWL.
3. Reduce respiratory water losses by using humidified gas mixtures.
4. Even with maximal reductions in IWL, fluid intake must occasionally be increased, especially in ELBW infants. Giving too much fluid in response to hypernatremic dehydration can aggravate hyperglycemia and increase the risk of heart failure, pulmonary edema, and central nervous system (CNS) injury. It is usually recommended to give just enough fluid to maintain the serum sodium in the high normal range (145 to 150 mEq/L) during the first 24 to 72 hours of life (Kerr et al., 2006).
5. Restrict sodium (unless the infant is hyponatremic), adding gradually when serum sodium level decreases and diuresis begins.
6. Monitor hydration closely. Weight loss may be accepted if other parameters indicate adequate hydration.

G. Complications.
1. Excessive weight loss.
2. Hypotension, tissue damage, or metabolic acidosis from hypoperfusion.
3. Impaired excretion of drugs when urine output is minimal.
4. Electrolyte imbalances from slow excretion of daily solute load.
5. Renal failure and vascular thrombosis: possible result of severe dehydration.

Fluid Excess

A. Pathophysiology: The spectrum of disease that can cause body fluid excess in the neonate is broad. Many of the disorders are characterized by edema, which is the abnormal accumulation of ECF within the interstitial spaces. Edema can be caused by the following:
1. Low colloid osmotic pressure (decreased plasma protein concentration).
2. Increased capillary permeability to water and protein (may be secondary to tissue hypoxia).
3. Increased hydrostatic pressure within the capillaries.
4. Impaired lymphatic drainage of interstitial fluids and proteins.
  With some of the disorders associated with these pathologic processes, a combination of venous congestion, renal failure, and edema suggests a state of fluid overload even when circulating blood volume is low.

B. Etiologies and precipitating factors.
1. Cardiac dysfunction: congenital heart disease, congestive heart failure, patent ductus arteriosus (PDA).
2. Respiratory distress syndrome and bronchopulmonary dysplasia (BPD). Therapeutic use of oxygen and positive-pressure ventilation causes endothelial injury with subsequent fluid leakage. In the first few days after birth, increased lung fluid complicates the picture of respiratory distress and failure to clear the fluid adds to the possibility of developing BPD (Adams et al., 2000, 2002).

   3. Perinatal asphyxia.
   4. Sepsis, necrotizing enterocolitis.
   5. Hydrops fetalis.
   6. Renal failure.
   7. Miscalculation of fluid needs or provision of too much fluid (possibly from failure to account for all sources of fluid, such as flush solutions, medications, and colloids).
   8. Use of neuromuscular blocking agents.
   9. Syndrome of inappropriate antidiuretic hormone (SIADH): usually associated with CNS infection or injury. ADH secretion is inappropriate to usual osmotic and volume stimuli. The result is fluid retention with hyponatremia, low serum osmolality, and high urinary sodium loss.
C. **Clinical presentation and assessment.**
   1. Weight gain, if there is a net increase in TBW.
   2. Urine output: possible decrease.
   3. Edema: peripheral, generalized, pulmonary.
   4. Hemodynamic changes: dependent on intravascular volume status. When increased, there may be symptomatic PDA, tachycardia, and increased pulses or blood pressure. With congestive heart failure, venous filling pressure is high.
D. **Diagnostic studies.**
   1. Serum osmolality is low (<280 mOsm/l); urine osmolality is normal.
   2. In SIADH, osmolalities and sodium levels of urine and serum are diagnostic (urine output is low with high specific gravity and high sodium levels; serum has low sodium level and low osmolality).
E. **Patient care management**: In addition to therapy aimed at the underlying disease process:
   1. Precise fluid management with fluid restriction is necessary. Daily fluid calculations must take into account renal function and the extra fluids given to administer medications and flush intravascular catheters.
   2. Diuretics may be useful.
   3. Infants with severe edema and low intravascular volume (shock) present a challenge. Maintenance of an adequate circulating blood volume may require volume expansion and vasoactive agents while minimizing maintenance fluid administration.
   4. Edema may predispose the infant to necrotic injury of the skin. The skin must be protected from pressure with careful repositioning, support, and the use of a nonrigid sleeping surface, such as a gel- or water-filled mattress.
F. **Complications.**
   1. Fluid sequestration in static body fluid compartments ("third spacing") can result in a loss of effective blood volume, compromising the delivery of oxygen and nutrients to tissues throughout the body. This can lead not only to serious metabolic imbalances but also permanent tissue damage.
   2. Excessive fluid administration early in life has been associated with worsening of respiratory distress syndrome and development of BPD, symptomatic PDA, and necrotizing enterocolitis.

ELECTROLYTE BALANCE AND DISORDERS

Sodium

A. **Sodium homeostasis:** Reference ranges vary slightly between laboratories. In general, a range of 135 to 145 mEq/l is acceptable.
   1. Functions of sodium (Na). Na, the major extracellular cation, is closely involved in water balance. Na and other electrolytes are found in varying concentrations in all body fluid compartments. Electrolytes determine the tonicity of the fluid compartment and influence the passage of water through the vascular and cell membranes, thereby controlling the osmotic equilibrium between compartments. With a surplus of Na, blood becomes hypertonic, causing a shift of fluid from intracellular to extracellular spaces, which results in

cellular dehydration. A deficit of Na causes hypotonicity and fluid shifts into the cells (cellular edema).

2. Regulation of Na. Cellular transport of Na is achieved by the sodium-potassium pump, which maintains the electrochemical sodium and potassium gradients across the cell membrane. Renal (GFR, tubular function) and hormonal (aldosterone, ADH) mechanisms influence the body content of Na. Although preterm infants can excrete sodium, a low GFR early in life may hamper this ability. In addition, minimal responsiveness to aldosterone and ADH contributes to a baseline salt-wasting tendency.

3. Positive Na balance. Na intake greater than Na losses. This is a prerequisite for the growth of new tissue.

B. Hyponatremia.

1. Pathophysiology. A serum Na below 130 mEq/dl. Reflects either an excess of body water relative to normal body Na content or a primary Na depletion. When urinary Na wasting occurs, a proportionate loss of water (isotonic dehydration) can reduce ECF volume and lead to oliguria.

2. Causes and precipitating factors.
   a. Prematurity (renal and hormonal immaturity, with tendency to excrete Na). Preterm infants are most vulnerable to hyponatremia just after the period of postnatal extracellular volume contraction (Kerr et al., 2006).
   b. Conditions associated with low intravascular volume (e.g., shock). Baroreceptor stimulation of ADH results in reduced renal water excretion and a dilutional hyponatremia.
   c. Dilutional hyponatremia from excessive free water intake.
   d. Renal losses related to prematurity or medications (furosemide, methylxanthines). Urine Na excretion rate should be measured to rule out excessive Na losses.
   e. Inadequate Na intake during period of rapid growth, especially in preterm infants fed exclusively human milk. Called *late hyponatremia* because it occurs after the first week of life.
   f. Serum Na can be factitiously low in the presence of hyperlipidemia.

3. Clinical presentation and assessment.
   a. Usually asymptomatic, but apnea, irritability, twitching, or seizures can occur if Na drops acutely or falls to less than 115 mEq/l.
   b. Infants with late hyponatremia may fail to gain weight.

4. Patient care management.
   a. Provide Na supplementation after postnatal diuresis begins (usually on day 2). Maintenance Na requirement is 1 to 4 mEq/kg/day and is usually given as sodium chloride, though sodium acetate or sodium bicarbonate may be used if the infant has metabolic acidosis. In very small infants, early Na supplementation has been associated with increased risk of BPD (Hartnoll et al., 2000).
   b. A chronic hyponatremic state is corrected gradually over 48 to 72 hours to prevent injury to brain cells (Seri et al., 2005).
   c. Monitor weight, urine output, parameters of hydration, and adequacy of intravascular volume (monitoring of central venous pressure, capillary refill time, and core-peripheral temperature differential).
   d. When hyponatremia is associated with an excess of body water, fluids are restricted. True SIADH is managed with fluid restriction and monitoring of Na, osmolality, and urine output.
   e. Commercial preparations designed to fortify human milk supply additional dietary sodium for this population.

5. Complications.
   a. Acute drops in the serum Na can lead to a shift of fluid into brain cells and cellular edema. This may result in apnea and seizures.
   b. The degree to which the infant's brain may be able to adapt to chronic hyponatremia is not known; however, chronic hyponatremia does impair skeletal and tissue growth.

C. Hypernatremia.
   1. Pathophysiology. A serum Na level >150 mEq/l. Usually reflects a deficiency of water relative to total body Na content and thus is actually a disorder of water balance rather than one of Na balance.
   2. Causes and precipitating factors.
      a. Excessive IWL with insufficient fluid intake (even without added Na).
      b. High inadvertent Na intake (saline infusions in arterial catheters, sodium bicarbonate [$NaHCO_3$], medications) or early addition of maintenance sodium chloride (NaCl).
      c. Breastfeeding malnutrition in term infants. Elevated human milk Na content accompanying insufficient lactation and decreased amount of free water contribute to the hyperosmolar state.
      d. Diabetes insipidus: deficiency of pituitary-secreted ADH, causing loss of water in excess of loss of Na.
   3. Clinical presentation and assessment.
      a. Signs of dehydration may be present.
      b. In severe hypernatremia, high-pitched cry, lethargy, irritability, and apnea can progress to seizures and coma.
   4. Patient care management.
      a. Gradually restrict Na to avoid sudden fall in plasma osmolality. If maintenance Na administration has not been started, it is usually delayed.
      b. Recalculate fluid intake. Fluids may have been restricted too much in light of insensible losses.
      c. Prevent hypernatremia in ELBW infants. Na supplementation may be withheld longer than usual after birth if serum Na level remains normal. In addition, measures to reduce TEWL will aid in the prevention of hypernatremia (Kerr et al., 2006; Seri et al., 2005).
      d. The need for saline solutions to maintain catheter patency presents a dilemma. Attempts to lower the infused Na concentration too far result in administration of hypotonic solutions, with risk of hemolysis.
   5. Complications. As hypernatremia develops, intracellular water can be drawn out, causing cells to shrink. If this process is rapid, this can affect the brain. Sudden increases in plasma osmolality can also contribute to intraventricular hemorrhage.

Potassium

A. Potassium homeostasis: A generally accepted reference range is 3.5 to 5.5 mEq/l.
   1. Functions of potassium (K): The major cation in ICF, K contributes to intracellular osmotic activity and in part determines ICF volume. K plays a fundamental role along with Na in regulating cell membrane potential.
   2. Regulation: K is distributed both intracellularly and extracellularly. The distribution of K between ICF and ECF is regulated by the sodium-potassium pump and is influenced by acid–base balance, insulin, and glucagon. The excretion of K from the body depends on kidney function, GFR, urine flow rate, and aldosterone sensitivity.
B. Hypokalemia: Serum K <3.5 mEq/l.
   1. Pathophysiology: Because K is 90% intracellular, it is assessed indirectly by measuring the quantity in the serum. A subnormal serum K implies insufficient K within the cells, which may impede their function. Muscle cells of the gastrointestinal system and the heart can be affected.
   2. Causes and precipitating factors.
      a. Loss of K in the urine (kaliuresis) during postnatal diuresis, before K supplementation is begun.
      b. Inadequate K intake.
      c. Increased gastrointestinal losses from an enterostomy or nasogastric tube output or vomiting.
      d. Metabolic alkalosis. A high serum pH drives K into cells, resulting in a low serum K.

      e. Medications including bicarbonate, diuretics, and insulin. Insulin increases cellular uptake of K through stimulation of activity of the sodium-potassium pump.

  3. Clinical presentation and assessment: cardiac effects (flattened T waves, prominent U waves, ST depression), hypotonia, abdominal distention, and ileus.

  4. Patient care management.

      a. Begin K supplementation when urine output is well established, usually on the second or third day of life. The maintenance K requirement is 2 to 3 mEq/kg/day.

      b. Correction of hypokalemic states must be done cautiously, with continuous cardiac monitoring.

  5. Complications.

      a. Rapid administration of K to correct hypokalemia can lead to fatal arrhythmias.

      b. Hypokalemia potentiates digitalis toxicity.

C. Hyperkalemia: Serum K >6.5 mEq/l.

  1. Pathophysiology: Heel-stick samples are often hemolyzed, rendering results unreliable. Venipuncture or arterial line sample must be obtained to determine level. In the ELBW infant, the normal postnatal shift of K from the intracellular to the extracellular compartment is intensified. During the prediuretic phase, this excess K is not efficiently excreted secondary to a low GFR and a low Na excretion rate (Eichenwald, 2005).

  2. Causes and precipitating factors.

      a. Extreme prematurity (nonoliguric, hyperkalemia).

      b. Endogenous release of K from tissue destruction, hypoperfusion, hemorrhage, and bruising.

      c. Metabolic acidosis. A low serum pH shifts K out of cells.

      d. Renal failure, with decreased K clearance. Tests of renal function: BUN, creatinine should be measured concomitantly.

      e. Adrenal insufficiency.

      f. Transfusion with blood stored longer than 3 days.

  3. Clinical presentation and assessment: Cardiac effects may be seen—ventricular tachycardia, peaked T wave, or a widened QRS complex. An electrocardiogram (ECG) should be obtained to detect cardiac arrhythmias. Serum ionized calcium should also be assessed as hypocalcemia may potentiate cardiac toxicity from hyperkalemia.

  4. Patient care management.

      a. For prevention of hyperkalemia, K is withheld from early IV fluids. Serum K is monitored as diuresis (and K excretion) begins; K is added when serum K stabilizes in the 4- to 4.5-mEq/l range.

      b. Acidosis is corrected.

      c. Diuretics and low-dose dopamine therapy may improve renal excretion of K. Dopamine also enhances K uptake by stimulation of activity of the sodium-potassium pump.

      d. Temporary measures may be needed to reduce the effects of circulating K until the total body K level can be reduced.

          (1) Administration of calcium gluconate will lower the cell membrane threshold transiently, antagonizing the effects on the heart muscle.

          (2) Glucose/insulin infusion to enhance cellular uptake of K.

          (3) $NaHCO_3$ (metabolic alkalosis shifts K into cells).

      e. When other measures fail to normalize K:

          (1) Cation exchange resin. Sodium polystyrene sulfonate (Kayexalate), a potassium-binding resin given by rectum or mouth, exchanges Na for K in the intestine to increase the excretion of K. Because the onset of action is within 2 to 24 hours, treatment with this medication alone may not be sufficient to rapidly correct severe hyperkalemia (Taketamo et al., 2002).

          (2) Exchange transfusion.

          (3) Peritoneal dialysis or continuous arteriovenous hemofiltration for severe, intractable hyperkalemia.

  5. Complications.

      a. Hyperkalemia is life threatening because of the risk of cardiac arrest.

   b. Sodium polystyrene sulfonate (Kayexalate) can cause hypocalcemia, hypomagnesemia, and hypernatremia.

Calcium

A. Calcium homeostasis: A reference range of 8.5 to 10.2 mg/dl is generally used for serum calcium (Ca). Some care providers prefer to follow the ionized calcium (iCa). An acceptable reference range for iCa is 4.4 to 5.3 mg/dl.

   1. Functions of Ca: Ca plays a central role in many physiologic processes, maintaining cell membrane permeability and activating enzyme reactions for muscle contraction, nerve transmission, and blood clotting. Ca is vital for normal cardiac function and development of the skeleton, where 99% of the body's Ca is stored.

   2. Regulation:
   a. Parathyroid hormone (PTH) increases serum Ca by mobilizing Ca from the bone and intestines and reducing renal excretion of Ca. PTH is stimulated by low serum Ca and magnesium (Mg) levels and is suppressed by high Ca and Mg levels.
   b. Vitamin D acts with PTH to restore Ca to normal levels by increasing absorption of Ca and phosphorus from the intestines and bone.
   c. Calcitonin, a Ca counterregulatory hormone secreted from thyroid C cells, lowers Ca levels primarily by inhibiting bone resorption.
   d. Phosphorus (P) also inhibits the absorption of Ca (the higher the P, the lower the absorption of Ca).

   3. Serum Ca is transported in three forms:
   a. Protein-bound calcium, accounting for 40% of total serum Ca.
   b. Inactivated Ca (complexed with anions such as bicarbonate, lactate, and citrate), accounting for 10% of total serum Ca.
   c. Free ionized calcium (iCa), the physiologically active form that can cross the cell membrane, accounting for 50% of the total serum Ca. Blood pH influences the amount of iCa: acidosis increases iCa, and alkalosis decreases iCa.

B. Fetal Ca metabolism: Fetal Ca needs are met by active transport of Ca across the placenta. Ca accretion increases during the last trimester as Ca is incorporated into newly forming bones. Because maternal PTH and calcitonin do not cross the placenta, the fetus is relatively hypercalcemic, which suppresses fetal PTH and stimulates fetal calcitonin.

C. Neonatal Ca metabolism: When the supply of Ca ceases at birth, the neonate depends on stored and dietary Ca to avoid hypocalcemia. After birth, the Ca level declines to its nadir by 24 hours of age, but PTH activity remains low. By 48 to 72 hours, PTH and vitamin D levels rise and the calcitonin level declines, allowing Ca to be mobilized. The serum Ca level returns to normal despite a low Ca intake. Approximately 16% of infants born less than 32 weeks of gestation develop nephrocalcinosis in the face of normal serum Ca levels (Narendra et al., 2001). Development is multifactorial but is associated with increased furosemide use, increased gentamicin levels, and extreme prematurity.

D. Hypocalcemia: Serum Ca <7 mg/dl or iCa <4.4.

   1. Pathophysiology: Failure to achieve Ca homeostasis after birth can result from inadequate Ca stores, immature hormonal control, inability to mobilize Ca, or interference with Ca use. Hypocalcemia increases cellular permeability to Na ions and increases cell membrane excitability.

   2. Causes and precipitating factors.
   a. "Early" hypocalcemia.
      (1) Prematurity: reduced Ca stores and relative hypoparathyroidism (blunted PTH response to hypocalcemia).
      (2) Infant of a diabetic mother (IDM): prolonged delay in PTH production by infant after birth.
      (3) Placental insufficiency: reduced Ca stores.
      (4) Perinatal asphyxia and stress, which precipitate a surge in calcitonin that suppresses Ca. In addition, tissue damage and glycogen breakdown release phosphorus into the circulation, which decreases Ca uptake.

(5) Maternal anticonvulsant therapy, which affects hepatic enzymes involved in vitamin D metabolism.

(6) Low intake of Ca.

(7) Factors that may decrease iCa even when the total serum Ca is normal: exchange transfusion, intravenous administration of lipid emulsion, alkalosis, or alkali therapy for acidosis.

   b. "Late" hypocalcemia.

     (1) Hypomagnesemia.

     (2) Transient congenital hypoparathyroidism or secondary hypoparathyroidism from maternal hyperparathyroidism. An increased PTH level in the mother raises the fetal Ca level and suppresses the fetal parathyroid gland. After birth, the suppressed gland cannot maintain a normal Ca level.

     (3) DiGeorge syndrome: absence of thymus and parathyroid glands.

     (4) High-phosphate formulas or cereals. The neonate cannot excrete the excess phosphate; the hyperphosphatemia suppresses Ca.

     (5) Intestinal malabsorption.

3. Clinical presentation and assessment.

   a. Early hypocalcemia is usually asymptomatic; signs of neuromuscular excitability (jitteriness, twitching) may be present.

   b. Severe hypocalcemia (neonatal tetany) is rare and presents with jitteriness, seizures, high-pitched cry, laryngospasm, stridor, and a prolonged QT interval.

4. Patient care management.

   a. Monitor serum Ca of infants at risk: premature, IDM, asphyxiated.

   b. Early, mild hypocalcemia often resolves without treatment.

   c. Serious hypocalcemia is treated with boluses and/or continuous infusions of calcium gluconate (can also be given orally).

   d. Treatment of late hypocalcemia depends on the underlying cause.

5. Complications.

   a. Rapid infusion of Ca can cause bradycardia or cardiac arrest. Infusions for rapid correction of hypocalcemia should be administered slowly, over 20 to 30 minutes by syringe pump, while the heart rate is monitored.

   b. Tissue necrosis and calcifications can result from extravasated Ca infusions.

   c. Intestinal necrosis and liver necrosis have been reported with Ca infusion given via incorrectly placed umbilical catheters.

E. Metabolic bone disease.

1. Pathophysiology: Infants born prematurely can miss all or most of the period of greatest intrauterine mineral accretion, which places them at risk of having inadequate postnatal bone mineralization. The primary cause of metabolic bone disease (MBD) is inadequate Ca and P intake, rather than vitamin D deficiency.

2. Causes and precipitating factors.

   a. Prematurity: the more immature the infant, the higher the MBD rate.

   b. Parenteral nutrition: low Ca and P intakes.

   c. Unsupplemented human milk feeding (inadequate Ca and P content) or use of formulas not designed for the preterm infant.

   d. BPD secondary to fluid restriction and use of diuretics, with renal Ca wasting.

3. Clinical presentation and assessment.

   a. MBD is asymptomatic; it is often detected initially on routine x-ray examination.

   b. Skeletal fractures may be seen in the thoracic cage or extremities.

   c. Other reported presentation is late-onset respiratory distress from "softening" of the ribs.

   d. Pain may occur with handling; close monitoring of response is necessary.

4. Diagnostic tests.

   a. Serum: normal Ca, low P, high alkaline phosphatase, and high 1,2,5-dihydroxyvitamin D levels. Ca and P levels alone are not good indicators of MBD.

   b. Urine: low or absent P excretion; increased urinary Ca.

   c. Radiologic bone examinations; wrist x-ray films at age 6 to 8 weeks may be used to monitor for MBD. Early evidence can be difficult to discern because bone mineral content must decrease by 30% to be visible. Photon absorptiometry may be done in centers where the necessary equipment is available.

    d. X-ray examination; findings may include "washed out" (undermineralized) bones, known as osteopenia, or epiphyseal dysplasia and skeletal deformities, known as rickets (Faerk et al., 2002).

  5. Patient care management and prevention of MBD.

    a. Maintain Ca/P ratio in parenteral nutrition at 1.3:1 to 1.7:1.

    b. For enteral feeding, use preterm formulas or human milk supplementation.

    c. Direct supplementation of Ca and P may be needed. Ca given without P will be inadequately used, resulting in hypercalciuria and possibly nephrocalcinosis.

    d. Gentle handling of infants at risk and avoidance of chest physiotherapy are warranted to prevent fractures.

F. Hypercalcemia: Serum Ca >11 mg/dl or iCa >5.8 mg/dl.

  1. Pathophysiology. A rise in the serum Ca level can rapidly overwhelm the infant's compensatory mechanisms for Ca equilibrium. An excess supply of Ca has multiple effects and is potentially lethal.

  2. Causes and precipitating factors.

    a. Iatrogenic: overtreatment with Ca or vitamin D.

    b. Hyperparathyroidism: primary neonatal disorder or secondary to maternal hypoparathyroidism, with chronic stimulation of the fetal parathyroid gland. In hyperparathyroidism the serum Ca level is high, phosphate levels may be low, and urinary Ca and phosphate excretion are high.

    c. Phosphate depletion: caused by low dietary intake; may be associated with low phosphate content in human milk.

    d. Subcutaneous fat necrosis: found over the back and limbs; associated with difficult delivery, hypothermia, and maternal diabetes. Pathogenic mechanism is unknown.

    e. Familial infantile hypercalcemia.

    f. Hypervitaminosis D: excessive maternal intake of vitamin D.

  3. Clinical presentation and assessment.

    a. Hypotonia, weakness, irritability, and poor feeding, all from a direct effect of Ca on the CNS.

    b. Bradycardia.

    c. Constipation.

    d. Polyuria, dehydration (associated with severe hypercalcemia).

  4. Patient care management.

    a. Hydrate infant and promote excretion of Ca (furosemide has calciuretic action).

    b. Restrict Ca and vitamin D intake; increase phosphate intake.

  5. Complications.

    a. Nephrocalcinosis from hypercalciuria, but may be seen with normal serum Ca levels.

    b. Metastatic calcification of damaged cells or tissues throughout the body, including the brain.

    c. Cardiac effects: bradycardia and arrhythmias.

Magnesium

A. Magnesium (Mg) homeostasis. A reference range of 1.5 to 2.5 mg/dl is usually accepted.

  1. Functions: Magnesium (Mg) is a catalyst for many intracellular enzyme reactions, including muscle contraction and carbohydrate metabolism, and is critical for normal parathyroid function and bone-serum Ca homeostasis. Mg is regulated primarily by the kidneys.

  2. Fetal and neonatal Mg homeostasis: The fetus receives its supply of Mg by active transport across the placenta. Maternal health and diet can influence the amount of Mg accrued by the fetus. After birth, Mg level falls along with Ca level, then rises to normal within 48 hours.

3. Serum total Mg versus the ionized form: Ionized Mg (iMg) is the biologically active fraction of Mg. Total Mg concentration in the serum does not necessarily reflect iMg activity.
4. Concurrent use of Mg and gentamicin potentiates the neuroblocking effect of the Mg, which may result in apnea. Clinical status must be monitored closely. Slow infusion times for gentamicin are indicated (Taketamo et al., 2002).

B. **Hypomagnesemia:** Serum Mg level <1.5 mg/dl.
  1. Pathophysiology: A low neonatal Mg level is directly related to the maternal level before birth. Although an acute decline in Mg stimulates PTH release, chronic Mg deficiency suppresses PTH and blocks the hormone's actions on the bone and kidneys. Hypocalcemia ensues.
  2. Causes and precipitating factors.
      a. Decreased Mg supply: prematurity, placental insufficiency and intrauterine growth restriction (IUGR), low dietary intake.
      b. Increased Mg losses: renal and intestinal disorders, including renal tubular acidosis, diarrhea, short bowel syndrome.
      c. Endocrine causes: neonatal hypoparathyroidism, maternal hyperparathyroidism.
  3. Clinical presentation and assessment.
      a. Tremors, irritability, and hyperreflexia, progressing to seizures.
      b. Failure to respond to therapy for hypocalcemia: hypomagnesemia a possibility.
  4. Patient care management.
      a. If hypomagnesemia is severe, administration of magnesium sulfate may be necessary to relieve symptoms until Ca balance is restored.
      b. Seizures are usually unresponsive to anticonvulsant agents.
  5. Complications. Overtreatment with magnesium sulfate can result in hypotonia and respiratory depression, hypotension, and cardiac arrhythmias.

C. **Hypermagnesemia:** Serum Mg >2.5 mg/dl.
  1. Pathophysiology: Excess Mg is slow to be excreted by the neonatal kidneys. Very high Mg levels can cause CNS and neuromuscular depression.
  2. Causes and precipitating factors.
      a. Excessive Mg load: magnesium sulfate treatment in labor, excess administration of Mg to neonate.
      b. Reduced excretion of Mg: renal failure, oliguria.
  3. Clinical presentation and assessment (may be asymptomatic).
      a. Respiratory depression, apnea.
      b. Neuromuscular depression: lethargy, poor suck, loss of reflexes, flaccidity, hypotonia.
      c. Gastrointestinal hypomotility, abdominal distention.
  4. Patient care management.
      a. Prepare to resuscitate infants born to mothers receiving large doses of magnesium sulfate.
      b. Hypermagnesemia usually resolves with adequate hydration and urine output. Mg excretion can be increased with furosemide.
      c. If infant is unresponsive to treatment, exchange transfusion may be necessary.
  5. Complications. Cardiac arrest and respiratory failure are possible.

ACID–BASE BALANCE AND DISORDERS

Acid–Base Physiology

A. **pH:** Acid–base balance is normal when the pH of the blood is between 7.35 and 7.45. The pH is determined by the hydrogen ion (H^+) concentration in the ECF. An acid is an H^+ donor; a base is an H^+ receptor. A complex system of buffers, compensation, and excretion regulates the H^+ concentration, thus keeping the pH in the normal range.

B. **Buffering system:** This is the first line of defense against excess H^+ concentration. Buffers, including bicarbonate (HCO_3^-), plasma proteins, and hemoglobin, act rapidly to pick up excess H^+. The major buffer, HCO_3^-, teams with H^+ to form carbonic acid, which dissociates into water and CO_2 to be eliminated. The normal HCO_3^- level in the neonate is 22 to 26 mEq/l, lower than in the adult.

C. **Lung regulation:** The lungs act to lower the H^+ level in the blood by removing CO_2, which is produced as a waste product of cellular metabolism. It is then transported to the lungs, where it is removed from the body by ventilation. The rate of CO_2 removal can be increased or decreased by altering minute ventilation.

D. **Kidney regulation:** The kidney acts to maintain equilibrium between acids and bases in the body by reabsorbing HCO_3^- and other buffers and by excreting H^+ and other acids. In this way, the body eliminates the daily load of nonvolatile acids produced by normal metabolism.

E. **Compensation:** When one or more of the body's regulatory systems fail, other systems have a limited ability to maintain the acid–base equilibrium. When the pH is outside the normal range (<7.35 or >7.45), compensation has failed.

   1. An acid–base deviation is respiratory if it is due to an abnormal P_{CO_2} and metabolic if it is due to an abnormal level of plasma HCO_3^-.
   2. The lungs attempt to compensate for a metabolic aberration, and the kidneys for a respiratory aberration. The result is a change in pH toward normal despite an abnormal blood P_{CO_2} or HCO_3^-. The lungs compensate much more quickly than the kidneys; however, neither can totally normalize the pH unless the underlying disorder is corrected.

Disorders of Acid–Base Balance

Only those disorders classified as primary metabolic problems are discussed here.

A. **Metabolic acidosis.**

   1. Pathophysiology: A pH of less than 7.35 or serum HCO_3^- of <22 mEq/l can result from the loss of HCO_3^- (buffering capacity) or from excess acid production. The immature kidneys contribute to acidosis by failing both to reabsorb HCO_3^- and to excrete H^+ when faced with an acid load. When cells do not receive enough oxygen (because of low blood oxygen levels or diminished perfusion), they must use anaerobic metabolism to meet energy needs. This results in the accumulation in the body of lactic acid (lactate), the level of which reflects the severity of tissue oxygen deficiency. Blood lactate may be a more sensitive indicator of tissue hypoxia than pH and base-excess values (Volpe, 2008). Calculation of the anion gap (difference between positive and negative ions) can be a useful tool to differentiate between excess acid and insufficient HCO_3^- as cause of acidosis. Anion gap = (serum Na + K) – (serum Cl + HCO_3^- [*or serum CO_2*]). Usual range is 8 to 16 mEq. If high (>20 mEq), acidosis is due to excess acid. If normal with elevated chloride level, acidosis is due to loss of HCO_3^-.

   2. Causes and precipitating factors.
      a. Loss of HCO_3^-: normal anion gap.
         (1) Prematurity: poor renal conservation of HCO_3^-.
         (2) Renal tubular acidosis: decreased proximal reabsorption.
         (3) Severe diarrhea or ileal drainage.
      b. Excess acid load: ingestion or endogenous production of acid, greater than the ability to excrete it; increased anion gap.
         (1) Lactic acidosis from conditions resulting in hypoxia or hypoperfusion: respiratory distress, congenital heart disease, PDA, sepsis, asphyxia, or shock/hypovolemia. Plasma lactate level greater than 2.5 mmol/l; may be elevated in some conditions, such as early sepsis, even when the pH is normal.
         (2) Inborn errors of metabolism: disorders of organic acid and carbohydrate metabolism.
         (3) Caloric deprivation: catabolism of protein or fat for energy.
         (4) Parenteral amino acid solutions.
         (5) "Late metabolic acidosis" of prematurity, caused by intolerance of cow's milk protein.

   3. Clinical presentation and assessment.
      a. Metabolic acidosis occurring early in life is primarily related to systemic illness (e.g., respiratory, cardiac); thus the signs and symptoms are those of the underlying condition(s).

    b. Late metabolic acidosis may present at 1 to 3 weeks of age by poor growth, hyponatremia, and persistent renal acid excretion (urinary pH <5). Urinary pH greater than 7 with systemic acidosis suggests renal tubular acidosis.

    c. Infants with profound acidosis (metabolic defects such as congenital lactic acidosis) may have respiratory compensation (tachypnea, hyperpnea) or neurologic depression (seizures, coma) reflecting CNS acidosis.

4. Patient care management.

    a. Treat the underlying cause of acidosis.

    b. Correction of severe acidosis (pH <7.2) is usually with $NaHCO_3$ (concentration of 0.5 mEq/ml), in a 1- to 2-ml/kg dose. Administer slowly by syringe pump or continuous drip; rapid increase in osmolality and pH may be dangerous.

    c. Late metabolic acidosis, if not self-correcting, is sometimes treated with oral $NaHCO_3$.

5. Complications.

    a. Severe acidosis: may depress myocardial contractility and cause arteriolar vasodilation, hypotension, and pulmonary edema.

    b. Impaired surfactant production.

    c. Electrolyte imbalance: decreased iCa, hyperkalemia.

    d. Adverse effects of HCO_3^-: cerebral hemorrhage or edema related to wide swings in plasma osmolality. Increased cerebral blood flow, more pronounced when infused rapidly (van Alfen-van der Velden et al., 2006). $NaHCO_3$ can also worsen acidosis by rapidly increasing CO_2 if lung disease is present and ventilation is inadequate. $NaHCO_3$ can aggravate hypernatremia and cause tissue injury in extravasation.

6. Outcome: In follow-up studies, metabolic acidosis was correlated with poor developmental outcome in VLBW infants (van Alfen-van der Velden et al., 2006).

B. Metabolic alkalosis.

1. Pathophysiology: Metabolic alkalosis, pH >7.45 or HCO_3^- >26 mEq/l, results from an excess of HCO_3^- or from a loss of acid.

2. Causes and precipitating factors.

    a. Gain of HCO_3^- from overcorrection of acidosis with $NaHCO_3$.

    b. Loss of H^+ during vomiting or nasogastric suction.

    c. Increased renal acid loss from diuretic therapy.

    d. Rapid ECF reduction (contraction alkalosis).

3. Patient care management.

    a. Decrease $NaHCO_3$ intake if alkali therapy is the cause of alkalosis.

    b. Restoring fluid and electrolyte balance is critical.

4. Complications: Severe alkalosis causes tissue hypoxia, neurologic damage, and electrolyte disturbances (increased iCa, hypokalemia).

(Please refer to chapter 26 for discussion of respiratory acidosis and respiratory alkalosis.)

REFERENCES

Adams, E., Counsell, S.J., Hajnal, J.V., et al.: Investigation of lung disease in preterm infants using magnetic resonance imaging. *Biology of the Neonate*, 77(Suppl 1):17-20, 2000.

Adams, E., Counsell, S.J., Hajnal, J.V., et al.: Magnetic resonance imaging of lung water content and distribution in term and preterm infants. *American Journal of Respiratory and Critical Care Medicine*, 166(3):397-402, 2002.

Davis, I.D. and Avner, E.D.: Fluid, electrolytes, and acid-base homeostasis. In A.A. Fanaroff and R.J. Martin (Eds.): *Neonatal-perinatal medicine: Diseases of the fetus and infant* (7th ed.). St. Louis, 2002, Mosby.

Eichenwald, E.C.: Care of the extremely-low-birth-weight infant. In H.W. Taeusch, R.A. Ballard, and C.

A. Gleason (Eds.): *Avery's diseases of the newborn* (8th ed.). Philadelphia, 2005, Saunders.

Faerk, J., Peitersen, B., and Michaelson, K.F.: Bone mineralisation in premature infants cannot be predicted from serum alkaline phosphatase or serum phosphate. *Archives of Disease in Childhood, Fetal Neonatal Edition*, 87(2):F133-F136, 2002.

Hartnoll, G., Betremieux, P., and Modi, N.: Randomised controlled trial of postnatal sodium supplementation on oxygen dependency and body weight in 25-30 week gestational age infants. *Archives of Disease in Childhood, Fetal Neonatal Edition*, 82(1):F19-F23, 2000.

Jain, A., Rutter, N., and Cartlidge, P.: Influence of antenatal steroids and sex on maturation of the epidermal barrier in the preterm infant. *Archives of Disease in*

Childhood, Fetal Neonatal Edition, 83(2):F112-F116, 2000.

Kerr, B.A., Starbuck, A.L., and Block, S.M.: Fluid and electrolyte management. In G.B. Merenstein and S.L. Gardner (Eds.): *Handbook of neonatal intensive care* (6th ed.). St. Louis, 2006, Mosby.

Lund, C.H. and Kuller, J.M.: Integumentary system. In C. Kenner and J.W. Lott (Eds.): *Comprehensive neonatal care: An interdisciplinary approach* (4th ed.). St. Louis, 2007, Saunders.

Modi, N., Betremieux, P., Midgley, J., and Hartnoll, G.: Postnatal weight loss and contraction of the extracellular compartment is triggered by atrial natriuretic peptide. *Early Human Development, 59*(3):201-208, 2000.

Narendra, A., White, M.P., Rolton, H.A., et al.: Nephrocalcinosis in preterm babies. *Archives of Disease in Childhood, Fetal Neonatal Edition, 85*(3):F207-F213, 2001.

Omar, S., DeCristofaro, J.D., Agarwal, B.I., and La Gamma, E.F.: Effects of prenatal steroids on water and sodium homeostasis in extremely low birth weight neonates. *Pediatrics, 104*(3 Pt 1):482-488, 1999.

Seri, I., Ramanathan, R., and Evans, J.R.: Acid-base, fluid, and electrolyte management. In H.W. Taeusch, R.A. Ballard, and C.A. Gleason (Eds.): *Avery's diseases of the newborn* (8th ed.). Philadelphia, 2005, Saunders.

Taketamo, C.K., Hodding, J.H., and Kraus, D.M.: *Pediatric Lexi-Comp Drugs* [online]. 2002. Available at www.lexi.com. Accessed November 8, 2008.

Van Alfen-van der Velden, A.A.E.M., Hopman, J.C.W., Klaessens, J.H.G.M., Feuth, T., Sengers, R.C.A., and Liem, K.D.: Effects of rapid versus slow infusion of sodium bicarbonate on cerebral hemodynamics and oxygenation in preterm infants. *Biology of the Neonate, 90*:122-127, 2006.

Vogt, B.A., Davis, I.D., and Avner, E.D.: The kidney. In M. Klaus and A. Fanaroff (Eds.): *Care of the high-risk neonate* (5th ed.). Philadelphia, 2001, Saunders.

Volpe, J.J.: Hypoxic-ischemic encephalopathy: Biochemical and physiological aspects. In J.J. Volpe (Ed.): *Neurology of the newborn* (5th ed.). Philadelphia, 2008, Saunders.

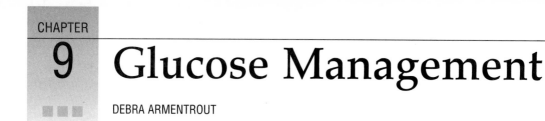

9 Glucose Management

DEBRA ARMENTROUT

OBJECTIVES
1. Describe the mechanisms of glucose homeostasis in the fetus and newborn.
2. Discuss hypoglycemia and hyperglycemia in the neonate.
3. Discuss infants of diabetic mothers.
4. Differentiate neonatal diabetes from hyperglycemia.

Organ systems, especially the human brain, are primarily dependent on glucose as their major energy source. Compared with adults, infants have a higher brain-to-body-weight ratio, resulting in a higher glucose demand in relation to glucose production capacity. Cerebral glucose utilization accounts for 90% of the neonate's total glucose consumption. Continuous glucose and energy delivery to the fetus is provided from the maternal circulation via the placenta so there is no need for fetal glucose production in utero. An essential part of the neonate's successful transition to extrauterine life therefore is the maintenance of euglycemia. Whereas most infants are indeed able to readily adapt to the metabolic demands of extrauterine life, newborns in general remain extremely susceptible to any condition that may impair their ability to establish normal glucose homeostasis during this transition process (Hume et al., 2005; Sunehag and Haymond, 2002).

GLUCOSE HOMEOSTASIS

Glucose is vital for cellular metabolism throughout the body. Blood glucose concentration is determined by the balance between intake/production of glucose and glucose use by the body.
A. **Glucose production.**
   1. Glucose taken in but not used for immediate energy needs is converted to glycogen via glycogenesis and stored in the liver, heart, and skeletal muscles. During fasting, glycogen is broken down to re-form glucose that is then released from the liver in a process known as glycogenolysis. The infant's ability for glycogenolysis varies according to fetal growth and maturity.
   2. The other main source of glucose is gluconeogenesis: production of glucose and glycogen in the liver by means of nonglucose precursors such as lactate, pyruvate, glycerol (fat), and amino acids (de Lonlay et al., 2004; Haninger and Farley, 2001; Hume et al., 2005; Kalhan and Parimi, 2000).
B. **Glucose metabolism (Blackburn, 2007; Ogata, 2005).**
   1. Glucose can be metabolized in the body in several ways: production of energy, storage as glycogen, and conversion to gluconeogenic precursors.
   2. In the brain, oxidized glucose provides 99% of the cerebral energy production, a process dependent on a number of important enzymes and reactions.
      a. Glucose molecules are transported across the blood-brain barrier and into the brain cells by glucose transporter proteins.
      b. Within the cytoplasm, glucose is metabolized by glycolysis to pyruvate. Pyruvate is then oxidized to acetyl-coenzyme A (acetyl-CoA), which is transported to the mitochondrion for entry into the citric acid cycle. The end products are carbon dioxide, water, and energy released in the generation of adenosine triphosphate (ATP).
      c. Of importance to the neonate is that during hypoglycemia other substrates (ketone bodies, lactate, glycerol, and amino acids) can also be converted to pyruvate, enter the citric acid cycle, and produce ATP, thus serving as a source of energy for the brain (Noerr, 2001).

C. **Hormonal regulation of glucose homeostasis (Blackburn, 2007; Ogata, 2005).**
   1. Insulin. Secreted by the pancreatic β cells in response to an increase in plasma glucose, insulin decreases the blood glucose level by promoting glycogen formation, suppressing hepatic glucose release, and driving the peripheral uptake of glucose. Insulin does not control the entry of glucose into the brain or liver.
   2. Glucagon. Secreted by the pancreatic β cells when blood glucose levels decrease, glucagon promotes glycogenolysis and gluconeogenesis. Glucagon is called a counterregulatory hormone because it opposes the effect of insulin by raising the blood glucose level. Other counterregulatory hormones include catecholamines, cortisol, and growth hormone. Although these hormones may not be important regulators in the fast-feed cycle of healthy neonates, minimum basal levels may be needed to maintain euglycemia.

D. **Fetal glucose homeostasis.**
   1. Glucose reaches the fetus by facilitated diffusion across the placenta at a concentration of about 60% to 80% of the mother's (Noerr, 2001).
   2. Glycogen storage for postnatal energy needs begins early in gestation, with most glycogen accumulating during the third trimester.
   3. Fetal insulin is detectable by 8 to 10 weeks of gestation, but the response to a glucose load is not fully developed even at term (Dunne et al., 2004; Stokowski, 2007).
   4. The fetus is capable of gluconeogenic activity, using substrates such as lactate if needed to meet metabolic demands in utero.

E. **Neonatal glucose homeostasis.**
   1. After cord clamping, the neonate's blood glucose concentration falls, reaching a nadir at 1 to 2 hours of age.
   2. In the first postnatal hours, the neonatal brain metabolizes lactate, which is abundant, so that even though the glucose concentration is low, the brain is not fuel deficient.
   3. The neonate gradually mobilizes glucose to meet energy needs by secreting glucagon and catecholamines and suppressing insulin release. Thus, even if a healthy term newborn infant is not fed soon after birth, blood glucose levels rise at 3 to 4 hours of age.
   4. Hepatic glycogen, however, is rapidly depleted if feeding is not established early and the infant is dependent on gluconeogenesis and lipolysis as the primary modes of maintaining euglycemia (Hume et al., 2005; Sunehag and Haymond, 2002).

HYPOGLYCEMIA

A. **Definition of hypoglycemia (Blackburn, 2007; Rozance and Hay, 2006).**
   1. Most clinicians believe that rather than a specific value, neonatal hypoglycemia lies on a continuum of low blood glucose values of varied duration and severity that is influenced by a number of different factors:
      a. Conceptual and postnatal age
      b. Adequacy of gluconeogenic pathways
      c. General health status
      d. Presence or absence of symptoms
   2. A widely used cutoff point for plasma glucose concentration is 40 mg/dl as the typical threshold for intervention in both premature and term neonates, with some authors advocating 55 to 70 mg/dl (Louis and Weinzimer, 2003; Rozance and Hay, 2006; Steinkrauss et al., 2005).
   3. The optimal range for plasma glucose is 70 to 100 mg/dl, and there is no evidence that neonates have a lower requirement for glucose concentrations, or that the neonatal brain can better tolerate hypoglycemia when compared to older infants and adults (Stanley and Pallotto, 2005).

B. **Incidence.**
   1. Overall incidence is 1 to 5/1000 live births.
   2. The incidence in at-risk infants may be as high as 30%, occurring in 8% of large-for-gestational-age (LGA) infants and in 15% of premature and small-for-gestational-age (SGA) infants (McGowan, 1999).

C. **Pathophysiology (Blackburn, 2007; Ogata, 2005; Stanley and Pallotto, 2005).**

1. The immediate postnatal drop in the blood glucose concentration is physiologic. Failure to increase glucose concentrations after 4 hours is pathologic. Subsequently, hypoglycemia is usually a result of inadequate hepatic glucose production that cannot meet peripheral demand or excessive insulin production (Cowett and Loughead, 2002; de Lonlay et al., 2004).

2. Glucose delivery is dependent on blood glucose concentration and blood flow rate. During hypoglycemia, the brain increases blood flow to improve glucose delivery that may predispose the neonatal brain to hemorrhagic and hyperoxic injury if there is diminished cerebral autoregulatory ability.

3. When glucose consumption exceeds delivery, the brain uses alternate fuels such as ketone bodies, lactic acid, free fatty acids, and glycerol if they are available. The production of energy from these sources involves the use of brain structural components such as proteins and phospholipids that may play a contributory role in neuronal damage.

4. Lactic acid becomes elevated in late fetal and early postnatal life and healthy term infants produce ketones effectively on days 2 and 3 of life, thus protecting their brains from fuel deficiency if the blood glucose level falls while feeding becomes established. However, the ability of preterm infants and of infants who are SGA to mount a counterregulatory ketogenic response at any time is severely limited, so these infants are heavily dependent on an adequate glucose supply (Cowett and Loughead, 2002; Rozance and Hay, 2006).

5. Prolonged hypoglycemia, when not compensated by a supply of alternative fuels, induces biochemical changes at the cell level that may damage the neuronal and glial cells of the brain. It is thought that an accumulation of excitatory amino acids, especially glutamate, during hypoglycemia leads to prolonged cellular depolarization with entry of water and calcium into the cell, first impairing neuronal growth and eventually causing cell death. In addition, the hypoglycemic brain may be more vulnerable to the damaging effects of ischemia. Degrees of ischemia and hypoglycemia that alone would not result in brain injury might do so in combination (Volpe, 2008).

D. **Etiologies and precipitating factors.**

1. Inadequate production or supply of glucose accounts for the more common causes of neonatal hypoglycemia. These conditions involve decreased substrate (glycogen, lactate, glycerol, amino acids) availability, immature or altered enzyme pathways, or altered responses to neural or hormonal factors (Blackburn, 2007; Ogata, 2005; Stanley and Pallotto, 2005).

    a. Prematurity: possible diminished oral and parenteral intake, immature counterregulatory response to low glucose concentration, and insufficient glycogen stores and release.

    b. Intrauterine growth restriction: low glycogen and fat stores, increased substrate utilization.

    c. Delayed feedings, insufficient breastfeeding, or fluid restriction.

    d. Inborn errors of metabolism: defective gluconeogenesis and/or glycogenolysis (e.g., galactosemia, amino acid disorders, organic acid deficiencies, fatty acid oxidation disorders).

    e. Glycogen storage disease: autosomal recessive defects characterized by a deficient or abnormally functioning enzyme involved with formation or degradation of glycogen in the liver.

    f. Perinatal stress/hypoxia, respiratory distress, hypothermia, polycythemia/hyperviscosity, infection, adrenal hemorrhage, congestive heart failure.

2. Increased uptake of glucose related to hyperinsulinism (De Leon and Stanley, 2007; Steinkrauss et al., 2005).

    a. Infant of diabetic mother (IDM).

    b. Persistent neonatal hyperinsulinism and nesidioblastosis: autosomal recessive disorders thought to be caused by regulatory defects in β-cell function. Surgical exploration may be necessary for definitive diagnosis, with subtotal pancreatectomy the required therapeutic measure.

    c. Beckwith-Wiedemann syndrome: of unknown cause; characterized by omphalocele, macroglossia, visceromegaly, and hypoglycemia. Pancreatic islet cell hyperplasia noted. The resultant hypoglycemia may be quite profound and difficult to treat.

    d. Rh incompatibility: severe cases can have associated β-cell hypertrophy and hyperinsulinemia.

    e. High glucose infusion and tocolytics used before delivery. β-Adrenergic agonists such as terbutaline can stimulate fetal pancreatic β cells.

    f. Iatrogenic: position of tip of umbilical artery catheter near the pancreas can cause glucose to be directly delivered to the pancreas via the celiac artery, resulting in excessive insulin secretion.

E. Clinical presentation and assessment (Blackburn, 2007; Ogata, 2005; Stanley and Pallotto, 2005; Volpe, 2008).

  1. Clinical signs of hypoglycemia are nonspecific and may be present at varying blood glucose concentrations in different infants or they may not be evident at all even though the infant is experiencing severe hypoglycemia. In addition, signs often linked with hypoglycemia may occur in conjunction with other clinical conditions.

    a. Tremors; jitteriness; irritability; exaggerated Moro reflex.

    b. Abnormal cry: high-pitched or weak.

    c. Respiratory distress: apnea, irregular respirations, tachypnea, cyanosis.

    d. Stupor, hypotonia, lethargy, refusal to feed.

    e. Hypothermia, temperature instability.

    f. Seizures.

F. Diagnostic studies.

  1. Point-of-care blood glucose screening.

    a. Enzymatic reagent strips. Their reliability is questioned because they:

      (1) may underestimate the true glucose level as whole blood gives a reading 10% to 15% lower than the plasma value;

      (2) may fail to detect clinically important hypoglycemia because of unpredictable measurement errors; and

      (3) are sensitive to error from technical and operator variables such as timing, blotting, and distribution of blood droplets.

    b. Absorption photometry and electrochemical glucose meters (Dollberg et al., 2001; Noerr, 2001).

    c. Subcutaneous microdialysis (Baumeister et al., 2001).

      (1) Decreases the need for frequent blood sampling.

      (2) Enables long-term glucose monitoring.

  2. All current techniques require laboratory confirmation for establishing a diagnosis of neonatal hypoglycemia; however, appropriate interventions should be initiated promptly and not wait on laboratory confirmation (Noerr, 2001).

  3. In suspected hyperinsulinism, additional testing may include concurrent insulin and glucose levels, ketone and free fatty acid levels, and cortisol and growth hormone levels.

G. Patient care management (McGowan et al., 2006).

  1. Identify infants at risk.

  2. Prevent hypoglycemia by providing glucose substrate.

    a. Early enteral feedings.

    b. Intravenous (IV) glucose at 4 to 6 mg/kg/minute.

  3. Assess glucose status with blood glucose screening.

    a. Perform blood glucose screening test on infants at risk on admission, frequently during the first 4 hours of life and then at 4-hour intervals until the risk period has passed (Ogata, 2005).

    b. Clinically unstable infants and any infant with signs of a possible low blood glucose concentration require regular monitoring.

    c. Early and exclusive breastfeeding will meet the nutritional and energy needs of healthy full-term infants, and routine blood glucose screening of these infants is not presently recommended.

4. If hypoglycemia persists despite feeding, correction is with IV glucose infusion. A mini-bolus (dextrose 10% in water, 2 ml/kg), followed by continuous infusion at a rate of 6 to 8 mg/kg/minute, rapidly raises the blood glucose level but does not treat the underlying hormonal and metabolic causes of the hypoglycemia.

5. Monitoring of blood glucose levels must then continue, for documentation of the resolution of hypoglycemia with IV therapy and subsequently during the transition to full enteral feedings. Oral feedings should be initiated once clinical symptoms have resolved (Rozance and Hay, 2006).

6. Persistent hypoglycemia raises the possibility of hyperinsulinism, although some infants without biochemical hyperinsulinism also have transiently high glucose requirements. Those with true hyperinsulinism may require the following:

    a. High IV glucose infusion rates (12 to 16 mg/kg/minute). Delivery of concentrated glucose (>12.5%) requires a central line for safe administration.

    b. Hormonal therapy, which may include the following:

        (1) Glucagon. Stimulates glycogen release from the liver. Glucagon, however, may also stimulate insulin release, so its use requires the presence of an IV glucose infusion.

        (2) Diazoxide. Suppresses pancreatic insulin secretion. Its use is reserved for situations of profound hyperinsulinism that have failed other therapies. It has been used for prolonged periods (years) without significant side effects noted (Cowett and Loughead, 2002).

        (3) Somatostatin. Suppresses insulin and glucagon secretion; however, its use is limited by its extremely short half-life (Cowett and Loughead, 2002).

    c. Corticosteroids, which stimulate gluconeogenesis from noncarbohydrate (protein) sources (McGowan et al., 2006).

        (1) Hydrocortisone or prednisone may be used when parenteral glucose therapy is greater than 15 mg/kg/minute.

        (2) Gradual decreases in corticosteroid dosage and decreases in parenteral glucose concentrations are required as oral intake is increased.

    d. Subtotal or total pancreatectomy if severe, persistent hyperinsulinism is unresponsive to medical therapy (De Leon and Stanley, 2007; Lindley and Dunne, 2005).

H. Complications.

1. Hypoglycemia will often recur when a bolus of glucose is not followed by a continuous infusion.

2. Extravasations of peripheral glucose infusions may cause necrosis of skin and other tissue (Lund et al., 2007).

    a. Hyaluronidase can be injected subcutaneously around the periphery of any extravasation site to prevent or limit tissue injury.

    b. Skin injury can be prevented by making multiple puncture holes using an aseptic technique over the involved area and allowing the fluid to be infiltrated.

    c. Elevation of the affected area, if an extremity, may limit the leakage of the exudate.

    d. Use of an occlusive dressing (hydrocolloid dressing; hydrogel sheets, and amorphous gel) will provide for exudate management, adherence without damaging the surrounding tissue, and a microbial barrier; debridement and compression should be used.

3. Reactive hypoglycemia with return of symptomatology may occur if the intravenous glucose infusion infiltrates or is stopped abruptly.

I. Outcome.

1. Potential long-term sequelae remain unclear since there often are coexisting medical conditions that also predispose to brain injury (Ogata, 2005).

2. In general, outcome studies show that neonates with seizure-associated and/or persistent hyperinsulinemic hypoglycemia have the worst neurologic prognosis (Rozance and Hay, 2006; Volpe, 2008).

3. Follow-up of infants who experienced persistent neonatal hyperinsulinism suggests that early events were responsible for the subsequent mental retardation (Menni et al., 2001).

INFANT OF DIABETIC MOTHER

A. **Incidence:** 20% of infants of women with gestational diabetes mellitus and 35% of infants of mothers with other forms of diabetes (Blackburn, 2007).

B. **Pathophysiology:** The hormonal and metabolic changes that complicate diabetic pregnancy can adversely affect the developing fetus and neonate in a number of ways (Blackburn, 2007; Stokowski, 2007).

1. Early in gestation during organogenesis, the abnormal metabolic milieu is teratogenic, resulting in a higher incidence of congenital malformations.

2. Throughout pregnancy and particularly in the third trimester, the pregnant diabetic woman is increasingly insulin resistant and often has hyperglycemia and hyperaminoacidemia. Excess glucose and amino acids are freely delivered to the fetus, but maternal insulin is not. These nutrients stimulate the fetal pancreas to produce insulin to use the excess fuels, resulting in β-cell hyperplasia and hyperinsulinemia. This fetal hyperinsulinemia, in turn, stimulates protein, lipid, and glycogen synthesis, causing a high rate of fetal growth, increased deposition of fat and visceral enlargement (especially heart and liver), and subsequent macrosomia. This fetal macrosomia does not involve the brain or kidneys.

3. After birth, the neonate's pancreas continues to produce insulin, and available glucose is rapidly used. The infant's ability to mobilize glycogen stores is decreased. The IDM may exhibit an exaggerated and persistent hypoglycemia. Maternal glucose homeostasis during pregnancy as well as maternal glycemia during delivery influences the degree of neonatal hypoglycemia.

4. The IDM is at risk of having neural impairment because, even with plentiful adipose tissue, ketogenesis and lipolysis are suppressed by hyperinsulinemia, leaving the brain without a supply of alternative fuels for metabolism during hypoglycemia.

C. **Clinical presentation and assessment (McGowan et al., 2006).**

1. Hypoglycemia: It may occur immediately after birth without symptoms. In one large retrospective series, hypoglycemia (defined as serum glucose <40 mg/dl) occurred in about one third of IDMs. The majority of those responded rapidly to treatment, but 10% had persistent hypoglycemia despite treatment.

2. Macrosomia/LGA (approximately 35% of IDMs): Some infants are SGA because of placental insufficiency in advanced stages of diabetes.

3. Increase in preterm births in association with diabetic pregnancy: Hyperbilirubinemia in IDMs may be secondary to prematurity.

4. Respiratory distress syndrome and other conditions such as transient tachypnea of the newborn infant: Fetal hyperinsulinemia may retard the maturation of various aspects of the pulmonary surfactant system and not just inhibit surfactant production, delaying lung maturation.

5. Polycythemia (venous hematocrit >65%): The insulin-induced high glucose uptake and high metabolic rate causes a cellular hypoxia, leading to an elevated erythropoietin level (Ogata, 2005). Newborns with polycythemia do not always look plethoric, so the hematocrit level must be measured.

6. Hypocalcemia, hypomagnesemia thought to result from a functional hypoparathyroidism due to maternal magnesium loss (Stanley and Pallotto, 2005).

7. Cardiomyopathy, visceromegaly possibly related to maternal diabetes control and to fetal/neonatal hyperinsulinemia.

8. Congenital malformations. Cardiac defects (especially transposition), neural tube defects, sacral agenesis, and caudal regression are 2 to 4 times more frequent than in the general population. The anomalies are thought to be due to the diabetic intrauterine environment during organogenesis frequently before the pregnancy is recognized and prenatal diabetic treatment initiated.

D. **Diagnostic studies.**

1. Blood glucose screening with laboratory confirmation of plasma glucose.
2. Other laboratory analyses, including calcium and magnesium levels and venous hematocrit.
3. X-ray examination if fractures from traumatic delivery are suspected.
4. Echocardiography.

E. **Patient care management (McGowan et al., 2006; Stokowski, 2007).**
   1. The main goal of the treatment of gestational diabetes is to achieve and maintain euglycemia. Tight control of intrapartum glucose levels may reduce the incidence of neonatal complications.
   2. Anticipate problems of IDM before delivery; prompt recognition and treatment of neonatal morbidities postdelivery.
   3. Provide early feeding of human milk or formula, orally or via gavage tube if the infant does not feed well. IV administration of glucose is necessary for infants too small or sick to tolerate enteral feeding.

F. **Complications.**
   1. Seizures resulting from cerebral fuel deficiency.
   2. Shoulder dystocia. Macrosomic infants delivered with forceps or vacuum extraction may have brachial plexus injury (Erbs palsy) or fractures.
   3. Renal vein thrombosis (secondary to polycythemia/hyperviscosity).
   4. Development of juvenile insulin-dependent diabetes with a 2% transmission risk for female IDM and 6% for male IDM (Stanley and Pallotto, 2005).

G. **Outcome (McGowan et al., 2006; Stokowski, 2007).**
   1. Increased perinatal mortality rate results from relatively high rates of congenital malformations, stillbirths, and premature delivery.
   2. Morbidities associated with IDM include neurologic sequelae, developmental delay, behavioral differences, obesity, and diabetes.
   3. Maternal complications, including poor glycemic control, vascular disease, infection, and pregnancy-induced hypertension, are associated with poorer perinatal outcome. Improved outcomes are seen in IDMs when maternal diabetes is metabolically controlled.
   4. The outcomes for SGA infants born to women receiving intensive therapy for gestational diabetes may be worse than those of appropriate-for-gestational-age (AGA) or LGA infants.

HYPERGLYCEMIA*

A. **Definition:** Whole blood glucose concentration greater than 120 to 125 mg/dl or a plasma glucose concentration greater than 150 mg/dl.
B. **Incidence:** Prevalence of 29% to 86% in low birth weight infants overall; 2% of infants weighing more than 2000 g; 45% of infants less than 1000 g; and up to 80% of infants weighing less than 750 g.
C. **Pathophysiology.**
   1. Normally an infant responds to an exogenous glucose supply with a rise in insulin, suppressing endogenous glucose production and enhancing peripheral uptake of glucose. Though clinically stable extremely low birth weight (ELBW) infants may be able to regulate glucose in this manner, many of them become hyperglycemic.
   2. Hepatic glucose production in this latter group continues in the presence of hyperglycemia and circulating insulin. This represents a failure of glucose autoregulation involving both the pancreas and liver of infants with hyperglycemia.
   3. Corticosteroid therapy stimulates glycogenolysis and gluconeogenesis and may block insulin secretion as well as inhibit its peripheral action.
D. **Etiologies and precipitating factors.**
   1. Low birth weight, extreme prematurity, and intrauterine growth restriction (IUGR).
   2. Excessive glucose load (>6 to 8 mg/kg/minute), with 50% of infants receiving a glucose infusion rate (GIR) of 11 mg/kg/minute and all infants receiving a GIR of 14 mg/kg/minute developing hyperglycemia.
   3. Stress related to clinical problems such as sepsis or infection.
   4. Transient or permanent neonatal diabetes mellitus (see p. 179).
   5. Side effects of medications such as corticosteroids.
   6. Lipid infusion, which may contribute to hyperglycemia.
   7. Release of catecholamines secondary to surgery/anesthesia.

---

*McGowan et al., 2006; Stanley and Pallotto, 2005.

E. Clinical presentation and assessment.
   a. Onset can be as early as 24 hours of age; usually before 3 days of life.
   b. No characteristic clinical presentation.
   c. Symptoms may include dehydration, weight loss, failure to thrive, fever, glycosuria, ketosis, and metabolic acidosis.
   d. Diagnosis is usually determined by measuring blood glucose concentration.
F. Diagnostic studies.
   1. Serum or plasma blood glucose levels greater than 125 mg/dl or 150 mg/dl, respectively.
   2. Urinary glucose. Very low birth weight (VLBW) infants have a low renal threshold for glucose and may spill sugar at blood glucose levels as low as 80 to 100 mg/dl.
   3. Investigation for possible underlying cause (sepsis workup to rule out infection or insulin level to rule out neonatal diabetes mellitus).
G. Patient care management.
   1. Monitor blood glucose of infants at risk for developing hyperglycemia, particularly when fluid intake is increased on day 2 or 3 of life.
   2. Decrease glucose load as much as possible to allow the blood glucose level to stabilize in a normal range (<125 mg/dl or plasma glucose <150 mg/dl).
   3. Monitor weight, urine output, fluid intake, GIR, electrolytes, and acid-base balance.
   4. Insulin is sometimes administered to ELBW infants along with parenteral nutrition in an attempt to normalize blood glucose levels without reducing the caloric intake. Insulin is also used to treat transient neonatal diabetes. Insulin normalizes blood glucose by suppressing hepatic glucose production and by increasing peripheral glucose utilization. However, premature infants have a very small mass of insulin-dependent tissue, with only 10% of their glucose utilization being insulin dependent. Severe hyperglycemia may occur in the VLBW infant despite decreased glucose infusion rates. Continuous insulin infusion may be used although routine use not advised because of adverse effects.
   5. Begin enteral feedings when feasible because the subsequent release of gut hormones may promote insulin secretion, allowing for improved blood glucose control.
H. Complications.
   1. Neonatal hyperglycemia may be accompanied by urinary loss of glucose and an osmotic diuresis with its risk of dehydration. In addition, possible resultant hyperosmolarity of extracellular fluid in the brain may increase the premature infant's chance for intraventricular hemorrhage (Sunehag and Haymond, 2002).
   2. Insulin management may be difficult in the ELBW infant; blood glucose levels can fluctuate widely. A precisely controlled continuous-infusion pump is essential. Priming of the tubing is required because insulin tends to adhere to the catheters. Whether insulin therapy promotes linear growth or just converts glucose into fat is not yet fully understood.
   3. Electrolyte abnormalities, elevated CO_2 retention, and an elevated triglyceride level.
I. Outcome.
   1. Controversy exists concerning the outcome of neonatal hyperglycemia.
   a. Hypothesized that hyperglycemia in the premature neonate may increase the risk of IVH because rapid fluctuations in osmolarity negatively impact the germinal matrix.
   b. There is a strong association between neonatal hyperglycemia and increased mortality rates or poor neurodevelopmental outcomes among survivors (Hays et al., 2006).
   c. Neonatal hyperglycemia is usually self-limiting and not associated with adverse outcomes.
   d. Possible association between hyperglycemia and severe retinopathy of prematurity in ELBW infants (Ertl et al., 2006)

TRANSIENT OR PERMANENT NEONATAL DIABETES

A. Definition: Hyperglycemia requiring insulin therapy occurring within the first month of life and lasting at least 2 weeks to several months can be lifelong (Ozlu et al., 2006).

B. **Incidence:** 1:500,000. Predominantly occurring in SGA infants, with 46% developing permanent diabetes in the neonatal period, 23% in childhood or adolescence; 31% are resolved in the neonatal period (Ogata, 2005).

   1. Appears in the first week of life and persists for greater than 2 weeks (Stokowski, 2007).

   2. Etiology is variable, including dysfunctional insulin molecule or receptor deficiencies and activating mutations of the K_{ATP} channel (Stokowski, 2007).

   3. Instances of transient neonatal diabetes are associated with abnormalities of an imprinted region on chromosome 6q24. Mutations in encoder genes have been attributed to instances of permanent and transient neonatal diabetes (Babenko et al., 2006).

C. **Pathophysiology.**

   1. Both transient and permanent neonatal diabetes mellitus (NDM) are due to a failure of pancreatic β cells causing an endogenous insulin deficiency with the exact pathogenesis involved not yet fully understood (Ozlu et al., 2006; Stokowski, 2007).

   2. The IUGR commonly seen with affected infants is due to insufficient insulin secretion (Stokowski, 2007).

D. **Clinical presentation.**

   1. The transient form appears within the first week of life, resolves within weeks or months and reappears in late childhood. The permanent form appears within days or months of birth and persists throughout life (Stokowski, 2007).

   2. Hyperglycemia (frequently >600 mg/dl), polyuria, glycosuria, weight loss, dehydration, fever, failure to thrive, ketosis, metabolic acidosis (may or may not be evident), and low levels of C-peptide and plasma insulin (Ozlu et al., 2006; Stokowski, 2007).

E. **Management.**

   1. Restore intravascular volume.

   2. Replace fluid and electrolyte losses as indicated and provide for ongoing needs.

   3. Correct the hyperglycemia; monitor glucose levels.

   4. Provide adequate nutrition for growth and development.

   5. Usually a daily dose of 0.2 to 3 units/kg/day of insulin is necessary to achieve plasma glucose levels of 100 to 180 mg/dl; however, individualization of insulin requirement is needed.

   6. Average length of insulin therapy varies from 2 weeks to 18 months. Tapering of insulin dose as requirement decreases lessens the risk of recurrent hyperglycemia (Ozlu et al., 2006; Stokowski, 2007).

F. **Complications:** See Hyperglycemia section above.

G. **Outcomes.**

   1. Course of disease is highly variable.

   2. Close follow-up is recommended after remission because of a high rate of recurrence later in childhood.

REFERENCES

Babenko A.P., Polak M., Cavé H., et al.: Activating mutations in the ABCC8 gene in neonatal diabetes mellitus. *New England Journal of Medicine, 355*(5):456-466, 2006.

Baumeister, F.A., Rolinski, B., Busch, R., and Emmrich, P.: Glucose monitoring with long-term subcutaneous microdialysis in neonates. *Pediatrics, 108*(5):1187-1192, 2001.

Blackburn, S.T.: *Maternal, fetal, & neonatal physiology: A clinical perspective* (3rd ed.). St. Louis, 2007, Saunders, pp. 598-625.

Cowett, R.M. and Loughead, J.L.: Neonatal glucose metabolism: Differential diagnoses, evaluation, and treatment of hypoglycemia. *Neonatal Network, 21*(4):9-19, 2002.

De Leon, D.D. and Stanley, C.A.: Mechanisms of disease: Advances in diagnosis and treatment of hyperinsulinism in neonates. *Nature Clinical Practice Endocrinology and Metabolism, 3*(1):57-68, 2007.

de Lonlay, P., Giurgea, I., Guy, T., and Saudubray, M.J.: Neonatal hypoglycaemia: Aetiologies. *Seminars in Neonatology, 9*:49-58, 2004.

Dollberg, S., Bauer, R., Lubetzky, R., and Mimouni, F.B.: A reappraisal of neonatal blood chemistry reference ranges using Nova M electrodes. *American Journal of Perinatology, 18*(8):433-439, 2001.

Dunne, M.J., Cosgrove, K.E., Shepherd, R.M., Aynsley-Green, A., and Lindley, K.J.: Hyperinsulinism in infancy: From basic science to clinical disease. *Physiological Reviews, 84*:239-279, 2004.

Ertl, T., Gyarmati, J., Gaal, V., et al.: Relationship between hyperglycemia and retinopathy of prematurity in very low birth weight infants. *Biology of the Neonate, 89*:56-59, 2006.

Haninger, N.C. and Farley, C.L.: Screening for hypoglycemia in healthy term neonates: Effects on breastfeeding. *Journal of Midwifery and Women's Health,* *46*(5):292-301, 2001.

Hays, S., O'Brian Smith, E., and Sunehag, A.: Hyperglycemia is a risk factor for early death and morbidity in extremely low birth-weight infants. *Pediatrics,* *118*(5):1811-1818, 2006.

Hume, R., Burchell, A., Williams, F., et al.: Glucose homeostasis in the newborn. *Early Human Development, 81*:95-101, 2005.

Kalhan, S. and Parimi, P.: Gluconeogenesis in the fetus and neonate. *Seminars in Perinatology, 24*(2):94-106, 2000.

Lindley, K.J. and Dunne, M.J.: Contemporary strategies in the diagnosis and management of neonatal hyperinsulinaemic hypoglycemia. *Early Human Development, 81*:61-72, 2005.

Louis, C. and Weinzimer, S.A.: A 12-day-old infant with hypoglycemia. *Current Opinion in Pediatrics, 15*(3):333-337, 2003.

Lund, C.H. and Kuller, J.M.: Assessment and management of the integumentary system. In C. Kenner and J.W. Lott (Eds.): *Comprehensive neonatal nursing: A physiologic perspective* (3rd ed.). Philadelphia, 2007, Saunders, pp. 700-724.

McGowan, J.E.: Neonatal hypoglycemia. *Pediatrics in Review, 20*(7): E6-E15, 1999. Retrieved August 10, 1999, from www.pedsinreview.org/

McGowan, J.E., Douglas, W.P., and Hay, W.W., Jr.: Glucose homeostasis. In G.B. Merenstein and S.L. Gardner (Eds.): *Handbook of neonatal intensive care* (6th ed.). St. Louis, 2006, Mosby, pp. 368-390.

Menni, F., de Lonlay, P., Sevin, C., et al.: Neurologic outcomes of 90 neonates and infants with persistent hyperinsulinemic hypoglycemia. *Pediatrics, 107*(3): 476-479, 2001.

Noerr, B.: State of the science: Neonatal hypoglycemia. *Advances in Neonatal Care, 1*(1):4-21, 2001.

Ogata, E.S.: Carbohydrate homeostasis. In M.G. MacDonald, M.D. Mullet, and M.M.K. Seshia (Eds.): *Avery's neonatology: Pathophysiology and management of the newborn* (6th ed.). Philadelphia, 2005, Lippincott Williams & Wilkins, pp. 876-891.

Ozlu, F., Tyker, F., and Yuksel, B.: Neonatal diabetes mellitus. *Indian Pediatrics, 43*:642-645, 2006.

Rozance, P.J. and Hay, W.W.: Hypoglycemia in newborn infants: Features associated with adverse outcomes. *Biology of the Neonate, 90*:74-86, 2006.

Stanley, C.A. and Pallotto, E.K.: Disorders of carbohydrate metabolism. In H.W. Taeusch, R.A. Ballard, and C.A. Gleason (Eds.): *Avery's diseases of the newborn* (8th ed.). Philadelphia, 2005, Saunders, pp. 1410-1422.

Steinkrauss, L., Lipman, T.H., Hendell, C.D., Gerdes, M., Thornton, P.A., and Stanley, C.A.: Effects of hypoglycemia on developmental outcome in children with congenital hyperinsulinism. *Journal of Pediatric Nursing, 20*(2):9-17, 2005.

Stokowski, L.: Endocrine system. In C. Kenner and J.W. Lott (Eds.): *Comprehensive neonatal care: An interdisciplinary approach* (4th ed.). St. Louis, 2007, Saunders, pp. 155-174.

Sunehag, A.L. and Haymond, M.W.: Glucose extremes in newborn infants. *Clinics in Perinatology, 29*(2):245-260, 2002.

Volpe, J.H.: *Neurology of the newborn* (5th ed.). Philadelphia, 2008, Saunders.

10 Nutritional Management

GEORGIA R. DITZENBERGER

OBJECTIVES

1. Describe the effects of prematurity on the gastrointestinal (GI) physiology of digestion and absorption.
2. Identify nutritional store deficiencies most common in premature and term infants.
3. Describe basic nutritional requirements for premature and high-risk term infants and factors that influence these requirements.
4. Identify nutritional components, uses, methods of delivery, complications, and nursing care issues for parenteral nutrition (PN).
5. Review the use of commercial preterm and full-term infant formulas for enteral nutrition management.
6. Review human milk feedings for premature and high-risk term infants and related nursing care issues.
7. Review the use of human milk supplements in enteral nutrition management for premature infants.
8. Describe the various methods of providing enteral feedings and the advantages and disadvantages of each.
9. Describe minimal enteral feedings and application in initiating enteral nutrition for premature infants.
10. Describe risks and interventions for feeding intolerances and nutritional deficiency states in premature infants.
11. Describe assessment of an infant's readiness for enteral nutrition.
12. Describe assessments used to determine premature and high-risk infant nutritional status.
13. Describe the standards used to assess growth in term and premature infants.

Neonatal nurses face challenges in helping to meet the basic nutritional requirements and support the growth needs of premature and high-risk infants. Tremendous advances in technology and pharmacology permit the survival of very premature infants who require intensive and specialized care and support for immature body systems. Nutritional care is of vital importance for premature infants, who are deprived of transplacentally acquired nutrient stores and have rapid extrauterine growth rates. Other high-risk infants have special needs related to illness-associated metabolic demands and physiologic instability.

Neonatal nurses with knowledge of the effects of prematurity on GI functioning, the special nutritional needs of premature and high-risk infants, and methods of delivering nutritional support can better assess infant status and contribute to nutritional management. This chapter reviews the nutritional requirements of premature and high-risk infants, methods for providing parenteral and enteral nutrition, and nursing interventions for optimal nutritional support.

ANATOMY AND PHYSIOLOGY OF THE PREMATURE INFANT'S GASTROINTESTINAL TRACT

A. **Anatomic and functional development of the GI tract.**
   1. Anatomic development (Berseth, 2006; Blackburn, 2007).
      a. Pylorus and fundus of stomach defined and gastric glands formed by 14 weeks of gestation.
      b. Esophageal sphincter present by 28 weeks of gestation.
      c. GI tract resembles that of a term newborn infant by 20 weeks of gestation.
      d. Gut lengthens to 250 to 300 cm by term; gastric capacity is about 30 ml.

2. Functional development (Berseth, 2004, 2006; Blackburn, 2007).
   a. Premature infants have limited production of gut digestive enzymes and growth factors.
   b. By 28 weeks, biochemical and physiologic capacities for limited digestion and absorption is present.
   c. Major gut-regulating polypeptides, gastrin, motilin, cholecystokinin, pancreatic polypeptide, and somatostatin, are present in limited amounts by the end of the first trimester; act locally to regulate growth and development of the gut; reach adult distribution by term gestation.
   d. Intestinal transport of amino acids seen by 14 weeks, glucose by 18 weeks, and fatty acid by 24 weeks of gestation.
   e. Lactose is a predominate source of carbohydrate in breast milk and formula. Lactase reduces lactose to glucose.
   f. Lactase activity is first seen at 9 weeks of gestation; at 24 weeks of gestation less than one fourth activity level of term infant; dramatically increases between 32 and 34 weeks of gestation to the activity level of term infant.
   g. Disaccharidases, such as salivary amylase and mucosal glucoamylase, are functionally active after 27 to 28 weeks of gestation (Blackburn, 2007). Some formulas contain glucose polymers, likely hydrolyzed by salivary amylase or absorbed directly at the mucosal level via mucosal glucoamylase.
   h. Fat (lipid) emulsification and hydrolyzation to free fatty acids and monoglycerides result from lipase and bile acid activity.
   i. Lingual and gastric lipases present by 26 weeks of gestation; limited in volume and function. Additional lipases also in breast milk; function well in conditions with low bile acid synthesis and stores such as seen in premature infants.
   j. Bile acid secretion observed by 22 weeks of gestation.
   k. Bile acid synthesis and stores of premature infant decreased when compared to term infant synthesis and stores, which is in turn one half that seen in adult synthesis and stores.
   l. Gastric gland secretion activity seen by 20 weeks of gestation; gastric acid secretion lower than adult levels even at term gestation; activated with introduction of enteral feeding.
   m. Ingested proteins are denatured by gastrin and cleaved by pepsin; further reduced by pancreatic proteolytic enzymes into oligopeptides and amino acids. Pepsin activity induced by increased gastric acid resulting from initiation of enteral feedings.
   n. GI motility refers to the coordinated facilitation of mechanical digestion, the movement of food from injection to elimination; includes suck-swallow and esophageal, stomach, and intestinal peristalsis. Immature GI motility is a major limitation to enteral digestion; presence of disorganized, random contractions between 25 and 30 weeks of gestation; motility improves after 30 to 32 weeks of gestation, gradually becomes more organized closer to term gestation (Berseth, 2004; Blackburn, 2007; Omari and Rudolph, 2004).

B. Postnatal development of the GI tract.
   1. GI motility is a major limitation in providing enteral nutrition for premature infants (Berseth, 2004; Omari and Rudolph, 2004).
      a. Nonnutritive suck coordination present around 28 weeks of gestation; suck-swallow coordination for adequate expression of milk from breast or nipple develops closer to 34 to 36 weeks of gestation; appears to be dependent on neuromaturation related to postmenstrual age rather than chronologic age (age in days since birth) (Berseth, 2006; Blackburn, 2007; Omari and Rudolph, 2004).
      b. Well-developed tone and swallow-related relaxation in the lower esophageal sphincter (LES), allowing food passage into the stomach from the esophagus; transient LES relaxation related to immaturity, allowing gastric contents to reenter the esophagus (gastroesophageal reflux [GER]); diminishes closer to term gestation (Omari and Rudolph, 2004).

    c. Delayed gastric emptying related to disorganized, random peristalsis contractions with immature duodenal response to food; duodenal contractions of premature infants cease rather than increase in response to food, delaying gastric emptying. Peristalsis becomes more organized, duodenal responses and gastric emptying time improves with increasing gestational age; regular enteral feeding for at least 10 days seems to have positive maturational effect on duodenal response for premature infants (Berseth, 2004; Kleinman, 2004).

  2. Influences on postnatal development of GI function include genetic endowment, gut trophic factors, and hormonal regulatory mechanisms, and enteral feeding initiation and feeding type (Blackburn, 2007).

    a. Gut trophic factors include nutrients, hormones, and peptides; principal nutrients: iron, zinc, vitamin B_{12}, vitamin A, and folate; principal hormones: insulin and growth factor; principal peptides: epidermal growth factor, transforming growth factor, insulin-like growth factors, and somatostatin.

    b. Hormonal regulatory mechanisms have a critical role in mediating gut development after birth. Gut development stimulated by increases in specific GI hormones and enteric neuropeptides such as enteroglucagon, promoting intestinal mucosa growth; gastrin, stimulating gastric mucosa and exocrine pancreas growth; motilin and neurotensin, stimulating development of gut motility; and gastric inhibitory peptide, promoting glucose tolerance.

    c. Initiation of enteral feeding is a major stimulus for hormonal regulatory mechanisms in both premature and term infants; response delayed in premature and high-risk infants receiving only PN without enteral feedings.

    d. Type of enteral feeding has an influence on gut maturation; breast milk contains high levels of GI trophic factors, which enhance the postnatal maturation of gut.

    e. Minimal enteral feeding, also known as trophic feeding, or gut or GI priming feeding, appears to stimulate hormonal regulatory mechanisms, with subsequent gut development; as little as 0.5 to 1 ml/kg/hour seems beneficial (Berseth, 2006; Blackburn, 2007).

C. Nutrient deficiencies of premature infants: cessation of transplacental transfer of nutrients during the third trimester, a critical period for somatic and brain growth (Limperopoulos et al., 2005; Schanler, 2005).

  1. Carbohydrate, lipid, and protein.

    a. Glucose is a primary source of carbohydrate; during the third trimester, glucose is stored as glycogen in the liver and cardiac and skeletal muscle, and to a lesser extent in the kidneys, intestines, and brain; glycogen stores of term infants are significantly greater than those of adults (Blackburn, 2007).

      (1) Glucose is the primary fetal energy source; accounts for 80% of fetal energy.

      (2) Carbohydrate in the form of lactose and glucose provides 40% of the postnatal caloric intake (Berseth, 2006).

    b. Lipid stores; significant lipid accretion and increased adipose tissue deposition occurs in the fetus between 24 and 40 weeks. At 26 to 28 weeks, fat stores account for approximately 3.5% of body composition, 30 to 34 weeks 8%, and by 35 to 38 weeks 16%; weight gain due to fat deposition is about 14 g/day (Moore and Persaud, 2008).

      (1) Adipose tissue: white and brown (Blackburn, 2007).

        (a) White adipose tissue: subcutaneous tissue; acts as a heat insulator, shock absorber, and calorie storage unit.

        (b) Brown adipose tissue: accumulates in the neck, scapulae, axillae, mediastinum, and perirenal tissues; critical for nonshivering thermogenesis, a major method of neonatal heat production.

      (2) Lipids contribute minimally to fetal energy needs; critical component of brain development (neuronal and glial membranes, and myelin sheath), retinal development, cell membrane formation, synthesis of surfactant and other phospholipids, bile, serum lipoprotein, and adipose tissue deposition (Blackburn, 2007; Un and Carlson, 2004).

(3) Lipids provide approximately 50% of the postnatal caloric intake; major postnatal energy source (Berseth, 2006; Blackburn, 2007; Putet, 2004).

c. Protein stores; major structural and functional components of all cells of the body; during the third trimester, fetal accretion rate is 3.6 to 4.8 g/kg/day (Blackburn, 2007; Hay and Regnault, 2004; Heird and Kashyap, 2004).

   (1) Amino acids and lactate secondary fetal energy source; critical in all organ development, growth, and function (Berseth, 2006).

   (2) Protein catabolism contributes approximately 10% of postnatal caloric intake (Berseth, 2006).

d. Premature infants have minimal adipose tissue and glycogen stores at birth; stores decrease with decreasing gestational age; at birth sources will be quickly exhausted if sufficient exogenous sources to meet energy needs are not provided (Blackburn, 2007).

e. Stable term infants have sufficient glycogen and fat stores to provide for energy demands during the relative state of low nutrient intake that normally occurs during the first few days of life (Blackburn, 2007).

   (1) Estimated 90% of liver and 50% to 80% cardiac and skeletal muscle glycogen stores used within the first 24 hours post birth (Blackburn, 2007).

   (2) Fat is a major source of stored calories for term infant; preferred energy source for high energy demands of such tissues as the heart and the adrenal cortex (Blackburn, 2007).

2. Vitamins and minerals.

   a. Fat-soluble vitamins A and E; stored in body fat and organs (Greer, 2006).

      (1) Vitamin A transferred throughout pregnancy, increases in the third trimester, adequate fetal level maintained despite variations in maternal diet; essential for epithelial cell growth and differentiation, vision, healing, reproduction, and immunocompetency (Greer, 2006; Shenai, 2004).

      (2) Vitamin E gradually increases throughout pregnancy with direct correlation between vitamin E level and body weight and adipose tissue; provides protection from oxidant free-radical damage (Johnson, 2004).

   b. Calcium, phosphorus, and magnesium.

      (1) Two thirds of the calcium accumulated in a term infant transplacentally transferred to the fetus during the third trimester; allows for rapid fetal bone mineralization (Husain et al., 2004).

      (2) Fetal phosphorus levels higher than maternal levels during the third trimester; important role in fetal intermediary metabolism and bone mineralization (Husain et al., 2004; Itani and Tsang, 2006).

      (3) Eighty percent of the magnesium in term infants is accrued in the third trimester; important to plasma membrane excitability, regulatory role in numerous biologic processes involved in energy storage, transfer, and production, significant in calcium and bone homeostasis (Itani and Tsang, 2006; Namgung and Tsang, 2004).

   c. Trace elements: copper, selenium, chromium, manganese, molybdenum, cobalt, fluoride, iodine, iron, and zinc provided during pregnancy; essential for various metabolic processes, cell and organ function and development (Hambidge, 2006; Jones and King, 2005).

      (1) Iron has a prominent role in oxygen transport, principally in the hemoglobin; a 28-week fetus has 64 mcg iron per gram of fat-free tissue, and a term infant has 94 mcg; in term infants, almost 80% of the iron is stored in the hemoglobin; required by virtually all cells for normal growth and metabolism; rapidly growing and differentiating cells have particularly high iron requirements; necessary for the development and functional integrity of the immune system (Georgieff, 2006; Hambidge, 2006).

      (2) Fetal zinc levels markedly increase midpregnancy, then decreases gradually over the third trimester; important biologic role in protein structure and function, enzymes, transcription factors, hormonal receptor sites, and cell membranes; and numerous central roles in DNA and RNA metabolism (Hambidge, 2006; Hambidge and Krebs, 2004).

NUTRITIONAL REQUIREMENTS

A. **Term Infants (Table 10-1).**
1. Fluid requirements.
   a. Parenteral: 100 to 120 ml/kg/day.
   b. Enteral: 120 to 150 ml/kg/day.

■ TABLE 10-1
■ ■ **Daily Nutritional Requirements for Term Infants**

Nutrient	Parenteral	Enteral
Fluid (ml/kg/day)*	100 to 120	120 to 150
Energy (kcal/kg/day)[†]	80 to 90	100 to 120
Protein (g/kg/day)[‡]	2 to 2.5	2 to 2.5
Carbohydrate (g/kg/day)	10 to 15	8 to 12
Fat (g/kg/day)	2 to 4	3 to 4
Sodium (mEq/kg/day)	2 to 3	2 to 3
Potassium (mEq/kg/day)	2 to 3	2 to 3
Chloride (mEq/kg/day)	2 to 3	2 to 3
Calcium (mg/kg/day)[§]	60 to 80	130
Phosphorus (mg/kg/day)[§]	40 to 45	45
Magnesium (mg/kg/day)	5 to 7	7
Iron (mg/kg/day)[‖]	0.1 to 0.2	1 to 2
Vitamin A (IU/day)[¶]	2300	1250
Vitamin D (IU/day)	400	300
Vitamin E (IU/day)**	7	5 to 10
Vitamin K (mg/day)	0.05	0.2
Vitamin C (mg/day)	80	30 to 50
Vitamin B_1 (mg/day)	1.2	0.3
Vitamin B_2 (mg/day)	1.4	0.4
Vitamin B_6 (mg/day)	1	0.3
Vitamin B_{12} (mcg/day)	1	0.3
Niacin (mg/day)	17	5
Folate (mcg/day)[††]	140	25 to 50
Biotin (mcg/day)	20	10
Zinc (mcg/kg/day)[‡‡]	250	830
Copper (mcg/kg/day)[‡‡,§§]	20	75
Manganese (mcg/kg/day)[§§]	1	85
Selenium (mcg/kg/day)[‖‖]	2	1.6
Chromium (mcg/kg/day)	0.2	2
Molybdenum (mcg/kg/day)	0.25	2
Iodine (mcg/kg/day)	1	7

Adapted from Blackburn, S.T.: *Maternal, fetal, & neonatal physiology: A clinical perspective* (3rd ed.). St. Louis, 2007, Saunders, p. 454.
*After immediate postnatal initiation of fluid therapy.
[†]Adjust according to weight gain and stress factors.
[‡]Requirements increase with increasing degree of prematurity.
[§]Inadequate amount in total parenteral nutrition solutions because of risk of precipitation.
[‖]Initiate between 2 weeks and 2 months of age. Delay initiation in preterm infants with progressive retinopathy.
[¶]Supplementation might reduce the incidence of bronchopulmonary dysplasia.
**Supplementation might reduce the severity of retinopathy of prematurity.
[††]Not present in oral multivitamin supplements.
[‡‡]Increased requirement in patients with excessive ileostomy drainage or chronic diarrhea.
[§§]Removed from total parenteral nutrition solutions in patients with cholestatic liver disease.
[‖‖]Not present in standard trace element solution for neonates.

   2. Energy (caloric) intake requirements.
      a. Parenteral: 80 to 90 kcal/kg/day.
      b. Enteral: 100 to 120 kcal/kg/day.
   3. Carbohydrate, fat, and protein (Berseth, 2004; Blackburn, 2007).
      a. Total caloric intake should be represented by the following:
        (1) Carbohydrate: approximately 40%; 8 to 12 g/kg/day.
        (2) Fat.
          (a) Parenteral: 2 to 4 g/kg/day; 20% intravenous (IV) lipid emulsion preferred over 10%, and has less phospholipid per gram of fat. High phospholipid levels associated with increased triglyceride, cholesterol, and low-density lipoprotein levels in neonates (Haumont et al., 1989).
          (b) Enteral: 3 to 4 g/kg/day.
        (3) Protein: both parenteral and enteral: 2 to 2.5 g/kg/day.
      b. Human milk and standard commercial infant formulas supply these nutrients within acceptable ratios (Blackburn, 2007).
   4. Vitamins, minerals, and trace elements.
      a. Dietary reference intakes for enteral and parenteral are summarized in Table 10-1.
      b. Pediatric parenteral vitamin, minerals and trace element solutions, human milk, and commercial infant formulas provide adequate amounts of most vitamins to meet the needs of infants (Greer, 2006; Kleinman, 2004).
      c. Newborn deficiencies in fat-soluble vitamins A, D, E, and K well described; countermanded with human milk and formulas; significant vitamin deficiency rare (Greer, 2006).
        (1) Vitamin K is the only vitamin routinely given at the time of birth, seems to sustain sufficient levels for the first 3 months of life for exclusively breastfeeding infants even though human milk does not meet dietary reference intakes; formulas have sufficient vitamin K to meet dietary reference intakes (Greer, 2006); oral forms of vitamin K not recommended, may not provide adequate vitamin K necessary to prevent hemorrhage later in infancy unless repeated doses given in the first 4 months of life (American Academy of Pediatrics, Section on Breastfeeding, 2005).
        (2) American Academy of Pediatrics (AAP) recommends vitamin D supplementation for breastfed or formula-fed infants unless taking at least 500 ml/day of vitamin D–fortified formula or milk, beginning in the first 2 months of life (AAP, Section on Breastfeeding, 2005; Greer, 2006; Kleinman, 2004).
        (3) Fluoride supplements should not be provided for the first 6 months of life for any infant; after 6 months, fluoride supplementation recommended only if the fluoride level in drinking water supply is <0.3 ppm; consideration should include other fluoride sources: food, toothpaste, other fluid sources (AAP, Section on Breastfeeding, 2005; Kleinman, 2004).
        (4) Iron supplements not recommended for healthy term infants until 6 months; recommended in the first 6 months of life only for infants with hematologic disorders, or infants with inadequate iron stores at birth (AAP, Section on Breastfeeding, 2005).
        (5) Vitamin B_{12} supplementation recommended for infants of vegan mothers with inadequate B_{12} intake (Greer, 2006).

B. Premature infants (Blackburn, 2007).
   1. General considerations.
      a. Recommendations for nutritional requirements and advisable intakes are used as guidelines.
      b. Individual premature infant nutritional needs vary with gestational age and health status.
      c. Recommendations for parenteral and enteral nutritional needs are summarized in Table 10-2.
   2. Fluid requirements.
      a. Parenteral: 100 to 150 ml/kg/day.
      b. Enteral: 150 to 200 ml/kg/day.
      c. Varies with hydration state (e.g., dehydration to overhydration/edematous states), estimated insensible water losses, gestational age, postmenstrual age, generalized

■ TABLE 10-2
■ ■ **Daily Nutritional Requirements for Premature Infants**

Nutrient	Parenteral	Enteral
Fluid (ml/kg/day)*	120 to 150	150 to 200
Energy (kcal/kg/day)[†]	80 to 100	110 to 130
Protein (g/kg/day)[‡]	2.5 to 3.5	3 to 3.8
Carbohydrate (g/kg/day)	10 to 15	8 to 12
Fat (g/kg/day)	2 to 3.5	3 to 4
Sodium (mEq/kg/day)	2 to 3.5	2 to 4
Potassium (mEq/kg/day)	2 to 3	2 to 3
Chloride (mEq/kg/day)	2 to 3	2 to 3
Calcium (mg/kg/day)[§]	60 to 90	210 to 250
Phosphorus (mg/kg/day)[§]	40 to 70	112 to 125
Magnesium (mg/kg/day)	4 to 7	8 to 15
Iron (mg/kg/day)[‖]	0.0 to 0.2	1 to 2
Vitamin A (IU/day)[¶]	700 to 1500	700 to 1500
Vitamin D (IU/day)	120 to 260	400
Vitamin E (IU/day)**	2 to 4	6 to 12
Vitamin K (mg/day)	0.06 to 0.1	0.05
Vitamin C (mg/day)	35 to 50	20 to 60
Vitamin B_1 (mg/day)	0.3 to 0.8	0.2 to 0.7
Vitamin B_2 (mg/day)	0.4 to 0.9	0.3 to 0.8
Vitamin B_6 (mg/day)	0.3 to 0.7	0.3 to 0.7
Vitamin B_{12} (mcg/day)	0.3 to 0.7	0.3 to 0.7
Niacin (mg/day)	5 to 12	5 to 12
Folate (mcg/day)[††]	40 to 90	50
Biotin (mcg/day)	6 to 13	6 to 20
Zinc (mcg/kg/day)[‡‡]	400	800 to 1000
Copper (mcg/kg/day)[‡‡,§§]	20	100 to 150
Manganese (mcg/kg/day)[§§]	1	10 to 20
Selenium (mcg/kg/day)[‖‖]	1.5 to 2	1.3 to 3
Chromium (mcg/kg/day)	0.2	2 to 4
Molybdenum (mcg/kg/day)	0.25	2 to 3
Iodine (mcg/kg/day)	1	4

Adapted from Blackburn, S.T.: *Maternal, fetal, & neonatal physiology: A clinical perspective* (3rd ed.). St. Louis, 2007, Saunders, p. 454.
*After immediate postnatal initiation of fluid therapy.
[†]Adjust according to weight gain and stress factors.
[‡]Requirements increase with increasing degree of prematurity.
[§]Inadequate amount in total parenteral nutrition solutions because of risk of precipitation.
[‖]Initiate between 2 weeks and 2 months of age. Delay initiation in preterm infants with progressive retinopathy.
[¶]Supplementation might reduce incidence of bronchopulmonary dysplasia.
**Supplementation might reduce severity of retinopathy of prematurity.
[††]Not present in oral multivitamin supplement.
[‡‡]Increased requirement in patients with excessive ileostomy drainage or chronic diarrhea.
[§§]Removed from total parenteral nutrition solutions in patients with cholestatic liver disease.
[‖‖]Not present in standard trace element solution for neonates.

health status, and underlying disease state of the infant (e.g., presence of patent ductus arteriosus, bronchopulmonary disease, postrecovery phase of necrotizing enterocolitis [NEC], and short gut syndrome).

3. Energy (caloric) intake requirements.
   a. Based on an estimation of the caloric need for premature infants as summarized in Table 10-3.

■ TABLE 10-3
■ ■ **Estimation of Caloric Requirements for the Low Birthweight Infant (kcal/kg/day)**

Physiologic Activity	kcal/kg/day
Energy expended	40 to 60
Resting metabolic rate	40 to 50
Activity	0 to 5
Thermoregulation	0 to 5
Synthesis	15
Energy stored	20 to 30
Energy excreted	15
Total energy intake	90 to 120

Adapted from American Academy of Pediatrics Committee on Nutrition: *Pediatric nutrition handbook* (5th ed.). Elk Grove Village, IL, 2004, American Academy of Pediatrics, p. 26.

    b. Parenteral: 90 to 100 kcal/kg/day.
    c. Enteral: 110 to 130 kcal/kg/day.
    d. Varies depending on day of life, fluid intake, thermal environment, activity, maturation, health status, underlying disease state, and growth rate.
  4. Carbohydrate, fat, and protein (Blackburn, 2007; Hay, 2006; Kashyap, 2007).
    a. Carbohydrate.
      (1) Parenteral: 10 to 15 g/kg/day; glucose IV infusion.
      (2) Enteral: 8 to 12 g/kg/day; primarily lactose.
      (3) Glucose intake must be adequate to maintain serum levels greater than 45 mg/dl.
      (4) Premature infants rapidly become hypoglycemic with inadequate glucose intake. Hyperglycemia can also be a problem with extremely premature infants. Hyperglycemia contributes to hyperosmolality and may be a risk factor for intracranial hemorrhage in those infants.
    b. Fat.
      (1) Parenteral: 2 to 3.5 g/kg/day.
      (2) Enteral: 3 to 4 g/kg/day.
      (3) Medium-chain triglycerides are easier to absorb than long-chain triglycerides; medium-chain triglycerides are absorbed by passive diffusion and do not require bile salts.
        (a) Premature infant formulas use a combination of medium-chain triglycerides and shorter-chain vegetable fatty acids.
        (b) Linoleic acid is an essential fatty acid and should account for at least 3% of total calories; achieved with adequate intake of human milk and commercial premature infant formulas.
        (c) Very-long-chain fatty acids—arachidonic acid and docosahexaenoic acid—which are derivatives of linoleic and linolenic acids and are found in human milk but not cow's milk; associated functionally with cognition and vision.
    c. Protein (Kashyap, 2007; Poindexter and Denne, 2004).
      (1) Parenteral: 3 to 4 g/kg/day
        (a) Extremely low birth weight (ELBW) infants, that is, <1000 g birth weight: 3.5 to 4.0 g/kg/day.
        (b) Very low birth weight (VLBW) infants, that is, 1000 to 1500 g birth weight: 3.0 to 3.5 g/kg/day.
      (2) Enteral: 2.9 to 4.3 g/kg/day; higher protein amounts for low birth weight (LBW) infants.

(3) Protein requirements for VLBW infants controversial owing to uncertainty related to ability to tolerate protein and what is actually needed to provide for growth and development.

   (a) Protein losses can be significant for VLBW infants when not receiving amino acids; ELBW infants lose 1.5 g/kg/day body protein, equaling approximately 1.5% body protein when they should be accumulating at a rate of 2% per day; 3 days of no protein intake results in 10% body protein deficit.

   (b) Good evidence that early amino acid intake compensates for potential protein losses; 1.5 to 2 g/kg/day as soon as possible after birth preserves limited body protein stores in ELBW infants even at low caloric intakes; increasing caloric intake will improve protein accretion.

   (c) Ultimate goal of parenteral amino acid administration is to achieve a rate of fetal protein accretion; recent evidence shows that 3.5 to 4.0 g/kg/day are tolerated for ELBW infants.

   (d) Protein and energy intakes should be determined concurrently to optimize nitrogen retention and promote proportionate body composition (lean-to-fat mass ratio) growth; protein-to-energy-intake ratio (P:E) recommendations for VLBW infants range from 2.25 to 3.6 g/100 kcal.

   (e) In addition to the eight essential amino acids necessary for cell growth, premature infants require four conditionally essential amino acids: histidine, taurine, cysteine, and tyrosine.

5. Vitamins, minerals, and trace elements.
   a. Dietary reference intakes for enteral and parenteral nutrition are summarized in Table 10-2.
   b. Pediatric parenteral vitamin, minerals and trace element solutions, and commercial premature infant formulas provide adequate amounts of most vitamins; premature infants on primarily human milk intake will require oral multivitamin supplement (Greer, 2006; Kleinman, 2004).
   c. Newborn deficiencies in fat-soluble vitamins A, D, E, and K are well described, countermanded with human milk and formulas; significant vitamin deficiency rare even for premature infants (Greer, 2006).
      (1) Vitamin K per intramuscular injection at birth; oral forms not recommended (Greer, 2006).
      (2) Vitamin D supplementation for breastfed or formula-fed infants until intake of vitamin D–fortified formula exceeds 500 ml/day (AAP, Section on Breastfeeding, 2005; Greer, 2006; Kleinman, 2004).
   d. Iron supplements recommended for premature infants, owing to inadequate iron stores at birth and iatrogenic blood losses; required for erythropoietin treatment for early physiologic anemia of prematurity (Blackburn, 2007; Georgieff, 2006; Greer, 2006).
6. Electrolytes (Blackburn, 2007).
   a. Sodium, potassium, and chloride: necessary for growth; significant role in water and acid-base balance.
   b. Premature infants, especially VLBW infants, have increased urine sodium and obligatory water loss during the transitional neonatal period.
   c. After reduction of the extracellular fluid, loss of body weight slows and urinary excretion of sodium chloride decreases. VLBW infants may require sodium supplements until renal tubular function matures.
   d. Premature infant formulas provide higher amounts of sodium, potassium, and chloride than term infant formulas; premature human milk has higher sodium and chloride levels than mature human milk (after 4 weeks); may still need to supplement until renal tubular function matures.

PARENTERAL NUTRITION (PN)

PN is indicated for initiation of nutrition support for premature and high-risk neonates; provides nutritional support when enteral intake is not possible or does not provide sufficient caloric requirements. The initial goal of PN is to minimize losses and preserve existing body stores; it progresses to provide nutrition to promote growth and development (Poindexter and Denne, 2005).

A. **Indications for PN in the neonatal period (Kleinman, 2004; Poindexter and Denne, 2005).**
   1. Congenital and/or surgical GI disorders: gastroschisis, tracheoesophageal fistula, malrotation, and intestinal obstruction.
   2. Short bowel syndrome.
   3. Acute GI conditions, such as NEC or intestinal perforation.
   4. Renal failure.
   5. Insufficient caloric or nitrogen (protein) content of enteral feeds.
   6. Severe respiratory or cardiac disease.

B. **PN administration.**
   1. Peripheral route (Kleinman, 2004).
      a. IV access may become problematic for prolonged PN use; limit dextrose concentrations to 12.5% or less to prevent irritation of small peripheral veins.
      b. Provides up to 90 kcal/kg/day with dextrose and lipid emulsions and adequate fluid intake.
   2. Central route (Kleinman, 2004).
      a. Prolonged dwell time for central catheters, decreases IV access problems; dextrose concentrations not restricted except by desired glucose infusion rate (GIR).
      b. Complications of central catheters: sepsis; thrombosis of large vessels; pleural or pericardial effusions due to malposition outside the vessel; hemorrhage associated with erosion of central vessels; thrombophlebitis.
      c. Peripherally inserted central catheters provide prolonged venous access; inserted at the bedside with a strictly aseptic technique by a qualified personnel.
      d. Surgically placed central venous catheters (i.e., Broviac or Hickman) provide long-term venous access; require anesthesia; and is recommended for home PN use.
      e. All central venous catheters require radiographic confirmation for placement prior to initiation of PN.

C. **Guidelines for determining appropriate intake, compositions of available preparations, and guidelines for IV administration.**
   1. Fluid (Blackburn, 2007).
      a. Minimum requirement approximately 100 to 150 ml/kg/day.
      b. Varies with gestational and postnatal age and environmental conditions, such as incubator versus radiant heat source and phototherapy. Incubators and heat shields can reduce insensible water losses, whereas radiant warmers and phototherapy increase these losses.
   2. Calories (Blackburn, 2007).
      a. Parenteral requirements are about 20% less than enteral intake, 90 to 100 kcal/kg/day.
         (1) Caloric values must be adjusted to meet activity levels, body temperature, and degree of stress.
         (2) Activity and catabolic states can cause a 25% to 75% increase in metabolic demands.
   3. Nutrients (see Table 10-1) (Poindexter and Denne, 2005).
      a. Carbohydrates: glucose monohydrate (dextrose), 3.4 kcal/g.
         (1) Dextrose preparations are made according to the infant's tolerance; standard dextrose concentrations are available in 5% or 10% solutions (percentage: grams of dextrose per deciliter of solution). Other concentrations may be tailored to the individual needs of the infant.
         (2) Guidelines for carbohydrate administration:
            (a) GIR of 4 to 6 g/kg/day (2.5 to 4 mg/kg/minute) is the starting point; provides for minimal caloric intake, protein metabolism, and growth; serves to preserve limited neonatal carbohydrate stores.
            (b) Gradual increase in GIR to 13 to 17 g/kg/day (9 to 12 mg/kg/minute) over 2 to 7 days usually tolerated in the presence of amino acid administration; maintain serum glucose 40 mg/dl to 150 mg/dl; maximum GIR recommended:

18 g/kg/day (12.5 mg/kg/minute); higher rates exceed glucose oxidative capacity, cause extensive lipogenesis.

(c) In some VLBWI, severe hyperglycemia may present and continue despite reduced carbohydrate intakes; continuous insulin infusion may be used; routine use not advised because of side effects. The usual infusion of insulin is 0.01 to 0.1 unit/kg/hour to maintain blood glucose levels between 100 and 200 mg/dl.

b. Fat: 20% lipid preparations, 2.2 kcal/ml.

(1) In United States, all IV lipid emulsions are derived from soybean oil or a combination of soybean and safflower oils, contain long-chain triglycerides.

(2) Intravenous lipid emulsions have a fatty acid profile substantially different from human milk.

(3) Lipid emulsions of 0.5 to 1 g/kg/day prevents deficiency of essential fatty acids; should be introduced as a component of PN by 24 to 48 hours of age; increase by 0.5 to 1 g/kg/day to 3 g/kg/day.

(4) Premature infants <28 weeks of gestational age have limited lipoprotein lipase activity and triglyceride clearance; may require slower advances in IV lipid infusion rate to improve tolerance.

(5) Although heparin releases lipoprotein lipase from the endothelium into circulation, there is no evidence that this increases lipid utilization in premature infants; therefore, routine addition of heparin into lipid infusion is not recommended (Poindexter and Denne, 2005).

c. Protein: amino acids, 4 kcal/g. Recommended intake: 2.25 to 4 g/kg/day.

(1) The smaller and less mature the infant, the higher the protein intake recommended; for example, infants of less than 1000 g weight may receive 4 g/kg/day protein intake (refer to the Nutrition Requirement, Premature Infant Section).

(2) Pediatric amino acid solutions designed to mimic plasma amino acid concentrations in healthy 20-day-old breastfed infant (Trophamine) or fetal or neonatal cord blood amino acid concentrations (Primine); no evidence to support superiority of one solution over the other.

(a) Glutamine, an amino acid abundant in breast milk, not included in available amino acid solutions owing to issues of stability.

(b) Tyrosine has limited solubility, and so a small amount is included; Trophamine contains a soluble derivative of tyrosine but appears to have poor bioavailability; current research suggests that tyrosine supply in amino acids is suboptimal for VLBW infants.

(c) Cysteine unstable for long periods; cysteine hydrochloride supplement can be added to PN just prior to administration; there is conflicting evidence as to whether cysteine improves protein accretion.

d. Calcium and phosphorus.

(1) PN preparations for infants receiving 100 to 150 ml/kg/day should contain 50 to 60 mg/dl (12.5 to 15 mmol/l) elemental calcium and 40 to 47 mg/dl (12.5 to 15 mmol/l) phosphorus; provides 50 to 90 mg/kg/day calcium and 40 to 70 mg/kg/day phosphorus; a calcium-to-phosphorus ratio of 1.7:1 by weight (1.3:1 by molar ratio) maintains optimal bone mineralization.

(2) Precipitation of calcium and phosphorus remains an issue in the United States owing to commercially available solutions; not possible to supply VLBW infants with adequate amounts of parenteral calcium and phosphorus to support optimal bone mineralization.

e. Vitamins and trace elements are summarized in Tables 10-1 and 10-2.

f. Suggestions for monitoring growth and biochemical laboratory tests during PN use are summarized in Table 10-4.

D. Complications associated with PN administration (Blackburn, 2007; Poindexter and Denne, 2004).

1. Increased risk of metabolic derangements (e.g., hyperglycemia, hypoglycemia, azotemia, acidosis, alkalosis), electrolyte imbalances; require close blood chemistry monitoring; alleviated with manipulation of PN constituents.

■ TABLE 10-4
■ ■ **Suggested Monitoring Schedule for Infants Receiving Parenteral Nutrition**

Parameter	Suggested Frequency per Week	
	Initial Period*	Later Period*
ANTHROPOMETRIC		
Weight	7	7
Length	1	1
Head circumference	1	1
METABOLIC (BLOOD OR PLASMA)		
Electrolytes	2 to 4	1
Calcium, magnesium, and phosphorus	2	1
Acid-base status	2	1
Blood urea nitrogen/creatinine	2	1
Albumin	2	1
Liver function tests	1	1
Hemoglobin/hematocrit	2	1
PREVENTION AND DETECTION OF INFECTION		
Clinical observations (e.g., activity, temperature)	Daily	Daily
White blood cell count, differential	As indicated	As indicated
Cultures	As indicated	As indicated

Adapted from Heird, W.C.: Intravenous feeding. In P.J. Thureen and W.W. Hay (Eds.): *Neonatal nutrition and metabolism* (2nd ed.). Philadelphia, 2006, Cambridge University Press, p. 325.
*Initial period refers to the time before full intake is achieved as well as any period during which metabolic instability is present or suspected (postoperative, symptoms of sepsis). Later period refers to any time there is metabolic stability.

2. Cholestasis and cholestatic jaundice result of hepatic dysfunction; initial intracellular and intracanalicular cholestasis, followed by portal inflammation; progressing to bile duct proliferation after several weeks of PN administration; may progress to portal fibrosis and cirrhosis. Most often resolves gradually with cessation of PN use when on full enteral nutrition; rare instances of irreversible liver failure documented after several months of continuous PN.
    a. Very little recent information regarding incidence of cholestasis; older studies suggest increased prevalence in ELBW infants; occurs predominantly in critically ill premature infants with prolonged PN administration who potentially experienced a variety of insults (e.g., hypoxia, hemodynamic instability, and/or infection); higher incidence of sepsis reported in infants with cholestasis.
    b. Precise cause unknown; probably multifactorial; growing body of evidence of association with prolonged lack of enteral nutrition; research evidence suggests that enteral feedings even at low caloric intakes can reduce the incidence of cholestasis.
    c. Clinical features: hyperbilirubinemia and jaundice.
        (1) Direct bilirubin (DB) level >1 mg/dl (17.1 μmol/l) and total serum bilirubin (TB or TSB) ≤5 mg/dl (85.5 μmol/l), or DB equal to 20% TB with TB >5 mg/dl.
        (2) Sensitive, nonspecific early indicator: increase in γ-glutamyl transferase.
        (3) Later: increase in aspartate transaminase (AST; serum glutamic-oxaloacetic transaminase [SGOT]) and alanine transaminase (ALT; serum glutamate-pyruvate transaminase [SGPT]).
3. PN-induced osteopenia: long-term PN associated with osteopenia and bone demineralization (Itani and Tsang, 2005).
    a. Hypercalciuria; several factors implicated in hypercalciuria: cyclic PN infusion, sulfur-containing amino acids, hypertonic dextrose infusions causing hyperinsulinemia and decreased tubular calcium resorption, acidosis, and low phosphate in PN.

   b. Aluminum-containing PN solutions; metabolic bone disease characterized by reduced bone formation and aluminum accumulation in bone correlating with decreased bone formation.

   c. Decreased mineral retention; inappropriate mineral ratio; suboptimal minerals in PN during periods of rapid growth rate.

   d. Vitamin D deficiency rare in infants receiving PN containing pediatric IV vitamins; does not contribute to PN-related metabolic bone disease.

4. Sepsis; infection is a major complication of PN; incidence higher in VLBW infants; increases with longer PN duration.

   a. Two most common bacterial pathogens: *Staphylococcus epidermidis* and *Staphylococcus aureus*.

   b. Two most common fungal pathogens: *Candida albicans* and *Malassezia furfur*.

5. Measures to prevent or minimize complications associated with PN.

   a. Standardized procedures/policies to facilitate a consistent methodology to prevent and/or minimize complications.

   b. Record intake and assess IV insertion site hourly.

   c. Readjust fluid volume, dextrose concentration, protein and/or fat intake, electrolytes, and minerals as needed in response to blood chemistry results.

   d. Initiate enteral feedings as soon as possible.

   e. Pharmacy preparation of PN under laminar airflow hood; nothing should be added to PN solution once it leaves the pharmacy; filter central PN with an in-line filter.

   f. Wash hands scrupulously before handling any PN tubing or IV sites; use sterile techniques for dressing changes.

ENTERAL FEEDINGS: HUMAN MILK AND COMMERCIAL FORMULAS FOR TERM, SPECIAL-NEEDS, AND PREMATURE INFANTS

A. Comparison of human milk and commercial infant formulas (Blackburn, 2007; Schanler, 2006).

   1. Human milk: host resistance factors and antimicrobial properties (e.g., lactoferrin, lysozyme, and sIgA), hormones (e.g., cortisol, somatomedin-C, insulin-like growth factors, insulin, thyroid hormone), and growth factors (e.g., epidermal and nerve growth factors); increased bioavailability of fat, amino acid, and carbohydrate with enhanced absorption, digestion, gastric motility, and gastric emptying; very-long-chain fatty acids (may be important for cognition, growth, and vision); increased absorption of zinc and iron; low renal solute load; optimal distribution of calories (7% protein, 55% fat, 38% carbohydrate); provides variability in nutrient amounts between feeds and/or time of day, which may enhance sensory development, acceptance of new flavors and foods later. A comparison of term and premature human milk summarized in Table 10-5.

   a. Contraindications for human milk consumption: relatively few true contraindications exist (Schanler, 2006).

   (1) Galactosemia; cannot ingest lactose-containing milk (e.g., human milk and commercial cow milk–based formulas).

   (2) Human immunodeficiency virus (HIV): in the United States, counseled regarding risks to infant of breastfeeding, recommend not breastfeeding. Globally, health risks of the infant need to be balanced against the risk for acquiring HIV.

   (3) Human T-cell lymphotropic virus: no breastfeeding.

   (4) Miliary tuberculosis: no breastfeeding while contagious (needs documentation, generally approximately 2 weeks).

   (5) Herpetic lesions: if localized to breast, no breastfeeding; vaginal herpetic lesions not a barrier to breastfeeding.

   (6) Varicella lesions on breast: provide expressed human milk until completely crusted over; infant should receive varicella immune globulin.

   (7) Breast cancer; treatment should not be delayed; no breastfeeding with antimetabolite chemotherapy.

■ TABLE 10-5
■ ■ Composition of Premature and Mature Human Milk

Component	Premature Human Milk (1 week)	Mature Human Milk (1 month)
Volume (ml)	100	100
Energy (kcal)	67	70
Protein (g)	2.4	1.8
% Whey/casein	70/30	70/30
Fat (g)	3.8	4
% MCTs/LCTs	2/98	2/98
Carbohydrate (g)	6.1	7
% Lactose	100	100
Calcium (mg)	25	22
Phosphorus (mg)	14	14
Magnesium (mg)	3.1	2.5
Sodium (mg)	50	30
Potassium (mg)	70	60
Chloride (mg)	90	60
Zinc (mcg)	500	320
Copper (mcg)	80	60
Vitamin A (IU)	560	400
Vitamin D (IU)	4	4
Vitamin E (mg)	1	0.3
Vitamin C (mg)	5.4	5.6

LCTs, Long-chain triglycerides; *MCTs*, medium-chain triglycerides.
Adapted from Blackburn, S.T.: *Maternal, fetal, & neonatal physiology: A clinical perspective* (3rd ed.). St. Louis, 2007, Saunders, p. 456.

      (8) Maternal use of prescription and/or over-the-counter medications; direct contraindications for breastfeeding include cytotoxic drugs; some drugs have strong associations with adverse effects in infants; need extra caution with premature infants (Kleinman, 2004; Schanler, 2006).

      (9) Illicit drug abuse: recommend counseling; no breastfeeding until free of abused drug(s) (Kleinman, 2004; Schanler, 2006).

  2. Commercially prepared term infant formulas; summarized in Table 10-6.

    a. Commercial infant formulas for term infants are cow milk or soy based; available in powder, concentrate, and ready-to-feed forms; all should be iron fortified. Both types support adequate weight gain for term infants.

    b. Cow milk–based formulas recommended except for infants with galactosemia, primary lactase deficiency, immunoglobulin E (IgE)-mediated reaction to cow milk–based formulas, or parents seeking vegan-based diet for term infant.

    c. Soy-based formulas may be allergenic in infants with cow milk allergy (O'Connor et al., 2006; Turck, 2007).

    d. Soy-based formulas not recommended for premature infants (Blackburn, 2007; Kleinman, 2004; O'Connor et al., 2006; Schanler, 2006; Turck, 2007).

B. Term infants

  1. Human milk is the ideal food for term infants. Exclusive breastfeeding should be encouraged for the first 6 months of life when complementary foods are introduced; breastfeeding should be encouraged for at least the first year of infant's life and beyond for as long as mutually desired by mother and child (AAP, Section on Breastfeeding, 2005; O'Connor et al., 2006).

  2. Commercial term infant formulas used primarily when breastfeeding is contraindicated, as a supplement to breastfeeding during inadequate human milk supply or poor infant growth, or maternal preference not to breastfeed (O'Connor et al., 2006).

■ TABLE 10-6
■ ■ **Commercially Prepared Formulas for Term Infants (Standard: 20 cal/oz)**

Manufacturer/Product	Comments	Supplements
MILK-BASED FORMULAS	Infants with intact GI function	Iron, 2 mg/kg/day if not iron fortified
Mead Johnson Nutritionals		
Enfamil		
Enfamil Lipil	Contains essential fatty acids DHA, ARA	
Lactofree	No lactose; fat blend with LCT; low renal solute load	
Abbott Laboratories (Ross)		
Similac with Iron		
Similac Advance	Contains DHA and ARA	
Carnation		
Gerber		
SOY-BASED FORMULAS	Term infants with lactase deficiency	Multivitamins 0.5 ml/day Galactosemia, or vegetarian preference.
Mead Johnson		
Enfamil Prosobee		
Enfamil Prosobee Lipil		
Abbott Laboratories (Ross)		
Similac Isomil		
Similac Isomil Advance		
Carnation		
Nursoy		
PROTEIN HYDROLYSATE FORMULAS	Term infants with cow's milk allergy Lactose intolerance, malabsorptive condition	
Mead Johnson		
Pregestimil		
Nutramigen		
Abbott Laboratories (Ross)		
Alimentum		
Portagen		
SHS		
Neocate	Does not contain sucrose, lactose, and galactose.	

ARA, Arachidonic acid; *DHA*, docosahexaenoic acid; *LCT*, long-chain triglycerides.
Adapted from Blackburn, S.T.: *Maternal, fetal, & neonatal physiology: A clinical perspective* (3rd ed.). St. Louis, 2007, Saunders, pp. 457-458.

C. **Infants with special nutritional requirements.**
   1. Infants with inborn errors of metabolism (IEM); also referred to as inherited metabolic disorders; disorders resulting from genetically inherited disruption of enzymatic activities that occur in normal metabolic processes (Thomas et al., 2006).
      a. Nutrition plays an important role in the management of treatable IEM disorders; modification of diet can alter biochemical imbalances to improve mental and physical development.
      b. Goals for nutritional support: provide all essential nutrients and supply the optimal amount of any nutrient that is restricted as a result of IEM to promote growth and correct metabolic imbalances.

c. Management depends on the specific biochemistry and pathophysiology of the diagnosed IEM; includes restriction of any compound or precursor of metabolites that could accumulate as a result of the missing or defective enzyme(s) and/or supplement deficient end products and cofactors not produced as a result of the missing or defective enzyme(s).

d. Premature infants have the same risk for IEM as term infants; may not be suspected when symptoms resemble more common problems expected in premature infants; diagnostic tests may be altered by common treatments (e.g., early blood transfusions producing false-negative newborn screen testing for galactosemia).

e. Examples of IEM with dietary restrictions, supplements requiring specialty formula compositions:

  (1) Phenylketonuria; restriction of the amino acid phenylalanine; supplement with tyrosine.

  (2) Maple syrup urine disease; restriction of branched-chain amino acids; supplement with valine and isoleucine.

  (3) Galactosemia: restriction of galactose/lactose; supplement with calcium.

  (4) Glycogen storage disease, type I (glucose-6-phosphate deficiency): restriction of galactose/fructose; modified fat and moderate protein; frequent feedings, nocturnal continuous feedings; cornstarch in feedings.

  (5) Urea cycle disorders: low protein diet with nonessential amino acid restriction; supplement with carnitine, biotin, folate, and pyridoxine.

2. Infants with altered fluid and/or calorie intake requirements.

  a. Bronchopulmonary disease (BPD); may have increased metabolic demands, respiratory workload, oxygen consumption; energy needs may increase by 20% to 40% above that of healthy infants (Blackburn, 2007). Postnatal growth failure common, extends beyond early neonatal life for several years; multifactorial causes of feeding difficulties related to fluid restriction, long-term PN, oral feeding intolerance, and gastroesophageal reflux; recover more quickly if given adequate caloric intake, yet metabolism of this energy results in increased CO_2 production and oxygen consumption in infants with compromised respiratory function (Atkinson, 2006; Thureen and Hay, 2005).

    (1) Relative fluid restriction to reduce pulmonary edema, appears to complicate the pathology of BPD.

    (2) Infants with BPD may have higher caloric requirements to meet the demands of healing tissue and growth requirements.

    (3) May benefit from specially developed nutritional products to allow for fluid restriction and support optimal growth; currently use increased caloric density formula and/or fortified human milk mixtures with variable results.

  b. Cardiac problems; poor growth may result from increased metabolic demands, higher metabolic rate and oxygen consumption secondary to increased cardiac and respiratory workload; tissue hypoxia, protein loss, increased associated frequency of infections, and decreased nutrient absorption owing to diminished splenic blood flow; might be fluid and sodium restricted to reduce overcirculation; infant may be easily fatigued and become tachypneic and stressed with feeding (Barry and Thureen, 2006; Blackburn, 2007)

    (1) Caloric requirements to improve growth may be met with increased caloric density of formula and/or breast milk mixtures (Kuzma-O'Reilly, 2000; Pye and Green, 2003).

    (2) Often described as poor feeders, give fewer cues, and are less responsive to caregivers during feeds (Barry and Thureen, 2006; Pye and Green, 2003).

  c. Formula and/or breast milk may be fortified to meet higher caloric needs and not exceed possible fluid restriction or normal fluid intakes with increased caloric densities (Kuzma-O'Reilly, 2000; Pye and Green, 2003).

    (1) Osmolarity of formulas and breast milk mixtures increases approximately by the same percentage as the caloric increase (Kuzma-O'Reilly, 2000).

    (2) Strict attention must be paid to the renal solute load and osmolarity when concentrating formulas and adding calories to breast milk beyond 24 cal/oz.

3. Infants with short bowel syndrome: intestinal length (normal small bowel length not clearly established; estimated 250 to 270 cm at term) reduced because of surgical resection resulting from congenital anomaly (e.g., gastroschisis, midgut volvulus, intestinal atresias) or NEC; results in reduction of the intestinal absorptive surface area; remaining sections of bowel may have been ischemic, resulting in villous atrophy; full enteral feedings might be achieved if at least 25 cm of the small bowel with ileocecal valve or 40 cm without ileocecal valve remains after surgical resection (Blackburn, 2007; Sondheimer, 2006).

   a. Depending on the length of the intestine, may need PN for prolonged period until linear growth occurs.

   b. Slow initiation of enteral feedings, similar to minimal feeding regimen of premature infants, may be beneficial (Sondheimer, 2006).

D. **Premature infants**.

1. Human milk from mothers of premature infants contain slightly higher concentrations of protein, sodium, and chloride; more lipid, energy, vitamins, and trace elements; lower concentrations of phosphorus and calcium; and has lower osmolality than breast milk from mothers of term infants; differences decline as lactation progresses, becoming similar in composition between 2 and 4 weeks (Blackburn, 2007; Hattner, 2005; Schanler, 2006). A comparison of premature and mature human milk is summarized in Table 10-5.

   a. The significant benefits of human milk for premature infants warrant encouraging and actively supporting mothers to pump and provide milk for their infants (Heiman and Schanler, 2006; Jones and Spencer, 2007; Neville and McManaman, 2006; Schanler, 2006).

      (1) Importance of human milk for premature infants should be discussed during the first visit with parents; counseling as early as possible increases the incidence of lactation initiation and does not seem to increase maternal stress and/or anxiety.

      (2) Important to begin expressing human milk at the earliest possible moment following delivery.

      (3) Initial volume may be few drops of colostrum for the first 24 to 48 hours postpartum; may have considerable delay before substantial production begins; increases from about 50 ml/day to 500 to 600 ml/day in subsequent 36 hours (the "coming in" period of milk).

      (4) Encourage expressing milk at least 8 times in 24 hours; break in frequency while establishing milk supply may seriously compromise potential of maximum production.

      (5) Goal of 600 to 750 ml/day by day 10 to 14; milk production typically plateaus by 14 days postpartum.

      (6) Once milk production is established, it can be maintained with >6 pumps per day (at least 45 pumping times per week); needs to be monitored for ongoing success.

      (7) Optimal milk expression technique includes the following:

         (a) Supportive environment for mother.

         (b) Regular breast massage with good technique.

         (c) Simultaneous pumping of both breasts with high-quality breast pump and properly fitting milk expression shield.

   b. Collection, storage, and handling of human milk (Kleinman, 2004).

      (1) Wash hands with soap and warm water.

      (2) Collection kits should be rinsed, cleaned with hot soapy water, and air-dried.

      (3) Glass or hard plastic containers for storage.

      (4) Freeze milk that is not to be used within 48 hours; single milk expressions in each container, labeled with name, date, and time of pumping; keeps from 3 to 6 months in the rear of freezer compartment.

         (a) Freezing preserves many of the nutritional and immunologic benefits of human milk.

         (b) Thaw rapidly with tepid running (not hot) water; never in microwave oven; once thawed, do not refreeze; use completely within 24 hours.

2. Human milk fortifiers provide additional protein, fat, carbohydrate, sodium, potassium, phosphorus, and calcium; 4 packets added to 100 ml human milk averages 24 cal/oz, 2.7 g protein, 4.5 g fat, and 7.5 g carbohydrate (Hattner, 2005).

■ TABLE 10-7
■ ■ **Commercially Prepared Human Milk Fortifiers and Formulas for Premature Infants (Standard: 24 cal/oz)**

Product/Manufacturer	Comments	Supplements
HUMAN MILK FORTIFIERS Mead Johnson Nutritionals	Whey predominates protein Iron fortified; may still need supplemental	Iron 2 mg/kg/day if not fortified
Abbott Laboratories MILK-BASED FORMULAS Mead Johnson Nutritionals	Whey predominates protein	Iron 2 mg/kg/day if not fortified
Enfamil Premature	20 and 24 cal/oz preparations	
Abbott Laboratories (Ross) Similac Special Care	20, 24, and 30 cal/oz preparations	
TRANSITIONAL FORMULAS	Used primarily as discharge formulas; 22 cal/oz	Iron 2 mg/kg/day if not fortified
Mead Johnson Nutritionals Enfacare		
Abbott Laboratories (Ross) NeoSure		

Adapted from Blackburn, S.T.: *Maternal, fetal, & neonatal physiology: A clinical perspective* (3rd ed.). St. Louis, 2007, Saunders, pp. 457-458.

3. Commercial premature infant formulas, 24 cal/oz, have increased amounts of protein, carbohydrate, fat, sodium, potassium, calcium, and phosphorus; supply these nutrients within acceptable ratios similar to breast milk with added human milk fortifier (Blackburn, 2007).
4. Transitional premature infant formulas provide 22 cal/oz and more calcium, phosphorus, and magnesium than term infant formulas but less than premature infant formulas and are designed for use after hospital discharge; studies vary as to how long to continue using the transitional formulas (Schanler, 2006).
5. Premature infant formulas can be mixed with human milk as a means of nutrient fortification; an alternative, preferable approach would be to feed human milk with fortifiers and use premature infant formula when human milk is not available (Atkinson, 2006; Schanler, 2006).
6. Available fortifiers, formulas for premature infants summarized in Table 10-7.

ENTERAL FEEDING METHODS

Enteral feedings are achieved via several routes, including nasogastric, orogastric, transpyloric, and gastrostomy tubes, and orally by bottle or breast. Decisions regarding enteral feeding are dependent on gestational age, birth weight, and clinical condition of the infant. When to initiate feeding, type of feeding, method of delivery, feeding frequency, concentration of feeding, and rate of advancement may vary according to unit practices (Kleinman, 2004).

A. **Minimal enteral feedings or trophic feeding (Blackburn, 2007; Kleinman, 2004; Neu and Bernstein, 2006; Neu and Zhang, 2005).**
  1. Have benefit without adverse consequences for most VLBW infants.
  2. Defined as ≤25 ml/kg/day of human milk or premature infant formula.
  3. Not intended for primary source of nutrition.
  4. Given concurrently with PN as primary nutrition.
  5. Intended to provide physiologic effects, including to stimulate and maintain digestive-absorptive, immunologic, and neuroendocrine functions of the GI tract.
    a. Promotion of gut mucosal development.
    b. Stimulation of intestinal motor activity.

    c. Increased secretion of GI hormones and peptides.

    d. Colonization of the gut with normal flora, limiting colonization by other pathogenic organisms, helps development of the innate immune system of the GI tract.

6. Does not increase the incidence of NEC.

7. Dilute formula or breast milk or sterile water does not stimulate GI motor activity as well as full-strength formula or breast milk.

8. Recommended length of minimal enteral nutrition: 1 to 5 days; longer period for more immature infants (Neu and Zhang, 2005).

B. **Potential contraindications for initiation of feedings, advancing feeds, and feeding tolerance/intolerance for VLBW infants (Neu and Zhang, 2005; Premji, 2004).**

1. Perceived contraindications for initiating and/or continuing feeds: hypoxic-ischemic insults at birth (low Apgar scores), apnea and/or bradycardia, sepsis, umbilical arterial catheters, indomethacin administration, inotropic agents (dopamine), heme-positive stools (Neu and Zhang, 2005).

    a. Presence of apnea and/or bradycardia: one reason given to not feed infant is that apnea causes transient ischemia to the intestine, may lead to NEC; epidemiologic investigations did not find this to be an increased risk.

    b. Presence of umbilical arterial catheters (UAC): implicated as a risk factor for NEC because of the observation that many UACs have thrombi that may dislodge and embolize to the intestine; also, frequent blood draws and flushes may compromise the hemodynamics of the intestine; theoretically, these possibilities exist but true cause-and-effect relationships or strong associations between the UAC and NEC have not been demonstrated.

    c. Minimal enteral nutrition does not appear to increase the incidence of NEC in the presence of apnea and/or bradycardia, UACs, indomethacin; caution must be used in advancing feedings while in the presence of these situations.

2. Evidence that advancing enteral feedings faster than 20 ml/kg/day is associated with increased incidence of NEC (Neu and Zhang, 2005).

3. Assessing for feeding tolerance/intolerance: feeding intolerance has no uniform definition, in premature infants refers to not digesting formula or breast milk rather than intolerance to the carbohydrate source of formulas (e.g., lactose intolerance). Manifestations of intolerance vary, based on prefeed gastric residual volume, color, and associated clinical manifestations such as abdominal distension, emesis, presence of blood in stool, apnea, and bradycardia (King, 2005; Neu and Bernstein, 2006; Neu and Zhang, 2005).

    a. Gastric aspirates; prefeed gastric residuals (King, 2005).

        (1) Fasting basal gastric residuals average 3 ml every 4 hours found in infants of 28 to 36 weeks of gestational age; >2 ml in <760-g infants and 3 ml in >750-g infants; volume of >30% of the milk given during previous feedings may be abnormal and requires more extensive evaluation; >10 to 15 ml is considered excessive (Gomella, 2004).

        (2) Bile-stained aspirate may not be sufficient reason to withhold feeds; may be due to immature gut motility, leading to periodic antiperistalsis.

        (3) Determination of significance of gastric aspirate may need to rely on what volume is reasonably expected at the infant's gestational age or what is "normal" for an individual infant, and the presence of clinical manifestations.

    b. Clinical manifestations: abdominal distension, emesis, blood in stool, apnea, and bradycardia (King, 2005; Neu and Bernstein, 2006).

        (1) Abdominal distention; visual examination for visible bowel loops, erythema, auscultate for bowel tones, palpate to assess whether soft, firm, and for tenderness; ascertain when last stool occurred (Gomella, 2004).

        (2) Emesis; may be result of LES or increased abdominal pressure resulting from NEC, obstruction, undigested milk feeding.

        (3) Blood in stools; trauma from nasogastric tube; swallowed maternal blood (if soon after delivery), bleeding disorder (such as vitamin K deficiency, disseminated intravascular coagulation, congenital coagulopathy); stress ulcer; severe fetal asphyxia; NEC; medications (such as indomethacin, corticosteroids) (Gomella, 2004).

(4) Apnea and bradycardia; generalized response to change in condition, sepsis, NEC (Gomella, 2004).

C. Nasogastric and orogastric tube feeding (Blackburn, 2007; Kleinman, 2004).

1. Most commonly used method in the NICU environment; used for very premature or critically ill infants to reduce risk of aspiration and conserve energy; determined by infant's lack of ability to coordinate a suck-swallow-breathe feeding pattern.

2. Procedure for gastric (nasal or oral) intubation (Gomella, 2004).

   a. Gather equipment: infant feeding tube, stethoscope, sterile water (lubricant), syringe (5 to 10 ml), adhesive tape, or transparent dressing, gloves, suctioning equipment.

   b. Monitor heart rate and respiratory function throughout the procedure.

   c. Place infant supine; head of bed may be elevated.

   d. Choose size of gastric tube: general guideline—for infants <1000 g, No. 5 French gastric tube; ≥1000 g, No. 8 French gastric tube.

   e. Determine the length of tubing required to reach the stomach: measure the distance from the nose to the earlobe to the xiphoid process, mark the tube at the appropriate length.

   f. Moisten the tip of the tube with sterile water and insert via nare or mouth.

      (1) Nasal insertion: flex neck, push nose up, insert the tube straight back into the nare, advance as tolerated to desired length.

      (2) Oral insertion: push the tongue down and insert the tube into the oropharynx, advance as tolerated to desired length.

   g. Verify correct positioning in the stomach.

      (1) Inject small amounts of air into the tube with a syringe, listen with a stethoscope for rush of air into the stomach. May be unreliable because rush of air can be auscultated as if entering the stomach when the tip of the tube is actually positioned in the distal esophagus; recommended to use concurrently with other methods of determination.

      (2) Aspirate contents from the tube with a syringe; may check acidity by pH tape and/or assess color and consistency of aspirate to determine stomach contents.

      (3) Definitive verification of tube placement with chest/abdominal radiographic imaging.

   h. Complications.

      (1) Apnea and bradycardia; vagal response; usually resolve without specific treatment beyond stimulation.

      (2) Hypoxia; resolves with correction of apnea and bradycardia response; may require oxygen to resolve; if severe, may need positive-pressure ventilation with bag and mask. If this continues, suspect misplacement of tube into the trachea and remove the tube immediately.

      (3) Perforation of the esophagus, posterior pharynx, stomach, or duodenum (rare); the tube should never be forced during the insertion procedure.

      (4) Aspiration: complication of misplacement into the trachea, esophagus, or hypopharynx; results from stomach distention or failure of feeding to continue through the GI tract. Verify position of tube and the presence of residuals prior to every bolus feeding or periodically with continuous feeding infusion.

3. Feeding may be accomplished by bolus or continuous infusion of human milk or formula (Blackburn, 2007; Kleinman, 2004).

   a. Bolus feeds every 2 to 3 hours similar to feeding pattern when bottle- or breast-feeding; associated with improved nutrient absorption and growth.

   b. Continuous infusions associated with increased feeding intolerance, reduced nutrient absorption, and decreased growth in premature infants; may be perceived to be necessary with early feeding initiation; should transition to bolus feeds as tolerated. Human milk fat and medium-chain triglyceride additives adhere to feeding tube surfaces, and nutrient loss from human milk fortifiers further reduces nutrient intake and energy density provided by continuous enteral tube feeding.

D. Transpyloric and gastrostomy tube feeding (Blackburn, 2007; King, 2005; Kleinman, 2004; Premji, 2004).

1. Transpyloric tube feeding bypasses the stomach and reduces the digestive capability of the GI tract.
    a. Feeds can only be by continuous infusion; placement confirmed with radiographic imaging.
    b. Associated with significant risks: abdominal distension, gastric bleeding, bilious vomiting, and mortality.
    c. Does not improve energy intake or growth.
    d. Should be used only in rare instances of prolonged gastroparesis or dysmotility.
    e. Gastric feedings should be resumed as soon as possible.
2. Gastrostomy tube feeding via a surgically placed tube through the abdominal wall directly into the stomach; can be bolus or continuous infusion; used primarily for infants unable to sustain full oral feeds or maintain sufficient caloric intake to promote growth, such as abnormal neurologic status, congenital anomalies of the GI tract (e.g., esophageal atresia), or other conditions requiring long-term gavage feedings.

E. **Oral feeding, breast or bottle:** determined by the infant's ability to coordinate a suck-swallow-breathe pattern, sustain an alert-awake behavior, and maintain cardiorespiratory stability; premature infants limited by weaker flexor control and immature musculature (Blackburn, 2007; Kirk et al., 2007; Kleinman, 2004; McGrath and Braescu, 2004).
1. Oral feeding readiness.
    a. Infant should be free of signs and/or symptoms of respiratory distress (e.g., respiratory rate <60 breaths per minute; blood gas values within normal limits); criteria may be modified for infants with BPD or CHD.
    b. Infant demonstrates suck-swallow-breathe coordination with an intact gag reflex.
        (1) Swallow reflex well developed by 28 to 30 weeks, easily exhausted; matures by 34 weeks.
        (2) Gag reflex matures by 34 weeks.
        (3) Suck maturation related to gestational not postnatal age; nonnutritive suck present in <32 to 33 weeks of gestation; nutritive suck appears by 32 to 33 weeks; matures by 37 weeks of gestation.
        (4) Suck-swallow reflexes are present by 28 weeks; synchrony of suck-swallow appears by 32 to 34 weeks; complete coordination develops by 36 to 37 weeks of gestation.
2. Oral feeding initiation: major goal of nurses and families: assist VLBW infants to develop safe and effective early oral feeding skills, improve breastfeeding outcomes (Thoyre, 2007).
    a. Healthy infants ≥34 weeks of gestation may have oral feedings initiated as soon after birth as indicated. Factors to be considered include infant behavior and maternal preference for breastfeeding or bottle-feeding (Blackburn, 2007).
    b. Transition from gastric tube feeding to oral feeding (breast or bottle) may be dependent on infant behavior, unit-specific feeding policy, and/or gestational age or weight criteria (Jones, 2005).
        (1) Use of infant state assessment and feeding cues shown to facilitate improved progression to full oral feedings (Kirk et al., 2007).
        (2) Careful monitoring must take place during feedings to ensure safe intake without complications of aspiration, desaturation (or increased requirement for fractional inspired oxygen), apnea, and bradycardia; reported to occur less frequently during breastfeeding than bottle-feeding (Jones, 2005; Kirk et al., 2007).
    c. Increasing number of VLBW infants are referred for treatment of significant, persistent feeding problems after discharge; during hospitalization, provide positive feeding experiences and identify feeding problems at an early stage when most amenable to change (Thoyre, 2007).

NURSING INTERVENTIONS TO FACILITATE TOLERANCE OF ENTERAL FEEDINGS

A. **Sensory-motor-oral stimulation and nonnutritive sucking provided during gavage feedings** (Boiron et al., 2007; Rocha et al., 2006).

1. May promote earlier oral feeding and decrease length of stay.
2. May enhance sucking patterns and coordination.
3. May support maturation of neural structures, which, in turn, may result from influences of learned experiences.
B. **Assessment of infant readiness.**
  1. May be defined in terms of readiness for the initiation of oral feedings in general and in terms of a specific feeding time in particular (McGrath and Braescu, 2004).
  2. May enhance oral feeding initiation and success (Kirk et al., 2007; Simpson et al., 2002).
  3. May promote infant engagement during bottle-feeding (Thoyre and Brown, 2004).
  4. May promote successful breastfeeding of premature infants (Nye, 2008).
    a. Premature infants have been able to breastfeed successfully as early as 32 weeks of gestation and may establish mature suck-swallow-breathe coordination earlier with breastfeeding than with bottle-feeding (Jones, 2005; Nye, 2008).
    b. Higher birth weight, less need of ventilator and oxygen, higher hemoglobin, no bottle-feeding, minimal apnea of prematurity, and no signs and symptoms of infection is associated with successful breastfeeding (Jones, 2005).
    c. Test-weighing of infants (before and after breastfeeding) with an electronic scale is a relatively reliable method of determining infant intake of human milk from the breast for in-hospital assessment (Jones, 2005).
C. **Position of infant during and after feedings.**
  1. Kangaroo care (skin-to-skin positioning of infant on mother's chest) during gavage feeding is associated with improved breast milk production and may improve breastfeeding rates (Nye, 2008).
  2. Supine posture, right lateral position, and infant car seat positioning may worsen GER (Jadcherla, 2006).
  3. Prone or left lateral positions with 30-degree elevation are associated with fewer GER-like episodes, improved gastric emptying (Corvaglia et al., 2007; Jadcherla, 2006).
  4. Recent research with small sample size supports a strategy that a right lateral position for the first hour post-feeding followed by a left lateral position change is associated with a reduction of GER and promotion of gastric emptying (van Wijk et al., 2007).

NUTRITIONAL ASSESSMENT AND STANDARDS FOR ADEQUATE GROWTH

Nutritional management is meant to improve growth and minimize harm; require nutritional assessment tools to provide for growth in an efficacious and safe manner (Ridout and Georgieff, 2006).

A. **Nutritional intake: ascertain whether the prescribed nutritional intake is provided (Ridout and Georgieff, 2006).**
  1. Monitor volume and caloric intakes daily: Follow current recommended intakes for gestational age and condition of infant; adjust intake accordingly to maintain nutritional goals.
  2. Periodically review all dietary intakes from birth; early nutrition has a profound impact on long-term growth and development.
B. **Laboratory assessment: serves a key role in the assessment of nutritional adequacy and toxicity (Ridout and Georgieff, 2006).**
  1. Electrolytes, sodium (Na^+), potassium (K^+), chloride (Cl^-), bicarbonate ($NaCO_3^-$)
    a. Provide information on renal function and fluid status.
    b. Results need to be assessed in relation to an infant's fluid status (intake and output), condition and previous trends in electrolyte results.
  2. Blood urea nitrogen (BUN) and creatinine (Cr) (Cooke, 2006; Heird, 2005; Ridout and Georgieff, 2006; Ridout et al., 2004).
    a. BUN may not be a good indicator of protein intake and/or tolerance in the first weeks of life for VLBW infants; should not be considered as a biochemical marker during this period; reflects more the fluid status.

    b. BUN level has improved validity for protein intake with serial levels in stable, older VLBW infants who are receiving enteral nutrition, if taken into consideration with GFR and renal function indicators (creatinine level) and anthropometric growth parameters; may have increased sensitivity and specificity for protein tolerance during this period.

    c. Creatinine and creatinine clearance are valid biochemical markers for renal function assessment for VLBW infants (Auron and Mhanna, 2006).

3. Calcium (Ca^+), magnesium (Mg^+), phosphorus (PO_4^-), and alkaline phosphatase (alk phos) (Demarini, 2005; Ridout and Georgieff, 2006).

    a. Followed for management and surveillance of metabolic bone disease, assess bone mineralization status. Decreased calcium and phosphorus levels or increased alkaline phosphatase levels may indicate bone demineralization; alkaline phosphatase levels greater than 500 to 700 mg/dl or radiologic evidence of rickets indicates need for increased calcium and phosphorus intake. Hypophosphatemia (serum concentration <4 mg/dl) considered an early warning sign of decreased bone mineralization.

    b. Calcium levels may remain within the normal range, preserved at the expense of bone calcium stores; serum alkaline phosphatase concentration is a more direct method to assess increased bone turnover.

    c. Medications that have a negative effect on calcium and phosphorus stores: furosemide, caffeine citrate, and glucocorticosteroids.

C. Anthropometric measurements (Ridout and Georgieff, 2006).

1. Daily approximate weight gains with recommended caloric intake (Blackburn, 2007; Kashyap, 2007).

    a. 24 to 32 weeks: 15 to 20 g/kg/day.

    b. 33 to 36 weeks: 14 to 15 g/kg/day.

    c. 37 to 40 weeks: 7 to 9 g/kg/day.

    d. 40 weeks to 3 months: 30 g/day.

2. Weekly length and head circumference measurements. Although it is common to discuss growth expectations of VLBW infants in terms of weight gain, gains in head circumference and lengths are just as necessary to determine optimal growth. Head circumference has a close relationship with the growth of brain volume (Brandt et al., 2003; Katrine, 2000; Poindexter et al., 2006). Length in comparison with weight gives good indication of body composition, if accurately measured (Gibson et al., 2006).

    a. Length measurement.

        (1) Typically crown to heel of naked infant.

        (2) For accurate measurement, two people perform the procedure with length board specific for premature infants (e.g., Premie Length Board [O'Leary, Ellard Instrumentation, Seattle, WA]); one person holding the head in place against board top and another providing gentle straightening of body and lower extremities with one hand while pushing the moveable footrest into place with the other hand; average of 2 to 3 measurements (Ehrenkranz et al., 2006; Moyer-Mileur, 2007).

        (3) Average gain in length from 24 to 40 weeks of gestation: 0.69 to 0.75 cm/week (Katrine, 2000).

    b. Head circumference, also known as occipital-frontal circumference.

        (1) Determined by applying paper or plasticized paper measurement tape firmly around the head above the supraorbital ridges, over the most prominent part of the frontal bulge anteriorly, and the part of the occiput that gives the maximum circumference; average of 2 to 3 measurements (Ehrenkranz et al., 2006).

        (2) Average gain in head circumference from 24 to 40 weeks of gestation: 0.1 to 0.6 cm/week (Katrine, 2000).

3. Plot weight, head circumference, and length on growth chart weekly.

D. Growth Charts.

1. Term infant growth charts include incremental growth curves and percentiles of weight, length, and head circumference; developed by the National Center for Health Statistics and the National Center for Chronic Disease Prevention and Health Promotion (2000); Web site: http://www.cdc.gov/growthcharts (Kleinman, 2004).

2. Premature infant growth charts include incremental growth curves and percentiles of weight, length, and head circumference.
   a. Adequate growth to genetic potential for premature infants implies lean mass accumulation, brain volume development, and somatic growth to maintain body composition comparable to that of a fetus of similar gestation (Kleinman, 2004).
   b. Typical growth curve charts with weight, length, and head circumference, used in the NICU to establish growth patterns and in current research, based on fetal and newborn growth and less frequently on the growth of former VLBW infants (Sherry et al., 2003).
   c. Example of a recommended growth chart: Fetal-Infant Growth Graph; includes meta-analysis results of data from globally published studies during 1982 to 2002; ethnically diverse sample of fetuses and newborns from 22 to 40 weeks of gestation and term infants to 50 weeks postmenstrual age; weekly increments for weight, head circumference, and length (Fenton, 2003).
3. Postnatal growth curves for premature infants based on actual growth of premature infants; controversy over appropriateness of using growth curves based on the actual postnatal growth of VLBW infants of the 1990s as references for assessment of current VLBW infants.
   a. Postnatal growth curves reflect a slower growth velocity than is seen with growth curves based on intrauterine and newborn growth curves (Sherry et al., 2003).
   b. Postnatal growth curves are a reflection of longitudinal growth for VLBW infants of the 1990s; recent studies of premature infants with similar postnatal growth restriction followed through to school age reflect neurologic and physical deficits that had been reported for VLBW infants of the 1980s (Fanaroff et al., 2007; Lemons et al., 2001; Peterson et al., 2006).
   c. Postnatal growth restriction is associated with poorer outcomes (Foulder-Hughes and Cooke, 2003; Latal-Hajnal et al., 2003).

REFERENCES

American Academy of Pediatrics, Section on Breast-feeding: Breastfeeding and the use of human milk. *Pediatrics*, 115(2):496-504, 2005.

Atkinson, S.: Nutrition for premature infants with bronchopulmonary dysplasia. In P.J. Thureen and W.W. Hay (Eds.): *Neonatal nutrition and metabolism* (2nd ed.). New York, 2006, Cambridge University Press, pp. 522-532.

Auron, A. and Mhanna, M.J.: Serum creatinine in very low birth weight infants during their first days of life. *Journal of Perinatology*, 26(12):755-760, 2006.

Barry, J.S. and Thureen, P.J.: Nutrition in infants with congenital heart disease. In P.J. Thureen and W.W. Hay (Eds.): *Neonatal nutrition and metabolism* (2nd ed.). Philadelphia, 2006, Cambridge University Press, pp. 533-543.

Berseth, C.L.: Developmental anatomy and physiology of the gastrointestinal tract. In H.W. Taeusch, R.A. Ballard, and C.A. Gleason (Eds.): *Avery's diseases of the newborn* (8th ed.). Philadelphia, 2004, Saunders, pp. 1071-1085.

Berseth, C.L.: Development and physiology of the gastrointestinal tract. In P.J. Thureen and W.W. Hay (Eds.): *Neonatal nutrition and metabolism*. New York, 2006, Cambridge University Press, pp. 67-75.

Blackburn, S.T.: *Maternal, fetal, and neonatal physiology: A clinical perspective* (3rd ed.). St. Louis, 2007, Saunders.

Boiron, M., Da Nobrega, L., Roux, S., Henrot, A., and Saliba, E.: Effects of oral stimulation and oral support on non-nutritive sucking and feeding performance in preterm infants. *Developmental Medicine & Child Neurology*, 49:439-444, 2007.

Brandt, I., Sticker, E., and Lentze, M.: Catch-up growth of head circumference of very low birth weight, small for gestational age preterm infants and mental development to adulthood. *Journal of Pediatrics*, 142:463-468, 2003.

Cooke, R.J.: Adjustable fortification of human milk fed to preterm infants. *Journal of Perinatology*, 26(10):591-592, 2006.

Corvaglia, L., Rotatori, R., Ferlini, M., Aceti, A., Ancora, G., and Faldella, G.: The effect of body positioning on gastroesophageal reflux in premature infants: Evaluation by combined impedance and pH monitoring. *Journal of Pediatrics*, 151:591-596, 2007.

Demarini, S.: Calcium and phosphorus nutrition in preterm infants. *Acta Paediatrica*, 94:87-92, 2005.

Ehrenkranz, R.A., Dusick, A.M., Vohr, B., Wright, L.L., Wrage, L.A., Poole, K., and the NICHD Research Network: Growth in the neonatal intensive care unit influences neurodevelopmental and growth outcomes of extremely low birth weight infants. *Pediatrics*, 117:1253-1261, 2006.

Fanaroff, A.A., Stoll, B.J., Wright, L.L., et al.: Trends in neonatal morbidity and mortality for very low birth-weight infants. *American Journal of Obstetrics and Gynecology*, 196(2):147.e141-147.e148, 2007.

Fenton, T.: A new growth chart for preterm babies: Babson and Benda's chart updated with recent data and a new format. *BMC Pediatrics*, 3(1):13-22, 2003.

Foulder-Hughes, L.A. and Cooke, R.W.I.: Motor, cognitive, and behavioral disorders in children born very preterm. *Developmental Medicine and Child Neurology,* 45(2):97-103, 2003.

Georgieff, M.K.: Iron. In P.J. Thureen and W.W. Hay (Eds.): *Neonatal nutrition and metabolism* (2nd ed.). New York, 2006, Cambridge University Press, pp. 291-298.

Gibson, A., Carney, S., and Wales, J.K.H.: Growth and the premature baby. *Hormone Research,* 65(Suppl. 3):75-81, 2006.

Gomella, T.L.: Neonatology: *Management, procedures, on-call problems, diseases, and drugs* (5th ed.). New York, 2004, Lange Medical Books/McGraw-Hill.

Greer, F.R.: Vitamins. In P.J. Thureen and W.W. Hay (Eds.): *Neonatal nutrition and metabolism* (2nd ed.). New York, 2006, Cambridge University Press, pp. 161-184.

Hambidge, K.M.: Trace minerals. In P.J. Thureen and W.W. Hay (Eds.): *Neonatal nutrition and metabolism* (2nd ed.). New York, 2006, Cambridge University Press, pp. 273-290.

Hambidge, K.M. and Krebs, N.F.: Zinc in the fetus and neonate. In R.A. Polin, W.W. Fox, and S.H. Abman (Eds.): *Fetal and neonatal physiology* (3rd ed., Vol. 1). Philadelphia, 2004, Saunders, pp. 342-347.

Hattner, J.T.: Part 2: Human milk and pediatric formula update 2006. *Nutrition Focus for Children with Special Health Care Needs,* 20(6):1-12, 2005.

Haumont, D., Deckelbaum, R.J., Richelle, M., et al.: Plasma lipid and plasma lipoprotein concentrations in low birth weight infants given parenteral nutrition with twenty or ten percent lipid emulsion. *Journal of Pediatrics,* 115(5 Pt 1):787-793, 1989.

Hay, W.: Nutritional requirements of the very preterm infant. *Acta Paediatrica,* 94:37-46, 2005.

Hay, W.W.: Early postnatal nutritional requirements of the very preterm infant based on a presentation at the NICHD-AAP Section on research in neonatology. *Journal of Perinatology,* 26(S2):S13-S18, 2006.

Hay, W.W. and Regnault, T.R.H.: Fetal requirements and placental transfer of nitrogenous compounds. In R.A. Polin, W.W. Fox, and S.H. Abman (Eds.): *Fetal and neonatal physiology* (3rd ed., Vol. 1). Philadelphia, 2004, Saunders, pp. 509-527.

Heiman, H. and Schanler, R.: Benefits of maternal and donor human milk for premature infants. *Early Human Development,* 82:781-787, 2006.

Heird, W.C.: Biochemical homeostasis and body growth are reliable end points in clinical nutrition trials. *Proceedings of the Nutrition Society,* 64:297-303, 2005.

Heird, W.C.: Intravenous feeding. In P.J. Thureen and W.W. Hay (Eds.): *Neonatal nutrition and metabolism* (2nd ed.). Philadelphia, 2006, Cambridge University Press, pp. 312-331.

Heird, W.C. and Kashyap, S.: Protein and amino acid metabolism and requirements. In R.A. Polin, W.W. Fox, and S.H. Abman (Eds.): *Fetal and neonatal physiology* (3rd ed., Vol. 1). Philadelphia, 2004, Saunders, pp. 527-539.

Husain, S.M., Mughal, M.Z., and Tsang, R.C.: Calcium, phosphorus, and magnesium transport across the placenta. In R.A. Polin, W.W. Fox, and S.H. Abman

(Eds.): *Fetal and neonatal physiology* (3rd ed., Vol. 1). Philadelphia, 2004, Saunders, pp. 314-322.

Itani, O. and Tsang, R.C.: Normal bone and mineral physiology and metabolism. In P.J. Thureen and W.W. Hay (Eds.): *Neonatal nutrition and metabolism* (2nd ed.). New York, 2006, Cambridge University Press, pp. 185-228.

Jadcherla, S.R.: Gastrointestinal reflux. In P.J. Thureen and W.W. Hay (Eds.): *Neonatal nutrition and metabolism* (2nd ed.). Philadelphia, 2006, Cambridge University Press, pp. 445-453.

Johnson, L.H.: Vitamin E nutrition in the fetus and newborn. In R.A. Polin, W.W. Fox, and S.H. Abman (Eds.): *Fetal and neonatal physiology* (3rd ed., Vol. 1). Philadelphia, 2004, Saunders, pp. 353-369.

Jones, E.: Transition from tube to breast. In E. Jones and C. King (Eds.): *Feeding and nutrition in the preterm infant.* Edinburgh, 2005, Churchill Livingstone, pp. 151-163.

Jones, E. and King, C.: *Feeding and nutrition in the preterm infant.* Edinburgh, 2005, Saunders.

Jones, E. and Spencer, S.A.: Optimizing the provision of human milk for preterm infants. *Archives of Diseases in Childhood, Neonatal Edition,* 92:F236-F238, 2007.

Kashyap, S.: Enteral intake for very low birth weight infants: What should the composition be? *Seminars in Perinatology,* 31:74-82, 2007.

Katrine, K.: Anthropometric assessment. In S. Groh-Wargo, M. Thompson, and J.H. Cox (Eds.): *Nutritional care for high-risk newborns* (3rd. ed.). Chicago, 2000, Precept Press.

King, C.: Enteral feeding. In E. Jones and C. King (Eds.): *Feeding and nutrition in the premature infant.* Edinburgh, 2005, Churchill Livingstone, pp. 103-116.

Kirk, A.T., Alder, S.C., and King, J.D.: Cue-based oral feeding clinical pathway results in earlier attainment of full oral feeding in premature infants. *Journal of Perinatology,* 27:572-578, 2007.

Kleinman, R.E.: *Pediatric nutrition handbook* (5th ed.). Elk Grove Village, IL, 2004, American Academy of Pediatrics.

Kuzma-O'Reilly, B.: Preparing formulas with various caloric densities. In S. Groh-Wargo, M. Thompson, J.H. Cox, and J.V. Hartline (Eds.): *Nutritional care of high-risk newborns* (3rd ed.). Chicago, 2000, Precept Press, pp. 651-656.

Latal-Hajnal, B., von Siebenthal, K., Kovari, H., Bucher, H.U., and Largo, R.H.: Postnatal growth in VLBW infants: Significant association with neurodevelopmental outcome. *Journal of Pediatrics,* 143(2):163-170, 2003.

Lemons, J.A., Bauer, C.R., Oh, W., et al., for the NNRN: Very Low Birth Weight Outcomes of the National Institute of Child Health and Human Development Neonatal Research Network, January 1995 through December 1996. *Pediatrics,* 107(1):e1, 2001.

Limperopoulos, C., Soul, J.S., Gauvreau, K., et al.: Late gestation cerebellar growth is rapid and impeded by premature birth. *Pediatrics,* 115:688-695, 2005.

McGrath, J.M. and Braescu, A.V.B.: State of the science: Feeding readiness in the preterm infant. *Journal of Perinatal and Neonatal Nursing,* 18(4):353-364, 2004.

Moore, K.L. and Persaud, T.V.N.: *The developing human: Clinically oriented embryology* (8th ed.). Philadelphia, 2008, Saunders.

Moyer-Mileur, L.J.: Anthropometric and laboratory assessment of very low birth weight infants: the most helpful measurements and why. *Seminars in Perinatology, 31*:96-103, 2007.

Namgung, R. and Tsang, R.C.: Neonatal calcium, phosphorus, and magnesium homeostasis. In R.A. Polin, W.W. Fox, and S.H. Abman (Eds.): *Fetal and neonatal physiology* (3rd ed., Vol. 1). Philadelphia, 2004, Saunders, pp. 323-341.

Neu, J. and Bernstein, H.: Minimal enteral nutrition. In P.J. Thureen and W.W. Hay (Eds.): *Neonatal nutrition and metabolism* (2nd ed.). Philadelphia, 2006, Cambridge University Press, pp. 369-376.

Neu, J. and Zhang, L.: Feeding intolerance in very low birthweight infants: What is it and what can we do about it? *Acta Paediatrica, 94*(Suppl. 449):93-99, 2005.

Neville, M.C. and McManaman, J.L.: Milk secretion and composition. In P.J. Thureen and W.W. Hay (Eds.): *Neonatal nutrition and metabolism* (2nd ed.). Philadelphia, 2006, Cambridge University Press, pp. 377-389.

Nye, C.: Transitioning premature infants from gavage to breast. *Neonatal Network, 27*(1):7-13, 2008.

O'Connor, D., Brennan, J., and Merko, S.: Formulas for preterm and term infants. In P.J. Thureen and W.W. Hay (Eds.): *Neonatal nutrition and metabolism* (2nd ed.). New York, 2006, Cambridge University Press, pp. 409-436.

Omari, T.I. and Rudolph, C.D.: Gastrointestinal motility. In R.A. Polin, W.W. Fox, and S.H. Abman (Eds.): *Fetal and neonatal physiology* (3rd ed., Vol. 2). Philadelphia, 2004, Saunders, pp. 1125-1135.

Peterson, J., Taylor, H.G., Minich, N., Klein, N., and Hack, M.: Subnormal head circumference in very low birth weight children: Neonatal correlates and school-age consequences. *Early Human Development, 82*(5):325-334, 2006.

Poindexter, B.B. and Denne, S.C.: Parenteral nutrition. In H.W. Taeusch, R.A. Ballard, and C.A. Gleason (Eds.): *Avery's diseases of the newborn* (8th ed.). Philadelphia, 2004, Saunders, pp. 1061-1070.

Poindexter, B., Langer, J., Dusick, A., and Ehrenkranz, R.: Early provision of parenteral amino acids in extremely low birth weight infants: Relation to growth and neurodevelopmental outcome. *Journal of Pediatrics, 148*:300-305, 2006.

Premji, S.S.: Enteral feeding for high-risk neonates: A digest for nurses into putative risk and benefits to ensure safe and comfortable care. *Journal of Perinatal and Neonatal Nursing, 19*(1):59-71, 2004.

Putet, G.: Lipids as an energy source for the premature and full-term neonate. In R.A. Polin, W.W. Fox, and S.H. Abman (Eds.): *Fetal and neonatal physiology* (3rd ed., Vol. 1). Philadelphia, 2004, Saunders, pp. 415-428.

Pye, S. and Green, A.: Parent education after newborn congenital heart surgery. *Advances in Neonatal Care, 3*(3):147-156, 2003.

Ridout, R.E. and Georgieff, M.K.: Nutritional assessment of the neonate. In P.J. Thureen and W.W. Hay (Eds.): *Neonatal nutrition and metabolism* (2nd ed.). Philadelphia, 2006, Cambridge University Press, pp. 586-601.

Ridout, E., Melara, D., Rottinghaus, S., and Thureen, P.: Blood urea nitrogen concentration as a marker of amino-acid intolerance in neonates with birthweight less than 1250 g. *Journal of Perinatology, 25*(2):130-133, 2004.

Rocha, A.D., Moreira, M.E.L., Pimenta, H.P., Ramos, J.R.M., and Lucena, S.L.: A randomized study of the efficacy of sensory-motor-oral stimulation and non-nutritive sucking in very low birthweight infant. *Early Human Development, 83*:385-388, 2006.

Schanler, R.: Human milk supplementation for preterm infants. *Acta Paediatrica, 94*:64-67, 2005.

Schanler, R.: Fortified human milk for premature infants. In P.J. Thureen and W.W. Hay (Eds.): *Neonatal nutrition and metabolism* (2nd ed.). New York, 2006, Cambridge University Press, pp. 401-408.

Shenai, J.P.: Vitamin A metabolism in the fetus and neonate. In R.A. Polin, W.W. Fox, and S.H. Abman (Eds.): *Fetal and neonatal physiology* (3rd ed., Vol. 1). Philadelphia, 2004, Saunders, pp. 347-353.

Sherry, B., Mei, Z., Grummer-Strawn, L., and Dietz, W.H.: Evaluation of and recommendations for growth references for very low birth weight (<1500 gram) infants in the United States. *Pediatrics, 111*(4): 750-758, 2003.

Simpson, C., Schanler, R.J., and Lau, C.: Early introduction of oral feeding in preterm infants. *Pediatrics, 110*(3):517-522, 2002.

Sondheimer, J.: Neonatal short bowel syndrome. In P.J. Thureen and W.W. Hay (Eds.): *Neonatal nutrition and metabolism* (2nd ed.). New York, 2006, Cambridge University Press, pp. 492-507.

Thomas, J.A., Tsai, A., and Bernstein, L.: Nutrition therapies for inborn errors of metabolism. In P.J. Thureen and W.W. Hay (Eds.): *Neonatal nutrition and metabolism* (2nd ed.). New York, 2006, Cambridge University Press, pp. 544-568.

Thoyre, S.M.: Feeding outcomes of extremely premature infants after neonatal care. *Journal of Perinatal and Neonatal Nursing, 36*(4):366-376, 2007.

Thoyre, S.M. and Brown, R.L.: Factors contributing to preterm infant engagement during bottle-feeding. *Nursing Research, 53*(5):304-313, 2004.

Thureen, P.J. and Hay, W.W.: Conditions requiring special nutritional management. In R.C. Tsang, R. Uauy, B. Koletzko, and S. Zlotkin (Eds.): *Nutrition of the preterm infant: Scientific basis and practical guidelines* (2nd ed.). Cincinnati, OH, 2005, Digital Educational Publishing, pp. 383-412.

Turck, D.: Soy protein for infant feeding: what do we know? *Current Opinions in Nutritional Metabolic Care, 10*:360-365, 2007.

Un, S. and Carlson, S.E.: Long chain fatty acids in the developing retina and brain. In R.A. Polin, W.W. Fox, and S.H. Abman (Eds.): *Fetal and neonatal physiology* (3rd ed., Vol. 1). Philadelphia, 2004, Saunders, pp. 429-440.

van Wijk, M.P., Benninga, M.A., Dent, J., et al.: Effect of body position changes on postprandial gastroesophageal reflux and gastric emptying in the healthy premature neonate. *Journal of Pediatrics, 151*:585-590, 2007.

11 Developmental Support

CAROL TURNAGE CARRIER

OBJECTIVES

1. Apply four standards of developmental care to guide practice in the neonatal intensive care unit (NICU).
2. Assess physiologic and behavioral organization of preterm and ill newborn infants using the neurobehavioral subsystems from Als' Synactive Framework.
3. Design a developmental care plan that respects and supports each infant's unique needs as related to the environment, direct caregiving, parent support, and consistency of care.
4. Practice pain management within a developmental framework that includes environmental modification, positioning, other evidence-based nonpharmacologic comfort measures, parent support, and sucrose.

Developmental support in the NICU integrates the developmental needs of infants within the context of medical care. The developmental continuum that nature designed is disrupted through parent-infant separation, prematurity, illness, anomalies, and the complex, atypical environment of the NICU. Randomized controlled trials have shown positive benefits of developmental care and clinical, neurobehavioral, cost, and parent outcomes (Als et al., 1986, 1994; Buehler et al., 1995; Fleisher et al., 1995; Westrup et al., 2000). Parent satisfaction with nursing care based on the developmentally supportive model is significantly more positive compared with traditional care (Wielenga et al., 2006). Although developmental care continues to have champions and skeptics, an evidence base is accumulating to guide practice. Developmental care is a philosophy of supporting newborns and their families that is integrated into neonatal intensive care routines, family-staff relationships, policies, and the overall NICU culture. It is a model of delivering individualized care to newborns within a family context.

BARRIERS TO INFANT DEVELOPMENT IN THE NICU SETTING

A. **The NICU environment lacks the developmentally nurturing physical and social components that normally occur for the maturing fetus and term newborn (Als, 1998; Anand, 2000; Glass, 1999; Goldberger and Wolfer, 1991).** Challenges in the NICU to developing preterm and newborn infants include some or all of the following (list not exclusive):
   1. Numerous caregivers—possibly as many as 30 to 40 nurses when primary teams of nurses are not provided.
   2. Mechanical challenges such as medically necessary equipment, i.e., endotracheal tubes, intravenous lines, arterial lines, drains, and monitor leads.
   3. Unpredictable schedules based on caregiver convenience for touch, care, and procedures.
   4. No sleep-wake cycle or familiar routine.
   5. Pain and discomfort.
   6. Separation from parents, minimal touch policies.
   7. Continuous sensory stimulation.
   8. Restraint, confinement.
   9. Alternative feeding practices without pleasure or enjoyment.
   10. Medications that cause sedation or irritability and agitation.
B. **Evaluating the challenges in each NICU allows for proactive changes in policy and practice that support a developmental philosophy for care delivery.**

For such a philosophical and cultural change to occur, the largest group essential for successful implementation of developmental care is the neonatal nurse at the bedside. Nurses' perceived barriers to implementation of developmental care is reported to include the following factors in decreasing order of importance (Hendricks-Munoz and Prendergast, 2007).

1. Staff nurses and physicians
2. Funding
3. Physician champion or leader
4. Facility limitations
5. Lack of parent involvement
6. Both physician and nursing leadership

Multidisciplinary team developmental care meetings positively impact implementation of developmental care. Perceived barriers are significantly decreased and staff nurses are less likely to perceive nursing leadership as an obstacle when team meetings are utilized.

DEVELOPMENTAL CARE STANDARDS

A. **Four standards of developmental care (Als and Gilkerson, 1997; Robison, 2003):** These standards provide guidance for a successful developmental program and assistance for program implementation and evaluating individual practice.
   1. **Standard 1:** Individualized care is based on observation and continuous feedback of each infant's cues with ongoing responsiveness to an infant's abilities, sensitivities, and thresholds of autonomic, motor, and state subsystem functioning.
   2. **Standard 2:** A developmentally supportive environment is provided for every infant and family based on continuous assessment and interaction.
   3. **Standard 3:** Parents are viewed as the most important relationship, with continual support of this bond starting with the birth of the infant(s).
   4. **Standard 4:** Collaborative and consistent caregiving is considered necessary for clinical and developmental support of infants and families.

Standard 1. Individualized care is based on observation and continuous feedback of each infant's cues with ongoing responsiveness to an infant's abilities, sensitivities, and thresholds of autonomic, motor, and state subsystem functioning.

A. **In order to provide individualized care, the caregiver must accurately assess infant behavior.** The framework for understanding premature infant behavior is based on the work by Heidelise Als (1995, 1998; Als and Gilkerson, 1997). Five subsystems within three channels of communication include observable behaviors in the autonomic, motor, and state systems. These five subsystems as defined in detail in Table 11-1 are used as a systematic assessment. Basic premises of the model are that:
   1. Infants continually strive to function in the smoothest manner at their current level of functioning. The infant's job is to maintain stability of all subsystem functioning but depending on their gestational age and individual abilities, their level of subsystem functioning may be poorly equipped for life outside the womb.
   2. Competence is seen in a hierarchic integration of subsystem competence:
      a. Stabilization of physiologic functioning. For example, premature infants 25 to 28 weeks old are most likely to demonstrate loss of stability or stress signals through physiologic destabilization.
      b. Restabilization of physiologic, motor, or state functioning as new skills or levels of functioning emerge. For example, Jacob, at 29 weeks, is able to maintain oxygen saturation and heart rate within normal limits during chest auscultation.
      c. Gradual development of a full range of behavioral (sleep-wake) states. For example, Sara's mother is delighted that her daughter, now 33 weeks of postmenstrual age, can focus briefly on her face with an interested gaze.
      d. Attaining alert states that are clear and robust; sustained alerting with the ability to interact with people and the environment without compromise of either physiologic or motor stability. For example, Tyrell follows the red ball smoothly for 60 degrees horizontally and 30 degrees vertically while maintaining physiologic stability and without squirming or extending his arms.

■ TABLE 11-1
■ ■ ■ **Synactive Theory of Development: Neurobehavioral Subsystems**

Subsystem	Signs of Stress	Signs of Stability
AUTONOMIC	**PHYSIOLOGIC INSTABILITY**	**PHYSIOLOGIC STABILITY**
Respiratory	Tachypnea, pauses, gasping, sighing	Smooth, stable respirations, regular rate and pattern
Color	Mottled, flushed, dusky, pale or gray	Pink, stable color
Visceral	Hiccups, gagging, choking, spitting up, grunting, and straining as if having a bowel movement. Coughing, sneezing, yawning	Absence of hiccups, gagging, spitting up, etc.
Autonomic	Tremors, startles, twitches	Absence of tremors, startles, twitches, etc.
MOTOR	**Fluctuating tone, lack of control over movement, activity, and posture**	**Consistent tone, controlled or improved movement, activity, and posture**
Flaccidity	Low tone in trunk, limp/floppy upper and lower extremities, limp drooping jaw (gape face)	Tone consistent and appropriate for postconceptional age
		Well-maintained posture
Hypertonicity	Arm and/or leg extensions, arm(s) outstretched with fingers splayed in salute gesture, fingers stiffly outstretched, trunk arching, neck hyperextended	Smooth, controlled movements
Hyperflexion	Trunk, extremities, fisting	Successful motor strategies for self-regulation (see Self-Regulation)
Activity	Squirming, frantic diffuse activity, or little or no activity or responsiveness	
STATE	**Disorganized quality to state behaviors including range of available states, maintenance of state control, and transition from one state to another**	**Easy to read state behaviors that are maintained; calm, focused alertness; well-modulated sleep**
Sleep	Whimpering sounds, facial twitching, irregular respirations, fussing, grimacing, appears restless	Clear, well-defined sleep states, periods of quiet, restful sleep
Awake	Glazed, unfocused look, staring, worried or pained expression. Hyperalert or panicked appearance, eye roving, crying, cry-face, actively averting gaze or closing eyes, irritability, prolonged awake periods, inconsolability, frenzy	Alert with bright, shiny eyes, focused attention on object or person, animated expression (e.g., cheek softening, frowning, "ooh face," cooing, smiling)
	Abrupt and/or rapid state changes	Robust crying
		Good calming, consolability
		Smooth changes between states
		Full range of sleep-wake states
Attention and interaction	**Efforts to attend and interact with environmental stimulation elicits signs of stress and disorganized subsystem functioning**	**Responsive to auditory, visual, and social stimuli**
Autonomic	Physiologic instability of varying degrees with autonomic, respiratory, color, and visceral responses	Responsiveness to stimuli is well maintained and prolonged
Motor	Fluctuating tone, increased motor activity, progressively frantic diffuse activity if stimulation continues	Actively seeks auditory stimulus, minimal motor activity
State	Roving eyes, gaze averting, glazed-unfocused look or worried, panicked expression, weak cry, cry-face, irritability	Bright, shiny-eyed alert and attentive expression
	Closed eyes and sleep-like withdrawal	
	Abrupt state changes	Sustained awake and alert state
	Signs of stress when presented with more than one type of stimulus at a time	Shifts attention smoothly to more than one type of stimulation

■ TABLE 11-1
■ ■ **Synactive Theory of Development: Neurobehavioral Subsystems—cont'd**

Subsystem	Signs of Stress	Signs of Stability

Self-Regulation: Infant's efforts to achieve, maintain, or regain a balanced, stable, and relaxed state of subsystem functioning and integration. Success of these efforts will vary among infants depending on maturity, available self-regulatory skills, and overall subsystem organization.

Examples of self-regulatory strategies include:

Motor	foot bracing against a boundary or blanket nest; hand holding; grasping hands together; hand to mouth or face; grasping blanket, tubing, etc.; tucking trunk; sucking; position changes
State	lowers state from high arousal to quiet alert or sleep state; releases energy by rhythmic, robust crying; focused attention; and orientation

Facilitation by caregivers through environmental modifications or developmental care techniques can aid the infant's own self-regulatory abilities when environmental challenges exceed the infant's capabilities.

Modified from Als, H.: Toward a synactive theory of development: promise for the assessment and support of infant individuality. *Infant Mental Health Journal, 3*:229-243, 1982; Als, H.: A synactive model of neonatal behavior organization: Framework for the assessment of neurobehavioral development in the premature infant and for support of infants and parents in the neonatal intensive care environment. *Physical and Occupational Therapy in Pediatrics, 6*:3-55, 1986; Hunter, J.G.: The neonatal intensive care unit. In J. Case-Smith, A.S. Allen, and P.N. Pratt (Eds.): *Occupational therapy for children*. St. Louis, 2001, Mosby, p. 593; Carrier C.T., Walden, M., and Wilson, D.: The high-risk newborn and family. In M.J. Hockenberry (Ed.): *Wong's nursing care of infants and children* (7th ed.). St. Louis, 2003, Mosby.

B. **Assessment is the key element for formulating moment-to-moment, as well as more global, changes (formal care plan) in care to meet the needs of individual infants.** Data on autonomic, motor, and state functioning are collected before, during, and after care or procedures and to gain perspective on the infant's abilities, sensitivities, thresholds, and unique communication repertoire. A nurse can learn so much about an infant's sensitivities and capabilities by watching a patient between care as the infant rests or interacts with the environment around the bedside. Watching how an infant responds to touch, handling, care, or procedures provides excellent information about physiologic/autonomic, motor, and state functioning when faced with challenges or when left alone. The gathered data helps the whole team come up with a developmental plan that is aligned with the clinical plan of care in supporting a stable, well-functioning, comfortable, and nurtured infant.

1. Neurobehavioral subsystems (see Table 11-1) provide information regarding the infant's vulnerabilities, thresholds, strengths, and abilities and are placed within a context whether it is during care, procedures, nurturing by parents, or when the infant is alone.

2. Newborn state system provides the context for any interaction between infant and environment; used by the infant to control the amount and kind of input received from the environment. The state system is an indicator of central nervous system maturation and organization. Before 28 weeks, the fetus or premature infant is in an indeterminate state without the electroencephalogram (EEG) characteristics of typical sleep states or the motor or eye movements related to rapid eye movement (REM) or non-REM (NREM) sleep. Even though an immature rest/activity cycle may be present, cellular events are occurring that are necessary for building the foundation for early neurodevelopment. After 28 weeks, NREM and REM emerge and gradually become more mature with physiologic, EEG, and behavioral characteristics that are almost mature by 5 to 8 months of age. Neuronal activity during REM sleep occurs in the neocortex, hippocampus, pons, thalamus, and midbrain reticular formation. REM and NREM sleep play a vital role in neurosensory development, learning, and memory formation. Another protective function during sleep is the protection of brain plasticity (Graven, 2006).

   All infants are developing organized sleep during the first year of life. Full-term newborn infants sleep from 16 to 18 hours, whereas preterm infants spend about 75% of their time in light sleep (Als, 1995, 1998; Als and Gilkerson, 1997; Holditch-Davis et al., 2003; Thoman et al., 1987).

C. **Individualized developmental care relies on both the moment-to-moment caregiver adaptations while in interaction with an infant and the formal plans based on infant assessment that provide overall guidance for care of that particular infant.** Both are flexible, in that changes may need to be made based on infant responses at any given moment.

1. Direct care adjustments and modified techniques are based on each infant's response to touch, handling, and routine care and procedures. This component may include therapeutic handling techniques, repositioning methods, nurturing, facilitation during exams and procedures (routine or painful), care clusters, timing of care, and recovery time or time-out techniques. This component is dependent on the caregiver being completely in tune and in interaction with the infant rather than performing care on the infant.

2. Developmental plans reflect all four developmental standards (environment and direct care, parent/family, collaborative practice, and consistency) and:
   a. Allow infant's family and primary nurse to make specific recommendations regarding environmental modifications, positioning techniques, calming measures, and the promotion of self-quieting abilities.
   b. Should incorporate input from appropriate members of the multidisciplinary team: parents, medicine, nursing, occupational therapy, physical therapy, respiratory therapy, and child life and social services.
   c. Communicate the plan developed between the family and health care providers that outlines environmental, direct care, parent, and consistency required by an individual infant for optimal behavioral organization and neurodevelopmental growth. The formal plan is communicated in writing and through direct report during medical and nursing rounds, shift report, and in family conferences.

3. Questions to consider when assessing an infant's level of behavioral stability or organization and planning developmental support include:
   a. How does the infant respond to the daily caregiving routine? How can the family be as involved in daily caregiving as they are comfortable?
   b. What therapeutic handling and positioning techniques best support this infant?
   c. What, if anything, in the environment has a negative impact on the infant?
   d. How much stimulation can the infant tolerate before losing the ability to stay organized?
   e. What facilitation or environmental support is necessary to help the infant maintain stability?
   f. Can the timing and organization of medical and nursing procedures be altered to help decrease the infant's level of stress and increase his or her organization?
   g. What is missing from the infant's environment and experiences that typically support stability and the natural developmental progression in utero or at home (e.g., dim light, touch, parent smell, breast milk odor, and taste)?

D. **Intervention strategies that can be used to help individual infants cope with NICU stress and support neurobehavioral organization must be carefully considered with the understanding that in developmental care "an intervention does not necessarily fit all."** Although intervention research is accumulating, the evidence base should be examined in light of its quality and strength before applying any practice in the NICU that has potential significant short- and long-term effects. There are available criterion lists for evaluating research (Melynk and Fineout-Overholt, 2005; Philbin and Klaas, 2000a). A team trained in developing evidence-based summaries of developmental literature, evaluating and rating the results, then making recommendations for practice can provide guidelines for care. The Cochrane Neonatal Database, Joanna Briggs Institute, and others are useful resources. In general, the nurse should think in terms of the most biologically relevant interventions based on the infant's stage of development (e.g., 26 weeks vs. 32 weeks) and experiences expected at that developmental and maturational level.

E. **Routine care.**

1. Providing a momentary time-out from incoming stimuli when an infant is stressed and disorganized allows him or her time to draw on self-regulatory abilities.

2. Observe for avoidance behaviors (e.g., gaze aversion, regurgitation, crying, increased extension patterns) in response to movement transitions or particular positions. Such patterns of behavior suggest repetitive responses that may evolve into heightened reactivity and agitation especially in infants with prolonged NICU stays or chronic conditions. These infants may need a referral for occupational therapy or an infant developmental specialist evaluation and intervention.

3. Simple modifications to routine care practices may be used to minimize stress for preterm infants such as swaddled bathing (Fern et al., 2002) or swaddled weighing (Neu and Browne, 1997).

4. "Clustered care" has been recommended to allow longer rest periods by clustering several routine or nursing care events together rather than spacing them out over time. Careful monitoring by staff during care clusters must take place to avoid overwhelming an immature or ill infant with too long or intense an episode of care (Peters, 1999).

5. Respect infant's sleep states as an important part of maturation and make every attempt not to disrupt sleep and provide care during naturally occurring awake periods.

6. Even when infants are lying alert in their beds, it is important to let them know care or touch is about to begin by soft speech, calling their name, smell, and finally touch so as not to startle them and elicit a disorganized response.

7. If an infant is demonstrating stress through the motor system, help him or her to reorganize by gently supporting extremities in flexion close to body with warmed hands until infant is calm, thereby decreasing unnecessary energy expenditure and encouraging self-regulation.

8. Containment by blanket swaddling or nesting is reported to decrease physiologic and behavioral stress cues during routine care such as eye examinations, weighing, or heel lance (Corff et al., 1995; Fearon et al., 1997; Graven, 2000; Peters, 1992; Slevin et al., 1999).

F. **Touch and handling.** With physiologically unstable high-risk infants, care must be taken to avoid further medical compromise and to help the infant conserve energy. The amount, type, and timing of touch require staff to consider each infant's current age, medical status, and sensitivity to stimulation and choose the most appropriate approach based on available evidence (Browne, 2000; Harrison et al., 1991, 1996; Harrison and Woods, 1991).

1. Stroking infants who are not physiologically stable has been shown to elicit gasping, grunting, averted gaze, and decreased transcutaneous oxygen levels (Browne, 2000; Harrison et al., 1991, 1996; Harrison and Woods, 1991).

2. Therapeutic touch may include a variety of tactile sensations:
   a. Gentle human touch (GHT) or hand containment. GHT is the gentle placement of warmed hands on the head and lower back or buttocks applying supportive containment for about 15 minutes. A few studies have shown GHT may be soothing and without risk, but no long-term evidence is available. It is recommended that close monitoring accompany any touch or handling of an NICU infant (Harrison et al., 1991, 1996, 2000; Modrcin-Talbott et al., 2003).
   b. Conventional holding involves holding clothed infants in the traditional semi-upright position while supporting extremities and head close to the caregiver's body; often used when infants are stable enough to transfer from bed to parent's arms.
   c. Kangaroo care (KC) or skin-to-skin holding (Charpak et al., 2001; Feldman and Eidelman, 2003; Feldman et al., 2002a; McGrath and Brock, 2002). NICU parents perform skin-to-skin contact with their diaper-clad infant who is resting prone and semi-upright against the mother or father's bare chest and covered by a blanket. Warmth, rise and fall of the chest (vestibular), tactile sensation of skin to skin, smell of parents (olfactory) and maternal breast, and the parent's tender, quiet, vocalizations, breathing sounds, and heartbeat (auditory) comprise the sensory modalities stimulated during KC. This intervention provides low-intensity stimulation to the earlier developing senses and is most appropriate for the NICU infant.
      (1) Controversial use with extremely premature infants during acute illness phase.
      (2) Maintaining physiologic and behavioral stability during transfer from bed to parent and back remains a challenge (Neu et al., 2000).
      (3) Positive benefits of KC include decreased incidence and severity of infections, longer duration of breastfeeding, increased weight gain, shorter length of stay,

increased maternal milk volume, less variable heart rate and oxygenation levels, decreased apnea and bradycardia, less crying, and increased frequency or duration of quiet sleep (Acolet et al., 1989; Anderson, 1991; Bauer et al., 1996, 1997; Chwo et al., 2002; Conde-Agudelo et al., 2000; Feldman and Eidelman, 2003; Fohe et al., 2000; Ludington-Hoe et al., 1999; McGrath and Brock, 2002; Messmer et al., 1997; Roberts et al., 2000; Tornhage et al., 1999).

    (4) Positive benefits of KC on preterm infant development include the following (Feldman and Eidelman, 2003; Feldman et al., 2002a, 2002b):

        (a) Better arousal modulation at 3 months when presented with increasingly complex stimulation.

        (b) Higher scores at 6 months on Bayley Scales of Infant Development mental and psychomotor index than controls without KC.

        (c) Improved state organization with longer quiet sleep, quiet alerting, and decreased amounts of active or light sleep.

        (d) Improved habituation and orientation skills.

  d. Massage. Positive benefits of massage such as weight gain, more active alert periods, more mature orientation, habituation, motor, and range of state behaviors on the Brazelton's Newborn Behavior Assessment Scale (BNBAS) have been reported in older, stable preterm infants greater than 31 weeks of gestation (Browne, 2000; Field et al., 1986; Vickers et al., 2000). Massage has also been shown to improve weight gain, decrease stress behaviors, reduce postnatal complications, and improve motor performance in infants prenatally exposed to cocaine (Wheeden et al., 1993).

    (1) Smaller, fragile preterm infants are at risk for physiologic compromise during massage.

    (2) Consider teaching parents rather than using a therapist to provide massage to older, stable preterm or term infants.

    (3) Determine infant eligibility for massage on an individual basis in consultation with care team.

    (4) Parent teaching should be performed by certified infant massage therapists working in the NICU such as occupational therapists or neonatal child life specialists.

  e. Other considerations for touch and handling in the NICU (Browne, 2000).

    (1) Synchronize touch with sleep-wake behavior.

    (2) Consider the risks and benefits of any touch or handling.

    (3) Balance aversive touch with therapeutic touch opportunities.

    (4) Consistent caregivers to provide nurturing touch.

    (5) Continually monitor autonomic and behavioral responses and modify or stop interaction as appropriate.

    (6) Consider parents the most appropriate providers of therapeutic touch.

    (7) Teach parents to evaluate their infant's responses to touch and handling and how to intervene as necessary.

    (8) Continually update evidence on touch, massage, and KC.

3. The literature is insufficient to support specific recommendation for vestibular stimulation alone (Symington and Pinelli, 2002). In theory it is reasonable to believe that vestibular input is important to the developing preterm infant. Skin-to-skin care has a vestibular component of the rise and fall of mother's chest during breathing. Gentle vestibular stimulation may be tolerated by stable infants with gentle swaying or rocking.

4. Repositioning has been associated with significant physiologic stress responses (Evans, 1991); therefore, sudden postural changes should be avoided. The impact of this procedure can be reduced by slowly repositioning while containing infant in a gentle, tucked midline position.

G. Positioning and containment. Provision of developmentally supportive positioning and containment interventions promote a calm state, physiologic stability, and prevent position-related deformities in the high-risk infant.

  1. Sequential patterns of neuromotor maturation (not timing, which is individual) are identified by examining the following (Sweeney and Gutierrez, 2002):

    a. Muscle development.

      (1) Muscle fiber development incomplete until term.

(2) Lower ratio of type 1 muscle fibers (high-oxidative type) to type 2 fibers (low-oxidative) predisposes preterm infants to muscle fatigue (includes respiratory muscles).

b. Muscle tone and reflex development proceeds caudocephalad (lower to upper extremities) and centripetal (distal to proximal).

c. Skeleton and joint articulation.

(1) Restricted movement and positioning in the NICU produce joint compression and poor refinement of mechanical receptors; these factors predispose fragile infants to skeletal deformation, shortening of muscles, and contractures.

(2) Poor ossification and density of bone establish susceptibility to rib fractures.

H. **Common "acquired positioning malformations"** occur in preterm infants related to maturational hypotonia unless appropriate positioning interventions take place (Sweeney and Gutierrez, 2002). Common positioning deformities include hip adduction and external rotation (frog leg), shoulder retraction and scapular adduction (W position of arms), neck extension, arching postures, and abnormal head molding.

I. **Prevention of positioning deformities** requires specialized knowledge, careful thought and planning, skilled use of positioning aids and supports, and adequate monitoring of infants following any change in position.

1. General considerations for positioning in the NICU:

a. Provide support for breathing and ventilation.

b. Promote skin integrity.

c. Provide proprioceptive input to facilitate containment and security as needed.

d. Facilitate developing flexion in both posture and movement.

e. Provide opportunities for midline skill development (hand to face or mouth).

f. Encourage alignment and symmetry.

g. Support rest/calming/comfort and neurobehavioral organization.

h. Counteract emerging stereotypical or abnormal postures.

i. Offer a variety of well-supported and tolerated positions with a plan to implement supine position prior to discharge necessary for SIDS prevention in the home sleep environment.

j. Assist in the progression toward balanced flexor/extensor tone and movement.

2. Monitor the infant's physiologic and behavioral response to positioning because benefits to motor and state control may be counterbalanced by destabilization of physiologic parameters (heart rate, breathing pattern, blood pressure, etc.).

3. Intentional movement by infants enhances neuromotor development and stability. Regulatory efforts such as pushing against boundaries are examples of such movement. Containment or nests should not restrict movement that is necessary for growth and development of the neuromotor system. Restraint should be avoided unless absolutely necessary and then should be used only for a short period of time.

4. General guidelines for positioning (Box 11-1).

5. Occupational and physical therapists (OT and PT) serve as excellent resources for staff and parents. They offer treatment for muscle toning, increasing touch and handling tolerance, improving oral-motor function, movement and motor patterns, equilibrium, relaxation, sensory integration, and in some units teach massage to parents.

J. **Comfort/Nonpharmacologic Pain Relief.** NICU infants are repeatedly exposed to painful procedures that may have serious neurologic and behavioral costs. Developmentally supportive interventions that provide comfort and reduce pain responses in NICU infants are shown to be effective. These nonpharmacologic techniques (Box 11-2) can be used alone or in combination for discomfort or procedural pain and as an adjunct with pharmacologic treatment for moderate to severe pain (Axelin et al., 2006; Boyle et al., 2006; Castral et al., 2008; Cignacco et al., 2007; Golianu et al., 2007; Goubet et al., 2003, 2007; Leslie and Marlow, 2006; Parry, 2008; Shah et al., 2006; Stevens et al., 2005).

K. **Positioning for home.** The American Academy of Pediatrics (AAP) recommends the supine position as the preferred sleep position during infancy (AAP, 2000, 2005b). Since 1992 and this change in sleeping pattern by many parents, the incidence of sudden infant death syndrome (SIDS) has been reduced by 40% (AAP, 2000). Prone positioning is recommended when infants

■ BOX 11-1
■ **POSITIONING GUIDELINES**

1. Bedding and positioning aids must be individually determined to meet the needs of the infant. Soft bedding, such as sheepskin, secure nesting, and boundaries or swaddling, is used for those infants requiring such devices to maintain comfortable positioning and to prevent skin problems. Waterbeds (Fowler et al., 1997) or gel or water pillows (Marsden, 1980) are recommended to avoid abnormal head molding.
2. Calm, organized behavior may be improved by use of the following strategies:
   a. Prone position to facilitate improved oxygenation and ventilation.
   b. Side-lying position, well supported with swaddling, commercial containment devices or a heavy blanket roll surrounding the infant's flexed back, to promote midline hands-together or hands-to-face movements.
   c. Swaddling to provide the most secure containment and to be used in combination with other positioning devices as needed.
3. Repositioning is usually indicated every 2 to 3 hours or when care must be provided. An infant may demonstrate behavioral cues that suggest discomfort and the need for positional change.
4. Oversized diapers may result in hips maintained in the externally rotated and abducted "frog leg" posture. Appropriately sized commercial diapers are available and should be used to preserve normal hip alignment.
5. Tension from lines or tubing such as endotracheal tubes, naso- or orogastric tubes, cardiac leads, or intravenous lines may result in deforming pressures or postures and should be avoided.
6. Repositioning is often stressful for sick or preterm infants. Caregivers can reduce the stress of this necessary procedure with slow, gentle rolling of the infant while containing the extremities and providing a pacifier for a brief time after moving the infant.
7. Once repositioned, the infant's breathing pattern, color, oxygen saturation, heart rate, respiratory rate and pattern, behavioral cues, and stability of position should be monitored and noted whether positioning principles have been followed.
8. Finally, a very important consideration is that caregivers continually observe each infant's emerging capabilities to determine appropriate positioning and bedding options. Infants who begin to fight containment or boundaries or those who have matured beyond the need for positioning devices and can maintain a flexed posture unassisted should be allowed to do so. Transitioning infants out of boundaries and positioning aids is required before discharge. Slow transition will ease the process and prepare infants for being without aids once they are home.
9. Daily physical activity has been shown to enhance bone growth and development in low birth weight preterm infants (Moyer-Mileur et al., 2000). It is important to avoid restrictive swaddling or nesting that inhibits infants from all movement or pushing against their boundaries. Such practice could prove detrimental to motor development.
10. Supine positioning at least 2 weeks before discharge should be initiated so that infants can adjust to the home sleeping position.

Modified from Hunter, J.: The neonatal intensive care unit. In J. Case-Smith (Ed.): *Occupational therapy for children* (4th ed.). St. Louis, 2001, Mosby; Carrier, C.T., Walden, M., and Wilson, D.: The high-risk newborn and family. In M.J. Hockenberry (Ed.): *Wong's nursing care of infants and children* (7th ed.). St. Louis, 2003, Mosby; Fowler, K., Kum-Nji, P., Wells, P.J., and Mangrem, C.L.: Water beds may be useful in preventing scaphocephaly in preterm very low birthweight neonates. *Journal of Perinatology, 17*(5):397, 1997; Marsden, D.J.: Reduction of head flattening in preterm infants. *Developmental Medicine and Child Neurology, 22*(4):308-314, 1980; Moyer-Mileur, L.J., Brunstetter, V., McNaught, T.P., et al: Daily physical activity program increases bone mineralization and growth in preterm very low birthweight infants. *Pediatrics, 106*(5):1088-1092, 2000.

are awake and being observed to promote acquisition of developmental milestones and prevent positional plagiocephaly. Parent teaching prior to discharge should include the AAP's recommendations and other recommended modifications identified by the AAP task force on infant sleep position and SIDS that include avoiding the following (AAP, 2000, 2005b):
1. Use of soft/loose bedding or objects such as pillows, quilts, comforters, sheepskins, stuffed toys.
2. Use of waterbeds, sofas, or soft mattresses as a bed.

■ BOX 11-2
■ **NONPHARMACOLOGIC PAIN MANAGEMENT**

Environmental Modification
Comfortable, low-stress environment
Flexed, containment with midline opportunities for hands to face/mouth
Positioning support as needed

Nonnutritive Sucking
Lower pain scores, deceased crying
Immediate effects; pain response resumes when pacifier is removed
In combination with sucrose may achieve more analgesic effects

Nutritive Sucking
Sucrose
Efficacy for single dosing demonstrated in more than 30 randomized controlled trials
Absolute effectiveness and safety for repeated dosing over time lacks sufficient evidence
Decreased pain scores, crying, facial grimacing
AAP recommends for use with eye exams

Breast Milk
Effects similar to both glucose and sucrose administration
Reduced pain scores, duration of crying
Effectiveness over time not established

Facilitated Tuck
Containment or nesting reduces pain response with retinopathy of prematurity exams
Decreased pain scores during suctioning
Decreases heart rate and variability, cry duration
More rapid return to baseline heart rate
Decreased sleep disruption time after heel lance
Effectively administered by parents

Swaddling
Decreased heart rate and crying time
Decreased pain scores
Facilitates return to sleep state after heel lance
Effects last longer in term infant

Kangaroo or Skin-to-Skin Holding
Decreased pain scores, heart rate, crying, and grimacing
Parent participation
Efficacy in preterm infants <32 weeks not well established

Olfactory Experience
Vanilla odor previously experienced shows pain-relieving effects
Effective during venipuncture; no analgesic/distraction response during heel-lance
Efficacy not yet established

Care Coordination/Technical Considerations
■ Reducing number and frequency of unnecessary procedures
■ Coordinating blood-sampling clusters
■ Reduce failed procedural attempts; improve staff technical skills
■ Enhance use of noninvasive bedside monitoring (e.g., oxygenation)
■ Avoid sleep disruption or painful events after care clusters
■ Consider venipuncture over heel-lance as less painful

3. Bed sharing or co-sleeping even with siblings.
4. Overheating by too many clothes and overly warm bedroom temperature.

New recommendation in 2005 suggest that offering a clean pacifier at sleep time may be a preventive measure against SIDS (AAP, 2005b). A meta-analysis of relevant studies has shown that providing a pacifier at all sleep times including naps may significantly reduce SIDS (Hauck et al., 2005). In addition, pacifier use is endorsed for up to 1 year of age, when both the highest risk of SIDS and NNS needs decline.

Surveys have shown that parents tend to practice what they observe NICU staff do in relation to positioning regardless of education on supine positioning for sleep. Nurse modeling of "back to sleep" supine positioning, including the "back to sleep" bed with only a mattress cover and no other items in the crib, seems to be essential in getting the message across that SIDS prevention is a critical part of routine care at home (Bullock et al., 2004).

Based on reports of parents and nurses, SIDS prevention education remains variable, sometime inappropriate, and modeling of recommendations in the NICU often nonexistent (Aris et al., 2006; Bullock et al., 2004; Colson et al., 2001; Rao et al., 2007). Predictors for prone positioning after discharge are (Colson et al., 2006; Vernacchio et al., 2003):

1. birthweight less than 1500 g,
2. sleep position at 1 month predictive of position at 3 months,
3. multiples,
4. single mother,
5. African American, and
6. perception of infant "preference."

Furthermore, it is critical to note there is racial disparity in SIDS prevention behaviors of parents postdischarge. Surveys/interviews show that black mothers are more likely to place their infant prone for sleep compared with nonblack parents and use soft bedding more frequently than white parents (Colson et al., 2006; Rasinski et al., 2003). Factors to consider when strategizing parent education related to SIDS prevention include identifying potential barriers that may affect compliance, such as the following (Aris et al., 2006; Colson et al., 2006; Rasinski et al., 2003):

1. Resource for SIDS information (health care provider, family members, friends—especially an important female friend).
2. Quality of advice (knowledge of AAP SIDS-prevention recommendations, experience, personal beliefs).
3. Trust in information provider.
4. Perception of infant comfort and safety (choking and aspiration, restlessness, irritability, prone more comfortable, etc.).

Standard 2. A developmentally supportive environment is provided for every infant and family based on continuous assessment and interaction.

A. **Environmental modifications** are made according to the infant's responses, vulnerabilities, and thresholds and includes lighting, sound, activity around the bedside, bedding, positioning aids, and other environmental inputs.

B. **Visual system.** Animal models have shown that early stimulation to an immature visual system can alter the developmental trajectory of the visual and other sensory systems, resulting in atypical behavioral responses (Banker and Lickliter, 1993; Casey and Lickliter, 1998; Foushee and Lickliter, 2002; Honeycutt and Lickliter, 2001; Lickliter, 2000b; Sleigh et al., 1996; Sleigh and Lickliter, 1995, 1998).

1. Although light has not been related to the development of retinopathy of prematurity (ROP), it remains to be seen what role early exposure to light may play in the development of cortical processes and visual-motor performance (Kennedy et al., 2001; Reynolds et al., 1998).
2. Studies using reduced lighting for premature infants have shown no negative visual impact or differences in medical outcomes and may be a safer, more conservative approach until more is known concerning the impact of illumination on early developing visual systems (Kennedy et al., 1997, 2001; Roy et al., 1999).
3. Phototherapy (Fielder and Moseley, 2000) is a known hazard that can negatively affect the visual system. The light exposure ranges from 200 to 280 foot-candles (ftc) (2400 to 3000 lux) with small amounts of ultraviolet radiation (UV) from 330 to 400 nanometers (nm)

that can damage the retina. Careful monitoring to ensure eye patches are in place will reduce about 90% of the phototherapy light exposure and minimize the risk of visual impairment.

4. Preterm infants cared for with day-night cycled lighting have shown significantly faster weight gain (Brandon et al., 2002); lower heart rate and activity during the reduced light cycle (Blackburn and Patterson, 1991); increased sleep time, improved feeding efficiency, and faster weight gain at 6 and 12 weeks after discharge (Mann et al., 1986); less time to oral feeding; and fewer ventilator days (Miller et al., 1995). None of the studies report visual function or long-term visual performance when cycled lighting is introduced at an earlier stage of development.

C. **Auditory environment.** Exposure to sound in the NICU can disrupt sleep patterns and alter physiologic and behavioral responses of premature and term infants (Anderssen, 1993; Gadeke et al., 1969; Long et al., 1980; Morris et al., 2000; Zahr and Balian, 1995). The NICU sound environment must be evaluated in order to make the acoustic and personnel behavior changes that support sleep, normal development, and optimal parent-infant interaction. Auditory intervention in the NICU consists of reduction of ambient noise levels, provision of appropriate auditory stimulation, and screening and treatment for hearing loss (see Chapter 37).

1. Physiologic responses to acoustic stimulation are reported as early as 23 to 25 weeks of gestation in the developing fetus (Abrams and Gerhardt, 2000; Crade and Lovett, 1988; Hall, 2000).

2. The intrauterine influence on the preterm infant's auditory system is primarily made up of sounds emanating from the mother, the most important being the mother's voice (Abrams and Gerhardt, 2000; Gerhardt and Abrams, 2000; Graven, 2000; Moon and Fifer, 2000).

3. The fetal sound experience is important to the normal development of the auditory system. The preterm infant developing in the NICU is subjected to an atypical sound environment that may influence later postnatal language perception and acquisition (Graven, 2000; Jennische and Sedin, 1998; Lickliter, 2000a; Moon and Fifer, 2000; Robertson et al., 1999b, 2001).

4. Undesirable effects associated with sudden, loud noise in the NICU have been reported in both term and preterm infants including increased heart rate; agitation, crying, and irritability; increased anterior fontanelle pressure; sleep disruption, irregular respirations, decreased oxygen saturation; mottling, apnea, and bradycardia; and increased motor activity (Anderssen et al., 1993; Gadeke et al., 1969; Graven, 2000; Morris et al., 2000; Philbin, 2000; Philbin and Klaas, 2000b; Wharrad and Davis, 1997; Zahr and Balian, 1995).

5. Speech delay, articulation, comprehension, receptive and expressive language, auditory memory, and processing problems have been reported at increased rates in preterm infants compared with full-term infants (Byrne et al., 1993; Davis et al., 2001; Jennische and Sedin, 1999, 2001; Whitfield et al., 1997).

6. Whether the NICU environment is directly related to later speech and language problems remains to be seen; however, the concern is that NICU noise can disrupt normal language development and communication processing by distorting socially relevant sounds during critical periods of speech and language development (Byrne et al., 1993; Davis et al., 2001; Dupin et al., 2000; Graven, 2000; Jennische and Sedin, 1999, 2001; Wharrad and Davis, 1997).

7. Quiet times scheduled in an NICU have been shown to increase duration of deep sleep (85% vs. 34%) and decrease crying (14% vs. 2%) in infants during "quiet hour" compared with control periods (Strauch et al., 1993). A general overall respect of the infant's sound environment is important at all times, keeping the noise levels low as to not disturb infant rest and providing stimulation at a level for infants who need it while not disturbing infants nearby.

8. Structural modifications with acoustics designed to support noise abatement in the NICU setting have been successful (Philbin and Gray, 2002; Robertson et al., 1998, 1999a; Smith, 1999; Strauch et al., 1993; Walsh-Sukys et al., 2001). Recommended changes to the environment include increased size of bed space and sound-absorbent surfacing for floors, walls,

and ceiling. The evaluation and recommendations of an acoustical engineer are valuable when renovating or designing new NICUs (Philbin and Gray, 2002).

9. There is little evidence in the literature that supports the need for supplemental auditory stimulation beyond that provided naturally by parents and family. In a report by the Sound Study Group of the National Resource Center of the Physical and Developmental Environment of the High Risk Infant, recommendations for the NICU sound environment based on available evidence are as follows (Graven, 2000):

    a. NICUs should create and maintain a program for controlling noise within specified noise criteria guidelines for continuous sound in the infant's surroundings.

    b. Parents and infants should be afforded opportunities for interaction in a quiet, ambient environment that does not interfere or mask speech sounds.

    c. The use of earphones placed in or over the ear is not recommended.

    d. Recorded music or speech is not supported in the available research evidence and not recommended. Provision of recorded sound should not replace the interactive experience provided by parents necessary for speech and language development.

Standard 3. Parents are viewed as the most important relationship with continual support of this bond starting with the birth of the infant(s).

A. Parental support strategies. The key to supporting mutually satisfying parent-infant interaction is to establish a family-centered approach on admission that will empower the parents to assume the natural parental role of advocating for their child's needs and desires and become the primary nurturer to their infant. Supporting the parents' ability to understand their infant's level of communication through the infant's behavior will place the parents in a better position to respond to and interact with their infant in a developmentally supportive manner.

1. Establish an atmosphere in the NICU that is welcoming to parents and does not treat them as "visitors" but as parents who deserve respect as important members of their infant's care team.

2. Help parents identify the most effective techniques for interacting with their infant (e.g., recognizing stress and time-out signs). Include information on temperament differences in infants and ways to modify daily interactions to support varying temperament traits (Carey, 1998).

3. Place parents in situations in which they will succeed in interacting positively with their infant.

4. Help parents identify both the consoling measures unique to their infant and how their child is providing feedback concerning the consoling measures.

5. Have the caregiving team work with the parents to plan specific activities (i.e., KC or skin-to-skin holding, biologically meaningful smells and tastes, verbal interaction, eye contact, use of toys, therapeutic touch) for parental interaction when appropriate (McGrath and Brock, 2002; Porter and Winberg, 1999).

6. Encourage parents to assume caregiving responsibilities when appropriate.

7. Discuss parents' expectations and goals for themselves and their infant. Encourage families to write down these expectations and goals. Writing down these dreams and goals or journaling will be the beginning of a lifelong care plan.

8. Encourage the parents to use their child's medical record as a communication tool.

9. Be aware of and involve the family's support system. Encourage parent-to-parent support if possible, either in a formal or an informal manner. Reports by families show that attending a parent support group helps them cope with their circumstances by feeling supported, learning about infant development, and understanding how to use the hospital and community resources. When unit staff have participated in these groups, they expressed gaining insights that influenced their interactions with parents and behaviors in the NICU (Pearson and Andersen, 2001).

10. Studies have shown three areas of parenting influenced by cultural differences: parents' emotional responses and understanding of their infant's condition, utilization of resources by minority cultures, and interaction with health professionals (Bracht et al., 2002).

11. Consider implementing a "Parent Buddy Program" with identified parents of different cultures or backgrounds who have experienced having a child in the NICU to serve as a

resource for parents who are not represented by support programs and educational opportunities already available (Bracht et al., 2002).

12. Request a qualified interpreter to assist with language and cultural implications whenever needed to reduce the impact of language barriers and cultural differences.

13. Document the family's goals and the interventions necessary to help them reach their objectives in an individualized family support plan (IFSP) (Robison, 2003).

14. As a professional caregiver, staff are accountable for incorporating the interventions from the IFSP or care plan with infants and families (Robison, 2003).

15. Recognize that the parents are the constant in the child's life and that the various health professionals will come and go. Family factors are more predictive of school performance at 10 years of age than perinatal conditions of low birth weight infants (Gross et al., 2001).

B. **Feeding within a developmental framework for nutrition and parent-infant interaction (Ancona et al., 1998; Ludwig and Waitzman, 2007; McGrath and Braescu, 2004).** The goal of feeding is more than an infant ingesting an adequate volume of food. A key concept is recognizing the difference between a successful feeding (volume and duration of feeding) and a successful feeder (infant competence and enjoyment). Within this context lies the difference between task-oriented or procedural feedings and a developmental feeding philosophy.

1. The framework for a developmental feeding involves three concepts (Ancona et al., 1998).
   a. Physiologic, motor, and state behavioral assessment before, during, and after feeding.
   b. Individualized feeding approach based on specific infant cues.
   c. Fostering parent competence, confidence, and enjoyment while feeding the infant.

2. Nurse's role in preparing infants for transition to oral feeding (Hunter, 2001).
   a. Support sleep-wake behavioral organization.
   b. Provide therapeutic positioning to promote neuromuscular control and postural alignment necessary for suck, swallow, and breathing (prevent hyperextended neck or trunk and shoulder retraction).
   c. Protect against aversive oral stimulation.
   d. Provide pleasurable oral experiences.
   e. Offer opportunities to smell breast milk or formula depending on parent choice of food type.
   f. Offer a pacifier for pleasure and not just as comfort during routine care or uncomfortable/painful procedures.

3. The nurse's role in feeding is not just to ensure safe and adequate transition to oral feeding. It is as important that consistent caregivers develop a relationship with infant and parents to gain familiarity that aids in guiding and monitoring feeding skill and progression.
   a. Recognize feeding readiness behaviors (Hunter, 2001).
      (1) Medical status.
      (2) Energy for feeding.
      (3) Capable of quiet, alert state behavior.
      (4) Gag response with orogastric tube insertion.
      (5) Rooting and sucking behaviors.
      (6) Functional sucking reflex.

C. **Nonnutritive sucking (NNS):** A meta-analysis of NNS literature demonstrated a significant effect on length of hospital stay for infants receiving NNS. No negative outcomes were observed in the 13 randomized, controlled trials reviewed in the meta-analysis. With such a small number of studies for each outcome, the results are inconclusive (Pinelli and Symington, 2000). More studies are needed; however, the positive cues provided by the infant as to enjoyment make this a valuable intervention.

D. **Nutritive sucking (Carrier et al., 2003; Hunter, 2001).**
   1. Greater coordination of the suck-swallow-breathe sequence is required than in NNS.
   2. To encourage as normal a suck-swallow pattern as possible while infant maintains physiologic, motor, and state stability, it is very important to hold the nipple still and allow the infant to pace the feeding. Allow rest between suck bursts. Manage environmental distractions so the infant can focus on the task of learning to feed.

3. Monitor infant for fatigue, especially with first oral feeding trials; forced feeding after an infant is tired may lead to:
   a. Prolonged feeding duration.
   b. Increased energy expenditure.
   c. Poor weight gain.
   d. Increasing incoordination during the feeding.
   e. Higher risk of aspiration.
   f. Deglutition apnea (deglutition is the sequence of moving a liquid or solid bolus in the mouth, through the pharynx and into the esophagus).
   g. Oxygen desaturation.
   h. Bradycardia.
   i. Oral aversion and defensiveness.
4. Intervene with infants who become fatigued by oral feeding:
   a. Stop feeding when infant shows fatigue.
   b. Continue feeding by nasogastric (NG) or orogastric (OG) tube to provide adequate intake.
   c. Decrease number of oral feedings per day or feeding duration per each feed.
   d. If feeding fatigue persists, discuss with care team for further evaluation and planning.

E. **Maturation and coordination** of suck, swallow, and breathing in preterm infants (Diaz and Valdebenito, 2007; Lau et al., 2000; Mizuno and Ueda, 2003; Pickler et al., 2006).
   1. There is a significant correlation in the maturity of the infant's sucking ability and post-menstrual age (PMA).
   2. Neurobehavioral maturation is a developmental sequence that supports feeding progression/abilities.
   3. Coordination of suck, swallow, and respiration is seen by 34 weeks of PMA.
   4. Maturation of the swallowing-respiratory pattern is not fully established even at 36 weeks of PCA.
   5. Sucking pressure, frequency, and duration are related to maturation. The first sucking burst is a positive indicator of successful feeding outcomes. The number of sucks in the first sucking burst of a feeding relates to an infant's maturity, behavioral state before feeding begins, and feeding experience.
   6. Milk flow volume is related to nipple hole size (Hill, 2002).
   7. Restricted milk flow facilitates oral feeding in preterm infants (Lau et al., 1997), allowing rest between suck and swallow with adequate time for bursts of respiration. Rapid-flow nipples may overwhelm preterm infants with milk flow they cannot handle, resulting in interference with respiration and stressful feeding.
   8. Increased milk consumed per feeding, duration of oral feedings, efficiency of feeding, and percentage of successful feedings are enhanced with the use of a vacuum-free bottle that eliminates both hydrostatic pressure and vacuum within the bottle, allowing the preterm infant at 34 to 35 weeks (26 to 29 weeks at birth) to self-pace initial bottle feedings by allowing milk to flow only during sucking (Lau and Schanler, 2000).
   9. Nipples advertised for use with premature infants are softer and allow for higher milk flow, which is inappropriate considering the immature ability and increase the risk of choking, coughing, and aspiration (Ross and Browne, 2002).
   10. Changing nipples frequently may affect feeding organization and adaptation; identifying an appropriate nipple and using it regularly as long as an infant is successfully feeding may be more supportive.
   11. Studies (Arvedson et al., 1994; Comrie and Helm, 1997) have shown that around 94% of aspiration in infants and children evaluated by video fluoroscopy is "silent" (without clinically observable signs).
   12. In general, gut motility follows the same sequence as oral-motor development and is improved by around 35 weeks (Lemons, 2001).
   13. Feeding success is directly related to an infant's ability to maintain physiologic stability, a flexed posture, and an alert state while feeding (Lemons, 2001).
   14. Infants with medical complications may achieve full oral feedings 2 to 5 weeks later than other hospitalized infants.

15. Chronic lung disease from prematurity is the most common medical condition that affects feeding.
16. Breast milk odor may increase NNS during gavage feedings (Bingham et al., 2003).
17. Infants provided 5 minutes of NNS prior to feeding demonstrate more alert and quiet awake states during feeding than those who do not receive the intervention; the NNS infants also demonstrated higher oxygen saturation levels before and after feeding (Hill, 2002; Pickler et al., 1996).
18. Ross and Browne (2002) suggest that oral cheek and jaw support removes the infant's own ability to pace the feeding and also increases milk volume; both experiences may lead to negative feedback during a feeding and ultimately increase the risk of oral defensiveness or aversion.
19. In a randomized controlled trial, preterm infants (32 to 34 weeks of PMA) receiving NNS prior to feeding, oral feedings based on feeding readiness cues, and amount by demand achieved full oral feeding an average of 5 days earlier than a control group on a standard time-based protocol (McCain et al., 2001).
20. Pacing is thought to support feeding success by regulating breathing breaks to slow sucking or successive swallowing and allow adequate breathing opportunity for infants who are having difficulty with stability during a feeding. Pacing is achieved by tilting the bottle slightly so that milk drains out of the nipple and does not continue to flow. This method is preferred to removing the nipple from the infant's mouth, resulting in frequent attempts to reestablish an appropriate latch onto the nipple.
21. Preterm infants randomized to receive early oral stimulation provided by occupational therapists attained full oral feeding about 7 days earlier than those who did not get the intervention. Overall volume and milk transfer rate was significantly greater in the experimental group (Fucile et al., 2002). Authors suggest that both nurses and parents can be taught to provide the oral stimulation to enhance feeding efficiency and performance.
22. Sucking rhythms become increasingly stable from 32 to 40 weeks and are comparable to term sucking patterns.
23. In a prospective study of weekly observations of infants around 35 to 36 weeks, infants with chronic lung disease demonstrated unstable sucking rhythms, decreased aggregation and duration of sucking bursts, and decreased percentage and duration of swallows compared with their healthy preterm counterparts (Gewolb et al., 2001). These infants will require carefully monitored feedings, and parents may need consultation from feeding experts to assist development of oral feeding skills.

F. **Assessment.** Feeding the preterm infant requires close monitoring and documentation of meaningful information to be used in planning the progression and nature of feedings (Ancona et al., 1998; Hunter, 2001; Ross and Browne, 2002). Physiologic stability provides the safe foundation for feeding with the overall integration of physiologic, motor, and state systems working together to support success. If the feeding experience is overwhelming to an infant, both motor and state disruption may occur rapidly and lead to physiologic compromise. Repeated negative feeding experiences may manifest in oral defensiveness or aversion.

1. The new demand of feeding may result in instability of the physiologic, motor, and state systems.
2. As the infant restabilizes and integrates new information, the caregiver must observe cues and pace feedings accordingly.
3. Physiologic assessment includes heart rate, respiratory pattern, oxygenation, color, vigor, and stable digestion.
   a. Physiologic stability while managing oral feeding.
   b. Maintenance of stability following feeding.
   c. Choking or gagging during feeding.
   d. Apnea or bradycardia.
   e. Oxygen saturation and work of breathing.
   f. Signs of fatigue.
   g. Weight gain with adequate caloric intake.

4. Motor assessment includes the following:
   a. General tone and posture.
   b. Changes in muscle tone, posture, and movements with handling.
   c. Quality and strength of suck.
   d. Maturity of sucking pattern (rhythmic and efficient).
   e. Coordination of suck-swallow, breathing (breathing pauses are adequate).
   f. Control of the milk bolus (no significant loss of milk from mouth).
5. Behavioral state assessment includes the following:
   a. Timing, duration, and quality of arousal.
   b. Sensitivity to environment and/or stimulation (shutdown or hyperalerting).
   c. Response to touch, handling, and position changes.
   d. Interest in feeding by facial expression or stress evidenced by frown, grimace, slack or limp jaw.
   e. State transitions (rapidity, frequency).
   f. Signs of "shutdown": closed eyes, generally unresponsive, appearance of sleep.
6. Endurance.
   a. Volume taken.
   b. Time frame for feeding.
   c. Vigor during feeding.
7. Evaluation of a successful feeding.
   a. Physiologic and behavioral cost of feeding is minimal (vital signs are maintained with good oxygenation, muscle tone stable/relaxed, and predominant state is quiet, alert, and interested).
   b. Little or no recovery time required for physical and behavioral return to baseline.
   c. Energy and vigor maintained during and after feeding.
   d. Infant participates in feeding experience with interest, energy, and enjoyment.
   e. Adequate intake by mouth and/or by mouth/gavage.
   f. Adequate weight gain.
   g. Tolerance of feeding observed by minimal residuals, soft abdomen with audible bowel sounds, and regular elimination.

G. **Interventions for oral feeding** are based on available evidence and clinical report using the four standards of developmental care as a guide (Ancona et al., 1998; Case-Smith and Humphrey, 1996; Comrie and Helm, 1997; Daley and Kennedy, 2000; Hunter, 2001; Pinelli and Symington, 2000; Premji et al., 2002a, 2002b; Ross and Browne, 2002) (Box 11-3).

H. **Parents and feeding (Thomas, 2007; Thoyre, 2001):** Safe oral feeding techniques and infant assessment are essential information required by parents prior to discharge. Essential to feeding success in the home setting is an infant who demonstrates identifiable feeding/satiety cues and has transitioned to ad lib feeding rather than the sometimes inflexible scheduled interval and volume routines of the NICU. Ample opportunity to observe infant feeding behaviors and practice in an environment of nursing/health provider support can facilitate success, confidence, competence, and enjoyment.

I. **Breastfeeding the preterm infant (AAP, 2005a; Hurst, 2007; Lau, 2001; Lau and Hurst, 1999; Merten et al., 2005; Reynolds, 2001; Schanler, 2001):** An important antecedent to breastfeeding is the opportunity for skin-to-skin holding or KC that includes eye contact, containment, olfactory, tactile, vestibular motion from rhythmic maternal respirations, and mother's voice that integrate the sensory components necessary for nonnutritive then nutritive breastfeeding. The AAP recommends human milk for all infants, including premature and sick newborn infants except in rare circumstances (AAP, 2005a). They also acknowledge that the choice of breast- or bottle-feeding is within the parents' right to choose and as such, they should be provided with accurate and current information on the benefits and techniques of breastfeeding. Developmentally, breastfeeding follows the natural course for promoting the connection between mother and child along with advantages related to immunity, improved digestion and absorption, gastrointestinal (GI) function, neurodevelopmental outcomes, maternal psychologic health, and emotional bonding or attachment. Support for the breastfeeding mother and infant includes the following (AAP, 2005a; Hurst, 2007; Lau and Hurst, 1999; Merten et al., 2005):

■ BOX 11-3
■ **FEEDING FACILITATION TECHNIQUES FOR PRETERM INFANTS**

Environment
- Prepare calm, quiet area with dim lighting and no distractions.
- Ensure restful environment between feedings.

Direct Care
- Begin preparing for oral feeding by providing NNS and milk odors with gavage feedings.
- Avoid trial PO feeds after stressful procedures.
- Allow adequate time for rest between caregiving and before feedings.
- Provide feedings on semidemand or demand basis depending on institutional feeding practices.
- Choose slightly firmer nipple with slower flow rather than a "preemie" nipple that may result in rapid milk flow (infant will gain strength of suck over time) that the infant cannot manage.
- Be prepared to focus on the infant and feeding with ongoing observation and adaptation.
- Gently arouse to alert state; may use NNS prior to feeding.
- Swaddle in gentle flexion with hands midline toward face.
- Support positioning with infant cradled close to body in semiupright or upright position with neck in neutral to slightly flexed position.
- Continually observe physiologic, behavioral, and oral-motor functioning, being careful to respond when subtle cues are demonstrated indicating the need for modification or termination of the feeding.
- Provide adequate breathing/rest periods for infants who cannot pace themselves by either gently removing nipple or if that is too stressful, tip bottle gently downward to drain milk from nipple.
- Provide gentle jaw and cheek support discriminately only when problems occur with latching onto nipple, weak seal, or loss of milk bolus and after determining whether infant is really ready for oral feeding because this intervention may be aversive and disable the infant's own control and pacing of the feeding.
- Institute "developmental burping" on shoulder with postural support and gentle back rubbing in an upward motion to stimulate burp; avoid sitting infant upright and leaning forward or patting the back because this is an unstable position with tactile stimulation that is often disorganizing for the preterm infant with immature motor subsystems.
- Recognize infant's limits and when to stop feeding to avoid potential fatigue, aversion, physical compromise, and aspiration (infant cues guide all feedings and progression of feedings).
- Gavage the rest of the feeding as needed according to infant cues.
  - Reduce energy expenditure.
  - Promote a positive feeding experience and minimize feeding aversion.
- Schedule plenty of undistracted rest between feedings.
- Evaluate feeding tolerance.
  - Soft abdomen without distention.
  - Normal bowel sounds.
  - Minimal or no gastric residual.
  - Usual frequency, color, and consistency of stools.
  - Little or no spitting or regurgitation.
  - Interest and pleasure in feeding observed.
  - Maintains quiet, awake state for most of feeding.
  - Stable physiologic, motor, and state functioning throughout and postfeeding.
  - Manages liquid without drooling or leaking.
  - Coordinated oral-motor abilities (suck-swallow-breathing).
  - Adequate growth for age on standard growth curve, length, and frontal-occipital circumference measurements.
- Document volume, duration of feeding, feeding behaviors (autonomic, state, and motor) and interventions required.
  - Avoid subjective qualifiers such as "infant fed well, fair, or poor."
  - Record stress/stability signs and predominant infant state during feeding.
  - Note type of nipple.
  - Identify nursing support needed by infant (pacing, rest, swaddling).
  - Describe specific feeding problems demonstrated by infant (fatigue, coordination of suck-swallow-breathing, leakage of milk, tongue thrust, loss of muscle tone, etc.).

■ BOX 11-3

■ **FEEDING FACILITATION TECHNIQUES FOR PRETERM INFANTS—CONT'D**

- Describe rationale for stopping a feeding (choking, fatigue, leakage, facial and body tone, coughing, color change, breathing pauses, etc.).
- Report any signs of feeding intolerance.
- Note duration of feeding and volume taken by mouth and by gavage if needed.
- Collaborate with team on feeding plan to make feeding both a pleasant learning experience and an opportunity to maintain adequate nutrition.
  - Decrease number of oral feedings per day or limit feeding duration each feed based on infant responses.
  - Complement feeding with gavage to preserve adequate nutrition rather than "force feed" infant.
  - Follow occupational therapist's plan (when involved) to promote therapeutic goals.
  - Ensure consistency with core team of nurses working with infants as individuals.

Family Support and Education
- Model appropriate feeding techniques.
- Discuss cultural preferences for feeding experiences and incorporate when possible.
- Provide ample opportunities for feeding practice (starting with feeding preparation with kangaroo or skin-to-skin care and milk odor if family desires).
- Educate on infant cues and measuring feeding success.
- Identify both enjoyment and adequate nutrition as feeding goals.

Consistency of Care
- Same caregivers consistently feed infant.
- Consistent feeding techniques are used between caregivers.
- Consistent use of appropriate feeding equipment.

Modified from Hunter, J.: The neonatal intensive care unit. In J. Case-Smith (Ed.): *Occupational therapy for children* (4th ed.). St. Louis, 2001, Mosby; Carrier, C.T., Walden, M., and Wilson, D.: The high-risk newborn and family. In M.J. Hockenberry (Ed.): *Wong's nursing care of infants and children* (7th ed.). St. Louis, 2003, Mosby.

1. Privacy and comfort of both infant and mother with the use of screens, comfortable chairs, pillows to support the infant, dim lighting, minimal activity around mother-infant dyad, decreased noise, and bottled water or fluids to quench thirst. Arm, back, and neck support with pillows and a footstool can help the mother relax during the breastfeeding session.
2. Easy access to pumping equipment and breast milk storage.
3. Lactation consultants available for education, evaluation, and personal support during breastfeeding.
4. Training in proper breastfeeding positions.
5. Share feeding readiness cues and prepare the mother for assessing stability and stress cues throughout a feeding; discuss and model appropriate interventions as indicated.
6. The most common problem observed in preterm infants is the difficulty in maintaining secure attachment to the nipple and areola. Lau and Hurst (2001) report successful use of silicone nipple shields over the breast to help the infant latch on and successfully maintain attachment (Lau and Hurst, 1999).
7. Methods of measuring milk intake: accurate measurement by test-weighing in which the clothed infant is weighed before and after feeding under the same conditions (no diaper or clothing changes) using electronic scales provide mothers with an objective assessment that may alleviate more anxiety concerning milk intake than subjective estimates.
8. Assist mother in evaluating breastfeeding success with objective rather than subjective measures that may leave her discouraged.
9. Prompt evaluation and correction of inadequate positioning or latch-on is recommended to facilitate breastfeeding success.

J. **Alternative feeding modalities** include gavage or gastrostomy feeding by gravity or by syringe pump. Developmental inputs associated with normalized feeding are extremely important for enhancing the pleasure of feeding associated with the feeling of fullness and stomach filling. Ways to enhance these alternative feeding methods include the following:

1. Environmental modification to minimize stress.
2. Nonnutritive sucking opportunity during feeding.
3. Human contact through holding and/or containment.
4. Olfactory stimulation from breast milk or formula as appropriate.
5. Feeding during KC or skin to skin.
6. Continual monitoring of infant cues during feeding by alternative methods.

K. **Cue-based feeding practices or infant-driven feedings** (Ludwig and Waitzman, 2007) depends on clinical decision making by the nurse or parent about when and by what method to feed an infant based on feeding readiness behaviors that indicate timing is appropriate to try nipple feeding. Infant-driven feeding readiness scales are available for evaluation and documentation but are not yet a validated tool. Components of the scale include readiness to nipple, quality of nippling, and caregiver techniques required during the feeding. The scales are simple enough for use by parents. As parents begin to transition toward going home, it becomes essential that they can recognize their infant's feeding readiness cues and quality of feeding, as well as the volume taken for that feeding. More important, parents will need to be able to relax and nurture their baby so the feeding is an enjoyable experience for both.

Standard 4. Collaborative and consistent caregiving is considered necessary for clinical and developmental support of infants and families.

A. **Collaboration fosters care that is consistent between caregivers.** Consistency and collaboration by caregivers who establish familiarity and predictable routine support trust with both infant and family. Consistency of caregivers is not only important for developmental planning and intervention but provides a measure of safety toward the recognition of clinical and behavioral changes requiring prompt intervention. The evolution of larger and larger NICUs requires critical appraisal of ways to maintain continuity, consistency, and communication to sustain safe clinical and developmental care (Goldschmidt and Gordin, 2006).

1. Consistency of care is a continuum that requires documentation of individual stress and stability cues, written plans of care based on individual assessment of each infant's response to the environment, care, procedures, and medical treatments.
2. Communication through the medical record, easily accessible assessment and care plans, and direct communication between and among caregivers at shift report and/or daily medical/nursing rounds foster collaborative practice and enhance consistent care.
3. A familiar group of people that care for individual infants provide reassurance that establishes trust and builds a partnership that is rewarding to the entire team, especially the family.

REFERENCES

Abrams, R.M. and Gerhardt, K.J.: The acoustic environment and physiological responses of the fetus. *Journal of Perinatology, 20*(8 Pt 2):S31-S36, 2000.

Acolet, D., Sleath, K., and Whitelaw, A.: Oxygenation, heart rate and temperature in very low birth-weight infants during skin-to-skin contact with their mothers. *Acta Paediatrica Scandinavica, 78*(2):189-193, 1989.

Als, H.: *Manual for the naturalistic observation of newborn behavior: Newborn individualized developmental care and assessment program.* Boston, MA, 1995, Harvard Medical School.

Als, H.: Developmental care in the newborn intensive care unit. *Current Opinion in Pediatrics, 10*(2):138-142, 1998.

Als, H. and Gilkerson, L.: The role of relationship-based developmentally supportive newborn intensive care in strengthening outcome of preterm infants. *Seminars in Perinatology, 21*(3):178-189, 1997.

Als, H., Lawhon, G., Brown, E., et al.: Individualized behavioral and environmental care for the very low birth weight preterm infant at high risk for bronchopulmonary dysplasia: Neonatal intensive care unit and developmental outcome. *Pediatrics, 78*(6):1123-1132, 1986.

Als, H., Lawhon, G., Duffy, F.H., et al.: Individualized developmental care for the very low-birth-weight preterm infant. Medical and neurofunctional effects. *Journal of the American Medical Association, 272*(11):853-858, 1994.

American Academy of Pediatrics: Breastfeeding and the use of human milk. *Pediatrics, 115:*496-506, 2005a.

American Academy of Pediatrics: The changing concepts of sudden infant death syndrome: Diagnostic coding shifts, controversies regarding the sleeping environment, and new variables to consider in reducing risk. *Pediatrics,* [serial online] Vol 116:1245-1255,

2005b. Retrieved November 5, 2007, from http://pediatrics.aappublications.org/cgi/content/abstract/pediatrics;116/5/1245

American Academy of Pediatrics: Changing concepts of sudden infant death syndrome: Implications for infant sleeping environment and sleep position (RE9946). *Pediatrics*, 105(3):650-656, 2000.

Anand, K.J.: Effects of perinatal pain and stress. *Progress in Brain Research*, 122:117-129, 2000.

Ancona, J., Shaker, C.S., Puhek, J., and Garland, J.S.: Improving outcomes through a developmental approach to nipple feeding. *Journal of Nursing Care Quality*, 12(5):1-4, 1998.

Anderson, G.C.: Current knowledge about skin-to-skin (kangaroo) care for preterm infants. *Journal of Perinatology*, 11(3):216-226, 1991.

Anderssen, S.H., Nicolaisen, R.B., and Gabrielsen, G.W.: Autonomic response to auditory stimulation. *Acta Paediatrica*, 82:913-918, 1993.

Aris, C., Stevens, T.P., LeMura, C., et al.: NICU nurses' knowledge and discharge teaching related to infant sleep position and risk of SIDS. *Advances in Neonatal Care*, 6(5):281-294, 2006.

Arvedson, J.C., Rogers, B., Buck, G., et al.: Silent aspiration prominent in children with dysphagia. *International Journal of Pediatric Otorhinolaryngology*, 28(2-3):173-181, 1994.

Axelin, A., Salantera, S., and Lehtonen, L.: Facilitated tucking by parents' in pain management of preterm infants-a randomized crossover trial. *Early Human Development*, 82:241-247, 2006.

Banker, H. and Lickliter, R.: Effects of early and delayed visual experience on intersensory development in bobwhite quail chicks. *Developmental Psychobiology*, 26(3):155-170, 1993.

Bauer, J., Sontheimer, D., Fischer, C., and Linderkamp, O.: Metabolic rate and energy balance in very low birth weight infants during kangaroo holding by their mothers and fathers. *Journal of Pediatrics*, 129(4):608-611, 1996.

Bauer, K., Uhrig, C., Sperling, P., et al.: Body temperatures and oxygen consumption during skin-to-skin (kangaroo) care in stable preterm infants weighing less than 1500 grams. *Journal of Pediatrics*, 130(2):240-244, 1997.

Bingham, P.M., Abassi, S., and Sivieri, E.: A pilot study of milk odor effect on nonnutritive sucking by premature newborns. *Archives of Pediatrics and Adolescent Medicine*, 157(1):72-75, 2003.

Blackburn, S. and Patterson, D.: Effects of cycled light on activity, state, and cardiorespiratory function in preterm infants. *Journal of Perinatal and Neonatal Nursing*, 4(4):47-54, 1991.

Boyle, E.M., Freer, Y., Khan-Orakzai, Z., Watkinson, M., et al.: Sucrose and non-nutritive sucking for the relief of pain in screening for retinopathy of prematurity: A randomised controlled trial. *Archives of Diseases in Childhood, Fetal Neonatal Edition*, 91:F166-F168, 2006.

Bracht, M., Kandankery, A., Nodwell, S., et al.: Cultural differences and parental responses to the preterm infant at risk: Strategies for supporting families. *Neonatal Network*, 21(6):31-37, 2002.

Brandon, D.H., Holditch-Davis, D., and Belyea, M.: Preterm infants born at less than 31 weeks' gestation

have improved growth in cycled light compared with continuous near darkness. *Journal of Pediatrics*, 140(2):192-199, 2002.

Browne, J.V.: Considerations for touch and massage in the neonatal intensive care unit. *Neonatal Network*, 19(1):61-64, 2000.

Buehler, D.M., Als, H., Duffy, F.H., et al.: Effectiveness of individualized developmental care for low-risk preterm infants: Behavioral and electrophysiologic evidence. *Pediatrics*, 96(5 Pt 1):923-932, 1995.

Bullock, L.F.C., Mickey, K., Green, J., and Heine, A.: Are nurses acting as role models for the prevention of SIDS. *Maternal Child Nursing*, 29(3):173-177, 2004.

Byrne, J., Ellsworth, C., Bowering, E., and Vincer, M.: Language development in low birth weight infants: The first two years of life. *Journal of Developmental and Behavioral Pediatrics*, 14(1):21-27, 1993.

Carey, W.B.: Communicating with parents and community involvement: Teaching parents about infant temperament. *Pediatrics*, 102(5):1311-1316, 1998.

Carrier, C.T., Walden, M., and Wilson, D.: The high-risk newborn and family. In M.J. Hockenberry (Ed.): *Wong's nursing care of infants and children* (7th ed.). St. Louis, 2003, Mosby, pp. 333-414.

Case-Smith, J. and Humphrey, R.: Feeding and oral motor skills. In J. Case-Smith (Ed.): *Occupational therapy for children*. St. Louis, 1996, Mosby, pp. 430-460.

Casey, M.B. and Lickliter, R.: Prenatal visual experience influences the development of turning bias in bobwhite quail chicks (*Colinus virginianus*). *Developmental Psychobiology*, 32(4):327-338, 1998.

Castral, T.C., Warnock, F., Liete, A.M., Haas, V.J., and Scochi, C.G.S.: The effects of skin-to-skin contact during acute pain in preterm newborns. *European Journal of Pain*, 12:464-471, 2008.

Charpak, N., Ruiz-Pelaez, J.G., Figueroa de, C.Z., et al.: A randomized, controlled trial of kangaroo mother care: Results of follow-up at 1 year of corrected age. *Pediatrics*, 108(5):1072-1079, 2001.

Chwo, M.J., Anderson, G.C., Good, M., et al.: A randomized controlled trial of early kangaroo care for preterm infants: Effects on temperature, weight, behavior, and acuity. *Journal of Nursing Research*, 10(2):129-142, 2002.

Cignacco, E., Hamers, J.P.H., Stoffel, L., et al.: The efficacy of non-pharmacological interventions in the management of procedural pain in preterm and term neonates. A systematic literature review. *European Journal of Pain*, 11:139-152, 2007.

Colson, E.R., Bergman, D.M., Shapiro, E., and Leventhal, J.H.: Position for newborn sleep: Associations with parents' perceptions of their nursery experience. *Birth*, 28(4):249-253, 2001.

Colson, E.R., Levenson, S., Rybin, D., et al.: Barriers to following the supine sleep recommendations among mothers at four centers for the women, infants, and children program. *Pediatrics*, 118(2):e243-e250, 2006. Retrieved from http://www.pediatrics.org/cgi/doi/10.1542/peds.2005-2517 November 25, 2008.

Comrie, J.D. and Helm, J.M.: Common feeding problems in the intensive care nursery: Maturation, organization, evaluation, and management strategies.

Seminars in Speech and Language, 18(3):239-260; quiz 261, 1997.

Conde-Agudelo, A., Diaz-Rossello, J.L., and Belizan, J.M.: Kangaroo mother care to reduce morbidity and mortality in low birthweight infants. *Cochrane Database of Systematic Reviews,* 4:CD002771, 2000.

Corff, K.E., Seideman, R., Venkataraman, P.S., et al.: Facilitated tucking: A nonpharmacological comfort measure for pain in preterm neonates. *Journal of Obstetric, Gynecologic, and Neonatal Nursing, 24*(2):143-147, 1995.

Crade, M. and Lovett, S.: Fetal response to sound stimulation: Preliminary report exploring use of sound stimulation in routine obstetrical ultrasound examinations. *Journal of Ultrasound in Medicine, 7*(9):499-503, 1988.

Daley, H.K. and Kennedy, C.M.: Meta analysis: Effects of interventions on premature infants feeding. *Journal of Perinatal and Neonatal Nursing, 14*(3):62-77, 2000.

Davis, N.M., Doyle, L.W., Ford, G.W., et al.: Auditory function at 14 years of age of very-low-birthweight. *Developmental Medicine and Child Neurology, 43*(3):191-196, 2001.

Diaz, P.F. and Valdebenito, M.R.: The transition from tube to nipple in the premature newborn. In C. Kenner (Ed.): "International Connections," *Newborn and Infant Nursing Reviews, 7*(2):114-119, 2007.

Dupin, R., Laurent, J.P., Stauder, J.E., and Saliba, E.: Auditory attention processing in 5-year-old children born preterm: Evidence from event-related potentials. *Developmental Medicine and Child Neurology, 42*(7):476-480, 2000.

Evans, J.C.: Incidence of hypoxemia associated with caregiving in premature infants. *Neonatal Network, 16*(3):33-40, 1991.

Fearon, I., Kisilevsky, B.S., Hains, S.M., et al.: Swaddling after heel lance: Age-specific effects on behavioral recovery in preterm infants. *Journal of Developmental and Behavioral Pediatrics, 18*(4):222-232, 1997.

Feldman, R. and Eidelman, A.I.: Skin-to-skin contact (kangaroo care) accelerates autonomic and neurobehavioural maturation in preterm infants. *Developmental Medicine and Child Neurology, 45*(4):274-281, 2003.

Feldman, R., Eidelman, A.I., Sirota, L., and Weller, A.: Comparison of skin-to-skin (kangaroo) and traditional care: Parenting outcomes and preterm infant development. *Pediatrics, 110*(1 Pt 1):16-26, 2002a.

Feldman, R., Weller, A., Sirota, L., and Eidelman, A.I.: Skin-to-skin contact (kangaroo care) promotes self-regulation in premature infants: Sleep-wake cyclicity, arousal modulation, and sustained exploration. *Developmental Psychology, 38*(2):194-207, 2002b.

Fern, D., Graves, C., and L'Huillier, M.: Swaddled bathing in the newborn intensive care unit. *Newborn and Infant Nursing Reviews, 2*(1):3-4, 2002.

Field, T.M., Schanberg, S.M., Scafidi, F., et al.: Tactile/kinesthetic stimulation effects on preterm neonates. *Pediatrics, 77*(5):654-658, 1986.

Fielder, A.R. and Moseley, M.J.: Environmental light and the preterm infant. *Seminars in Neonatology, 24*(4):291-292, 2000.

Fleisher, B.E., VandenBerg, K., Constantinou, J., et al.: Individualized developmental care for very-low-birth-weight premature infants. *Clinical Pediatrics (Phila), 34*(10):523-529, 1995.

Fohe, K., Kropf, S., and Avenarius, S.: Skin-to-skin contact improves gas exchange in premature infants. *Journal of Perinatology, 20*(5):311-315, 2000.

Foushee, R.D. and Lickliter, R.: Early visual experience affects postnatal auditory responsiveness in bobwhite quail (*Colinus virginianus*). *Journal of Comparative Psychology, 116*(4):369-380, 2002.

Fucile, S., Gisel, E., and Lau, C.: Oral stimulation accelerates the transition from tube to oral feeding in preterm infants. *Journal of Pediatrics, 141*(2):230-236, 2002.

Gadeke, R., Doring, B., Keller, F., and Vogel, A.: The noise level in a children's hospital and the wake-up threshold in infants. *Acta Paediatrica Scandinavica, 58*:164-170, 1969.

Gerhardt, K.J. and Abrams, R.M.: Fetal exposures to sound and vibroacoustic stimulation. *Journal of Perinatology, 20*(8):S21-S30, 2000.

Gewolb, I.H., Bosma, J.F., Taciak, V.L., and Vice, F.L.: Abnormal developmental patterns of suck and swallow rhythms during feeding in preterm infants with bronchopulmonary dysplasia. *Developmental Medicine and Child Neurology, 43*(7):454-459, 2001.

Glass, P.: The vulnerable neonate and the neonatal intensive care environment. In M.G. MacDonald (Ed.): *Neonatology: Pathophysiology and management of the newborn.* Philadelphia, 1999, Lippincott Williams & Wilkins.

Goubet, N., Rattaz, C., Pierrat, V., Bullinger, A., and Lequien, P.: Olfactory experience mediates response to pain in preterm newborns. *Developmental Psychobiology, 42*:171-180, 2003.

Goubet, N., Strasbaugh, K., and Chesney, J.: Familiarity breeds content? Soothing effect of a familiar odor on full-term newborns. *Journal of Developmental and Behavioral Pediatrics, 28*:189-194, 2007.

Golianu, B., Krane, E., Seybold, S., Almgren, C., and Anand, K.J.S.: Non-pharmacological techniques for pain management in neonates. *Seminars in Perinatology, 31*:318-322, 2007.

Goldberger, J. and Wolfer, J.: An approach for identifying potential threats to development in hospitalized toddlers. *Infants and Young Children, 3*(3):74-83, 1991.

Goldschmidt, K.A. and Gordin, P.: A model of nursing care: Microsystems for a large neonatal intensive care unit. *Advances in Neonatal Care, 6*(2):81-88, 2006.

Graven, S.: Sleep and brain development. *Clinics in Perinatology, 33*:693-706, 2006.

Graven, S.N.: Sound and the developing infant in the NICU: Conclusions and recommendations for care. *Journal of Perinatology, 20*(8 Pt 2):S88-S93, 2000.

Gross, S.J., Mettleman, B.B., Dye, T.D., et al.: Impact of family structure and stability on academic outcome in preterm children at 10 years of age. *Journal of Pediatrics, 138*(2):169-175, 2001.

Hall, J.I.: Development of the ear and hearing. *Journal of Perinatology, 20*(8):S12-S20, 2000.

Harrison, L., Olivet, L., Cunningham, K., et al.: Effects of gentle human touch on preterm infants: Pilot study results. *Neonatal Network, 15*(2):35-42, 1996.

Harrison, L.L., Leeper, J., and Yoon, M.: Preterm infants' physiologic responses to early parent touch. *Western*

Journal of Nursing Research, 13(6):698-707; discussion 708-713, 1991.

Harrison, L.L., Williams, A.K., Berbaum, M.L., et al.: Physiologic and behavioral effects of gentle human touch on preterm infants. *Research in Nursing and Health*, 23(6):435-446, 2000.

Harrison, L.L. and Woods, S.: Early parental touch and preterm infants. *Journal of Obstetric, Gynecologic, and Neonatal Nursing*, 20(4):299-306, 1991.

Hauck, F.R., Omojokun, O.O., and Siadaty, M.R.: Do pacifiers reduce the risk of Sudden Infant Death Syndrome? A meta-analysis. *Pediatrics*, 116:e716-e723, 2005. Retrieved from http://www.pediatrics.org/cgi/doi/10.1542/peds.2004-2631 November 25, 2008.

Hendricks-Munoz, K.D. and Prendergast, C.C.: Barriers to provision of developmental care in the neonatal intensive care unit: Neonatal Nursing Perceptions. *American Journal of Perinatology*, 24(2):71-77, 2007.

Hill, A.S.: Toward a theory of feeding efficiency for bottle-fed preterm infants. *Journal of Theory Construction & Testing*, 6(1):75-81, 2002.

Holditch-Davis, D., Blackburn, S.T., and VandenBerg, K.A.: *Newborn and infant neurobehavioral development*. St. Louis, 2003, Saunders.

Honeycutt, H. and Lickliter, R.: Order-dependent timing of unimodal and multimodal stimulation affects prenatal auditory learning in bobwhite quail embryos. *Developmental Psychobiology*, 38(1):1-10, 2001.

Hunter, J.: The neonatal intensive care unit. In J. Case-Smith (Ed.): *Occupational therapy for children* (4th ed.). St. Louis, 2001, Mosby, pp. 636-707.

Hurst, N.M.: The 3 M's of breast-feeding the preterm infant. *Journal of Perinatal and Neonatal Nursing*, 21(3):234-239, 2007.

Jennische, M. and Sedin, G.: Speech and language skills in children who required neonatal intensive care. I. Spontaneous speech at 6.5 years of age. *Acta Paediatrica*, 87(6):654-666, 1998.

Jennische, M. and Sedin, G.: Speech and language skills in children who required neonatal intensive care: Evaluation at 6.5 y of age based on interviews with parents. *Acta Paediatrica*, 88(9):975-982, 1999.

Jennische, M. and Sedin, G.: Linguistic skills at 6½ years of age in children who required neonatal intensive care in 1986-1989. *Acta Paediatrica*, 90(2):199-212, 2001.

Kennedy, K.A., Fielder, A.R., Hardy, R.J., et al.: Reduced lighting does not improve medical outcomes in very low birth weight infants. *Journal of Pediatrics*, 139(4):527-531, 2001.

Kennedy, K.A., Ipson, M.A., Birch, D.G., et al.: Light reduction and the electroretinogram of preterm infants. *Archives of Disease in Childhood, Fetal and Neonatal Edition*, 76(3):F168-F173, 1997.

Lau, C.: Effects of stress on lactation. *Pediatric Clinics of North America*, 48(1):221-234, 2001.

Lau, C., Alagugurusamy, R., Schanler, R.J., et al.: Characterization of the developmental stages of sucking in preterm infants during bottle feeding. *Acta Paediatrica*, 89(7):846-852, 2000.

Lau, C. and Hurst, N.: Oral feeding in infants. *Current Problems in Pediatrics*, 29(4):105-124, 1999.

Lau, C. and Hurst, N.: *Oral feeding of the preterm infant*. Nutrition Conference, Texas Children's Hospital, Houston, TX, Nov. 15, 2001.

Lau, C. and Schanler, R.J.: Oral feeding in premature infants: Advantage of a self-paced milk flow. *Acta Paediatrica*, 89(4):453-459, 2000.

Lau, C., Sheena, H.R., Shulman, R.J., et al.: Oral feeding in low birth weight infants. *Journal of Pediatrics*, 130(4):561-569, 1997.

Lemons, P.K.: From gavage to oral feedings: Just a matter of time. *Neonatal Network*, 20(3):7-14, 2001.

Leslie, A. and Marlow, N.: Non-pharmacological pain relief. *Seminars in Fetal and Neonatal Medicine*, 11:246-250, 2006.

Lickliter, R.: Atypical perinatal sensory stimulation and early perceptual development: Insights from developmental psychobiology. *Journal of Perinatology*, 20(8 Pt 2):S45-S54, 2000a.

Lickliter, R.: The role of sensory stimulation in perinatal development: Insights from comparative research for care of the high-risk infant. *Journal of Developmental and Behavioral Pediatrics*, 21(6):437-447, 2000b.

Long, J.G., Lucey, J.F., and Philip, A.G.: Noise and hypoxemia in the intensive care nursery. *Pediatrics*, 65(1):143-145, 1980.

Ludington-Hoe, S.M., Anderson, G.C., Simpson, S., et al.: Birth-related fatigue in 34-36-week preterm neonates: Rapid recovery with very early kangaroo (skin-to-skin) care. *Journal of Obstetric, Gynecologic, and Neonatal Nursing*, 28(1):94-103, 1999.

Ludwig, S.M. and Waitzman, K.A.: Changing feeding documentation to reflect infant-driven feeding practice. *Newborn and Infant Nursing Review*, 7(3):155-160, 2007.

Mann, N.P., Haddow, R., Stokes, L., et al.: Effect of night and day on preterm infants in a newborn nursery: Randomised trial. *British Medical Journal (Clinical Research Edition)*, 293(6557):1265-1267, 1986.

McCain, G.C., Gartside, P.S., Greenberg, J.M., et al.: A feeding protocol for healthy preterm infants that shortens time to oral feeding. *Journal of Pediatrics*, 139(3):374-379, 2001.

McGrath, J.M. and Braescu, A.V.B.: State of the science: Feeding readiness in the preterm infant. *Journal of Perinatal and Neonatal Nursing*, 18(4):353-368, 2004.

McGrath, J.M. and Brock, N.: Efficacy and utilization of skin-to-skin care in the NICU. *Newborn and Infant Nursing Reviews*, 2(1):17-26, 2002.

Melnyk, B.M. and Fineout-Overholt, E.: *Evidence-based practice in nursing & healthcare: A guide to best practice*. Philadelphia, 2005, Lippincott Williams & Wilkins.

Merten, S., Dratva, J., and Ackermann-Liebrick, U.: Do baby-friendly hospitals influence breastfeeding duration on a national level? *Pediatrics*, 116:e702-e708, 2005. DOI: 10.1542/peds.2005-0537. Retrieved from http://www.pediatrics.org/cgi/content/full/116/5/e702 November 25, 2008.

Messmer, P.R., Rodriguez, S., Adams, J., et al.: Effect of kangaroo care on sleep time for neonates. *Pediatric Nursing*, 23(4):408-414, 1997.

Miller, C., White, R., Whitman, T., et al.: The effects of cycled versus noncycled lighting on growth and development in preterm infants. *Infant Behavioral Development*, 18:87-95, 1995.

Mizuno, K. and Ueda, A.: The maturation and coordination of sucking, swallowing, and respiration in preterm infants. *Journal of Pediatrics*, 142(1):36-40, 2003.

Modrcin-Talbott, M.A., Harrison, L.L., Groer, M.W., and Younger, M.S.: The biobehavioral effects of gentle human touch on preterm infants. *Nursing Science Quarterly*, 16(1):60-67, 2003.

Moon, C.M. and Fifer, W.P.: Evidence of transnatal auditory learning. *Journal of Perinatology*, 20(8):S37-S44, 2000.

Morris, B.H., Philbin, M.K., and Bose, C.: Physiological effects of sound on the newborn. *Journal of Perinatology*, 20(8 Pt 2):S55-S60, 2000.

Neu, M. and Browne, J.V.: Infant physiologic and behavioral organization during swaddled versus unswaddled weighing. *Journal of Perinatology*, 17(3):193-198, 1997.

Neu, M., Browne, J.V., and Vojir, C.: The impact of two transfer techniques used during skin-to-skin care on the physiologic and behavioral responses of preterm infants. *Nursing Research*, 49(4):215-223, 2000.

Parry, S.: Acute pain management in the neonate. *Anaesthesia and Intensive Care Medicine*, 9(4):147-151, 2008.

Pearson, J. and Andersen, K.: Evaluation of a program to promote positive parenting in the neonatal intensive care unit. *Neonatal Network*, 20(4):43-48, 2001.

Peters, K.: Infant handling in the NICU: Does developmental care make a difference? An evaluative review of the literature. *Journal of Perinatal and Neonatal Nursing*, 13(3):83-109, 1999.

Peters, K.L.: Does routine nursing care complicate the physiologic status of the premature neonate with respiratory distress syndrome? *Journal of Perinatal and Neonatal Nursing*, 6(2):67-84, 1992.

Philbin, M.K.: The influence of auditory experience on the behavior of preterm newborns. *Journal of Perinatology*, 20(8 Pt 2):S77-S87, 2000.

Philbin, M.K. and Gray, L.: Changing levels of quiet in an intensive care nursery. *Journal of Perinatology*, 22(6):455-460, 2002.

Philbin, M.K. and Klaas, P.: Evaluating studies of the behavioral effects of sound on newborns. *Journal of Perinatology*, 20(8 Pt 2):S61-S67, 2000a.

Philbin, M.K. and Klaas, P.: Hearing and behavioral responses to sound in full-term newborns. *Journal of Perinatology*, 20(8 Pt 2):S68-S76, 2000b.

Pickler, R.H., Chiaranai, C., and Reyna, B.A.: Relationship of the first suck burst to feeding outcomes in preterm infants. *Journal of Perinatal and Neonatal Nursing*, 20(2):157-162, 2006.

Pickler, R.H., Frankel, H.B., Walsh, K.M., and Thompson, N.M.: Effects of nonnutritive sucking on behavioral organization and feeding performance in preterm infants. *Nursing Research*, 45(3):132-135, 1996.

Pinelli, J. and Symington, A.: How rewarding can a pacifier be? A systematic review of nonnutritive sucking in preterm infants. *Neonatal Network*, 19(8):41-48, 2000.

Porter, R.H. and Winberg, J.: Unique salience of maternal breast odors for newborn infants. *Neuroscience and Biobehavioral Reviews*, 23(3):439-449, 1999.

Premji, S., Paes, B., Jacobson, K., et al.: Evidence-based feeding guidelines for very-low-birthweight infants. *Advances in Neonatal Care*, 2(1):5-18, 2002a.

Premji, S.S., Chessell, L., Paes, B., et al.: A matched cohort study of feeding practice guidelines for infants weighing less than 1500 g. *Advances in Neonatal Care*, 2(1):27, 2002b.

Rao, H., May, C., Hannam, S., Rafferty, G.F., and Greenough, A.: Survey of sleeping position recommendations for prematurely born infants on neonatal intensive care unit discharge. *European Journal of Pediatrics*, 166:809-811, 2007.

Rasinski, K.A., Kuby A., Bzdusek, S.A., Silvestri, J.M., and Weese-Mayer, D.E.: Effect of a sudden infant death syndrome risk reduction education program on risk factor compliance and information sources in primarily black urban communities. *Pediatrics*, 111:e347-e354, 2003. Retrieved from http://www.pediatrics.org/cgi/content/full/111/4/e347 November 25, 2008.

Reynolds, A.: Breastfeeding and brain development. *Pediatric Clinics of North America*, 48(1):159-171, 2001.

Reynolds, J.D., Hardy, R.J., Kennedy, K.A., et al.: Lack of efficacy of light reduction in preventing retinopathy of prematurity. Light Reduction in Retinopathy of Prematurity (LIGHT-ROP) Cooperative Group. *New England Journal of Medicine*, 338(22):1572-1576, 1998.

Roberts, K.L., Paynter, C., and McEwan, B.: A comparison of kangaroo mother care and conventional cuddling care. *Neonatal Network*, 9(4):31-35, 2000.

Robertson, A., Cooper-Peel, C., and Vos, P.: Contribution of heating, ventilation, and air conditioning airflow and conversation to the ambient sound in a neonatal intensive care unit. *Journal of Perinatology*, 19(5):362-366, 1999a.

Robertson, A., Cooper-Peel, C., and Vos, P.: Sound transmission into incubators in the neonatal intensive care unit. *Journal of Perinatology*, 19(7):494-497, 1999b.

Robertson, A., Kohn, J., Vos, P., et al.: Establishing a noise measurement protocol for neonatal intensive care units. *Journal of Perinatology*, 18(2):126-130, 1998.

Robertson, A., Stuart, A., and Walker, L.: Transmission loss of sound into incubators: Implications for voice perception by infants. *Journal of Perinatology*, 21(4):236-241, 2001.

Robison, L.D.: An organizational guide for an effective developmental program in the NICU. *Journal of Obstetric, Gynecologic, and Neonatal Nursing*, 32(3):379-386, 2003.

Ross, E.S. and Browne, J.V.: Developmental progression of feeding skills: An approach to supporting feeding in preterm infants. *Seminars in Neonatology*, 7(6):469-745, 2002.

Roy, M.S., Caramelli, C., Orquin, J., et al.: Effects of early reduced light exposure on central visual development in preterm infants. *Acta Paediatrica*, 88(4):459-461, 1999.

Schanler, R.J.: The use of human milk for premature infants. *Pediatric Clinics of North America*, 48(1):207-219, 2001.

Shah, P.S., Aliwalas, L.L., and Shah, V.: Breastfeeding or breast milk for procedural pain in neonates. *Cochrane Database of Systematic Reviews*, 3:CD004950, 2006. DOI: 10.1002/14651858.CD004950.pub.2

Sleigh, M.J., Columbus, R.F., and Lickliter, R.: Type of prenatal sensory experience affects prenatal auditory learning in bobwhite quail (*Colinus virginianus*). *Journal of Comparative Psychology*, 110(3):233-242, 1996.

Sleigh, M.J. and Lickliter, R.: Augmented prenatal visual stimulation alters postnatal auditory and visual responsiveness in bobwhite quail chicks. *Developmental Psychobiology*, 28(7):353-366, 1995.

Sleigh, M.J. and Lickliter, R.: Timing of presentation of prenatal auditory stimulation alters auditory and visual responsiveness in bobwhite quail chicks (*Colinus virginianus*). *Journal of Comparative Psychology*, 112(2):153-160, 1998.

Slevin, M., Murphy, J.F.A., Daly, L., et al.: Retinopathy of prematurity screening, stress related responses, the role of nesting. *British Journal of Ophthalmology*, 81(9):762-764, 1999.

Smith, D.: Facility profile. Noises off: Nursery pumps down the volume. *Health Facilities Management*, 12(5):20-21, 1999.

Strauch, C., Brandt, S., and Edwards-Beckett, J.: Implementation of a quiet hour: Effect on noise levels and infant sleep states. *Neonatal Network*, 12(2):31-35, 1993.

Stevens, B., Yamada, J., Beyene, J., et al.: Consistent management of repeated procedural pain with sucrose in preterm neonates: Is it effective and safe for repeated use over time? *Clinical Journal of Pain*, 21(6):543-548, 2005.

Sweeney, J.K. and Gutierrez, T.: Musculoskeletal implications of preterm infant positioning in the NICU. *Journal of Perinatal and Neonatal Nursing*, 16(1):58-70, 2002.

Symington, A. and Pinelli, J.: Distilling the evidence on developmental care: A systematic review. *Advances in Neonatal Care*, 2(4):198-221, 2002.

Thoman, E.B., Davis, D.H., and Denenberg, V.H.: The sleeping and waking states of infants: Correlations across time and person. *Physiology and Behavior*, 41(6):531-537, 1987.

Thomas, J.A.: Guidelines for bottle feeding your premature baby. *Advances in Neonatal Care*, 7(6):311-318, 2007.

Thoyre, S.M.: Challenges mothers identify in bottle feeding their preterm infants. *Neonatal Network*, 20(1):41-50, 2001.

Tornhage, C.J., Stuge, E., Lindberg, T., et al.: First week kangaroo care in sick very preterm infants. *Acta Paediatrica*, 88(12):1402-1404, 1999.

Vernacchio, L., Corwin, M.J., Lesko, S.M., et al.: Sleep position of low birth weight infants. *Pediatrics*, 111:633-640, 2003. Retrieved from http://www.pediatrics.org/cgi/content/full/111/3/633 November 25, 2008.

Vickers, A., Ohlsson, A., Lacy, J.B., et al.: Massage for promoting growth and development of preterm and/or low birth-weight infants. *Cochrane Database of Systematic Reviews*, 2:CD000390, 2000.

Walsh-Sukys, M., Reitenbach, A., Hudson-Barr, D., et al.: Reducing light and sound in the neonatal intensive care unit: An evaluation of patient safety, staff satisfaction and costs. *Journal of Perinatology*, 21(4):230-235, 2001.

Westrup, B., Kleberg, A., von Eichwald, K., et al.: A randomized, controlled trial to evaluate the effects of the newborn individualized developmental care and assessment program in a Swedish setting. *Pediatrics*, 105(1 Pt 1):66-72, 2000.

Wharrad, H.J. and Davis, A.C.: Behavioural and autonomic responses to sound in pre-term and full-term babies. *British Journal of Audiology*, 31(5):315-329, 1997.

Wheeden, A., Scafidi, F.A., Field, T., et al.: Massage effects on cocaine-exposed preterm neonates. *Journal of Developmental and Behavioral Pediatrics*, 14(5):318-322, 1993.

Whitfield, M.F., Grunau, R.V., and Holsti, L.: Extremely premature (< or = 800 g) schoolchildren: Multiple areas of hidden disability. *Archives of Disease in Childhood, Fetal Neonatal Edition*, 77(2):F85-F90, 1997.

Wielenga, J.M., Smit, B.J., and Unk, L.K.A.: How satisfied are parents supported by nurses with the NIDCAP model of care for their preterm infant? *Journal of Nursing Care Quality*, 21(1):41-48, 2006.

Zahr, L.K. and Balian, S.: Responses of premature infants to routine nursing interventions and noise in the NICU. *Nursing Research*, 44(3):179-185, 1995.

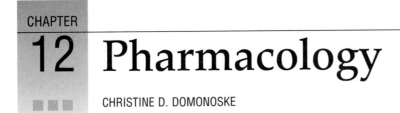

CHRISTINE D. DOMONOSKE

OBJECTIVES

1. Define the concepts of (a) pharmacology, (b) pharmacodynamics, and (c) pharmacokinetics.
2. Describe the developmental changes that affect medication absorption, distribution, metabolism, and elimination.
3. Identify specific considerations when one is administering medications of the following types to a neonate: (a) antimicrobial agents, (b) cardiovascular agents, (c) central nervous system agents, (d) diuretics, and (e) immunizations.
4. Describe nursing responsibilities and interventions when administering medication to the neonate.

■
■■ The study and clinical application of neonatal pharmacology can facilitate safe medication administration in the neonate. The application of pharmacologic principles involves evaluating existing knowledge related to the pharmacodynamic and pharmacokinetic responses of the neonate to specific medications. Unfortunately, this body of knowledge is extremely limited in the neonatal population owing to a lack of controlled clinical trials with these patients. Confounding factors relative to gestational and chronologic age, weight, fluid status, and the health-illness state of individual organ systems make dosing medications in this population a challenging and perpetual learning process. The decision to administer a medication should be evaluated for the desired response and the potential for an undesirable reaction. The nurse is in the ideal position to observe and evaluate both response and reaction and to intervene if necessary.

This chapter provides pharmacologic information specific to the neonate. Information on medication dosages and implications for medication administration is provided in individual clinical chapters. Additional current reference materials should also be available in the neonatal intensive care unit (NICU).

PRINCIPLES OF PHARMACOLOGY

Terminology

A. **Pharmacology:** the science of the properties of medications and their effects in the body.
   1. **Pharmacotherapy:** the administration of a medication to a patient with the intent of preventing, diagnosing, or treating disease.
   2. **Medication:** any substance or mixture of substances intended to be used for the cure, mitigation, or prevention of disease in human beings or animals.
   3. **Pharmacodynamics:** the relationship between medication concentrations at the site of action and the pharmacologic response (intensity and time course of therapeutic and adverse effects). This is what the drug does to the body.
   4. **Pharmacokinetics:** the fate of a medication in the body from the time it enters until it and all of its metabolites are removed. This includes medication absorption, distribution, metabolism, and excretion. It is also the specialized study of the mathematical relationship between a medication dosage regimen and the resulting serum concentration. This is what the body does to the drug.
   5. **Bioavailability:** the portion of the administered dose that reaches the site of action in the body. This is usually the amount entering the circulation and may be reduced when medications are given by mouth versus when given intravenously.
   6. **Therapeutic range:** a range of medication concentrations within which the probability of the desired clinical response is relatively high and the probability of unacceptable toxicity or subtherapeutic response is relatively low.

7. **Therapeutic drug monitoring (TDM):** determinations of plasma medication concentrations to optimize medication therapy. TDM is valuable when:
   a. A good correlation exists between the pharmacologic response and plasma concentration.
   b. Wide intersubject variation in drug plasma levels results from a given dose.
   c. The medication has a narrow therapeutic range.
   d. The medication's desired pharmacologic effects cannot be readily assessed by other simple means.
8. **Steady state:** a term used to refer to a situation in which the amount of medication administered is equal to the amount of medication eliminated. When steady state is reached in a patient, the blood concentrations remain "steady." Therefore at steady state, all peak drug levels and all trough drug levels should be the same.
9. **Half-life:** the time necessary for a measured medication concentration to fall to half its original value. A medication's duration of action is often related to its half-life and may also indicate when another dose should be given. It takes approximately five half-lives to reach steady state.
10. **Types of medication levels:**
    a. *Peak level:* a drug level that is drawn after the dose is given and after adequate time is allowed for the drug to distribute throughout the body. The time for the drug to distribute varies with each medication and the route of administration.
    b. *Trough level:* a drug level that is drawn just prior to the dose.
    c. *Random level:* a drug level that is drawn at any time after a dose is given. These levels are often used to follow drug levels in patients with changing renal function or changing volume status.

PHARMACODYNAMICS

A. **Receptor concept:** The principle that medications act by forming a complex with a specific macromolecule in a way that produces a given response. This response may include inhibition or potentiation of the macromolecule's activity to create the desired medication effect. Receptor effects are as follows:
   1. The medication's affinity for binding to the receptor plays a large part in the determination of the concentration of the medication required to achieve the desired response.
   2. The individual characteristics of the receptor are responsible for the selective nature of medication response.
   3. Receptor theory of medication action allows an explanation of medication antagonists. The antagonist medication may alter the characteristics of the receptor molecule in a way that limits or inhibits the response to the original medication (e.g., naloxone and morphine) or stimulus (e.g., a β-blocker such as propranolol).
   4. Some medications do not appear to act through receptors. Their action is related to a direct response in the recipient.
B. **General mechanisms of medication action.**
   1. Based on the nature of the receptor–medication complex.
   2. Types of receptor–medication complexes.
      a. Receptor–medication complexes that regulate gene expression.
         (1) One common class of medications acts by mediating a response that ultimately involves gene expression and new protein synthesis.
         (2) These medications generally do not have a rapid effect after initial administration (e.g., epoetin alfa).
      b. Receptor–medication complexes that change cell membrane permeability.
         (1) Many clinically useful medications act by changing the cell membrane permeability and therefore altering membrane characteristics.
         (2) These medications may have a relatively short lag time between administration and response (e.g., penicillin).
      c. Receptor–medication complexes that increase the intracellular concentration of a second messenger molecule.

      (1) These medications increase production and activity of enzyme systems within the cell.

      (2) These medications may stimulate a rapid response in changing cell characteristics (e.g., dopamine).

C. **Relationship between medication dose and clinical response.**

  1. Individuals in a population receiving a medication may have a wide range of responses to a medication dose. An idiosyncratic medication response is an abnormal response to a medication that is not usually observed. These unpredictable responses include the following:

    a. Low sensitivity: a patient who, on receiving the usual medication dose, exhibits a clinical or biologic response that is less intense than expected (e.g., inadequate pain relief with usual doses of analgesic medications).

    b. Extreme sensitivity: a patient whose response to a medication is more intense than is expected (e.g., severe hypotension from an antihypertensive agent).

    c. Unpredictable adverse reaction: a patient whose medication reaction is substantially different from what would have been predicted and may differ from the usual response in most patients (e.g., an anaphylactic reaction).

    d. Tolerance: a diminished response to a given medication dose that is related to long-term administration of a medication (e.g., fentanyl doses must be increased as the length of therapy increases to achieve the same effects).

    e. Tachyphylaxis: a rapidly diminished medication response without a medication dosage change. This may be caused by any of a number of factors, including a limited number of receptor sites or limited numbers of transmitter chemicals (e.g., response to albuterol may diminish if given frequently).

  2. Factors that may affect individual medication response are as follows:

    a. Alterations in medication concentration: a change from the expected norm in the amount of medication that reaches the receptor molecule.

    b. Variation in amounts of antagonistic substances: an unusually large or limited amount of antagonistic substances that alter receptor molecule response.

    c. Alterations in numbers or function of receptor molecules: an increased or diminished number of receptor molecules changes the number of potential medication–receptor complexes.

    d. Changes in concentration of molecules other than receptor molecules: if medication response is ultimately dependent on an effect on molecules other than those of the medication–receptor complex, medication response may be limited by the amount of the third molecule type (e.g., prodrugs such as fosphenytoin).

D. **Desired versus undesired effects of medications.**

  1. No medication causes only one effect; all medications have several effects, which can be divided into four groups:

    a. Desired, or therapeutic, effects: those effects that are the desired outcome of the medication administration (e.g., reduction in apnea episodes with theophylline treatment).

    b. Subtherapeutic effect: those effects that are less than the desired outcome of the medication administration (e.g., continued apnea episodes with low theophylline levels).

    c. Side effects: those medication effects that result from medication administration and that are in addition to the desired effects. All medications have some side effects, varying from minor and clinically insignificant to major side effects that are sufficiently adverse to require discontinuation of the medication therapy (e.g., tachycardia with theophylline treatment).

    d. Toxic effects: medication response that results from a medication overdose or unexpected high serum medication concentrations (e.g., seizures from a high theophylline level).

  2. It is the responsibility of the health care provider to weigh the benefits of the therapeutic effect against the risk of undesirable side effects and toxic effects or subtherapeutic responses and make adjustments accordingly.

PHARMACOKINETICS

A. Principles of medication absorption (Fig. 12-1).

1. General principles of medication absorption.
   a. The movement of a medication from the site of administration to the bloodstream.
   b. Regardless of the route of administration, most medications must cross cell membranes to reach their site of action.
      (1) Most medications cross cell membranes by passive diffusion. Physiochemical properties of the medication molecule have a major impact on the ease of diffusion.
      (2) Medications can enter the cell through other mechanisms also, such as active transport or facilitated diffusion.
   c. The absorption of a medication is dependent, in large part, on the route of administration. The common sites of administration are as follows:
      (1) **Gastrointestinal (GI):** commonly used because of minimal infection risk, decreased cost, and convenience.
         (a) Gastric emptying and intestinal transit times: prolonged and irregular; approaches adult values at 6 to 8 months of age. Gastric and intestinal motility are reduced with prematurity, asphyxia, gastroesophageal reflux, and respiratory distress syndrome. Administration of hypocaloric feeds, human milk, or prokinetic agents (e.g., metoclopramide, bethanechol) can increase motility. Prolonged transit times and enterohepatic recirculation may also increase the bioavailability and pharmacologic effect of some substances (Chemtob, 2004).

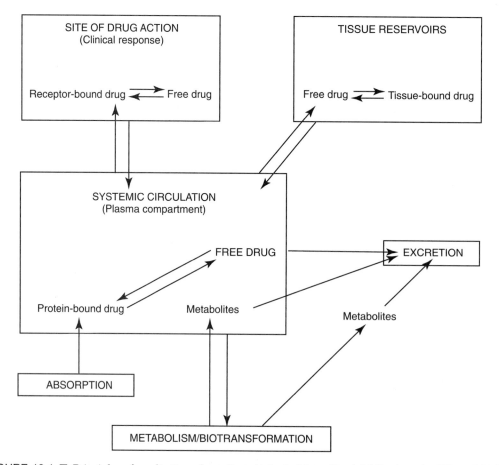

FIGURE 12-1 ■ Principles of medication absorption. (Adapted from Reed, M.D., Aranda, J.V., and Hales, B.F.: Developmental pharmacology. In R.J. Martin, A.A. Fanaroff, and M.C. Walsh [Eds.]: *Fanaroff and Martin's neonatal-perinatal medicine: Diseases of the fetus and infant* [8th ed.]. Philadelphia, 2006, Mosby.)

However, the bioavailability of the medication may decrease because of increased first-pass loss, increased GI destruction of medication or shortened transit times from diarrhea or emesis.

(b) GI tract acidity: the presence of marked changes in pH from the stomach through the distal portion of the GI tract may affect absorption. The pH of the GI tract is nearly neutral or slightly alkaline at birth owing to the presence of amniotic fluid in the stomach. Gastric acid increases secretion rapidly such that it doubles by 2 months, even in the extremely low birth weight neonate (Blackburn, 2007a; Stewart and Hampton, 1987). The net effect of GI acidity on the absorption of medications is dependent on the pH characteristics of the medication and preparation. Medications that normally may not be absorbed well in the stomach may be absorbed at a higher rate in the neonate because of decreased stomach acidity. The absorption of acidic drugs will be reduced (e.g., phenobarbital, phenytoin) and the absorption of basic drugs will be enhanced (e.g., penicillin, erythromycin) as compared with adults (Kraus and Pham, 2005).

(c) GI enzyme activity: neonates are deficient in pancreatic enzymes at birth. This deficiency may inhibit absorption of some medications that require pancreatic enzymes for efficient absorption. One compensating mechanism that neonates have is an increased β-glucuronidase secretion. This is an enzyme produced by organisms normally present in the small intestine that are capable of metabolizing some medications. It is up to seven times the adult amounts (Blackburn, 2007a).

(d) Bacterial flora: composition and rate of colonization of the GI tract by the normal bacterial flora may affect both GI tract motility and the metabolism of some medications. Colonization is dependent on oral intake, antibiotic administration, or disease states such as necrotizing enterocolitis or infectious gastroenteritis. Normal colonization in vaginally born term neonates occurs by 4 to 6 days of age. Intestinal flora are required for the production of vitamin K (Chemtob, 2004).

(e) GI tract perfusion: in very ill neonates, hypoperfusion of the gut may decrease medication absorption.

(f) Underlying disease states: underlying disease states such as diarrhea, emesis, or the presence of nasogastric suction may reduce the time available for medication absorption. Diseases of genetic (e.g., cystic fibrosis) or circulatory (e.g., necrotizing enterocolitis) origin will alter pancreatic enzymes or intestinal mucosa, decreasing GI absorption.

(2) **Rectal:** may be a very rapid and efficient means of medication absorption.

(a) Useful when rapid IV access is not available (e.g., patients in status epilepticus in need of anticonvulsant agents).

(b) Serum levels of some medications may be as high as levels obtained through the IV route of administration (Kraus and Pham, 2005).

(c) Routine administration by rectal route is discouraged. Relative volume and fragility of the neonatal rectum must be considered.

(d) The retention time is the rate-limiting step.

(3) **Inhalation:** useful for gaseous or easily vaporized medications.

(a) Absorption is favored owing to the large surface area of the alveolar membranes and the generous blood flow. Medication response may be very rapid.

(b) Medications administered by this route have a particular advantage when the site of desired action is the tracheobronchial tree (e.g., albuterol).

(c) There is a potential for fewer side effects when medications are administered this way, because much of the medication may not be systemically absorbed (e.g., inhaled corticosteroids).

(d) Most frequently used in neonatal intensive care for the administration of various surfactant preparations.

(e) Certain medications (e.g., epinephrine and lidocaine) can be given through the endotracheal tube in emergency situations when IV access is not readily available.

(f) This route may be less effective in a neonate with pulmonary hypertension and poor or abnormally distributed pulmonary blood flow.

(4) **Topical/percutaneous:** utility is limited to medications whose absorptive characteristics allow permeation through the skin or mucous membranes. Percutaneous absorption has particular advantages as well as risks in the neonate.

(a) The rate of absorption is inversely related to skin thickness and directly related to skin hydration. With increasing gestational age, skin thickness increases and water content decreases, thus reducing the amount of absorption from this route. Maturation of the epidermis occurs between 23 and 33 weeks of gestation. The stratum corneum forms after 23 to 24 weeks of gestation. Formation of this layer of the skin greatly decreases the permeability of the skin to water and infection (Hoath, 2004). This allows much more efficient percutaneous absorption of medications in neonates of lower birth weight and younger gestational age. However, this poses a particular hazard in care, because substances that may be safely applied to the skin of a more mature patient may be absorbed in dangerous amounts in the immature neonate (Nahata & Taketomo, 2005).

(b) The ratio of body surface area to body weight is higher in neonates than adults, providing a relatively larger absorptive surface in comparison with body mass.

(c) The absorptive response time is variable and may be limited to the local area of application; however, some topically applied medications (e.g., nitroglycerin) can have a systemic effect. As a result, products that contain alcohol and hexachlorophene skin washes should be avoided. Any treatment with topical steroids should be limited to less than 2 weeks to prevent adrenal suppression. On the other hand, antibiotic ointments will be more readily absorbed to treat infections, povidone-iodine (Betadine) absorption can prevent iodine deficiency, and topical safflower oil may prevent essential fatty acid deficiency.

(d) Occlusive dressings will increase the extent of absorption.

(5) **Intramuscular/subcutaneous:** administration into muscle or subcutaneous tissue.

(a) Minimal subcutaneous tissue and muscle mass significantly limit these two routes of administration, particularly in the low birth weight neonate.

(b) These routes are limited to medications that do not cause tissue damage at the administration site and are soluble at physiologic pH.

(c) These routes will achieve slower responses as compared with the IV route because of the lag time between administration and achievement of blood concentration.

(d) Response time is dependent on blood flow to muscle and may be greatly delayed in hypoperfused tissue. Poor peripheral blood flow and low blood pressure are common in neonates. These problems become less common with increasing gestational age but can occur in the presence of many neonatal disease states. Poor cardiac output frequently occurs with many illness states in the neonatal period. Subsequent increases in the peripheral perfusion after resolution of the primary illness states may put the neonate at risk of having an increase in the rate and amount of medication absorption.

(e) Diminished muscle activity in the ill neonate decreases muscle perfusion and consequently may limit absorption of medications administered by this route.

(6) **Intravenous:** direct administration into the bloodstream.

(a) Bypasses all absorptive barriers.

(b) Most effective and reliable method of medication administration because the medication is delivered directly to the circulating plasma volume.

(c) Significant medication serum concentrations are reached rapidly, allowing for immediate medication response. This includes both desired and undesired or toxic reactions.

(d) Adequate and equal distribution to all organs or compartments is not guaranteed. Characteristics of some biologic membranes may limit medication distribution to body compartments (e.g., blood-brain barrier).

(e) Rapid achievement of potentially dangerous serum medication concentrations may require administration of the intravenous medication over a prolonged period rather than by intravenous push (e.g., vancomycin, amphotericin, and aminoglycosides).

B. Principles of medication distribution.

1. **Distribution:** movement of the medication to and through various body compartments. The extent of this movement, the "size" of the compartment, the number and character of the binding sites, and the amount of the medication administered determine the amount of medication at the desired site of action. When medication movement reaches a steady state, the volume of distribution is defined as the hypothetical volume of body fluid that would be required to dissolve the total amount of medication as found in the serum. This volume is sometimes described as apparent volume of distribution. This volume may be larger than the total body volume if the medication is highly protein- or tissue-bound.

2. **Body compartments.**

   a. *Total body water:* as age increases, total body water, as a percentage of total body mass, decreases. Total body water in adults comprises approximately 55% of total body weight; in term infants it is 75%, and in preterm infants it is 85% (Kerr et al., 2006).

   (1) As body water increases, as a percentage of body mass, water-soluble medications have a larger volume of distribution.

   (2) Because of increased total body water, a less mature neonate may require a larger per-kilogram dose to achieve the same peak medication concentration and effect as an older patient (e.g., aminoglycosides).

   (3) In the first several days after birth, total body water decreases, causing the volume of intracellular fluid to be increased relative to the amount of extracellular water (Kerr et al., 2006). This leads to rapid changes in the volume of distribution for water-soluble medications, in relation to normal physiology and illness states.

   (4) Body water loss is divided into two main categories: sensible and insensible. Sensible losses can be measured and quantified. In term neonates, insensible losses occur in a strong relationship to metabolism. In extremely premature neonates, insensible losses occur primarily through evaporative loss, independent of metabolic rate. Insensible losses are difficult to quantify (Kerr et al., 2006).

   (5) Medications frequently administered to the neonate (e.g., diuretics, indomethacin) may have a major impact on body water volume and, as a side effect, may alter the volume of distribution (Chemtob, 2004).

   (6) Neonates with disease states that alter water excretion (e.g., primary renal disease, secretion of inappropriate antidiuretic hormone [SIADH], congestive heart failure, capillary leak syndromes) may have expansion of body water as a result of this dysfunction.

   (7) The preceding alterations make dosing medications that are primarily distributed in body water (e.g., aminoglycosides) difficult.

   (8) Frequent monitoring of medication levels may be required as the mentioned changes in body compartment volumes occur.

   b. *Fat:* wide variability of neonatal values, based on gestational age, intrauterine, and postnatal growth patterns. This percentage increases from 1% of body weight at 28 weeks of gestation to approximately 15% in a term neonate (Blackburn, 2007b).

   (1) Medications with more lipid solubility have affinity for this tissue.

   (2) Reduced amounts of the percentage of body fat may make the volume of distribution smaller for medications distributed primarily in fatty tissue. Hence the plasma levels of these medications will be higher because less drug will be bound in the fat tissue, resulting in a greater potential for side effects and toxicity (e.g., morphine, lorazepam).

   c. *Blood components:* potential sites for medication binding.

   (1) Erythrocytes: neonates have 2.5 times more binding sites for digoxin as compared with the erythrocytes in adults. This results in the need for much higher doses per total body weight in neonates than adults (Stewart and Hampton, 1987).

(2) Plasma protein concentrations: medications may form a complex with large circulating molecules (usually proteins).

(a) The amount of medication that binds to these sites has a direct effect on the amount of medication available for the desired pharmacologic effect. This binding may result in a limited medication response because only the unbound medication can be distributed to active receptor sites. When more of the medication is protein-bound, less is available for the desired medication effect: serum concentration = protein-bound medication + unbound medication.

(b) The primary binding protein for acidic medications (e.g., phenytoin, indomethacin, and furosemide) in the serum is albumin (Chemtob, 2004).

(c) Serum albumin levels may be markedly decreased in the ill extremely low birth weight neonate.

(d) The primary binding protein for basic molecules (e.g., lidocaine, propranolol) are lipoproteins, glycoproteins, and β-globulins (Chemtob, 2004).

   d. *Unconjugated bilirubin:* many neonates have increased plasma unconjugated bilirubin levels. Fetal albumin has an increased affinity for bilirubin and a decreased affinity for medications. This causes the unconjugated bilirubin to displace some medications from the albumin-binding sites, making more free medication available for action. In contrast, some medications (e.g., ceftriaxone, sulfonamides) may displace unconjugated bilirubin from albumin-binding sites. This may lead to the deposition of unconjugated bilirubin in the neonatal brain, causing kernicterus (Frank and Frank, 2006). These medications should be avoided if possible in patients younger than 2 months of age or in patients with high unconjugated bilirubin levels.

   e. *Free fatty acids:* increased serum-free fatty acid concentrations have been shown to displace some medications from plasma albumin-binding sites (Chemtob, 2004).

   f. *Blood pH:* acidosis is a common finding associated with many neonatal disorders. Changes in blood pH have been shown to change albumin-binding characteristics. This may cause medication displacement from albumin. Changes in blood pH may also cause medications to displace unconjugated bilirubin (see above).

   g. *Blood-brain barrier:* incomplete in the neonate, causing a greater permeability to lipophilic medications (e.g., phenytoin, benzodiazepines). This incomplete barrier may be beneficial when treating neonatal meningitis because the antibiotics penetrate the cerebrospinal fluid more readily (Kraus and Pham, 2005).

3. **Medication movement:** an important part of medication distribution involves medication movement from the site of administration to sites throughout the body. It is dependent on the blood flow and medication solubility.

   a. *Blood flow:* amount and distribution of blood flow to the target organ or cell affect the delivery of a medication absorbed into the bloodstream. Continued adequate blood flow and serum medication concentration are required to maintain an adequate concentration of the medication at the target organ. Several neonatal conditions affect blood flow:

   (1) Hypotension: may affect peripheral medication absorption and/or distribution.

   (2) Distributive shock: caused by inappropriate vasodilatation; seen with sepsis. Medication distribution to specific organs may be limited by local hypoperfusion.

   (3) Pulmonary hypertension: may impede medication delivery to the pulmonary vascular bed.

   (4) Patent ductus arteriosus: blood flow may be distributed preferentially to either the pulmonary or systemic circulation, depending on the pressure differential.

   (5) Congestive heart failure: may affect peripheral medication absorption or distribution.

   b. *Medication solubility:* in biologic tissues, the relative ability of the medication to dissolve in biologic fluids.

   (1) Medications with low lipid solubility do not distribute well through lipid membranes, though they may be distributed well through the body water spaces. Highly lipid-soluble medications are distributed readily through most lipid membranes but are not distributed well through body water spaces.

(2) The relative medication solubility may make some medication use inappropriate. A medication with low lipid solubility may not reach therapeutic concentrations in an organ that is primarily fat tissue (e.g., aminoglycosides do not readily cross the blood-brain barrier).

C. Principles of medication metabolism.

1. **General principles of medication metabolism.** Many medications must be converted into more water-soluble compounds before they can be removed from the body. Metabolism (biotransformation) is the *chemical change* of a medication into another form. This transformed medication may be pharmacologically active or inactive. The liver, kidney, gastrointestinal tract, lung, adrenal gland, blood, and skin are tissues capable of biotransforming certain compounds. Of these sites, the liver is the principal organ for medication metabolism.

   a. Liver.

      (1) Metabolic activity is divided into two main types.

          (a) Phase I (nonsynthetic) metabolism of medications: primarily oxidation, reduction, hydrolysis, or demethylation reactions, which generally occur in the smooth endoplasmic reticulum of the hepatocyte. The function of these enzymes in the full- and preterm neonate is approximately 50% to 70% of adult values (Stewart and Hampton, 1987). Maturation occurs as a function of chronologic rather than postconceptional age, with a wide range of variability. Maturation of nonsynthetic enzyme systems during the first several days of life requires careful monitoring of serum levels of some classes of medications (e.g., anticonvulsants). For instance, at term gestation, neonates have approximately 30% of adult ability to metabolize phenytoin. Hence the half-life is significantly prolonged. Within several weeks of medication exposure, metabolic enzyme activity for phenytoin surpasses adult activity.

          (b) Phase II (synthetic) metabolism of medications: primarily involves the acetylation, methylation, or conjugation of the medication with another substance. The function of these enzymes is also immature, and they may not reach adult levels in concentration and function until well after the neonatal period.

      (2) Hepatic uptake of the medication is dependent on the concentration of the medication in the liver (dependent on hepatic blood flow) and the hepatocyte concentration of ligandin (Y-protein). This protein is responsible for substrate uptake by hepatic cells.

      (3) In the first-pass effect, hepatic biotransformation may markedly alter medication availability by directly metabolizing medications absorbed from the GI tract, before those medications reach other organs. Slow GI motility may increase the potential for first-pass effect. Prolonged GI transit times may increase potential for hepatic metabolism and eventual excretion of orally administered medications.

      (4) Certain medications (e.g., phenobarbital) are thought to induce enzyme maturity in the fetus and neonate, resulting in increased rates of medication elimination.

      (5) Both hepatic enzyme systems may be vulnerable to hypoxic/ischemic insult.

      (6) Maturational changes in medication metabolism can have a major clinical significance. Careful monitoring of serum levels of some medication classes (e.g., anticonvulsants) is necessary in the first weeks of life.

D. Principles of medication excretion.

1. **General principles of medication excretion.** Excretion is the final elimination of medication from the body. The process of excretion begins with administration of the medication and ends when the medication is completely eliminated from the body. There are several important organs of excretion:

   a. **Salivary, sweat, and mammary glands:** small amounts of medication may be excreted through these minor organs. Very limited sweat production makes excretion by this mode insignificant in the neonate.

   b. **Lungs:** the lungs are an important route of excretion of gaseous anesthetics but are relatively less important for other medications. Excretion by the lungs is not well studied in the neonatal population. Because lung disease is common in newborn infants, adult data indicate that this may affect or limit the ability to excrete medications by this method.

c. **GI tract:** the large, lipid-soluble surface of the GI tract allows diffusion of medications into the bloodstream. The limited motility in neonates affects excretion and increases the potential for reabsorption of medications or metabolites back into the circulation.

d. **Liver:** the most important site of medication biotransformation also serves as an important site of medication excretion. The excretion of bile is an important means of medication elimination.

   (1) Limited oral intake, long-term parenteral nutrition, or intrinsic hepatic disease may reduce bile flow. This may reduce the efficacy of this route of elimination.

   (2) Metabolite or medication elimination in bile is dependent on the solubility characteristics of that substance in bile.

e. **Kidneys:** the most important site for medication excretion.

   (1) *Renal blood flow:*

      (a) Clamping of the umbilical cord is a significant event that signals a major increase in renal blood flow.

      (b) As a percentage of cardiac output, renal blood flow is limited in neonates in comparison with older children and adults. Limited renal blood flow as an absolute value and as a percentage of cardiac output restricts medication or metabolite delivery to the kidney for excretion.

      (c) Renal blood flow increases with increasing gestational and postnatal age.

      (d) High umbilical artery catheter placement may reduce the renal blood flow.

   (2) *Glomerular filtration rate (GFR):* the removal, by passive filtration, of small unbound medication molecules at the glomerulus. Glomerular filtration is dependent on renal blood flow, the characteristics of the glomerular membranes, and the water solubility of the medication.

      (a) The GFR function is extremely limited in neonates as compared with adult values (30% of adult values, per unit of body surface area; reaches adult values by 3 to 5 months of age) (Blackburn, 2007a).

      (b) GFR is related to gestational age; the lower the gestational age, the lower the GFR. Neonates born at less than 34 weeks of gestation have fewer glomeruli, with total glomerular mass proportional to gestational age (Blackburn, 2007a). Nevertheless, glomerular filtration has been shown to mature with postnatal age, independent of gestational age at birth.

      (c) GFR can be further compromised with asphyxia, hypoxia, or indomethacin treatment. Limited glomerular filtration reduces removal of medications or metabolites at the glomerulus.

      (d) Medication excretion dependent on glomerular filtration includes indomethacin, digoxin, aminoglycosides, and vancomycin.

   (3) *Tubular secretion:* the active secretion of molecules into the tubular urine. Tubular secretion is dependent on the efficiency of tubular function.

      (a) Neonates have a relatively small mass of functional tubular cells, as well as an immaturity of tubular function. This functional limitation is thought to be caused in part by a decrease of renal blood flow to the renal tubular region and by shortened renal tubules (Blackburn, 2007b).

      (b) The limitation in tubular mass and function causes poor excretion of medications and metabolites removed by this method.

      (c) Tubular secretion matures much more slowly than glomerular filtration.

      (d) Tubular secretion is also vulnerable to hypoxic-ischemic insult.

      (e) Medications dependent on tubular secretion for excretion include penicillins, morphine, and thiazide diuretics.

   (4) *Tubular reabsorption:* reabsorption, for some medications, back into the circulating plasma.

      (a) May occur through either passive diffusion or active transport.

      (b) Passive diffusion appears to be the most important process.

(c) Tubular reabsorption matures much more slowly than glomerular filtration.

(d) Substances dependent on tubular reabsorption include caffeine, glucose, phosphate, and sodium.

(5) *Urinary output:*

(a) Because of changes in renal blood flow, glomerular filtration, and tubular secretion in the neonate, urinary output is not a reliable sign of renal excretion of medications.

(b) Blood level monitoring is required to ensure safe serum levels of renally excreted medications.

MEDICATION CATEGORIES

Antimicrobial Agents

A. **Introduction.** The use of a larger variety of antimicrobial agents in the neonatal population has occurred in the past several years for several reasons. As the threshold of viability is pushed, the length of stay of NICU infants is increasing. The additional numbers of antibiotic courses, coupled with increasing antibiotic resistance patterns, necessitate more broad-spectrum antibiotic usage as well as increased use of antifungal agents.

B. **Definitions.**

1. **Antimicrobial medications:** medications that inhibit the growth of or kill microorganisms such as bacteria, fungi, viruses, protozoa, and amebae.

   a. Bacteriostatic medications: agents that inhibit the growth of microorganisms, preventing their growth and allowing normal body defense mechanisms to control spread of the organism (e.g., clindamycin, fluconazole).

   b. Bactericidal medications: agents that kill microorganisms. At lower concentrations they may be bacteriostatic (e.g., aminoglycosides, penicillin, cephalosporins).

2. **Minimal inhibitory concentration (MIC):** the lowest concentration of a medication that stops visible organism growth in a laboratory setting. In the body this cannot be directly measured and is dependent on achieved tissue concentration and bacterial count. This is easily measured in the microbiology laboratory and is used to measure the susceptibility of the microorganism to antimicrobial agents.

3. **Minimal bactericidal concentration (MBC):** the lowest concentration of a medication that results in an equal to or more than 99.9% decline in microbial number, measured in the laboratory setting. It is useful when compared with known potential toxic concentration levels to choose the antimicrobial regimen that does the greatest good with the fewest adverse or toxic effects.

4. **Resistance:** the ability of microorganisms to counteract the bacteriostatic or bactericidal effects of an antimicrobial agent.

   a. Resistance interferes with the medication's action either through changes in the microorganism's cellular structure or through production of enzymes that reduce antimicrobial activity.

   b. Microorganisms develop resistance by:

      (1) Enzymes: microorganisms produce various enzymes to inactivate antimicrobial agents (e.g., β-lactamase inactivates penicillins and cephalosporins).

      (2) Decreased cellular penetration: microorganisms alter their cell wall permeability to prevent penetration of antimicrobial agents into the cell (e.g., *Pseudomonas aeruginosa* alters porin channels to limit the entry of ceftazidime, imipenem-cilastatin).

      (3) Altered target proteins: microorganisms change target proteins so that antimicrobial agents cannot bind and elicit antimicrobial activity (e.g., *Streptococcus pneumoniae*'s resistance to penicillin).

      (4) Efflux pump: microorganisms pump the antimicrobial agent out of the cell before the antimicrobial agent can kill the microorganism (e.g., *Streptococcus pneumoniae*'s resistance to erythromycin).

C. **Basic principles of antimicrobial use.**

1. Antibiotics must reach the target tissue in a concentration adequate to inhibit the growth of or to kill the desired microorganism. This concentration:

      a. Ideally would be such that it would have limited side effects or toxic effects on target tissues or the patient as a whole.

      b. Must be readily achievable and sustainable for the desired duration of antimicrobial therapy.

  2. The choice of antimicrobial agent(s) must be taken into account:

      a. Microorganism susceptibility to available antimicrobial agents.

      b. Relative permeability of the target tissue to agent of choice (e.g., blood-brain barrier).

      c. Bioactivity of chosen antimicrobial agent in target tissue (e.g., bactericidal or bacteriostatic).

      d. Known MIC/MBC in relation to existing body of knowledge concerning side effects and toxic effects in the specific population.

      e. Specific characteristics of the individual patient in relation to the chosen antimicrobial's toxicities (e.g., the blood levels of a nephrotoxic antimicrobial such as gentamicin should be closely monitored in patients with impaired renal function).

D. Specific considerations in the neonatal population.

  1. Pharmacodynamics.

      a. Tissue concentration of medication may be altered by clinical and physiologic conditions that may increase or decrease bioavailability of the medication in the target tissue (e.g., cerebrospinal fluid penetration by antibiotics may be excellent early in meningitis. As meningeal inflammatory response subsides, penetration into the cerebrospinal fluid diminishes).

      b. Differences in response or potential for toxic effects may result from immaturity and/or illness state.

  2. Pharmacokinetics.

      a. To optimize the probability of response to antibiotics, the unpredictable pharmacokinetic influences should be minimized; hence, the intravenous (IV) route is preferred for septic patients.

      b. Absorption.

         (1) Changes in GI-tract pH affect absorption of oral medication: may be increased or decreased (e.g., oral penicillin G is absorbed better in neonates than in older infants and children because of increased gastric pH).

         (2) Changes in skin permeability in the extremely immature neonate may allow topically applied antimicrobial agents to be absorbed systemically.

         (3) Blood flow changes may affect absorption and distribution of antimicrobials administered intramuscularly or subcutaneously (e.g., repeated intramuscular administration of aminoglycosides to premature neonates may result in local tissue damage and unacceptably variable rates of absorption).

      c. Distribution: Decreasing body water and increasing body fat concentration in more mature neonates affect the volume through which the antimicrobial agent is distributed. This may make dosage adjustments necessary in the first days of life.

      d. Metabolism: Limited hepatic function, because of immaturity or illness state, may affect dosage regimen of some antibiotics, requiring smaller or less frequent doses of some antibiotics (e.g., nafcillin, erythromycin).

      e. Excretion: Limited renal function with lower gestational age may prolong the half-life of antimicrobials excreted by the kidneys (e.g., aminoglycosides, cephalosporins, penicillins, vancomycin). This limited renal function (GFR and tubular secretion) commonly improves significantly in the first few days of life and with advancing chronologic age. For this reason, serum antibiotic levels must be monitored closely and dosage adjustments made accordingly.

Cardiovascular Agents

A. Introduction.

  1. A broad group of medications that affect the regulation, inhibition, or stimulation of the cardiovascular system.

  2. The use of cardiovascular agents is increasing in the care of neonates.

B. **Basic principles of cardiovascular medication use.**
   1. The wide range of pharmacologic actions of this class of medications requires specific in-depth knowledge about each medication and about concurrent medication therapy.
   2. Knowledge of the pathophysiologic basis of neonatal cardiovascular disease is necessary to ensure proper application of this class of medications.
   3. Many of these medications have overlapping or synergistic effects. This overlap in clinical response makes the optimal choice of a medication and dose difficult.
   4. Extensive knowledge and application of invasive and noninvasive cardiovascular monitoring techniques in the neonatal population are necessary to allow titration of the medication dose to the clinical response.
C. **Types of cardiovascular medications.**
   1. Inotropic/vasopressive agents.
      a. Includes a broad range of medications that act to improve cardiac output by increasing the heart rate (chronotropic effect), increasing the force of myocardial contraction (inotropic effect) and the vascular tone.
      b. Used both for cardiovascular resuscitation and long-term support of the myocardium.
      c. Specific inotropic agents:
         (1) Digitalis glycosides (e.g., digoxin). Inhibits the sodium/potassium pump to increase intracellular calcium, thus increasing myocardial contractility. It also decreases conduction through the sinoatrial (SA) and atrioventricular (AV) nodes to slow the ventricular rate in tachyarrhythmias.
         (2) Sympathomimetic amines (e.g., epinephrine, dopamine, dobutamine, isoproterenol).
            (a) Clinical responses stimulated by this group of medications are classified according to their effects on the "receptors" in the body. These receptors are categorized as either α-, β-, or dopamine types.
               (i) α_1-adrenergic receptor response: contractions of vascular smooth muscle and constriction of blood vessels.
               (ii) α_2-adrenergic receptor response: activation of central nervous system (CNS) receptors in the brain to suppress outflow of the sympathetic nervous system activity from the brain. Results in decreased motility and tone of intestine and stomach.
               (iii) β_1-adrenergic receptor response: increased strength and rate of myocardial contraction.
               (iv) β_2-adrenergic receptor response: vascular smooth muscle dilation and bronchial muscle relaxation.
               (v) Five different dopamine receptors are located in multiple organs and have mixed actions involving motor function, cardiovascular (e.g., vasodilating properties), renal (e.g., intrarenal vasodilator), behavioral, and hormonal (e.g., prolactin secretion) systems.
            For example, epinephrine increases blood pressure by stimulating the α_1- and β_1-receptors. Dobutamine increases cardiac output by stimulating the β_1-receptors.
            (b) Response to each of these medications depends on relative amounts of α-, β-, and dopamine effects.
            (c) Prolonged administration of sympathomimetic amines may result in diminished clinical efficacy secondary to diminished responses of α- and β-receptors, referred to as tachyphylaxis.
   2. Antihypertensives/vasodilators.
      a. Used to normalize blood pressure in patients with hypertension, reduce vascular resistance in patients with poor myocardial function, and reduce pulmonary vascular resistance in conditions associated with pulmonary hypertension.
      b. May be used to inhibit pathophysiologic changes that cause increased blood pressure (e.g., captopril, propranolol) or directly reduce blood pressure through changes in intravascular volume (e.g., diuretics) or vascular resistance (e.g., hydralazine).

    3. Antiarrhythmics.
        a. Used to treat cardiac dysrhythmias causing adverse effects on cardiovascular stability.
        b. Includes adenosine, digoxin, esmolol, and lidocaine.

D. Specific considerations in the neonatal population.
    1. Pharmacodynamics.
        a. Specific in-depth knowledge about neonatal cardiovascular physiology and pathophysiology is required to determine the need for these medications.
        b. Cardiovascular medications are commonly used in conjunction with other medications that may affect the neonate's response to the medication regimen (e.g., the digoxin-furosemide combination may result in electrolyte loss with the diuretic, which in turn may potentiate a toxic response to the digoxin).
    2. Pharmacokinetics.
        a. Absorption: Many cardiovascular medications cannot be given effectively through any significant absorptive barrier. For this reason, IV administration is necessary in many cases (e.g., pressors, inotropes).
        b. Distribution.
            (1) Poor cardiac output/shock states may affect the distribution of medication to all tissues.
            (2) Medication administered for a desired response to one target organ may cause an undesirable systemic response (e.g., dobutamine increases cardiac output but may cause decreased blood pressure, furosemide reduces pulmonary edema but may decrease blood pressure).
            (3) Some cardiovascular medications are highly albumin-bound; this raises the possibility of unconjugated bilirubin displacement from albumin.
        c. Metabolism.
            (1) Hepatic metabolic activity may markedly affect the bioavailability of the medication (e.g., the high rate of first-pass metabolism of oral propranolol causes the IV and oral dosing to be significantly different).
            (2) Medication metabolites may cause a toxic response (e.g., cyanide liberation as a result of nitroprusside metabolism).
            (3) Rapid metabolism and serum clearance may require continuous IV infusion (e.g., dopamine, dobutamine).
        d. Excretion: Impaired renal function will markedly affect the excretion of some medications (e.g., captopril, furosemide). This requires careful monitoring of the clinical response and serum medication levels.

CENTRAL NERVOUS SYSTEM (CNS) MEDICATIONS

A. Introduction.
    1. In adult patients, these are the most widely used group of medications.
    2. The value of pain control and mood alteration in the neonatal population has only recently been recognized.
    3. Recent increased interest in the use of CNS medications in the neonatal population has caused a recognition that the body of knowledge about these medications is limited.
    4. The use of these medications is increasing as neurobehavioral assessment skills increase among neonatal caregivers.

B. Definitions.
    1. Analgesic medication: a medication (e.g., morphine, acetaminophen) that provides diminished sensation of pain. These help to promote control of undesirable responses to a painful event.
    2. Anesthetic medication: a medication that removes pain sensation either through peripheral nerve block (e.g., lidocaine) or through CNS effects (e.g., high-dose fentanyl). Not all anesthetic medications provide pain relief (e.g., inhalation gases, propofol).
    3. Sedative/hypnotic medications: medications that provide mood alteration in patients with anxiety. These are divided into two groups: barbiturates (e.g., phenobarbital) and nonbar-

biturates (e.g., chloral hydrate, lorazepam). These medications do not provide relief from pain.

4. Addiction: a lifestyle change that occurs in a medication-dependent person. This lifestyle change involves a focus on medication use. This behavior cannot occur in a neonate.

5. Tolerance: a condition that may occur with many types of medications. Tolerance exists when larger doses and higher serum concentrations of the medication are required to achieve the desired response, and commonly occurs in conjunction with physical dependence.

6. Dependence: a physiologic state in which the individual requires regular medication administration for continued physiologic well-being. Patients who develop dependence to a medication may need a dosage-tapering regimen rather than abruptly discontinuing the medication in order to prevent withdrawal symptoms. In neonates, dependence can develop from either placental transfer of medications or iatrogenically due to long-term infusions of sedatives and/or narcotics.

C. **Basic principles of CNS medication use.**
1. Mechanism of action of most CNS medications is not clearly understood.
2. Assessment of need for these medications must be carefully performed as an ongoing process.
   a. Close attention must be paid to differentiation of need for sedation, pain relief, or both.
   b. These medications may cause the development of medication tolerance and/or dependence.
3. Consideration must be made for the risks and benefits of the medication in relation to potential side effects or toxicities.
4. The science of the study of neonatal neurologic development is still emerging, and much is yet to be learned. The effect that CNS medications may have on that development is largely unknown.

D. **Specific considerations in the neonatal population.**
1. Pharmacodynamics.
   a. Limited knowledge of CNS development in premature and term neonates mandates a special need for caution in the use of CNS-active medications.
   b. Specific physiologic characteristics in the neonatal population require careful observation for harmful side effects or toxicities (e.g., reduction in blood pressure with IV bolus doses of morphine, chest wall rigidity with fentanyl).
   c. Narcotic analgesics may cause respiratory depression and may precipitate respiratory failure in neonates. Therefore the lowest possible dose that relieves the patient's pain should be used.
   d. Careful assessment of clinical response is necessary to determine the most safe and effective dose and interval.
2. Pharmacokinetics.
   a. Absorption.
      (1) Poor GI motility and high first-pass clearance may make oral administration highly unpredictable for many medications (e.g., morphine).
      (2) Oral or rectal absorption of mild analgesics and sedatives is often adequate (e.g., acetaminophen).
   b. Distribution.
      (1) Because these agents work in the CNS, they must be lipid soluble in order to cross the blood-brain barrier.
      (2) As neonates increase their proportion of body fat, the doses required will increase.
      (3) Because these agents are stored in the body fat, patients must be monitored for the accumulation of these agents and hence prolonged effects.
   c. Metabolism.
      (1) Slower hepatic metabolism may cause a prolonged half-life.
      (2) Hepatic disease may markedly increase the risk of toxic effects (e.g., chloral hydrate).

(3) Hepatic metabolism may convert medications to either toxic metabolites or active metabolites (e.g., theophylline converts to caffeine).
   d. Excretion.
      (1) Limited renal function or failure may cause toxic effects as a result of accumulation of medication or metabolites (e.g., seizures from penicillin, nephrotoxicity from aminoglycosides).
      (2) Medication may have a direct effect on renal function.
         (a) Blood flow to kidney may be diminished (e.g., amphotericin can cause renal artery vasospasms).
         (b) Urinary output may be diminished (e.g., indomethacin reduces the glomerular filtration rate).

Diuretics

A. **Introduction.**
   1. Commonly used in neonatal patients to promote the removal of excessive extracellular fluid.
   2. Site of action of nearly all diuretic agents is the luminal surface of the renal tubular cell.
B. **Basic principles of diuretic use.**
   1. Use must be based on a thorough understanding of the functions of the various segments of the nephron in the neonatal population.
   2. Diuretic medications whose primary purpose is to cause the excretion of excess extracellular fluid commonly cause a secondary or side effect of loss of electrolytes, along with the desired water loss. Knowledge of the specific action of each diuretic medication will assist the clinician in monitoring electrolytes for undesirable losses.
   3. The pharmacologic response is dependent on the existing level of renal function and the medication's ability to reach the target tissue in amounts adequate to produce the desired diuretic effect.
   4. Any medication or therapy that increases the glomerular filtration rate may have an indirect diuretic effect. Some medications that act on the cardiovascular system to increase cardiac output or increase renal blood flow through vasodilation may cause diuresis (e.g., dopamine). Maximal water and electrolyte excretion usually occurs in the first days of use. Later, decreased GFR and hyperaldosteronism resulting from diuretic-induced hypovolemia limit these losses.
C. **Specific considerations in the neonatal population.**
   1. Pharmacodynamics.
      a. Many diuretic medications are dependent on reaching the lumen of the proximal tubule to achieve diuresis.
      b. The renal tubular function is limited in all neonates and is more limited in less mature neonates.
      c. The clinical response to diuretic agents is commonly decreased because of existing poor renal tubular absorption. Therefore a larger dose is needed to achieve the response.
      d. Limited tubular function potentiates electrolyte loss with many diuretic agents (e.g., furosemide, hydrochlorothiazide).
   2. Pharmacokinetics.
      a. Absorption. Oral absorption may be limited, requiring a larger per-kilogram dose as compared with the IV dose to achieve the desired effect (e.g., furosemide). Other diuretics (e.g., hydrochlorothiazide, spironolactone) are well absorbed orally.
      b. Distribution. Some diuretic medications are strongly protein-bound. Some concern has been raised over the displacement of bilirubin from albumin-binding sites (e.g., furosemide, spironolactone).
      c. Metabolism. Some diuretics are primarily metabolized by the liver (e.g., spironolactone).
      d. Excretion.
         (1) Low renal blood flow and low glomerular filtration rate, along with limited renal tubular function, may delay excretion and limit the effectiveness of the medication

(e.g., the plasma clearance of furosemide is prolonged in extremely premature neonates and in neonates with renal failure).

(2) Some diuretics are primarily eliminated unchanged in the urine (e.g., furosemide, hydrochlorothiazide).

Immunizations

A. **Introduction.**
  1. Vaccines are commonly given to the hospitalized neonatal patient.
  2. Each year in January, the Centers for Disease Control and Prevention (CDC)'s Advisory Committee on Immunization Practices publishes an updated version of the recommended immunization guidelines. Each nurse should be familiar with these guidelines.
  3. The following documentation is required when vaccines are given:
     a. Name, title, and business address of person administering the vaccine.
     b. Vaccine administered.
     c. Manufacturer of the vaccine.
     d. Lot number of the vaccine.
     e. Expiration date of vaccine.
     f. Date of administration.
     g. Site of administration.
     h. Route of administration.
     i. Documentation that the vaccine information statement (VIS) has been given to the parents/guardians.
     j. Documentation of the VIS publication date (the most current version must be used).

B. **Basic principles of immunization use.**
  1. The goal of immunization is to prevent many viral and bacterial diseases and their sequelae.
  2. For maximum effectiveness, the immunizations must be given at specific ages before the recipients have been exposed to the diseases.
  3. Live vaccines (e.g., measles-mumps-rubella [MMR], rotavirus, varicella) should NOT be administered in the NICU.
  4. All adverse events associated with immunization should be reported in detail in the patient's medical record and also on the vaccine adverse event reporting system (VAERS) form found on the U.S. Food and Drug Administration (FDA) Web site.

C. **Types of immunizations.**
  1. Active immunization.
     a. Involves the administration of all or part of a microorganism or a modified product of that microorganism to evoke an immunologic response mimicking that of natural infection. This usually presents little or no risk to the recipient.
     b. Some immunizing agents provide complete protection against disease for life (e.g., polio vaccine), some provide partial protection (e.g., influenza vaccine), and some must be readministered at intervals (booster doses) (e.g., tetanus vaccine).
     c. Vaccines may be either live (attenuated) or killed (inactivated). Inactivated vaccines may not elicit the range of immunologic response provided by attenuated agents.
  2. Passive immunization.
     a. Involves the administration of preformed antibody to a recipient.
     b. Most often used when a person exposed to a disease has a high likelihood of complications from that disease and time does not permit adequate protection by active immunization alone.
     c. Can be used when a disease is already present with the hope of reducing the reaction to the disease.
     d. Accomplished through the use of immune globulin preparations (e.g., hepatitis B immune globulin, palivizumab, varicella immune globulin).
     e. There are strict indications for the use of these products (American Academy of Pediatrics [AAP], 2006).

D. Specific considerations in the neonatal population.
  1. Pharmacodynamics.
     a. Most immunizations are usually given starting at 2 months of age; the immune response to the vaccines may be limited if given before this age. Resistance to certain diseases before this time may be provided from the mother's antibodies that are transferred across the placenta.
     b. Preterm infants who are medically stable should receive the immunizations at the recommended chronologic age as long as the following are met:
        (1) The infant does not require ongoing treatment for serious infections or metabolic disease.
        (2) The infant does not have acute renal, cardiovascular, or respiratory illness.
        (3) The infant demonstrates a clinical course of sustained recovery and pattern of steady growth (AAP, 2006).
     c. The dose should NOT be decreased in preterm infants.
     d. Antibody titers may be measured to prove adequate immune responses.
  2. Pharmacokinetics.
     a. Absorption.
        (1) Injectable vaccines should be administered in sites that limit the risk of neural, vascular, or tissue injury.
        (2) The preferred site for administration is the anterolateral aspect of the upper thigh.
        (3) The deltoid area of the upper arm can be used in older infants (> 1 year).
        (4) The upper, outer aspect of the buttocks should not be routinely used because of the possibility of damaging the sciatic nerve and reduced immunogenicity.
        (5) When necessary, two vaccines can be given in the same limb but should be separated by at least 1 inch if possible so that local reactions are not likely to overlap.
        (6) The recommended routes of administration are included in the package inserts of the vaccines (e.g., intramuscular [IM], subcutaneous [SC]).
     b. Distribution. Vaccines should be held when the neonate is on pressor agents because the blood flow to the muscle and subcutaneous tissues may be limited.
     c. Metabolism/Excretion: Kidney and/or liver failure should not prevent the administration of vaccines.
E. Misconceptions about vaccine contraindications: The nurse should be familiar with the specific contraindications listed in the package inserts of the vaccines so that immunizations are not withheld unnecessarily (AAP, 2006).

NURSING IMPLICATIONS FOR MEDICATION ADMINISTRATION IN THE NEONATE

There are several areas in which the nursing staff are an invaluable resource for the patient in helping to prevent errors in this fragile patient population.
A. Correct order-writing policies should be followed to reduce the potential for error. Unapproved abbreviations should be avoided, trailing zeros should be avoided (e.g., 1.0), leading decimals should be used (e.g., 0.1), and all verbal orders should be read back to the physician for clarification.
B. Standard concentrations for IV continuous infusions should be used rather than relying on concentrations based on weight.
C. Double check of medication doses involves recalculating the weight-based doses and comparing written doses with current medication dosing reference books to prevent potential medication dosing errors. In addition, new technology that involves dosing ranges for continuous IV infusions should be used with the IV pumps to avoid programmable errors.
D. Cross-checking on a regular basis is a nursing responsibility. Because of the very small volumes of medications commonly given to the NICU patient, a system for regular cross-checking of medications' volume accuracy with medication concentration before administration should be established for all medications and especially with high-risk medications.

E. **Monitoring renal function through intake and output measurements** may alert the care team to potential changes in medication metabolism and/or excretion.

F. **Meticulous medication dosing and precise documentation** involves giving the medication at the correct time and at the correct time interval, which is essential for the maximal desired effect by many medications, with minimal undesired effects. Documenting the medication administration date, time, dose, route, and interval and the time medication levels are obtained are important in interpreting patient response to therapy.

G. **Facilitation of medication serum level monitoring with absolute accuracy** makes safe administration of medications—with a narrow margin between effective and toxic levels—possible.

H. **Careful assessment of vital sign parameters and clinical responses** may assist in the evaluation of desirable or undesirable medication responses.

I. **Careful observation of the neonate for therapeutic and toxic medication effects** will allow medication administration to achieve the maximal desired response while minimizing toxic responses.

J. **Monitoring renal function through intake and output measurements** may alert the care team to potential changes in medication metabolism and/or excretion.

K. **Medication precautions** must be observed. Any medication or medication preparation known to have a high risk of adverse effects in the neonate should be removed from the patient care area (e.g., concentrated potassium vials) or should be specifically labeled to avoid inadvertent administration.

L. **Facilitation of or participation in clinical trials** designed to evaluate a medication's efficacy does much to advance the body of knowledge related to neonatal pharmacology.

M. **Recognition of established clinical experience with individual medications in the neonatal population is essential.** Because some medications are introduced into the clinical area after only minimal study of specific medication response in the neonate, early observation of potential toxic effects may avert a later disaster.

REFERENCES

American Academy of Pediatrics: Active and passive immunization. In L.K. Pickering (Ed.): *2006 Red Book: Report of the Committee on Infectious Diseases* (27th ed.). Elk Grove Village, IL, 2006, American Academy of Pediatrics, pp. 1-103.

Blackburn, S.T.: Gastrointestinal and hepatic systems and perinatal nutrition. In *Maternal, fetal, & neonatal physiology: A clinical perspective* (3rd ed.). St. Louis, 2007a, Saunders, pp. 443-472.

Blackburn, S.T.: Renal system and fluid and electrolyte homeostasis. In *Maternal, fetal, & neonatal physiology: A clinical perspective* (3rd ed.). St. Louis, 2007b, Saunders, pp. 395-410.

Chemtob, S.: Basic pharmacologic principles. In R.A. Polin, W.W. Fox, and S.H. Abman (Eds.): *Fetal and neonatal physiology*. Philadelphia, 2004, Saunders, pp. 179-190.

Frank, C.G. and Frank, P.H.: Jaundice. In G.B. Merenstein and S.L. Gardner (Eds.): *Handbook of neonatal intensive care* (6th ed.). St. Louis, 2006, Mosby, pp. 548-568.

Hoath, S.B.: Physiologic development of the skin. In R.A. Polin, W.W. Fox, and S.H. Abman (Eds.): *Fetal and neonatal physiology*. Philadelphia, 2004, Saunders, pp. 597-611.

Kerr, B.A., Starbuck, A.L., and Block S.M.: Fluid and electrolyte management. In G.B. Merenstein and S.L. Gardner (Eds.): *Handbook of neonatal intensive care* (6th ed.). St. Louis, 2006, Mosby, pp. 351-367.

Kraus, D.M. and Pham, J.T.: Neonatal therapy. In M. Koda-Kimble and L. Young (Eds.): *Applied therapeutics: The clinical use of drugs*. Baltimore, 2005, Lippincott Williams & Wilkins, pp. 94-1–94-53.

Nahata, M.C. and Taketomo, C.: Pediatrics. In J.T. Dipiro, R.L. Talbert, G.C. Yee, et al. (Eds.): *Pharmacotherapy: A pathophysiologic approach*. New York, 2005, McGraw-Hill, pp. 91-101.

Stewart, C.F. and Hampton, E.M.: Effect of maturation on drug disposition in pediatric patients. *Clinical Pharmacy*, 6(7):548-564, 1987.

13 Laboratory Concepts and Test Interpretation

DIANE M. SZLACHETKA

OBJECTIVES

1. Identify the types of laboratory testing in the neonatal intensive care unit (NICU).
2. Discuss the purpose of laboratory testing and diagnostics.
3. Review the process of specimen collection and the principles of test utilization.
4. Review the principles of laboratory interpretation.
5. Describe iatrogenic sequelae associated with laboratory testing and diagnostic procedures.
6. Discuss strategies to minimize iatrogenic sequelae associated with laboratory testing and diagnostic procedures.
7. Discuss the decision-making process of ordering and interpreting laboratory values—a decision tree.

Newborns delivered in the United States receive an average of one or two laboratory tests, typically in the form of screening for genetic disorders and birth defects. In addition, all infants admitted to the NICU require laboratory testing to assess their clinical status. Given the U.S. birth rate of 4.28 million infants (CDC, 2007) and average NICU admission rates of 8% to 12% of live births (Ferguson, 2001; Schwartz et al., 2000), this translates to a minimum of 8 million screening/laboratory tests per year.

It has been estimated that 10% to 15% of the U.S. national health budget is spent on laboratory testing, constituting 15% to 20% of each patient's hospital bill (Sacher et al., 2000a). The impact of laboratory testing on the patient, health care, and its cost is significant.

Because all health care workers in the NICU are in some way involved in obtaining laboratory samples, understanding the principles of laboratory testing and the contribution of laboratory tests to patient care and cost is essential. Developing skills in laboratory interpretation at the NICU bedside provides a key element in comprehensive patient care.

This chapter features a review of the types and purposes of laboratory testing in the NICU, describes principles of laboratory testing and interpretation, and discusses potential iatrogenic sequelae. Included is a discussion of strategies to avoid sequelae, when to obtain laboratory testing, and a strategy to interpret results for patient care. A decision-making process for laboratory testing and interpretation is presented.

LABORATORY TESTS IN THE NICU

A. Laboratory testing occurs daily in the NICU. Why and when laboratory testing is performed is driven by patient history and presenting symptoms. By one estimate, 70% of all medical decisions are based on laboratory results (Kurec and Lifshitz, 2006). Data obtained from laboratory analysis assist clinicians in determining diagnosis, measuring success of treatment, and monitoring trends in an infant's clinical course. The common laboratory tests performed in the NICU include the following (see Table 13-1):

1. Chemistry analysis: serum tests that measure the chemical activity or state of the body. Serum is the byproduct of clotted blood that is centrifuged to remove the clot and any other cells (Laposata, 2002). Chemical substances reflect metabolic processes and disease

■ TABLE 13-1
Common Laboratory Tests in the NICU by System

Fluids Electrolytes Nutrition	Respiratory	Cardiac	Gastrointestinal	Renal	Endocrine/ Metabolic	Neurologic	Hematologic	Other
Electrolytes (serum)	Blood gas	Isoenzymes	Alkaline phosphatase	BUN (serum)	Thyroxine level	Phenobarbital level	CBC w/differential	Chromosome levels
Calcium (serum)	pH		Triglyceride levels	Creatinine (serum)	Thyroid-stimulating hormone level	Dilantin level	Hct	Buccal smear
Magnesium (serum)	$PaCO_2$		AST (SGOT)	Specific gravity	Cortisol level	Ammonia (serum)	Plt	CRP
Phosphorus (serum)	Pao_2		ALT (SGPT)	Urine sodium	Insulin level	Amino acid (serum)	Plt antibody	Drug levels
Alkaline phosphorus	Bicarbonate (HCO_3)		GGT (GGTP)	Urine potassium	Growth hormone level	Amino acid (urine)	Reticulocyte count	Urine toxicology screen
Glucose (serum) level	Base excess		Bilirubin (total and direct)	Urine osmolality	Testosterone level	Organic acids (urine)	Direct Coombs'	Cultures (all sources)
Vitamin levels	Theophylline level		Ammonia (serum)	Drug levels	Aldosterone (serum and urine) level	Glycine (serum and CSF)	Blood type	RPR
Serum osmolality	Caffeine level		α_1-antitrypsin	Uric acid (serum)	17-hydroxy corticosteroids	Pyridoxine level	G6PD	Occult blood (fecal)
Albumin (serum)			Trypsin (stool)	Urinalysis	Parathyroid hormone level	Lactic acid	Sedimentation rate	PCR (serum)
Total protein			Pyridoxine level				Folic acid	
							Fibrinogen	
							PT	
							PTT	
							Immunoglobulins	
							Methemoglobin	

ALT, Alanine aminotransferase (SGPT); *AST*, aspartate aminotransferase (SGOT); *BUN*, blood urea nitrogen; *CBC*, complete blood count; *CRP*, C-reactive protein; *CSF*, cerebrospinal fluid; *GGT*, gamma-glutamyl transferase; *G6PD*, glucose-6-phosphate dehydrogenase; *Hct*, hematocrit; *PCR*, polymerase chain reaction; *Plt*, platelet; *PT*, prothrombin time; *PTT*, partial thromboplastin time; *RPR*, rapid plasma reagin.

states in the body. Measuring changes in chemical concentrations (chemical substances) is useful in diagnosis, planning care, monitoring of therapy, screening, and determining the severity of disease and response to treatment.

   a. Four categories (Sacher et al., 2000b).

     (1) Chemical substances normally present with function in the circulation. Laboratory examples: electrolytes, calcium, magnesium, phosphorus, total proteins, albumin, hormones, and vitamins.

     (2) Metabolites: nonfunctioning waste products in process of being cleared. Laboratory examples: bilirubin, ammonia, blood urea nitrogen (BUN), creatinine, and uric acid.

     (3) Substances released from cells as a result of cell damage and abnormal permeability or abnormal cellular proliferation. Laboratory examples: alkaline phosphatase, alanine aminotransferase (ALT), aspartate aminotransferase (AST), and creatinine kinase.

     (4) Drug and toxic substances. Laboratory examples: antibiotics, theophylline, caffeine, digoxin, phenobarbital, and substances of abuse.

2. Hematologic tests: study of the blood and blood-forming tissues of the body such as the bone marrow and reticuloendothelial system (Sacher et al., 2000c). This area of testing also includes the study of hemoglobin structure, red cell membrane, and red cell enzyme activity. Whole blood is composed of blood cells suspended in plasma fluid (see also Chapter 31). Plasma is unclotted blood that has been centrifuged to remove any cells (Laposata, 2002). Plasma contains the protein fibrinogen, which is converted to the substance composing the fibrin clot (Farmer and Kee, 2005).

   a. Blood cells: erythrocytes (red blood cells), leukocytes (white blood cells), and thrombocytes (platelets). Laboratory examples: hematocrit (Hct), reticulocyte (Retic) count, platelet (Plt) count, peripheral blood smear, complete blood count (CBC), Kleihauer-Betke test, white blood cell (WBC) count, and WBC differential count.

   b. Plasma: plasma proteins, coagulation factors I through XIII, immunoglobulins. Laboratory examples: total protein, albumin, fibrinogen (factor I), prothrombin (factor II), partial thromboplastin time (factor III), factors IV through XIII assays, immunoglobulin G (IgG), A (IgA), and M (IgM).

3. Microbiology tests: identification of infectious microorganisms causing disease. Tests include diagnostic bacteriology, mycology, virology, parasitology, and serology. Laboratory examples: culture of any body fluid, bacterial stain, and bacteria antigen detection.

4. Microscopy tests: examination of body fluids and tissues under a microscope. Laboratory examples: cell counts, fecal blood, fecal fat, Apt test, and urinalysis.

5. Blood bank tests (transfusion medicine): area of blood component preparation, blood donor screening and testing, blood compatibility testing, and blood and stem cell banking.

   a. Commonly used blood components in the NICU:

     (1) Whole blood: hematocrit (approximately 35%) typically low for infants.

       (a) Used for large-volume replacement in surgery.

       (b) Used for extracorporeal membrane oxygenator (ECMO) pump.

     (2) Packed red blood cells: spun blood with supernatant removed to concentrate red blood cells, approximately Hct 70%.

       (a) Reconstituted to an average Hct 50% and used for blood transfusions in the treatment of anemia.

       (b) Used in exchange transfusions.

     (3) Platelets: platelets separated from donor blood and stored suspended in plasma.

       (a) Often spun to concentrate platelets in smaller volume.

       (b) Used for platelet replacement in thrombocytopenia.

     (4) Fresh frozen plasma: plasma separated from blood cells and stored frozen. Has some fibrinogen but cryoprecipitate is a better source.

       (a) Used for clotting factor replacement, rich in factors VIII and IX and contains other stable and labile coagulation factors.

       (b) Used in the treatment of disseminated intravascular coagulopathy (DIC).

(5) Granulocytes: WBCs removed from fresh donor blood.

(a) Used to replace WBCs in cases of severe neutropenia.

(6) Cryoprecipitate: a plasma preparation rich in factor VIII and XIII, and fibrinogen.

(a) Used in the treatment of hemophilia.

(b) Used in the treatment of DIC.

b. Common blood bank tests:

(1) Blood typing and crossmatch.

(2) Direct antiglobulin test (DAT).

(3) Indirect antiglobulin test (IAT).

(4) Erythrocyte Rosette test, Kleihauer-Betke test for fetomaternal hemorrhage.

6. Immunoassays: laboratory method based on antigen-antibody reactions employed in therapeutic drug monitoring, toxicology screening, detection of plasma proteins, and certain endocrine testing. Laboratory examples: urine and meconium toxicology test for "street drugs," latex agglutination test, and drug levels.

7. Cytogenetic tests: testing used to determine genetic composition by chromosome analysis. Laboratory examples: simple karyotype (blood, amniotic fluid, tissue, bone marrow, buccal swab), chromosome-specific probes, and fluorescence in situ hybridization (FISH).

8. Immunology tests: laboratory evaluation measuring immune system activity (Sacher et al., 2000d). This consists of complement activity and its cascade of activation, humoral, and cell-mediated immunity. Tests are used to diagnose inflammatory responses, immunodeficiency, and autoimmune disorders. Laboratory examples: C-reactive protein, cytokine measurement, complement C3 and C4, IgG, IgM, and IgA.

PURPOSE OF LABORATORY TESTING

A. Laboratory testing in the NICU is multidimensional. The rationale for selecting, ordering, and interpreting laboratory tests needs to be scrutinized (considered) in order to maximize patient care, minimize patient risk, and contain health care costs. The purpose of laboratory testing is to:

1. Determine the health state of the patient.

2. Monitor the clinical status, trends, and disease severity.

3. Assist in a differential diagnosis.

4. Confirm a diagnosis or cure.

5. Screen for common disorders and disease prevention.

6. Measure the effect of therapy.

7. Assist in the management of disease.

8. Establish a prognosis.

9. Assist in genetic counseling.

10. Evaluate specific events—example: medication errors, sudden clinical decompensation, medical–legal problems, and postmortem tests.

PROCESS OF LABORATORY COLLECTION

A. Collection of laboratory specimens requires meticulous technique to ensure the best possible results. Proper technique, source of laboratory sample, use of collection tubes, labeling, and laboratory processing combine to play a key role in patient treatment, in minimizing blood loss and painful stimuli, and in reducing the costs of NICU care. Anticipatory pain management is needed prior to heel sticks, venipuncture, and arterial puncture (American Academy of Pediatrics [AAP], 2007; Folk, 2007; see also Chapter 16) as well as other specimen collection procedures such as lumbar puncture and suprapubic bladder tap.

1. Types of laboratory collection (see also Chapter 15).

a. *Capillary blood sampling*: admixture of arterial, venous, and capillary blood and tissue fluid obtained from a well-perfused heel. Heel sticks should not be performed on infants whose feet are edematous, injured, bruised, infected, or anomalous (Folk, 2007). Note: Finger-stick sampling is contraindicated in infants, because distance from skin surface to bone is less than 1.5 mm (Olsowka and Garg, 2001).

(1) Most common route for obtaining small blood samples in the infant.

(2) Heel stick no deeper than 2 mm (Garza and Becan-McBride, 2005b and Garza and Becan-McBride, 2005d), and with heel stick devices ranging from 0.65 to 2 mm depending on infant size (Folk, 2007).

(3) Avoid squeezing or milking site to obtain blood (Folk, 2007; Garza and Becan-McBride, 2005d).

(4) Cell counts such as WBC, platelet count, or blood gas Po_2 may not be accurate.

(5) Anticipatory pain management should be considered (see also Chapter 16).

  b. *Venipuncture*: venous blood typically obtained from the hand, arm, foot, leg, or scalp. Venous blood can also be obtained from an umbilical vein catheter, tunneled central venous catheter or percutaneously inserted central catheter (PICC) (Folk, 2007). In term infants, venipuncture has been shown to be less painful a procedure than heel stick when performed by skilled personnel (Shah and Ohlsson, 2007).

(1) May need use of tourniquet to distend peripheral veins. Recommended time for tourniquet application is ≤1 minute. Tourniquet application ≥3 minutes may alter laboratory test results (Garza and Becan-McBride, 2005a; Garza and Becan-McBride, 2005e).

(2) Venipuncture may be difficult to obtain in small infants.

(3) May wish to ration available veins for future intravenous sites vs. use for laboratory drawing (Folk, 2007; Miller and Lifshitz, 2006).

(4) Anticipatory pain management should be considered (see also Chapter 16).

  c. *Arterial puncture* (see also Chapter 15): arterial blood typically obtained from an artery stick of the radial, tibial, or temporal arteries. Brachial artery stick is performed less often due to potential for arteriospasm of brachial artery supplying the lower arm. Femoral artery stick is rarely performed in the NICU population. Arterial blood can also be obtained from an umbilical artery catheter or percutaneous arterial line.

(1) Allen test (modified) should be done prior to radial artery stick (Garza and Becan-McBride, 2005; Miller and Lifshitz, 2006).

(2) Anticipatory pain management should be considered (see also Chapter 16).

  d. *Point-of-care testing* (POCT), alternate-site testing (AST), near-patient testing (NPT), patient-focused testing (PFT): tests done in a variety of settings, often at the bedside (Threatte, 2007).

(1) Uses whole blood obtained from capillary stick, arterial, or venous sources.

(2) Provides "real-time," rapid testing.

(3) Uses small blood volumes, less than 0.5 ml.

(4) Common POCT assays obtained in the NICU include levels of electrolytes, ionized calcium, BUN, creatinine, Hct, hemoglobin (Hgb), blood gases, and glucose.

(5) Anticipatory pain management should be considered (see also Chapter 16).

  e. *Lumbar puncture* (see Chapter 15): procedure done to remove cerebrospinal fluid (CSF) from the spinal canal.

(1) CSF evaluated in the laboratory for:

    (a) Infection.

    (b) Hemorrhage.

    (c) Demyelinating diseases.

    (d) Malignancy.

  f. *Urine sampling* (see also Chapter 15): urine obtained for chemical analysis, bacterial cultures, or microscopic examination.

(1) Techniques for obtaining samples include:

    (a) Bag collection.

    (b) Straight catheterization.

    (c) Suprapubic bladder tap.

  g. *Thoracentesis* (see also Chapter 15): procedure using a needle tap or chest tube to remove abnormal collection of fluid (effusion) from the thoracic cavity.

(1) Thoracic cavity fluid evaluated in laboratory for:

    (a) Microorganisms: cultures, Gram stains.

(b) Chemistries: levels of electrolytes, total protein, albumin, glucose, and triglycerides.

(c) Hematology: WBC count and WBC differential count.

h. *Peritoneal tap*: procedure using a needle tap to remove an abnormal collection of fluid (ascites) from the abdomen.

(1) Peritoneal cavity fluid evaluated in laboratory for:

(a) Microorganisms: cultures, Gram stains.

(b) Chemistries: levels of electrolytes, total protein, albumin, glucose, and triglycerides.

(c) Hematology: WBC count and WBC differential count.

2. **Process of laboratory collection.**

a. Order request for test.

b. Check for appropriateness of order.

c. Cluster laboratory drawing as much as possible.

d. Check patient identification prior to laboratory sampling per hospital protocol.

e. Prepare infant for laboratory test, for example:

(1) Wrap foot for capillary specimen—a wrapped foot arterializes specimen and helps promote blood flow (Blackburn, 2007; Garza and Becan-McBride, 2005d; Kaplan and Tange, 1998; Olsowka and Garg, 2001). Some studies suggest that heel warming has not resulted in greater blood volume yield (Folk, 2007).

(2) Provide pain management.

f. Observe strict aseptic technique per institution guidelines.

g. Observe Standard Precautions per institution guidelines.

h. Obtain laboratory test using an appropriate route, for example:

(1) Capillary vs. arterial vs. venous.

i. Discard the initial few drops of blood after lancing the heel—along with prewarming the heel this reduces the magnitude of capillary and venous lab value differences (Blackburn, 2007).

j. Obtain blood cultures first, hematology specimens next to minimize platelet clumping, then chemistry and blood bank samples (Folk, 2007; Garza and Becan-McBride, 2005c; Miller and Lifshitz, 2006) or per institution protocol.

k. Insert proper amount of specimen into proper specimen container.

l. Label specimen.

m. Place specimen in biohazard container or bag.

n. Promptly send specimen to laboratory.

3. **Specimen tubes**: standardized, color-coded containers indicating whether they contain whole blood, plasma (which contains fibrinogen), or serum (Farmer and Kee, 2005). Specimen tubes can be glass or plastic, with many labs converting to plastic collection tubes to increase occupational safety (Miller and Lifshitz, 2006). Tube colors in the NICU typically come in red, blue, green, lavender, and yellow. Plastic microtainers are the most common types of specimen collection tubes in the NICU. Microtainers allow use of smaller blood volumes to obtain laboratory results. Blood culture tubes, sterile swabs, and glass slides are also used in the NICU for specimen collection. Tubes with anticoagulant coating should be gently inverted, end over end, 7 to 10 times for proper anticoagulant-blood mixing (Farmer and Kee, 2005; Fischbach, 2002).

a. *Red tube (plain)*: no additives or anticoagulant. Clotted blood for *serum* testing. Hemolysis should be avoided. Laboratory examples: electrolytes, serology, blood bank, proteins, hormones, and drug monitoring.

b. *Blue tube (light)*: contains sodium citrate, an anticoagulant that removes calcium to prevent clotting (Fischbach, 2002). Unclotted blood-*plasma* specimens. Laboratory specimens: prothrombin time (PT), partial thromboplastin time (PTT), factor assays. Another light-blue tube containing thrombin and soybean trypsin inhibitor is good for measurement of fibrin-degradation products (Miller and Lifshitz, 2006).

c. *Green tube*: contains anticoagulant heparin (sodium, lithium, ammonium) that inhibits thrombin activation to prevent clotting. Unclotted blood-*plasma* specimens. Laboratory examples: chromosome analysis (use sodium heparin tube), ammonia levels, and hormone levels.

d. *Lavender tube*: contains ethylenediaminetetraacetic acid (EDTA) that removes calcium to prevent clotting. Tube used for whole blood and *plasma* specimens. Laboratory examples: CBC, reticulocyte count, platelet count, Hct.

e. *Yellow tube/bottle cap* (SPS)—sterile, contains sodium polyanetholesulfonate (SPS) that aids in bacterial recovery by inhibiting complement, phagocytes, and certain antibiotics (Miller and Lifshitz, 2006). Whole blood used for blood cultures. These cultures should be processed quickly to minimize the potential for decreased yield owing to storage or prolonged exposure to SPS (Olsowka and Garg, 2001). A yellow, acid citrate dextrose (ACD) tube is not typically used in NICU but used for human leukocyte antigen (HLA) phenotyping and paternity testing (Miller and Lifshitz, 2006).

CONCEPTS OF LABORATORY TEST INTERPRETATION

A. **It is important to be familiar with the limitations and applications of the laboratory data as they apply to patient care.** Many factors influence blood values and their interpretation in the newborn including timing, site and amount of blood sample, placental transfusion, and infant growth rate (Blackburn, 2007). A laboratory test has certain characteristics that influence how it is interpreted and used in the clinical setting. The following concepts are integral in the process of laboratory interpretation:

1. **Accuracy:** synonymous with "correctness," this term refers to how close a test result is to the true value (Laposata, 2002; Oxley et al., 2001).
  a. Point-to-point variability in test results.
  b. Variation in value may be more reflective of an analytic variation of automated chemistry systems than actual patient status.

2. **Precision:** synonymous with "reproducibility," this term describes the distribution of results when a sample is analyzed repeatedly.
  a. Imprecision is known as random error.
  b. Test precision is a more desirable test characteristic than accuracy in measuring treatment response or clinical changes.

3. **Sensitivity:** the ability of a test to correctly identify an individual with disease and not miss anyone by falsely testing "healthy." It refers to a test's ability to generate more true-positive results and fewer false-negative results.
  a. Sensitive test has a low threshold for abnormality.
  b. Sensitive test usually has a low specificity.
  c. Certain testing requires sensitivity over specificity—example: blood bank donors screened for infectious diseases when it is better to err in excluding donors who are falsely positive than include donors who are falsely negative.

4. **Specificity:** the ability of a test to identify only those individuals with disease as opposed to individuals testing positive when there is no disease. It refers to a test's ability to generate more true-negative results and fewer false-positive results.
  a. Specific test has a high threshold for "normal" or negative test results.
  b. Specific test usually has low sensitivity.
  c. Certain testing requires specificity over sensitivity—example: urine toxicology screen to detect presence of cocaine, cardiac isoenzymes to rule out a myocardial infarct.

5. **Reference range:** established upper and lower boundary levels of a laboratory value by which a patient's result will be measured for presence of disease. The range of normality (mathematical) is dependent on population subsets such as age, gender, pregnancy, and other patient attributes.
  a. Often referred to as "normal" range.
  b. Term *normal* is misleading—reference range determined based on specific attributes of a population subset, not due to "normalcy" (Oxley et al., 2001).
  c. Approximately 5% of "healthy" laboratory results fall outside the reference range.
  d. Reference range can vary from laboratory to laboratory.

PRINCIPLES OF TEST UTILIZATION

A. **Patient management depends on good clinical skills, judicious use of laboratory testing, and careful interpretation of laboratory data.** Once a laboratory value is determined and the patient's clinical status evaluated, the combined information is used to direct treatment. In an effort to optimize care, minimize patient discomfort, and contain health care costs, Wallach (2007) identifies key principles of test utilization:

1. Even under the best of circumstances, no test is perfect.
   a. Results can be misleading.
   b. Specificity or sensitivity of a test is never 100%.
2. Choice of tests should be based on the prior probability of the diagnosis being sought, which affects the predictive value of the test.
   a. History, physical examination, and prevalence of a disease determine the probability of diagnosis.
   b. Patient history and examination should precede choice of laboratory tests.
3. The combination of short-term physiologic variation and analytical error is sufficient to render the interpretation of single determinations difficult when the concentrations are in the borderline range.
   a. Despite the high quality of a laboratory, any laboratory result may be incorrect.
   b. Laboratory tests may need to be rechecked or redrawn, at times in another laboratory.
4. Reference ranges vary from one laboratory to another.
   a. Age, gender, race, size, and physiologic status must be considered.
   b. 5% of test results will be outside the reference range in the absence of disease.
5. Tables of reference values represent statistical data for 95% of the population; values outside these ranges do not necessarily represent disease.
   a. Test results falling within the reference range may be abnormal from the patient's baseline range.
   b. Certain conditions warrant serial testing.
6. An individual's test values when performed in a good laboratory tend to remain fairly constant over a period of years.
   a. Comparing patient laboratory values obtained when not ill are often a better reference value than "normal" ranges.
7. Multiple test abnormalities are more likely to be significant than single test abnormalities.
   a. Two or more positive tests for a given disease reinforce diagnosis.
8. The greater the degree of abnormality of a test result, the more likely that a confirmed value is clinically significant or represents a real disorder.
9. Characteristic laboratory test profiles representing full-blown or advanced disease may all be present in only one third of patients with said condition.
   a. Other disorders or conditions may produce exactly the same combination of laboratory test changes.
10. Excessive repetition of tests is wasteful, and the excess burden increases the possibility of laboratory errors.
    a. Patient's acuity should dictate testing interval.
11. Tests should be performed only if they will alter the patient's diagnosis, prognosis, treatment, or management.
12. Clerical errors are far more likely than technical errors to cause incorrect results.
13. The effect of drugs on laboratory test values must never be overlooked.
    a. Certain drugs can produce false-negative and false-positive results; examples: anticonvulsants, antihypertensives, and antiinfectives.
14. The effect of artifacts can cause spurious values and factitious disorders, especially in the face of discrepant laboratory results.
15. Negative laboratory tests (or any other type of tests) do not necessarily rule out a clinical disease.

IATROGENIC SEQUELAE OF LABORATORY TESTING—PREVENTIVE STRATEGIES

A. **The goal of laboratory testing is to help diagnose and guide management of disease.** Inadvertently, laboratory testing can complicate patient care by creating additional illness, stress, injury, and/or cost. An understanding of the potential sequelae associated with laboratory sampling and strategies that can be used to minimize sequelae is integral to patient care.

   1. **Physiologic stress.**

      a. Adverse physical symptoms triggered by pain stimuli, sensory stimuli, and/or disease state.

      b. Laboratory sampling via skin puncture elicits a painful stimuli creating physiologic stress.

      c. Common physiologic stress symptoms include the following (AAP, 2007) (see also Chapter 11):

        (1) Tachycardia or bradycardia.

        (2) Hypertension or hypotension.

        (3) Apnea or crying.

        (4) Cyanosis or respiratory distress.

        (5) Changes in skin color and temperature.

      d. An event creating physiologic stress can potentially alter a laboratory sample result; example:

        (1) Change in Pco_2 and Po_2 reading when infant cries (Kaplan and Tange, 1998).

        (2) Altered blood pH if infant becomes hypothermic.

      e. Strategies to minimize sampling-induced physiologic stress include the following:

        (1) Minimize skin punctures for laboratory sampling by minimizing or combining labwork.

        (2) Utilize existing indwelling catheters (when available) to obtain laboratory samples.

        (3) Use noninvasive pain management techniques to assist infant in coping with painful stimuli (AAP, 2007; see also Chapter 16).

        (4) Use spring-loaded lancets for heel stick sampling (Folk, 2007; Walden and Franck, 2003).

        (5) Ensure quick, efficient execution of laboratory sampling.

        (6) Apply warm compress to the heel, which might promote blood flow and improve testing accuracy, thus avoiding repeat laboratory sampling.

        (7) Venipuncture may be preferable to the heel stick procedure in minimizing procedure-related pain in term neonates (Shah and Ohlsson, 2007).

        (8) Careful specimen collection, handling, and labeling can decrease repeat laboratory draws.

   2. **Pain** (see also Chapter 16).

      a. An unpleasant sensory and emotional experience associated with actual or potential tissue invasion (Walden and Franck, 2003).

      b. Laboratory sampling by skin puncture evokes pain.

      c. Pain causes adverse physiologic stress (see number 1 c, this section), including potential central nervous system (CNS) alterations (AAP, 2007).

      d. It is difficult to differentiate between acute and chronic pain in the infant (AAP, 2007).

      e. Strategies to minimize sampling-induced pain include the following:

        (1) Strategies that minimize physiologic stress (see number 1 e, this section).

        (2) Nonpharmacologic pain management strategies; examples: swaddling, facilitated tucking, nonnutritive sucking, skin-to-skin contact (AAP, 2007; Folk, 2007).

        (3) Pharmacologic pain management strategies; examples: 24% sucrose, local anesthetic, and opioid and nonopioid analgesics.

        (4) Usefulness of topical local anesthesia for pain control in infants can be helpful for procedures such as venipuncture, lumbar puncture, and intravenous catheter insertion. It is not effective for heel sticks (AAP, 2007).

(5) Using venipuncture when obtaining blood samples may be less painful and have less potential sequelae (i.e., nerve damage, arterial spasm) compared with arterial puncture.

(6) In term infants, venipuncture has been shown to be less painful a procedure than heel stick when performed by skilled personnel (Shah and Ohlsson, 2007).

3. **Skin injury.**

   a. Alteration in normal barrier function of skin as a result of invasive procedures, adhesives to skin, reaction to skin antiseptics, and/or disease states (Lund and Kuller, 2003).

   b. Arterial punctures, venipunctures, and capillary heel sticks used to obtain laboratory samples may potentially create skin injury (LeFrak and Lund, 2001).

   c. Potential skin injury from peripheral laboratory samples includes:

      (1) Bruising.
      (2) Hematoma.
      (3) Abrasion from antiseptic solutions, friction, or tape application.
      (4) Dermal stripping from friction or tape application.
      (5) Scarring from multiple punctures.
      (6) Calcifications.
      (7) Burns secondary to prewarming heel with a soak that is too hot; warm soak should not exceed 44°F.
      (8) Chemical burns secondary to antiseptic skin-cleansing agents.

   d. Strategies to minimize sampling-induced skin injury from skin puncture include:

      (1) Minimize labwork.
      (2) Avoid excessive "squeeze" when obtaining capillary blood work.
      (3) Apply adequate pressure to puncture sites to minimize bleeding and formation of hematoma.
      (4) Use nonadhering products to apply as a dressing to puncture site; example:
         (a) Loose elastic wrap (Coban) around extremity holding gauze in place.
      (5) Thoroughly wash skin of antiseptic solutions.
      (6) Use proper skin puncture devices when obtaining blood; example:
         (a) Spring-loaded lancet of proper length (no deeper than 2 mm) (Garza and Beacon-McBride, 2005a) and with heel stick devices ranging from 0.65 to 2 mm depending on infant size (Folk, 2007).
         (b) Butterfly needle of proper gauge and length for site.

4. **Infection.**

   a. An important skin function is to provide a barrier to infection.

   b. Any break in skin barrier creates potential for infection.

   c. Common infections associated with altered skin barrier include:

      (1) Bacterial/candidal skin surface infection.
      (2) Cellulitis.
      (3) Abscess formation at puncture site.
      (4) Septicemia.
      (5) Osteomyelitis.
      (6) Urinary tract/bladder infection.
      (7) Meningitis.

   d. Strategies to minimize sampling-induced infection include:

      (1) Minimize laboratory sampling.
      (2) Avoid sampling in area of existing skin injury.
      (3) Avoid repeated sampling from dedicated central lines (Folk, 2007); example: routine laboratory sampling via PICC or Broviac catheter.
      (4) Meticulous aseptic technique when obtaining a laboratory sample.
      (5) Use of nursing strategies to maintain optimal skin integrity (see Chapter 36).

5. **Organ/nerve injury.**

   a. Needle puncture for laboratory sampling can potentially contribute to organ injury.

   b. Potential organ injury associated with needle puncture includes:

    (1) Damage to nerve and/or tissues in wrist or brachial area from arterial puncture.
    (2) Damage to lung and/or breast tissue from thoracentesis.
    (3) Damage to abdominal organs from peritoneal tap.
    (4) Damage to bladder or nearby intestine from suprapubic bladder tap.
    (5) Damage to nerves or tissue of spine from lumbar puncture.
    (6) Damage to skin as mentioned in number 3, this section.
    (7) Tissue ischemia from arterial vasospasm secondary to arterial puncture.
  c. Strategies to minimize sampling-induced organ/nerve injury include the following:
    (1) Prudent use of laboratory sampling.
    (2) Proper technique for needlestick sampling (see also Chapter 15).
    (3) Ultrasound guidance as needed for pleural and peritoneal aspiration.

6. **Anemia.**
  a. Iatrogenic anemia owing to blood loss from laboratory sampling (Kaplan and Tange, 1998; Shaw, 2003).
  b. Iatrogenic anemia, along with physiologic anemia, constitutes the most common causes of chronic anemia in infants (Shaw, 2003).
  c. Despite micro-sampling and conservative laboratory sampling, sick infants can lose more than 5 ml of blood per day (Clapp et al., 2001).
  d. Removal of 1 ml of blood from a 1 kg infant equals removal of 70 ml of blood from an adult (Blackburn, 2007).
  e. Iatrogenic blood loss correlates with degree of illness.
  f. Laboratory sample overdraws (19% ± 1.8% more than needed) is common in the NICU (Blackburn, 2007).
  g. Strategies to minimize sampling-induced anemia include:
    (1) Judicious use of laboratory sampling.
    (2) Micro-sampling when possible.
    (3) Accurate documentation of blood loss.
    (4) Avoiding overdrawing of blood samples.

7. **False diagnosis.**
  a. Even under the best circumstances, no test is perfect.
  b. Excess repetition of a test increases the possibility of laboratory error.
  c. The more laboratory samples drawn, the more likely one or more results will be outside the reference range.
  d. Clinical decision making should be based on trends or multiple laboratory values pointing to disease vs. spurious results.
  e. Strategies to minimize sampling-related false diagnosis include:
    (1) Obtain laboratory samples only when necessary to assist in diagnosis, prognosis, treatment, or management.
    (2) Verify spurious laboratory values.
    (3) Draw laboratory samples using proper technique and conditions.

8. **Cost factor.**
  a. 15% to 20% of a patient's hospital bill results from laboratory sampling.
  b. If the average ancillary cost of a NICU stay is $13,873, a patient spends $3,308 for laboratory testing.
  c. Cost of hospitalization in the NICU is inversely related to gestational age.
  d. Rising cost of medical care is complicating delivery of care.
  e. Strategies to minimize sampling-related laboratory costs include:
    (1) Minimize laboratory sampling.
    (2) Prudent medical and nursing decision making regarding laboratory sampling.
    (3) Minimizing laboratory errors precipitating repeat sampling.

DECISION—QUESTIONS TO ASK PRIOR TO OBTAINING A LABORATORY TEST

A. **Judicious use of laboratory testing is critical in any setting, particularly in the NICU, where acuity is high.** Below are questions to consider prior to ordering and/or obtaining a laboratory

■ BOX 13-1
■ QUESTIONS TO ASK *BEFORE* OBTAINING A LABORATORY TEST

- Does the patient require the laboratory test?
  Are the patient examination results abnormal, whereby a laboratory test will help in diagnosis?
  Is the medical history helpful in directing which laboratory test to order?
- Will the laboratory test requested answer the "so what" question?
  Is the laboratory result integral to the immediate clinical management of the infant?
  Is the laboratory result contributory to a patient's diagnosis?
- Is the laboratory test requested still applicable to the current clinical status?
  Has the outcome of the infant's clinical examination changed?
  Has the infant recovered?
- Is the timing of the laboratory test appropriate?
  When should the labwork be obtained?
- Is the laboratory test ordered the "best" test to answer the clinical question?
- Does the laboratory test require too much blood volume?
- Does the potential benefit of the laboratory test outweigh the risk of sequelae in the patient?
- If the laboratory sample is inadequate, faulty, or "lost," is it necessary to redraw?
  Has the clinical status changed?
  Has the infant recovered?

sample. Asking oneself these questions will assist in refining critical thinking skills and aid in selective use of labwork (Box 13-1). To simplify the discussion process, one presenting symptom—*jittery infant*—will be used and applied to all phases of critical thinking.

1. **Does the patient require the laboratory test?**
    a. **Are the patient examination results abnormal, whereby a laboratory test will help in diagnosis?**
        (1) Example:
            (a) Abnormal finding: model-jittery infant.
            (b) Possible laboratory tests: glucose, calcium, and urine toxicology screen.
    b. **Is the medical history helpful in directing which laboratory test to order?**
        (1) *Example: model-jittery infant.*
            (a) Infant of a gestational, class A1, diabetic mother (IDM-A1). Might choose to obtain a serum glucose and/or serum calcium level vs. a urine toxicology screen.
            (b) Infant with delayed drying of skin after birth and axilla/skin temperature of 96° F? Might choose to place infant under heat source and not obtain labwork.
            (c) Infant 1800 g, IDM-A1, and mother with minimal prenatal care? Might choose to obtain all possible laboratory tests.
2. **Will the laboratory test requested answer the "so what" question?** Model-*jittery infant.*
    a. **Is the laboratory result integral to the immediate clinical management of the infant?**
        (1) Hypoglycemia in an IDM-A1 will mandate increasing the carbohydrate intake to treat the problem.
        (2) Mild hypothermia in an otherwise healthy infant will not require a change in management directed by labwork.
    b. **Is the laboratory result contributory to a patient's diagnosis?**
        (1) Serum glucose test result will help diagnose hypoglycemia as a cause of jitteriness.
        (2) Serum glucose test result will not help diagnose respiratory distress syndrome.
3. **Is the laboratory test requested still applicable to current clinical status?**
    a. *Example: model-jittery infant.*
        (1) **Has the infant's clinical examination changed?**
            (a) 1-hour-old IDM-A1 whose jitteriness has changed to tonic–clonic movements of extremities—in addition to serum glucose and calcium levels—will need to consider a urine toxicology screen and electrolytes.

(b) 3-hour-old IDM-A1 who breastfed for 20 minutes and is no longer jittery may not require further testing, particularly if the original serum glucose level was normal.

(c) Hypothermic infant who continues to remain hypothermic after 2 hours under heat source may need serum glucose test and sepsis evaluation.

b. *Example: model-jittery infant.*

(1) **Has the infant recovered?**

(a) Infant with multiple normal glucose test results: may no longer require frequent glucose testing.

(b) Infant no longer jittery after acquiring a normal body temperature—may need to cancel labwork ordered to evaluate jitteriness.

4. **Is the timing of the laboratory test appropriate?**

a. *Example: model-jittery infant.*

(1) **When should the labwork be obtained?**

(a) IDM-A1 at birth—might wait to check serum glucose level at 30 minutes of age when the result would reflect infant's status vs. that of the maternal environment.

(b) Jittery infant with normal serum glucose and calcium levels—might obtain first voided specimen for a urine toxicology screen.

5. **Is the laboratory test ordered the "best" test to answer the clinical question?**

a. *Example: model-jittery infant.*

(1) Should the jittery infant have a serum glucose sample sent to the laboratory or should a whole blood glucose level be obtained at the bedside by POCT, NPT? A POCT glucose result is available in seconds, allowing for rapid clinical intervention.

(2) Should the jittery infant with polycythemia have a POCT whole blood glucose test or should a serum glucose sample be sent to the laboratory? A POCT glucose result may not be accurate in the face of polycythemia.

6. **Does the laboratory test require too much blood volume?**

a. *Example: model-jittery infant.*

(1) A 500-g infant with q2h serum glucose—POCT whole blood glucose testing requires average sample size of one drop to 0.1 ml of blood, whereas serum glucose test requires an average sample size of 0.5 ml.

(2) A 5-ml sample of blood is required for metabolic screening in a 500-g infant—10% blood volume loss may not be tolerated; need to prioritize labwork and draw in stages based on most common to least common disorders.

7. **Does the potential benefit of the laboratory test outweigh the risk of sequelae in the patient?**

a. *Example: model-jittery infant.*

(1) A 500-g infant with hypoglycemia—frequent glucose testing needed to monitor treatment; benefit outweighs potential harm of blood loss. Also, POCT use can minimize blood loss.

(2) A 5-ml blood sample for metabolic screening in a 500-g, symptomatic infant—potential harm of an acute 10% blood loss outweighs the need to simultaneously obtain all the ordered metabolic screening laboratories.

8. **If the laboratory sample is inadequate, faulty, or "lost," is it necessary to redraw?**

a. *Example: model-jittery infant.*

(1) **Has the clinical status changed?**

(2) **Has the infant recovered?** (See number 3, this section.) If the status improves or the infant recovers while waiting for sample, repeat sampling may not be indicated.

LABORATORY INTERPRETATION—DECISION TREE

A. **Careful laboratory data interpretation is essential in providing accurate therapeutic interventions.** Asking focused questions will assist in refining critical thinking skills related to

■ BOX 13-2
■ **LABORATORY INTERPRETATION: IS IT RELIABLE? IS IT BELIEVABLE?**

Laboratory test result. Is it *reliable*? Is it *believable*?

Yes	No
■ Implement an appropriate clinical intervention, if needed.	■ Consider repeating the laboratory test when the appropriate correction is made.
	■ Consider repeating the laboratory test if the clinical status continues to warrant a laboratory test.

Laboratory test result. Is it *reliable*? Is it *believable*?

If Result too Low	If Result too High
■ Is the sample diluted?	■ Was the laboratory specimen drawn too early?
■ Was the sample handled correctly?	■ Was the sample handled correctly?
■ Was the timing of the test an issue?	■ Was medical therapy not implemented or inadequate?
■ Was medical therapy not implemented or inadequate?	■ Was the source of the laboratory sample not appropriate?
■ Was the specimen site condition a factor?	■ Was the POCT device calibrated?
■ Was the POCT device calibrated?	
■ Was there interference from a past medical therapy?	

POCT, Point-of-care testing.

utilization of laboratory values in patient management. Below are questions to consider when using laboratory results to direct patient care.

1. **Laboratory test result. Is it reliable? Is it believable? (Box 13-2) A question tree *if result too low*.**
   a. **Is the sample diluted?** Examples:
      (1) A laboratory specimen can be contaminated with or diluted by fluids infusing through indwelling arterial and/or venous lines if the initial few drops of blood are incorporated into the sample.
      (2) A laboratory specimen can be diluted by interstitial fluid from the skin tissues if heel stick puncture is not fresh, the puncture site is not prewarmed, or the infant is exceedingly edematous.
   b. **Was the sample handled correctly?** Examples:
      (1) A serum bilirubin count can be falsely low if obtained while the infant is under phototherapy or if exposed too long in the daylight unanalyzed.
      (2) A serum glucose level can be falsely low if left in a microtainer and not processed and analyzed promptly.
      (3) An overfilled or underfilled hematology sample can precipitate clotting and falsely decrease platelet count.
   c. **Was the timing of the test an issue?** Examples:
      (1) A serum gentamicin, vancomycin, or theophylline level will be too low if drawn too early in the drug treatment.
      (2) A serum glucose or POCT glucose level obtained too soon after feeding the infant may remain falsely low due to lack of digestion time.
      (3) Electrolyte levels may remain falsely low if obtained too soon after electrolyte replacement.
   d. **Was medical therapy not implemented or inadequate?** Examples:
      (1) A blood gas level obtained prior to weaning the ventilator for a P_{CO_2} of 25.
      (2) A serum glucose or POCT glucose level obtained prior to medical intervention for hypoglycemia.
      (3) A serum gentamicin, vancomycin, or theophylline level will be too low if the dose is inadequate or dose interval too long.

(4) A theophylline level may be low because intermittent doses are held as a result of tachycardia in the infant.

   e. Was the specimen site condition a factor? Examples:

     (1) A capillary blood sample from an edematous infant can be falsely low due to excessive tissue fluids.

     (2) A nonwarmed heel can falsely lower a capillary blood gas pH, Po_2.

   f. Was the POCT device calibrated? Examples:

     (1) Laboratory test results may be unreliable if the:

       (a) POCT device was not calibrated recently.

       (b) POCT device was calibrated by an untrained individual.

       (c) Reagent used for calibration had expired.

       (d) Sample cartridge expired or was not kept at room temperature.

   g. Was there interference from past medical therapy? Examples:

     (1) An infant's blood culture result may be falsely negative if a mother was treated with antibiotics during labor.

     (2) Phenobarbital use may decrease theophylline concentrations.

2. **Laboratory test result. Is it** *reliable?* **Is it** *believable?* **A question tree** *if result too high.*

   a. Was the laboratory specimen drawn too early? Examples:

     (1) A triglyceride level may be falsely elevated if drawn too soon after lipid infusion.

     (2) A serum calcium level may be falsely increased if drawn soon after a calcium gluconate bolus.

     (3) Electrolytes can remain elevated if drawn too soon after IV fluids increased.

   b. Was the sample handled correctly? Examples:

     (1) A serum potassium level may be falsely elevated due to hemolysis from squeezing the heel for capillary laboratory sampling.

     (2) A serum protein or potassium level may be falsely elevated if a tourniquet is applied too tightly or too long ($\geq$3 minutes).

     (3) An Hct count can be falsely elevated if drawn from a poorly perfused heel.

   c. Was medical therapy not implemented or inadequate? Examples:

     (1) A serum bilirubin count can remain elevated if phototherapy is not instituted long enough to measure change.

     (2) A Pco_2 can remain elevated if ventilator setting changes are not sufficient to correct for the respiratory ailment or the sample is drawn too soon after corrective intervention.

   d. Was the source of the laboratory sample not appropriate? Examples:

     (1) An Hct can be falsely elevated from a capillary sample vs. an arterial or venous sample.

     (2) An ammonia level can be falsely elevated if hemolyzed, so needs to be drawn via an artery or vein.

   e. Was the POCT device calibrated? Examples:

     (1) Laboratory result may be unreliable if the POCT device was not recently calibrated or was calibrated by an untrained individual, if the reagent for calibration had expired, or the sample cartridge either expired or was not kept at room temperature.

3. **Laboratory test result. Is it** *reliable?* **Is it** *believable?* **YES**

   a. Implement appropriate clinical intervention, if needed. Examples:

     (1) Alert physician or midlevel practitioner of laboratory result and implement appropriate medical or nursing corrective intervention as needed:

       (a) Medication dose change for inadequate drug level.

       (b) Ventilator setting change for under- or overventilation.

       (c) Blood product transfusion for anemia, thrombocytopenia.

       (d) Change in IV fluid concentration or rate for electrolyte imbalance or dehydration.

       (e) Change feeding interval for hypoglycemia.

4. **Laboratory test result. Is it** *reliable?* **Is it** *believable?* **NO**

   a. Consider repeating laboratory test when the appropriate correction is made. Example:

(1) Repeat laboratory test at an appropriate time for drug level measurement.

(2) Warm heel prior to obtaining capillary sample.

(3) Wait 2 to 3 hours after a milk feeding to test a postfeed serum glucose level.

b. **Consider repeating laboratory test if clinical status continues to warrant laboratory test.** Examples:

(1) A clotted CBC sample after red blood cell transfusion or after antibiotic therapy: may not require a repeat sample or might wait for redraw until another blood sample is needed.

(2) A high Hct value taken from an acrocyanotic heel in a hypoglycemic infant would need a central Hct to determine if polycythemia is a cause of hypoglycemia.

5. **Laboratory test result. Is it *normal*? YES** (Box 13-3).

a. **Consider a change in medical management.** Examples:

(1) Normal electrolyte results in the face of electrolyte replacement may signal a need to decrease or stop the electrolyte supplementation.

(2) A normal Hct may warrant cancellation of a projected red blood cell transfusion.

b. **Consider implementing surveillance plans.** Examples:

(1) Normal serum calcium, phosphorus, and alkaline phosphatase may need weekly surveillance in very low birth weight infants to monitor for potential rickets.

(2) Normal electrolytes may need frequent monitoring when initiating diuretic therapy.

6. **Laboratory test result. Is it *normal*? NO** (see Box 13-3).

a. **Consider calling the laboratory to verify specimen.** Examples:

(1) See numbers 1, 2, and 4 of this section.

(2) Call laboratory to verify that the result is indeed that of the patient in question.

(3) Ascertain that the abnormal laboratory value was taken from the patient in question.

b. **Is the laboratory result in the appropriate reference range?** Examples:

(1) A critical Hct value differs with age. An Hct of 55% in a newborn is normal as compared with an adult.

(2) Laboratory methods and equipment vary among different laboratories; need to confirm laboratory result with the laboratory that analyzed the sample.

c. **Review patient care practice at time of laboratory specimen sampling.** Examples:

(1) See numbers 1, 2, and 4 of this section.

d. **Consider medication interactions as etiology.** Examples:

(1) Heparin in a blood sample will prolong PT and PTT.

(2) Narcotic sedation may depress respirations and increase Pco_2 level.

(3) Sulfonamides can increase serum bilirubin.

(4) Stool Hematest can be falsely positive when patient is on iron supplement, indomethacin, potassium preparations, or steroids.

■ BOX 13-3
■ **LABORATORY INTERPRETATION: IS IT NORMAL?**

Laboratory Test Result. Is it *normal*?	
Yes	**No**
■ Consider a change in medical management.	■ Consider calling the laboratory to verify the specimen.
■ Consider implementing surveillance plans.	■ Is the laboratory result in the appropriate reference range?
	■ Review patient care practice at the time of laboratory specimen sampling.
	■ Consider medication interactions as etiology.
	■ Institute corrective medical and/or nursing action.

■ BOX 13-4
■ **LABORATORY INTERPRETATION: TEST FOLLOW-UP**

Laboratory Test *Follow-up*	
Normal Test Result	**Abnormal Test Result**
Continue to watch for potential sequelae of treatment.	Consider a change in clinical practice.
Consider a plan for implementing maintenance laboratory surveillance.	Allow time for corrective action then repeat laboratory test to measure effective therapy.

    e. Institute corrective medical and/or nursing action. Example:

      (1) See number 3 of this section.

7. **Laboratory test** *follow-up*—**normal test result** (Box 13-4).

    a. Continue to watch for potential sequelae of treatment. Examples:

      (1) Periodic monitoring of electrolytes is needed when the patient is on diuretic therapy.

      (2) Periodic monitoring of renal function and electrolytes is needed when the patient is on antifungal therapy.

    b. Consider a plan for implementing maintenance laboratory surveillance. Examples:

      (1) Routine weekly monitoring of electrolytes, liver function, and renal function when the infant is on prolonged hyperalimentation.

      (2) Routine monitoring of skeletal integrity of the premature infant susceptible for rickets.

8. **Laboratory test** *follow-up*—**abnormal test result** (see Box 13-4).

    a. Consider a change in clinical practice. Examples:

      (1) See number 3 of this section.

    b. Allow time for corrective action, then repeat laboratory test to measure effective therapy. Examples:

      (1) Weaning from ventilatory support may warrant blood gas analyses every half hour to every 4 hours for an overventilated infant recovering from primary atelectasis.

      (2) Repeated serum glucose level checks every half hour to every hour may be necessary after a hypoglycemic infant receives an IV glucose bolus.

      (3) Weekly or biweekly serum electrolyte tests may be necessary when adjusting oral electrolyte supplementation for borderline low serum electrolyte levels in infants on diuretics for chronic lung disease.

REFERENCES

American Academy of Pediatrics and Canadian Paediatric Society: Prevention and management of pain in the neonate. An update. *Advances in Neonatal Care*, 7(3):151-160, 2007.

Blackburn, S.T.: Hematologic and hemostatic systems. In S.T. Blackburn (Ed.): *Maternal, fetal and neonatal physiology: A clinical perspective* (3rd ed.). St. Louis, 2007, Saunders, pp. 227-266.

Clapp, D.W., Shannon, K.M., and Phibbs, R.H.: Hematologic problems. In M.H. Klaus and A.A. Fanaroff (Eds.): *Care of the high-risk neonate* (5th ed.). Philadelphia, 2001, Saunders, pp. 447-479.

Farmer, L.S. and Kee, J.L.: The importance of specimen collection. In J.L. Kee (Ed.): *Laboratory and diagnostic tests with nursing implication* (7th ed.). New Jersey, 2005, Prentice Hall, pp. xvii-xxii.

Ferguson, C.C. (June 2001). *RIte Stats, Analysis of RIte care utilization data.* Rhode Island Department of Human Services, Center for Child and Family Health, 1 (1), 1-4. Retrieved February 6, 2008, from www.ritecare.ri.gov/documents/reports_publications/RIteStats_vol1_iss1.pdf

Fischbach, F.: Diagnostic testing: Intratest phase: Elements of safe, effective, informed care. In F. Fischbach (Ed.): *A manual of laboratory & diagnostic tests* (7th ed.). Philadelphia, 2002, Lippincott Williams & Wilkins, pp. 19-25.

Folk, L. A.: Guide to capillary heelstick blood sampling in infants. *Advances in Neonatal Care*, 7(4):171-178, 2007.

Garza, D. and Becan-McBride, K.: Arterial, intravenous (IV), and special collection procedures. In D. Garza and K. Becan-McBride (Eds.): *Phlebotomy handbook: Blood collection essentials* (7th ed.). New Jersey, 2005, Pearson Prentice Hall, pp. 361-394.

Garza, D. and Becan-McBride, K.: Blood collection equipment. In D. Garza and K. Becan-McBride (Eds.):

Phlebotomy handbook: Blood collection essentials (7th ed.). New Jersey, 2005a, Pearson Prentice Hall, pp. 207-244.

Garza, D. and Becan-McBride, K.: Pediatric procedures. In D. Garza and K. Becan-McBride (Eds.): *Phlebotomy handbook: Blood collection essentials* (7th ed.). New Jersey, 2005b, Pearson Prentice Hall, pp. 327-359.

Garza, D. and Becan-McBride, K.: Preanalytical complications in blood collection. In D. Garza and K. Becan-McBride (Eds.): *Phlebotomy handbook: Blood collection essentials* (7th ed.). New Jersey, 2005c, Pearson Prentice Hall, pp. 303-326.

Garza, D. and Becan-McBride, K.: Procedures for collecting capillary blood specimens. In D. Garza and K. Becan-McBride (Eds.): *Phlebotomy handbook: Blood collection essentials* (7th ed.). New Jersey, 2005d, Pearson Prentice Hall, pp. 289-302.

Garza, D. and Becan-McBride, K.: Venipuncture procedures. In D. Garza and K. Becan-McBride (Eds.): *Phlebotomy handbook: Blood collection essentials* (7th ed.). New Jersey, 2005e, Pearson Prentice Hall, pp. 245-285.

Kaplan, L.A. and Tange, S.M. (Eds.): *Standards of laboratory practice.* Washington, DC, 1998, National Academy of Clinical Biochemistry (monograph).

Kurec, A.S. and Lifshitz, M.S.: General concepts and administrative issues. In R.A. McPherson and M.R. Pincus (Eds.): *Henry's clinical diagnosis and management by laboratory methods* (21st ed.). Philadelphia, 2006, Saunders Elsevier, chap. 1. Retrieved January 24, 2008, from www.mdconsult.com

Laposata, M.: *Laboratory medicine: Clinical pathology in the practice of medicine.* Chicago, 2002, American Society for Clinical Pathology, p. 14.

LeFrak, L. and Lund, C.H.: Nursing practice in the neonatal intensive care unit. In M.H. Klaus and A.A. Fanaroff (Eds.): *Care of the high-risk neonate* (5th ed.). Philadelphia, 2001, Saunders, pp. 223-242.

Lund, C.H. and Kuller, J.M.: Assessment and management of the integumentary system. In J. Kenner and J.W. Lott (Eds.): *Comprehensive neonatal nursing: A physiologic perspective* (3rd ed.). St. Louis, 2003, Saunders, pp. 700-724.

Miller, H. and Lifshitz, M.S.: Pre-Analysis. In R.A. McPherson and M.R. Pincus (Eds.): *Henry's clinical diagnosis and management by laboratory methods* (21st ed.). Philadelphia, 2006, Saunders, chap. 3. Retrieved January 24, 2008, from www.mdconsult.com

National vital statistics reports, CDC: Births, marriages, divorces, and deaths: Provisional data for February 2007. *National Vital Statistics Reports,* 56(2). Retrieved October 9, 2007, from www.cdc.gov

Olsowka, E.S. and Garg, U.: Specimen collection and point-of-care testing. In D.S. Jacobs, D.K. Oxley, and W.R. DeMott (Eds.): *Jacobs & DeMott laboratory test handbook* (5th ed.). Hudson, Ohio, 2001, Lexi-Comp Inc, pp. 35-48.

Oxley, D.K., Garg, U., and Olsowka, E.S.: Maximizing the information from laboratory tests—The Ulysses syndrome. In D.S. Jacobs, D.K. Oxley, and W.R. DeMott (Eds.): *Jacobs & DeMott laboratory test handbook* (5th ed.). Hudson, Ohio, 2001, Lexi-Comp Inc, pp.15-23.

Sacher, R.A., McPherson, R.A., and Campos, J.M.: Principles of interpretation of laboratory tests. In R.A. Sacher, R.A. McPherson, and J.M. Campos (Eds.): *Widmann's clinical interpretation of laboratory tests* (11th ed.). Philadelphia, 2000a, F.A. Davis, pp. 3-27.

Sacher, R.A., McPherson, R.A., and Campos, J.M.: General chemistry. In R.A., Sacher, R.A. McPherson, and J.M. Campos, (Eds.): *Widmann's clinical interpretation of laboratory tests* (11th ed.). Philadelphia, 2000b, F.A. Davis, pp. 445-446.

Sacher, R.A., McPherson, R.A., and Campos, J.M.: Hematological methods. In R.A. Sacher, R.A. McPherson, and J.M. Campos (Eds.): *Widmann's clinical interpretation of laboratory tests* (11th ed.). Philadelphia, 2000c, F.A. Davis, pp. 31-32.

Sacher, R.A., McPherson, R.A., and Campos, J.M.: Principles of immunology and immunology testing. In R.A. Sacher, R.A. McPherson, and J.M. Campos (Eds.): *Widmann's clinical interpretation of laboratory tests* (11th ed.). Philadelphia, 2000d, F.A. Davis, p. 325.

Schwartz, R.M., Kellogg, R., and Muri, J.H.: Specialty newborn care: Trends and issues. *Journal of Perinatology,* 20(8 Pt 1):520-529, 2000.

Shah, V. and Ohlsson, A.: Venipuncture versus heel lance for blood sampling in term neonates. *Cochrane Database of Systematic Reviews,* 4:CD001452, 2007. DOI: 10.1002/14651858.CD001452.pub3. Retrieved November 5, 2007, from www.cochrane.org/reviews/.

Shaw, N.: Assessment and management of the hematologic system. In C. Kenner and J.W. Lott (Eds.): *Comprehensive neonatal nursing: A physiologic perspective* (3rd ed.). St. Louis, 2003, Saunders, pp. 580-623.

Threatte, G.A.: Point of care and physician office laboratories. In R.A. McPherson and M.R. Pincus (Eds.): *Henry's clinical diagnosis and management by laboratory methods* (21st ed.). Philadelphia, 2007, Saunders, chap. 6. Retrieved January 24, 2008, from www.mdconsult.com

Walden, M. and Franck, L.S.: Identification, management, and prevention of newborn/infant pain. In C. Kenner and J.W. Lott (Eds.): *Comprehensive neonatal nursing: A physiologic perspective* (3rd ed.). St. Louis, 2003, Saunders, pp. 844-856.

Wallach, J.: Introduction to normal values (reference ranges). In J. Wallach (Ed.): *Interpretation of diagnostic tests* (8th ed.). Philadelphia, 2007, Wolters Kluwer/Lippincott Williams & Wilkins, pp. 3-7.

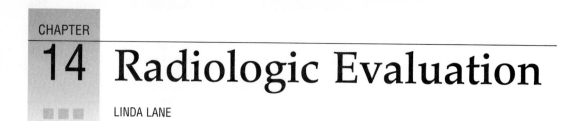

14 Radiologic Evaluation

LINDA LANE

OBJECTIVES

1. Define common radiologic terms used to describe an x-ray.
2. Differentiate various densities that are evident on an x-ray.
3. Describe radiologic findings that are commonly seen in neonatal disease states.
4. Differentiate normal from abnormal findings on a chest x-ray.
5. Recognize findings on an x-ray that are consistent with congenital heart disease.
6. Describe an x-ray consistent with necrotizing enterocolitis.
7. Review correct line and endotracheal tube placement on an x-ray.

Radiographic interpretation of abnormalities in a sick newborn infant is an established part of diagnostic evaluation. This evaluation assists the clinician in determining a diagnosis or formulating a differential diagnosis for treatment of the patient. Rarely is a newborn infant admitted to the neonatal intensive care unit (NICU) without having at least one x-ray taken, and frequently several additional films are needed during the course of treatment. Nurses need to become familiar with common radiographic findings to add to the knowledge base on which patient care is founded. This chapter reviews essentials of radiologic interpretation, discusses pathologic findings, and presents x-rays with common findings.

BASIC CONCEPTS

A. Radiographs are images produced on a radiosensitive surface, such as film, when x-ray beams are passed through an object to the surface below (Haller et al., 2004).
B. By comparing densities and shapes from the image produced on the film, information can be deduced or inferred regarding anatomy, pathology, and function.

TERMINOLOGY

A. **Air bronchogram:** air in the bronchial tree visualized against a background of generalized alveolar atelectasis (AHD Editors, 2007).
B. **Artifact:** an unnaturally occurring silhouette that is artificially reproduced on an x-ray and is not a part of the patient (e.g., electrocardiogram [ECG] leads, temperature probes).
C. **Cardiothoracic ratio:** computed by dividing the maximum cardiac width by the maximum thoracic width to determine the heart size (AHD Editors, 2007).
D. **Carina:** bifurcation of the trachea, usually about the level of the third and fourth thoracic vertebrae (AHD Editors, 2007). Used in determining location of the endotracheal tube.
E. **Expiratory film:** obtained when the infant is in expiration; appears to increase cardiac size, accentuate lung markings, and decrease normal lung expansion.
F. **Exposure:** amount of radiation used, producing a film ranging from light to dark. An underpenetrated (underexposed) film causes images to appear light and hazy. Overpenetration (overexposure) causes the film to be dark and to lack contrast, in comparison with an appropriately penetrated and exposed film.
G. **Hyperexpanded lungs:** lungs expanded to greater than the ninth rib.
H. **Hypoexpanded lungs:** lungs expanded to less than the seventh rib.

I. **Inspiratory film:** obtained when infant is in full inspiration and the lungs project to the eighth rib above the right diaphragmatic dome, with the trachea shown in a straight projection. This is the most desirable for chest film interpretation.

J. **Interlobar fissure:** accumulation of fluid in the pleural space between the lung lobes. The fissure may be fluid filled and may appear as a distinctive line.

K. **Perihilar:** pertaining to radiographic area bordering mediastinal structures.

L. **Pleural effusion:** abnormal collection of fluid in the pleural space (AHD Editors, 2007).

M. **Radiolucent:** pertaining to substances with varying degrees of transparency (AHD Editors, 2007).

N. **Radiopaque:** pertaining to substances that are dense and nonpenetrable to x-rays (AHD Editors, 2007).

O. **Rad:** fundamental unit of radiation measurement (Haller et al., 2004).

P. **Roentgen:** unit of exposure (Haller et al., 2004).

Q. **Rotation:** turned from the midline. Chest structures closest to the beam are magnified, making their shadows appear enlarged and distorted.

R. **Skinfold:** the most common artifact seen in the neonate. Manifests as a straight line of variable length that can travel across or outside the chest or across the diaphragm and into the abdomen. Results from folding of excessive skin; may mimic a pneumothorax. However, the obliquity of the line produced by a skinfold is opposite to that produced by the edge of the lung in pneumothorax (AHD Editors, 2007).

S. **Proper technique:** signifies correct exposure, positioning, and timing in relation to inspiration and proper labeling of a film.

T. **X-ray:** a form of electromagnetic radiation with shorter wavelengths than normal light. X-rays can penetrate most structures (Haller et al., 2004).

X-RAY VIEWS COMMONLY USED IN THE NEWBORN INFANT (Fig. 14-1)

A. **Anteroposterior view.** X-ray tube is positioned above the infant's chest, with the x-ray beam passing through from front to back. Most common view used in the neonate for general assessment.

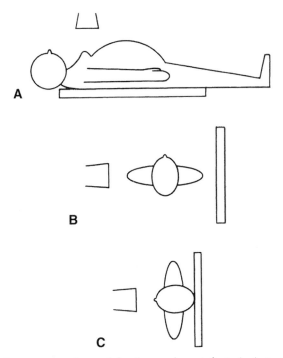

FIGURE 14-1 ■ X-ray views commonly used for the newborn infant. **A,** Anteroposterior view. **B,** Cross-table lateral view. **C,** Lateral decubitus view.

  B. Cross-table lateral view. X-ray beam passes horizontally through infant in the supine position. Used to verify line placement, for assessment of free air in the chest, and for general assessment.

  C. Lateral decubitus view. X-ray beam passes horizontally through the patient, who is positioned with suspect side uppermost. The film is placed on the infant's back, and the patient is placed perpendicular to the bed, facing the x-ray tube. The patient is usually elevated on diapers or blankets, with the arm positioned above the head and out of the field of view. Free air will rise to the highest portion of the thorax if a pneumothorax is present. If an abdominal perforation is present, free air will also rise above the liver when the patient is positioned with the left side down.

RADIOGRAPHIC DENSITIES

A. Radiodensities of various substances and tissues differ according to their composition.
1. The least dense (radiolucent) substance will radiograph black or dark gray because the sparse molecules offer no obstacle to the rays.
2. A very dense (radiopaque) object such as a lead will radiograph gray or white because no rays or few rays will penetrate it, so the film underneath will remain unchanged.
3. Subcutaneous fat is very radiolucent and produces a dark gray shadow on the x-ray film.
4. Blood, muscle, and liver are of similar densities and will be seen as white and medium gray. Moist solid or fluid-filled organs and tissue masses have about the same radiodensity—greater than air but less than bone or metal.
5. Bone is composed of an organic matrix into which the complex bone mineral (primarily calcium) is precipitated. Organic substances will reduce the radiodensity of bone and will be seen as white with a tinge of gray.
6. Metal such as the surgical clip used for patent ductus arteriosus ligation is very dense and radiopaque. All the x-rays are absorbed by the metal, producing a white image on the film.

B. Differentiation of densities is the basis for interpretation of an x-ray film. For example, because of the contrast in densities between the fluid-filled heart, which radiographs white, and the air-filled lungs, which radiograph black, the heart can be seen against the lungs. Organs of the same density that are located side by side, such as the heart and the thymus, may be difficult to distinguish from each other. Changes in normal density can indicate a pathologic process, such as severe respiratory distress syndrome. Surfactant-deficient lungs will appear on the film completely white instead of black, indicating areas of alveolar collapse.

RISKS ASSOCIATED WITH RADIOGRAPHIC EXAMINATION IN THE NEONATE

A. Early radiation effects (Haller et al., 2004).
1. Adverse effects of x-rays do not occur unless a threshold amount of radiation is delivered.
2. Threshold amounts are far in excess of the radiation delivered during an x-ray examination.

B. Delayed effects of x-rays. The risk of radiation-induced childhood cancer is dependent on age at exposure and the lifelong cumulative effect (Haller et al., 2004).

C. Risks to personnel.
1. Risks to personnel in the area where studies are properly done are too small to be of serious concern.
2. At 2 m from the patient, the risk to personnel from an abdominal radiograph of the neonate is much less than the equivalent risk from 1 day of natural background radiation.

APPROACH TO INTERPRETING AN X-RAY

A. Develop a systematic approach and a definite order for assessing a film to ensure that no pathology is missed.

B. **Labeling.** Note name or identification of the patient, date and time of the film, and radiographic labeling on the right or left side of the film.

C. **Assess for correct exposure of the film.**

D. **Note positioning.** Clavicles and ribs should be even on both sides of the chest. Rotation distorts structures.

E. **Individually assess all anatomic and pathologic changes on each film.**

1. Lung fields.
   a. Normal lung expansion: eight ribs projecting above the right diaphragmatic dome, with the trachea in a slightly curved, near-midline position (Haller et al., 2004).
   b. Lung volume, determined by noting the number of ribs expanded on an inspiratory film.
   c. Pulmonary vascularity: vessels branching from the lung root (hilum) and decreasing in size, with extension into the lung fields. Vascularity will be increased or diminished depending on the pathologic state.
   d. Presence of free air: pneumothorax, pneumoperitoneum, pneumopericardium, and pneumomediastinum.

2. Mediastinum.
   a. Heart.
      (1) Size.
      (2) Malposition: any inappropriate position of the heart—that is, any position other than the usual position in the hemithorax.
      (3) Contour: variable because of the influence of patient position and angulation of the x-ray beam.
      (4) Shape: may indicate pathologic change—for example, boot-shaped heart in tetralogy of Fallot and egg-shaped heart in transposition of the great vessels (Haller et al., 2004).
      (5) Pulmonary vascular markings: may be significantly diminished, as in pulmonary atresia, or increased, as in congestive heart failure (CHF) (Haller et al., 2004).
   b. Trachea.
      (1) Normally located within the mediastinum.
      (2) Assessment on x-ray film for presence and position of endotracheal tube.
   c. Thymus.
      (1) Size.
      (2) Presence or absence.
      (3) Presence of "sail sign" when mediastinal air lifts the thymus upward.
   d. Diaphragm.
      (1) General pattern: two smooth, curved shadows on either side of the heart, taking off from the midline at the origin of the 10th and 11th ribs (Haller et al., 2004).
      (2) Contour: possibly flattened with lung overdistention or elevated if there is abdominal distention.
      (3) Diaphragmatic hernia: abdominal contents passing through a hole in the diaphragm.
      (4) Eventration: herniation of bowel and liver against a weakened hemidiaphragm.
   e. Gastrointestinal (GI) tract.
      (1) Esophagus: Distended, air-filled esophageal pouch may be visible in an esophageal atresia.
      (2) Tracheoesophageal fistula: Fistula is present if an esophageal atresia exists and if air is visible in the stomach and intestine.
      (3) Passage of air through the stomach and intestines.
      (4) Location of stomach bubble.
      (5) Bowel gas pattern.
      (6) Presence of pneumatosis intestinalis.
      (7) Presence of calcifications as a result of bowel perforation in utero.
      (8) Fluid, seen as a gasless abdomen. It is necessary to distinguish fluid from masses.
      (9) Pneumoperitoneum: Free air is seen within the peritoneal cavity.

(10) Obstructions: Gaseous distention of the bowel is seen at various levels, depending on the location of the obstruction.
f. Skeletal system.
(1) General skeletal assessment. Assess for symmetry, size, continuity, intactness, and abnormalities.
(2) Fractures of long bones, clavicles, ribs, and skull. A dark line is seen along any portion of a fractured bone because of the air or tissue that settles between the bone fragments (Haller et al., 2004).
g. Tubes and catheters.
(1) Position of endotracheal, gastric, or chest tube.
(2) Umbilical catheter placement.
(3) Central venous line placement.

RESPIRATORY SYSTEM

A. **The normal chest (Fig. 14-2).**
1. Complete aeration of the chest occurs within a few breaths after onset of respirations at delivery (Haller et al., 2004).
2. Residual fluid may be present in the alveoli after delivery. Early films (<6 hours after delivery) may show increased bronchovascular markings because of this fluid.
3. Normal lung pattern.
   a. Uniform radiolucent appearance.
   b. Hilar and perihilar regions show some increased density because of vascular, bronchial, and hilar structures, which produce some increase in density.
   c. Periphery shows few, if any, markings.
   d. Fluid in the various interlobar fissures represents a normal variation.
B. **Thymus.**
1. Occupies the anterior part of the superior portion of the mediastinum and consists of right and left lobes (Haller et al., 2004).
2. Appears as a smoothly rounded outline superior to the cardiac shadow and blending imperceptibly with the cardiac silhouette.
3. Definite notch visible in some cases at the junction of the cardiac silhouette and the thymus.
4. Generally more prominent on the right.
5. Shape may alter markedly with degree of inspiration.

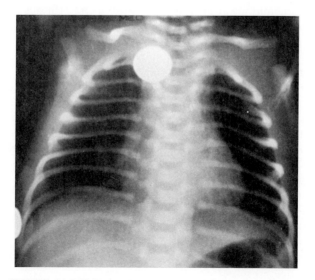

FIGURE 14-2 ■ Normal appearance of chest on x-ray film.

6. Rapid involution during times of stress.
7. Aplasia of the thymus (DiGeorge syndrome).
8. Creation of "sail sign" when mediastinal air lifts the thymus upward.
C. **Trachea.**
   1. Trachea is normally displaced slightly to the right by the left aortic arch.
   2. Deviated trachea supports a mediastinal shift.
   3. On inspiration, the trachea dilates and lengthens.
   4. On expiration, the trachea constricts and shortens.
   5. On deep inspiration, the trachea and major bronchi are well distended and are easily identifiable.

PULMONARY PARENCHYMAL DISEASE

A. **Respiratory distress syndrome (hyaline membrane disease) (Fig. 14-3, *A*).**
   1. Pronounced under aeration. Fewer than eight ribs expand on inspiration on the antero-posterior film, with doming of the hemidiaphragms on lateral view.
   2. Bilateral diffuse alveolar infiltrates. Reticulogranular (ground-glass) appearance is due to microatelectasis of the alveoli (Haller et al., 2004).
   3. Homogeneous pattern throughout both lung fields.
   4. Air bronchograms. Air-filled bronchi (black) are contrasted against the more radiopaque (whiter) lung fields (AHD Editors, 2007).
   5. With severe disease a generalized opacity or frank "white-out" appearance (see Fig. 14-3, *B*).
   6. Reticulogranular pattern and air bronchograms. May resemble those seen in group B streptococcal pneumonia and may be impossible to distinguish from respiratory distress syndrome.
   7. X-ray findings after surfactant administration (Fig. 14-4).
      a. Improvement in pulmonary aeration on x-ray.
      b. Asymmetric distribution of surfactant, showing areas of improved lung alternating with areas of unchanged respiratory distress syndrome (RDS).
      c. Poor prognosis with pulmonary interstitial emphysema after surfactant therapy.
B. **Pulmonary interstitial emphysema (Fig. 14-5).**
   1. Alveolar overdistention is due to assisted ventilation, visualized as multiple small, cystlike radiolucencies that are bilateral, unilateral, localized, or in a diffuse pattern (Kenner and Lott, 2007).
   2. Condition may lead to a pneumothorax or other air leak.

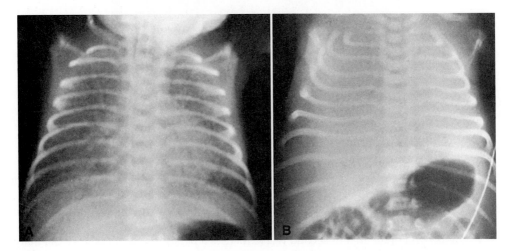

FIGURE 14-3 ■ **A,** Hyaline membrane disease. Note reticulogranular lung pattern and air bronchograms. **B,** Severe hyaline membrane disease. Note "white-out" appearance bilaterally with faint air bronchograms visible.

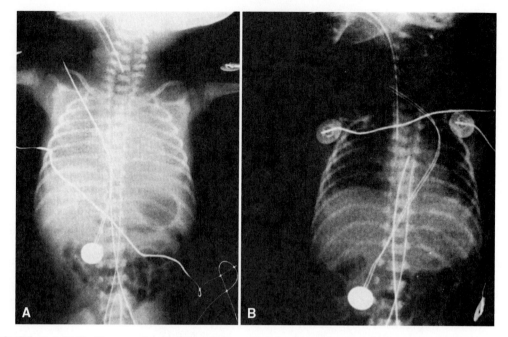

FIGURE 14-4 ■ Hyaline membrane disease before administration of surfactant **(A)** and significant clearing after administration **(B)**.

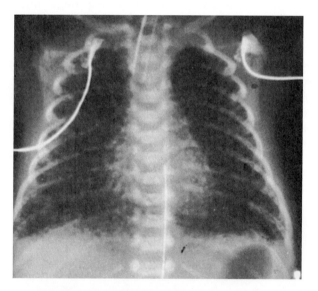

FIGURE 14-5 ■ Pulmonary interstitial emphysema. Note hyperexpansion bilaterally and pinpoint dark bubbles throughout both lung fields.

C. Bronchopulmonary dysplasia (BPD) (Fig. 14-6).
   1. Initial x-ray picture shows lung disease (e.g., respiratory distress syndrome, meconium aspiration syndrome).
   2. Radiologic appearance and course of BPD have changed since Northway and Rosan (1968) described their four stages (Martin et al., 2006).
       a. By the end of the first or second week, there is a persistent haziness of vessel margins, progressing to linear densities that persist into the third or fourth week of life.
       b. Subsequently, there is gradual development of a bubbly appearance of the lungs in association with hyperaeration, which is more pronounced at the lung bases. This

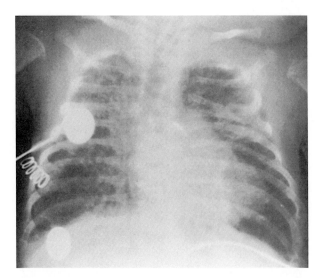

FIGURE 14-6 ■ Bronchopulmonary dysplasia. Note ill-defined densities bilaterally. Also note fractured rib in the upper-left portion of chest and pale-appearing ribs.

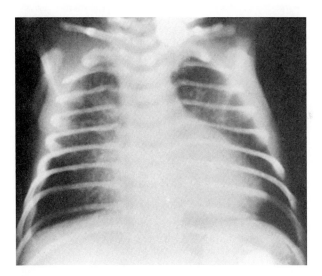

FIGURE 14-7 ■ Transient tachypnea of neonate. Note mild hyperexpansion and perihilar streakiness. A small pleural effusion is also present on the right side.

persists after 1 month of age and represents a modified form of stage IV BPD (Martin et al., 2006).
D. **Transient tachypnea of the newborn (TTN) (retained fetal lung fluid, wet lung disease) (Fig. 14-7).**
   1. Bilateral, symmetric perihilar streakiness due to increased interstitial and alveolar fluid (Martin et al., 2006).
   2. Mild to moderate overaeration of the lungs and strand-like densities (Haller et al., 2004).
   3. Possible fluid in minor (or horizontal) fissure and major (or oblique) lobar fissure.
   4. Mildly enlarged cardiothymic silhouette (Haller et al., 2004).
   5. Lung fields begin to clear in 24 to 48 hours.
E. **Meconium aspiration syndrome (Fig. 14-8).**
   1. Mild cases may show a normal lung pattern to mild infiltrates with overexpanded lungs.
   2. Bilateral asymmetric areas of atelectasis; hyperaeration of the lungs with flattened hemi-diaphragms (Haller et al., 2004).

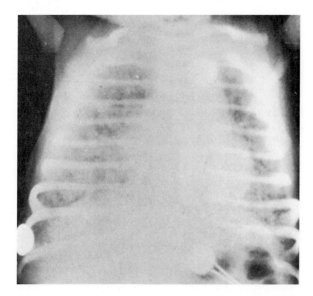

FIGURE 14-8 ■ Meconium aspiration syndrome. Note coarse, patchy infiltrates bilaterally.

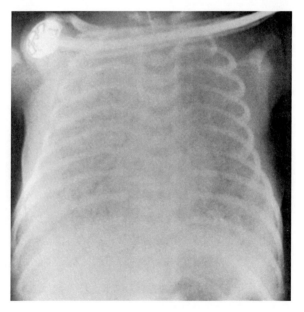

FIGURE 14-9 ■ Group B streptococcal pneumonia. Note reticulogranular appearance seen with hyaline membrane disease.

   3. Possible atelectasis if airway is obstructed because of debris.
   4. Possible air leaks (pneumothorax or pneumomediastinum) resulting from overdistention and rupture of the alveoli.
F. Pneumonia.
   1. Patchy, occasionally asymmetric, radiating, bilateral interstitial infiltrate. A nodular pattern may predominate in hazy lungs, and an effusion is a common occurrence (Haller et al., 2004).
   2. Reticulogranular pattern similar to that of respiratory distress syndrome. Some alveoli contain inflammatory exudate, which will appear more opaque and reticulogranular on x-ray than those filled with air (Haller et al., 2004).
   3. Group B streptococcal pneumonia is often difficult to diagnose using x-ray because of variable lung volumes and variable densities. May be indistinguishable from RDS (Haller et al., 2004; Kenner and Lott, 2007) (Fig. 14-9).

PULMONARY AIR LEAKS

A. Pneumothorax (Fig. 14-10, *A*).
 1. Accumulation of air in the pleural space. Air can outline the lung circumferentially or can accumulate.
 2. Mediastinal shift of structures away from the affected side as air accumulates (tension pneumothorax) (Kenner and Lott, 2007).
 3. Outline of the collapsed lung, with a band of hyperlucency between the chest wall and the underlying lung (Kenner and Lott, 2007).
 4. Other findings related to a pneumothorax.
    a. Pneumothorax not under tension may not exhibit a mediastinal shift.
    b. Diaphragm on the affected side of a pneumothorax under tension will be flattened because of the tensile force acting on it as a result of air accumulation superior to it (Kenner and Lott, 2007).
    c. Skinfold may mimic a pneumothorax (Kenner and Lott, 2007) (see Fig. 14-10, *B*).
B. Pneumomediastinum (Fig. 14-11).
 1. Mediastinal air collection, which produces irregular gas collections within the soft tissues of the superior mediastinum, with air frequently outlining the undersurface of the thymus gland and thus creating a "sail sign" (Kenner and Lott, 2007).
 2. Can accompany a pneumothorax.
 3. On cross-table lateral film, a radiolucent area of hyperlucency in the superior retrosternal space.
C. Pneumopericardium (Fig. 14-12).
 1. Radiolucent halo of free air surrounds the heart as air accumulates within the pericardial space (Kenner and Lott, 2007).
 2. Width of air around the heart is proportional to the amount of air present. Air is limited to the pericardium and cannot extend beyond the origins of the aorta and pulmonary artery.
 3. Decreased cardiac size may indicate cardiac tamponade.
 4. Other pulmonary air leaks and/or pulmonary interstitial emphysema are generally present.
 5. Pneumopericardium is rare in the absence of assisted ventilation.

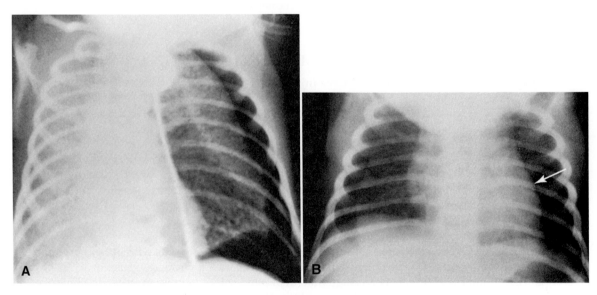

FIGURE 14-10 ■ **A,** Left tension pneumothorax. Note mediastinal shift toward right side. **B,** Note skinfold on right *(arrow)*. It can be mistaken for a pneumothorax. It extends beyond the chest and crosses over the diaphragm.

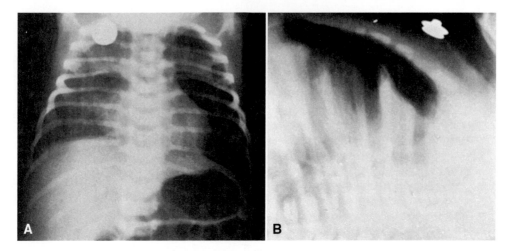

FIGURE 14-11 ■ **A,** Pneumomediastinum with thymus lifted, demonstrating the "sail sign." **B,** Pneumomediastinum on lateral view. Note air in anterior chest outlines thymus.

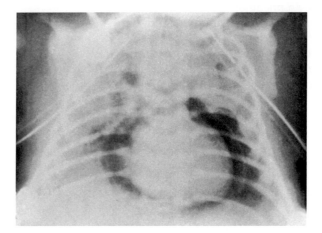

FIGURE 14-12 ■ Pneumopericardium. Note that the air completely encircles the heart. Bilateral chest tubes are also in place.

MISCELLANEOUS CAUSES OF RESPIRATORY DISTRESS

A. **Diaphragmatic paralysis (phrenic nerve injury)** (Fig. 14-13).
   1. Elevation and fixation of a diaphragmatic leaflet (Haller et al., 2004).
   2. More common on the right than the left side and usually unilateral.
   3. Mediastinum may be shifted away from the affected side.
   4. Most often results from obstetric injury to the brachial plexus.
   5. Erb palsy an associated finding.
B. **Eventration of the diaphragm** (Fig. 14-14).
   1. Weakness of the hemidiaphragm, with abdominal organs pushing up against it but not entering the chest because no opening exists.
   2. Either partial or complete; usually right-sided (Haller et al., 2004).
C. **Pulmonary edema** (Fig. 14-15).
   1. Increased pulmonary permeability is common in premature infants with lung injury that can manifest as diffuse haziness of the lungs to a white-out appearance (Haller et al., 2004).
   2. Significant association between high fluid intake and subsequent occurrence of a clinically significant patent ductus arteriosus and BPD (Kenner and Lott, 2007).
   3. Also common with certain congenital heart defects as a result of increased pulmonary blood flow (coarctation of the aorta, hypoplastic left heart syndrome).

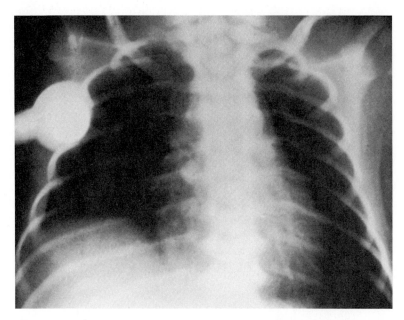

FIGURE 14-13 ■ Paralysis of right side of the diaphragm. Note that the right side of the diaphragm is markedly elevated in comparison with the left side of the diaphragm.

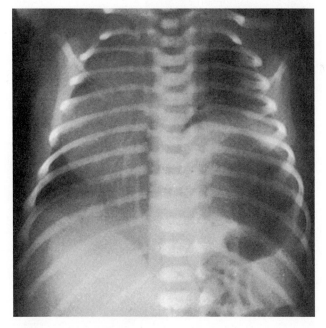

FIGURE 14-14 ■ Eventration of the diaphragm. Note the left side of the diaphragm bulging upward, with the stomach pushing upward against it.

THORACIC SURGICAL PROBLEMS

A. **Congenital diaphragmatic hernia** (Fig. 14-16, *A*).
  1. Herniation of abdominal contents through various portions of the diaphragm into the thoracic cavity, most commonly through the foramen of Bochdalek (Kenner and Lott, 2007).
  2. The majority occur on the left side.
  3. Hemithorax filled with loops of bowel, stomach, and often liver; displaces the mediastinal structures away from the affected side.
  4. Abdomen relatively gasless and may be scaphoid.

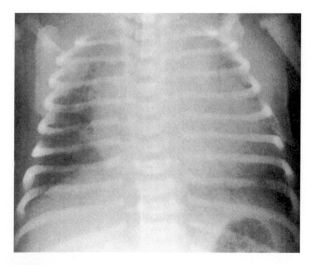

FIGURE 14-15 ■ Pulmonary edema. Note congested lung fields and cardiomegaly.

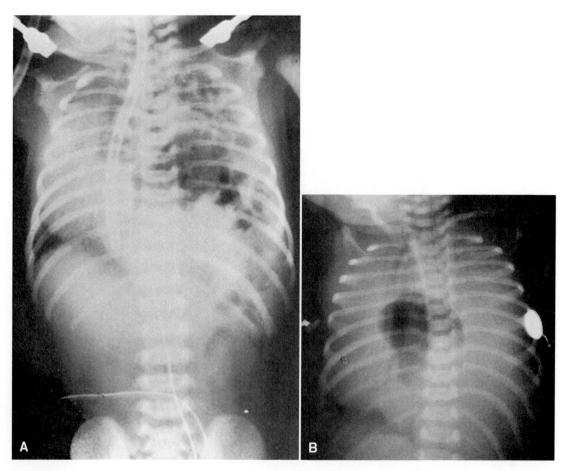

FIGURE 14-16 ■ **A,** Left diaphragmatic hernia. Note presence of bowel in the left side of the chest, a mediastinal shift to the right, and lack of bowel in the abdomen. **B,** Left diaphragmatic hernia before much air has expanded the bowel. Note that the trachea and heart have shifted to the right.

5. Contralateral pneumothorax possible with assisted ventilation or as a result of pulmonary hypoplasia on the unaffected side.
6. If the x-ray is obtained before the bowel is expanded with air, the affected hemithorax may appear entirely opacified with the mediastinal structures shifted to the opposite side (Kenner and Lott, 2007) (see Fig. 14-16, *B*).

B. **Congenital lobar emphysema** (Fig. 14-17).
 1. Most common cause of cystic malformation of the lung.
 2. Air trapped within one or more lung lobes at birth, resulting in obstructive emphysema.
 3. Overdistended affected lobe, with the mediastinum shifted to the contralateral side.
 4. Possibly hyperlucent but may also be opaque because of fluid accumulation distal to the obstruction (Haller et al., 2004).
 5. Generally limited to the upper lobes.

C. **Cystic adenomatoid malformation** (Fig. 14-18).
 1. Overdistention of affected lobe, with mediastinal shift to the contralateral side.

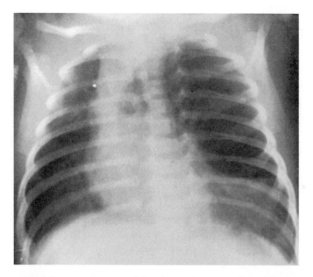

FIGURE 14-17 ■ Congenital lobar emphysema. Note hyperlucency of the left upper lung lobe, with mediastinal shift toward the right.

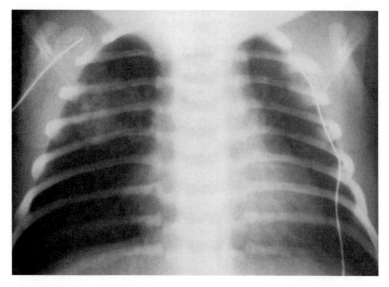

FIGURE 14-18 ■ Cystic adenomatoid malformation in the right lung.

2. Lobar overdistention, caused by air and fluid.
3. Upper lobes most frequently affected (Haller et al., 2004).
4. X-ray findings: multiple air-filled cysts, mediastinal shift, and compression of opposite lung. Diaphragmatic hernia must be ruled out.

CARDIOVASCULAR SYSTEM

A. **Size of the heart.**
   1. Difficult to assess on anteroposterior film because of a large thymus. Lateral film assessing a specific chamber enlargement may be more useful (Haller et al., 2004).
   2. Enlargement suggested by cardiothoracic ratio greater than 65% (Haller et al., 2004) (Fig. 14-19).
   3. Malpositioning: may represent cardiac displacement, developmentally abnormal cardiac position, or ambiguous rotation or site.
   4. Possible transient enlargement as a result of polycythemia, perinatal anoxia, or normally increased fluid present at birth.
B. **Pulmonary vascularity.**
   1. Normal vascular markings are seen in the middle one third of the lung fields (Fig. 14-20).

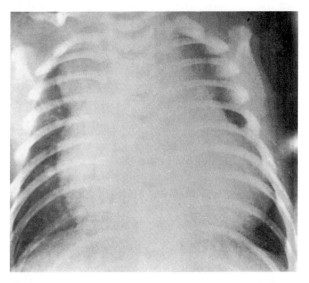

FIGURE 14-19 ■ Cardiomegaly. Note that the enlarged heart occupies the majority of the thorax.

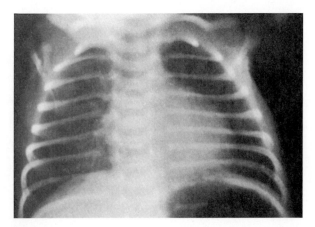

FIGURE 14-20 ■ Normal pulmonary vascularity. Note the presence of vascularity radiating from the perihilar region.

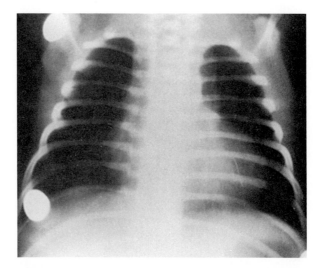

FIGURE 14-21 ■ Hyperlucent lung fields because of decreased blood flow to the lungs.

2. Decreased vascular markings occur with obstruction along the right ventricular outflow tract of the heart and are manifested as hyperlucency in both lung fields (Fig. 14-21).
3. Increased pulmonary vascularity occurs when excess blood flow causes congestion in the blood vessels and is manifested as increased streakiness, hazy lung fields, and increased densities as the condition worsens.

C. **Positional anomalies of the heart.**
   1. Types of malposition are as follows:
      a. Dextrocardia: right-sided heart.
      b. Mesocardia: midline heart.
      c. Extrathoracic: ectopia cordis.
   2. Position of other organs in relation to the heart is also incorporated into the definition of cardiac malposition. Positions of the abdominal organs are as follows:
      a. Situs solitus: normal abdominal organ position.
      b. Situs inversus: stomach and spleen on right, liver on left, and left atrium on right.
      c. Situs ambiguus: abdominal organs and atrial position are anatomically uncertain. The liver may be symmetric and at midline, and the stomach may be central. There may be duplication or absence of unilateral structures such as the spleen (asplenia or polysplenia).
   3. "Mirror image" dextrocardia with situs inversus is the most common type of malposition; congenital heart disease is unlikely (Martin et al., 2006) (Fig. 14-22).
   4. Dextrocardia with situs solitus—dextrocardia is an isolated finding with all other organs in their normal position. Incidence of congenital heart disease is 95% to 98% (Martin et al., 2006).
   5. Cardiac malposition caused by shift of the heart within the thorax must be differentiated from extracardiac causes, such as pneumothorax, hypoplastic lung, diaphragmatic hernia, decreased lung volume, and lung mass.

D. **Lesions with increased pulmonary vascularity.**
   1. Left-to-right shunt or intracardiac mixing.
      a. Transposition of the great vessels: Plain film shows "egg on a string" appearance. Cardiac silhouette of normal size or mild cardiomegaly may be seen (Haller et al., 2004). Pulmonary vascularity is variable, depending on the presence or absence of a ventricular septal defect or a patent ductus arteriosus.
      b. Total anomalous pulmonary venous return: X-ray film shows cardiomegaly; increased pulmonary vascularity; and enlargement of the right atrium, right ventricle, and pulmonary artery. The "snowman" appearance of the heart, caused by a characteristic widening of the superior mediastinum due to the connecting blood vessels, is rarely

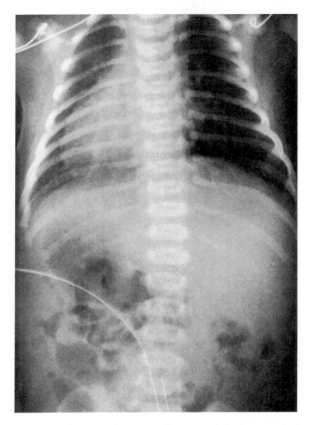

FIGURE 14-22 ■ "Mirror image" dextrocardia. Note the apex of the heart pointing to the right, with the stomach located on the right and the liver on the left.

      seen in the neonate because of the slow development of excessive pulmonary blood flow (Haller et al., 2004).

   c. Atrioventricular (AV) canal defect (endocardial cushion defect): Pulmonary vascular resistance usually remains high enough to delay the onset of CHF until after the first 1 to 2 weeks, after which marked cardiomegaly and vascular congestion are evident.

   d. Truncus arteriosus: Right and left ventricles are prominent, with left atrial dilation. As CHF develops, pulmonary vessels become indistinct and obscured by pulmonary edema.

   e. Atrial septal defect: Chest x-ray may be normal, with small defects. With large left-to-right shunts, there is a moderate cardiac enlargement and increased pulmonary vascularity. The right atrium and right ventricle are enlarged.

   f. Ventricular septal defect: With small defects the heart size and vascularity may be normal. With moderate-sized defects, the heart size may be enlarged, with increased pulmonary vascular markings. With large defects and increased blood flow, cardiomegaly is evident because of right and left ventricular enlargement. Pulmonary vascularity is markedly increased. CHF, interstitial edema, and alveolar fluid may be present.

   g. Patent ductus arteriosus: Pulmonary vasculature and cardiac silhouette may be obscured by underlying lung disease of RDS. Lung fields may show pulmonary edema and increasing heart size compared with heart size on previous x-ray films (Haller et al., 2004).

 2. Left-sided obstruction: Outflow of blood from the left side of the heart or return of blood from the lungs is obstructed, which will eventually cause CHF.

   a. Hypoplastic left heart syndrome (aortic atresia, mitral atresia): Pulmonary vascularity may appear normal until significant cardiac decompensation is present, and then cardiomegaly and CHF become evident. Right atrial enlargement may also be seen (Haller et al., 2004). This is the most common cause of CHF in the first few days of life.

  b. Coarctation of the aorta: Heart size is normal, but left ventricular enlargement may subsequently be seen on lateral views (Haller et al., 2004). X-ray findings vary according to the degree of patency of the patent ductus arteriosus and the severity of the obstruction at the coarctation site. CHF occurs, with ductal closure resulting in cardiomegaly and pulmonary venous congestion.

  c. Aortic stenosis: Normal cardiac size and vasculature may be seen, with mild stenosis of the aortic valve. Left ventricular enlargement occurs, with cardiac decompensation or associated aortic regurgitation resulting in cardiomegaly and venous congestion (Haller et al., 2004).

3. Lesions with decreased pulmonary vascularity. All these lesions involve some form of obstruction to the normal flow of blood through the right outflow tract. They can be located anywhere from the tricuspid valve to the pulmonary artery.

  a. Pulmonary valve atresia with an intact ventricular septum: Pulmonary vascularity is reduced or normal, depending on alternative sources of pulmonary blood flow, such as a patent ductus arteriosus. A shallow or concave pulmonary artery is evident (Haller et al., 2004). Closure of the ductus arteriosus and obstruction of the right ventricular outflow tract cause decreased pulmonary blood flow. Pulmonary vessels are underfilled and appear small and thin, which results in dark, hyperlucent lung fields. Heart size is variable, but cardiomegaly is usually present because of right atrial and left ventricular enlargement.

  b. Tricuspid atresia: Tricuspid valve has complete atresia, and the right ventricle and right outflow tract are underdeveloped. Chest x-ray shows a normal or small heart and diminished pulmonary blood flow (Haller et al., 2004).

  c. Tetralogy of Fallot: Cardiac size and shape are frequently normal. Pulmonary vascular markings are decreased. A "boot-shaped" contour may occur from a small, concave pulmonary artery and a prominent cardiac apex as a result of right ventricular hypertrophy (Haller et al., 2004).

  d. Pulmonary stenosis: Severe valvular obstruction is associated with hypoxemia because of a right-to-left shunt at the foramen ovale. This is referred to as critical pulmonary stenosis. Neonate's chest x-ray is normal, but cardiomegaly with predominant right atrium and right ventricle, decreased pulmonary vascularity, and dilation of the pulmonary artery eventually occur.

GASTROINTESTINAL SYSTEM

A. **Characteristics of the normal abdomen (Fig. 14-23).**

  1. Air is present in the stomach immediately after birth because of respiratory movement of the thorax and swallowing of air. By 24 hours of life, air should appear in the rectum (Haller et al., 2004).

  2. A gasless abdomen may be seen in infants with decreased swallowing, decreased GI motility (i.e., with intubation or chemical paralysis), vomiting, or gastric decompression from suctioning.

  3. Resuscitation may increase the amount of bowel gas seen on an x-ray.

B. **The esophagus.**

  1. May show indentations near the aortic arch and left mainstem bronchus.

  2. May assume peculiar configurations because of flexibility during the respiratory cycle.

  3. Air in the esophagus is a normal finding on regular chest films.

C. **Esophageal abnormalities.**

  1. Esophageal atresia (Fig. 14-24, *A*). A portion of the esophagus is atretic, and both distal and proximal portions of the esophagus end in blind pouches.

    a. On x-ray a radiolucent, air-filled, distended proximal esophageal pouch is present. The abdomen is gasless because no air can enter. The proximal pouch can be identified by passing a radiopaque tube and obtaining a chest film. The tube will not advance beyond 9 to 11 cm (Merenstein and Gardner, 2006).

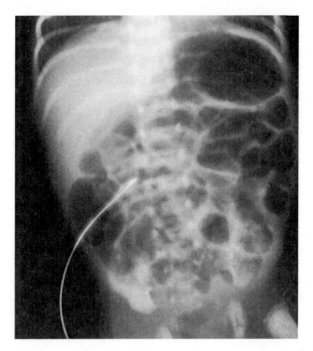

FIGURE 14-23 ■ Normal bowel gas pattern. Note the presence of stomach bubble and air through the entire abdomen to the rectum.

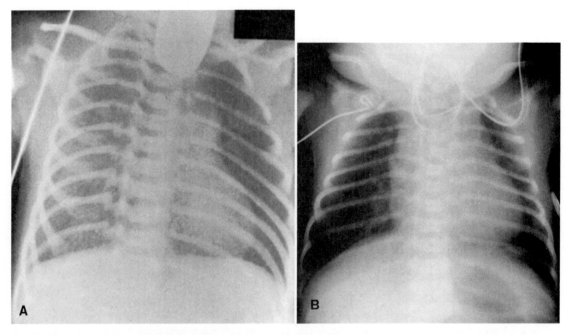

FIGURE 14-24 ■ **A,** Esophageal atresia. Contrast medium outlines the esophagus, which ends in the blind pouch. **B,** Esophageal atresia with tracheoesophageal fistula. The gastric tube cannot be advanced because of esophageal atresia. Air is in the abdomen, confirming the presence of a tracheoesophageal fistula.

      b. Aspiration pneumonitis of the upper lobes, especially the right upper lobe, is a common finding.

  2. Esophageal atresia with tracheoesophageal fistula (see Fig. 14-24, *B*).

      a. Esophageal atresia with fistulous connection to the distal esophageal pouch is the most common esophageal anomaly.

  b. Excessive dilation of the stomach and/or small bowel, resulting from distal fistula communication between the lungs and the stomach, may occur.

  c. Chest film should be obtained with a radiopaque tube in place. The tube will not advance into the stomach, and air will be present in the GI tract.

 3. Tracheoesophageal fistula with no esophageal atresia (H type of fistula).

  a. Difficult to identify without a contrast study.

  b. Fistula characteristically assumes an upwardly oblique configuration on contrast study.

  c. Widespread pulmonary infiltrates are commonly present because of constant aspiration through the fistula into the lungs.

D. The stomach.

 1. Visible directly beneath the left diaphragm.

 2. Often appears large in the neonate as a result of dilation with air.

 3. Mucosal folds are absent. Stomach wall appears smooth.

 4. Begins to empty moments after being filled.

E. Abnormalities of the stomach.

 1. Pyloric stenosis.

  a. Symptoms develop 2 to 8 weeks after birth (Kenner and Lott, 2007).

  b. Plain films demonstrate a distended stomach and duodenum, with disproportionately less gas in the small bowel.

  c. Ultrasonography is the study of choice for the diagnosis.

 2. Gastric perforation.

  a. Uncommon, but may result from gastric ulcers, hypoxia-induced focal necrosis, gastric tubes, or indomethacin therapy for closure of ductus arteriosus.

  b. Possible overinflation due to distal obstruction, as with mechanical ventilation.

  c. Common finding of free air (pneumoperitoneum) with absence of gastric gas.

F. Duodenal abnormalities (Fig. 14-25).

 1. Duodenal atresia and stenosis.

  a. Infants with duodenal atresia present with vomiting in the first few hours of life. Those with stenosis present at variable times, depending on the degree of stenosis.

  b. Duodenal atresia and stenosis are present in approximately 33% of infants with Down syndrome (trisomy 21) (Mandell, 2007).

  c. X-ray demonstrates dilation of the stomach and proximal duodenum, producing the characteristic "double bubble" pattern. No air is present distal to the duodenum (Kenner and Lott, 2007).

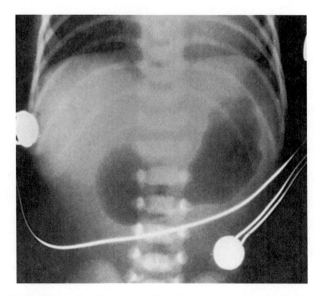

FIGURE 14-25 ■ Duodenal atresia with a characteristic "double bubble" pattern.

2. Annular pancreas.
   a. Pancreas grows in the form of an encircling ring around the duodenum (Kenner and Lott, 2007).
   b. Presentation is similar to that of duodenal atresia or stenosis.
   c. X-ray findings are generally indistinguishable from duodenal atresia or stenosis. Identification is made with ultrasonography.

G. **Abnormalities of the small bowel.**
   1. Small-bowel atresia and stenosis.
      a. Single or multiple areas of atresia or stenosis may exist.
      b. Clinically abdominal distention and bile-stained vomiting are apparent early on.
      c. Types of small-bowel atresia.
         (1) High jejunal obstruction. One or two loops of bowel are visible on x-ray.
         (2) Midjejunal obstruction. More dilated loops are visible on x-ray.
         (3) Distal ileal atresia. Many dilated loops are visible on x-ray.
   2. Meconium ileus (Fig. 14-26).
      a. Approximately 16% to 20% of infants with cystic fibrosis present with meconium ileus at birth (Irish, 2006).
      b. Obstruction results from impaction of thick, tenacious meconium in the distal portion of the small bowel. Ileal atresia or stenosis, ileal perforation, meconium peritonitis, and volvulus are common complications (Irish, 2006).
      c. Clinical presentation includes bile-stained vomiting, abdominal distention, and failure to pass meconium.
      d. X-ray shows a low small-bowel obstruction with numerous, variably sized air-filled loops of bowel (Irish, 2006). There is a "soap bubble" appearance in the right lower quadrant as a result of trapping of air in the meconium.
      e. A contrast-enema study will demonstrate a microcolon. A water-soluble contrast agent draws large amounts of fluid into the intestine and lubricates the meconium, allowing it to pass without surgical intervention. This technique is successful 35% of the time (Irish, 2006).
   3. Midgut volvulus.
      a. Most common form of small-bowel volvulus.
      b. Twisting and spiraling of entire gut around the superior mesenteric artery, resulting in vascular compromise, necrosis, perforation, and gangrene.
      c. May present with bilious vomiting.

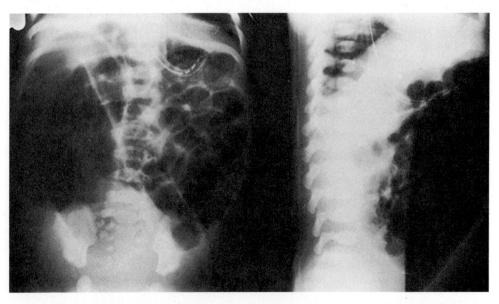

FIGURE 14-26 ■ Meconium ileus with perforation and free air visible on the lateral film.

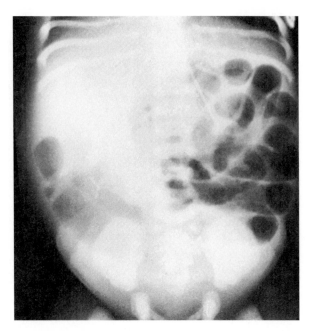

FIGURE 14-27 ■ Hirschsprung disease. Note the abdominal distention with dilated loops of bowel and lack of air in the distal portion of the bowel.

    d. May be difficult to determine on x-ray because findings are variable, from a normal abdomen to one suggesting a gastric outlet obstruction, partial obstruction of the duodenum, or small-bowel obstruction (Kenner and Lott, 2007).

    e. Ultrasonography, barium enema, or x-ray of upper GI tract may be needed for diagnostic purposes or to demonstrate complete obstruction of the third portion of the duodenum.

H. Abnormalities of the colon.

  1. Hirschsprung disease (aganglionosis of the colon) (Fig. 14-27).

    a. Typical presentation is vomiting, obstruction, and failure to pass meconium within the first 24 to 36 hours of life.

    b. Commonly involves the distal colonic segment—rectal and rectosigmoid areas.

    c. Plain films show some degree of low small-bowel or colonic obstruction, air-fluid levels, and distention of the bowel (Kenner and Lott, 2007). Rectal gas may be absent or sparse.

    d. Barium enema will support the findings, and a rectal biopsy will show absence of ganglion cells.

  2. Meconium plug syndrome/small left colon syndrome.

    a. Normal meconium becomes impacted in the distal portion of the colon. In meconium plug syndrome, the obstruction is generally in the sigmoid colon. In small left colon syndrome, the site of obstruction is the splenic flexure.

    b. Functional immaturity of the colon is thought to be the cause of the initial inability to pass meconium (Kenner and Lott, 2007).

    c. Condition is manifested within the first 23 to 36 hours of life with abdominal distention, bilious vomiting, and failure to pass meconium.

    d. Diagnosis is by contrast-enema examination. The examination may also be therapeutic by dislodgment of the meconium (Merenstein and Gardner, 2006).

    e. Plain films are nonspecific and usually show a low small-bowel obstruction with distention of the bowel.

  3. Necrotizing enterocolitis (Fig. 14-28).

    a. X-ray findings include generalized distention caused by paralytic ileus, asymmetric distribution of bowel gas, and localized distention of bowel loops.

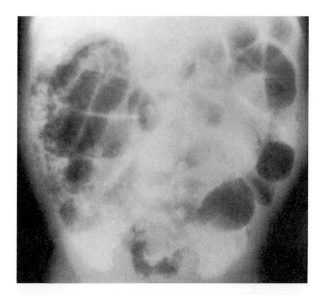

FIGURE 14-28 ■ Necrotizing enterocolitis. Note the presence of distended bowel loops and pneumatosis intestinalis.

    b. X-ray films are obtained every 6 to 8 hours to follow the progression of the disease in the acute phase. A cross-table lateral view, along with plain film, should be obtained to detect free air.

    c. Subsequently, individual loops may become tubular, with thickened bowel walls.

    d. Persistently dilated loops may be evident on consecutive films.

    e. At any point, pneumatosis cystoides intestinalis can be seen. This represents gas formed in the intestinal wall by bacteria. The typical picture is linear or of a bubbly or foamy appearance. Air may be located in the submucosal or subserosal layer and can enter the GI tract or portal venous system (Haller et al., 2004).

    f. Right segment of colon and terminal ileum are most likely to be affected, although the entire colon may be affected.

    g. The most common cause of intestinal perforation; it is seen as free abdominal gas on plain film or in the left lateral decubitus view.

I. **Pneumoperitoneum** (see Fig. 14-26).

    1. Most commonly a result of perforation of the GI tract because of perinatal asphyxia, indomethacin therapy, gastric overdistention, iatrogenic perforation with a thermometer, and as a complication of necrotizing enterocolitis and GI obstruction (Kenner and Lott, 2007).

    2. Air may dissect from the neonate's chest during positive-pressure ventilation.

    3. Presents with abdominal distention and respiratory distress, or abdominal wall erythema.

    4. Supine x-ray may not reveal free air (Kenner and Lott, 2007), necessitating lateral decubitus or cross-table view.

    5. Abdomen is distended and radiolucent on x-ray (Kenner and Lott, 2007). Individual loops of bowel are visible because of air inside and outside the bowel wall. Falciform ligament (an opaque stripe) may be visualized in the right upper quadrant or upper mid portion of the abdomen.

J. **Meconium peritonitis.**

    1. Results from intrauterine GI perforation due to obstruction (atresia, stenosis, imperforate anus) and/or volvulus associated with meconium ileus (Irish, 2006).

    2. Calcifications, which are easily identifiable on x-ray, assume a focal or diffuse, patchy, irregular pattern. Multiple white-speckled areas are seen in one area or throughout the abdomen and may be present in the scrotum (Irish, 2006).

    3. Calcifications will slowly disappear.

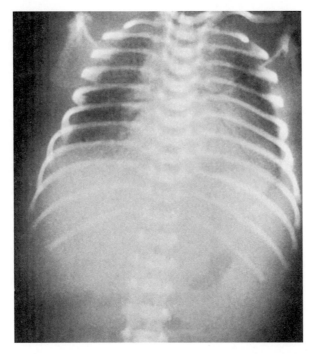

FIGURE 14-29 ■ Abdominal ascites with bilateral pleural effusions.

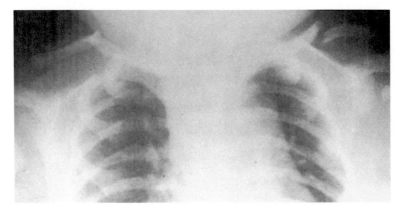

FIGURE 14-30 ■ Fractured left clavicle.

K. Abdominal ascites (Fig. 14-29).
1. Cases include infants with fetal hydrops, GI obstruction with perforation, and peritonitis.
2. Uniform density to the distended abdomen is noted with a gasless or centralized bowel gas pattern. Body wall edema may also be present in infants with fetal hydrops.

SKELETAL SYSTEM

A. Fractures: occur most often during delivery with an increased incidence during breech deliveries. In breech deliveries, fractures can occur in both upper and lower extremities.
1. Clavicle: fractured during delivery (Fig. 14-30). Fractures occur at the midclavicle most commonly. Fractured clavicle is common in large infants during difficult vaginal delivery (Kenner and Lott, 2007).

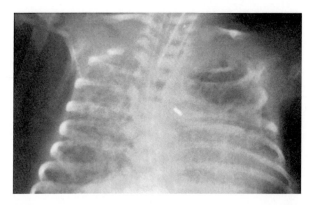

FIGURE 14-31 ■ Fractured rib on the left, with pale, "washed out" ribs.

2.   Rib fractures: may occur at delivery and be asymptomatic. With multiple fractures the infant may show signs of respiratory distress and pain. Premature infants may have rib fractures as a result of osteopenia of prematurity 8 to 16 weeks after birth (Fig. 14-31) (Haller et al., 2004). These bones are fragile and will fracture with handling and chest physiotherapy. Fractures may be preceded by a thin, "washed out" appearance of the ribs or extremities.

3.   Skull fractures.
a.   Can be linear, buckled, or frankly depressed.
b.   Linear and buckling fractures most often occur in the parietal bone and may be suspected in the presence of cephalhematoma or other skull trauma.
c.   Computed tomography (CT) scan is more helpful than plain films for evaluation of skull fractures.

B.   **Bony dysplasias.**
1.   Osteogenesis imperfecta (see Chapter 36).
2.   Dwarfism (common types).
a.   Achondroplasia: short extremities and marked flaring of the metaphyses. Classic signs include spinal curvature and narrowed spinal canal; short, squared-off iliac wings; deep-set sacrum; flat acetabular roofs; and bulky proximal femurs.
b.   Thanatophoric dwarfism (type I) (Fig. 14-32): marked underdevelopment of the skeleton; extremely short, bent, or curved long bones; and flaring of the metaphyses. Vertebral bodies are very flat and underdeveloped. Thorax is small and narrow, with pulmonary hypoplasia. Condition is uniformly fatal in the perinatal period.

INDWELLING LINES AND TUBES

A.   **Endotracheal tube.**
1.   Placement is 1.2 cm below the vocal cords and 2 cm above the carina, with the neonate's head in the neutral position (Haller et al., 2004).
2.   Placement beyond the carina results in occlusion of a bronchus (usually the right mainstem bronchus), with subsequent atelectasis and clinical deterioration (Fig. 14-33).

B.   **Umbilical artery catheter (Fig. 14-34, A):** Proceeds from the umbilicus down toward the pelvis, making an acute turn into the internal iliac artery and common iliac artery advancing into the aorta (Merenstein and Gardner, 2006).
1.   Low placement: at third and fourth lumbar vertebrae.
2.   High placement: at sixth through tenth thoracic vertebrae.

C.   **Umbilical venous catheter (see Fig. 14-34, B):** Proceeds from the umbilicus cephalad to join the left portal vein.
1.   On lateral view the catheter is directly distal to the abdominal wall until it passes through the ductus venosus.
2.   Correct placement is above the diaphragm, below the junction of the right atrium (Merenstein and Gardner, 2006).

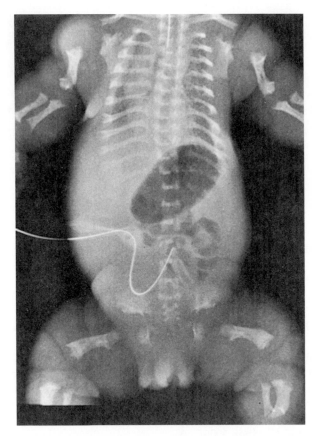

FIGURE 14-32 ■ Thanatophoric dwarf. Note the small, narrow thorax and shortness of long bones.

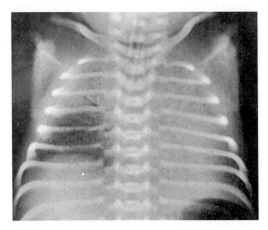

FIGURE 14-33 ■ Endotracheal tube is down the right mainstem bronchus, causing atelectasis of the right upper lobe and entire left lung.

D. Chest tube (see Fig. 14-12).
  1. X-rays are obtained to determine placement and effectiveness in reinflating the lung.
  2. Lateral chest x-ray film will determine anterior or posterior placement. For air evacuation, anterior placement is desirable. For fluid evacuation, posterior placement is most effective.
  3. Correct placement will show the tube in the midclavicular line, with the distal chest tube hole inside the thoracic space.

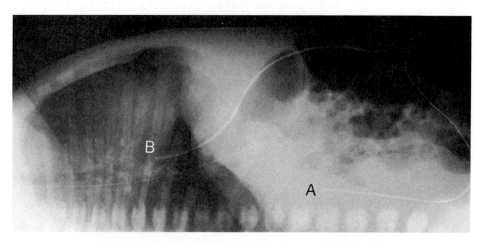

FIGURE 14-34 ■ Umbilical artery catheter **(A)** enters the abdomen and proceeds distally as it enters the aorta. Umbilical venous catheter **(B)** proceeds toward the head, passes through the ductus venosus, and lies in the inferior vena cava.

E. **Central venous line:** Tip should be located in the superior vena cava or right atrium above the tricuspid valve.

F. **Percutaneous central venous line:** If placed in an upper extremity, the tip of the catheter should be located in the superior vena cava and is considered central once it crosses the mid-clavicular line and is above the right atrium of the heart (Merenstein and Gardner, 2006). If placed in a lower extremity, the line should be positioned in the inferior vena cava and is considered central once it crosses to the pelvic cavity and rests below the right atrium of the heart (Merenstein and Gardner, 2006).

　1. A chest x-ray is obtained to confirm placement of a catheter placed in an upper extremity. Arm placement will affect the position of the line. The arm should be extended and at a 45-degree angle from the body to best represent normal arm position.

　2. An abdominal x-ray is obtained to confirm placement of a catheter placed in a lower extremity. Lower extremities should be extended and held in place for the abdominal x-ray.

DIAGNOSTIC IMAGING

A. **Ultrasound.**

　1. Uses sound waves to depict anatomic and functional motion of tissue. The sound waves evaluate varying density of tissues, the movement of tissue, and blood flow. The sound waves can be directed in a variety of planes and angles to enhance imaging (Merenstein and Gardner, 2006).

　2. Used to evaluate internal anatomic structures and some function. Unlike conventional radiography, ultrasound does not emit radiation. The images are typically recorded on videotape or magnetic disks (Merenstein and Gardner, 2006).

　3. Ultrasound is less expensive than CT or magnetic resonance imaging (MRI), is portable, and therefore more convenient for the evaluation of the unstable patient.

　4. Ultrasound is painless and generally does not require sedation. The procedure is performed at the bedside and the infant's environment is minimally disrupted. Peripheral IVs placed in the area of the anterior fontanelle may need to be relocated if brain imaging is required.

　5. Poor imaging technique, presence of bone and air in the imaging area, and patient position adversely affect the quality of the exam. Infant should be supine; for cranial imaging, the head should be in the midline position.

　6. The nurse's role during an ultrasound exam is to correctly position infant, offer comfort measures if necessary, and monitor vital signs and infant's tolerance of the procedure.

7. Ultrasound is commonly used to evaluate brain parenchyma and ventricular size, myocardial function and structure, urinary tract anatomy and pathology, pelvic masses, liver anatomy, and blood flow in major vessels.

B. **Computed Tomography (CT).**
   1. Obtains cross-sectional images of structures by emitting multiple x-ray beams through tissue. CT passes multiple fan x-ray beams through the same cross-sectional slice of tissue at different angles during different time intervals. The beams rotate about the infant, pass through the body, and the exit transmission of x-ray beams is monitored by a series of detectors (Merenstein and Gardner, 2006).
   2. CT provides a two-dimensional visualization of anatomy and can be further enhanced by the use of a radiographic contrast agent. Contrast enhancement can assist in the evaluation of blood flow and help define pathologic abnormalities.
   3. CT can distinguish changes in density in very small areas of tissue and allows identification of a variety of soft tissues. This allows for superior anatomic detail and precise clarity of tissue structure (Merenstein and Gardner, 2006).
   4. CT requires the infant to be transported to the radiology department, so the infant's environment is disrupted. CT is painless but may require sedation depending on the infant's state.
   5. Used to evaluate structure, function, malformation, and extent of disease process. Used commonly in the NICU to evaluate brain anatomy, intraventricular hemorrhage, and extent of parenchymal disease and subgaleal, subarachnoid, and subdural bleeds (Merenstein and Gardner, 2006).
   6. The nurse's role in caring for an infant undergoing a CT examination is to swaddle the infant to decrease movement while in the scanner, thus diminishing artifacts from the scan. The nurse must also provide comfort measures, evaluate the need for sedation, and monitor vital signs and infant's tolerance of procedure.

C. **Magnetic Resonance Imaging (MRI).**
   1. Uses radio waves to image protons and hydrogen ions within the body (Merenstein and Gardner, 2006). The image quality is excellent and the increased sensitivity allows for more precise imaging of even the smallest of structures (Haller et al., 2004).
   2. Does not use ionizing radiation and has less artifact to obscure visualization.
   3. Is costly and has limited availability. The magnetic field can interfere with monitoring devices and may restrict the availability to unstable infants.
   4. Requires that the infant be transported to the MRI department, so the infant's environment is disrupted. MRI is painless but heavy sedation may be required for an optimal study, which may require mechanical ventilation.
   5. May be useful in the early diagnosis of periventricular leukomalacia, or when a more accurate definition of tissue structures is needed for evaluation and diagnosis (Merenstein and Gardner, 2006).
   6. The nurse's role in MRI includes swaddling the infant and positioning in the scanner. The infant must be placed on a monitor designed to function within a magnetic field; specialty ventilators are also available for use with MRI. The nurse provides comfort measures and sedation as ordered, as well as monitors vital signs and infant's tolerance of procedure.

D. **Echocardiogram (ECHO).**
   1. Noninvasive diagnostic tool to evaluate cardiac structure and function.
   2. High-frequency sound waves send vibrations through the heart, which reflect energy, and this energy is transmitted into a visual image.
   3. Poor imaging technique and infant movement adversely affect the ECHO quality. It is portable and therefore available for even the unstable infant.

E. **Barium enema.**
   1. Used to evaluate the structure and function of the large intestine and diagnose disorders such as Hirschsprung disease, malrotation, and meconium plug syndrome (Kenner and Lott, 2007).
   2. A water-soluble contrast solution is instilled and a series of x-rays are taken under fluoroscopy. A series of follow-up x-rays may be taken at timed intervals to evaluate the evacuation of the solution from the bowel.

F. Upper GI series with small-bowel follow-through.
1. Used to evaluate the structure and function of the upper GI tract. The three main areas examined are (1) the esophagus (for size, patency, reflux, and presence of fistula or swallowing abnormalities), (2) stomach (abnormalities and motility), and (3) the small intestine (for strictures, patency, and function).
2. A water-soluble contrast solution is swallowed and a series of x-rays are taken under fluoroscopy. A series of follow-up x-rays are obtained to evaluate the emptying ability of the stomach, intestinal motility, and potential obstruction (Kenner and Lott, 2007). Complications include reflux of the contrast solution, vomiting, and potential for aspiration.

G. Voiding cystourethrogram (VCUG).
1. Used to evaluate the structure and function of the kidneys, bladder, and lower urinary tract.
2. The infant's bladder is emptied by catheterization and then filled with a contrast solution. A series of x-rays are taken under fluoroscopy in a variety of positions during voiding. After voiding, follow-up x-rays are taken to evaluate residuals in the bladder and any reflux into the kidneys (Merenstein and Gardner, 2006).
3. The infant should be monitored for hematuria and signs of infection related to a contaminated catheterization.

REFERENCES

AHD Editors: *The American Heritage Medical Dictionary,* 2007. Retrieved from www.medical-dictionary.thefreedictionary.com

Haller, J.O., Slovis, T.L., and Joshi, A.: *Pediatric radiology* (3rd ed.). Chicago, London, 2004, Springer.

Irish, G.: Surgical aspects of cystic fibrosis and meconium ileus, 2006. Retrieved January 14, 2008, from www.emedicine.com

Kenner, C. and Lott, J.W.: *Comprehensive neonatal care: An interdisciplinary approach* (4th ed.). St. Louis, 2007, Saunders.

Mandell, G.: Duodenal atresia. 2007. Retrieved January 14, 2008, from www.emedicine.com

Martin, R.J., Fanaroff, A.A., and Walsh, M.C.: *Fanaroff and Martin's neonatal-perinatal medicine: Diseases of the fetus and infant* (8th ed.). Philadelphia, 2006, Mosby.

Merenstein, G.B. and Gardner, S.L.: *Handbook of neonatal intensive care* (6th ed.). St. Louis, 2006, Mosby.

Northway, W.H., Jr. and Rosan, R.C.: Radiographic features of pulmonary oxygen toxicity in the newborn: Bronchopulmonary dysplasia. *Radiology, 91*(1):49-58, 1968.

15 Common Invasive Procedures

GINA M. HEISS-HARRIS and TERESA BAILEY

OBJECTIVES

1. Understand the indications for common procedures performed in the neonatal intensive care unit (NICU) such as endotracheal tube (ETT) intubation and suctioning, vascular access methods, blood sampling methods, bladder catheterization, bladder aspiration, thoracentesis, and lumbar puncture.
2. Know the equipment and supplies needed to perform common fundamental and advanced invasive procedures in the neonate.
3. Identify pertinent anatomic landmarks for commonly performed invasive procedures in the NICU.
4. Describe the precautions and contraindications for each invasive procedure.
5. Describe potential complications associated with each invasive procedure.

■■ Approximately 250,000 to 350,000 newborn infants are admitted into the NICU in the United States annually. These infants undergo hundreds of diagnostic and/or therapeutic procedures during their hospitalization (Porter et al., 1999). This chapter incorporates many of the diagnostic and therapeutic interventions that are commonly performed in the NICU. These procedures are crucial to the infant's survival; however, they expose the infant to pain and stress that can result in harmful long-term consequences. Therefore, pain management is essential when performing interventions in the NICU.

In many NICUs today, qualified registered nurses or advanced practice nurses perform many invasive procedures rather than physicians. Prior to performing any procedure it is essential that one must have knowledge of the indications, precautions, and complications associated with each procedure. Infants are extremely vulnerable; therefore, the ability to perform the procedure proficiently is a major requirement to prevent harm.

The details pertaining to each of the covered procedures make up this chapter. Aspects that are common to each include the crucial issues listed below.

■ Know your institution's protocols about the qualifications needed to perform any procedure.
■ Know your institution's protocols about any specific ways in which procedures differ from the descriptions included here.
■ Obtain informed consent whenever required for an invasive procedure. Discussion with family is key, even if signed informed consent is not required.
■ Always use standard infection control precautions and implement aseptic technique whenever indicated.
■ Provide for pain and comfort control before, during, and after the procedure.
■ Monitor the patient's clinical status during the procedure. Minimally, monitoring will include oxygenation, ventilation, temperature, and reaction to the procedure.
■ Make written documentation about pertinent aspects of the procedure and enter this into the medical record.
■ Perform time out before procedure to ensure patient safety.

AIRWAY PROCEDURES

Endotracheal Tube Suctioning: Fundamental Procedure

A. **Indications.**
   1. Facilitate oxygenation and ventilation.

2. Maintain patent airway.
3. Clearance of tracheobronchial secretions.
4. Obtain tracheal aspirate specimens.

B. **Contraindications.**
1. Recent surgical procedure to area.
2. Recent surfactant administration.
3. Pulmonary hemorrhage—suction only if needed to maintain tube patency.

C. **Precautions.**
1. Suctioning should be done only when the infant needs it and not on a routine schedule.
2. Maintain aseptic technique.
3. Monitor vital signs and for adverse responses to procedure such as bradycardia and oxygen desaturations.
4. Avoid hyperoxygenation, hyperinflation, and hyperventilation techniques if possible. Hyperoxygenation in preterm neonates is discouraged owing to risk of retinopathy of prematurity (ROP). If the infant easily becomes hypoxic or oxygenation status is critical, oxygen can be increased by 10% to 20% above baseline to maintain adequate oxygenation. Hyperinflation should be avoided as this places the neonate at risk for air leaks. The effects of hyperventilation alone in neonates is unclear and therefore discouraged (Davis and Rosenfeld, 2005).
5. Loss of lung volume can occur with suctioning. Increased loss of lung volume and hypoxia are associated with open catheters versus closed "inline" catheters (Tingay et al., 2007).
6. Keep infant's head midline during suctioning to prevent jugular vein distention, which can increase intracranial pressure (ICP).
7. Pulmonary hemorrhage may be exacerbated by suctioning. However, suctioning may be needed to clear the blood from the airway or tube.
8. Always suction ETT before suctioning mouth.
9. When feasible, use two caregivers to perform endotracheal suctioning if the closed (inline) system is not in use. This may minimize adverse responses and shorten procedure time.

D. **Equipment and supplies.**
1. Sterile gloves.
2. Choose the appropriate-sized catheter. Catheter should be no larger than half the inside diameter of the ETT.
   a. Use 8 Fr for ETT >3.5 mm.
   b. Use 6 Fr for ETT <3.5 mm.
3. Resuscitation bag with 100% oxygen source and oxygen blender.
4. Suction source with vacuum control setting.
5. Manometer.
6. Stethoscope.
7. Specimen trap (if applicable).

E. **Procedure.**
1. Determine the need to suction and suction only when indicated. Suctioning should be individualized based on changes in the patient's physical assessment and not on a routine schedule (Hagedorn et al., 2006). The following situations may warrant suctioning:
   a. Falling oxygen saturations.
   b. Increasing oxygen requirements.
   c. Diminished breath sounds.
   d. Changes in vital signs.
   e. Changes in blood gases.
   f. Changes in respiratory rate and pattern.
   g. Agitation.
   h. Visible secretions in ETT.
   i. Pattern change in ventilator graphics.
   j. Loss of or poor chest wall excursion with ventilator breaths.
2. Wash hands and ensure that equipment is in working order.

3. Shallow suctioning technique is the preferred method. Deep suctioning should be avoided as this has been shown to cause tissue damage and inflammation.
   a. Determine suction catheter insertion depth by summing the length of the ETT and its adapter. The catheter should not be inserted more than 1 cm beyond the total distance determined (Hagler and Traver, 1994).
4. Gather supplies.
   a. Commercially prepared suction catheter kit or sterile suction catheter and sterile gloves. Closed-system (inline) suction catheter kits are available that remain attached to the ETT adapter and should be used per manufacturer's recommendations. The closed-system suction technique is preferred as it allows the infant to be suctioned without being removed from the ventilator. Closed-system suction devices may decrease respiratory contamination and pulmonary infections and have been shown to have decreased physiologic consequences such as bradycardia and desaturation (Choong et al., 2003; Kalyn et al., 2003; Tan et al., 2005).
   b. Appropriate-sized suction catheter with measurement markings.
   c. If using a commercially prepared suction kit, open package and maintain sterility of contents. Remove and don sterile gloves, then remove catheter. If using separate gloves and catheter supplies, open suction catheter package, maintaining sterility of catheter, then open and don gloves. Continue to maintain aseptic technique and remove catheter from package.
5. While maintaining aseptic procedure, attach suction catheter to suction tubing with nondominant hand (now considered contaminated). With sterile dominant hand hold suction catheter and maintain sterility of catheter.
6. Release suction tubing from nondominant hand and remove infant from ventilator. Provide oxygen and ventilation at necessary levels to maintain the heart rate and provide adequate oxygen saturation. Infant may be ventilated by hand or by providing manual breaths from ventilator. If manual breaths are provided by the ventilator, use caution to avoid hyperinflation and to allow adequate exhalation times.
7. Suction at 60 to 100 mm Hg or with just enough suction to extract secretions through catheter.
8. Advance catheter only to a predetermined distance. If a cough reflex is initiated, catheter distance is too far.
9. Apply suction only when withdrawing catheter and limit suction duration to 5 to 10 seconds. Ventilate patient between suction passes while monitoring vital signs, oxygen saturation, and chest wall movement.
10. Routine NS irrigation is not recommended as this may dislodge viable bacteria from colonized ETT into the lower airway (Hagedorn et al., 2006).
11. Limit the number of suction passes. Suction until secretions are removed or infant shows signs of intolerance. Clear suction catheter with NS between suction passes. Most secretions can be cleared in one or two passes.
12. If obtaining tracheal specimen, attach sterile specimen trap to suction catheter and suction tubing prior to suctioning.
13. Return infant to previous oxygen requirement as tolerated if applicable.
14. Label and send tracheal specimen to laboratory, if applicable.
15. Document patient's tolerance, character of secretions (amount, color, and consistency), and breath sounds.
16. If using a closed-system (inline) catheter device, change per manufacturer's recommendation or per institution's policy if sooner.

F. **Complications.**
   1. Hypoxia.
   2. Bradycardia.
   3. Apnea.
   4. Accidental extubation or malpositioning of tube.
   5. Trauma to trachea or bronchi.
   6. Hemorrhage.
   7. Loss of lung volume.

8. Atelectasis.
9. Infection/pneumonia.
10. Pneumothorax.
11. Increased ICP.
12. Granular tissue formation.
13. Bronchial stenosis.
14. Tracheal laceration.

Oral Endotracheal Intubation: Advanced Practice Procedure

A. **Indications.**
1. To perform resuscitation.
2. Bag-and-mask ventilation is ineffective or undesirable.
3. Need for mechanical ventilation.
4. Tracheal suctioning or lavage is required, such as to remove meconium from the trachea.
5. Obtain sterile tracheal aspirate specimen.
6. Protection of the airway is required.
7. Diaphragmatic hernia is present.
8. Administration of exogenous surfactant.
9. Relieve critical upper-airway obstruction.

B. **Precautions.**
1. Select oral intubation for emergent intubations. Nasal intubations should be used for elective procedures, in infants with copious secretions, or when defects of the oral anatomy are present (MacDonald and Ramasethu, 2007).
2. Patient's heart rate and oxygen saturation should be monitored continuously during the procedure and stabilized with bag-and-mask ventilation if possible prior to intubation.
3. Hypoxia during the procedure should be minimized.
4. Use free-flow oxygen held near the mouth and nose of any infant with respiratory effort, to maximize oxygenation during the procedure.
5. Limit intubation attempts to 20 seconds. The infant's condition should be stabilized with bag-and-mask ventilation between attempts.
6. Have all equipment necessary for intubation prepared and in working order prior to initiating procedure.
7. Consider sedation of infant prior to procedure for nonemergent intubation, using institutional protocol.
8. Maintain thermal homeostasis and developmental care.

C. **Equipment and supplies.**
1. Pediatric laryngoscope handle.
2. Laryngoscope blade with functioning secure bulb.
   a. Size 00 blade for preterm infants weighing less than 1000 g.
   b. Size 0 blade for infants weighing 1000 to 3000 g. Most infants weighing 3000 to 4000 g can be successfully intubated with a size 0 blade. However, if unable to visualize landmarks, a size 1 blade may be necessary.
   c. Size 1 for infants weighing more than 4000 to 5000 g.
   d. Types of blades:
      (1) Miller straight blade
      (2) Macintosh curved blade
3. ETT size:
   a. Internal diameter (ID) 2.5 mm for infants weighing less than 1000 g or less than 28 weeks of gestation.
   b. ID 3 mm for 1000- to 2000-g infant or infants with a gestational age of 28 to 34 weeks.
   c. ID 3.5 mm for 2000- to 3000-g infant or infants with a gestational age of 34 to 38 weeks.
   d. ID 3.5 to 4 mm ETT for infants weighing more than 3000 g or greater than 38 weeks of gestation.

4. Stylet (though use is optional, it should be available).
5. Suction catheters (size 5F to 10F) and suction source set at 60 to 100 mm Hg of negative pressure.
6. Resuscitation bag and mask of appropriate sizes. Alternatively, availability of infant ventilation device, such as a T-piece (i.e., NeoPuff).
7. 100% oxygen source with blender set minimally at a flow rate of 5 to 10 l/minute with attached manometer.
8. Tape and other supplies to secure ETT according to hospital policy.
9. Cardiorespiratory monitor and oxygen saturation monitor.
10. Stethoscope.
11. Meconium aspirator, if applicable.
12. End-tidal CO_2 (EtCO$_2$) detector, colorimetric device such as the Pedi-Cap or Easy-Cap to confirm intubation.
   a. Limitations of Neonatal Colormetric EtCO$_2$ Detection Devices (DeBoer and Seaver, 2004).
      (1) Decreased peripheral perfusion—adapter may not change color quickly if at all when the neonate has little to no perfusion.
      (2) False-positive readings—verify ETT placement after at least 6 breaths have been given via ETT with attached EtCO$_2$ device.
      (3) Detector contamination—detector may be contaminated with bodily fluids or medication and limit ability to display color change. False-positive color change has been reported with atropine, epinephrine, calfactant (Infasurf) and naloxone (Narcan) (Hughes et al., 2007).
      (4) Limited time accuracy—sufficient exhalation time must be allowed for device to detect CO_2 and display color change (may take up to six ventilations with a resuscitation bag), device is good for up to 24 hours of intermittent use or 2 hours of continuous use.

D. **Procedure.**
   1. Gather ancillary personnel and ensure that all equipment is in working order, i.e., stethoscope, bag and mask at bedside, suction on and functioning, laryngoscope with secured working light source, etc.
   2. Wash hands and verify patient and procedure to be performed.
   3. Premedicate if applicable, for example, in nonemergent controlled situations (Carbajal et al., 2007; DeBoer and Peterson, 2001; Oei et al., 2002). Continuous cardiorespiratory and pulse oximetry is highly recommended during intubation procedure, especially with use of pharmacologic agents. Administer anticholinergic, sedation/analgesic followed by neuromuscular blockade if applicable. Common medications used in intubation:
      a. Analgesics
         (1) Morphine
            (a) Action—opioid, narcotic analgesic, sedation.
            (b) Dose—0.05 to 0.2 mg/kg/dose intravenously over 5 minutes.
            (c) Considerations—analgesic effects and sedation, reversed with naloxone.
         (2) Fentanyl (Sublimaze)—use with caution; even low doses (3 to 5 mcg/kg/dose) can lead to thoracic rigidity and laryngospasm.
            (a) Action—opioid, narcotic analgesic.
            (b) Dose—1 to 4 mcg/kg/dose intravenously over 5 minutes.
            (c) Considerations—100 more times potent than morphine; give slowly as rapid infusion may cause thoracic and skeletal muscle rigidity; reversed with naloxone. Analgesic effects and sedation, reversed with naloxone.
      b. Sedation
         (1) Midazolam (Versed)
            (a) Action—sedation, amnesia, antianxiety.
            (b) Dose—0.1 to 0.2 mg/kg/dose intravenously over 5 minutes.
            (c) Considerations—has not been established as safe for use in very preterm infants, dystonic reactions and seizures have been reported and significantly

decreases cerebral blood flow in preterm infants. Effects reversed with flumazenil.

    c. Neuromuscular blocking agents (optional)—muscle relaxants are contraindicated in situations where intubation may be difficult, such as micrognathia and cleft lip/palate or with health care providers with limited neonatal intubations. Sensation remains intact with neuromuscular blockade, and thus, analgesia should be used in combination. If neuromuscular blocking agent is used for intubation give medications in order of anticholinergic → analgesic → neuromuscular blocking agent.

       (1) Suxamethonium (succinylcholine, Anectine)

          (a) Action—muscle relaxation/paralysis.

          (b) Dose—1.5 to 3 mg/kg/dose intravenously over 30 seconds.

          (c) Considerations—do not use in neonates with hyperkalemia, suspicion of muscular dystrophy, increased ICP, or a family history of hyperthermia; monitor for bradycardia (pretreatment with Atropine minimizes bradycardia).

       (2) Vecuronium bromide (Norcuron)

          (a) Action—skeletal muscle relaxation/paralysis.

          (b) Dose—0.1 mg/kg/dose intravenously over 1 to 2 minutes.

          (c) Considerations—minimal cardiovascular side effects; however, decrease in heart rate and blood pressure has been observed when used concurrently with narcotics. Reversed with neostigmine and atropine.

       (3) Mivacurium (Mivacron)

          (a) Action—skeletal muscle relaxation/paralysis in infants requiring endotracheal intubation.

          (b) Dose—0.2 mg/kg/dose intravenously over 30 seconds.

          (c) Considerations—hypotension and bronchospasm has been reported in children with asthma. Use single dose vial only, as multidose vials contain benzyl alcohol, which is contraindicated in neonates. Reversed with neostigmine.

       (4) Pavulon is not recommended as a neuromuscular blocking agent owing to a long duration of action (1 to 4 hours). It should be used with extreme caution as an intubation agent.

  4. Select ETT of the appropriate size.

  5. Insert stylet (optional) and shape the ETT as desired. The stylet must be secured so that its tip does not extend below the tip of the ETT and also so the stylet cannot advance during the procedure. Keep the tube and stylet as clean as possible.

  6. Determine ETT insertion depth. A variety of methods has been reported for predicting insertional length such as nasal-tragus length, sternal length, foot length, and weight. The American Heart Association Neonatal Resuscitation Program (NRP) uses the 7-8-9 Rule (AAP and AHA, 2006).

    a. 6 plus the weight in kilograms (e.g., in a 2-kg neonate the ETT should be inserted to the 8 cm marking, 2 kg + 6 = 8 cm)

       (1) The 7-8-9 Rule has been associated with overestimated depth insertion in infants weighing <750 g (Peterson et al., 2006).

  7. Aspirate gastric contents and suction the oropharynx.

  8. Position the patient supine on a flat surface, with the head midline and the neck slightly extended (optional: place a soft flat roll under neck) in a "sniffing" position. The person performing intubation must have easy access to the airway and equipment while positioned at the patient's head.

  9. Hold the laryngoscope in the left hand between the thumb and first finger, with the blade pointing away. The laryngoscope is designed to be held with the left hand only (Fig. 15-1).

10. Open the patient's mouth with the fingers of the right hand and gently slide the blade into the right side of the mouth.

11. Stabilize the left hand against the left side of the patient's face, advance the blade tip to the base of the tongue, and move the blade to the midline, pushing the tongue to the left.

12. Expose the pharynx by lifting the entire blade upward in the direction in which the handle is pointing. Do not rock the tip of the blade upward or use the upper gum as a fulcrum.

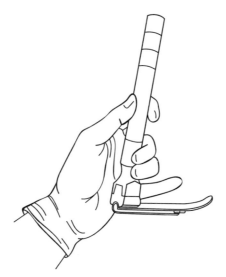

FIGURE 15-1 ■ Correct hand position when holding a laryngoscope for neonatal intubation. (From American Academy of Pediatrics and American Heart Association: *Textbook of Neonatal Resuscitation* [5th ed.]. Elk Grove Village, IL, 2006, American Academy of Pediatrics and American Heart Association.)

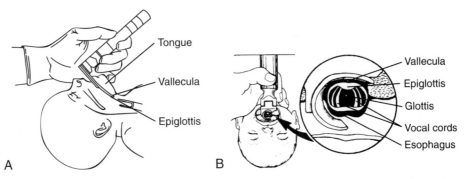

FIGURE 15-2 ■ Identification of landmarks before placing endotracheal tube through glottis. (From American Academy of Pediatrics and American Heart Association: *Textbook of Neonatal Resuscitation* [5th ed.]. Elk Grove Village, IL, 2006, American Academy of Pediatrics and American Heart Association.)

13. If unable to see the glottis, apply gentle external tracheal pressure (cricoid pressure) with the fifth finger of the left hand or have an assistant perform this and withdraw the blade slowly until the glottis is visible.
14. Remove any secretions that interfere with visualization by suctioning. Direct suctioning under laryngoscopy is ideal.
15. Identify anatomic landmarks (Fig. 15-2).
    a. Epiglottis is uppermost.
    b. Glottis is anterior, with vocal cords closing side to side.
    c. Esophagus is posterior.
16. After identifying the vocal cords, and with the cords in clear view, place the ETT into the right side of the patient's mouth with the right hand.
17. Keeping the cords in view, pass the ETT between the cords 1 to 2 cm into the trachea on inhalation (level of the vocal cord guide mark on the ETT). This should position the tip of the tube midway between the thoracic inlet and the carina, approximately at the second and third thoracic vertebra.
    a. If the vocal cords are closed or will not open, wait for spontaneous breath.

18. With the right hand, firmly grasp the ETT at the level of the patient's lip, stabilize the right hand against the patient's face, and carefully remove the laryngoscope with the left hand.
19. Carefully remove the stylet, if used, from the ETT.
20. Attach the resuscitation bag and $EtCO_2$ detector if applicable and assess tube placement.
    a. Auscultate both sides of the chest for the presence and intensity of breath sounds.
    b. Assess chest movement with inflationary breaths.
    c. Auscultate over the epigastrium and visually assess for distention.
    d. Check for condensation in tube during exhalation.
    e. Check for color change on CO_2 detector, if available.
21. Following confirmation of successful intubation, attach ETT to bag or special ventilation device such as a T-piece resuscitator and deliver breaths.
22. If the tube is in too far and placed in a right or left mainstem bronchus, auscultation may reveal unilateral or unequal breath sounds. The tube should be withdrawn in increments of 0.5 cm until, and assessed until, equal bilateral breath sounds are auscultated. If the tube is in the esophagus:
    a. Air may be heard entering the stomach with inflationary breaths.
    b. The stomach may become distended.
    c. No breath sounds will be heard on auscultation of the chest during inflationary breaths, though air movement may be heard, especially over the lower portion of the chest.
    d. No color change with $EtCO_2$ detector.
    e. Remove the ETT and discard it and hand ventilate with bag and appropriate-sized mask.
23. In very small infants, breath sounds may seem audible even with an ETT in the esophagus.
24. When the tube is assessed to be in good position, note the markings and secure the tube according to hospital policy.
25. Position of the tube must be confirmed by chest radiograph.
    a. Obtain chest x-ray in anteroposterior (AP) view with head midline and not in a flexed position.
    b. Tip of ETT should lie approximately 0.5 to 1 cm above the carina.
26. After confirming tube placement by chest radiograph, any length of tube that extends more than 4 cm beyond the lip should be cut off to limit dead space and to prevent kinking.
27. Document according to hospital policy: date, time, ETT size, centimeter marking at lip, $EtCO_2$ results, chest radiograph, and patient's tolerance of procedure. Sedation interventions performed, if any, should also be documented.

E. **Complications.**
   1. Hypoxia.
      a. During the procedure.
      b. Due to misplacement of tube.
   2. Bradycardia.
      a. Due to hypoxia.
      b. Due to vagal stimulation from the laryngoscope, ETT, or suction catheter.
   3. Infection.
   4. Perforation of esophagus or trachea.
   5. Trauma/edema to oropharyngeal and laryngeal tissues.
   6. Vocal cord injury.
   7. Subglottic stenosis associated with long-term (>3 to 4 weeks) intubation.
   8. Palatal grooves from prolonged intubation.
   9. Misplacement of tube into esophagus or bronchus.
   10. Interference of oral development caused by oral ETT.
   11. Defective dentition.

12. Ingestion of laryngoscope bulb.
13. Tube obstruction or kinking.
14. Pain, agitation, or discomfort.

Thoracentesis: Advanced Practice Procedure

A. **Indications.**
   1. Emergency evacuation of pneumothorax.
   2. Emergency evacuation of pleural fluid.
B. **Equipment and supplies.**
   1. Skin antiseptics according to hospital policy.
   2. Large-bore over-the-needle IV catheter (14 to 22 gauge).
   3. Three-way stopcock.
   4. Syringe, 20 to 35 ml.
   5. Local anesthetic, tuberculin (TB) syringe with small-bore needle, if medical condition permits.
C. **Procedure.**
   1. Position the infant supine and restrain limbs if necessary.
   2. Provide pharmacologic pain management if medical condition permits.
   3. Identify entry site. Use second or third intercostal space along the midclavicular line.
   4. Prepare skin with antiseptic as per hospital policy.
   5. Infiltrate the area with 1 ml of local anesthetic using a TB syringe and 25- to 27-gauge needle.
   6. Puncture skin at 45-degree angle, angling over third or fourth rib, and advance needle/catheter at a 90-degree angle. Inserting the catheter over the top of the rib will avoid blood vessels and nerves that run along the bottom of the rib. If thoracentesis is being done because of pleural fluid or effusion, the thorax should be punctured between the fifth and sixth intercostal spaces, midaxilla.
   7. Remove needle from IV catheter while sliding the catheter into the pleural space.
   8. Attach catheter hub to stopcock and syringe. The stopcock allows for aspiration of free air or fluid into the syringe and emptying of the syringe while maintaining a closed system.
   9. When free air or fluid is obtained, stabilize the catheter and continue to aspirate until preparation for chest tube insertion is complete, or until the air leak or fluid accumulation is evacuated.
   10. Document according to hospital policy: date, time, catheter size, location, amount of air/fluid evacuated, patient's tolerance of procedure. Pharmacologic interventions performed should also be documented.
D. **Complications.**
   1. Hemorrhage.
   2. Infection.
   3. Needle injury to lung or adjacent structures.
   4. Damage to breast tissue.
   5. Pain.

CIRCULATORY ACCESS PROCEDURES

Peripheral Intravenous Line Placement: Fundamental Procedure

A. **Indications.**
   1. Administration of medications.
   2. Administration of fluids, volume expanders, or blood products.
   3. Administration of parenteral nutrition.
B. **Precautions.**
   1. Avoid areas of infection or loss of skin integrity near selected puncture site.
   2. Use caution in infants with coagulation disorders, which may result in bleeding into surrounding tissues.

3. Padded armboard is to be used only if necessary to maintain line placement and must be of an appropriate size for gestational age.
4. Avoid sites that may be needed for possible central venous cannulation, such as the basilic, cubital, and saphenous veins.
5. Differentiate between veins and arteries.
6. Recommended for short-term intravenous therapy (<6 days).
7. Avoid infusion of hyperosmolar fluids because of the risk of injury.

C. **Equipment and supplies.**
1. 22- to 27-gauge over-the-needle catheter.
2. Tape and dressing supplies as per hospital policy.
3. Skin antiseptics as per hospital policy.
4. Tourniquet (a sanitized rubber band will suffice).
5. NS flush solution in a 3-ml syringe.
6. T-connector device, if applicable.
7. Transilluminator, if necessary.
8. Small scissors or safety razor, if necessary.
9. Warm compress (i.e., heel warmer), if necessary.
10. Appropriately sized padded armboard, if necessary.
11. Nonsterile gloves.
12. Pain/developmental management: pacifier, sucrose pacifier, blankets for developmental swaddling, eye protection from bright lights.

D. **Procedure.**
1. Gather supplies, wash hands, and don gloves.
2. Provide pain management such as pacifier for nonnutritive sucking, sucrose pacifier, and/or developmental care with facilitated tucking or swaddling. Shield eyes from bright lights.
3. Flush T-connector device with NS flush solution.
4. Determine vein for cannulation (Fig. 15-3). Accomplish distention of the vessel by applying a gentle tourniquet proximal to the selected insertion site. Alternatively, an assistant may encircle the proximal extremity with hand/fingers and apply direct pressure for the same effect.
   a. Transilluminate to locate vein, if necessary (use caution to avoid skin burns from heated device).
   b. Apply warm compress for 5 minutes to help dilate veins and make them more visible.
   c. If a scalp vein will be cannulated, trim hair with scissors preferably over shaving to help visualize and secure IV.
5. Choose appropriate-sized catheter for patient's size and vein.
6. Prepare skin at selected puncture site with antiseptic as per hospital policy.
7. Position and stabilize puncture site keeping skin taut.
8. Beginning a few millimeters distal to the anticipated site of the vessel puncture, insert the needle bevel up, at a 10- to 20-degree angle, depending on location of vein. Puncture skin in the direction of blood flow and advance needle in 1- to 2-mm increments.
9. If resistance is met or vein is not punctured, withdraw needle slowly to just below the level of the skin, relocate vein, and advance the needle again.
10. If a hematoma develops or bleeding occurs, occlude the vessel with pressure just proximal to the puncture site, remove tourniquet, withdraw the needle or catheter, and apply pressure until hemostasis has occurred.
11. If cannulation appears to be successful (i.e., flash back-blood in hub), remove the tourniquet and catheter needle (if using over-the-needle catheter), connect the T-connector to the catheter hub, and inject some of the flush solution gently to evaluate patency of the catheter. If flush solution infiltrates the tissues surrounding the catheter tip, occlude the vessel with pressure just proximal to the puncture site, withdraw the needle or catheter, and apply pressure until hemostasis has occurred.
12. If cannulation was successful and flush solution infuses without complications, connect T-connector and IV tubing with appropriate fluid to catheter, if applicable.

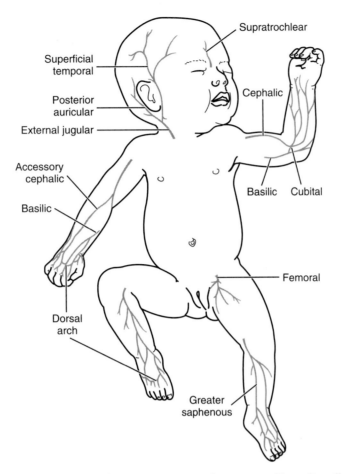

FIGURE 15-3 ■ Frequently used sites for venous access in the neonate. (From Gomella, T.L.: *Neonatology: Management, procedures, on-call problems, diseases, and drugs* [4th ed.]. New York, 1999, Lange Medical Books/ McGraw-Hill.)

13. Tape catheter in position that is developmentally appropriate and per hospital policy. Tape, dressing, and restraint must allow for easy inspection of insertion site, circulation of the distal extremity, and patency of the IV tubing. Avoid occlusion of the IV tubing with the tape or dressing.
14. Dispose of needle(s) in appropriate sharps container.
15. Document date, time, catheter size, site location, and patient's tolerance of procedure, according to hospital guidelines. Pain management interventions should also be documented.
16. Monitor for tissue infiltration or device dislodgment. If signs of infiltration are present, stop infusion immediately. Adverse signs may include the following:
    a. Redness, blanching, or discoloration at or near IV insertion site.
    b. Edema or swelling of extremity.
    c. Blistering at site.
    d. Pain with flushing.
    e. Resistance with flushing.
    f. Leaking at site.
    g. Coolness of skin around insertion site/extremity.
17. Treatment for infiltration/extravasation (MacDonald and Ramasethu, 2007; Ramasethu, 2004; Thigpen, 2007):
    a. Elevation of affected extremity.
    b. Avoid cold or warm compresses.

c. Pharmacologic intervention:
   (1) Hyaluronidase (Amphase)—indicated for the treatment of severe infiltration of intravenous solutions, especially hypertonic solutions or those containing calcium (examples: total parenteral nutrition [TPN], sodium bicarbonate, potassium chloride, and aminophylline). Do not use for infiltrations of vasoactive drugs such as dopamine, epinephrine, or norepinephrine. For best results use hyaluronidase within 1 hour of infiltration but may be given up to 3 hours after infiltration. Reconstitute product with NS. The recommended dose is 150 units/ml. Inject five 0.2-ml injections subcutaneously around the periphery of the infiltration (do not inject directly into affected area), using a different 25- to 27-gauge needle for each injection. Not recommended for IV use.
   (2) Phentolamine (Regitine)—indicated for treatment of infiltration of vasoactive drugs. For best results use within 12 hours of infiltration. Reconstitute product with NS. The recommended dose has been reported as 0.01 to 0.02 mg/kg per dose diluted to 1 mg/ml or up to 5 ml of a 1-mg/ml solution. Injected subcutaneously into the area of infiltration using multiple small injections with a 25- to 27-gauge needle, changing the needle between each skin entry. Use cautiously in hemodynamically unstable infants. Monitor for hypotension, tachycardia, cardiac arrhythmias, flushing.
   (3) Nitroglycerin 2%—indicated for infiltration of vasoactive drugs. Apply 4 mm/kg to affected area (or 2 mg measured as 0.1 ml in a syringe). Use cautiously in preterm infants less than 14 to 21 days of age because of enhanced absorption through the thin immature skin, which may put them at risk for overdosage and toxicity. Monitor heart rate and blood pressure as it may cause tachycardia and hypotension.
d. Multiple Puncture Technique
   (1) To be used to express fluid in extreme infiltrations to reduce pressure and prevent skin necrosis.
   (2) Prepare skin at site with antiseptic technique as per hospital policy.
   (3) Provide pain management with sucrose pacifier and/or pain medication.
   (4) Use a large-bore (18-gauge) sterile needle and make multiple perforations over the greatest area of swelling with strict aseptic technique.
   (5) Allow for free flow of infiltrated fluid. May gently massage affected area.
   (6) Cover skin with room-temperature saline-soaked dressing and elevate affected extremity.
E. **Complications.**
   1. Hematoma.
   2. Infection.
   3. Air, clot, or particle embolus.
   4. Tissue injury (phlebitis, infiltration) and possible necrosis after infiltration of infused solutions and/or medications.
   5. Injury to extremity from restraint.
   6. Compromised distal circulation.
   7. Pressure necrosis over bony areas.
   8. Limb deformity after prolonged immobilization.
   9. Pressure injury of peripheral nerves.
   10. Inadvertent arterial line placement.
   11. Blood loss from inadvertent catheter or tubing dislodgment.
   12. Pain from infiltration or ruptured blood vessel from unsuccessful cannulation.

Peripherally Inserted Central Catheter and Midline Catheter: Advanced Practice Procedure

A midline catheter (MLC) is a peripherally inserted catheter that dwells deeper in the vein than those used for standard peripheral intravenous therapy but never enters the abdominal-thoracic cavity. Midline catheters are a form of intermediate intravenous therapy and should not be used in infants who require the use of a peripherally inserted central catheter (PICC). The CDC recommends insertion of an MLC or PICC if intravenous therapy is expected to exceed 6 days (CDC, 2002). Insertion of an MLC is the same as for a PICC (i.e., equipment, use of strict aseptic technique, need for continuous heparinized carrier fluid); however, their use is strictly that of a peripheral intravenous device. A midline catheter can remain in place for 2 to 4 weeks. Midline catheter studies in neonates have reported MLC mean dwell times from 4 to 11 days (Dawson, 2002; Leike-Rude and Haney, 2006; Lesser et al., 1996; Reynolds, 1993; Wyckoff, 1999). The longer MLC dwell time therefore minimizes the frequent painful intravenous insertions associated with standard peripheral IV lines for neonates.

Note: Polyurethane catheters with a guidewire are available. However, because of the potential risk of perforation to vessels or organs, the discussion below will be limited to the more common Silastic catheters that do not use a guidewire.

A. **Indications.**
   1. Intermediate or long-term intravenous therapy (>6 days).
   2. Parenteral nutrition.
   3. Antibiotic or other medicinal therapy.
   4. Difficult venous access.
   5. Irritating drug therapy.
   6. Very low birth weight (<1500 g).

B. **Contraindications.**
   1. Active bacteremia or sepsis.
      a. Defer placement for at least 24 to 48 hours after antibiotic therapy is initiated.
   2. Inadequate vessel for cannulation.
   3. Anatomical irregularities in infant's extremities or chest that could interfere with proper insertion.
   4. The infant can be adequately treated with a peripheral IV access.
   5. Parental refusal.

C. **Precautions.**
   1. Avoid areas of infection or loss of skin integrity near selected puncture site.
   2. Avoid placement of a PICC in an extremity with inadequate or poor circulation.
   3. Obtain parental informed consent for PICC insertion prior to the procedure per institutional policy.
   4. Use caution in infants with coagulation disorders.
   5. Use caution with high-frequency ventilation as pressure changes within the chest may lead to catheter migration, particularly with upper body insertions.
   6. Do not measure blood pressure or perform venipuncture on the extremity containing the PICC/MLC.
   7. Use aseptic technique during insertion and care of PICC/MLC.
   8. Ensure attention to pain management, developmental care, and thermal homeostasis.
   9. Infuse medication via medication infusion pump; avoid "pushes."
   10. Use larger-bore syringes (>5 ml) that generate less pressure. Do not use a TB syringe.
   11. Avoid tension on catheter and tubing.
   12. Never pull catheter back through needle introducer because of the risk of damage or shearing of catheter.
   13. Monitor for bradycardia and hypoxia during procedure.
   14. Do not infuse blood products or obtain blood specimens from PICC or MLC.
   15. Never infuse hyperosmolar infusates through an MLC.

D. **Equipment and supplies.**
   1. Commercially prepared catheter insertion kit, or the following:
      a. Antiseptic per hospital policy or alcohol swabs (3) and povidone-iodine swabs (3).
      b. Forceps.
      c. Sterile measuring tape.
      d. Sterile gown and gloves, mask and surgical cap.
      e. Sterile heparin flush solution per institutional policy.
      f. Sterile gauze pads.

  g. Sterile drapes and towels.
  h. Sterile tourniquet (optional with preterm infants).
   (1) Sterile 5- or 10-ml syringes.
  i. Transparent, semipermeable dressing.
  j. Sterile adhesive strips.
  k. Luer-Lock or T-connector device.
  l. Select a neonatal percutaneous catheter of appropriate size. Catheter sizes include 1.2 Fr, 1.9 Fr (single- or double-lumen), 2 Fr, and 3 Fr (MacDonald and Ramasethu, 2007).
  m. Select an introducer of appropriate size. Introducer sizes include 19, 20, 22, and 24 gauge (MacDonald and Ramasethu, 2007).
   (1) Two types of catheter introducers are available:
    (a) Breakaway needle—this technique uses a breakaway introducer needle. The vessel is cannulated and the catheter advanced through the needle to the pre-measured distance. The catheter needle is then retracted and pulled apart along its longitudinal axis and discarded.
    (b) Peel-away plastic cannula—this technique uses a needle with a plastic cannula. The vessel is cannulated and the needle is removed, leaving the plastic cannula in the vessel for catheter insertion. Advance the catheter to the premeasured distance, then retract the plastic cannula from the vessel and pull the catheter apart along its longitudinal axis and discard.

E. Procedure.
 1. Verify order for PICC/MLC.
 2. Check to ensure informed consent is obtained per institutional policy.
 3. Gather equipment and supplies.
 4. Provide sedation/analgesia.
 5. Maintain thermoregulation and developmental positioning. Also provide environmental support by protecting infant's eyes from bright lights.
 6. Select vein (Fig. 15-3). Most common sites for neonates include the cephalic, basilic, and greater saphenous. A right-sided basilic or cephalic approach is preferred because of the shorter distance between the insertion site and the superior vena cava. Other sites include popliteal, temporal, and axillary veins.
 7. Position infant so selected vein is accessible. Restrain infant if necessary to prevent contamination of sterile field.
 8. Measure length of catheter to be inserted.
  a. For PICC (central venous access) insertion (MacDonald and Ramasethu, 2007; Becton, Dickinson and Co., 2000):
   (1) Upper body insertion: Tip should be in the superior vena cava above the T2 vertebra.
    (i) Measure from insertion site to the third or intercostal space, with the arm at a 90-degree angle for upper-extremity placement.
   (2) Lower body insertion: Tip should be in the inferior cava above the L4-L5 vertebra or iliac crest and below the right atrium.
    (ii) Measure from insertion site to xyphoid process for lower extremity placement.
   (3) The catheter tip should be about 1 cm outside the cardiac silhouette in preterm infants and 2 cm in the term infant.
  b. For MLC (peripheral venous access) insertion:
   (1) Upper body insertion: Tip should end in the upper arm just below the shoulder. The catheter tip should not be in the midclavicular region because this has been associated with complications due to catheter whip and thrombosis.
    (i) Measure from the insertion site to the desired site of catheter tip.
   (2) Lower body insertion: Tip should end in the upper leg below the femoral/inguinal fold.
    (i) Measure from the insertion site to the desired site of catheter tip.
 9. Don mask and cap and perform a 3- to 5-minute scrub.

10. Don sterile gown and gloves. Set up sterile field and open catheter kit, maintaining sterility of contents. Assemble equipment using an aseptic technique.
11. Trim catheter to predetermined length per manufacturer's recommendations and institution's policy.
12. Attach flush-syringe and prime catheter.
13. Have an assistant place on sterile gloves and elevate extremity. Prepare insertion site with povidone-iodine or antiseptic per hospital policy and allow to dry.
14. Change into new sterile gloves and hold elevated extremity with sterile gauze.
15. Drape infant with sterile towels.
16. Apply sterile tourniquet (optional) and stabilize vein.
17. Take introducer and puncture vessel at an approximately 5- to 15-degree angle for shallow veins and approximately 15 to 30 degrees for deeper veins. After skin puncture pause and let infant relax to prevent vasoconstriction. Entry into the vessel is signaled by blood leaking from puncture site or from the introducer needle/cannula.
18. Loosen tourniquet (if applicable) after advancing catheter a short distance. Remove needle, leaving peel-away plastic cannula in place if using this method.
19. Advance flushed catheter with forceps in 0.5- to 1-cm increments to predetermined distance. Catheter should advance smoothly, that is, without resistance.
20. Once catheter is advanced 7 to 8 cm or to the predetermined distance, remove introducer. Catheter may be pulled out slightly during splitting technique and may need to be advanced slightly when complete. Gentle pressure with finger distal to puncture site may reduce blood loss.
21. Aspirate on catheter to confirm blood return. If blood is obtained, flush catheter.
22. Temporarily secure catheter with sterile adhesive strips and obtain chest radiograph for central catheter placement while maintaining sterile field and aseptic technique. Radiograph for MLC is optional.
23. Radiographically confirm placement is central prior to any infusions. Pull back or advance catheter, if necessary, to appropriate distance. Check for blood return and obtain another chest radiograph to confirm satisfactory position.
24. Remove antiseptic from surrounding skin with sterile water.
25. Secure and dress catheter per manufacturer's recommendations.
26. Document procedure including catheter lot number, catheter size, catheter type, catheter length if trimmed, location and insertion distance, location of catheter tip on radiograph, and sedation/analgesia provided.
27. It is recommended for 1.1 to 2 Fr catheters to maintain patency and prevent thrombus to have a continuous infusion of 0.5 to 1 units of heparin per milliliter of infusion solution at a minimum rate of at least 1 ml/hour (Becton, Dickinson and Co., 2000).
28. Change dressing per manufacturer's recommendations.
29. Monitor for infiltration or extravasation:
    a. Redness.
    b. Edema.
    c. Difficulty with flushing or fluid infusion.

F. **Complications.**
   1. Cardiac arrhythmias.
   2. Pericardial effusion with cardiac tamponade.
   3. Atrial perforation with cardiac tamponade.
   4. Intravascular catheter shearing, followed by embolization of catheter fragment.
   5. Thrombus formation.
   6. Infection, local or systemic.
   7. Nerve damage.
   8. Air embolism.
   9. Rupture of catheter from using excessive infusion pressure (e.g., from using small-bore syringes).
   10. Infiltration/extravasation.
   11. Hemorrhage.
   12. Vascular perforation.

Removal of Peripherally Inserted Central Catheter: Fundamental Procedure

A. **Indications.**
1. No longer needed or indicated.
2. Septicemia, especially fungal.
3. Malfunctioning.

B. **Precautions.**
1. Avoid catheter disruption.
2. Venospasm (if resistance is met, do not force catheter; apply warm compress for 20 to 30 minutes and reattempt).

C. **Equipment and supplies.**
1. Sterile gauze.
2. Measuring tape.
3. Transparent dressing.
4. Nonsterile gloves.

D. **Procedure.**
1. Verify order for removal.
2. Wash hands and don gloves.
3. Remove securing tape and dressing carefully to avoid skin trauma.
4. Cleanse site with povidone-iodine or antiseptic per hospital policy and allow to dry.
5. Slowly and carefully retract catheter 1 cm at a time, grasping the catheter near the insertion site until the catheter has been removed. Do not apply pressure over insertion site during catheter removal.
6. Apply sterile gauze over insertion site as withdrawal is complete.
7. Continue to apply pressure with gauze until hemostasis is obtained. Once hemostasis is confirmed, cover site with transparent dressing. Dressing should remain in place for at least 24 hours.
8. Measure and inspect removed catheter and compare that distance with the recorded insertion depth.
    a. If any part has broken off during removal or the length of the catheter differs from the recorded insertion length, place a tourniquet on the affected extremity above the insertion site, such as upper arm or upper leg, to prevent advancement of the catheter piece into the right atrium. Check for pulses. If no pulse or the extremity is dusky, loosen the tourniquet. Immediately notify health care provider as catheter embolization is an emergency and may require removal via cardiac catheterization or via surgery.
9. Document date, time, site location, measurement of catheter removed in comparison to recorded insertion depth, patient's tolerance of procedure, and any complications according to hospital guidelines.

E. **Complications.**
1. Shearing of catheter inside patient, before complete removal.
2. Dislodgment of thrombus from tip.

Umbilical Vessel Catheterization: Advanced Practice Procedure

A. **Indications.**
1. Arterial catheterization.
    a. Frequent arterial blood sampling.
    b. Continuous arterial blood gas monitoring.
    c. Continuous arterial blood pressure monitoring.
    d. Vascular access for intravenous fluids when other sites are not available or suitable.
    e. Exchange transfusion.
    f. Cardiac catheterization.
2. Venous catheterization.
    a. Emergency administration of drugs.
    b. Emergency measurement of Pco_2 and pH.
    c. Fluid administration (hypertonic solutions or inadequate peripheral access).
    d. Exchange transfusion.

     e. Central venous pressure monitoring.

     f. Blood sampling.

B. Contraindications.

    1. Abdominal wall defects.

    2. Necrotizing enterocolitis (controversial).

    3. Vascular compromise below level of umbilicus.

    4. Omphalitis.

    5. Peritonitis.

C. Precautions.

    1. Maintain thermal homeostasis.

    2. Monitor heart rate and oxygen saturation throughout the procedure.

    3. Maintain aseptic technique.

    4. Dilate artery before attempting vessel cannulation.

    5. Do not force catheter past obstruction.

D. Equipment and supplies.

    1. Commercially prepackaged sterile umbilical catheter tray or sterile instrument tray for umbilical catheterization to include the following:

      a. 4 × 4 gauze pads.

      b. Sterile drapes.

      c. Small container for antiseptic solution.

      d. Scissors.

      e. Umbilical tape.

      f. Measuring tape.

      g. Syringes, 10 ml.

      h. No. 11 scalpel with handle.

      i. Mosquito hemostats (2).

      j. Curved, nontoothed iris forceps (2).

      k. Toothed iris forceps (1).

      l. Needle holder.

      m. Umbilical catheter of either argyle or Silastic material. Silastic catheters may be more difficult to insert owing to their lack of rigidity.

      n. Determine appropriate-size catheter with either a single, double, or triple lumen or as desired by your institution's medical staff.

        (1) Size 3.5F for infants weighing less than 1500 g.

        (2) Size 3.5F, 4.0F, or 5.0F for infants weighing more than 1500 g.

        (3) A 2.5F argyle catheter is available for use in the extremely premature infant.

      o. 3-0 silk suture.

      p. 4-0 silk suture with curved needle.

      q. Three-way Luer–Lock stopcock.

      r. Dressings for securing (clear occlusive dressing and a hydrocolloid skin barrier).

      s. Sterile heparin-flush solution (1 unit/ml).

    2. Sterile antiseptic solution.

    3. Mask, surgical cap, and sterile gown and gloves.

    4. Standardized premeasurement graph or access to a formula to determine insertion depth.

E. Procedure.

Umbilical artery catheterization (UAC). Note: *Low position*, catheter tip placed between the third and fourth lumbar vertebrae (L3-L4). *High position*, catheter tip placed between the sixth and tenth thoracic vertebrae (T6-T10). Either position is accepted practice currently. Consult your institution's guidelines for desired positioning of UACs.

    1. Inspect lower extremities for bruising and palpate pulses.

    2. Assess umbilical cord to rule out umbilical anomaly, such as a small omphalocele.

    3. Place infant supine and restrain limbs.

    4. Calculate insertion depth.

      a. Measure shoulder to umbilical distance (adding length of umbilicus stump) and multiply by 0.66 to arrive at insertion depth for a "low" placement (L3-L4), or

  b. 2.5 times body weight in kilograms plus 9.7 cm ($2.5 \times$ weight $+ 9.7$) for a "high" placement (T6-T10).
5. Don mask and cap and perform a 3- to 5-minute scrub.
6. Don sterile gown and gloves.
7. Have assistant hold heparin flush vial and draw up flush into sterile syringe.
8. Prepare catheter by attaching Luer-Lock stopcock to catheter and connect flush-filled syringe to stopcock and flush catheter.
9. Turn stopcock off to catheter.
10. Have assistant hold umbilical cord up and out of procedure area while you prepare cord with antiseptic solution. Scrub in a circular manner moving from the cord to approximately 5 cm in radius on surrounding abdomen. Do not let antiseptic drip down infant's side because this may cause burns, especially in extremely premature infants.
11. Drape procedure area with sterile towels.
12. Tie umbilical tape using a single hand knot tight enough to prevent bleeding at base of cord, not on the skin. Umbilical tape may have to be loosened to advance catheter or tightened to control bleeding.
13. Using a scalpel, cut through the umbilical cord 1 to 1.5 cm from skin.
14. Identify cord vessels.
  a. Arteries: two small, thick-walled, and white constricted vessels that may stick out slightly and typically located at the 4 and 8 o'clock positions.
  b. Vein: single, large, thin-walled vessel, often open and typically located at the 12 o'clock position.
15. Stabilize cord stump.
  a. Grasp portion of cut edge of cord with hemostat and apply gentle traction.
  b. Apply hemostats to opposite sides of the cord and roll them away from each other, causing the arteries to protrude from the cut surface of the cord.
16. Dilate artery.
  a. Insert one tip of curved iris forceps into selected artery and probe gently to a depth of about 0.5 cm.
  b. With tips of forceps together, gently probe artery to a depth of about 0.5 cm.
  c. Gently spread forceps apart, and then slowly withdraw forceps from artery, dilating lumen as forceps is withdrawn.
  d. Continue to dilate lumen (approximately 15 to 60 seconds) until forceps can easily be inserted to a depth of about 1 cm.
17. Insert catheter.
  a. Insert catheter into dilated artery.
  b. Thread catheter to predetermined depth.
  c. If resistance is met, do not force catheter. Apply gentle, steady pressure to catheter while applying gentle traction on cord.
  d. If catheter cannot be advanced to the desired distance, discontinue attempts and catheterize second artery.
  e. Observe for blanching of legs, toes, and/or buttocks.
18. Aspirate blood to ensure placement in vessel after catheter advanced approximately 5 cm. If blood is obtained, clear catheter by injecting 0.5 ml flush solution. If blood cannot be aspirated, remove catheter and attempt catheterization of second artery.
19. Obtain radiograph to confirm catheter position.
  a. If the catheter tip is too high, pull the catheter back to its proper position and obtain another radiograph.
  b. If the catheter tip is too low for "high position," pull back to "low position," if your institutional guidelines allow this.
  c. If catheter tip is too low for "low position," it should be adjusted to an acceptable position. Keep in mind that a catheter that is no longer sterile should not be advanced.
20. Suture catheter in place.
  a. Place pursestring suture around cord. Avoid piercing the vessels and catheters. Secure to umbilical skin or cord depending on your institution's guidelines.

     b. Knot suture securely in cord close to catheter per manufacturer's recommendations.

     c. If suture around catheter, it must be tight to prevent catheter from sliding, but not so tight that flow through catheter is obstructed.

21. Loosen umbilical tape.

22. Remove antiseptic as soon as possible from the skin to prevent burns.

23. Secure catheter per hospital policy. The following are various securing techniques used to secure catheters:

     a. Commercially manufactured securing devices.

     b. "Bridge" or "goalpost" taping technique.

     c. Hydrocolloid skin barrier to umbilical area with clear occlusive dressing.

24. Document procedure according to hospital policy noting type of catheter, catheter size, distance catheter threaded, location of catheter tip on radiograph, adjustments made to catheter to correct malpositioned catheter, and assessment of color, pulses, and perfusion to lower extremities.

Umbilical Vein Catheterization. Note: Equipment for umbilical vein catheterization is the same as that for UAC insertion with the exception that an 8F catheter may occasionally be used for infants weighing greater than 3500 g.

1. Maintain aseptic technique.

2. Prepare cord as for umbilical artery catheter and identify the thin-walled vein.

3. Grasp the base of the cord with curved hemostats or toothed forceps, hold upright, and dilate vessel with the tip of iris forceps.

4. Insert the catheter to predetermined distance.

     a. Emergency placement (temporary catheter, low position): Insert 2 to 3 cm into vessel until blood is obtained. Once emergency medications and fluids have been administered and the infant is stabilized, remove the catheter.

     b. Indwelling umbilical venous catheter:

        (1) Measure shoulder to umbilical distance and multiply by 0.75 to arrive at insertion depth, or

        (2) Calculate insertion depth with the formula 1.5 times body weight in kilograms plus 5.6 cm ($1.5 \times$ weight + 5.6).

5. If resistance is met, withdraw the catheter 2 to 3 cm and attempt to reinsert. If cannulation remains unsuccessful, remove the catheter.

6. If cannulation is successful, connect and secure catheter and confirm position by radiograph. Correct radiographic position is 0.5 to 1 cm above the diaphragm.

7. Secure catheter per hospital policy.

8. Document procedure according to hospital policy, noting type of catheter, catheter size, distance catheter threaded, location of catheter tip on radiograph, and adjustments made to catheter to correct malpositioned catheter.

F. **Complications of using umbilical catheters.**

    1. Vasospasm, embolism, thrombosis, and distal ischemia:

      a. Blanching, cyanosis, and mottling of skin.

      b. Sloughing of skin.

      c. Necrosis of extremities, possibly leading to loss of toes.

      d. Paraplegia.

      e. Intestinal necrosis and perforation.

    2. Infection.

    3. Mechanical complications:

      a. Perforation of vessels.

      b. Perforation of peritoneum.

      c. False aneurysm.

      d. Knot in catheter or breaking of catheter.

    4. Malpositioned catheter:

      a. Cardiac arrhythmias.

      b. Pericardial effusion.

      c. Cardiac tamponade

      d. Hydrothorax.

    5. Necrotizing enterocolitis (controversial).
    6. Perforation of colon.
    7. Hepatic necrosis.
    8. Skin burns from antiseptics.
    9. Hemorrhage, exsanguination.
   10. Portal hypertension.
   11. Death.

Radial Artery Catheterization: Advanced Practice Procedure

A. Indications.
    1. Need for frequent blood sampling and umbilical artery catheterization cannot be done or has been removed.
    2. Need for continuous blood pressure monitoring.

B. Precaution.
    1. Avoid areas of skin breakdown or infection.
    2. Use caution in infants with coagulopathy, who may bleed excessively.
    3. Inadequate ulnar artery blood flow.
    4. Limb malformation.

C. Equipment and supplies.
    1. 22 to 27 gauge over the needle IV catheter.
    2. Antiseptic solution per institution policy.
    3. 0.25 to 0.5 normal saline flush.
    4. Occlusive dressing and tape per institution policy.
    5. Transilluminator if needed.
    6. Appropriately sized padded armboard.
    7. Plastic IV cover if available.
    8. Arterial pressure transducer and extension tubing per institution policy.
    9. Nonsterile gloves.
   10. 4-0 sutures if needed per institution policy.
   11. T-connector as needed per institution policy.
   12. Pain/development management: pacifier, sucrose, blankets for swaddling, and eye protection from bright lights.

D. Procedure.
    1. Select site for catheterization:
      a. Palpate radial artery pulse.
      b. Transillumination may assist in identifying vessel.
    2. Take care not to hyperextend wrist, as this will occlude artery flow.
    3. Perform modified Allen's test to ensure adequate collateral circulation:
      a. Elevate hand.
      b. Occlude both radial and ulnar arteries.
      c. Massage the palm toward wrist to blanch hand.
      d. Release pressure on the ulnar artery.
      e. Perfusion to hand should return in less than 10 seconds; if longer than 15 seconds, do not puncture artery.
    4. Position and secure wrist as shown in Figure 15-4.
    5. Provide pain management and developmental support.
    6. Prepare site with antiseptic solution per institution policy.
    7. Puncture the skin proximal to the wrist crease with the needle at a 30- to 45-degree angle (a deeper angle may be needed for larger babies).
    8. Cannulate the artery using one of the following methods (Fig. 15-5):
      a. Puncture both walls of the artery with the needle bevel up (blood return may be delayed). Remove the stylet and withdraw the catheter until blood return is noted. When blood return is seen, advance the catheter into the artery and flush. Flushing while advancing may stabilize the catheter and make advancing easier.

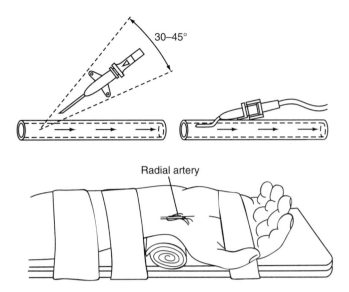

FIGURE 15-4 ■ Peripheral arterial line insertion. (From Gomella, T.L.: *Neonatology: Management, procedures, on-call problems, diseases and drugs* [5th ed.]. New York, 2004, Lange Medical Books/McGraw-Hill.)

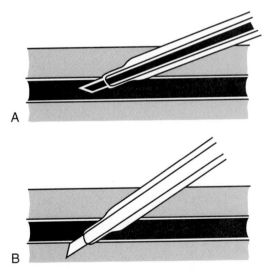

FIGURE 15-5 ■ Arterial cannulation methods A and B. (From MacDonald, M.G. and Ramasethu, J.: *Atlas of Procedures in Neonatology* [4th ed.]. Philadelphia, 2007, Lippincott Williams & Wilkins.)

  b. Puncture the anterior wall of the artery until blood return is seen, at this point the catheter is in the artery. Advance the catheter while simultaneously withdrawing the stylet and flush.
 9. Secure cannula with sutures or tape per institution policy.
10. Attach T-connector per institution policy and flush line.
11. Secure line with armboard and dressing per institution policy. Ensure visibility of insertion site and all fingers.
12. Attach pressure transducer and extension tubing per institution policy and ensure unobstructed flow of fluids by pump. Secure all connection sites to avoid backflow of blood into line.
13. Maintain patency of catheter with heparinized fluids.
14. Dispose of needle in designated sharps container.
15. Document date, time, location, catheter size, distal perfusion, and pain response to placement of catheter.

16.   Monitor site for extravasation or leakage of fluids and/or blood.

17.   Monitor fingers for adequate perfusion of all digits.

E. **Complications.**

1.   Arteriospasm.

2.   Infection.

3.   Extravasation of fluids.

4.   Hematoma or hemorrhage.

5.   Embolism or thrombus formation leading to tissue ischemia or necrosis and possible loss of hand or digits.

6.   Damage to surrounding tissues or structures.

BLOOD SAMPLING PROCEDURES

Capillary Blood Sampling: Fundamental Procedure

A. **Indications**

1.   Small amount of blood collection is needed (<1 to 1.5 ml) (Folk, 2007; MacDonald and Ramasethu 2007).

2.   Venous or arterial blood sample is not possible or necessary.

3.   Collection of blood specimen for blood gas sampling, routine laboratory sampling, state newborn metabolic screens.

B. **Contraindications.**

1.   Impaired circulation in selected limb or at puncture site.

2.   Infection near puncture site.

C. **Precautions.**

1.   Consider venipuncture if impaired skin integrity noted at selected puncture site (edema, bruising, multiple puncture marks).

2.   Consider venipuncture as an alternative to capillary sampling in term neonates, as it may be less painful (Shah and Ohlsson, 2007).

3.   Hyperviscous blood may render sampling difficult. Consider venipuncture in infants with polycythemia.

4.   Use caution in infants with coagulation disorders.

5.   Avoid using the center or back of the heel.

6.   Avoid finger sticks.

7.   Avoid excessive squeezing that may cause hemolysis.

D. **Equipment and supplies.**

1.   Alcohol swabs or other site preparation material, as per institutional guideline.

2.   Spring-loaded lancet with tip not longer than 2.4 mm or manufactured lancets based on infant size.

3.   Sterile gauze pad.

4.   Warm compress. Caution: maximum temperature of 40° C.

5.   Nonsterile gloves.

6.   Appropriate specimen collection containers.

7.   Pain management: pacifier, sucrose pacifier, and blankets for developmental swaddling.

E. **Procedure.**

1.   Select puncture site on the lateral or medial aspect of the heel. Avoid other areas because of the possibility of nerve damage or osteomyelitis (Fig. 15-6).

2.   Warm heel with compress for 5 to 10 minutes to improve blood flow.

3.   Provide pain management: use spring-loaded lancets, consider venipuncture in term newborns, pacifier for nonnutritive sucking, sucrose pacifier, dim and quiet environment, skin-to-skin holding, and/or hand or blanket swaddling with selected extremity exposed.

4.   Gather supplies, wash hands, and don gloves.

5.   Prepare area selected for skin puncture with site prepping material or alcohol and allow to dry.

6.   Puncture heel perpendicular to the skin.

7.   Wipe away first drop of blood with sterile gauze pad.

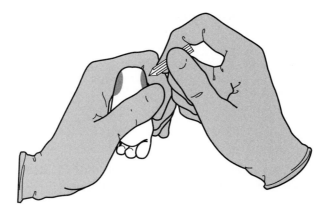

FIGURE 15-6 ■ Use shaded areas when performing heel stick in infant. (From Gomella, T.L.: *Neonatology: Management, procedures, on-call problems, diseases, and drugs* [5th ed.]. New York, 2004, Lange Medical Books/ McGraw-Hill.)

8. Collect specimen from free-flowing drops at puncture site.
   a. Blood flow is increased if the puncture site is dependent relative to the extremity.
   b. Gentle "pumping" of the extremity above the puncture site may encourage blood flow.
9. After specimen is collected, elevate foot and apply pressure with sterile gauze pad until hemostasis has occurred.
10. Dispose of lancet in appropriate sharps container.
11. Label specimen per institutional policy.
12. Document the heel-stick procedure, specimen obtained, date and time, nonpharmacologic interventions, and patient's tolerance.

F. **Complications.**
   1. Bruising or loss of skin integrity.
   2. Infection.
   3. Scarring.
   4. Calcified nodules.
   5. Cellulitis.
   6. Osteomyelitis.
   7. Nerve damage (Folk, 2007).
   8. Pain.
   9. Erroneous laboratory values may result from the following:
      a. Contamination of specimen with tissue fluid.
      b. Contamination of specimen with alcohol.
      c. Inadequate warming or poor circulation at puncture site.
      d. Hemolysis of specimen.

Venipuncture (Phlebotomy): Fundamental Procedure

A. **Indications.**
   1. Large quantity of blood required.
   2. Arterial sample not possible or necessary.
   3. Capillary sample not possible or sufficient.
   4. Sterile collection for blood culture.
   5. Specific laboratory tests requiring venous sampling.
B. **Contraindications.**
   1. Inadequate or impaired circulation in selected limb.
   2. Infection or loss of skin integrity near selected venipuncture site.
C. **Precautions.**
   1. Use caution in infants with coagulation disorders.

2. Avoid sites that may be needed for possible central venous cannulation.
3. Differentiate between arteries and veins.

D. **Equipment and supplies.**
   1. Antiseptic skin preparation per hospital policy.
   2. 23- to 25-gauge butterfly needle or hypodermic needle attached to syringe.
   3. Syringe(s) for specimen collection.
   4. Appropriate specimen collection tubes.
   5. Sterile gauze pad.
   6. Tourniquet or rubber band.
   7. Nonsterile gloves.
   8. Pain management: pacifier, sucrose pacifier, blankets for swaddling leaving venipuncture site accessible, and/or cloth to protect eyes from bright lights.

E. **Procedure.**
   1. Gather supplies, wash hands, and don gloves.
   2. Choose vein to be used. Accomplish distention of the vessel by applying a gentle tourniquet proximal to the selected insertion site. Alternatively, an assistant may encircle the proximal extremity with his or her hand or fingers and apply direct pressure for the same effect.
   3. Provide pain-relieving measures and developmentally position/swaddle with selected venipuncture site accessible.
   4. Stabilize and position the selected puncture site to allow puncture in direction of blood flow.
   5. Prepare skin at selected puncture site with antiseptic per hospital policy.
   6. Puncture skin at a 15- to 45-degree angle, bevel up, just distal to anticipated vessel entry site, using shallow angle for smaller infants or superficial vessels.
   7. Advance needle until blood appears in the tubing.
      a. If resistance is met or vessel is not punctured, withdraw needle slowly to just below level of the skin, relocate vessel, and advance the needle again.
      b. If a hematoma develops or bleeding occurs, occlude the vessel with pressure just proximal to the puncture site, remove tourniquet, and withdraw needle. Apply pressure until hemostasis has occurred.
   8. On entrance of blood into tubing, attach syringe and gently aspirate to obtain specimen. If a hypodermic needle with an intact hub was used, blood specimen may drip into laboratory collection container.
   9. After specimen is obtained, using a gauze pad just proximal to puncture site, occlude vessel with pressure over entry site while removing tourniquet and withdrawing needle.
   10. Apply pressure to site until hemostasis has occurred.
   11. Dispose of needle in appropriate sharps container.
   12. Label specimens per institution policy.
   13. Document date, time, site location, specimen collected, amount of blood removed, nonpharmacologic interventions, patient's tolerance of procedure, and any complications according to hospital guidelines.

F. **Complications.**
   1. Hematoma.
   2. Infection.
   3. Hemorrhage.
   4. Needle injury to adjacent structures.
   5. Pain.

Radial Artery Puncture: Advanced Practice Procedure

A. **Indications.**
   1. Venous and/or capillary sites are not satisfactory.
   2. Other arterial line is unavailable for sampling.

3. Arterial blood gas sampling.
4. Need to sample large quantities of blood.

B. **Precautions.**
1. Avoid area of infection or loss of skin integrity near selected puncture site.
2. Use caution in infants with coagulation defects.
3. Avoid puncture in extremity with inadequate or impaired circulation.
4. Consider need to preserve arterial site for possible cannulation.
5. Avoid extremity with inadequate collateral circulation distal to the selected puncture site.
6. Use of small-gauge needle reduces potential complications.

C. **Equipment and supplies.**
1. Antiseptic supplies to prepare for arterial puncture per hospital policy.
2. 23- to 25-gauge butterfly needle or 23- to 25-gauge needle attached to a 3-ml syringe.
3. Extra syringes.
4. Sterile gauze pad.
5. Arterial blood gas (ABG) syringe, other applicable lab specimen containers.
6. Transilluminator (optional).

D. **Procedure.**
1. Determine puncture site.
   a. Transillumination may assist in vessel location.
   b. Extend wrist, do not hyperextend, which may occlude vessel.
   c. Palpate artery at distal crease of wrist.
2. Perform modified Allen test to assess collateral circulation.
   a. Elevate hand.
   b. Apply pressure to occlude both radial and ulnar arteries.
   c. Massage the palm to blanch hand.
   d. Release pressure on ulnar artery.
   e. If color returns to hand in less than 10 seconds, adequate collateral circulation is suggested. If color returns in greater than 15 seconds, do not puncture artery because of poor collateral circulation.
   f. Doppler-flow evaluation of ulnar, radial, and palmar circulation can also help determine adequacy of collateral flow.
3. Provide pain management such as pacifier for nonnutritive sucking, sucrose pacifier, and/or developmental care with facilitated tucking or blanket swaddling.
4. Position and stabilize extended wrist to allow puncture against direction of arterial flow.
5. Prepare area with antiseptic for skin puncture (middle to outer third of wrist) per hospital policy.
6. Puncture skin with needle (bevel up) at a 15- to 45-degree angle, using shallower angle for smaller infants or more superficial arteries (Fig. 15-7).
7. Advance needle slowly to puncture artery.
   a. If resistance is met or blood is not obtained, withdraw needle slowly to just below skin level, palpate artery, and advance needle again in the direction of the artery.
   b. If hematoma or bleeding develops, occlude artery with gauze and pressure just proximal to the puncture site, withdraw needle, and apply pressure until hemostasis has occurred (approximately 5 minutes of direct pressure).
8. If arterial cannulation is successful, when blood enters the butterfly tubing, attach syringe and aspirate gently to obtain sample.
9. Apply firm, but not occlusive, pressure to artery with gauze just proximal to puncture site and withdraw needle. Apply pressure to site for 5 minutes or until hemostasis has occurred.
10. Ensure distal circulation after puncture.
    a. Evaluate color and temperature.
    b. Check capillary refill time.
    c. Palpate arterial pulse.

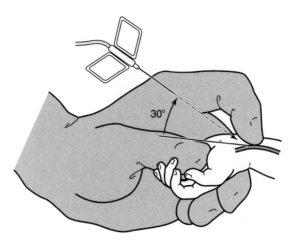

FIGURE 15-7 ■ Arterial puncture technique in the neonate. (From Gomella, T.L.: *Neonatology: Management, procedures, on-call problems, diseases, and drugs* [5th ed.]. New York, 2004, Lange Medical Books/ McGraw-Hill.)

11. Document the following or according to hospital policy: Date, time, site location, Allen test result prior to procedure, pain management interventions, tolerance to procedure, specimen obtained, amount of blood drawn, hemostasis, distal circulation, and any complications if encountered.
E. **Complications.**
   1. Hematoma.
   2. Hemorrhage.
   3. Infection.
   4. Thrombosis, embolism.
   5. Arteriospasm, tissue necrosis, possibly leading to loss of hand.
   6. Needle injury to adjacent structures.
   7. Pain.

MISCELLANEOUS PROCEDURES

Bladder Catheterization: Fundamental Procedure

A. **Indications.**
   1. To obtain urine specimen/culture when suprapubic aspiration cannot be obtained.
   2. To monitor urinary output.
   3. To monitor bladder residuals.
   4. To relieve urinary retention.
   5. To accomplish genitourinary testing such as cystogram or voiding cystourethrogram.
B. **Contraindications.**
   1. Anatomic malformations.
C. **Precautions.**
   1. Use caution in infants with coagulation disorders.
   2. Maintain an aseptic technique.
   3. Do not force the catheter, as this may lead to trauma to the urethra and bladder.
   4. Remove catheter as soon as possible to minimize infection.
   5. Use the smallest-diameter catheter to avoid trauma.
D. **Equipment and supplies.** Note: All equipment is sterile and is available in commercially prepared kits.
   1. Urethral catheters.
      a. Size 3.5F umbilical artery catheter for infants weighing less than 1000 g may be used.

    b. Size 6F Foley catheter or 5F feeding tube for infants weighing 1000 to 1800 g.

    c. Size 8F feeding tube or Foley catheter for infants weighing greater than 1800 g.

  2. Urinary catheter tray.

    a. Sterile gloves.

    b. Povidone-iodine solution swabs.

    c. Sterile drapes.

    d. Lubricant.

    e. Sterile specimen container or closed-urinary drainage system.

E. Procedure.

Male Catheterization.

  1. Place infant supine and restrain legs or have assistant hold legs.

  2. Don sterile gloves.

  3. Clean penis:

    a. Hold the penis perpendicular to the body with the nondominant hand (which is now considered contaminated) and gently retract the foreskin (if not circumcised).

    b. Starting at the meatus and moving down the penis, clean with povidone-iodine solution swabs three times, using a new swab each time.

  4. Drape sterile towels across infant's lower abdomen and across legs.

  5. Apply sterile lubricant to appropriately sized catheter tip with the sterile dominant hand.

  6. Place the catheter (held by the still sterile dominant hand) into the meatus while maintaining perpendicular position of the penis with the nondominant hand. Advance catheter along the urethra until urine appears. Slight resistance may be felt as the catheter passes through the external bladder sphincter. Steady, gentle pressure is usually needed to pass beyond this area; however, never force the catheter (Fig. 15-8).

  7. Advance catheter slightly past the point where urine flow began. Inflate the balloon per hospital policy and manufacturer's recommendations, if applicable. Usually the catheter will function satisfactorily if simply taped in place. Balloon inflation may injure the urethra if the catheter is not properly positioned in the bladder.

  8. If catheter is to remain indwelling, tape it to lower abdomen or to penile shaft.

  9. Collect urine specimen in the sterile container and send to the laboratory or attach to a closed urinary drainage system.

  10. Document procedure, catheter type and size, patient's tolerance, quantity, and characteristics of sample obtained, and any difficulties encountered.

Female Catheterization.

  1. Place infant on back and secure legs in "frog-leg" position. You may secure with restraints or have an assistant hold the legs.

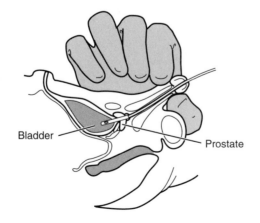

Bladder — Prostate

FIGURE 15-8 ■ Male bladder catheterization. (From Gomella, T.L.: *Neonatology: Management, procedures, on-call problems, diseases, and drugs* [5th ed.]. New York, 2004, Lange Medical Books/McGraw-Hill.)

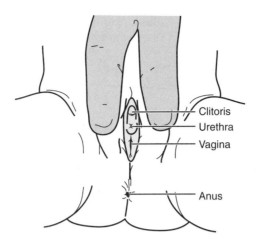

FIGURE 15-9 ■ Landmarks used in female bladder catheterization. (From Gomella, T.L.: *Neonatology: Management, procedures, on-call problems, diseases, and drugs* [5th ed.]. New York, 2004, Lange Medical Books/ McGraw-Hill.)

2. Don sterile gloves.
3. Separate the labia with the nondominant hand (which is no longer sterile). With the sterile dominant hand, clean the area around the meatus with the povidone-iodine solution swabs, using front-to-back strokes, repeating with three separate swabs.
4. Drape sterile towels across infant's lower abdomen and across legs.
5. Spread the labia and identify the meatus and urethra (Fig. 15-9).
6. Apply sterile lubricant to an appropriately sized catheter tip using the sterile dominant hand.
7. Insert the catheter into the urethra and advance until urine appears.
8. Advance catheter slightly past the point where urine flow began. Inflate balloon per hospital policy and manufacturer's recommendations, if applicable. Usually the catheter will function satisfactorily if simply taped in place. Balloon inflation may injure the urethra if the catheter is not properly positioned in the bladder.
9. If catheter is to remain indwelling, secure to inner thigh.
10. Collect urine specimen in the sterile container and send to the laboratory or attach to a closed urinary drainage system.
11. Document procedure, catheter type and size, patient's tolerance, quantity, and characteristics of sample obtained, and any difficulties encountered.

F. **Complications.**
1. Infection.
2. Hematuria.
3. Trauma to urethra.
4. Stricture of urethra or at meatus.
5. Possible knotting of catheter.
6. Pain.

Bladder Aspiration: Advanced Practice Procedure

A. **Indications.**
1. To obtain sterile urine sample for culture.
B. **Contraindications.**
1. Recent void or dehydration.
2. No clinical evidence or ultrasound evidence of urine in bladder (Chen et al., 2005).
3. Infection or loss of skin integrity over puncture site.

    4. Distention or enlargement of abdominal viscera.

    5. Genitourinary anomaly or enlargement of pelvic structures.

    6. Use caution in infants with coagulation disorders.

    7. Acute enteropathy such as necrotizing enterocolitis (NEC).

C. Precautions.

    1. Use aseptic technique.

    2. Consider catheterization as a primary attempt to collect urine, as suprapubic aspiration may be more painful (Kozer et al., 2006).

    3. Consider catheterization as an alternative for infants with coagulation defects or when previous needle aspirations were unsuccessful.

    4. Avoid inserting the needle directly over the pubic bone or away from the midline.

    5. Aspirate using gentle suction. Too much suction can occlude the needle, with the bladder mucosa preventing urine collection and increasing the risk of bladder injury.

D. Equipment and supplies. All equipment is sterile, except transillumination light or ultrasound equipment that may be covered with a sterile glove.

    1. Gloves.

    2. Povidone-iodine solution swabs or antiseptic per hospital policy.

    3. 3- to 6-ml syringe.

    4. 22- or 25-gauge needle.

    5. Sterile specimen container.

    6. Use of volumetric bladder ultrasound guidance may improve the success rate (Chen et al., 2005).

E. Procedure.

    1. Provide pain management, such as a pacifier for nonnutritive sucking, sucrose pacifier, and/or developmental positioning, with blanket swaddling of upper extremities.

    2. Determine the presence of urine in the bladder:

        a. Verify that the diaper has been dry for at least 1 hour.

        b. Use ultrasound guidance (optional).

        c. Consider prehydrating prior to procedure if medical condition permits.

    3. Have the assistant restrain the infant in the supine frog-leg position.

    4. Reflex urination may occur. Optimally, ask the assistant to pinch the base of the penis gently in a male infant.

    5. Perform a 3-minute scrub and don gloves.

    6. Locate the puncture site:

    7. Prepare the puncture site with hospital-approved antiseptic three times, using separate swabs each time.

        a. Palpate the symphysis pubis and locate a puncture site that is approximately 1 cm above symphysis pubis.

    8. Puncture bladder:

        a. Using the syringe with attached needle, maintain the needle at a 90-degree angle. Puncture skin and tissues over the bladder area and advance needle 2 to 3 cm and simultaneously aspirate with syringe. A slight decrease in resistance may be felt when the bladder is penetrated. Once urine has been obtained, do not advance the needle farther to avoid perforation of the posterior wall of the bladder.

    9. Do not probe with the needle or attempt to redirect it to obtain urine.

    10. Withdraw the needle if no urine is obtained and wait at least 1 hour before reattempting the procedure.

    11. If urine is obtained, withdraw the needle and apply gentle pressure over the puncture site with sterile gauze.

    12. Transfer the urine to a sterile specimen container. Send for culture and/or other diagnostic studies.

    13. Dispose of needle in an appropriate sharps container.

    14. Document procedure, patient's tolerance, laboratory samples obtained, amount and characteristics of urine, and any pain/developmental interventions performed.

F. **Complications.**
  1. Bleeding.
     a. Transient hematuria.
     b. Bladder wall hematoma.
     c. Abdominal wall hematoma.
     d. Pelvic hematoma.
  2. Infection.
     a. Abdominal wall abscess.
     b. Sepsis.
     c. Osteomyelitis of pubic bone.
     d. Peritonitis.
  3. Perforation of bowel or other pelvic organ.

Lumbar Puncture: Advanced Practice Procedure

A. **Indications.**
  1. To obtain cerebrospinal fluid (CSF) to diagnose central nervous system (CNS) disorders such as infections or subarachnoid hemorrhage.
  2. To monitor the efficacy of antibiotic therapy in the presence of CNS infection (rare).
  3. To drain CSF in communicating hydrocephalus associated with intracranial hemorrhage.
  4. To administer medication.
  5. To assist in the diagnosis of certain metabolic disorders.
B. **Contraindications.**
  1. Evidence of increased ICP. Performance of the procedure could cause herniation.
  2. Lumbosacral anomalies.
  3. Infants with uncorrected thrombocytopenia or coagulopathies.
  4. Severe cardiorespiratory instability.
C. **Precautions.**
  1. Avoid areas of infection or loss of skin integrity at puncture site.
  2. Monitor for and be prepared to respond to cardiorespiratory instability.
  3. Avoid flexion of the neck and ensure that a patent airway is maintained.
  4. Always maintain aseptic technique.
  5. Always use a needle with a stylet to avoid development of intraspinal epidermoid tumor.
  6. To prevent traumatic tap caused by overpenetration, insert the needle slowly while removing the stylet at frequent intervals to detect CSF as soon as the subdural space is entered.
  7. Never aspirate CSF with a syringe. Even a small amount of negative pressure can increase the risk of subdural hemorrhage or herniation.
  8. Palpate landmarks accurately to prevent puncture above the L4 interspace.
D. **Equipment and supplies.**
  1. Prepackaged lumbar puncture kit.
  2. If a prepackaged kit is not available, gather the following supplies:
     a. Sterile gloves and gown, mask, and surgical cap.
     b. Sterile cup with povidone-iodine.
     c. Sterile gauze pads.
     d. Sterile towels or transparent aperture drape.
     e. Spinal needle with short bevel and stylet (22-gauge needle).
     f. Three or more sterile specimen tubes with caps.
     g. Adhesive bandage.
  3. Cardiorespiratory monitor and pulse oximeter and emergency equipment such as suction and oxygen source.
  4. Analgesic agents and/or sedatives.
  5. Pressure-monitoring equipment, if planning to obtain CSF pressures.
E. **Procedure.**
  1. Obtain informed consent per institution's policy.
  2. Gather equipment and supplies.

3. Provide anxiety/pain management by considering the following:
   a. Oral sucrose solution to minimize pain (Leef, 2006).
   b. Topical anesthetics such as EMLA, Ametop, or LMX4 over puncture site in term newborns per institution's policy and manufacturer's recommendations (Kaur et al., 2003; O'Brien et al., 2005). Use of local anesthetic has shown to increase success rates (Baxter et al., 2006).
   c. Nonnarcotic relief such as acetaminophen.
   d. Local anesthesia: 1% lidocaine drawn up in a 1-ml syringe with a 27- to 25-gauge needle for injection.
   e. Opioid (fentanyl or morphine) or a benzodiazepine (Versed not recommended in premature infants).
4. Examine and determine puncture site:
   a. Grasp both iliac crests at their highest points, and following an imaginary line (that passes across the level of the fifth lumbar vertebra) palpate the interspace of the spinous process that falls immediately above or below the imaginary line drawn between the iliac crests (Fig. 15-10).
   b. The preferred puncture site is between L3-4 and L4-5 (MacDonald and Ramasethu, 2007).
   c. The puncture site can be marked by making a small nail print impression or using a surgical marker.
5. Don mask and cap and perform a 3-minute scrub and then don gown and sterile gloves.
6. Have an assistant open tray while maintaining the sterility of its contents.
7. Have assistant restrain the infant with hips flexed and back arched in the lateral decubitus (knee-chest) or sitting position, with spine flexed. An intubated infant must be positioned in the lateral decubitus position. Avoid flexion of the neck and ensure that a patent airway is maintained.
8. Clean the lumbar area three times with antiseptic using a new swab each time.
   a. Begin at the desired interspace, using a circular motion from puncture site outward to up and over the iliac crests.
   b. Allow antiseptic to dry.
9. If used, inject a wheal of local anesthetic at the puncture site. After several minutes, infiltrate the deeper tissues also.

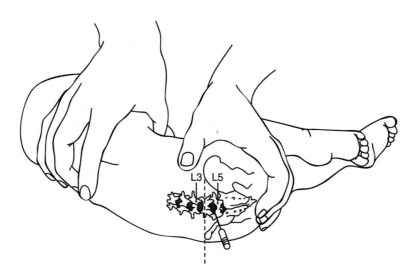

FIGURE 15-10 ■ Lumbar puncture positioning and landmarks. (From Gomella, T.L.: *Neonatology: Management, procedures, on-call problems, diseases, and drugs* [5th ed.]. New York, 2004, Lange Medical Books/ McGraw-Hill.)

10. Place one sterile drape under the infant and another that covers the patient, with the exception of the puncture site and the infant's face. Transparent aperture drapes are available and recommended because they permit better observation of the infant.
11. Relocate the desired interspace and insert the needle in the midline.
    a. Angle slightly cephalad to avoid the vertebral bodies.
    b. If resistance is met, withdraw the needle slightly and redirect more cephalad.
    c. Hold a finger on the vertebral process above or below the interspace to aid in locating the puncture site if the infant moves.
12. Advance the needle slowly to a depth of approximately 1.0 to 1.5 cm depending on infant's size, in small increments (2 to 3 mm) to avoid puncture of posterior wall.
    a. Remove the stylet frequently to observe the needle hub for fluid. Always replace the stylet before readvancing the needle.
    b. A pop may be felt when the ligamentum flavum and dura are penetrated. Penetration of the dura may also be detected when a loss of resistance is met.
    c. Once fluid is noted in the needle hub, patiently wait for CSF, which may be slow.
13. Obtain pressure measurement reading, if desired.
    a. Opening pressure measurements are difficult and often unreliable, but possible in a quiet infant in the lateral decubitus position. If measuring pressure, attach the manometer and wait for the fluid oscillations to stabilize in the tube before recording the pressure. Normal mean lumbar CSF pressures in neonates and preterm infants are 100 and 95 mm H_2O, respectively (Marra et al., 2004).
14. Allow CSF to collect dropwise into the collection tubes; never aspirate with a syringe.
15. If no fluid is obtained, try gently rotating the needle. If no fluid is obtained after repositioning the needle, replace the stylet, remove the needle, and try one interspace above or below, using a new needle for each attempt.
16. Allow the CSF to drop from the needle hub to collect 0.5- to 1-ml aliquots of CSF in three or four of the specimen tubes for the following diagnostic studies:
    a. Tube 1: culture, Gram stain, and sensitivity studies.
    b. Tube 2: protein and glucose.
    c. Tube 3: cell count and differential.
    d. Tube 4: other diagnostic studies such as Venereal Disease Research Laboratory (VDRL) and/or viral studies.
    e. Note: If a traumatic (bloody) tap was performed, send the clearest specimen for cell count and differential. Bloody CSF can be differentiated from venous blood by dropping a sample onto filter paper. Bloody CSF will form a "water ring" around a central patch of erythrocytes.
17. For treatment of hydrocephalus remove 10 to 15 ml/kg, or until CSF flow ceases.
18. Once specimens have been obtained, replace stylet and remove needle–stylet unit in a single outward motion to prevent injury to the spinal cord and nerves.
19. Apply local pressure to the puncture site for 3 to 5 minutes to minimize the risk of CSF leakage. Then place an adhesive bandage over the puncture site.
20. Remove the surrounding antiseptic with sterile water to avoid skin injury.
21. Document procedure according to hospital policy noting position of the patient during procedure, needle size used, complications or difficulties encountered, CSF characteristics, pain management interventions, patient's tolerance, and specimens sent to laboratory for analysis.

F. **Complications.**
   1. Infection from nonsterile conditions:
      a. Use of poor sterile technique.
      b. Bacteremia if blood vessel punctures during procedure, having passed through infected CSF.
   2. Intraspinal epidermoid tumor from lack of stylet use.
   3. Spinal cord and/or nerve damage if puncture performed above L4.
   4. Cerebral herniation.
   5. Apnea and/or bradycardia.
   6. Hypoxia.

7. Spinal cord or epidural abscess.
8. Spinal or intracranial subdural hematoma.
9. Spinal or intracranial subarachnoid hematoma.
10. Spinal fluid leakage into epidural space.
11. Vertebral body osteomyelitis.
12. Persistent bleeding, especially in patients with an underlying coagulopathy.
13. Pain.

REFERENCES

American Academy of Pediatrics and American Heart Association: *Textbook of neonatal resuscitation* (5th ed.). Elk Grove Village, IL, 2006, American Academy of Pediatrics and American Heart Association.

Baxter, A.L., Fisher, R.G., Burke, B.L., et al.: Local anesthetic and stylet styles: Factors associated with resident lumbar puncture success. *Pediatrics, 177*(3): 876-881, 2006.

Becton, Dickinson and Co: Workshop for midline and peripherally inserted central catheters. *Clinical education manual*. Franklin Lakes, NJ, 2000.

Carbajal, R., Eble, B., and Anand, K.J.: Premedication for tracheal intubation in neonates: Confusion or controversy. *Seminars in Perinatology, 31*(5):309-317, 2007.

Centers for Disease Control and Prevention: Guidelines for the prevention of intravascular-catheter related infections. *MMWR Morbidity and Mortality Weekly Report, 51*:1-38, 2002.

Chen, L., Hsiao, A.L., Moore, C.L., Dziura, J.D., and Santucci, K.A.: Utility of bedside bladder ultrasound before uretheral catheterization in young children. *Pediatrics, 115*(1):108-111, 2005.

Choong, K., Chatrkaw, P., Frndova, H., et al.: Comparison of loss in lung with open versus in-line catheter endotracheal suctioning. *Pediatric Critical Care Medicine, 4*(91):69-73, 2003.

Davis, J.M. and Rosenfeld, W.N.: Bronchopulmonary dysplasia. In M.G. MacDonald, M.D. Mullett, and M.M.K. Seshia (Eds.): *Avery's neonatology. Pathophysiology and management of the newborn* (6th ed.). Philadelphia, 2005, Lippincott Williams & Wilkins, pp. 578-599.

Dawson, D.: Midline catheters in neonatal patients evaluating a change in practice. *Journal of Vascular Access Devices*, Summer: 17-19, 2002.

DeBoer, S.L. and Peterson, L.V.: Sedation for nonemergent neonatal intubation. *Neonatal Network, 20*(7):19-23, 2001.

DeBoer, S. and Seaver, M.: End-tidal CO_2 verification of endotracheal tube placement in neonates. *Neonatal Network, 23*(3):29-38, 2004.

Folk, L.: Guide to capillary heelstick blood sampling in infants. *Advances in Neonatal Care, 7*(4):171-178, 2007.

Gomella, T.L.: *Neonatology: Management, procedures, on-call problems, diseases and drugs* (5th ed.). New York, 2004, Lange Medical Books/McGraw-Hill.

Hagedorn, M.I.E., Gardner, S.L., Dickey, L.A., and Abman, S.H.: Respiratory diseases. In G.B. Merenstein and S.L. Gardner (Eds.): *Handbook of neonatal intensive care* (6th ed.). St. Louis, 2006, Mosby, pp. 595-698.

Hagler, D.A. and Traver, G.A.: Endotracheal saline and suction catheters: Sources of lower airway contamination. *American Journal of Critical Care, 3*(6):444-447, 1994.

Hughes, S., Blake, B., Woods, S., et al.: False-positive results on a colorimetric carbon dioxide analysis in neonatal resuscitation: Potential for serious patient harm. *Journal of Perinatology, 27*(12):800-801, 2007.

Kalyn, A., Blatz, S., Feuerstake, S., et al.: Closed suctioning of intubated neonates maintains better physiologic stability: A randomized trial. *Journal of Perinatology, 23*(3):218-222, 2003.

Kaur, G., Gupta, P., and Kumar, A.: A randomized trial of eutectic mixture of local anesthetics during lumbar puncture in newborns. *Archives of Pediatric and Adolescent Medicine, 157*(11):1065-1070, 2003.

Kozer, E., Rosenbloom, E., Goldman, D., et al.: Pain in infants who are younger than 2 months during suprapubic aspiration and transurethral bladder catheterization: A randomized, controlled study. *Pediatrics, 118*(1):e51-e56, 2006.

Leef, K.H.: Evidence-based review of oral sucrose administration to decrease the pain response in newborn infants. *Neonatal Network, 25*(4):275-284, 2006.

Leike-Rude, M.K. and Haney, B.: Midline catheter use in the intensive care nursery. *Neonatal Network, 25*(3):189-199, 2006.

Lesser, E., Chhabra, R., Brion, L., et al.: Use of midline catheters in low birth weight infants. *Journal of Perinatology, 16*(3):205-207, 1996.

MacDonald, M.G. and Ramasethu, J.: *Atlas of procedures in neonatology* (4th ed.). Philadelphia, 2007, Lippincott Williams & Wilkins.

Marra, C., Whitley, R., and Scheld, M.: Approach to the patient with central nervous system infection. In W. Michael Scheld, Richard J. Whitley, and Christina M. Marra (Eds.): *Infections of the central nervous system.* Lippincott, 2004, Philadelphia, p. 13.

O'Brien, L., Taddio, A., Lyszkiewicz, D., et al.: A critical review of the topical anesthetic amethocaine (Ametop) for pediatric pain. *Paediatric Drugs, 7*(1):41-54, 2005.

Oei, J., Hari, R., Butha, T., and Lui, K.: Facilitation of neonatal nasotracheal intubation with premedication: A randomized controlled trial. *Journal of Paediatrics and Child Health, 38*(2):146-150, 2002.

Peterson, J., Johnson, N., Deakins, K., et al.: Accuracy of the 7-8-9 Rule for endotracheal tube placement in the neonate. *Journal of Perinatology, 26*(6):333-336, 2006.

Porter, F., Grunau, R., and Anand, K.J.: Long-term effects of pain in infants. *Journal of Developmental and Behavioral Pediatrics, 20*(4):253-261, 1999.

Ramasethu, J.: Prevention and management of extravasation injuries in neonates. *NeoReviews*, 5(11):e491-e497, 2004.

Reynolds, J.: Comparison of percutaneous venous catheters and Teflon catheters for intravenous therapy in neonates. *Neonatal Network*, 12(5):33-39, 1993.

Shah, V. and Ohlsson, A.: Venipuncture versus heel lance for blood sampling in term neonates (Review). *The Cochrane Collaboration*, 4:CD001452, 2007.

Tan, A.M., Gomez, J.M., Mathews, J., et al.: Closed versus partially ventilated endotracheal suction in extremely preterm neonates: Physiologic conse-quences. *Intensive Critical Care Nurse*, 21(4):234-242, 2005.

Thigpen, J.L.: Peripheral intravenous extravasation: Nursing procedure for initial treatment. *Neonatal Network*, 26(6):379-384, 2007.

Tingay, D.G., Copnell, B., Mills, J.F., et al.: Effects of open endotracheal suction on lung volume in infants receiving HFOV. *Intensive Care Medicine*, 33:689-693, 2007.

Wyckoff, M.M.: Midline catheter use in the premature and full-term infant. *Journal of Vascular Access Devices*, 4(3):26-29, 1999.

16 Pain Assessment and Management

MARLENE WALDEN

OBJECTIVES

1. Review the physiology of acute pain in preterm neonates.

2. Discuss current standards for assessing and managing pain in neonates.

3. Identify behavioral and physiologic responses that are indicative of pain in the neonate.

4. Select a valid and reliable composite measure for assessment of pain in neonates.

5. Discuss the evidence base for nonpharmacologic and pharmacologic approaches to the management of pain in neonates.

Advances in neonatal care during the past two decades has led to the increased survival of extremely preterm and sick neonates who regularly are subjected to numerous diagnostic and therapeutic procedures that are painful but medically necessary to their care. The prevention of pain in these critically ill neonates not only is an ethical obligation but may also minimize the immediate and cumulative effects of repeated painful experiences on the developing brain of these vulnerable neonates. Despite impressive gains in the knowledge related to the assessment and management of pain in neonates during the past 20 years, a large gap still exists between routine clinical practice and scientific evidence. This chapter will review pain pathways, identification of pain, and interventions to alleviate pain in the neonate.

DEFINITION OF PAIN

The International Association for the Study of Pain (IASP) defines pain as "unpleasant sensory and emotional experience associated with actual or potential tissue damage, or described in terms of such damage" (1979, p. 250). The IASP definition implies that the meaning of pain must be learned through experience and articulated within the context of verbal language. This conceptualization of pain perpetuates the misconceptions that infants, who lack linguistic skills, do not experience pain (Anand and Craig, 1996). In neonates, physiologic, behavioral, and hormonal indicators provide objective and quantifiable information about the location, intensity, and duration of painful stimuli. These responses can be used in conjunction with other contextual indicators to infer the existence of pain.

NEONATAL INTENSIVE CARE UNIT PROCEDURES THAT CAUSE PAIN

A. Many activities and interventions in the neonatal intensive care unit (NICU) cause pain. The most frequently occurring painful procedures include nasal and endotracheal suctioning, heel stick, adhesive removal, and venous and arterial punctures (Carbajal et al., 2008).

B. Frequency of invasive procedures is inversely related to gestational age and severity of illness. Therefore, the smaller and sicker neonates are those subject to the greatest numbers of most painful procedures.

1. Simons and colleagues (2003) found that infants born at 25 to 42 weeks of gestation experienced an average of 14 painful procedures per day during the first 2 weeks of life.

2. Carbajal and colleagues (2008) found that infants born between 24 and 42 weeks of gestation experienced on average a mean of 98 painful procedures during the first 14 days of admission, with one neonate having 364 painful procedures.

C. **The number of procedures encountered by infants in the NICU is partially due to a substantial number of failed attempts.**
   1. In the study by Simons and colleagues (2003), the failure rate for placement of central venous catheters, peripheral arterial catheters, and intravenous cannulae were 45.6%, 37.5%, and 30.9%, respectively.
   2. In the study by Carbajal et al. (2008), some of the most painful procedures needed as many as 10 to 15 attempts for completion.

D. **Despite safe, effective pharmacologic and nonpharmacologic interventions to prevent or minimize pain and distress, many painful procedures in the NICU are performed without analgesia.**
   1. In the study by Simons et al. (2003), many of the procedures were rated by physicians and nurses to be painful (>4 on a 10-point scale); however, very few infants received any pharmacologic or nonpharmacologic procedural pain management.
   2. In the study by Carbajal and colleagues, only 20.8% of painful procedures were performed with pharmacologic and/or nonpharmacologic therapy.

E. **The International Evidence-Based Group for Neonatal Pain, and more recently, the Association of Paediatric Anaesthetists of Great Britain and Ireland provides guidelines for preventing and treating neonatal procedural pain** (Anand and International Evidence-Based Group for Neonatal Pain, 2001; Howard et al., 2008).
   1. Heel stick
      a. Pain resulting from the heel-stick procedure is caused not only by the lancing procedure but also by the squeezing of the heel to obtain the blood sample.
      b. Spring-loaded mechanical lancets result in less bruising, less need for repeat punctures, and fewer behavioral and physiologic signs of pain.
      c. Heel warming has no effect on infant response to pain during the heel-stick procedure.
      d. Evidence-based interventions include pacifier with sucrose, swaddling, containment, facilitated tucking, breastfeeding, and skin-to-skin contact with mother.
   2. Circumcision
      a. Although the procedure is not medically necessary, procedural analgesia should always be used when parents or caregivers elect to have their infant circumcised (American Academy of Pediatrics Task Force on Circumcision listed, 1999).
      b. Subcutaneous ring block appears to provide superior analgesia. However, dorsal penile nerve blocks and EMLA cream (lidocaine 2.5% and prilocaine 2.5%) may also be used for pain associated with circumcision.
      c. Evidence-based interventions to decrease the infant's distress include containment, facilitated tucking, hand-to-mouth opportunities, and flexed positioning.
      d. The use of sucrose during the procedure and acetaminophen administered before or immediately following can be used to supplement the above analgesic approaches.
   3. Venipuncture may be preferable to heel stick in minimizing procedure-related pain in full-term infants. However, frequent venipuncture for blood sampling is not feasible for most infants in the NICU, necessitating the continued use of heel sticks. Evidence-based interventions include swaddling, facilitated tucking, sucrose, and topical anesthetic cream in infants ≥37 weeks of gestation.
   4. Technician expertise such as the skill of the operator influences pain responses in infants and should be monitored. Ensuring staff competence to perform required procedures may reduce the number of painful procedures to which an infant is exposed by reducing the number of failed attempts (Simons et al., 2003).

PHYSIOLOGY OF ACUTE PAIN IN PRETERM NEONATES

A. **An understanding of the physiology of acute pain in preterm neonates is essential for optimal pain management in the NICU.** Pain responses exhibited by neonates are the result of a concurrent set of reactions within the peripheral nervous system, spinal cord, and higher centers involved at the supraspinal/integrative level, including the thalamus and cerebral cortex (Melzack, 1996).

1. Peripheral nervous system (Evans, 2001).
   a. Fully mature and functional by 20 weeks of gestation.
   b. Consists of two types of neuronal afferent fibers.
      (1) A-delta fibers: thinly myelinated, rapid-conducting fibers associated with sharp pain or "first pain" (e.g., sharp, localized, pricking).
      (2) C fibers: polymodal, unmyelinated, slow-conducting fibers associated with aching, burning, poorly localized, or "second pain."
   c. Density of nociceptors is equal to or greater than those in adult skin.
   d. Local tissue injury such as heel stick or venipuncture activates nociceptors of sensory afferent fibers to:
      (1) Transmit pain impulses to spinal cord and central nervous system (CNS).
      (2) Release biochemical mediators such as substance P and prostaglandins that results in hyperalgesia (increased sensitivity to painful stimuli) or allodynia (pain caused by a stimulus that ordinarily does not cause pain). This decreased pain threshold may persist for days or weeks.
      (3) Cause dendritic sprouting and hyperinnervation that result in hypersensitivity and lower pain threshold that may persist into adulthood.
2. Spinal cord (Evans, 2001).
   a. During the first postnatal week, weak linkages exist between the peripheral nervous system and the dorsal horn, resulting in either prolonged pain responses or no reaction to the painful stimuli.
   b. Receptive fields of the dorsal horn cells are larger than those of adults and begin to diminish 2 weeks after birth.
   c. Local spinal cord response to pain impulses from peripheral afferent fibers stimulates efferent somatomotor neurons in the anterior horn and produce reflex withdrawal.
   d. Afferent fiber neurotransmitters stimulate N-methyl-D-aspartate and tachykinin receptors in the dorsal horns, producing central sensitization (increased excitability of dorsal horn neurons that spreads to several adjacent segments of the spinal cord), "wind-up" (perceived increase in intensity or duration of painful stimuli), or secondary hyperalgesia (hypersensitivity elicited by both painful and nonpainful stimuli that extends to areas beyond the site of injury).
   e. Increases in autonomic responses such as heart rate and respiratory rate and facial responses such as brow bulge, eye squeeze, and nasolabial furrow in response to heelstick procedures provide evidence of maturity of ascending pathways by 20 weeks of gestation.
   f. Preterm infants have a limited ability to modulate pain. Dopamine and norepinephrine are not available to modulate pain before 36 to 40 weeks of gestation. Serotonin is first released at approximately 6 to 8 weeks after birth.
3. Supraspinal/integrative level (Evans, 2001).
   a. Cerebral cortex has a full complement of neurons by 20 weeks of gestation.
   b. Cerebral cortex is functionally mature by 22 weeks of gestation and bilaterally synchronous by 27 weeks of gestation.
   c. Somatosensory-evoked potentials are slow and simple before 29 weeks of gestation, but short and complex by 40 weeks of gestation.
   d. Cortical cell migration is complete at approximately 24 weeks of gestation. However, the support structure of the germinal matrix remains highly vascular until 28 weeks. Therefore, the neonate is vulnerable to intraventricular hemorrhage related to increases in blood pressure associated with pain.
   e. Maximum number of cortical neurons is reached at 28 weeks of gestation, and then approximately 70% cortical neurons are lost before birth through apoptosis.
   f. Neonates as early as 27 weeks of gestation can differentiate touch (sham heel stick) from a noxious stimuli (heel stick) as evidenced by physiologic and facial response patterns.
   g. Neurologic connections are in place for the perception of, reaction to, and memory of pain on the cortical level as evidenced by mature visual and auditory response patterns

on electroencephalogram in infants younger than 30 weeks of gestation and by measurements of in vivo cerebral glucose in the sensory areas of the brain.

B. Repetitive, unrelieved pain can lead to serious and adverse consequences for neonates.
1. Short-term physiologic consequences of painful procedures include decreased oxygen saturations and increased heart rates that can place increased demands on the cardiorespiratory system.
2. Pain can cause elevation in intracranial pressure, thereby increasing risk of intraventricular hemorrhage in preterm neonates.
3. Pain and stress may also depress the immune system and contribute to increased susceptibility of neonates to infections.
4. The long-term effects of pain in animals are clear, with changes observed in pain thresholds, social behaviors, stress responses, and pain responses to nonpainful stimuli (Fitzgerald and Anand, 1993; Plotsky et al., 2000; Reynolds et al., 1997; Ruda et al., 2000). Preliminary human data suggest that early pain experiences may alter future pain responses. Johnston and Stevens (1996) reported that neonates who were born at 28 weeks of gestation and were hospitalized in an NICU for 4 weeks (32 weeks of postconceptional age) had decreased behavioral response and significantly higher heart and lower oxygen saturation during a heel-stick procedure compared with newly born neonates at 32 weeks of gestation. In another study, Taddio and colleagues (1995) reported that males circumcised within 2 days of birth had significantly longer crying bouts and higher pain intensity scores at immunization at 4 or 6 months of age than males who were not circumcised.

STANDARDS OF PRACTICE

A. Recognition of the widespread inadequacy of pain management promoted various professional organizations to issue position statements and clinical recommendations in an effort to promote effective pain management in undertreated populations. Organizations that support the importance of optimal pain assessment and management in hospitalized neonates include the National Association of Neonatal Nurses (Walden and Gibbins, 2008) and the American Academy of Pediatrics/Canadian Paediatric Society (2000, 2006). There is considerable consistency in the recommendations set by these professional organizations. Core principles contained within these guidelines and standards that are applicable to pain assessment and management in the NICU include the following:
1. Assess education and competency in pain assessment and management of new and current employees.
2. Regularly assess and reassess pain using a valid and reliable multidimensional pain assessment instrument.
3. Use both nonpharmacologic and pharmacologic approaches to prevent and/or manage pain.
4. Health care team members should collaborate together and with the infant's family in developing an approach to pain assessment and management.
5. Documentation should facilitate regular reassessment and follow-up intervention.
6. Policies and procedures should be established to provide consistency and quality of pain assessment and management practices.
7. Data should be collected to monitor the appropriateness and effectiveness of pain management practices.

B. The clinical challenge remains on how to implement these standards in various institutional settings based on patient types, frequently occurring clinical procedures performed, and current staffing patterns.

PAIN ASSESSMENT

A. Pain assessment has been advocated as the "fifth vital sign" and should be assessed routinely.

B. "The 'golden rule' of pain assessment must be: What is painful to an adult is painful to an infant until proven otherwise" (Franck, 1989). This rule, along with the use of valid and reliable tools, must be used for the assessment and intervention of pain.

C. Because previous painful experiences may modify pain expression, further research is needed to develop and test an instrument to assess chronic pain in the infant requiring prolonged hospitalization who has been subjected to multiple painful clinical procedures.

D. Pain assessment is an essential prerequisite to optimal pain management.

E. Behavioral responses.

1. Facial activity offers the most specificity as an indicator of pain, namely brow bulge, eye squeeze, and nasolabial furrow.

2. Acoustic and temporal characteristics of pain cries are different than other cry types in both preterm and full-term infants, including increases in peak fundamental frequency (pitch), peak spectral energy, cry duration, and intensity. However, differences in cry types are difficult to discriminate in the clinical setting.

3. Many preterm infants do not cry in response to a noxious stimulus. The absence of response may only indicate the depletion of response capability and not lack of pain perception.

4. Healthy full-term newborns use swiping motions by the unaffected leg to the lanced foot, as if trying to push away the noxious stimulus.

5. Preterm infants demonstrate an increase in motor extension patterns, including finger splay, saluting, and sitting on air during painful clinical procedures. These hyperextension motor patterns are quickly replaced with flaccidity in infants at younger postconceptional ages.

F. **Physiologic responses.**

1. Preterm infants respond to noxious stimuli in patterns similar to that of full-term neonates, including increases in heart rate and decreases in oxygen saturation.

2. Although physiologic measures provide greater objectivity in the assessment of pain, they also reflect the body's nonspecific response to stress and thus are not specific to pain (Ranger et al., 2007). Therefore, physiologic measures should be converged with behavioral measures that have been demonstrated to be more consistent and specific to pain in neonates.

3. Physiologic measures should be used to assess pain in infants who are paralyzed for mechanical ventilation or who are severely neurologically impaired. Increases in heart rate and blood pressure during handling generally indicate the need for more analgesia and/or sedation in the pharmacologically paralyzed infant.

4. If the infant is sedated, variability in heart rate and blood pressure decreases. However, it is important to remember that although sedatives may mask physiologic and behavioral signs of pain, sedatives do not provide pain relief.

G. **Contextual factors modifying pain responses.**

1. Developmental maturity, health status, and environmental factors may all contribute to an inconsistent, less robust pattern of pain responses between infants and even within the same infant over time and situations. Therefore, contextual factors that have been demonstrated to modify the pain experience must be considered when assessing for the presence of pain in neonates.

2. Infants in awake or alert states demonstrate a more robust reaction to painful stimuli than infants in sleep states.

3. Research examining facial as well as bodily activity has demonstrated that the magnitude of infant response has been observed to be less vigorous and robust with decreasing postconceptional age. Craig and colleagues (1993) suggest that the less vigorous responses demonstrated by preterm infants "should be interpreted in the context of the energy resources available to respond and the relative immaturity of the musculoskeletal system" (p. 296).

4. Less mature behavioral responses to noxious stimuli are also noted with increased number of painful procedures to which the infant is exposed, increased postnatal age of the infant at time of observation, and shorter length of time since last painful procedure (Ranger et al., 2007).

5. When pain stimuli or pain persists for hours or days without intervention, the infant exhibits a decompensatory response. The sympathetic nervous system, or the fight-or-flight mechanism, can no longer compensate. As a result, the physiologic parameters return to baseline (Hummel and van Dijk, 2006). *Return to baseline* does not indicate that

pain is no longer felt or is tolerated, but it does make the infant's pain more difficult to evaluate.

PAIN ASSESSMENT INSTRUMENTS

A. **Select a composite or multidimensional instrument that incorporates both physiologic and behavioral measures of pain.** Caregivers should select instruments with tested reliability, validity, and clinical utility. Infant population, setting, and type of pain experienced should also guide selection of a pain instrument (Duhn and Medves, 2004).

B. **CRIES: a postoperative pain tool** (Table 16-1) (Krechel and Bildner, 1995).
   1. Acronym for five behavioral and physiologic parameters: C = crying; R = requires oxygen to maintain saturation at greater than 95%; I = increased vital signs; E = expression; and S = sleeplessness.
   2. Demonstrates validity and interrater reliability for use in infants born at 32 weeks of gestation and later. Initial establishment of clinical utility.

■ TABLE 16-1
■ ■ **CRIES: Neonatal Postoperative Pain Measurement Score***

	Score			
	0	**1**	**2**	**Tips for Scoring CRIES**
Crying	No	High pitched	Inconsolable	Score 0: no cry or cry not high pitched Score 1: high-pitched cry, but consolable Score 2: high-pitched cry, inconsolable
Requires O$_2$ for saturation >95%	No	<30%	>30%	Score 0: no oxygen required from baseline Score 1: oxygen requirement <30% from baseline Score 2: oxygen requirement >30% from baseline
Increased vital signs	HR and BP ≤ preoperative values	HR or BP <20% of preoperative values	HR or BP ≥20% of preoperative values	Score 0: HR and BP are both unchanged or at less than baseline Score 1: HR or BP is increased by <20% Score 2: HR or BP is increased by >20% *Note:* Measure BP last so as not to wake the infant.
Expression	None	Grimace	Grimace/grunt	Score 0: no grimace Score 1: grimace only is present Score 2: grimace and inaudible grunt present *Note:* Grimace consists of lowered brow, eyes squeezed shut, deepening nasolabial furrow, and open lips and mouth.
Sleepless	No	Wakes at frequent intervals	Constantly awake	Score 0: continuously asleep Score 1: awakens at frequent intervals Score 2: awake constantly *Note:* Based on infant's state during previous hour.

BP, Blood pressure; *HR*, heart rate.
*Neonatal pain assessment tool developed at the University of Missouri–Columbia.
From Krechel, S. and Bildner, J.: CRIES: A new neonatal post-operative pain measurement score: Initial testing of validity and reliability. *Paediatric Anaesthesia, 5*(1):53-61, 1995.

3. Tool scoring system, 0 to 10, is structured in the same fashion as the Apgar score and was designed to make the tool easy to use and remember.
4. Score was originally developed to assess postoperative pain, but recently has been used in research related to procedural pain (Ahn, 2006; Belda et al., 2004).
5. A score of 4 or above indicates pain, and any assessment of 4 or above should receive pain intervention. The neonate should then be reevaluated 15 to 30 minutes after analgesia to assess for pain relief.
C. **The Premature Infant Pain Profile** (Stevens et al., 1996) (Table 16-2).
   1. Seven-item, four-point scale for assessment of pain in premature infants through term gestation.
   2. Score was originally developed to assess procedural pain, but recently has been used in research to assess postoperative pain in neonates (El Sayed, et al., 2007; McNair et al., 2004; Suraseranivongse et al., 2006).
   3. Multidimensional: includes heart rate, oxygen saturation, brow bulge, eye squeeze, and nasolabial furrow.
   4. Unique in that it includes two contextual modifiers (i.e., gestational age and behavioral state).

■ TABLE 16-2
■ ■ **Premature Infant Pain Profile**

Infant Study Date/time: _____   Number: _____
Event: _____

Process	Indicator	0	1	2	3	Score
Chart	Gestational age	36 weeks and more	32 to 35 weeks, 6 days	28 to 31 weeks, 6 days	Less than 28 weeks	
Observe infant 15 s	Behavioral state	Active/awake, eyes open, facial movements	Quiet/awake, eyes open, no facial movements	Active/sleep, eyes closed, facial movements	Quiet/sleep, eyes closed, no facial movements	
Observe baseline Heart rate _____	Heart rate Max _____	0 to 4 beats/minute increase	5 to 14 beats/minute increase	15 to 24 beats/minute increase	25 beats/minute or more increase	
Oxygen saturation _____	Oxygen saturation Min _____	0% to 2.4% decrease	2.5% to 4.9% decrease	5% to 7.4% decrease	7.5% or more decrease	
Observe infant 30 s	Brow bulge	None 0% to 9% of time	Minimum 10% to 39% of time	Moderate 40% to 69% of time	Maximum 70% of time or more	
	Eye squeeze	None 0% to 9% of time	Minimum 10% to 39% of time	Moderate 40% to 69% of time	Maximum 70% of time or more	
	Nasolabial furrow	None 0% to 9% of time	Minimum 10% to 39% of time	Moderate 40% to 69% of time	Maximum 70% of time or more	
					Total Score	_____

From Stevens, B., Johnston, C., Petryshen, P., and Taddio, A.: Premature infant pain profile: Development and initial validation. *Clinical Journal of Pain, 12*(1):13-22, 1996.

	Before Time		During Time					After Time		
	1	2	1	2	3	4	5	1	2	3
Facial expression 0—Relaxed 1—Grimace										
Cry 0—No cry 1—Whimper 2—Vigorous										
Breathing patterns 0—Relaxed 1—Change in breathing										
Arms 0—Relaxed/restrained 1—Flexed/extended										
Legs 0—Relaxed/restrained 1—Flexed/extended										
State of arousal 0—Sleeping/awake 1—Fussy										
Total										

Note: Time is measured in 1-minute intervals.

FIGURE 16-1 ■ Neonatal Infant Pain Scale. (From Lawrence, J., Alcock, D., McGrath, P., et al.: The development of a tool to assess neonatal pain. *Neonatal Network, 12*[6]:59-66, 1993.)

5. Good establishment of reliability and validity. Beginning establishment of clinical utility.
6. Total pain score of 7 to 12 indicates mild pain, and infant may benefit from use of non-pharmacologic comfort measures. Total pain score greater than 12 indicates moderate to severe pain and will most likely require pharmacologic intervention in conjunction with comfort measures.

D. **Neonatal Infant Pain Scale** (Lawrence et al., 1993) (Fig. 16-1).
   1. Six-item scale. Five behavioral items (facial expression, crying, arms, legs, and state of arousal) and one physiologic indicator (breathing pattern). Each behavior except cry has descriptors for the two possible scores of 0 and 1. Cry is scored on a three-point scale (0, 1, 2).
   2. Originally tested in preterm and full-term neonates who required capillary, venous, or arterial punctures, but more recently has also been used in research related to postoperative pain in neonates (Rouss et al., 2007; Suraseranivongse et al., 2006).
   3. Total score can range from 0 to 7.

E. **Neonatal Pain Agitation and Sedation Scale** (Hummel et al., 2008) (Fig. 16-2).
   1. Measures both pain/agitation and sedation in preterm and term neonates with prolonged pain postoperatively and during mechanical ventilation.
   2. Five-item scale. Four behavioral items (crying/irritability, behavior state, facial expression, extremities/tone) and one physiologic indicator (vital signs).
   3. Includes gestational age as a contextual modifier of pain.
   4. Total pain scores range from 0 to 10. Sedation scores range from 0 to –10.

NURSING CARE OF THE INFANT IN PAIN

Skilled observation, assessments, and interventions are the responsibility of the care providers. Pain intervention may be provided by both nonpharmacologic and pharmacologic methods.

Assessment criteria	Sedation		Normal	Pain/Agitation	
	−2	−1	0	1	2
Crying, Irritability	No cry with painful stimuli	Moans or cries minimally with painful stimuli	Appropriate crying Not irritable	Irritable or crying at intervals Consolable	High-pitched or silent-continuous cry Inconsolable
Behavior state	No arousal to any stimuli No spontaneous movement	Arouses minimally to stimuli Little spontaneous movement	Appropriate for gestational age	Restless, squirming Awakens frequently	Arching, kicking Constantly awake or arouses minimally/no movement (not sedated)
Facial expression	Mouth is lax No expression	Minimal expression with stimuli	Relaxed Appropriate	Any pain expression intermittent	Any pain expression continual
Extremities Tone	No grasp reflex Flaccid tone	Weak grasp reflex ↓ muscle tone	Relaxed hands and feet Normal tone	Intermittent clenched toes, fists, or finger splay Body is not tense	Continual clenched toes, fists, or finger splay Body is tense
Vital signs HR, RR, BP, SaO₂	No variability with stimuli Hypoventilation or apnea	<10% variability from baseline with stimuli	Within baseline or normal for gestational age	10%-20% from baseline SaO₂ 76%-85% with stimulation—quick recovery	>20% from baseline SaO₂ ≤75% with stimulation—slow recovery Out of sync with vent

Notes: 1) Pain and sedation scores are recorded separately
2) Points are added to the premature infant's pain score based on their gestational age:
   • +3 if <28 weeks of gestation/corrected age
   • +2 if 28-31 weeks of gestation/corrected age
   • +1 if 32-35 weeks of gestation/corrected age
3) Sedation assessment requires an assessment of response to stimuli

FIGURE 16-2 ■ Neonatal Pain Agitation and Sedation Scale. (From Hummel, P., Puchalski, M., Creech S.D., and Weiss, M.G.: Clinical reliability and validity of the N-PASS: neonatal pain, agitation, and sedation scale with prolonged pain. *Journal of Perinatology, 28*(1), 2008.)

A. Nonpharmacologic approaches to pain management.
  1. Goals.
     a. To help minimize pain and stress while maximizing the infant's ability to cope with and recover from clinical procedures.
     b. To provide additive or synergistic benefits to pharmacologic therapy (Franck and Lawhon, 1998).
  2. Preventive measures.
     a. Reduce the total number of painful procedures to which the infant is exposed by
        (1) Evaluating all aspects of caregiving,
        (2) Evaluating the number and grouping of laboratory and diagnostic procedures,
        (3) Scheduling clinical procedures based on medical necessity versus a routine schedule,
        (4) Using minimal amounts of tape/adhesives and using skin barrier products when possible,
        (5) Ensuring proper premedication prior to invasive procedures,
        (6) Using noninvasive monitoring devices when possible,
        (7) Establishing central venous/arterial access to minimize skin-breaking procedures, and
        (8) Involving parents in caregiving by teaching signs and symptoms of pain and comfort that they can provide.
     b. Painful procedures should not be performed at the same time as other, nonemergency routine care (e.g., taking vital signs, changing a diaper) as it can cause sensory hypersensitivity (referred to as wind-up phenomenon) causing nonnoxious stimuli to be perceived as painful (Holsti et al., 2005).
     c. Handling and immobilization in preparation for painful procedures should be minimized before a painful procedure as this may heighten activity in nociceptive pathways and accentuate the infants' pain responses.
     d. Use environmental interventions such as reduced lighting and noise levels to minimize infant stress.
  3. Behavioral measures.
     a. Facilitated tucking (hand-swaddling technique that holds the infant's extremities flexed and contained close to the trunk) during a painful procedure may significantly reduce pain responses in preterm infants.
     b. Blanket swaddling following a painful procedure may help reduce physiologic and behavioral pain and distress in preterm neonates.
     c. Pacifiers ranked by NICU nurses as the first choice of pain intervention.
        (1) Nonnutritive sucking (NNS) is thought to modulate the transmission or processing of nociception through mediation by the endogenous nonopioid system.
        (2) The efficacy of NNS is immediate but appears to terminate almost immediately upon cessation of sucking.
        (3) Pain relief is greater in infants who receive both NNS and sucrose.
     d. Studies demonstrate that a single 0.05- to 2-ml dose of 0.24 to 0.50 g (12% to 25%) sucrose given orally approximately 2 minutes before painful stimulus is associated with statistically and clinically significant reductions in crying after a painful stimulus.
        (1) Interval coincides with endogenous opioid release triggered by the sweet taste of sucrose.
        (2) Safety of implementing repeated doses of sucrose in very low birth weight infants has not been confirmed; therefore, caution is advised before widespread use of repeated doses in preterm and critically ill neonates. However, in a study by Stevens and colleagues (1999), no immediate adverse effects were noted when administering a 24% sucrose-dipped pacifier during four random, consecutively administered, routine heel-stick procedures.
     e. Breastfeeding may be used to alleviate procedural pain in neonates undergoing a single painful procedure.

B. **Pharmacologic approaches to pain management.**
1. Pharmacologic approaches to pain management should be used when moderate, severe, or prolonged pain is assessed or anticipated.
2. Intravenous opioids remain the most common class of analgesics administered in the NICU, particularly that of morphine sulfate and fentanyl citrate.
   a. Systemic opioids induce analgesia by acting at various levels of the CNS.
      (1) Spinal cord: Opioids impair or inhibit the transmission of nociceptive input from the periphery to the CNS.
      (2) Basal ganglia: Opioids activate a descending inhibitory system.
      (3) Limbic system: Opioids alter the emotional response to pain, making it more tolerable.
   b. Special considerations in neonates are as follows:
      (1) Longer dosing intervals are often required in neonates less than 1 month of age because of longer elimination half-lives and delayed clearance of opioids as compared with adults or children greater than 1 year of age.
      (2) Neonates should be monitored closely during opioid therapy and for several hours after opioids have been discontinued because enterohepatic recirculation in preterm and full-term neonates may result in higher plasma concentrations of opioids for longer periods as compared with older children.
      (3) Because of immature descending pain pathways, preterm infants may require significantly higher opioid concentrations to achieve adequate analgesia as compared with older children (Evans, 2001).
      (4) Efficacy of opioid therapy should be assessed using a valid and reliable neonatal pain scale. Sedation level should also be assessed regularly, monitoring for the attainment of desired sedation level or inadvertent oversedation.
      (5) Opioid-induced cardiorespiratory side effects in neonates are uncommon.
   c. Fentanyl is used as follows (Young and Mangum, 2008):
      (1) Bolus dose: 1 to 4 mcg/kg/dose every 2 to 4 hours by slow IV push.
      (2) Continuous infusion: 1 to 5 mcg/kg/hour.
      (3) Onset is almost immediately after IV administration.
      (4) Adverse effects include respiratory depression, chest wall rigidity, tolerance and dependence, and urinary retention.
   d. Morphine is used as follows (Young and Mangum, 2008):
      (1) Bolus dose: 0.05 to 0.2 mg/kg/dose by IV slow push, intramuscularly, or subcutaneous route. Repeat as required, usually every 4 hours.
      (2) Continuous infusion: give loading dose of 0.1 to 0.15 mg/kg over 1 hour followed by a continuous infusion of 0.01 to 0.02 mg/kg/hour.
      (3) Onset of action: beginning a few minutes after IV administration, with peak analgesia occurring at 20 minutes.
      (4) Adverse effects: respiratory depression, hypotension, bradycardia, transient hypertonia, ileus, delayed gastric emptying, urinary retention, tolerance and dependence, and seizures.
      (5) The potential for increased adverse neurologic outcomes exists in ventilated infants with hypotension receiving morphine. Therefore, all infants receiving morphine should be closely monitored for hypotension (Anand et al., 2004; Aranda et al., 2005; Hall et al., 2005).
   e. Managing opioid tolerance and dependence.
      (1) Tolerance is decreasing pain relief with the same dosage over time and is exhibited by increased wakefulness and increased sympathetic responses such as high-pitched crying and tremors when handled or disturbed. Tolerance to opioids is usually managed by increasing the dose, although adjunctive analgesics or sedatives may also be clinically beneficial.
      (2) Neonates who require opioid therapy for more than several days should be weaned slowly to prevent withdrawal symptoms such as signs of neurologic excitability, gastrointestinal dysfunction, autonomic signs, poor weight gain, and skin excoria-

tion due to excessive rubbing. The prevalence of opioid withdrawal is greater in infants who have received fentanyl as opposed to morphine. Similarly, infants who receive higher total doses or longer duration of infusion are significantly more likely to experience withdrawal (Dominguez et al., 2003). Data are insufficient to determine the optimal weaning rate of opioids to prevent withdrawal symptoms in neonates on opioid therapy. Ducharme and colleagues (2005) reported that adverse withdrawal symptoms in children who received continuous infusions of opioids and/or benzodiazepines could be prevented when the daily rate of weaning did not exceed 20% for children who received opioids/benzodiazepines for 1 to 3 days, 13% to 20% for 4 to 7 days, 8% to 13% for 8 to 14 days, 8% for 15 to 21 days, and 2% to 4% for more than 21 days. An opioid weaning scale such as the Finnegan Scoring System should be used to manage opioid withdrawal in neonates exposed to prolonged opioid therapy (Finnegan et al., 1975).

3. Nonopioid analgesics (Young and Mangum, 2008).
   a. Acetaminophen is a nonsteroidal antiinflammatory drug commonly used for short-term use with mild to moderate pain in neonates.
      (1) Oral dose: 20 to 25 mg/kg loading dose followed by 12 to15 mg/kg/dose.
      (2) Rectal dose: 30 mg/kg loading dose followed by 12 to 18 mg/kg/dose.
      (3) Maintenance intervals are every 6 hours for term infants, every 8 hours for preterm infants greater or equal to 32 weeks, and every 12 hours for preterm infants younger than 32 weeks.
      (4) Adverse effects: liver toxicity, rash, fever, thrombocytopenia, leukopenia, and neutropenia.
4. EMLA cream (eutectic mixture of local anesthetics, lidocaine and prilocaine).
   a. Approved in children at birth with a gestational age of 37 weeks or greater.
   b. EMLA cream reduces pain during venipuncture, circumcisions, arterial puncture, and percutaneous venous catheter placement but is not effective for management of pain associated with the heel-stick procedure.
   c. Local/topical dose: 1 to 2 g under occlusive dressing 60 to 90 minutes before procedure (Young and Mangum, 2008).
   d. Adverse effects: methemoglobinemia, redness, and blanching.
5. Liposomal lidocaine cream (LMX 4%; Ferndale Laboratories, Michigan)
   a. Relatively new topical anesthetic for use in newborns.
   b. LMX may be a better choice than EMLA because of its faster onset of action and no risk of methemoglobinemia (Lehr et al., 2005)
   c. Further studies in neonates are needed to establish the safety and efficacy of LMX for management of procedural pain in neonates.
6. Sedatives suppress the behavioral expression of pain and have no analgesic effects. Sedatives should only be used when pain has been ruled out. When administered with opioids, sedatives may allow more optimal weaning of opioids in critically ill, ventilator-dependent neonates who have developed tolerance from prolonged opioid therapy. The two most commonly used sedatives in neonates include midazolam and chloral hydrate. However, no research has been done to determine the safety or efficacy of combining sedatives and analgesics for the treatment of pain in infants.
7. Neuromuscular blocking agents. Chemical paralysis is often used for severely ill neonates. Because the use of paralytic agents masks the behavior signs of agitation and pain, sedatives or analgesics should be used in conjunction with paralytics.

PAIN MANAGEMENT AT END OF LIFE

A. Although dying adults commonly receive opioids to relieve suffering at end of life, opioids are not routinely administered to critically ill or dying infants when life support is being withdrawn or withheld (Partridge and Wall, 1997).
B. As it is often difficult to accurately assess pain in neonates at end of life, caregivers should consider risk factors for pain and use physiologic measures to guide pain management decisions.

C. Opioid doses well beyond those described for standard analgesia are often required for infants who are in severe pain or who have developed tolerance after the prolonged use of opioids (Partridge and Wall, 1997). Therefore, continuous infusions of opioids should be titrated to desired clinical response (analgesia).

D. Physiologic comfort measures may palliate pain and distress in infants at end of life and include reduction of noxious stimuli, organization of caregiving, and positioning and containment strategies.

PARENTS' ROLE IN PAIN ASSESSMENT AND MANAGEMENT

A. Parents have many concerns and fears about their infant's pain and about the medications used in the treatment of pain (Gale et al., 2004; Franck et al., 2005). Parents may fear the effects of pain on their child's development. They may also fear that their infant may become "addicted" to the analgesics (Franck et al., 2004).

B. Parents and healthcare professionals must talk openly and honestly about acute and chronic pain associated with medical diseases, as well as about pain associated with operative, diagnostic, and therapeutic procedures.

C. Parents should receive accurate and unbiased information about the risks and benefits of (as well as alternatives to) analgesia and anesthesia, so that they can make informed treatment choices (Harrison, 1993).

D. Parents' cultural and religious beliefs about pain should be taken into consideration when determining a pain management plan.

E. Parents should have the right to seek another medical opinion or to refuse a burdensome course of therapy (Harrison, 1993).

F. Parents should be taught to observe how their infant expresses pain through physiologic and behavioral cues.

G. Parents should be educated on how they can assist caregivers in providing nonpharmacologic pain relief during minor painful procedures their infant experiences.

REFERENCES

Ahn, Y.: The relationship between behavioral states and pain responses to various NICU procedures in premature infants. *Journal of Tropical Pediatrics, 52*(3):201-205, 2006.

American Academy of Pediatrics/Canadian Paediatric Society: Prevention and management of pain in the neonate: An update. *Pediatrics, 118*(5):2231-2241, 2006.

American Academy of Pediatrics/Canadian Paediatric Society: Prevention and management of pain and stress in the neonate. *Pediatrics, 105*(2):454-461, 2000.

American Academy of Pediatrics Task Force on Circumcision: Circumcision policy statement. *Pediatrics, 103*:686-693, 1999.

Anand, K.J., Hall, R.W., Desai, N., et al.: Effects of morphine analgesia in ventilated preterm neonates: Primary outcomes form the NEOPAIN randomized trial. *Lancet, 363*(9422):1673-1682, 2004.

Anand, K.J. and Craig, K.D.: New perspectives on the definition of pain [editorial]. *Pain, 67*(1):3-6, 1996.

Anand, K.J. and International Evidence-Based Group for Neonatal Pain: Consensus statement for the prevention and management of pain in the newborn. *Archives of Pediatrics and Adolescent Medicine, 155*(2):173-180, 2001.

Aranda, J.V., Carlo, W., Hummel, P., et al.: Analgesia and sedation during mechanical ventilation in neonates. *Clinical Therapeutics, 27*(6):877-899, 2005.

Belda, S., Pallas, C.R., De la Cruz, J., and Tejada, P.: Screening for retinopathy: Is it painful? *Biology of the Neonate, 86*(3):195-200, 2004.

Carbajal, R., Rousset, A., Danan, C., et al.: Epidemiology and treatment of painful procedures in neonates in intensive care units. *Journal of the American Medical Association, 300*(1):60-70, 2008.

Craig, K.D., Whitfield, M.F., Grunau, R., et al.: Pain in the preterm neonate: Behavioral and physiological indices. *Pain, 52*(3):287-299, 1993.

Dominguez, K.D., Lomako, D.M., Katz, R.W., and Kelly, H.W.: Opioid withdrawal in critically ill neonates. *Annals of Pharmacotherapy, 37*(4):473-477, 2003.

Ducharme, C., Carnevale, F.A., Clermont, M.S., and Shea, S.: A prospective study of adverse reactions to the weaning of opioids and benzodiazepines among critically ill children. *Intensive and Critical Care Nursing, 21*(3):179-186, 2005.

Duhn, L. and Medves, J.: A systematic integrative review of infant pain assessment tools. *Advances in Neonatal Care, 4*(3):126-140, 2004.

El Sayed, M.F., Taddio, A., Faliah, S., et al.: Safety profile of morphine following surgery in neonates. *Journal of Perinatology, 27*(7):444-447, 2007.

Evans, J.C.: Physiology of acute pain in preterm infants. *Newborn and Infant Nursing Reviews, 1*(2):75-84, 2001.

Finnegan, L., Connaughton, J., and Kron, R.: A scoring system for evaluation and treatment of the neonatal abstinence syndrome: A new clinical and research tool. In P. Marselli, S. Garanttini, and F. Sereni (Eds.): *Basic and therapeutic aspects of perinatal pharmacology.* New York, 1975, Raven, pp. 139-152.

Fitzgerald, M. and Anand, K.J.S.: Developmental neuroanatomy and neurophysiology of pain. In N. Schechter and D.B. Berde (Eds.): *Pain in infants, children and adolescents.* Baltimore, 1993, Wilkins, pp. 11-32.

Franck, L.S.: Pain in the nonverbal patient: Advocating for the critically ill neonate. *Pediatric Nursing,* 15(1):65-68, 90, 1989.

Franck, L.S., Allen, A., Cox, S., and Winter, I.: Parent's views about infant pain in neonatal intensive care. *Clinical Journal of Pain,* 21(2):133-139, 2005.

Franck, L.S., Cox, S., Allen, A., and Winter, I.: Parental concern and distress about infant pain. *Archives of Disease in Childhood Fetal and Neonatal Edition,* 89(1): F71-F75, 2004.

Franck, L.S. and Lawhon, G.: Environmental and behavioral strategies to prevent and manage neonatal pain. *Seminars in Perinatology,* 22(5):434-443, 1998.

Gale, G., Franck, L.S., Kools, S., and Lynch, M.: Parents' perceptions of their infant's pain experience in the NICU. *International Journal of Nursing Studies,* 41(1):51-58, 2004.

Hall, R.W., Kronsberg, S.S., Barton, B.A., et al.: Morphine, hypotension, and adverse outcomes among preterm neonates: Who's to blame? Secondary results from the NEOPAIN trial. *Pediatrics,* 115(5):1351-1359, 2005.

Harrison, H.: The principles for family-centered neonatal care. *Pediatrics,* 92:643-650, 1993.

Holsti, L., Grunau, R.E., Oberlander, T.F., and Whitfield, M. F.: Prior pain induces heightened motor responses during clustered care in preterm infants in the NICU. *Early Human Development,* 81(3):293-302, 2005.

Howard, R., Carter, B., Curry, J., et al.: Medical procedures. *Paediatric Anaesthesia,* 18(Supplement 1):19-35, 2008.

Hummel, P., Puchalski, M., Creech, S.D., and Weiss, M. G.: Clinical reliability and validity of the N-PASS: Neonatal pain, agitation, and sedation scale with prolonged pain. *Journal of Perinatology,* 28(1):55-60 2008.

Hummel, P. and van Dijk, M.: Pain assessment: Current status and challenges. *Seminars in Fetal & Neonatal Medicine,* 11:237-245, 2006.

International Association for the Study of Pain Subcommittee on Taxonomy: Pain terms: A list with definitions and notes on usage. *Pain,* 6(3):249-252, 1979.

Johnston, C.C. and Stevens, B.J.: Experience in a neonatal intensive care unit affects pain response *Pediatrics,* 98(5):925-930, 1996.

Krechel, S. and Bildner, J.: CRIES: A new neonatal postoperative pain measurement score: Initial testing of validity and reliability. *Paediatric Anaesthesia,* 5(1):53-61, 1995.

Lawrence, J., Alcock, D., McGrath, P., et al.: The development of a tool to assess neonatal pain. *Neonatal Network,* 12(6):59-66, 1993.

Lehr, V.T., Cepeda, E., Frattarelli, D.A., Thomas, R., et al.: Lidocaine 4% cream compared with lidocaine 2.5% and prilocaine 2.5% or dorsal penile block for circumcision. *American Journal of Perinatology,* 22(5): 231-237, 2005.

McNair, C., Ballantyne, M., Dionne, K., et al.: Postoperative pain assessment in the neonatal intensive care unit. *Archives of Disease in Childhood Fetal and Neonatal Edition,* 89(6):F537-F541, 2004.

Melzack, R.: Gate control theory: On the evolution of pain concepts. *Pain Forum,* 5:128-138, 1996.

Partridge, J.C. and Wall, S.N.: Analgesia for dying infants whose life support is withdrawn or withheld. *Pediatrics,* 99(1):76-79, 1997.

Plotsky, P., Bradley, C., and Anand, K.: Behavioral and neuroendocrine consequences of neonatal stress. In K.J.S. Anand, B.J. Stevens, and P.J. McGrath (Eds.): *Pain in neonates* (2nd revised and enlarged edition). Amsterdam, 2000, Elsevier Science, pp. 77-101.

Ranger, M., Johnston, C.C., and Anand, K.J.S.: Current controversies regarding pain assessment in neonates. *Seminars in Perinatology,* 31:283-288, 2007.

Reynolds, M., Alvares, D., Middleton, J., and Fitzgerald, M.: Neonatally wounded skin induces NGF-independent sensory neurite outgrowth in vitro. *Developmental Brain Research,* 102:275-283, 1997.

Rouss, K., Gerber A., Albisetti, M., et al.: Long-term subcutaneous morphine administration after surgery in newborns. *Journal of Perinatal Medicine,* 35(1):79-81, 2007.

Ruda, M., Ling, Q., Hohmann, A., et al.: Altered nociceptive neuronal circuits after neonatal peripheral inflammation. *Science,* 289:628-630, 2000.

Simons, S.H., van Dijk, M., Anand, K.S., et al.: Do we still hurt newborn babies? A prospective study of procedural pain and analgesia in neonates. *Archives of Pediatric Adolescent Medicine,* 157:1058-1064, 2003.

Stevens, B., Johnston, C., Franck, L., et al.: The efficacy of developmentally sensitive interventions and sucrose for relieving procedural pain in very low birth weight neonates. *Nursing Research,* 48(1):35-43, 1999.

Stevens, B., Johnston, C., Petryshen, P., and Taddio, A.: Premature infant pain profile: Development and initial validation. *Clinical Journal of Pain,* 12(1):13-22, 1996.

Suraseranivongse, S., Kaosaard, R., Intaking, P., et al.: A comparison of postoperative pain scales in neonates. *British Journal of Anaesthesia,* 97(4):540-544, 2006.

Taddio, A., Goldbach, M., Ipp, M., et al.: Effect of neonatal circumcision on pain responses during vaccination in boys. *Lancet,* 345(1):291-292, 1995.

Walden, M. and Gibbins, S.: *Pain assessment and management: Guideline for practice* (2nd ed.). Glenview, IL, 2008, National Association of Neonatal Nurses.

Young, T.E. and Mangum, B.: *Neofax: A manual of drugs used in neonatal care* (21st ed.). Montvale, NJ, 2008, Thomson Healthcare.

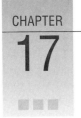

17 Families in Crisis

CAROLE KENNER*

OBJECTIVES

1. Define the concept of crisis.
2. Recognize the psychologic tasks that the mother and family must accomplish to establish a healthy parent-child relationship after the crisis of the birth of a premature or sick infant.
3. Describe assessment strategies for identifying a family in crisis.
4. Identify the risks of teenage parenting on the adolescent and the infant.
5. Identify nursing interventions to support a family coping with stressful events surrounding the birth of their infant.
6. Evaluate maternal behaviors found to be predictive of specific parenting outcomes.
7. Recognize emotional characteristics related to grief.
8. Identify strategies for working with families experiencing perinatal or neonatal end-of-life (EOL) issues.
9. Identify specific behaviors to be assessed in determining parental attachment to their infant.
10. Describe the nursing strategies to promote parental attachment.
11. Identify cultural influences that impact on parenting a sick or dying neonate.

With the current technologic and genomic advances, even the most acutely ill or most premature infant has a good chance of going home. Neonates born as prematurely as 23 weeks of gestation are surviving. For parents, although these advances are increasing the odds of having a live neonate, they also have brought on tremendous stress (Howland, 2007). The result may be a family that views the infant as medically fragile and vulnerable. This view changes the relationship between the family and child, especially the mother (Kenner and Ellerbee, 2007).

When an infant requires health care at birth because of prematurity, illness, or congenital malformations or when an infant dies, the effects of these unexpected events on the parents can be overwhelming. The families of these infants may experience multiple crisis events during the infant's hospitalization (Kenner and Ellerbee, 2007). Assessment skills are critical for the neonatal nurse who is caring for an infant and family at this period of crisis. The parents usually display signs of anxiety, fear, and powerlessness. They also may exhibit physiologic signs of stress such as cardiovascular or cognitive problems (Howland, 2007). It is the nurse who is viewed as the advocate for the family and who has the most continual interactions with them. Nursing care is generally concerned with both the physiologic and psychosocial needs of the patient and the family. However, the focus of this chapter is the psychosocial aspects of supporting parents who must cope with stressful events surrounding the birth of their infant. The chapter highlights various types of families who may experience a crisis when their infant undergoes a neonatal intensive care unit (NICU) stay or a perinatal/neonatal death. Many of the strategies or interventions are the same for all groups of parents because they represent parenting needs. Cultural influences must also be considered.

CRISIS AND THE BIRTH OF THE SICK OR PREMATURE INFANT

Pregnancy and transition to parenthood have been recognized as periods of stress and change during which mothers and fathers are attempting to master the normal developmental process of parenthood. These major life changes have been referred to as developmental or maturational stressors. In contrast, the birth of a premature or sick infant and the death of an infant are unex-

*The author wishes to thank Marina Boykova, MSc, RN, Children's Hospital #1, Saint Petersburg, Russia, for her assistance in revising this manuscript.

pected stressful life events for which a person or family is often psychologically unprepared. Such events are referred to as situational or accidental stressors. When such maturational and situational stressors occur simultaneously, the resulting pressure can overwhelm a person's usual coping resources and support systems. Rolland (1994) suggests there is a family life cycle that accompanies chronic illnesses. The five elements of psychosocial demands of this framework are onset, course, outcome, incapacitation, and uncertainty (Rolland, 1994; Street and Soldan, 1998). As health care professionals we need to recognize these stages of demands that families face. If they do not successfully work through these demands, ineffective coping may result. Ineffective coping causes personal and family psychologic disequilibrium or crisis, which continues until new ways of coping can be developed and maintained. Coping, however, is intimately tied to cultural values and beliefs and, in some instances, spirituality (Berg and Upchurch, 2007), so these must be taken into account.

A. **Several psychologic tasks** have been identified that the mother and family must accomplish to cope with the crisis of a premature birth or the birth of a sick infant and to establish a basis for a healthy parent-child relationship. These must take into consideration the psychological health of the mother and its impact on parent-infant interactions (McGrath, 2007).

   1. Preparation for the possible loss of the infant. Parents must consider the possibility of disability or death of the infant while simultaneously hoping for the infant's survival.

   2. Acknowledgment of failure to deliver a term infant. The mother struggles with feelings of guilt and failure and searches for causes of the infant's condition. Family members may actually be, or be perceived as, blaming the mother for the premature infant. Family members may also feel guilty as if they too have contributed to the infant's condition. These feelings must be acknowledged.

   3. Adaptation to the intensive care environment. Parents must be helped to develop secure relationships in an unfamiliar and stress-provoking setting.

   4. Resumption of interaction with the infant once the threat of loss has passed. Parents must participate in the infant's care and gain confidence in their abilities. Parental interaction may be adversely affected because of the effects of posttraumatic stress and fear that something might still happen to the infant. Taking part in their infant's care can ease the crisis, decrease guilt, and increase psychologic health (McGrath, 2007).

   5. Preparation for taking the infant home. Parents must understand the special needs and characteristics of the premature or sick infant and the necessary precautions that must be taken and yet maintain a positive relationship with the infant, realizing that these needs are only temporary. Failure to resolve these tasks can contribute to such maladaptive parenting as being overprotective, resulting in the "vulnerable child syndrome" and in other negative child outcomes such as failure to thrive, emotional deprivation, and battering. Mothers and health care professionals may view the child as medically fragile when this may or may not be the case. The psychologic impact of having a sick infant can continue even after a successful discharge, resulting in maternal psychologic distress (Kenner and Ellerbee, 2007). Whereas most of the current research focuses on the maternal role and the mother's level of distress, fathers must be considered too. The father's perception of a crisis is just as important as the mother's, and interventions to ease their distress must be part of the preparation for taking an infant home (Pohlman, 2004).

B. **Definition of *crisis:*** a temporary disequilibrium that occurs when people face an important problem or transitional phase so stressful that they are unable to cope by using their customary problem-solving resources (Howland, 2007). It usually lasts from 4 to 6 weeks. This period is the optimal time for effective interventions with the family.

C. **Discussion.** During the early stages of a crisis, parents are more receptive to overtures of help from other family members, friends, and the health care team. Nurses are in a key position because they work so directly with the parents to anticipate a family crisis and to promote positive coping and effective use of social supports (Howland, 2007). A family in crisis cannot effectively interact with their newly born infant because all their energies are going toward the crisis. When interventions are put into place to promote effective coping and positive social support, the crisis will resolve and psychologic equilibrium, a necessary step toward the establishment of a healthy parent-child relationship, will be restored. Factors that influence a family's return to equilibrium include the following:

1. Understanding of the infant's problem and the need for NICU care and understanding of their parental role.
2. Resolving or at least lessening of the family's grief reaction to the need for NICU care.
3. Viewing parents as partners in care, having a voice, and not as visitors.
4. Using positive coping and social supports (Kenner and Ellerbee, 2007).

SPECIFIC POPULATION OF PARENTS: ADOLESCENTS

Parents who are adolescent have some unique needs. They undergo the crises of parenthood and of having an infant in the NICU. In addition, these parents are dealing with the normal developmental tasks of adolescence. Sometimes these tasks seem to be in conflict with their needs as new parents. The nurse must be aware of these conflicts and realize their unique blending needs of taking on a new role and being at their developmental stage.

Adolescence is a turning point, or change period. It moves a child from childhood toward the maturation of the adult. Many physiologic changes are occurring, first at puberty and then in the move toward adulthood. Physical appearance changes, and the adolescent is capable of childbearing. Maturation of the reproductive system now occurs much earlier than in the past. In the United States, girls are reaching menarche as young as 8 years of age. Adolescence is the time when childbearing becomes a potential reality for most individuals.

Development of the personality is tied to role attainment, much as for parents and the parenting role. Adolescents strive to have an identity unique from those of other family members. They are developing their self-concept and self-esteem. The peer group becomes important for validation of attitudes, values, and beliefs. But adults can model this peer validation to enhance positive developmental outcomes for adolescent parents (Dishion et al., 2002). Adolescence is a time of constant change and usually turmoil—a period of maturational crisis.

A. **Some developmental tasks of this period are**
   1. Independence from adults,
   2. Preparation for financial security,
   3. Gender identification, and
   4. A stable, realistic, positive sense of self.
B. **In addition, adolescence**
   1. Is characterized by high anxiety;
   2. Can be anticipated and therefore preparation can be made;
   3. Requires normal social support for a successful transition;
   4. Is relatively easy to resolve because the individual's values usually do not conflict with societal expectations for the outcome, which is adult behavior; and
   5. Is a period of vulnerability to a crisis occurrence if a traumatic event is added to the transitional state.

While adolescents have unique needs, they also are unique individuals. As health professionals we often make assumptions of what they need or what type of parents they will be. The reality is they need to be assessed for their knowledge, level of crisis, and supports the same as any other individual or family. Perception is all there is—right or wrong—and we cannot or should not perceive that all adolescents will be bad parents, or immature in their actions, or be more concerned with peers than with their child. We must evaluate their needs certainly within the context of their developmental stage but also with consideration of their own personal, individualized needs.

THE FAMILY IN CRISIS

Assessment

A. **Determine parents' understanding of the situation** (i.e., realistic vs. distorted). The parents' ability to resolve the crisis depends on their realistic perception of their situation: they need to be fully informed about their infant's condition and expected progress. An inability to understand the crisis may be related to low socioeconomic status, educational level, or cultural values and beliefs. Parents of a lower socioeconomic status or educational level may not fully understand what to expect of their infant or their role because they may lack good role models for themselves or the financial means to provide adequate, safe care for themselves or their infant. Older mothers may have difficulty in coping as they are used to being in control of their situations. They may actually blame the health professionals for the adverse outcomes of their pregnancy and delivery. Cultural values and beliefs also may play a role because different cultures view the infant in relationship to parents in different ways and their view of health and death may be different from the typical U.S. views. In some countries, such as in India or China, only male offspring are valued, and girl babies are dismissed as nonessential. Whereas we often crave control over the environment in Western culture, other cultures may view this as fate. Native Americans usually accept what is; blacks are more oriented to specific situations than time; Latinos value the inclusion of the extended family and view death as having rituals associated with it; touching an infant's head is seen as threatening by some Southeast Asians, Buddhists, and native Hawaiians; and Middle Eastern children make few independent decisions (consideration when working with adolescent parents if their extended family is not present). When crucial conversations are necessary, the family's cultural values must be considered (Cone, 2007).

B. **Determine parents' grief response.** The extent to which they are experiencing a grief reaction must be determined. This grief may be in the form of anticipatory grief because they fear the infant might die, even though the physical condition does not appear to warrant this fear. Consider this within the cultural context of the family, because it may not be acceptable to express grief or worries to outsiders. If the child is dying, then consider EOL issues such as advance directives from the parents' perspectives and what they want or need from us as health professionals. Consider too that dressing the infant in a diaper or loose clothing will allow the parents to have at least one image of their child as a baby and not a dying infant.

C. **Determine parents' adaptation to and coping** with the stressful event.
   1. Are the parents maintaining responsibilities related to activities of daily living (e.g., eating, personal grooming)?
   2. To what degree has the family's normal lifestyle been affected by the crisis? (Are they able to return to work? Keep house? Care for other children in the household?)
   3. Are the parents exhibiting positive coping skills within the context of their cultural values and beliefs?
   4. To what extent has the financial status of the family been affected?

D. **Determine what support systems exist** for the parents and whether they are being used. It is also important to determine whether these supports are positive. The parents may have several people in their support network, but if these people are critical of how the parents are conducting themselves, then they may not be viewed as positive supports.
   1. Who are the significant others in the lives of the parents? Consider biologic kinship (family) and/or emotional kinship (friends).
   2. What professional supports are available?
   3. Is a parent support group available?

E. **Understanding the origins of a crisis** and their links with the normal "ups and downs" of life is crucial to successful assessment and intervention. Events that stimulate the occurrence of a crisis, such as those of the teenage parent in the NICU, can originate from:
   1. Being in a transitional state, such as
      a. Adolescence to adulthood, and
      b. Childhood to parenthood.
   2. Being a part of a social-cultural structure and
      a. Violating customs or cultural norms embedded in that structure, such as a teenager's becoming pregnant and having a newborn, or
      b. Behaving outside the accepted teenage social norms, as the role of parent would demand (although these examples are culture-specific): for example, being tied down to taking care of a newborn or having to arrange for child care at a time when peers are freely going to sports, games, and dances and having fun.
      c. Being exposed to hazardous or disturbing situations:
         (1) Birth of a first child. This is a disturbing situation because no one knows exactly what to expect of parenthood—a role never before experienced.

(2) Lack of experience with parenthood.

(3) Bearing of a sick newborn infant.

Problems Associated with Adolescent Pregnancy

When teens become pregnant, they often experience the following problems:

A. **Loss of peer group.** Adolescents' peers often disappear, leaving them without support and feeling socially isolated. Their self-concept changes as they approach parenthood because before the pregnancy the peer group helped shape their self-perception.

B. **Disruption of family ties.** The pregnant adolescent and her boyfriend often bring on direct conflict with their parents. The rationale for this conflict is that the parents of the adolescents often believe that adolescence is an inappropriate time to start a family and that the adolescents need to live by the parental house rules. At the same time, the adolescent parents may be trying to take on adult responsibilities while feeling that they are being treated as children. This conflict removes a possible positive social support. It also disrupts the effort to assume a parental role if the adolescents' parents try to make decisions regarding the coming infant.

C. **Maternal health problems.** The pregnant female adolescent often has engaged in risky behaviors besides being sexually active. She may smoke, drink, or use drugs. She is at risk of having human immunodeficiency virus (HIV) infection and other sexually transmitted infections (STIs). This risk is not unique to adolescents but is possible because of the feelings of invincibility that accompany this age. The pregnant adolescent may be emotionally immature and may have to interrupt her education to bear the child. She may be forced into a marriage she does not want or is not ready for at this time. She may lack knowledge about normal fetal and infant growth and development. She may have very unrealistic expectations of an infant and of herself as a parent. She may have sought pregnancy as a way to have someone need her. She may not seek prenatal care or may try to hide the pregnancy by limiting weight gain. These actions may put her health and her infant's health at risk. She also often lacks parenting skills.

D. **Paternal problems.** The adolescent father may have engaged in risky sexual behaviors. He may have been smoking or used alcohol or drugs. He also may be at risk of having HIV infection or other STIs. If he is infected, the pregnant adolescent and the fetus are also at risk because these infections can be passed on to the maternal-fetal unit. The male adolescent may be generally stable psychologically, but he may not be thinking about future consequences of his sexual behavior, such as his inability to fulfill his parenting role. For example, because of his risky behaviors, he may have contracted HIV, which will take him away from the pregnant adolescent and his future child. If his family, his significant other, or her family views his behaviors as irresponsible, he may be isolated from an active role in future parenting. He may feel excluded from decisions regarding the continuation of the pregnancy or the placement of the child after birth. He may interrupt his own education to provide financial support to his new "family." He may be forced into a marriage he neither wants nor is ready for at present.

E. **Risks to the infant.** The infant is at risk of having a faulty, or negative, parent-infant interaction, generally because of the parents' lack of understanding of the normal growth and development process. The parents also often have unrealistic expectations of the child and their role as parents and may lack parenting skills. The infant may be small for gestational age or premature and may require an expensive hospitalization that the parents are not ready financially or cognitively to accept. The infant may be less responsive or organized in cues for care by the parents. He or she may be more at risk of having slowed or delayed growth because of the parents' lack of understanding of normal infant care and feeding practices. The infant may not receive the type and amount of stimulation necessary for positive cognitive or behavioral development. An infant who is premature tends to be more irritable, to feed poorly, to have poor self-regulatory behaviors, and to be difficult to console. This seeming lack of responsiveness to parenting efforts often reinforces the adolescent parents' poor self-esteem and poor self-concept, which often accompany adolescent pregnancy. The infant may also be at risk of experiencing abuse or neglect.

1. Prematurity, birth between 23 and 27 weeks of gestation, is more common among infants of adolescent mothers. The risk factors for delivering early are (Bowers, 2007):
   a. Low pregnancy weight.
   b. Lower socioeconomic status.
   c. Marital status: single.
   d. Tobacco use (smoking).
   e. Narcotic or other substance use.
   f. Anemia (hemoglobin concentration <11 g/dl).
   g. First child.
   h. Poor prenatal care.
2. Low birth weight (<2500 g) is also a risk factor for an adolescent's offspring. The risk can be as much as 6 times greater for 14-year-old and younger mothers.

Intervention

A. **Be present with the physician or nurse practitioner at the initial meeting with the parents.**
B. **Talk with the mother and father together whenever possible.** Consider cultural values of each family. In some cultures the father must receive the information first (Kenner and Ellerbee, 2007).
C. **Determine and address the parents' perceptions of the infant's condition** (Kenner and Ellerbee, 2007).
D. **Be consistent with information given to parents by the staff.** If in an academic health care setting where the physicians or nurse practitioners rotate frequently, be sure that any changes in care that are reflective only of these staff changes are explained within that context. If parents do not understand the basis of these changes or are not told when their infant's condition really changes, then mistrust begins. Then the chance that the crisis will escalate is highly probable (Kenner and Ellerbee, 2007).
E. **Do not overload parents with detailed information about their infant during their initial visits to the NICU;** provide basic facts and allow the parents some time to process the information. Repeat information that is given either verbally or written so the parents understand and really hear what is said. Give them information on the disease process their infant is experiencing so they know what to expect.
F. **Assess the grief response.** Males and females express their grief in different ways. However, most, if not all, parents experience some form of grief by just having an infant who requires specialized care (Kenner and Ellerbee, 2007). This reaction must be assessed throughout the hospital stay. Sometimes this response is directly tied to their understanding of the infant's condition. Other times it is related to cultural beliefs and values.
G. **Acknowledge any feeling of guilt that might be expressed** about the unexpected birth outcome. Let the parents know that these feelings are normal (Siegel et al., 2006).
H. **Facilitate adaptation of the parents' new role** by being a very good listener, by observing body language, and by helping them verbalize their feelings (Siegel et al., 2006).
I. **Periodically assess the parents' understanding** of their infant's condition and their interpretation of the information that has been given to them. Information must be reinforced throughout the hospital stay. Whenever anyone is anxious, little information is actually heard or retained.
J. **Write notes from the infant to the parents** concerning current status (e.g., equipment, feedings, oxygen concentration) and take pictures of the infant periodically. A notebook containing the notes and pictures can be kept at the infant's bedside for the parents. These can be memory books or scrapbooks that become especially important if the child dies. This intervention should be individualized because not all parents want this form of "communication." However, for some parents it is one strategy that promotes positive attachment.
K. **Encourage the parents to keep a journal** concerning their experience of delivering a premature or sick infant. This action can assist families to work through their feelings as well as having memories to review what happened and reflect on issues that have been or have not been resolved (Howland, 2007).

L. **Give parents the freedom to express negative ideas without being judged.** Fear and frustration over the inability to control their infant's circumstances are often the basis for parental anger displaced to staff. Remember that control is not acceptable in all cultures, so it is important to ask what is making them uncomfortable. Also a positive way to approach this and possibly decrease their anger is to ask them what would help them to feel more comfortable.

M. **Encourage parents to participate in the care as they desire.** Parents need to understand and develop their roles as parents. If professionals provide all the care, a clear message is conveyed to the parents that they are not capable of helping their infant. They must understand all the things they have to contribute to the team approach to care. Parents must be a part of the health care team and as such should have a say in health care decisions. Dr. Bernadette Melynk's COPE Program—Creating Opportunities for Parent Empowerment—has decreased stress, shortened length of stay, and increased coping by involving parents in their infant's care (National Institute of Nursing Research, 2006).

N. **Do not refer to parents as visitors.** Parents are not visitors. They are parents and are partners in the care of the infant. They are an integral part of the infant's care and should be a focus of nursing care. Parents as partners is a concept that is growing as part of the patient safety movement from the Institute of Medicine (IOM) toward patient-focused care. Many hospitals are creating Family Advisory Councils (FACs) that are either unit or hospital based (Sullivan and Altimier, 2007). These councils are composed of parents of former patients and interdisciplines, which may include clergy and administration. The FACs guide the administration by giving input into policies that support family voices (Halm et al., 2006).

O. **Promote a developmentally supportive environment for the family.** Use of individualized family-centered care is important if the family is to be helped through this crisis (Kenner and McGrath, 2004). For example, kangaroo care (skin-to-skin contact, done by placing the naked infant next to the parent's naked chest, with a blanket or gown draped over the parent and infant), dimmed lights or cycled lights, private areas for parent interaction with the infant, and swaddling or cuddling of the infant promote positive development of the infant and family (McGrath, 2007).

P. **Determine parents' network of social support.** The social support network may include family, friends, clergy, and health professionals. Also determine whether the level of support is adequate from the parents' and the health professionals' standpoint. When possible, use new technologies such as mypatientline (www.mypatientline.com; by Jaduka, Dallas, Texas), which allows family a toll-free service with voice mail and connects the family to friends and other family members even at a distance.

Q. **Encourage parents to share their concerns and fears with each other.** Often it is not until the infant is discharged that parents share their feelings with each other. This is another area where culture plays a role. In some Asian cultures, expressions of concern are acceptable within the family unit but not with others. Health professionals may be viewed as authority figures and not ones to whom fears should be confided. It is important too to find out what this illness and hospitalization mean to the family and to what degree they are viewed as stress (Howland, 2007).

R. **Assist parents in maintaining their relationship with one another.** Reinforce with them that they must take time for themselves as a couple. If the mother is alone, encourage her to maintain ties with other family members and her friends.

S. **Assist parents in maintaining their relationship with the infant's siblings** by helping them recognize the needs of the other children and identify how the needs can be met. Use resources from www.premiecreations.com such as coloring and activity books to help the siblings express their feelings.

T. **Assist the adolescent parents in defining their role with their own parents** by helping them learn how to talk with their parents.

U. **Encourage parents to attend a parent support group if desirable.** Involvement in a parent support group has been demonstrated to facilitate parental grieving, reduce fears, and increase feelings of parental competence. This intervention must be culture specific. In some cultures it is not acceptable to discuss family problems openly. It is also important to include the father's perspective. Some groups are for fathers only because this is a recognized growing need.

V. **Assist families of dying infants to tell you what they need.** EOL issues are never easy but are especially difficult in this population when celebration of a birth is the expectation. Asking the family what they need from us as health care professionals is important. Understanding what this death means to them is critical to plan individualized care. Finding out if they want siblings and extended family involved, if clergy or spiritual healers are important, as well as what for them constitutes a good death are all important aspects of helping families cope (Kavanaugh and Wheeler, 2007). Use of consistent information and the same message from all health care providers is important too. The use of a palliative care protocol is one method to ensure more consistency (Catlin and Carter, 2002). Consideration of cultural differences once again is important (McGrath, 2007).

Evaluation of Maternal Parenting Outcomes

A. **Predictors of good maternal parenting outcomes (Kenner and Ellerbee, 2007).**
   1. Anxiety level is moderate to high: she worries about the infant's chances of surviving, the possibility of abnormality, and her competence as a mother.
   2. Seeks information about the infant.
   3. Demonstrates warmth toward infant and in other relationships.
   4. Has a support system (i.e., father of the infant, her mother, friends).
   5. Has had a previous successful experience with a premature infant (i.e., previous child, a sibling, other relative), which enables her to feel more experienced and confident.
   6. Recognizes positive attributes of the child (i.e., smiling).
   7. Views self positively.
   8. For an adolescent, has a centralized locus of behavioral control.
   9. Exhibits effective caregiving.
  10. Makes positive eye contact with the infant.

B. **Predictors of poor maternal parenting outcomes (Kenner and Ellerbee, 2007).**
   1. Exhibits an inappropriately low anxiety level.
   2. Demonstrates passivity—does not actively seek out information related to infant's condition.
   3. Has limited verbal interaction.
   4. Visits infrequently and for short periods in the NICU. (Remember that sometimes infrequent visits are due to a lack of transportation and not true parenting problems.)
   5. Is unaware of the infant's needs.
   6. Has unrealistic expectations of the infant or the parenting role.
   7. Personalizes the infant's behavior as a failure of her ability to parent or that the infant is "bad."
   8. During pregnancy, expressed little desire to have a child.
   9. Is more likely to express disappointment about the sex of the infant.
  10. Has no support system.
  11. Is an adolescent with little or no social supports.
  12. Exhibits role confusion.

Grief and Loss

A. **Introduction.** Unfortunately, not all pregnancies result in a healthy term infant. When adverse neonatal events occur, often the parents are overwhelmed by grief. As the parents realize that their newborn is "less than perfect" and not the infant of their fantasies, acute grief reactions occur. One of the early tasks of parenting is to resolve the discrepancy between the idealized infant and the real infant. In the case of neonatal death, the parents also grieve for the lost opportunity to parent the child. To assist parents therapeutically in working through the feelings associated with loss, nurses working with high-risk infants must understand the grief process, recognize typical parental behaviors associated with grief, and provide appropriate nursing interventions. It also may be appropriate to help the parents actively plan the care of their yet to be born or dying infant through use of an advance directive (Catlin, 2005). Much like in the adult, the advance directive during either the prenatal period or the neonatal one allows the parents to say what they wish to be done and whether or not they want to allow a natural death (AND), a term much more acceptable than a do not resuscitate (DNR) order.

B. Definitions.
1. Grief: the response of sadness and sorrow to the loss of a valued object (Kenner and Sudia-Robinson, 2007).
2. Anticipatory grief: grieving that occurs before an actual loss. If the outcome for the infant is healthy, then anticipatory grieving can lead to difficulties in attachment and problems in the parent-infant relationship.
3. Chronic grief: unresolved or blocked grief; frequently seen in parents of a disabled child, who is a constant reminder of loss.

C. Assessment.
1. Grief responses to death, premature birth, or the birth of an infant with a malformation are similar. These responses do not necessarily occur in the same sequence for all people. They are mediated by cultural beliefs and values as well as the parents' developmental stage. In addition, the responses may overlap and recur. Posttraumatic stress disorder (PTSD) often results from just having an infant in an NICU but is exacerbated if the child actually dies. Stages of grief such as shock, denial, anger, and acceptance may or may not be followed. Grief is very individualized.
2. One of the goals of the staff working with parents is to encourage the development of attachment, or an affectional tie, between the parent and infant. However, because the birth of a premature or a physically, psychologically, or neurologically challenged infant creates a sense of loss, the parents must first resolve their grief before attachment can be fully achieved.

Interventions for Facilitating Grief
A. Listen: parents need to be given the opportunity to express their feelings.
B. Acknowledge the pain of their loss: gives the parents permission to talk about their loss and provides support for acknowledging and working through their grief.
C. Convey an attitude of acceptance, openness, and availability to the family: grieving people need permission to experience their feelings, regardless of how uncomfortable or unpleasant.
D. Help the parents understand the individuality of the grieving process. Mothers and fathers usually have "incongruent grieving": they do not grieve at the same pace. This incongruence frequently leads to marital discord because of misconceptions about feelings and an inability to communicate.

Interventions for Parents Experiencing a Perinatal Loss
A. Encourage the family to see, hold, and spend time with the infant before and after death (Catlin and Carter, 2002; Kenner and Sudia-Robinson, 2007).
1. Be sensitive to individual and cultural differences in rituals of saying goodbye.
2. Physically bring the family together and offer privacy. Some hospitals have a neonatal hospice program in which the family is involved with the infant's care (Catlin and Carter, 2002; Kavanaugh and Wheeler, 2007; Kenner and Sudia-Robinson, 2007).
B. Provide the parents with the following mementos if culturally acceptable: photograph of the infant, identification bracelet, footprints, completed crib card, blanket, wisp of hair, and birth certificate. Keep these mementos in a file in the nursery for future retrieval should parents choose not to take the items at the time of the infant's death. This intervention must be individualized according to the needs and desires of each family (Catlin and Carter, 2002; Kavanaugh and Wheeler, 2007; Kenner and Sudia-Robinson, 2007). This is a very culturally sensitive topic and must be explored with the family.
C. Provide information about support groups and/or grief counseling. Consideration for individual family wishes is important. Not all families want or would benefit from support groups. Family follow-up even if just a phone call from an NICU nurse or hospice nurse a few weeks after the loss is very helpful to many families.
D. Encourage the parents to name the infant.

E. **Provide a booklet about perinatal loss for the parents and siblings.** Pediatric hospice and palliative care programs have a number of resources for parents and the left-behind siblings. There are many books and videos that are age appropriate. A good resource is Children's Hospice International at www.chionline.org or 1101 King Street, Suite 360, Alexandria, VA 22314; phone 800-242-4453.

F. **Discuss options for autopsy, disposition of the body, and a memorial or funeral service.** It is important to ask what they need and what they would like. For some parents they wish to be an active participant in the plans. Other families want these arrangements to be done for them. Rituals surrounding death are culturally driven; for example, the taking of pictures after death is not acceptable to Native Americans, Eskimos, Amish, Russians, Hindus, and Muslims. It is the family's choice (Kavanaugh and Wheeler, 2007).

G. **Offer the option for the infant to be baptized.** This option is not acceptable in all cultures.

H. **Assist parents in understanding the importance of informing siblings about the death of the infant.** Suggest that they use simple statements based on the children's level of understanding. Many times the siblings take the death much better than adults expect. Allowing them to see the infant after death may make the infant real to them. Of course parental wishes are always to be the guiding principle for how the siblings are informed of the death and what part they play in the rituals following the death. Again, this is a culturally sensitive issue and beliefs must be explored with the family.

I. **Talk with parents about possible responses** from family and friends, who often minimize the infant's death in an attempt to offer comfort. Encourage them to delegate or give tasks to those that call them. If they need the laundry done or groceries bought, then these are simple tasks that can be delegated to others who truly want to help and do not know what to do. More information on EOL issues can be obtained through the joint project of American Association of Colleges of Nursing (AACN) and the City of Hope (COH) End-of-Life Nursing Education Consortium (ELNEC) found at www.aacn.nche.edu/ELNEC/index.htm. A pediatric-specific program is available.

Interventions for Parents With a Preterm or Physically, Developmentally, or Psychologically Challenged Infant. These interventions have been incorporated into the interventions listed in the previous section (The Family in Crisis) and in the next section (Family-Infant Bonding).

Family-Infant Bonding

Parents who have an infant who is born ill, prematurely, or physically or psychologically challenged are at risk of having parenting difficulties. These stressful events around the time of the infant's birth generate feelings of anxiety, disappointment, and grief in the parents. Moreover, early disruptions in the acquaintance and attachment process between parent and infant place these parents in a state of increased vulnerability for establishing a nurturing relationship with their infant. Opportunities for parents to learn to interpret their infant's unique needs and to develop reciprocal interaction through sensitivity to behavioral cues are also interrupted (Kenner and Ellerbee, 2007). The relationship between parent-infant attachment and later parenting behaviors has been well established. In addition, the parent-infant attachment is the basis for all the infant's subsequent attachments and is the relationship through which a sense of self is developed. Therefore an important component of nursing care of the high-risk infant is facilitation of parent-infant interaction and attachment.

A. **Definitions.**

1. *Bonding:* a gradual, reciprocal process that begins with acquaintance. It is a unique and specific relationship between two people and endures across time. Bonding occurs on a different timetable for mothers than for fathers. Although mothers experience a sharp increase in bonding around the fifth month of pregnancy and have intensifying feelings throughout the pregnancy, the father's feelings usually tend to develop more slowly than the mother's and become congruent after birth, when infant caretaking begins (McGrath, 2007).

   2. *Attachment:* the quality of the bond, or affectional tie, between parents and their infant, which begins early in the prenatal period, appears to increase when fetal movement is felt and is intensified with interaction between the parent and the infant after birth.
B. Discussion. The development of a warm, nurturing, and reciprocal relationship between infant and parent is essential for a healthy psychologic outcome to the crisis of the birth of a premature, sick, or malformed infant (Kenner and Ellerbee, 2007). "The parent 'at risk' cannot resolve a crisis surrounding birth of their infant and simultaneously establish warm attachment bonds while retaining his or her self-esteem without the support of others in the social system" (Mercer, 1977, p. 5). Neonatal nurses can provide this support by assessing the parents' responses to their infant and facilitating their acquaintance and attachment process with the infant.
C. Assessment.
   1. Note pattern of parental visiting to the NICU, duration of visits, and frequency of phone calls. This pattern, if abnormal, is predictive of maternal parenting difficulties. If parents are not visiting frequently, be careful to determine the reasons (i.e., cultural practices after childbirth, conflicting obligations between work and family roles, or lack of transportation to the hospital) before assuming that the parents are unconcerned or that parenting difficulties exist.
   2. Identify the development of attachment behaviors. Mothers' activity with their infants has been found to be indicative of the initial adjustment to the infant, important past and present interpersonal relationships, and involvement in taking care of the infant. Examples of attachment behaviors include the following:
      a. Touching: typical maternal progression of touching the premature infant is from fingertip touching of the infant's extremities to palmar stroking of the infant's trunk, to holding and embracing the infant. This progression of touch usually occurs during a period of several visits to the NICU.
      b. Looking en face: aligning head with infant's head in the same plane to make eye-to-eye contact with the infant.
      c. Talking to the infant, calling the infant by name.
      d. Bringing pictures, toys, and/or clothes to the hospital.
      e. Participating in caretaking activities, such as feeding, bathing, and clothing the infant.

Interventions to Encourage Family-Infant Bonding

A. If at all possible, show the infant to the parents in the delivery room and allow them to touch the infant, if only for a few moments. This helps to establish the reality of the infant for the parents (Kenner and Ellerbee, 2007).
B. Encourage the parents to visit their infant in the intensive care nursery as soon as possible.
   1. Before the first visit to the nursery, prepare the parents for what to expect by giving them written information about the unit, describing the atmosphere of the nursery (i.e., noise, high activity level, infants attached to various kinds of equipment) and discussing the normal aspects of their infant as well as deviations.
   2. If the mother is unable to visit because of conditions such as ordered bed rest or transport of the infant to another hospital, the father can be given pictures of the infant for the mother. In addition, the mother should be given the phone number of the nursery and encouraged to call as often as desired.
   3. For the parents of an infant born with a malformation, encourage the parents to see the infant together as soon as possible, but do not force them to interact. Point out to the family the normal qualities of the infant as well as the abnormalities (Kenner and Ellerbee, 2007).
C. Ensure that during the family's first visit the nurse assigned to the infant stays at the bedside to explain equipment and the infant's condition, as well as to answer questions, provide emotional support, and encourage touching of the infant.

D. **Convey a positive, realistic attitude about the infant** rather than a negative or fatalistic viewpoint, which may alienate the parents and impair attachment (Kenner and Ellerbee, 2007).

E. **Assist the parents with holding and cuddling their infant** as soon as possible, taking into consideration the infant's condition and the parents' readiness (e.g., assist in managing respiratory and monitoring equipment and intravenous [IV] lines). Some nurseries are implementing skin-to-skin care (also called kangaroo care) by parents as an alternative to the traditional modes of providing care to stable, hospitalized premature infants. This care consists of positioning the infant, dressed only in diapers, upright and prone between the mother's breasts. This vertical position in skin-to-skin contact provides tactile stimulation and warmth from the mother, as well as opportunities for eye-to-eye contact, auditory stimulation, and breastfeeding. Mothers usually wear their own front-opening blouses or dresses that are loosely fitted. Fathers can also be encouraged to engage in kangaroo care.

F. **Encourage the parents to participate in caretaking activities** as warranted by the infant's condition and tolerance for input. Explain to parents of very premature infants the relationship between neurologic maturity and the capacity for handling stimulation (Holditch-Davis and Blackburn, 2007).

G. **Model nurturing parenting behavior** such as stroking, touching, and talking to the infant for parents who may need assistance in developing positive parenting behaviors.

H. **Give positive reinforcement** to parents as they interact with their infant. For example, say that "He seems to calm down when you talk with him," or "He really seems to sleep better after you have held him" (Kenner and McGrath, 2004). Assisting parents to recognize positive changes in the infant in response to their caretaking has a strong impact on the parents and increases their feelings of success (Kenner and Ellerbee, 2007).

I. **Use consistent caregivers for the premature or sick infant** to establish a rapport with the parents.

J. **Role-model caregiving techniques—one on one**, if possible, especially for adolescent parents.

K. **Avoid power struggles with parents by defining their role** and recognizing that they are the parents and that the infant is theirs, not the staff's.

L. **Suggest that the parents or siblings bring something for the infant**, such as a small toy, pictures of the family members to be taped on the infant's bed, and/or a tape recording of the parents' voices to be played for the infant. Share personalized information about the infant with the parents. This information can include statements such as "She really enjoys sucking on her pacifier" or "She was really active while I was giving her a bath," to assist the parents in individualizing and accepting the infant.

M. **Encourage sibling visitation** in the unit or window observation of the infant (Kenner and Ellerbee, 2007; McGrath, 2007).

N. **Promote individualized family-centered developmental care that includes the family unit** in the plan of care and an environment that supports the parents. Provide a private area, or a transitional care area, to encourage parental stays within a more homelike environment, and encourage developmental care that includes parents as an integral part of the health care team (Kenner and McGrath, 2004).

O. **After the mother's discharge from the hospital, maintain communication** with the parents by providing them with the phone number of the unit. For parents of transported infants, sending pictures and cards from their infant to show current status, arranging for transportation assistance through social service agencies for parents who lack means of travel (Kenner and Ellerbee, 2007), and maintaining frequent phone contact with parents can be helpful in promoting parent-infant attachment.

P. **Give the mother the opportunity to provide breast milk** for the infant should she so desire, and support her in this endeavor. However, be careful not to overemphasize the importance of breastfeeding. The rationale is that if she should be unsuccessful or decide to stop breastfeeding, feelings of guilt or disappointment may occur if breastfeeding has been touted as the ideal infant feeding method.

Q. **Identify situations in which there are difficulties in parent-infant interaction or problems in the family's functioning.**

R. **Be sensitive to cultural practices** that may influence parent-infant behaviors while bonding and attachment remain strong.
S. **Identify infants who are at risk of having developmental difficulties** (Kenner and McGrath, 2004).
T. **Identify the unique needs of the parent with lower socioeconomic status.** This parent may want to provide the best possible care to the infant but either may not know how to do so (poor role models) or may not have the means to provide for the infant's perceived needs.
U. **Assess the cultural needs of minority parents.** This means to be culturally sensitive to what the parenting role means in that culture and then gear the interventions toward these cultural values and beliefs.

Evaluation of Parent-Infant Bonding

Evaluation of parental behaviors should be based on ongoing patterns rather than on isolated incidents (Mercer, 1977).
A. **Positive attachment behaviors.** The parent
   1. Visits frequently,
   2. Has named the infant,
   3. Makes positive comments when talking to or about the infant,
   4. Demonstrates increasing skill in holding the infant, and
   5. Displays increasing eye and body contact between parent and infant (i.e., kissing, fondling, stroking, nuzzling).
B. **Behaviors of concern.** The parent
   1. Is overly optimistic;
   2. Appears unconcerned about the infant's condition;
   3. Does not ask questions;
   4. Is passive or indifferent;
   5. Avoids close body contact by holding the infant at a distance, props the bottle whether or not the infant is held, positions the bottle in such a way that milk is unable to flow from the nipple;
   6. Is unable to describe any physical or behavioral features unique to the infant; and
   7. Attributes inappropriate characteristics to the infant, such as "she's lazy and stubborn just like her father."
C. **Make sure these areas of concern are considered within the context of the culture of the parents.** Different cultures approach parenthood and parent-infant interaction in different ways.

SUMMARY OF PARENTAL NEEDS TO BE MET BY NICU STAFF

A. **Help the mother reconceptualize her image** of an "ideal" infant to the image of her premature, acutely ill, or malformed infant.
B. **Help the mother deal with feelings of guilt.**
C. **Help parents develop affectionate ties** with the infant through the infant's features (e.g., soft eyes; pretty, soft skin) and learn to read the infant's behavioral cues.
D. **Assist parents in gaining confidence** in holding the infant by encouraging them to participate in caretaking tasks.
E. **Promote communication** between the parents and if they desire extended family members.
F. **Be sensitive to the unique needs** of the individual families.
G. **Assist families in preparing for the transition** to home care after discharge (Kenner and Ellerbee, 2007).
H. **Provide support for parents during the transition phase** after discharge of their infant from the NICU (Kenner and Ellerbee, 2007).
I. **Assist parents in dealing with neonatal death** in a personally meaningful way.
J. **Assist parents in describing their cultural values and beliefs,** if applicable, to understand their views of the infant and their role as parents.

REFERENCES

Berg, C.A. and Upchurch, R.: A developmental-contextual model of couples coping with chronic illness across the adult life span. *Psychological Bulletin, 133*(6):920-954, 2007.

Bowers, B.: Prenatal, antenatal and postpartal risk factors. In C. Kenner C and J.W. Lott (Eds.). *Comprehensive neonatal care: An interdisciplinary approach* (4th ed.), St. Louis, 2007, Saunders Elsevier, pp. 648-656.

Catlin, A.: Thinking outside the box: Prenatal care and the call for a prenatal advance directive. *Journal of Perinatal & Neonatal Nursing, 19*(2):169-176, 2005.

Catlin, A. and Carter, B.: Creation of a neonatal end-of-life palliative care protocol. *Journal of Perinatology, 22*(3):184-195, 2002.

Cone, S.: The impact of communication and the neonatal intensive care unit environment on part involvement. *Newborn & Infant Nursing Reviews, 7*(1):33-38, 2007.

Dishion, T.J., Bullock, B.M., and Granic, I.: Pragmatism in modeling peer influence: Dynamics, outcomes, and change processes. *Development and Psychopathology, 14*(4):969-981, 2002.

Halm, M.A., Sabo, J., and Rudiger, M.: The patient-family advisory council: Keeping a pulse on our customers. *Critical Care Nurse, 26*(5):58-67, 2006.

Holditch-Davis, D. and Blackburn, S.T.: Neurobehavioral development. In C. Kenner and J.W. Lott (Eds.): *Comprehensive neonatal care: An interdisciplinary approach* (4th ed.). St. Louis, 2007, Saunders, pp. 448-479.

Howland, L.C.: Preterm birth: Implications for family stress and coping. *Newborn & Infant Nursing Reviews, 7*(1):14-19, 2007.

Kavanaugh, K. and Wheeler, S.R.: When a baby dies: Caring for bereaved families. In C. Kenner and J.W. Lott (Eds.): *Comprehensive neonatal care: An interdisciplinary approach* (4th ed.). St. Louis, 2007, Saunders, pp. 522-542.

Kenner, C. and Ellerbee, S.: Postdischarge care of the newborn and infant. In C. Kenner and J.W. Lott (Eds.): *Comprehensive neonatal care: An interdisciplinary approach* (4th ed.). St. Louis, 2007, Saunders, pp. 551-562.

Kenner, C. and McGrath, J.M.: *Developmental care of newborns and infants: A guide for health professionals.* St. Louis, 2004, Mosby.

Kenner, C. and Sudia-Robinson, T.: Palliative and end-of-life care. In C. Kenner and J.W. Lott (Eds.): *Comprehensive neonatal care: An interdisciplinary approach* (4th ed.). St. Louis, 2007, Saunders, pp. 510-521.

McGrath, J.M.: Family: Essential partner in care. In C. Kenner and J.W. Lott (Eds.): *Comprehensive neonatal care: An interdisciplinary approach* (4th ed.). St. Louis, 2007, Saunders, pp. 491-509.

Mercer, R.T.: *Nursing care for parents at risk.* Thorofare, NJ, 1977, Charles B. Slack.

National Institute of Nursing Research: Neonatal intensive care unit program reduces premature infants' length of stay and improves parents' mental health outcomes. Retrieved November 25, 2007, from http://www.nih.gov/news/pr/nov2006/ninr-01.htm2006.

Pohlman, S.: Father's role in NICU care: Evidence-based practice. In C. Kenner and J.M. McGrath (Eds.): *Developmental care of newborns and infants: A guide for health professionals.* St. Louis, 2004, Mosby, pp. 359-372.

Premie Creations, LLC: Retrieved November 25, 2007, from http://preemiecreations.com/main.sc

Rolland, J.S.: Chronic illness and the life cycle: A conceptual framework. *Family Process, 26*(2):229-244, 1994.

Siegel, R., Gardner, S.L., and Merenstein, G.B.: Families in crisis: Theoretical and practical considerations. In G.B. Merenstein and S.L. Gardner (Eds.): *Handbook of neonatal intensive care* (6th ed.). St. Louis, 2006, Mosby, pp. 647-672.

Street, E. and Soldan, J.: A conceptual framework for the psychosocial issues faced by families with genetic conditions. *Families, Systems & Health, 16*(3):217-232, 1998.

Sullivan, P. and Altimier, L.: Creating a family advisory council. *Newborn & Infant Nursing Reviews, 7*(1):3-6, 2007.

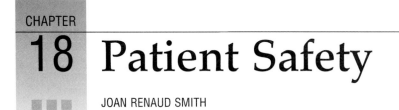

CHAPTER

18 Patient Safety

JOAN RENAUD SMITH

OBJECTIVES

1. Define and discuss organizational and individual approaches to developing a culture of safety.

2. Discuss the importance of teamwork, communication, and technology in providing safe care.

3. Discuss the role families have in promoting patient safety.

4. Discuss human factors and the relation to common errors.

5. Describe specific neonatal errors and recommended improvement strategies.

6. Describe the importance of discharge teaching to promote patient safety at home.

Patient safety has become a national priority and improvement in patient safety has accelerated since an Institute of Medicine's (IOM's) report concluded that up to 98,000 lives are lost annually in U.S. hospitals as a result of error (Kohn et al., 1999). Many of these errors are preventable and have resulted in both death and an economic consequence as high as $29 billion annually (Kohn et al., 1999). Medically fragile infants are at high risk for encountering errors during their stay in the neonatal intensive care unit (NICU) and are defenseless compared with physiologically more mature newborns, leaving little margin for error. It is the responsibility of health care organizations and neonatal care providers to ensure the safety of these vulnerable infants. While some errors occur at the point of service (e.g., a nurse administering the wrong medication), most errors occur as a result of flaws within the health care system or facility design (e.g., excessive noise levels or miscommunication) (Joseph, 2006). Identifying and mitigating sources of patient harm are critical in delivering safe patient care. Mitigating harm is best accomplished by designing reliable health care processes and developing an appropriate culture of safety (Luria et al., 2006).

Using evidence-based clinical practice interventions and strict adherence to protocols every time care is delivered, errors can be substantially reduced (Pronovost et al., 2006). It is now possible to eliminate or nearly eliminate adverse events (AE), and neonatal nurses are on the forefront of providing safe and efficient quality care. As neonatal nurses recognize and understand the causes of errors and rely on strict adherence to evidence-based interventions and improvement strategies, dramatic reduction of errors are possible. The knowledge and skills associated with safety must become routine nursing practice. Improving patient safety requires assimilation of knowledge from other disciplines and industries, and application of safety knowledge to health care.

The following chapter offers an introduction of basic patient safety principles and includes selected improvement strategies and resources for neonatal nurses to build a patient safety toolkit. Selected neonatal errors and improvement strategies are included and are by no means an exhaustive list. Box 18-1 includes definitions of selected improvement strategies. Neonatal nurses need to equip themselves with the best possible safety resources and knowledge in order to provide a safe and caring environment.

A. Organizational and Individual Approaches to Developing and Sustaining a Culture of Safety.

    1. Establish patient safety as a strategic priority (Botwinick et al., 2006). The senior leaders of health care organizations are responsible for establishing safe culture. Each organization should have a Patient Safety Officer (PSO) who is a senior leader and should report directly to the organization's top executive (e.g., Chief Executive Officer [CEO], Chief Operating Officer [COO], Chief Medical Officer [CMO], etc.). The Board of Directors should be actively involved in patient safety reports and routinely track patient safety goals and areas

▨ BOX 18-1
▨ **SELECTED NONTECHNOLOGICAL IMPROVEMENT STRATEGIES DEFINITIONS**

1. **Five rights:** rules traditionally thought to safeguard against errors. The five rights of medication administration (right patient, right drug, right dose, right route, and right frequency) are the basis of most education on drug administration and considered the "safe" way to administer medications. The five rights do not safeguard against major sources of error and may limit critical thinking.
2. **Forcing functions:** interventions that prevent error by "forcing" a safe action, such as removing concentrated potassium from the medication carts. Forcing functions are the strongest of interventions against human failure. A common example of a forcing function is designing oral syringes such that they cannot be connected to an intravenous port.
3. **Medication reconciliation:** the process of avoiding such inadvertent inconsistencies across transitions in care by reviewing the patient's complete medication regimen at the time of admission/transfer/discharge and comparing it with the regimen being considered for the new setting of care.
4. **Read-backs:** includes the listener repeating the key information, so that the transmitter can confirm its correctness.
5. **TALLman lettering:** highlights the dissimilar letters in two names to aid in distinguishing between the two. For example, the name pair epinephrine and ephedrine would be written epINEPHrine and epHEDrine.
6. **"Time Outs":** planned periods of quiet and/or interdisciplinary discussion focused on ensuring that key procedural details have been addressed. For example, the identification of a patient, for a surgical procedure, site, and other key aspects, often stating them aloud for double-checking by other team members.
7. **Executive walk rounds:** used for the sole purpose of discussing safety with frontline staff.
8. **Storytelling:** a tool used to share events in the form of a story. It helps listeners remember facts and details that otherwise might be forgotten.
9. **Safety briefings:** an efficient tool used to share information and to increase safety awareness among frontline staff and foster a culture of safety into the daily routine, 24 hours a day 7 days a week.

Adapted from Agency for Healthcare Research and Quality: AHRQ's Glossary (http://psnet.ahrq.gov/glossary.aspx). Accessed February 7, 2008.

needed for improvement. For safety to be seen as a priority for all staff members, senior leaders need to make safety a key focus for the organization. Senior leaders and front-line staff need to discuss AEs and near misses and develop strategic plans for future safety.

a. Selected strategies for incorporating a safe culture within the organization. See Box 18-1 for selected definition of strategy terms.
   ■ Executive walk rounds (Used for the sole purpose of discussing safety with front-line staff.)
   ■ Storytelling (Inspires cultural change using real-life clinical experiences.)
   ■ Safety briefings (Used to increase staff awareness of patient safety issues by creating an environment in which staff share information without fear of reprisal, and integrate the reporting of safety issues into daily work.)
   ■ Placing patient safety on executive meeting agendas
   ■ Assign executives to performance improvement teams
   ■ Include safety in orientation programs
   ■ Design a communication plan when successful patient safety projects are implemented
   ■ Connect executive performance and compensation to improvements in patient safety

   Senior leaders are key individuals in promoting and establishing a culture of safety. Promoting a safe culture can begin by integrating multidisciplinary patient safety teams into preexisting committees both at the departmental and unit levels to implement safety initiatives at the bedside. NICU safety teams may include front-line professional and support staff, medical and nursing leadership, advanced practice nurses

(APN), pharmacy, and respiratory therapy. These teams are responsible for identifying and responding to unit-specific safety concerns and risks, ensuring that safety efforts are integrated into the overall unit structure, as well as educating staff and faculty about the science of safety (Alton et al., 2006). As senior leaders strive to promote a safe culture, methods of improvement should be clearly outlined and a planned process in place to accelerate the improvement (Botwinick et al., 2006).

2. **Establish a culture that supports safety** (Botwinick et al., 2006). It is the responsibility of individual health care organizations to assess their current state of patient safety. Fostering a culture of safety involves understanding and anticipating human limitations, anticipating the unexpected, and creating a nonpunitive learning environment for improvement and error reduction. Traditionally, health care organizations responded to errors by naming and blaming individuals, known as a *person-centered approach.* This approach is focused on the individual and does not help to prevent future errors. An organization that seeks to blame and punish and lacks teamwork, communication, and transparency of errors is a culture that places patients in harm's way. A *systems approach* recognizes that the system is complex and that most errors reflect predictable human failings in the context of poorly designed systems. A shared accountability among health care organizations and individual practitioners is promoted in a just culture. A *just culture* recognizes that individuals should not be held responsible for system failures and that competent professionals make mistakes and may even adopt unhealthy shortcuts in their practice, but has a zero tolerance for their reckless behavior (Marx, 2001). It also provides a safe environment in which errors may be reported without fear of retribution in events in which there was no harm intended. In a just culture, individuals are encouraged to report errors that result in harm to patients as well as near misses, resulting in an environment in which to learn. Staff must experience a just culture in order to sustain self-disclosure of AEs. Although a just culture seeks potential system failures and does not seek to blame individuals, it does include a well-established system of shared accountability.

3. **Engage key stakeholders.** Senior leaders need to engage key stakeholders in establishing a safe culture.
   a. **Nurses.** Neonatal nurses, APNs, and clinicians are highly educated, organized, skilled, and experienced and are typically the first line of defense in keeping patients safe. Front-line staff can identify firsthand the issues affecting patient safety and are the primary source of care. Their inclusion in the process is essential to the success of implementing patient safety factors.
   b. **Physicians.** Neonatologist and other physicians caring for infants should be involved in the process of establishing a safe culture. Physicians are highly trained, autonomous individuals with many time constraints. Engaging physicians early on with improvement projects related to their area of interest and encouraging active participation is important to establishing a culture of safety.
   c. **Additional stakeholders.** All members of the health care team are extremely valuable in improving quality and safety and it is everyone's responsibility to promote a safe culture. Individual NICUs need to identify their own key members as part of their safety team. Clinical pharmacists; respiratory therapists; social workers; chaplains; dieticians; support staff; laboratory technicians; lactation consultants; discharge coordinators; physical, occupational, and speech therapists; housekeeping; and any other members of the organization who have direct or indirect impact on patient care. A culture of safety requires effective communication and teamwork from all disciplines.
   d. **Board of trustees** (Botwinick et al., 2006). The Board plays a crucial role in moving the organization toward a higher level of patient safety and effectiveness. Board members may establish goals for organization improvements; integrating patient safety goals into the organization's strategic goals and business plans; review adverse reports and root cause analyses, and provide monetary resources for patient safety education and staffing.
   e. **Patients and families.** Patient-centered care is pivotal in the prevention of medical errors. Families are at the core of delivering patient-centered care in the NICU and

family-centered care (FCC) is vital to promoting patient safety. Families should be invited to collaborate with the health care team as partners. Improving quality and safety by bringing families into the planning, delivery, and evaluation of health care is the foundation of FCC (Institute for Family-Centered Care, 2008). The American Academy of Pediatrics' (AAP's) policy statement, *Family-Centered Care and the Pediatrician's Role* (2003, reaffirmed in 2007), provides a summary of the core principles of FCC and includes specific recommendations for how pediatricians can integrate FCC in hospitals, clinics, and their community. Studies have shown that when health care providers and administrators partner with patients and families, the quality and safety of health care rise, the costs decrease, and provider and patient satisfaction increase (Institute for Family-Centered Care, 2008). The core concepts of FCC as outlined by the Institute for Family-Centered Care (2008) include the following:

(1) *Dignity and respect:* Health care professionals (HCPs) need to listen, honor, value, and respect families as partners in the daily planning and delivery of care.

(2) *Information sharing:* HCP need to provide families with unbiased, complete, accurate, and timely information in ways that are affirming and useful.

(3) *Participation:* HCP should encourage and support families to participate in decision making and care at the level the family chooses.

(4) *Collaboration:* Families, practitioners, and organizational leaders should collaborate in policy and program development; implementation, and evaluation; facility design; professional education; and delivery of care.

Establishing a family-centered environment and empowering families to promote patient safety and quality takes a long-term commitment. This approach requires a transformation of the health care organization, including infusing FCC principles into the organization's mission statement and philosophy. Health care organizations can promote FCC by inviting families to participate in hospital and unit committees; patient and family advisory councils; creating an environment that is welcoming and inviting to families and provides privacy, comfort, and the ability to access information; include families in education and training programs as well as research; and develop human resources policies to promote a family-friendly environment. Specific steps to assist health care organizations in developing an FCC environment are available (Institute for Family-Centered Care, 2008).

Both the AAP (2003, reaffirmed 2007) and the Vermont Oxford Network's (VON) Neonatal Intensive Care Quality Improvement Collaborative (NIC/Q) (Dunn et al., 2006) provide recommendations supporting the integration of families into high-quality patient care delivery. Families are encouraged to report concerns and to be actively involved in their infant's care as part of a patient safety strategy supported by the Joint Commission's 2008 National Patient Safety Goals (see Table 18-1). National initiatives outlining strategies to encourage family participation in error prevention are also available. Some of these initiatives include The Joint Commission's "Speak-Up" initiatives, the National Patient Safety Foundation's "Agenda for Action," and the Agency for Healthcare Research and Quality's "20 Tips."

4. **Teamwork and communication.**

According to the IOM, health care providers tend to be trained as individuals even though they function almost exclusively as teams, and patient safety programs that promote team training and functioning need to be adopted (Kohn et al., 1999). Neonatal care has become increasingly complex, requiring teamwork and collaboration among multiple disciplines in order to achieve a common goal, to improve patient outcomes. Communication and teamwork are vital to creating and sustaining a culture of safety. More than two thirds of sentinel events reported to The Joint Commission were primarily caused by failures in communication (Joint Commission, 2007). Communication among team members must flow freely regardless of their authority gradient. Patient care decision making should be shared among all members of the health care team. Mutual respect, trust, confidentiality, responsiveness, empathy, effective listening, and communication among all clinical team members are necessary for promoting shared decision making (Roberts and Perryman, 2007). Organizations need to adopt a zero-tolerance policy for abusive behaviors among any member of the health care team.

■ TABLE 18-1
■ ■ **The Joint Commission's Hospital National Patient Safety Goals**

Patient Safety Goal	Recommendations
Identify patients correctly	Use at least two ways to identify patients. For example, use the patient's name and date of birth. This is done to make sure that each patient gets the medicine and treatment meant for him. Make sure that the correct patient gets the correct blood type when he gets a blood transfusion.
Improve staff communication	Read back spoken or phone orders to the person who gave the order. Create a list of abbreviations and symbols that are not to be used. Quickly get important test results to the right staff person. Create steps for staff to follow when sending patients to the next caregiver. The steps should help staff tell about the patient's care. Make sure there is time to ask and answer questions.
Use medicines safely	Create a list of medicines with names that look alike or sound alike. Update the list every year. Label all medicines that are not already labeled. For example, medicine in syringes, cups, and basins. Take extra care with patients who take medicines to thin their blood.
Prevent infection	Use the hand cleaning guidelines from the World Health Organization or Centers for Disease Control and Prevention. Report death or injury to patients from infections that happen in hospitals. Use proven guidelines to prevent infections that are difficult to treat, and to prevent infections of the blood. Use safe practices to treat the part of the body where surgery was done.
Check patient medicines	Find out what medicines each patient is taking. Make sure that it is OK for the patient to take any new medicines with his current medicines. Give a list of the patient's medicines to the next caregiver or regular doctor and to the patient and family before the patient goes home. Explain the list. Some patients may get medicine in small amounts or for a short time.
Prevent patients from falling	Find out which patients are most likely to fall. For example, is the patient taking any medicines that might make him weak, dizzy, or sleepy? Take action to prevent falls for these patients.
Help patients to be involved in their care	Tell each patient and family how to report complaints about safety.
Identify patient safety risks	Find out which patients are most likely to try to kill themselves.
Watch patients closely for changes in their health and respond quickly if they need help	Create ways to get help from specially trained staff when a patient's health appears to worsen.
Prevent errors in surgery	Create steps for staff to follow so that all documents needed for surgery are on hand before surgery begins. Mark the part of the body where the surgery will be done. Involve the patient in doing this.

From The Joint Commission: *2009 hospital national patient safety goals.* Http://www.jointcommission.org/patientsafety/nationalpatientsafetygoals/. © The Joint Commission, 2009. Reprinted with permission.

a. **Simulation and debriefing.** The IOM suggests the use of simulation exercises focused on improving teamwork as one of the mechanisms to improve patient safety (Kohn et al., 1999). "Simulation refers to the recreation of an actual event that has previously occurred or could potentially occur" (Hunt et al., 2007, p. 306). Debriefing after a team simulation experience allows recognition of areas of appropriate performance and lessons learned from where and how the errors could potentially be prevented. Simulation in conjunction with debriefing is necessary so errors can be identified and team members are made aware of their role in the error. Simulation can provide a replication of the neonatal environment, equipped with the technology and the models of equipment that will be encountered in the NICU as well as complex scenarios that require successful team interactions. Procedural and technical skills can also be simulated, allowing for teamwork and competency checks. Leadership skills during emergent situations can also be enhanced through the use of role simulation by improving communication skills as it relates to discussions about the futility of medical care, end-of-life decision making, and the chronicity of medical care. Rapid-response teams, transport teams, and trauma teams are all high-functioning teams that rely on effective communication and have benefited from the use of simulation.

Incorporating simulation and debriefing methods into NRP training can promote effective communication and teamwork and potentially reduce the rate of errors (Thomas et al., 2007). Despite the high interest in improving teamwork using simulation in health care, few health care studies exist demonstrating that enhanced teamwork improves quality of care. Knowledge about how to improve team behavior and its ability to promote patient safety and improve outcomes is still in its infancy; more research is warranted.

b. **Effective methods of teamwork and communication.**

(1) *Crew resource management (CRM).* CRM is a communication methodology used to promote team-centered decision making learned from the aerospace industry to promote effective communication and teamwork (Sundar et al., 2007). CRM teaches team communication and highlights errors in a simulated setting in the hope of avoiding the same error in a real-life setting involving humans. It teaches that all members of a team are vital and that if a team member at any level believes that something is not being done appropriately or in the best interest of the team or other people who have put their trust in the team, then that member must speak up (Hunt et al., 2007).

(2) *SBAR (situation, background, assessment, and recommendation)* (Haig et al., 2006). SBAR is a method to improve hand-offs. The NICU is often chaotic and hurried, critical information can fall through the cracks at hand-offs, and communication can also be misunderstood. For example, a potential for error can occur with verbal orders for medication when it is written down by someone other than the order giver and transcribed onto an order form by a third person. Used extensively in medicine, and originating from the nuclear submarine service, SBAR is a communication tool to standardize discussion and information sharing among caregivers to ensure that patient information is consistently and accurately being delivered, especially during critical events, shift hand-offs, and patient transfers. As part of the National Patient Safety Goals, the Joint Commission (2008) (see Table 18-1) requires organizations to implement a standardized approach to hand-off communications. SBAR provides a shared mental model for all clinicians to use during hand-offs or transfers:

Situation: What is happening at the present time?

Background: What are the circumstances leading up to this situation?

Assessment: What do I think the problem is?

Recommendation: What should we do to correct the problem?

5. **Human factor engineering and the environment.**

a. **Fatigue and shift work.** The Institute of Medicine of the National Academies (IOM) report *Keeping Patients Safe—Transforming the Work Environment of Nurses* identifies that research findings on overtime practices indicate that long work hours, without adequate and quality rest time, is associated with impaired performance and human errors (2004). The effects of fatigue as a result of long work hours, working at night, and insufficient sleep are often underestimated. Studies linking fatigue with medical errors have been reported for critical care nurses (Scott et al., 2006) and residents (Jagsi et al., 2005). Nurses who have good sleep habits, minimize their shift rotations and excessive work hours, and use strategic naps can reduce the adverse effects of fatigue that could potentially put patients at risk (Dean et al., 2006). Although limited research has been conducted in the area of fatigue, specifically related to neonatal nurses and neonatal nurse practitioners (NNPs), the National Association of Neonatal Nurses and the National Association of Neonatal Nurse Practitioners have developed position statements recommending all health care employers implement guidelines to minimize staff fatigue (2007; 2008). These recommendations encourage close collaboration between staff and and their employers in order to develop and implement risk-reduction strategies to reduce the risk of fatigue-related incidents.

  b. **NICU environment.** Human factors that have contributed to errors include fatigue, communication failure, poor hand-offs, problems with cross-coverage, workload, and staffing patterns. Addressing these factors can aid in reducing medical errors. The NICU environment is a complex adaptive system conducive to human error. Frequently, the NICU is chaotic and prone to many unanticipated and life-threatening interruptions, leaving care providers with very little time to make thoughtful and sound decisions. Patients in the NICU often require complex multidisciplinary care; each layer of this complex system presents additional opportunities for error (Morriss, 2008).

    (1) The physical environment (Joseph, 2006; White, 2005). The NICU directly affects not only the highly vulnerable and sensitive preterm infant but also the caregiver within the environment. Overcrowded and poorly designed workspaces and work flow areas, excessive noise, inadequate lighting, poor ventilation and air flow filtration systems, and insufficient family space can all affect patient and staff health and safety. Inadequate lighting, excessive noise, and a disorganized environment are likely to compound the burden of stress for nurses and lead to errors. Providing caregivers with a physical environment that lowers stress and improves job performance, safety, and satisfaction is the key for health care organizations. Lighting and sound levels often conflict for the neonate and caregiver. While dim lighting is appropriate for night-time circadian cycles for the infant, dim lighting is difficult for night staff to provide direct physical care as well as to maintain a level of alertness and comfort. Providing night-shift workers with task lighting or short periods of bright-light exposure levels can improve mood, sleep, and levels of alertness. Many NICUs are designing or redesigning their units; efforts should focus on the individual needs of babies, families, and caregivers. Human engineers should be included in the design process to promote a safe environment.

  c. **Aging workforce.** Nurses are aging and their work is becoming more complex with changing technology, evolving work practices, and increasing documentation requirements. There is a need to redesign workplaces using ergonomic work principles in order to reduce the physical demands on nurses (Joseph, 2006). The mean age of a nurse in the United States is 46.8 years (47 years for females, 44.6 years for males) (U.S. Department of Health and Human Services, 2006). Advanced age may also negatively impact performance due to fatigue (Dean et al., 2006). Ergonomic evaluation of the work area specific to the NICU may provide solutions to problems encountered by neonatal care providers. For instance, an ergonomic evaluation of the work area at an infant's bedside to reduce a care provider's neck and back problems may include a height-adjustable footstool and better monitor placement as potential solutions. More ergonomics research is needed in the area of computer workstations as they affect nurses' posture, readability, and level of fatigue (Joseph, 2006).

  d. **Staffing** (Kane et al., 2007). Increases in staff workload and age, coupled with a decrease in the number of registered nurses (RN), can threaten patient safety. Nurses are vital in providing patients with high-quality and safe care. In a meta-analysis of 94 observational studies, greater nursing staff members was associated with better patient outcomes in ICUs and in surgical patients, but this association did not show a causal relationship and the majority of participating centers cared for adults (Kane et al., 2007). In a staffing study of two U.S. NICUs, researchers examined the impact of nurse staffing and bloodstream infections for all infants admitted ($N = 2675$) between 2001 and 2002; greater nurse-hours per patient day significantly reduced the incidence of infection in one NICU but not the other (Cimiotti et al., 2006). Staffing levels vary greatly across facilities, and methods for promoting safer staffing are needed. Skill mix and acuity are two additional factors that contribute to nurse staffing and its relationship to patient outcomes. A validated neonatal acuity tool is needed to determine appropriate nurse-patient ratios followed by a large neonatal multicentered rigorous trial to conclude whether a relationship exists between increased nurse staffing (including skill mix and acuity) and improved patient outcomes.

6. **Health information technology (HIT)** (Shekelle et al., 2006). In its 2001 report, *Crossing the Quality Chasm*, the Institute of Medicine (IOM) identified health information technology (HIT) as one of the most significant intervention to improve health care quality in the United States. Many national agencies support the use of HIT because of its promising improvement in the efficiency, cost-effectiveness, quality, and safety of medical care and delivery in the nation's health care system. Despite these recommendations, the majority of health care organizations have been slow to adopt HIT. Information technology strategies have proven effective in reducing human errors in industries such as aviation and banking. Technology eliminates duplicate work and illegible handwriting. HIT may improve care providers' decision-making with integrating relevant automated decision-making and knowledge acquisition tools along with evidence-based clinical practice guidelines. Communication among caregivers, accessibility and availability of patient information, medication prescribing and use, and adherence to clinical practice guidelines can all be improved through the use of HIT. Some of the technologies that improve medication delivery and provide decision support for medication therapy include computerized provider order entry (CPOE), bar coding, handheld computers, and first generation of smart pumps and automated dispensing machines (ADM).

   Limited evidence exists to support the use of HIT in the NICU and its effectiveness in reducing errors. Technology alone does not eliminate medication errors, and there are also concerns about the potential introduction of new errors or unintended consequences (Cochran et al., 2007). The cost of implementing HIT is a significant barrier for many health care organizations. Besides cost, there is also an element of human interface between good technology and user-friendly equipment. Health care professionals who adopt workaround strategies to override an inflexible system in order to achieve the desired task defeat the software-designed safeguards. Although HIT has grown exponentially, it may contribute to system complexity and additional opportunities for errors. Further research is needed to evaluate the efficacy of HIT and its impact on neonatal patient safety outcomes.

   a. **Clinical Decision Support System (CDSS).** A software program designed to help health care professionals make clinical decisions (Musen et al., 2006). CDSS is a system that can bring standardized, evidence-based practice (EBP) resources to the point of care and promote patient safety without having to rely on memory (Jenkins et al., 2006). Human errors increase when care providers rely on memory to complete a task. According to the IOM, the growing amount of information required to make sound clinical and reliable decisions is surpassing unassisted human capacity, and CDSS offers a practical solution as an EBP resource (Institute of Medicine, 2007).

   b. **Computerized Provider Order Entry (CPOE).** CPOE is an electronic application for writing orders that provides clinical guidance during the ordering process and intercepts potential errors at the point of order origination. Implementation of a CPOE system has been identified as one of the 30 safe practices identified by the National Quality Forum (NQF) to facilitate transfer of clear communication (2006). The majority of CPOE systems interface with CDSS and provide alerts and triggers as part of the clinical guidance. Both CPOE and CDSS promote safety by improving legibility; reducing transcription errors; using standard names, catalogs, and dictionaries; linking patient-specific data and clinical information; using evidence-based order sets; automating calculations; providing alerts and reminders; monitoring for adherence to best practice; and screening for populations at risk (Lehmann and Kim, 2006). CPOE is one of the most frequently used systems for reducing error and managing patient care more safely. Many national organizational bodies recommend CPOE as a strategy to reduce medication errors; however, there is limited pediatric and neonatal-specific evidence with adequate power to support its ability to reduce errors and prevent adverse drug events (ADEs) in the NICU (Miller et al., 2007; Morriss, 2008).

There are barriers in adopting CPOE within an organization. Barriers include cost for start-up and maintenance, changes to work flow process and design affecting all health care personnel and departments throughout the organization, and the challenge of implementing a system that is reliable and user-friendly. The majority of CPOE systems are designed for adult patients and require alteration in order to address the special needs of the NICU population. Many medications prescribed in the NICU are off-label or unlicensed (Cuzzolin et al., 2006), making it difficult to determine a CPOE standard based on best evidence. Although CPOE may decrease the frequency of ADEs, evidence suggests that computerized systems cannot prevent all errors or ADEs and may, in some cases, be responsible for new types of errors (Koppel et al., 2005; Nebeker et al., 2005). A newly designed evidence-based methodology for evaluating CPOE systems implemented and operating in hospitals does exist (Kilbridge et al., 2006). More research is needed to evaluate the efficacy of implementing CPOE in the NICU.

c. **Smart infusion pumps.** Medication errors related to intravenous (IV) infusion present the greatest potential for harm. Neonatal nurses program infusion pumps routinely in order to deliver parenteral fluids and high-risk medications such as dopamine, morphine, fentanyl, and insulin. Decimal point errors of 10 and even as high as 1000 times the intended dose can be easily programmed into these infusion pumps. In a comparison study examining the actual medication, dose, and rate of infusion with the prescribed medication, dose, and rate, investigators found that two thirds had some discrepancy (Husch et al., 2005). IV pumps rely heavily on human factors and depend on error-free programming. Smart pump technology contains computerized medication software to ensure appropriate dosage and flow rates based on safety parameters and are designed to reduce human fallibility and ADEs. Smart pump technology incorporates multiple comprehensive libraries of drugs, usual concentrations, dosing units (e.g., mcg/kg/min, units/hour), and dose limits. Both continuous and bolus infusions can be programmed with the expanded drug dose calculator. The libraries are designed and managed by the hospital pharmacy department but require interdisciplinary collaboration to ensure safe and appropriate parameters are programmed.

d. **Automated drug-dispensing units (ADUs) or automated dispensing machines (ADMs).** ADMs are computerized cabinets containing stock medications and supplies and are located on the patient unit. These automated machines provide quick access and tracking from the point-of-care entry to removal from the cabinet, leading to an elimination of possible errors within the phases of medication administration (from ordering, transcribing, dispensing, and administering). They are used for the purpose of automating access, distribution, management, and control of medications, fluids, and supplies. There are workaround or override concerns with the use of ADUs and ADMs; limiting the use of workarounds is necessary, otherwise the safety features become ineffective and staff may become complacent and not read the alert information when selecting overrides (Kester et al., 2006). Drug dose errors related to stocking are also a concern requiring the need for double-checks.

e. **Bar-code medication administration technology (BCMA) or barcode scanning medication administration (BSMA)** is used to prevent medication errors by placing a unique identifier (bar code) that is machine readable by an optical scanner on each medication. The effectiveness of BCMA to prevent medication errors before they reach the patient have been documented (Cochran et al., 2007). Before the medication is administered, BCMA matches the right medication with the right patient at the right time. BCMA has not yet been installed in many hospitals and no reports exist regarding its effectiveness in preventing ADEs in the NICU.

Bar coding is associated with fewer patient identification errors by using a system of machine-readable codes that uniquely identify an item (Gray et al., 2006). Misidentification errors are not only limited to medication; these errors affect diagnosis and therapeutics and are also commonly seen when mother's expressed breast milk (EBM) has been given to the wrong infant (Suresh et al., 2004). The use of point-of-care bar coding systems has been identified as a technology used to decrease patient identification error. Radio frequency identification systems, which do not require line-of-sight access to patient identification bands, may also be reliable. Despite the potential benefits of either of these autoidentification technologies, it is the responsibility of the clinician to ensure that such technologies are adequately tested in the NICU environment (Gray et al., 2006).

f.   **Radio frequency identification (RFID)** is expected to replace bar code scanning because of its ability to read identification tags with greater versatility. RFID tags are used in newborn security systems and have the capability to track individuals in order to identify their location. Infant security systems are crucial to the design of both maternity and neonatal units, with the alarming mechanism at every point of entry to prevent infant abduction.

g.   **Additional HIT.** Personal digital assistants (PDAs), handheld computers, and cellular phones can integrate with electronic health records (EHRs). Care providers work in a mobile environment, and these hand-held devices can document and retrieve information at the point of care without delay, including evidence-based clinical practice guidelines (CPGs), pharmacy database and assessment guides, and diagnostic tests (McCartney, 2006).

7.   **Evidence-based practice (EBP).** According to the IOM's *Roundtable on Evidence-Based Medicine* (2007), EBP serves as a necessary and valuable tool for future progress and as a projected goal, by the year 2020, 90% of all clinical decisions will be supported by accurate, timely, and up-to-date clinical information that is supported by the best available evidence. EBP is the integration of the best available evidence with clinical expertise and patient values (Sackett et al., 2000). All three of these components are vital to the process. While nurses may feel confident in their clinical expertise and, to some extent, patient/family values, many nurses are not aware of the most recent research findings available to optimize their nursing care (Brady and Lewin, 2007; Pravikoff et al., 2005). Neonatal nurses are encouraged to use EBP to guide daily decision making in order to provide the highest quality of care for individual patients and to decrease variations in practice (Smith et al., 2007). The EBP process requires nurses to be able to search for the evidence and apply the findings to practice. For nurses to integrate EBP into their practice, they need to value the importance of research and health care organizations need to commit to promoting EBP by allowing nurses time and the wherewithal to foster an EBP culture. Neonatal nurses need to be taught how to implement EBP and health care organizations need to accommodate convenient computer access to on-line EBP resources, including on-line journal articles and clinical practice guidelines (CPG) Web sites.

a.   **Clinical practice guidelines.** One form of evidence increasing in volumes internationally, mainly in the adult population, is the use of CPGs (Kent and Fineout-Overholt, 2007). Evidence-based CPGs are systematically developed based on the strongest evidence, contain statements to guide practitioners, and include recommendations to assist in decision making (Kent and Fineout-Overholt, 2007). These evidence-based guidelines assist practitioners by reducing variability in practice and standardizing treatment. This standardization has been shown to improve quality in health care settings. Librarians or APNs trained in EBP can champion or mentor individual clinicians in using the EBP process.

The following organizations foster development of high-quality evidence-based CPGs, Best Practice Sheets or Potentially Better Practices (PBPs):

■   The Association of Women's Health, Obstetric and Neonatal Nursing (AWHONN) provides CPGs specific to newborns and their families, including breastfeeding support and neonatal skin care (www.awhonn.org/awhonn/category.products. do?catid=6).

■   The National Guideline Clearinghouse (NGC) is an initiative of the Agency for Healthcare Research and Quality (AHRQ) and is a free public resource for evidence-based CPGs. The NGC site contains abstracts and full-text CPGs, guideline comparisons, a searchable bibliography database for literature citations, and a discussion forum for exchanging ideas about guidelines (www.guideline.gov).

■ The Joanna Briggs Institute (JBI) is an interdisciplinary, not-for-profit, international research and development agency in Australia. The role of the JBI is to improve the feasibility, appropriateness, meaningfulness, and effectiveness of health care practices and health care outcomes by facilitating international collaborating centers, groups, expert researchers, and clinicians. Although their Web site targets the adult population, it does include good resources for neonatal nurses. Multiple EBP tools and resources as well Best Practice Sheets (or clinical practice guidelines) are also available on this Web site (www.joannabriggs.edu.au/pubs/best_practice.php).

■ The American Academy of Pediatrics offers an online practice management Web site, including a brief description of CPGs, their own developed CPG (specifically, *Management of Hyperbilirubinemia in the Newborn Infant 35 or More Weeks of Gestation*) and a list of CPG resources (http://practice.aap.org/content.aspx?aid=1430&nodeID=4001).

■ The Vermont Oxford Network offers PBPs, which are practices that are developed and tested by multidisciplinary neonatal teams that participate in the VON. The practices are considered "potentially better" because VON members believe that until the practices can be evaluated, customized, and implemented into individual NICUs, it is unknown whether they are the best possible practice. Some practices may be controversial because there is limited or no evidence available. Members of the VON are given tools to assess the quality and strength of each PBP. PBPs are published and topics include, but are not limited to, neonatal pain management, family-centered care, reduction of bronchopulmonary dysplasia in very low birth weight infants, staffing in the NICU, and more. A list of publications related to the VON can be found at www.votxford.org/home.aspx?p=about/references.htm.

■ The National Association of Neonatal Nurses offers guidelines on the topics of pain, skin care, genetics, and peripherally inserted central catheters. A list of publications can be found at www.nann.org.

8. **Reporting methods.**

A number of reporting methods exist and have been used to identify medical errors and adverse events (AEs), including chart review (both focused or trigger-based and nonfocused), direct observation, voluntary reporting by health care providers, and review of medical malpractice claims. Multiple methods may be necessary to effectively measure harm associated with hospital-based health care.

a. **Voluntary reporting** systems are used by many health care organizations although it is limited owing to its voluntary nature. Reporting systems can be performed at the unit level (incident reports) or at the national level (multiinstitutional specialty-based reports). The majority of incident-reporting systems in the NICU use a voluntary, nonpunitive approach to incidents and these reporting systems elicit many more incidents in the NICU than a mandatory system (Snijders et al., 2007). Voluntary is key to reporting medical errors and AEs because health care providers may fear being stigmatized or punished for their actions. However, once a culture of safety is developed, reporting of errors by health care providers should begin to increase. It is important to include near misses when reporting in order to learn how to prevent errors. Automated reporting systems that allow quick and easy access are necessary for busy clinicians. Although voluntary reporting only provides a glimpse into a complex cause of error, system factors responsible for many errors can be identified in a voluntary reporting system. Using an Internet-based, voluntary, anonymous reporting system from 54 NICUs, members of the VON revealed large numbers of errors in virtually all domains in NICUs and identified factors contributing to the occurrence of errors. These identifying factors found that nearly half (47%) of reports were associated with a failure to follow a hospital policy or protocol, 27% with inattention, 22% with a communication problem, and 12% with distraction (Suresh et al., 2004). These findings suggest that adding new policies or protocols do not improve patient safety but the responsibility lies within the system itself, monitoring processes, and identifying systemwide improvements to effectively understand errors and improve patient safety. Once errors are identified, improvement strategies are implemented, and future errors are prevented, health care providers will recognize the benefit of reporting.

b. **Patient triggers.** Measuring the overall level of harm within a health care organization has been performed through the identification of "triggers," or clues, of AEs during manual chart review. A trigger is defined as an "occurrence, prompt, or flag" found on review of the medical chart that "triggers" a further investigation to determine the presence or absence of an AE. Historically, efforts to identify AEs have relied on voluntary reporting and tracking of errors. This method is often limited and may be unreliable because of a small percentage of errors ever being reported. Trigger methodology provides a more focused and efficient review of charts that may lead to identifying more AEs (Sharek et al., 2006). An example of a neonatal trigger would be the patient's use of naloxone, prompting a focused chart review for opioid-induced respiratory depression. In an effort to develop and test an NICU-specific trigger tool, members of the VON and the CHCA participated in a collaborative funded by the Agency of Healthcare Research and Quality. In a retrospective chart review, 749 charts from 15 different NICUs were examined for NICU-associated AEs. Results of this study identified low birth weight and early gestational-age infants as most susceptible to AEs, with the most common AEs being nosocomial infections (27.8%), catheter infiltrates (15.5%), abnormal cranial imaging (10.5%), and accidental extubations requiring reintubation (8.3%) (Sharek et al., 2006). More than half of all identified AEs were classified as preventable, with 40% falling into the severe-harm group. Specific limitations of this study exist; however, the authors conclude that the NICU trigger tool is superior to identifying AEs compared with nontrigger methods, and the NICU trigger tool can potentially be automated, allowing identification of AEs in real time as well as the ability to track AE rates (Sharek et al., 2006). This kind of proactive search for problems is more effective than responding to reports of injuries and accidents after they occur.

c. **Additional methods of identifying errors.** Traditional chart reviews or health care provider interviews are additional methods of identifying errors. Often these methods are labor intensive, costly, inefficient, and variable. Direct observation using real-time audits during team rounds or routine nursing care can provide immediate feedback to frontline staff, which is key to behavior change for focused improvements in patient safety (Ursprung et al., 2005). Checklist with real-time surveillance methods identify care processes especially prone to error that are important safety areas, including mislabeled medications (tubing or syringes), absence of wristbands for patient identification, failure to follow hand hygiene practices, and inappropriate pulse oximeter settings (Ursprung et al., 2005). A culture of safety involves promoting practices that are evidence-based and safe and should be part of any NICU's quality improvement efforts. Families are also encouraged to participate in the process of identifying errors in order to provide a different perspective from most health care providers and to enhance the opportunity to learn about error prevention.

9. **Transparency and full disclosure** (Massachusetts Coalition for the Prevention of Medical Error [MCPME], 2006).

Transparency is a process in which errors are fully disclosed to patients/families. It is a process that can be very challenging for health care providers. Disclosure refers to providing information to a patient and/or family about an incident. Data suggest that most patients/families wish to be informed of AEs. Nurses and physicians may find it difficult to acknowledge their mistakes, whether it is fear of litigation or just an intense shame or guilt. Health care professionals hold themselves to very high standards and as a result, may find it difficult to deal with failure. Because of the emotional effects of these events on both the patients/families and the caregiver, communication failures are often the reason patients/families file malpractice suits. Support to both families and caregivers is essential in disclosing errors. The Harvard teaching institutions have developed a consensus statement for use at the Harvard hospitals that provides a template for responding consistently and ethically to medical errors (MCPME, 2006).

a. Strategies to support families after an AE through disclosure by care providers:
- Prompt (within 24 hours after the event is discovered), compassionate, and honest communication with families following an incident telling them what happened.
- Take responsibility and openly acknowledge the incident, be sensitive, and provide good and skillful communication. The reactions of families to incidents are influenced both by the incident itself and the manner in which the incident is handled.
- The initial communication should be by, or at least in the presence of, a caregiver with a prior relation of trust with the patients. (This may be the attending physician or primary nurse.)
- Apologize when there has been an error. The attending physician responsible for the patient's care is the person most suitable to make the apology along with the clinician responsible for caring out the incident. However, in some situations, other health care professionals or administrators may be more appropriate for disclosing the error and apologizing. The apology helps to restore the family's dignity and begin the healing process.
- Open communication by individual clinicians should be strongly supported by institutional leaders and strongly supported by the health care team as a whole (It is difficult for the clinician to be open and honest about problems that have occurred if he or she does not feel supported by management/leadership.)
- Initial communication should focus on what happened and how it will affect the patient, including immediate effects and prognosis.
- Commit to finding out why the event occurred, how recurrences will be prevented from happening to others, and to conducting an ongoing investigation.
- Follow-up care should also be provided for the families after the initial incident with continued ongoing communication and support.

b. Support of caregivers following an AE. Similar to patients/families, caregivers are also affected, emotionally and functionally, following an AE and are frequently unrecognized as the "second victim." Caregivers should be provided with institutional support that enables them to recover. Adverse medical events are a time of charged emotions and hectic activity involving a variety of clinical services. A clearly defined process is required to assess, activate, and oversee an effective support response for clinicians in these situations. A trained group of individuals to provide emotional support to the caregivers who were involved in the AEs is recommended. Organizations need to offer caregivers professional help to manage the stress of the AE so healing can occur and they can comfortably return to work and take better care of their patients. Caregivers should have structured assistance in debriefing the AE as a team and should be given instruction on documenting the event. Coaching in communicating with the family during the emotionally intense period immediately following an incident can be critical for maintaining the relationship of compassion and trust. Training programs, including simulation training, need to be developed to teach nurses, physicians, and other clinicians, as well as department chairmen and managers, how to communicate AEs and how to provide support after experiencing an AE.

B. **Selected types of health care errors in the NICU.** Many selected improvement strategies are identified throughout this next section. This is not an exhaustive list and many of the same strategies can be used for each identified error. It is important to remember that the safety and efficacy of a new practice, protocol, or piece of equipment should be examined carefully prior to implementation.

1. **Patient misidentification** (Gray et al., 2006). Misidentification is a specific area of concern for NICU patients. Accurate patient identification is necessary for providing safe and effective services specifically related to medication and blood product administration, laboratory specimen collection, performance of diagnostic procedures, and administration of treatments. Unlike adults and many pediatric patients, neonates cannot participate in the process of identifying themselves. Methods used to differentiate individuals (age, size, sex, and hair color) are not readily available in the neonatal population. Frequently, names are similar and, in some cases, identical along with similar medical record numbers, resulting

in an increased chance for misidentification. Wristbands are another tool used to verify patient identification in the NICU. However, wristbands are often inaccurate, incomplete, missing, or are affixed to the patient's bedside because of concern for the preterm infant's fragile skin that can lead to lacerations or abrasions.

   a. Improvement strategies to reduce misidentification include:
- Two patient identifiers
- "Time out" immediately before starting the procedure
- Bar codes
- Radio frequency identification

2. **Wrong administration of expressed breast milk (EBM) and blood products.** Multiple steps are involved in the process of administering EBM and blood products. Both EBM and blood products are body fluids and can carry infectious agents; because of the risk associated with potentially administering the wrong breast milk or blood products, methods need to be identified in order to reduce wrong administration.

   a. Improvement strategies (use the same strategies as used for misidentification and medication errors). Six Sigma is a process improvement strategy and has been used to reduce the incidence of incorrectly administering EBM (Drenckpohl et al., 2007). The Six Sigma methodology has been used in the manufacturing industry for years and its goal is performance excellence, stating that perfection is possible. The Six Sigma approach reduces variability within a process, ultimately reducing opportunities for failures. The steps are to define, measure, analyze, improve (DMAI), and control a problem (Benbow and Kubiak, 2005). Administration of EBM is complex and involves many people handling, transporting, storing, preparing, and administering the milk, resulting in the potential for error. The primary goal of Six Sigma is to eliminate the number of defects that can occur in a process (Woodward, 2005). This same method can be used as an effective strategy for improving other processes related to errors within an organization.

3. **Medication errors.** Neonates are highly vulnerable to medication errors because of their extensive exposure to medications in the NICU, the lack of evidence on pharmacotherapeutic interventions in neonates, and the lack of neonate-specific formulations (Chedoe et al., 2007). Medication errors can occur throughout any stage of drug delivery and include preventable and nonpreventable ADEs. More research is needed regarding the epidemiology of medication errors in the NICU and evidence-based interventions are needed to reduce medication errors and improve patient safety. In an effort to reduce the rate of pediatric medication errors, the AAP has developed recommendations uniquely pertinent to children and/or neonates (Stucky, 2003; reaffirmed 2007).

   a. Common stages of medication ordering and delivery where errors occur.

      (1) *Prescribing.* Incorrect dosing is the most common medication error in the NICU, either related to the prescribing phase or the administration phase (Chedoe et al., 2007). Deficiencies in prescribing and monitoring of medications contribute to nearly three fourths of ADEs in hospitalized children (Lesar et al., 2006). The most common cause of medication errors at the prescribing stage is the deficiency in performance or knowledge of the prescriber, the physician, or nurse practitioner. Neonates are a heterogeneous group, and prescribing decisions must be made on an individual basis. Pharmacokinetic and pharmacodynamic parameters change continuously because of changes in the neonate's weight, length, and renal function (Chedoe et al., 2007; Rakhmanina and van den Anker, 2006). Incorrect recording of the patient's weight, dosage regimen, units (e.g., milligrams and micrograms), and misplacement of decimal points when calculating, resulting in 10- or 100-fold overdoses, all contribute to dose errors at the prescribing phase (Chedoe et al., 2007). Specific to the NICU population is the rapid change in weights requiring frequent dosing recalculations in order to maintain therapeutic drug levels. The use of abbreviations, verbal orders, and poor handwriting can also lead to medication errors at the prescribing stage. Reviewing the prescribed orders, by a nurse or pharmacist, is critical at this stage of the medication process in order to detect or prevent an ADE (Lesar et al., 2006).

■ TABLE 18-2
■ ■ "Do Not Use" Abbreviations

Do Not Use	Potential Problem	Use Instead
U (unit)	Mistaken for "0"(zero), the number "4" (four) or "cc"	Write "unit"
IU (International Unit)	Mistaken for IV (intravenous) or the number 10 (ten)	Write "International Unit"
Q.D., QD, q.d., qd (daily)	Mistaken for each other	Write "daily"
Q.O.D., QOD, q.o.d., qod (every other day)	Period after the Q mistaken for "I" and the "O" mistaken for "I"	Write "every other day"
Trailing zero (X.0 mg)	Decimal point is missed	Write X mg
Lack of leading zero (.X mg)		Write 0.X mg
MS	Can mean morphine sulfate or magnesium sulfate	Write "morphine sulfate"
MSO_4 and $MgSO_4$	Confused for one another	Write "magnesium sulfate"

Adapted from The Joint Commission: The Official "Do Not Use" List. Retrieved February 13, 2008, from www.jointcommission. org/PatientSafety/DoNotUseList. © The Joint Commission, 2009. Reprinted with permission.

(2) *Transcribing.* Multiple errors occur during the transcription process, from prescriber to clerk to pharmacist technician and pharmacist, to nurse, increasing the risk of error (Lehmann and Kim, 2006). Poor handwriting and errors in transcription account for many errors in administration, including delay in administration. Systems that rely on multiple transcriptions and "hand-offs" of written information increase the chance of an error in the transcription phase. In handwritten processes, each transcription is an opportunity for error (Lehmann and Kim, 2006). Errors related to similarly spelled drug names and similarly sounding drug names are common. Equally problematic are ambiguous abbreviations. The Joint Commission (2005) affirmed its Official "Do Not Use" List of abbreviations (see Table 18-2). Prior to dispensing medications, it is the responsibility of the pharmacist to review all orders confirming the name of the drug, patient, dose, quantity, directions for use, and route and time of administration.

(3) *Dispensing.* Control of drug preparation and dispensing is important in safeguarding children. Errors can arise from inadequate medication order review; incorrect pharmacy computer order entry; incorrect drug selection; preparation and labeling; wrong dose, patient route, and formulation; and failure to note allergies or contraindications. Wrong base solution or diluents are also an issue when preparing parenteral drugs as well as multiple preparation procedures (Lesar et al., 2006). Labeling and storage of look-alike and sound-alike drug names, or look-alike packaging coupled with frequent interruptions and distractions can lead to dispensing errors (Joint Commission, 2008). Pharmacist workload is another increased risk of dispensing a potentially unsafe medication (Malone et al., 2007). Ambiguous names, mistaken abbreviations, and miscommunication can also lead to adverse errors at this stage of the process.

(4) *Administration.* One third of all medication errors in the NICU occur at the point of drug administration (Suresh et al., 2004). Errors in the administration process could stem from administration to the wrong patient, incorrect administration technique, administration of expired drugs, incorrect preparation administered, or omission of a dose. Multiple distractions in the NICU, high workloads, and poor communication among health care providers can all lead to dosage calculation errors and delayed or missed drug administration. Errors in the route of administration, including IV infusions connected to nasogastric tubes have also been reported (Joint Commission, 2006). Unfamiliarity or inexperience of medications and infusion

■ BOX 18-2
■ **HIGH-ALERT MEDICATIONS**

- Insulin (subcutaneous and intravenous [IV])
- Concentrated potassium chloride injections
- Anticoagulants (e.g., heparin)
- Adrenergic agonists, IV (e.g., epinephrine, phenylephrine, norepinephrine)
- Adrenergic antagonists, IV (e.g., propranolol, metoprolol, labetalol)
- Anesthetic agents, general, inhaled, and IV (e.g., ketamine and propofol)
- Antiarrhythmics, IV (e.g., lidocaine and amiodarone)
- Dextrose, hypertonic, 20% or greater
- Hypertonic sodium chloride for injection (greater than 0.9% concentration)
- Inotropic medications, IV (e.g., digoxin and milrinone)
- Liposomal forms of drugs (e.g., liposomal amphotericin B)
- Moderate sedation agents, IV (e.g., midazolam)
- Moderate oral sedation agents, for children (e.g., chloral hydrate)
- Narcotics/opiates, IV, transdermal, and oral (e.g., fentanyl and morphine)
- Neuromuscular blocking agents (e.g., vecuronium, succinylcholine, rocuronium)
- Total parenteral nutrition solutions

Adapted from Institute for Safe Medication Practices: ISMP's high-alert medications. Available at www.ismp.org/tools/highalertmedications.pdf (accessed February 8, 2008).

devices along with poorly designed programming functions can also contribute to errors in administration.

b. High-alert medication: The ISMP created a list of high-alert medications that bear a heightened risk of causing significant patient harm (2007). The list provides health care professionals with specific medications that require special safeguards to reduce the risk of errors. Selected specific high-risk medications in the NICU (not an exhaustive list) are found in Box 18-2. The most commonly reported products to be associated with an error in the pediatric population are opioid analgesics (e.g., morphine and fentanyl), antimicrobial agents (gentamicin, vancomycin, and ceftriaxone), and antidiabetic agents (insulin) (Hicks et al., 2006).

(1) Selected safety measures to prevent high-alert medication errors
- Limiting access to the high-alert medications
- Special labeling of syringes and pumps infusing high-alert medications (e.g., color-coded)
- Standardize ordering, storage, preparation, and administration of products
- Double checking/redundancies mechanisms (automated or independent double checks)
- Smart pump technology
- System alerts
- Standard concentrations

c. Off-label medications (Conroy and McIntyre, 2005). Licensing procedures are performed to ensure the safety, effectiveness, and quality of medications. However, many medications intended to treat neonates are either prescribed outside the terms of the product license (off-label) or are not licensed (unlicensed) for this age group. Approximately 50% of medications prescribed in the NICU are used off label. Reference standards for doses of off-label and unlicensed medications are lacking and clinicians are faced with different published reference standards for a single medication. As a result of the limited range of licensed medications in appropriate dosage forms and the need for weight-based dosing in neonates, more calculations and dilutions are involved prior to administration compared with those required in adults, leading to an increased number of opportunities for errors (Chedoe et al., 2007).

   d. Selected medication improvement strategies:
- Instruct staff and practice mathematical calculations specific to neonates.
- Independently check calculations.
- Follow the 5 Rights of medication safety.
- Ensure medication reconciliation.
- Have a clinical pharmacist on the unit.
- Implement a CPOE/CDSS with "forcing functions" (functions that limit routes and frequencies of drugs that are ordered and are specific to neonates, such as weight in kilograms and age in days of life).
- Use barcode medication administration (BCMA) and automated drug-dispensing units (ADUs).
- Standardize all medication infusions.
- Order sets or preprinted orders.
- Avoid or eliminate dangerous abbreviations; spell out dosage units.
- Use TALLman lettering.
- Remove certain high-alert drugs from "ward stock" and require dispensing only by pharmacy.
- Restrict verbal order.
- Require double-checking by a second professional at each step of the medication process.
- Use a zero left of a dose less than 1 (e.g., use 0.1 rather than .1) and avoid trailing zero (e.g., use 1 rather than 1.0).
- Requirement for hand-off verification checks from one caregiver to the next for a patient receiving a high-alert drug infusion.
- Labeling precautions—labels on each medication dose should be specific to that single dose and contain all appropriate information. At a minimum, the label should include the patient name, room number, identification number, the medication's generic and trade names when applicable, dosage, route, frequency, and any alerts relating to the medication.
- Packaging—separate drugs that look or sound alike and reduce or eliminate the availability of multiple drug strengths.
- Drug standardization—all drugs should have a standardized order.
- Storage and stocking—limit the number of floor stock IV solutions. Remove all concentrated electrolytes from floor stock and never dispense them from the pharmacy.
- Use standardized abbreviations.
- Use standardized formulary.
- Ensure that the medication reference manual includes multiple dilutions of the same drug.
- Store neonatal doses away from adult doses.
- Increase the availability of dilute forms of drugs used in neonatal areas.
- Preferred use of "neonatal" intravenous pumps.

4. Health care–associated infections (nosocomial infections). (For detailed infectious disease information, see Chapter 34.)

   Health care–associated infections (HAIs) remain a major cause of morbidity, mortality, and cost for both adults and neonates despite concerted efforts of the Centers for Disease Control and Prevention (CDC) and infectious disease professionals (Klevens et al., 2007; Sharek et al., 2006; Siegel et al., 2007). An estimated 1.7 million HAIs occur in U.S. hospitals, of which 33,269 newborns in high-risk nurseries are affected (Klevens et al., 2007). Reducing the number of HAI is a Joint Commission National Patient Safety Goal (2008) (Table 18-1) and one of the 30 safe practices identified by the NQF (2006). Treatment of these infections have become more complex because of an alarming rise in antibiotic resistance. Multidrug-resistant organisms, including methicillin-resistant *Staphylococcus aureus* (MRSA) and vancomycin-resistant enterococci (VRE), and certain gram-negative bacilli (GNB) are problematic because they both are associated with increased mortality and their incidence has risen inexorably over the past decade. According to the CDC, MRSA now accounts for greater than 50% of hospital-acquired *S. aureus* infections, and there have been similar increases in VRE (Siegel et al., 2007). Selected improvement strategies have been effective in reducing the incidence of VAPs; however, additional prevention and surveillance efforts are needed along with strict adherence to these strategies in order to eliminate HAI.

a. **Central line–associated bloodstream infections (CLABSIs).** CLABSIs are primary bloodstream infections typically associated with the presence of a central line or an umbilical catheter in neonates at the time of or before the onset of the infection, resulting in an increased length of hospital stay, cost, and risk of mortality. Preterm infants are especially prone to infection, and the presence of a central line increases the odds of an infection; the longer the catheter duration, the higher the odds of an infection (Brady, 2005; Perlman et al., 2007). The most common organism associated with catheter-related sepsis is coagulase-negative *Staphylococcus*. Neonatal nurses can prevent CLABSI through proper central line management. Specific techniques are addressed in the CDC's *Guidelines for the Prevention of Intravascular Cather-Related Infections* (2002).

b. **Ventilator-associated pneumonia (VAP).** VAP is the second most common acquired HAI in the United States and is associated with significant morbidity and mortality (National Healthcare Safety Network [NHSN], 2006). VAP is a serious and common complication among intubated infants in the NICU, especially very low birth weight infants, and is associated with increased length of days in the NICU and death. Neonatal nurses can help eliminate VAPs by following the CDC's *Guideline for Prevention of Nosocomial Infections* (2003).

c. **Surgical site infections (SSIs).** SSIs are the third most common nosocomial infection among hospitalized patients and contribute greatly to the mortality and morbidity associated with surgery, resulting in longer hospital stays and higher costs (NHSN, 2006). Compounding the problem of SSIs are the increased acuity of in-hospital surgical patients and the increasing numbers of patients with MRSA and VRE, leading to a greater morbidity, mortality, and cost (Barnett, 2007). The CDC's guidelines for the prevention of SSI were published a decade ago (Mangram et al., 1999).

d. **Selected recommended improvement strategies reduce the risk of HAI.** The key to preventing transmission of organisms is highly correlated with the compliance rate to all practice interventions (Siegel et al., 2007). The majority of improvement strategies are taken from adult studies, and more research is needed to determine the effectiveness of these interventions in neonates.

- Educate health care workers about multidrug-resistant organisms, CLABSI, VAPs, and SSIs and the necessity of prevention.
- Educate families about basic infectious disease prevention, including the importance of adhering to hand hygiene practices and mode of transmission.
- Maintain strict adherence to hand hygiene practices and use of contact precautions.
- Implement a surveillance program to identify and track patients.
- Aim for aggressive detection of carriers. Measure infection rates, monitor compliance with best practices, and evaluate the effectiveness of prevention efforts.
- Share information with hospital senior leadership, physicians, nursing staff, and other clinicians.
- Employ NICU-based infectious disease personnel.
- Ensure rigorous isolation of colonized patients.
- Make sure that the environment and personal equipment are thoroughly disinfected.
- Elevate the head of bed to a 35- to 40-degree angle.
- Assess extubation readiness daily and the need for sedation.
- Ensure proper oral and ETT secretion care.
- Change the ventilator circuit of drained and accumulated condensed water.
- Evaluate central lines daily and remove nonessential catheters.
- Limit the number of times a central line is opened for access.

- Use a catheter checklist and a standardized protocol for central venous catheter insertion and daily maintenance (including routine cleaning and dressing changes).

5. **Unplanned extubations** (Veldman et al., 2006)

Unplanned endotracheal extubations requiring reintubation was in the top five of AEs reported using the NICU trigger methodology (Sharek et al., 2006). High-risk infants are at risk for hypoxia and hypercarbia with unintended extubation of the endotracheal tube (ETT), resulting in very dangerous and unsafe conditions and potentially a prolonged hospitalization. Limited data are available on the outcomes of unplanned ETT extubations in the NICU. Insufficient fixation of the ETT is reported as the primary rationale for unexplained ETT extubations followed by vigorous movement in the crib or incubator. However, limited evidence suggest that the majority of infants who experience unplanned ETT extubations do not require reintubation, signifying that many infants are remaining intubated who are ready for extubation. Additional research is needed to examine the relationship between unplanned ETT extubation and infant outcomes and potential strategies to reduce the incidence of unplanned ETT extubations.

a. Improvement strategies for unplanned extubations:
   - Frequently assess ETT stability.
   - Secure ETT (without over securing/taping).
   - Use two people when transferring or during excessive handling.
   - Avoid excessive jarring or movement of incubator or crib.

C. **Discharge safety instruction.** Proactively implementing a comprehensive formalized discharge process is recognized as one of the 30 safe practices outlined by the NQF to reduce readmissions, promote more satisfied and informed patients/families, and to promote better use of primary care services in the community after a hospital stay (NQF, 2006). Transitioning NICU families and their infants from hospital to home can be complex and challenging (Mills et al., 2006). Families need to be instructed on how to provide a safe environment at home (Forsythe and Kirchick, 2007). In addition to providing families with CPR instruction, immunization scheduling information, and developmental follow-up care, families also need to be aware of environmental and home safety precautions. Determining infant and family readiness for discharge and complete discharge instructions are provided in Chapter 19.

1. **Selected safety discharge topics** include the following:
   - *Medication reconciliation.* According to the Joint Commission's (2008) National Patient Safety Goals (Table 18-1), patients/families should be given a complete list of medications on discharge. The infant's primary care provider should also have a complete list of medications.
   - *Environmental checklist.* To assess patient/family safe home environment (water, electricity, heat, smoke detectors, phone, heat/air source, fire evacuation plan, etc.).
   - *Crib and furniture safety.* Parents should be alerted to standards of the Consumer Product Safety Commission and the importance of never leaving a baby unattended with the crib rails down.
   - *Home safety topics.* Topics should include, but are not limited to, car seat, bathing, medication storage, preparation, and administration (both for the neonate going home and for any other children at home), general baby care (including oral feeding), and emergency phone numbers (e.g., pediatrician, 9-1-1, or the Poison Control Center).
   - *Sudden infant death syndrome (SIDS) reduction strategies.* SIDS reduction strategies need to be included as part of families' discharge teaching. The majority of neonatal nurses are not providing specific back-to-sleep instructions and have identified a nonsupine position as the best position for hospitalized preterm infants (Aris et al., 2006). Neonatal nurses need to incorporate SIDS reduction strategies and safe sleep instructions into their discharge teaching for both term and preterm infants, especially because of the increased risk of SIDS among infants born preterm (AAP, 2005).
     a. Neonatal nurses need to model behavior practices prior to discharge.
     b. Place baby on a firm sleeping surface. No soft bedding, including sheepskin, pillows, stuffed animals, and other soft products should be in the crib.

   c. Avoid overheating; babies should be clothed for sleep with a bedroom temperature that is comfortable for an adult with a light layer of clothing.

   d. Avoid the use of sleep aid devices that are designed to keep babies in the side-lying position. There is no evidence to support the use of these devices and the prevention of SIDS. Consider using a sleeper or Halo SleepSack instead of blankets.

   e. Encourage a smoke-free environment.

   f. Avoid bed sharing. Babies should sleep in their own bed and in close proximity to their mother to promote breastfeeding.

Additional SIDS resources can be found at the National Institute of Child Health & Human Development (NICHD) at http://www.nichd.nih.gov/publications/pubs/safe_sleep_gen.cfm (Retrieved February 10, 2008) and the National Sudden Infant Death Resource Center at www.sidscenter.org (Retrieved February 10, 2008).

REFERENCES

Agency for Healthcare Research and Quality (AHRQ): 20 tips to help prevent medical errors in children. Patient fact sheet. Retrieved February 9, 2008, from www.ahrq.gov/consumer/20tipkid.htm

Alton, M., Frush, K., Brandon, D., and Mericle, J.: Development and implementation of a pediatric patient safety program. *Advances in Neonatal Care*, 6(3):104-111, 2006.

American Academy of Pediatrics: *The changing concept of sudden infant death syndrome: Diagnostic coding shifts, controversies regarding the sleep environment, and new variables to consider in reducing risk policy statement.* Washington, DC, 2005, American Academy of Pediatrics.

American Academy of Pediatrics and the Committee on Hospital Care (2003, reaffirmed): *Family-centered care and the pediatrician's role policy statement.* Washington, DC, 2007, American Academy of Pediatrics and the Committee on Hospital Care.

Aris, C., Stevens, T.P., Lemura, C., et al.: NICU nurses' knowledge and discharge teaching related to infant sleep position and risk of SIDS. *Advances in Neonatal Care*, 6(5):281-294, 2006.

Barnett, T.E.: The not-so-hidden cost of surgical site infections. *AORN Journal*, 86(2):249-256, 2007.

Benbow, D.W. and Kubiak, T.M.: *The certified Six-Sigma black belt handbook.* Milwaukee, WI, 2005, ASQ Quality Press.

Botwinick, L., Bisognano, M., and Haraden C.: *Leadership guide to patient safety. IHI Innovation Series white paper.* Cambridge, MA, 2006, Institute for Healthcare and Improvement.

Brady, M.T.: Health care-associated infections in the neonatal intensive care unit. *American Journal of Infection Control*, 33(5):268-275, 2005.

Brady, N. and Lewin, L.: Evidence-based practice in nursing: Bridging the gap between research and practice. *Journal of Pediatric Health Care*, 21(1):53-56, 2007.

Centers for Disease Control and Prevention: Guidelines for the prevention of intravascular catheter-related infections. *MMWR Morbidity and Mortality Weekly Report*, 51(No. RR-10):1-26, 2002.

Centers for Disease Control and Prevention: Guidelines for preventing health-care-associated pneumonia, 2003. Recommendations of CDC and the Healthcare Infection Control Practices Advisory Committee. *MMWR Morbidity and Mortality Weekly Report*, 53(No. RR-3): 2004.

Chedoe, I., Molendijk, H.A., and Dittrich, S.T.: Incidence and nature of medication errors in neonatal intensive care with strategies to improve safety. *Drug Safety*, 30(6):503-513, 2007.

Cimiotti, J.P., Haas, J.P., Saiman, L., et al.: Impact of staffing on bloodstream infections in the neonatal intensive care unit. *Archives of Pediatrics and Adolescent Medicine*, 160(8):832-836, 2006.

Cochran, G.L., Jones, K.J., Brockman, J., et al.: Errors prevented by and associated with bar-code medication administration systems. *Joint Commission Journal on Quality and Patient Safety*, 33(5):293-301, 2007.

Conroy, S., and McIntyre, J.: The use of unlicensed and off-label medicines in the neonate. *Seminars in Fetal and Neonatal Medicine*, 10(2):115-122, 2005.

Cuzzolin, L., Atzel, A., and Fanos, V.: Off-label and unlicensed prescribing for newborns and children in different settings: A review of the literature and a consideration about drug safety. *Expert Opinion on Drug Safety*, 5(5):703-718, 2006.

Dean, G., Scott, L., and Rogers, A.: Infants at risk: When fatigue jeopardizes quality care. *Advances in Neonatal Care*, 6(3):120-126, 2006.

Drenckpohl, D., Bowers, L., and Cooper, H.: Use of the Six Sigma methodology to reduce incidence of breast milk administration errors in the NICU. *Neonatal Network*, 26(3):161-166, 2007.

Dunn, M.S., Reilly, M.C., Johnston, A.M., et al.: Development and dissemination of potentially better practices for the provision of family-centered care in neonatology: The family-centered care map. *Pediatrics*, 188(Suppl 2):S95-S107, 2006.

Forsythe, P.L. and Kirchick, C.: Infant safety at home. *Advances in Neonatal Care*, 7(2):78-79, 2007.

Gray, J.E., Suresh, G., Ursprung, R., et al.: Patient misidentification in the neonatal intensive care unit: Quantification of risk. *Pediatrics*, 117(1):43-47, 2006.

Haig, K.M., Sutton, S., and Whittington, J.: A shared mental model for improving communication between clinicians. *Joint Commission Journal on Quality and Patient Safety*, 32(3):167-175, 2006.

Hicks, R.W., Becker, S.C., and Cousins, D.D.: Harmful medication errors in children: A 5-year analysis of data from USP's MEDMARX program. *Journal of Pediatric Nursing*, 21(4):290-298, 2006.

Hunt, E.A., Shilkofski, N.A., Stavroudis, T.A., et al.: Simulation: Translation to improved team performance. *Anesthesiology Clinics*, 25(2):301-319, 2007.

Husch, M., Sullivan, C., Rooney, D., et al.: Insights from the sharp end of intravenous medication errors: Implications for infusion pump technology. *Quality and Safety in Health Care*, 14(2):80-86, 2005.

Institute for Family-Centered Care: *Advancing the practice of patient- and family-centered care: How to get started*. Bethesda, MD, 2008, Author.

Institute for Safe Medication Practices: ISMP's list of high-alert medications. 2007. Retrieved February 8, 2008, from www.ismp.org/tools/highalertmedications.pdf

Institute of Medicine: *Crossing the quality chasm of national academies: Crossing the quality chasm*. Washington, DC, 2001, National Academies Press.

Institute of Medicine: *The learning healthcare system: Workshop summary*. Washington, DC, 2007, National Academies Press.

Institute of Medicine and the Committee on the Work Environment for Nurses and Patient Safety: In A. Page (Ed.): *Keeping patients safe: Transforming the work environment for nurse*. Washington, DC, 2004, National Academies Press.

Jagsi, R., Kitch, B.T., Weinstein, D.F., et al.: Residents report on adverse events and their causes. *Archives of Internal Medicine*, 265(22):2607-2613, 2005.

Jenkins, M.L., Hewitt, C., and Bakken, S.: Women's health nursing in the context of the national health information infrastructure. *Journal of Obstetric, Gynecologic and Neonatal Nursing*, 35(1):141-150, 2006.

Joint Commission: *National patient safety goals*. Oakbrook Terrace, IL, 2008, Joint Commission.

Joint Commission. Speak up initiatives. Retrieved February 9, 2008, from www.jointcommission.org/PatientSafety/SpeakUp/

Joint Commission: Tubing misconnections: A persistent and potential deadly occurrence. Sentinel Event Alert (Issue 36), 2006. Retrieved February 11, 2008, from www.jointcommission.org/SentinelEvents/SentinelEventAlert/

Joint Commission: Sentinel event Statistics. 2007. Retrieved February 15, 2008, from www.jointcommission.org/SentinelEvents/Statistics/

Joint Commission: The official "Do Not Use" list. 2005. Retrieved February 17, 2008, from www.jointcommission.org/PatientSafety/DoNotUseList

Joseph, A., and The Center for Health Design: *The role of the physical and social environment in promoting health, safety, and effectiveness in the healthcare workplace* (Issue paper #3). Concord, CA, 2006, Author.

Kane, R.L., Shamliyan, T., Mueller, C., et al.: Nurse staffing and quality of patient care. *Evidence Report/Technology Assessment*, 151: 1-115, 2007.

Kent, B. and Fineout-Overholt, E.: Teaching EBP: Part 1. Making sense of clinical practice guidelines. *Worldviews on Evidence-Based Nursing*, 4(2):106-111, 2007.

Kester, K., Baxter, J., and Freudenthal, K.: Errors associated with medications removed from automated dispensing machines using override function. *Hospital Pharmacy*, 41(6):535-537, 2006.

Kilbridge, P.M., Welebob, E.M., and Classen, D.C.: Development of the Leapfrog methodology for evaluating hospital implemented inpatient computerized physician order entry systems. *Quality and Safety in Health Care*, 15(2):81-84, 2006.

Klevens, R.M., Edwards, J.R., Richards, C.L., et al.: *Estimating healthcare-associated infections and Deaths in U.S. hospitals, 2002*. Atlanta, 2007, Centers for Disease Control and Prevention.

Kohn, L.T., Corrigan, J.M., and Donaldson, M.S.: *To err is human: Building a safer health system*. Washington, DC, 1999, National Academies Press.

Koppel, R., Metlay, J.P., Cohen, A., et al.: Role of computerized physician order entry systems in facilitating medication errors. *Journal of the American Medical Association*, 293(10):1197-1203, 2005.

Lehmann, C.U. and Kim, G.R.: Computerized provider order entry and patient safety. *Pediatric Clinics of North America*, 53(6):1169-1184, 2006.

Lesar, A., Mitchell, P., and Sommo, P.: Medication safety in critically ill children. *Clinical Pediatric Emergency Medicine*, 7(4):215-225, 2006.

Luria, J.W., Muething, S.E., Schoettker, P.J., et al.: Reliability science and patient safety. *Pediatric Clinics of North America*, 53(6):1121-1133, 2006.

McCartney, P.R.: Using technology to promote perinatal patient safety. *Journal of Obstetric, Gynecologic and Neonatal Nursing*, 35(3):424-431, 2006.

Malone, D.C., Abarca, J., Skrepnek, G.H., et al.: Pharmacist workload and pharmacy characteristics associated with dispensing of potentially clinically important drug-drug interactions. *Medical Care*, 45(5):456-462, 2007.

Mangram, A.J., Horan, T.C., Pearson, M.L., et al.: Guideline for prevention of surgical site infection. *American Journal of Infection Control Epidemiology*, 27(2):97-132, 1999.

Marx, D.: *Patient safety and the "Just Culture": A primer for health care executives*. Columbia University Press, 2001, New York. Retrieved February 11, 2008, from merstm.net/support/marx_primer.pdf

Massachusetts Coalition for the Prevention of Medical Error: *When things go wrong: Responding to adverse events*. Burlington, MA, 2006, Massachusetts Coalition for the Prevention of Medical Error.

Miller, M.R., Robinson, K.A., Lubomski, L.H., et al.: Medication errors in paediatric care: A systematic review of epidemiology and an evaluation of evidence supporting reduction strategy recommendations. *Quality and Safety in Health Care*, 16(2):116-126, 2007.

Mills, M.M., Sims, D.C., and Jacob, J.: Implementation and case-study results of potentially better practices to improve the discharge process in the neonatal intensive care unit. *Pediatrics*, 118(Suppl. 2):S124-S133, 2006.

Morriss, F.H.: Adverse medical events in the NICU: Epidemiology and prevention. *NeoReviews*, 9(1):e8-e22, 2008.

Musen, M.A., Shahar, E.H., and Shortliffe, E.H.: Clinical decision-support systems. In E.H. Shortliffe and J.J. Cimino (Eds.): *Biomedical Informatics: Computer applications in health and biomedicine* (3rd ed.). New York, 2006, Springer, pp. 698-736.

National Association of Neonatal Nurses: Bedside registered staff nurse shift length, fatigue, and impact on patient safety. Position Statement #3044. http://www.nann.org/pdf/810ps3044.pdf, August 28, 2008, pp. 1-5, Accessed December 14, 2008.

National Association of Neonatal Nurses and National Association of Neonatal Nurse Practitioners: Neonatal advanced practice nurses shift length, fatigue, and impact *on patient safety.* Position Statement #3043. *Advances in Neonatal Care,* 7(6):326-329, 2007.

National Healthcare Safety Network: *Patient safety component protocol.* Atlanta, 2006, Centers for Disease Control and Prevention.

National Patient Safety Foundation's Patient and Family Advisory Council: National agenda for action: Patients and families in patient safety; nothing about me, without me. Retrieved February 9, 2008, from www.npsf.org/paf/

National Quality Forum: *Safe practices for better healthcare: A consensus report.* Washington, DC, 2006, National Quality Forum.

Nebeker, J.R., Hoffman, J.M., Weir, C.R., et al.: High rates of adverse drug events in a highly computerized hospital. *Archives of Internal Medicine,* 165(10): 1111-1116, 2005.

Perlman, S.E., Saiman, L., and Larson, E.L.: Risk factors for late-onset health care-associated bloodstream infections in patients in neonatal intensive care units. *American Journal of Infection Control,* 35(3):177-182, 2007.

Pravikoff, D.S., Tanner, A.B., and Pierce, S.T.: Readiness of US nurses for evidence-based practice. *American Journal of Nursing,* 105(9):40-51, 2005.

Pronovost, P., Needham, D., Berenholtz, S., et al.: An intervention to decrease catheter-related bloodstream infections in the ICU. *New England Journal of Medicine,* 355(26):2725-2732, 2006.

Rakhmanina, N.Y. and van den Anker, J.N.: Pharmacological research in pediatrics: From neonates to adolescents. *Advanced Drug Delivery Reviews,* 58(1):4-14, 2006.

Roberts, V. and Perryman, M.M.: Creating a culture for health care quality and safety. *The Health Care Manager,* 26(2):155-158, 2007.

Sackett, D.L., Straus, S.E., Richardson, W.S., et al.: *Evidence-based medicine: How to practice and teach EBM.* Edinburgh, 2000, Churchill Livingstone.

Scott, L.D., Rogers, A.E., Hwang, W.T., et al.: Effects of critical care nurses' work hours on vigilance and patients' safety. *American Journal of Critical Care,* 15(1):30-37, 2006.

Sharek, P.J., Horbar, J.D., Mason, W., et al.: Adverse events in the neonatal intensive care unit: Development, testing, and findings of an NICU-focused trigger tool to identify harm in North American NICUs. *Pediatrics,* 118(4):1332-1340, 2006.

Shekelle, P.G., Morton, S.C., and Keeler, E.B.: *Costs and benefits of health information technology.* Evidence Report/Technology Assessment No. 132. Rockville, MD, 2006, AHRQ.

Siegel, J.D., Rhinehart, E., Jackson, M., et al.: *Guideline for isolation precautions: Preventing transmission of infectious agents in healthcare settings.* Surveillance. Atlanta, 2007, Centers for Disease Control and Prevention.

Smith, J.R., Donze, A., and Magliaro, B.: A tool for guiding clinical decisions. *Neonatal Network,* 26(1):63-69, 2007.

Snijders, C., van Lingen, R.A., Molendijk, A., et al.: Incidents and errors in neonatal intensive care: A review of the literature. *Archives of Disease in Childhood Fetal and Neonatal Edition,* 92(5):391-398, 2007.

Stucky, E.R., American Academy of Pediatrics Committee on Drugs, and American Academy of Pediatrics: Prevention of medication errors in the pediatric inpatient setting. *Pediatrics,* 112(2):431-436, 2003.

Sundar, E., Sundar, S., Pawlowski, J., et al.: Crew resource management and team training. *Anesthesiology Clinics,* 25(2):283-300, 2007.

Suresh, G., Horbar, J.D., Plsek, P., et al.: Voluntary anonymous reporting of medical errors for neonatal intensive care. *Pediatrics,* 113(6):1609-1618, 2004.

Thomas, E.J., Taggart, B., Crandell, S., et al.: Teaching teamwork during the Neonatal Resuscitation Program: A randomized trial. *Journal of Perinatology,* 27(7):409-414, 2007.

Ursprung, R., Gray, J.E., Edwards, W.H., et al.: Real time patient safety audits: Improving safety every day. *Quality and Safety in Health Care,* 14(4):284-289, 2005.

U.S. Department of Health and Human Services, Health Resources and Services Administration: The registered nurse population. Findings from the March 2004 National Sample Survey of Registered Nurses. 2006. Retrieved February 15, 2008, from http://bhpr.hrsa.gov/healthworkforce/rnsurvey04

Veldman, A., Trautschold, T., Weib, K., et al.: Characteristics and outcome of unplanned extubation in ventilated preterm and term newborns on a neonatal intensive care unit. *Pediatric Anesthesia,* 16(9):968-973, 2006.

White, R.D.: The physical environment of the neonatal intensive care unit: Implications for premature newborns and their care-givers. Business Briefing US Pediatric Care. 2005. Retrieved February 13, 2008, from www.touchbriefings.com/pdf/1268/White.pdf

Woodward, T.D.: Addressing variation in hospital quality: Is Six Sigma the answer? *Journal of Healthcare Management,* 50(4):226-236, 2005.

19 Discharge Planning and Transition to Home Care

PAT HUMMEL

OBJECTIVES

1. Describe current trends in the discharge of the high-risk infant.
2. Identify individualized clinical criteria for discharge.
3. Discuss the role of the family in the discharge of a high-risk infant
4. Describe discharge planning and the transition to home process for the high-risk neonate.
5. Identify discharge teaching needs for parents of a high-risk infant.
6. Identify key components of infant and family care postdischarge.

INTRODUCTION

Preterm birth rates have risen more than 20% since 1990. More than half a million babies—one of every eight—are born preterm each year, and the numbers have risen steadily. The National Center for Health Statistics released final birth data for 2005, showing that the preterm birth rate, the percentage of babies born at less than 37 weeks of gestation, is continuing to rise, with more than 525,000 babies, or 12.7%, born prematurely. The preterm birth rate has increased from 12.5% in 2004, and is projected to continue its upward trend and reach 12.8% or approximately 543,000 babies annually (Table 19-1).

- 71.2% are born between 34 and 36 weeks of gestation, and are termed late-preterm births.
- 13% are born between 32 and 33 weeks of gestation.
- 10% are born between 28 and 31 weeks of gestation.
- 6% are born at less than 28 weeks of gestation.
- The infant mortality rate fell to 6.8 deaths per 1000 live births in 2005, with prematurity the leading cause of death in the first month of life (Table 19-2).

Preterm birth cost the nation more than $26.2 billion in medical and educational costs and lost productivity in 2005. Average first-year medical costs were about 10 times greater for preterm than for term infants (Darmstadt et al., 2005; Kirkby et al., 2007). Many infants are discharged from the neonatal intensive care unit (NICU) with chronic conditions requiring ongoing medical care and increasing societal burden. Major morbidities tend to be highest in the smallest survivors (<1000 g at birth) and can include significant life-long conditions such as cerebral palsy, mental retardation, and visual or hearing loss (Wilson-Costello, 2007).

GENERAL PRINCIPLES

A. **Coordinated, comprehensive discharge planning with a safe transition to home is critical for the health and well-being of high-risk infants and their families.**
B. **Discharge planning begins on admission to the intensive care nursery and continues throughout the hospitalization.**
C. **An interdisciplinary team of skilled professionals ensures successful transition to home** (Box 19-1).
D. **Parent-infant relationships and family dynamics are altered by emotional and financial stressors.** Maternal depression is common and negatively affects the parent-child relationship (Beck, 2003).

■ TABLE 19-1
■ ■ **Percentage of Preterm Births: United States, Final 1990, 2000, and 2005; and Preliminary 2006**

Year	Preterm <37 weeks	Late Preterm 34 to 36 Weeks	32 to 33 Weeks	Very Preterm <32 weeks
2006	12.80	9.14	1.62	2.04
2005	12.73	9.09	1.60	2.03
2000	11.64	8.22	1.49	1.93
1990	10.61	7.30	1.40	1.92

Source: National Center for Health Statistics: Final natality data. Retrieved February 10, 2008, from www.marchofdimes.com/peristats.

■ TABLE 19-2
■ ■ **Birth Weight Specific Mortality, 2004**

Birth Weight	Mortality Rate Deaths/1000 Live Births
<500 g	849.56
500 to 749 g	480.49
750 to 999 g	155.91
1000 to 1249 g	67.81
1750 to 1999 g	45.11
2000 to 2249 g	27.35
2250 to 2499 g	11.01
2500 and over	2.26

Source: National Center for Health Statistics, final natality data. Retrieved February 10, 2008, from www.marchofdimes.com/peristats.

■ BOX 19-1
■ **MEMBERS OF INTERDISCIPLINARY DISCHARGE PLANNING/TRANSITION TO HOME TEAM**

Parents
Neonatologist/neonatal nurse practitioner (NNP)/resident/bedside nurse
Primary pediatrician
Subspecialty physicians and advanced practice nurses, as applicable
Primary nurse
Social worker
Discharge planning coordinator/case manager
Developmental assessment and early intervention/follow-up team member
Home care nurse
Infant-specific support services as needed: occupational or physical therapist, nutritionist, lactation
    support, respiratory therapist, pharmacist
Durable medical equipment representative

E. Parents, as the primary caregivers, must be educated to provide complex care for their infant and be empowered to advocate for their infant, facilitating transition to home and optimizing their child's health and development.

HEALTH CARE TRENDS

A. **Medical costs are rising rapidly.**
  1. The newborn period is a major source of uncompensated care and accounts for a high proportion of catastrophic cost cases, an increasing problem with the increased incidence and survival of premature infants (Kirkby et al., 2007).

2. Economic pressures, including equitable reimbursement for services, and the utilization of costly medical resources continue to be challenges health care systems face when caring for the very low birthweight (VLBW, <1000 g) infant in the hospital and home settings.

B. **Infants are discharged earlier from the NICU, requiring care of varying complexity, from nasogastric feedings, multiple medications, apnea monitors, and oxygen to ventilators, dialysis, and parenteral nutrition.**

C. **Infants are discharged with special needs on the premise that the home environment, as opposed to the hospital environment, is beneficial for the child and the family, and that health care costs will be decreased** (Hummel and Cronin, 2004).

D. **Early discharge of the VLBW infant can be accomplished in a safe and positive manner, benefiting the infant and family** (Sajous et al., 2007a, 2007b; Sturm, 2005).
   1. The infant must be physiologically stable before discharge.
   2. The parents must be able and willing to care for their infant in the home.
   3. Parental education must be complete before discharge, with parents demonstrating competency in the care of the infant.
   4. Skilled home nursing care by neonatal nurses contributes to the successful discharge of the high-risk infant. Sajous et al. (2007a, 2007b) describe an integrated neonatal home care program where preterm infants are discharged home safely to transition from nasogastric to oral feedings, and readmission rates were decreased for infants with bronchopulmonary dysplasia discharged with supplemental oxygen.

E. **Discharge planning includes the role of the case manager, whose roles include care coordination, utilization review, insurance reimbursement, and discharge planning.**

F. **Clinical pathways and care maps are effective tools for discharge planning and tracking outcomes.**

G. **NICU design is moving toward private rooms, enhancing family interaction and caregiving, facilitating preparation for discharge.**

H. **Electronic medical records are increasingly used, allowing improved documentation, retrieval, and interdisciplinary communication.**

I. **Evidence-based care is provided in the NICU and home care setting.**
   1. Resources include the Cochrane Neonatal Reviews, the Vermont-Oxford Network, and the National Institute of Child Health and Development (NICHD) Neonatal Research Group.
   2. Additional organizations that publish guidelines for transition of the preterm infant to home include the American Academy of Pediatrics (AAP); the National Association of Neonatal Nurses; Association of Women's Health, Obstetric and Neonatal Nurses; the March of Dimes; and the National Guideline Clearinghouse.

DISCHARGE CRITERIA MUST BE ESTABLISHED AND INDIVIDUALIZED TO THE INFANT AND FAMILY (BOX 19-2)

A. **Careful discharge planning, ensuring medical stability of the infant before discharge, is essential to the successful discharge and home care experience.** Medical stability is essential for a predetermined length of time before discharge. An infant that requires increasing support is not stable for discharge. Response to changes in care may not be apparent immediately in a child with a chronic illness; weaning and other major changes should not occur close to discharge.

B. **The required period of stability before discharge has not been studied or standardized.** Controversy and wide variations in practice exist in the apnea- or bradycardia-free length of time that an infant is observed before discharge (Hummel and Cronin, 2004; Zupancic et al., 2003). Discharge of a technology-dependent infant should be anticipated and planned, with the team agreeing on an end point and a stability point for discharge (Hummel and Cronin, 2004). Support should then be maintained and the infant prepared for discharge without changes.

C. **Assessment of the home and parental capabilities guide a safe discharge.** A multitude of factors contribute to the ability of a family to care for a medically complex infant in the home. Parent health, siblings, family support, financial difficulties, home facilities, proximity to

■ BOX 19-2
■ **INFANT READINESS FOR HOSPITAL DISCHARGE**

- Sustained pattern of weight gain of sufficient duration.
- Adequate maintenance of normal body temperature.
- Competent feeding by breast or bottle without cardiorespiratory compromise.
- Physiologic maturity and stable cardiorespiratory function of sufficient duration.
- Appropriate immunizations administered.
- Appropriate metabolic screening performed.
- Hematologic status assessed and appropriate therapy instituted if indicated.
- Nutrition risks assessed and therapy and dietary modifications instituted if indicated.
- Hearing evaluation complete.
- Funduscopic examinations complete.
- Neurodevelopmental and neurobehavioral status assessed and demonstrated to parents.
- Car seat evaluation complete.
- Review of hospital course complete, unresolved medical problems identified, plans for follow-up monitoring and treatment instituted.
- Home care plan developed.

From The American Academy of Pediatrics Committee on Fetus and Newborn: Hospital discharge of the high-risk neonate. *Pediatrics 122*(5):1119-1126, 2008.

health care, transportation options, child care or day care considerations, and other issues may prohibit discharge to the parent's home. Infant and parent needs must be balanced to achieve a safe discharge.

PARENTAL NEEDS AND ROLE IN THE DISCHARGE AND TRANSITION TO HOME PROCESS

A. **Parents need emotional support as they struggle to cope with the ups and downs and uncertainties that accompany parenting an ill newborn** (Eiser et al., 2005). Social work, pastoral care, and parent-to-parent support groups may benefit parents and should be tailored to meet the family's needs.

B. **Parenting an infant after discharge from the NICU presents many challenges, including multiple physician appointments, complex infant care, and the uncertainties of their infant's future** (Bakewell-Sachs and Gennaro, 2004; Hummel and Cronin, 2004). Effective interventions to promote mothering the high-risk infant include home nurse visits, skin-to-skin contact, individual infant-focused education and counseling, and theory-based group intervention (Gardner and Deatrick, 2006).

C. **Postpartum depression is common and exacerbated by mothering a high-risk infant** (Beck and Indman, 2005). NICU and home care nurses must remain vigilant, referring mothers for further care when depression is recognized (Beck, 2003).

D. **Cultural differences should be considered, as some cultures may expect that the infant stay in the hospital until the special needs are resolved.**

E. **The family is the constant in the infant's life and should be an active participant in care, starting at admission.** Continuing parental education involves assessment of knowledge and readiness to learn. Most parents desire an understanding of their infant's disease process and status. Caregivers should assist parents in learning their infant's behaviors and providing individualized care based on the responses (Heermann et al., 2005; Kleberg et al., 2007; Vandenberg, 2007; Westrup, 2007). Parents learn about parenting by observing caregivers and actively participating in their infant's care.

F. **Assessment of parental knowledge base and previous infant care experience contributes to an individualized teaching plan, established weeks prior to anticipated discharge.** Family educational, social, emotional, and financial needs must be assessed; discharge plans are individualized according to these needs (Giebe, 2007).

1. Barriers to parental learning and participation in care need to be assessed and resources identified to alleviate the barriers. Recognition of parental needs and addressing each area in the discharge plan will ease the transition to home. Current caregiver knowledge level is assessed prior to teaching sessions and each session is individualized according to the needs of the infant and family.

2. Learning experiences can be offered through hands-on care, demonstration of specific care practices, and verbal reinforcement. Information can be obtained from a variety of sources, including individual demonstration, group teaching sessions with other parents, published teaching tools, videos, written materials, and Internet resources.

G. **Parents are active participants in care conferences and involved in discharge planning.**

H. **Parents should contact and meet a health care provider in the community and make follow-up appointments prior to the infant discharge from the hospital.** The case manager, social worker, discharge coordinator, staff registered nurse, or advanced practice nurse can assist with the process.

I. **Parents should be provided an opportunity to care for their infant in an overnight/transition room prior to discharge.** This is particularly important when the care is complex or questions remain regarding parental capabilities in caring for the infant.

DISCHARGE PLANNING AND TRANSITION TO HOME

A. **Discharge planning begins at birth or when the infant's condition is no longer critical.**
   1. A long-term view of the infant's hospitalization is essential to discharge planning.
   2. A care map may assist in this process by cueing the team at specific intervals to plan for discharge.
   3. See Table 19-3 for planning for discharge with technology, related to complex medical issues.

B. **Discharge teaching should begin weeks prior to the projected discharge date.**
   1. Discharge education and home transition plans should be clearly outlined (see Fig. 19-1).
   2. Planning should include a timeline to complete parent education and all steps necessary for home transition.
   3. Written information regarding the infant's care should be provided, particularly with complex discharges (Menghini, 2005).

C. **Family members are active participants in the home transition plan.** Parents should participate in infant care from birth and are essential team members in the care of their infant.

D. **Discharge planning and the transition to home process requires a multidisciplinary approach.** Consistency in care providers is critical. Parents should be empowered to make decisions about their infant's care and discharge. The case manager, discharge planner, primary nurse, and social worker often coordinate the discharge process.

E. **Intermittent care conferences with the family throughout hospitalization ensure open communication, facilitating a smooth transition to home.** These can be formalized, including all team members, or simplified to include the parents and a few key team members.

F. **A comprehensive discharge-focused care conference should be completed several weeks prior to discharge.**
   1. Parents are encouraged to bring a list of questions and needs to the conference.
   2. All community providers should be invited to participate in the discharge care conference. If key personnel are unable to attend this conference, contact should be made to ensure that the practitioner is willing to care for the infant, and to communicate ongoing health issues and needs.
   3. Criteria for discharge are discussed and the teaching plan is reviewed. The anticipated course of recovery and ongoing problems are outlined, and the home care/durable medical equipment needs are discussed.
   4. Strategies to prevent rehospitalization are discussed (Smith et al., 2004).

G. **A comprehensive discharge summary including resolved and ongoing problems is given to the family on discharge, and sent to postdischarge caregivers.** See Box 19-3 for a list of

■ TABLE 19-3
■ ■ Planning for Discharge with Technology

Potential Technology	Stability Criteria	Diagnosis/Problem	Teaching Required	Home Nursing Needs	Supplemental Services
Oxygen Apnea Monitor Pulse Oximeter	Stable oxygen flow without changes for a defined number of days prior to discharge (varies from 5 to 10 days, per unit discretion)	BPD Other CLD	Signs or symptoms of respiratory distress Durable medical equipment CPR demonstration Medication administration	Intermittent skilled nursing visits	Occupational and physical therapy Speech therapy Nutrition
Nasogastric or gastrostomy tube feedings	Stable pattern of weight gain (15 to 30 g/day)	FTT Severe GERD Oral aversion	Nasogastric tube placement Gastrostomy tube care Tube feeds High caloric formula preparation Bolus (gravity feedings) Pump feedings	Intermittent skilled nursing visits	Speech therapy Nutrition
Apnea monitor	Free of apnea/bradycardia events requiring intervention, beyond gentle, tactile stimulation, for a defined number of days prior to discharge (varies from 2 to 7 days, per unit discretion)	Apnea of prematurity GERD Intrauterine growth restriction	Durable medical equipment CPR demonstration Medication administration Thickened formula as ordered Positioning	Intermittent skilled nursing visits	
Tracheostomy (with or without gastrostomy tube)	Stable oxygen requirement (room air or trach collar)	BPD Pierre–Robin syndrome Tracheomalacia Various disorders affecting airway competence	Signs or symptoms of respiratory distress Durable medical equipment CPR demonstration Medication administration Suction equipment Tracheostomy change	Private duty nursing (approximately 8 hours/day)	Speech therapy Occupational or physical therapy Respiratory therapy (usually provided by DME vendor)
Ventilator	Stable respiratory condition without changes in ventilator support* or medication for an agreed upon period prior to discharge (varies from 2 to 4 weeks, per unit discretion)	BPD Central hypoventilation	Signs or symptoms of respiratory distress Durable medical equipment CPR demonstration Medication administration Gastrostomy tube placement and feeds High caloric formula preparation Ventilator problem solving Ventilator setting adjustments	Private duty nursing (approximately 12 to 24 hours/day)	Occupational or physical therapy Speech therapy Respiratory therapy (usually provided by DME vendor) Nutrition Apply for handicap parking

BPD, Bronchopulmonary dysplasia; CPR, cardiopulmonary resuscitation; CLD, chronic lung disease; DME, durable medical equipment; FTT, failure to thrive; GERD, gastroesophageal reflux disease.
*Using a ventilator approved for in-home use.

NEONATAL DISCHARGE CHECKLIST

Things to do 1 week before discharge:

- Mother's maiden name _____

- Father's name _____

- Pediatrician's name and phone number _____
  **Remind parents with HMOs that they need a referral from their primary physician for
  any specialty appointments.
- Prescriptions (including for specialty formulas such as
  Neocate, Elecare, Pregestimil, Neosure, Enfacare) _____

- Car seat testing _____ • WIC form (if needed) _____
- Home health equipment (DME) form/order and training
  scheduled (by Case Manager or Social Worker) _____

Things to do 1–3 days before discharge:

- Blood pressure _____   • Head circumference _____

- Chest circumference _____   • Weight _____

- Length _____   • Newborn screen _____

- Appointments _____

- Home health referral (if needed) _____

- Discharge follow-up instructions _____

- Medication schedule _____

Things to do the day of discharge:

- Delayed infant discharge form
  (if infant is discharged home with mother) _____

- Release of patient to person other than natural mother form
  (if infant is discharged home without mother) _____

- EPIC discharge note _____

Things to send home with parents:

• Gift pack	• Discharge folder to include the following:
• Patient's belongings	☐ Discharge instructions
• Digital thermometer	☐ Scheduled appointments
• Bulb syringe	☐ Medication schedule
• Oral medication syringes	☐ Medication teaching sheets
• Additional supplies if necessary	☐ Formula preparation sheets
	☐ Completed immunization card
	☐ Admission and discharge summaries for parents
	☐ Additional teaching materials as needed

FIGURE 19-1 ■ Neonatal Discharge Checklist. (Copyright Loyola University Medical Center, Maywood, Illinois.)

information to be included in the summary. An electronic summary and information can be provided on a disc or flash drive for computerized use.

H. Infant care specifics to be completed prior to discharge including:

1. Parent and home evaluation, which may include a home visit if the infant has extensive needs.

2. Establish a realistic plan for care at home including feeding schedules, medication schedules, and treatments.

3. Medications: Provide prescriptions several days before discharge for parents to fill and bring to the hospital for verification and teaching.

   a. Some medications need to be compounded by the pharmacy and may not be immediately available.

■ BOX 19-3
■ **PERTINENT INFORMATION FOR PARENTS AND CARE PROVIDERS AT TIME OF DISCHARGE**

Comprehensive discharge summary, including resolved and ongoing problems
List of follow-up appointments with timing, location, and phone numbers specified
Immunizations given
RSV prophylaxis given
Written plan of care, particularly for complex discharge (could be electronic)
Medication schedule
Nutrition plan and formula recipe
Testing/imaging results: Head ultrasound, renal ultrasound, computed tomography (CT), electroencephalo-
    gram (EEG), electrocardiogram (ECG); echocardiogram, magnetic resonance imaging (MRI), other
    pertinent testing
Additional test results such as pneumograms, eye examination findings, hearing screen results, newborn
    metabolic/state screen results
Pertinent laboratory values: recent complete blood count with hematocrit, hemoglobin, and reticulocyte
    count, bone health, medication levels

b. Assess that the parent is able to afford the medication.
c. Ensure that the medication is ordered and filled with the correct concentration, and that the container is properly labeled. Problems also occur when the generic name is used on the bottle and the trade name is mentioned in the medication list—be sure names match, or provide both names.
d. Home medication doses should be rounded to the nearest $\frac{1}{10}$ (0.1) ml (except in extraordinary circumstances) to reduce the chance for error.
e. Verify that the medication label and instructions are documented in milliliters to be given, not with milligrams only.
f. Complete a medication sheet for home use, providing dosing and timing of each medication.

4. Feeding/formula (Cooke, 2007; Pridham et al., 2004).
   a. Facilitate acquisition of breast pump early in hospitalization.
   b. Encourage breastfeeding; provide lactation consultation to promote continued breast-feeding and/or pumping of breast milk (Isaacson, 2006; Vohr et al., 2006).
   c. Provide prescriptions for formulas well before discharge. Special formulas may be difficult to find in the store and may need to be ordered.
   d. Women, Infants, and Children (WIC) nutritional program may not provide special formulas, or may not provide enough formula for the infant's needs; this should be ascertained well before discharge.
   e. Assess the parent's ability to buy formula, especially expensive elemental formulas; provide assistance as needed with letters of necessity for payor coverage.

5. Primary care practitioner chosen and follow-up appointments are made.
6. Subspecialty appointments are made.
7. Home care agency/nursing care ordered and arranged.
8. Durable medical equipment ordered and teaching sessions arranged.
9. Arrange circumcision per parental choice.
10. Audiology testing.
11. Safe sleep practices are in place (see Box 19-4).
12. Car seat testing is completed (see Box 19-5).
13. Overnight stay in the transition room.
14. Respite care is explored, including strategies to deal with stress.
15. Emergency plan is formulated.

I. **Selection of a primary health care practitioner, home nursing agency, and durable medical equipment company that will meet the needs of the infant and the family.**
   1. The discharge team should ideally be able to recommend a primary health care practitioner who is willing and able to care for the infant's complex medical needs (Kelly, 2006b).

▨ BOX 19-4
▨ **SAFE SLEEP GUIDELINES**

1. Place infants to sleep on their backs, even though they may sleep more soundly on their stomachs. Infants who sleep on their stomachs and sides have a much higher rate of sudden infant death syndrome (SIDS) than infants who sleep on their backs.
2. Place infants to sleep in a baby bed with a firm mattress. There should be nothing in the bed but the baby—no covers, no pillows, no bumper pads, no positioning devices, and no toys. Soft mattresses and heavy covering are associated with the risk for SIDS.
3. Keep your baby's crib in the parents' room until the infant is at least 6 months of age. Studies clearly show that infants are safest when their beds are close to their mothers.
4. Do not place your baby to sleep in an adult bed. Typical adult beds are not safe for babies. Do not fall asleep with your baby on a couch or in a chair.
5. Do not overclothe the infant while it sleeps. Just use enough clothes to keep the baby warm without having to use cover. Keep the room at a temperature that is comfortable for you. Overheating an infant may increase the risk for SIDS.
6. Avoid exposing the infant to tobacco smoke. Don't have your infant in the same house or car with someone who is smoking. The greater the exposure to tobacco smoke, the greater the risk of SIDS.
7. Breastfeed babies whenever possible. Breast milk decreases the occurrence of respiratory and gastrointestinal infections. Studies show that breastfed babies have a lower SIDS rate than formula-fed babies do.
8. Avoid exposing the infant to people with respiratory infections. Avoid crowds. Carefully clean anything that comes in contact with the baby. Have people wash their hands before holding or playing with your baby. SIDS often occurs in association with relatively minor respiratory (mild cold) and gastrointestinal infections (vomiting and diarrhea).
9. Offer your baby a pacifier. Some studies have shown a lower rate of SIDS among babies who use pacifiers.
10. If your baby has periods of not breathing, going limp or turning blue, tell your pediatrician at once.
11. If your baby stops breathing or gags excessively after spitting up, discuss this with your pediatrician immediately.
12. Thoroughly discuss each of the above points with all caregivers. If you take your baby to daycare or leave him with a sitter, provide a copy of this list to them. Make sure they follow all recommendations.

Copyright American SIDS Institute, 2009, Marietta, Georgia.

▨ BOX 19-5
▨ **CAR SEAT GUIDELINES AND TESTING**

Discharge policies for newborns should include the following:
1. Determination of the most appropriate car safety seat for each newborn according to maturity and medical condition by a designated hospital employee.
2. Provision of information and training for parents and guardians should be presented before discharge on the generic issues related to correct use of car safety seats. Hands-on teaching including "return demonstration" should be a part of this instruction. The installation of a specific car seat in a specific car must be the parent's responsibility. Resources to address these issues are available from the AAP.
   ▪ A period of observation in a car safety seat before hospital discharge should be provided to each infant born at <37 weeks of gestation to monitor for possible apnea, bradycardia, or oxygen desaturation.

From American Academy of Pediatrics Committee on Injury and Poison Prevention: Safe transportation of newborns at hospital discharge. *Pediatrics, 104*(4):986-987, 1999.

Parental requests and third-party payor restraints should be equally considered in this process. Ideally, parents should meet with the primary health care practitioner before discharge. Identify home nursing needs—intermittent or private duty.

2. Plan home care after verification of third-party payor requirements and restraints.
3. Home care personnel should be familiar with the infant's medical issues, with skilled, experienced personnel available for home visitation. An example of a successful home care program in place for more than 10 years includes NICU nurses cross-trained to provide intermittent home care nursing visits (Sajous et al., 2007a, 2007b).
4. Criteria for selecting a durable medical equipment agency include (Gracey et al., 2004) the following:
    a. Third-party payor restraints.
    b. Availability of appropriate supplies.
    c. Ability to respond to emergencies.
    d. Availability of back-up equipment.
    e. Experience of care providers.
    f. Location of the agency.

J. **Discharge to an alternative setting may be necessary because of medical necessity, social problems, or family dynamics.** If the NICU and parents are unable to coordinate and complete the discharge process, transfer to an interim facility that routinely transitions children with special needs into the home, or a facility geographically closer to the parent may be optimal. Alternatives vary but can include specialized foster care, pediatric rehabilitation hospitals, pediatric nursing homes, or inpatient hospice care. Verify that the facility is able to provide care that meets the infant's needs.

NEONATAL TEACHING NEEDS

Teaching should be incorporated throughout the infant's stay. Written materials should be provided as much as possible, written at the sixth-grade reading level (Menghini, 2005). Teaching topics to be completed prior to discharge include the following:

A. **Back to sleep/safe sleep practices** (see Box 19-4).
B. **Car seat use.**
C. **Shaken baby syndrome prevention** (see Box 19-6).
D. **Basic infant care practices such as bathing, feeding, and diapering.**
E. **Medication teaching:**
    1. Observe the parent drawing up the medication.
    2. Provide a medication schedule, avoiding medication administration more than three times daily, and avoid nighttime dosing.
    3. Schedule medications carefully, as some medications cannot be mixed together or given concurrently.
F. **Formula/feeding teaching:**
    1. Observe the parent mixing the formula—verify that the parent has correct measuring cups/spoons, blender, pitcher; these may need to be provided.
    2. Written recipes for mixing formulas should be provided.
    3. Observe parent feeding the infant, oral or by nasogastric or gastrostomy tube (Gracey and Morton, 2002; Thomas, 2007).
G. **Home oxygen teaching** (Gracey et al., 2003):
    1. Hospital flow is usually in decimals (0.25 l/minute), home flow meters are in fractions ($\frac{1}{4}$ l/minute). Clarify hospital flow rate and verify in the home. Oxygen flow in the hospital should be rounded up to the next home flowmeter setting; increase, rather than decrease the oxygen flow in the home.
    2. Increased flow may be needed in the home because of the long tubing, or when using a concentrator since the output is of slightly lower concentration than that from the tank.
    3. Clarify that the parent knows how to adjust oxygen in case of an emergency; parents may think that they are increasing the oxygen when they are turning the flow $\frac{1}{2}$ to $\frac{1}{4}$ l/minute, since the denominator number is larger.

■ BOX 19-6
■ **SHAKEN BABY PREVENTION**

WHAT IS SHAKEN BABY SYNDROME?

When a baby is vigorously shaken, the head moves back and forth. This sudden whiplash motion can cause bleeding inside the head and increased pressure on the brain, causing the brain to pull apart and resulting in injury to the baby. This is known as shaken baby syndrome and is one of the leading forms of fatal child abuse. A baby's head and neck are susceptible to head trauma because his or her muscles are not fully developed and the brain tissue is exceptionally fragile. Head trauma is the leading cause of disability among abused infants and children.

Shaken baby syndrome occurs most frequently in infants younger than 6 months of age, yet can occur up to the age of 3. Often there are no obvious outward signs of inside injury, particularly in the head or behind the eyes. In reality, shaking a baby, if only for a few seconds, can injure the baby for life. These injuries can include brain swelling and damage, cerebral palsy, mental retardation, developmental delays, blindness, hearing loss, paralysis, and death. When a child is shaken in anger and frustration, the force is multiplied 5 or 10 times than it would be if the child had simply tripped and fallen.

HOW DOES IT HAPPEN?

Often frustrated parents or other persons responsible for a child's care feel that shaking a baby is a harmless way to make a child stop crying. The number one reason a baby is shaken is because of inconsolable crying. Almost 25% of all babies with shaken baby syndrome die. It is estimated that 25% to 50% of parents and caretakers are not aware of the effects of shaking a baby.

WHAT CAN YOU DO TO PREVENT A TRAGEDY?

If you or someone else shakes a baby, either accidentally or on purpose, call 9-1-1 or take the child to the emergency room immediately. Bleeding inside the brain can be treated. Immediate medical attention will save your baby many future problems . . . and possibly the baby's life.

OTHER SUGGESTIONS FOR PARENTS

Never throw or shake a baby	Always provide support for the baby's head and neck	Place the baby in a crib, leave the room for a few minutes	Sit down, close your eyes and count to 20
Take the baby for a stroller ride	Play music, or sing to the baby	Ask a friend to "take over" for a while	Do not pick the baby up until you feel calm
Make sure the baby is fed, burped, and dry	Gently rock or walk the baby	Check for discomfort of diaper rash, teething, or fever	Call the doctor if you think the baby is sick
Make sure clothing is not too tight	Give the baby a pacifier	Offer a noisy toy or rattle	Hug and cuddle the baby gently

National Exchange Club Foundation: *National shaken baby syndrome campaign.* Available at www.preventchildabuse.com/sbs/shtml. Accessed January 14, 2009 ⊛**EXCHANGE**.

H. **Apnea monitor teaching:**
   1. Monitor use, troubleshooting.
   2. Alarm response and CPR.
   3. Parents may remove the monitor when they are directly attending to the infant.
I. **Specialized teaching topics such as tracheostomy care, suctioning, ventilator, ostomy care, central line care, feeding alternatives, and any special equipment** (Fiske, 2004).
J. **Anticipatory guidance, educating parents regarding expectations postdischarge and tips on adapting to home** (see Box 19-7).
K. **Infection prevention** (see Box 19-8).
L. **Infant temperament, developmental tasks, and milestones reviewed, including sleep patterns, feeding patterns, and infant state regulation.**
M. **Care issues such as vaccinations, traveling, and visitors should be reviewed.**

■ BOX 19-7
■ **TIPS FOR PARENTS**

HOME READINESS FOR SPECIAL-NEEDS INFANT
Place for infant to sleep safely
Car seat
Heat, electricity, telephone, running water
Normal baby supplies: diapers, clothing, bottles
Formula, measuring cups and spoons, blender, pitcher
Medications and syringes
Equipment—monitor, oxygen, etc.
Emergency phone numbers and plan
Flashlight with extra batteries
Thermometer and bulb syringe (provided on discharge)
Pediatrician appointment arranged within 1 week
Other appointments made before discharge

TAKE CARE OF YOURSELF
Ask for help, from family, friends, and health care providers
Depression is common, get treatment—you want to be the best parent you can be
Enjoy your infant

INFANT ADJUSTING TO THE HOME
Realize that your baby will notice a difference in surroundings
Try to get into a routine
The baby may sleep better initially if there is a constant background noise (fan, soft music). Try to gradually lower the volume until your baby can sleep without noise.
Put your baby in bed when awake, when possible; allow him or her to learn how to get himself or herself to sleep rather than depending on you. This will help him or her sleep through the night.
Some babies cry more in the evening because they have received too much stimulation during the day—try decreasing the noise.

HELPING YOUR INFANT GROW AND DEVELOP
Hold your baby and respond to cries. Do not hold your baby constantly. Short periods of crying are fine if he or she is not hungry, or needs other attention. This helps your baby learn that you are there for him or her, but that she or he can also calm herself or himself.
Talk to your baby often.
Read books to your baby.
Turn off the television and videos—these hurt your baby's ability to pay attention for longer periods, and decrease their ability to calm themselves. Children should not watch TV until they are 2 years old.
Get therapies for your baby as the NICU or care provider recommends. Many infants need extra help for development. Therapies help your baby to develop the best they can, and therapy keeps your baby from developing or keeping abnormal developmental skills.
Avoid walkers, exersaucers, jumpers. These place a baby upright before they are ready and keep the baby from developing normally.
Babies need as much time as possible on their tummy, on a firm surface (playpen, floor), when they are awake and you are with them.
Make feeding time pleasant. Do not force-feed your baby. Ask for help if you have problems feeding your baby.

WEB SITES FOR PARENTS
www.tracheostomy.com
www.preemies.org
www.preemie-l.org
www.prematurity.org

■ BOX 19-8
■ **INFECTION PREVENTION AFTER DISCHARGE**

Routine infant immunizations
Respiratory syncytial virus (RSV) protection: monthly injections November through March for certain
  preterm infants
Influenza injections: for infants more than 6 months old, given in the fall in 2 doses 1 month apart
Influenza injections: for all caregivers, all people in the home
Handwashing—the best method to prevent infection
Disinfectant hand gels used by caregivers
Avoid contact with ill people, especially children

FAMILY AND INFANT CARE POSTDISCHARGE (see Box 19-9)

A. **A successful discharge plan and transition to home facilitates collaborative care postdischarge.**
  1. Encourage the parents to choose a pediatrician or health care provider that has experience with the ongoing problems of premature infants (Kelly, 2006a). Coordination of care is essential for infants with complex medical needs and should be approached comprehensively and systematically.
  2. Primary health care provider and specialty follow-up appointments need to be coordinated and scheduled without conflicts, with the infant and family in mind. Medically complex infants can have four or more specialist appointments in addition to a primary care provider.
  3. Transportation should be planned for visits to the primary provider and subspecialists after discharge.
  4. Ongoing assessment and assistance with family financial needs should be addressed before discharge, with referrals to the appropriate agencies (i.e., WIC, Social Security, state governmental assistance, private charities). Families should be aware of community resources available to them, such as early intervention services, case management services, counseling, and transportation assistance. Volunteer agencies, local and national parent support groups, and Internet resources may be recommended, as appropriate.
  5. Immunizations, including respiratory syncytial virus (RSV) prophylaxis are arranged for postdischarge care.
  6. Routine follow-up phone calls after discharge from the NICU can help with the transition and improve the discharge process as identified problems are addressed.
B. **Home care nursing may include intermittent home visits or in-home care for infants requiring complex around-the-clock care.**
  1. Transition from high-tech hospital setting to home environment may be facilitated by home care nursing.
  2. It is helpful if the home care nurse has met with the parents and infant before hospital discharge.
  3. The home care nurse reinforces the teaching and clarifies discharge instructions as needed.
  4. Intermittent home care is useful for infants that are medically stable, with parents able to provide care 24 hours a day without in-home direct nursing care. The home nurse assesses the infant, educates the parent, monitors medications and feedings, and communicates with the medical provider and the payor. Status updates are provided to the medical provider and a plan of care is formed in conjunction with the multidisciplinary team. The nurse assesses responses to changes in care on subsequent visits. Intermittent nursing visits conclude when the parent is independent with care and when the infant is stable medically and nutritionally, is not home-bound, and does not require frequent monitoring.
  5. Continuous in-home nursing care is another form of home care reserved for infants with complex needs that the parents cannot manage 24 hours a day. Continuous nursing care is usually required for infants with a tracheostomy or home ventilation, or an infant requiring

■ BOX 19-9
■ **PREMATURITY-RELATED PROBLEMS THAT PRESENT OR CONTINUE AFTER DISCHARGE**

RESPIRATORY
Ongoing oxygen dependency
Apnea
Reactive airway disease
Infections

CARDIAC
Right ventricular hypertrophy
Cor pulmonale/pulmonary hypertension
Uncorrected congenital heart disease with cyanosis and/or congestive heart failure

GASTROINTESTINAL
Emesis
Gastroesophageal reflux
Constipation
Strictures and bowel obstruction
Hernias (umbilical and inguinal)

NUTRITIONAL
Slow growth
Weight less than the 10th percentile on preterm growth curve
Feeding fatigue
Oral aversion
Need for nutritional supplements or hypercaloric formula
Need for adjunct feeding devices (e.g., tube feeding or gastrostomy)

HEMATOLOGIC
Anemia

DENTITION
Delayed tooth eruption
Altered oral and dental structures with arched palate secondary to dolichocephaly, exacerbated by pro-
    longed oral intubation
Enamel defects

SENSORY
Visual deficits secondary to retinopathy of prematurity (ROP): myopia, hyperopia, blindness
Strabismus and amblyopia
Hearing deficits
Speech and language delays
Hydrocephalus, ongoing shunt problems, such as infection and blockage

CENTRAL NERVOUS SYSTEM AND NEURODEVELOPMENTAL DIFFERENCES
Difficult temperament and behavior
Sensory integration problems
Tone and movement abnormalities
Cerebral palsy
IQ deficiencies
Learning disabilities
Attentional deficits
School problems

constant monitoring or care owing to special medical or nursing needs. Continuous nursing care may be provided 24 hours a day, or in shorter segments as needed. Twenty-four-hour-per-day nursing care is rarely possible because of financial and staffing constraints.

6. The primary long-term goal of home care nursing is to foster independence. This is achieved by educating the parent and by facilitating resource use and support services.

C. **Links to community agencies and resources facilitate coping with the changing needs of the child.** These links can start before discharge and are facilitated by the home care nurse and the primary provider.

D. **Problems related to prematurity often continue after discharge from the NICU** (Gracey et al., 2003). Hospital readmissions are not uncommon. Parents need education to recognize risk factors leading to readmission to the hospital and for the potential for ongoing problems (Kelly, 2006a, 2006b).

E. **Neurologic, developmental, neurosensory, and functional morbidities increase with decreasing birth weight.** Risk factors significantly associated with increased neurodevelopmental morbidity include a complicated NICU course, intracranial hemorrhage or cysts, and ongoing chronic illnesses such as BPD (Broitman et al., 2007; Kobaly et al., 2008). Preterm infants have a higher incidence of cerebral palsy, mental retardation, disorders of cortical function, including language disorders, visual perception problems, attention deficits, and learning disabilities. In addition, virtually all infants less than 1000 g at birth have weights at less than the 10th percentile at 36 weeks of postmenstrual age. Particular attention needs to be focused on postnatal growth and developmental assessment postdischarge.

F. **Referrals to a developmental follow-up clinic and to the state early intervention program are essential components of follow-up care.** Follow-up clinics often have criteria that qualify the infant for inclusion, such as gestational age, birth weight, neurologic abnormalities, or other risk factors. The goals of the follow-up clinic include early identification of developmental disability, parent counseling (anticipatory guidance), and identification and treatment of medical complications. Clinics are usually staffed by a multidisciplinary team of professionals, including physician, nurse practitioner, occupational therapist, physical therapist, audiologist, psychologist, ophthalmologist, speech and language specialist, respiratory therapist, nutritionist, neurologist, or subspecialists. The first visit usually occurs 1 to 4 months after discharge; follow-up continues for months to years. The goals of a follow-up program may include the following:

1. Developmental assessment, screening and/or diagnostic, is essential for the infant's well-being and for evaluation of NICU outcomes.
2. Management of sequelae.
3. Consultant follow-up assessment.
4. Parent support.

REFERENCES

American Academy of Pediatrics Committee on Fetus and Newborn: Hospital discharge of the high-risk neonate—proposed guidelines. *Pediatrics, 102*(2 Pt 1):411-417, 1998.

Bakewell-Sachs, S. and Gennaro, S.: Parenting the post-NICU premature infant. *MCN American Journal of Maternal Child Nursing, 29*(6):398-403, 2004.

Beck, C.T.: Recognizing and screening for postpartum depression in mothers of NICU infants. *Advances in Neonatal Care, 3*(1):37-46, 2003.

Beck, C.T., and Indman, P.: The many faces of postpartum depression. *JOGNN—Journal of Obstetric, Gynecologic, and Neonatal Nursing, 34*(5):569-576, 2005.

Broitman, E., Ambalavanan, N., Higgins, R.D., et al.: Clinical data predict neurodevelopmental outcome better than head ultrasound in extremely low birth weight infants. *Journal of Pediatrics, 151*(5):500-505, 2007.

Cooke, R.J.: Postdischarge nutrition of preterm infants: More questions than answers. *Nestle Nutrition Workshop Series. Paediatric Programme, 59*:213-224; discussion 224-228, 2007.

Darmstadt, G.L., Bhutta, Z.A., Cousens, S., et al.: Evidence-based, cost-effective interventions: How many newborn babies can we save? *Lancet, 365*(9463):977-988, 2005.

Eiser, C., Eiser, J.R., Mayhew, A.G., and Gibson, A.T.: Parenting the premature infant: Balancing vulnerability and quality of life. *Journal of Child Psychology & Psychiatry & Allied Disciplines, 46*(11):1169-1177, 2005.

Fiske, E.: Effective strategies to prepare infants and families for home tracheostomy care. *Advances in Neonatal Care, 4*(1):42-53, 2004.

Gardner, M.R. and Deatrick, J.A.: Understanding interventions and outcomes in mothers of infants. *Issues in Comprehensive Pediatric Nursing, 29*(1):25-44, 2006.

Giebe, J.M.: Safe discharge for infants with high-risk home environment. *Advances in Neonatal Care, 7*(4):167-172, 2007.

Gracey, K., Hummel, P., and Cronin, J.: Family teaching toolbox. Choosing a home care provider. *Advances in Neonatal Care, 4*(6):365-366, 2004.

Gracey, K. and Morton, J.A.: Family teaching toolbox. Guide for breastfeeding your premature baby at home. *Advances in Neonatal Care, 2*(5):283-284, 2002.

Gracey, K., Talbot, D., Lankford, R., and Dodge, P.: Family teaching toolbox. Nasal cannula home oxygen. *Advances in Neonatal Care, 3*(2):99-101, 2003.

Heermann, J.A., Wilson, M.E., and Wilhelm, P.A.: Mothers in the NICU: Outsider to partner. *Pediatric Nursing,* 31(3):176-181, 2005.

Hummel, P., and Cronin, J.: Home care of the high-risk infant. *Advances in Neonatal Care,* 4(6):354-364, 2004.

Isaacson, L.J.: Steps to successfully breastfeed the premature infant. *Neonatal Network,* 25(2):77-86, 2006.

Kelly, M.M.: The medically complex premature infant in primary care. *Journal of Pediatric Health Care,* 20(6):367-373, 2006a.

Kelly, M.M.: Primary care issues for the healthy premature infant. *Journal of Pediatric Health Care,* 20(5):293-299, 2006b.

Kirkby, S., Greenspan, J.S., Kornhauser, M., and Schneiderman, R.: Clinical outcomes and cost of the moderately preterm infant. *Advances in Neonatal Care,* 7(2):80-87, 2007.

Kleberg, A., Hellstrom-Westas, L., and Widstrom, A. M.: Mothers' perception of newborn individualized developmental care and assessment program (nidcap) as compared to conventional care. *Early Human Development,* 83(6):403-411, 2007.

Kobaly, K., Schluchter, M., Minich, N., et al.: Outcomes of extremely low birth weight (<1 kg) and extremely low gestational age (<28 weeks) infants with bronchopulmonary dysplasia: Effects of practice changes in 2000 to 2003. *Pediatrics,* 121(1):73-81, 2008.

Menghini, K.G.: Designing and evaluating parent educational materials. *Advances in Neonatal Care,* 5(5):273-283, 2005.

National Association of Neonatal Nurses: *Discharge guidelines for the technology dependent infant.* Unpublished manuscript, Glenview, IL, 1999.

Pridham, K., Saxe, R., and Limbo, R.: Feeding issues for mothers of very low-birth-weight, premature infants through the first year. *Journal of Perinatal & Neonatal Nursing,* 18(2):161-169, 2004.

Sajous, C.H., Chybik, M.F., and Weiss, M.G.: *Can infants be discharged home earlier from the neonatal intensive care unit without increasing their readmission?* Paper presented at the Pediatric Academic Societies' Annual Meeting, Toronto, Canada, 2007a.

Sajous, C.H., Chybik, M.F., and Weiss, M.G.: *Safety of home nasogastric feedings for healthy premature infants.* Paper presented at the Pediatric Academic Societies' Annual Meeting, Toronto, Canada, 2007b.

Smith, V.C., Zupancic, J.A., McCormick, M.C., et al.: Rehospitalization in the first year of life among infants with bronchopulmonary dysplasia. *Journal of Pediatrics,* 144(6):799-803, 2004.

Sturm, L.D.: Implementation and evaluation of a home gavage program for preterm infants. *Neonatal Network—Journal of Neonatal Nursing,* 24(4):21-25, 2005.

Thomas, J.A.: A parent's guide to bottle feeding your premature baby. *Advances in Neonatal Care,* 7(6):319-320, 2007.

Vandenberg, K.A.: Individualized developmental care for high risk newborns in the NICU: A practice guideline. *Early Human Development,* 83(7):433-442, 2007.

Vohr, B.R., Poindexter, B.B., Dusick, A.M., et al.: Beneficial effects of breast milk in the neonatal intensive care unit on the developmental outcome of extremely low birth weight infants at 18 months of age. *Pediatrics,* 118(1):e115-e123, 2006.

Westrup, B.: Newborn individualized developmental care and assessment program (NIDCAP)—Family-centered developmentally supportive care. *Early Human Development,* 83(7):443-449, 2007.

Wilson-Costello, D.: Is there evidence that long-term outcomes have improved with intensive care? *Seminars in Fetal and Neonatal Medicine,* 12(5):344-354, 2007.

Zupancic, J.A., Richardson, D.K., O'Brien, B.J., Eichenwald, E.C., and Weinstein, M.C.: Cost-effectiveness analysis of pre-discharge monitoring for apnea of prematurity. *Pediatrics,* 111(1):146-152, 2003.

20 Genetics: From Bench to Bedside

JULIEANNE SCHIEFELBEIN

OBJECTIVES

1. Define birth defects and possible causes.
2. Become familiar with genetic terminology.
3. Identify the number of chromosomes in a normal human cell.
4. Describe the characteristics and causes of structural and numeric chromosomal abnormalities, modes of inheritance of single-gene disorders, and multifactorial inheritance.
5. Describe what prenatal diagnostic tests are available and which anomalies they detect.
6. Describe the components and benefits of genetic counseling.
7. Identify three patient care management issues in genetic counseling.
8. Verbalize the systematic process used to evaluate the malformed infant.
9. List common congenital malformations and possible mechanisms of cause.

The neonate born with a genetic defect or fetal anomaly presents a challenge to the neonatal intensive care unit (NICU) team. A definitive diagnosis is essential for management and care of the neonate and the neonate's family.

Congenital malformations commonly have multiple causes. This chapter includes information on basic genetics, characteristics, and causes of some common fetal anomalies, and a systematic process for the evaluation of the malformed infant. Commonalities of patient care management issues are addressed, with the understanding that every family requires individualized care.

BASIC GENETICS

Terminology

A. **Allele:** one of a series of alternate forms of a gene at the same locus on a chromosome (Jones, 2005; Jorde et al., 2005).
B. **Autosome:** one of 22 chromosomes that do not determine the sex of the individual.
C. **Birth defect:** an abnormality of structure, function, or metabolism, whether genetically determined or a result of environmental interference during embryonic or fetal life. A congenital defect may cause disease from the time of conception through birth or later in life (March of Dimes Foundation, 2006).
D. **Chromosome:** structural elements in a cell nucleus that carry the genes and convey genetic information.
   1. Each cell (except erythrocytes) in the body contains all the chromosomes received from both parents within its nucleus.
   2. There are 23 pairs of chromosomes, for a total of 46 chromosomes, with one maternal and one paternal chromosome creating each pair.
E. **Diploid:** containing a set of maternal and a set of paternal chromosomes, for a total of 46 chromosomes.
F. **Gamete:** one of two cells, containing 23 chromosomes (haploid number), with the union of a male gamete and a female gamete required during sexual production to create a new individual (with the diploid number of chromosomes).

G. **Gene:** the smallest unit of inheritance of a single characteristic, responsible for a physical, biochemical, or physiologic trait and located with other genes in linear sequence along the chromosome.

H. **Genotype:** hereditary composition of an individual.

I. **Haploid:** having half the number of chromosomes found in the person's cells; characteristic of the gametes.

J. **Locus:** the position that the gene occupies on a chromosome.

K. **Karyotype:** pictorial representation of the chromosomal characteristics of an individual or species.

L. **Penetrance:** The degree to which an inherited trait is manifested in the person who carries the affected gene (Nussbaum et al., 2007).

M. **Sex chromosomes:** the X and Y chromosomes, which are responsible for sex determination—XX for female and XY for male.

Dominance and Recessiveness

A. **Phenotype:** observable characteristics of an individual.

B. **Heterogeneous chromosomes:** differing pair of chromosomes, one from each parent, arraying differing genes for specific traits. When there are unlike genes on a locus, one gene dominates.

C. **Homologous chromosomes:** a matched pair of chromosomes, one from each parent, carrying the genes for the same traits.

D. **Dominant gene:** a gene that is expressed in the heterozygous state. In a dominant disorder, the mutant gene overshadows the normal gene. A dose of this gene is needed for expression.

E. **Recessive gene:** a gene whose effect is masked or hidden unless both genes of a set of homologous chromosomes at a given locus are abnormal, thus showing the disease. In a heterozygote (carrier), the normal gene overshadows the mutant gene.

F. **Possible combinations of chromosomes.**
   1. Both genes can be dominant—AA (homozygous).
   2. Both genes can be recessive—aa (homozygous).
   3. One gene can be dominant and one can be recessive—Aa (heterozygous).

Autosomal Disorders Total 13,807 (OMIM, 2003)

A. **Autosomal dominant disorders.**
   1. Characteristics of autosomal dominant disorders.
      a. Males and females are both affected equally; either parent can pass the gene on to sons or daughters.
      b. An affected offspring has an affected parent if the mutation is not new.
      c. Half the sons and half the daughters of an affected parent can be anticipated to have the disorder. There is a 50% chance with each pregnancy.
      d. Unaffected offspring of an affected parent will have all normal offspring if the mate is an unaffected person (assuming complete penetrance).
      e. If two affected people mate, three fourths of their offspring will be affected. A double dose of the mutant gene in any of the offspring will result in a lethal anomaly (except in the case of Huntington disease).
      f. Family history of an anomaly indicates a vertical route of transmission through successive generations on one side of the family (if not a new mutation).
   2. Examples of autosomal dominant disorders: myotonic dystrophy, neurofibromatosis, and coronary artery disease (Allanson and Cassidy, 2005; Jones, 2005).

B. **Autosomal recessive disorders.**
   1. Characteristics of autosomal recessive disorders.
      a. Both males and females are affected equally.
      b. Parents of affected offspring are rarely affected and are usually heterozygous carriers.

    c. After the birth of an affected offspring, there is a 25% chance, with each pregnancy, of having another affected offspring and a 50% chance that the offspring will be a carrier.

    d. There may be a distant relative with the disorder.

    e. Affected people who mate with unaffected people will have offspring who will be heterozygous carriers.

    f. If two affected people mate, all offspring will be affected.

    g. No family history indicates a horizontal route of transmission in the same generation.

    h. There can be a difference in expression of the disorder: very mild in one member and extremely severe in another.

  2. Examples of autosomal recessive disorders: cystic fibrosis, sickle-cell anemia, Tay–Sachs disease, thalassemia major (Jones, 2005).

X-Linked Disorders: 819 Identified

A. X-linked dominant disorders.

  1. Characteristics of X-linked dominant disorders.

    a. Both sexes can be affected; because females have a double chance of receiving the mutant X chromosome, they have twice the risk of being affected.

    b. Affected males will have all affected daughters and no affected sons.

    c. Affected females will transmit the disorders in the same manner as with autosomal dominant patterns.

    d. Two thirds of the time, affected females have an affected mother; one third of the time, they have an affected father.

    e. Family history shows no father-to-son transmissions.

  2. Example: vitamin D–resistant rickets.

B. X-linked recessive disorders.

  1. Characteristics of X-linked recessive disorders.

    a. Only male offspring are affected, with rare exceptions. A female offspring will be affected if she has both a carrier mother and an affected father.

    b. Carrier females transmit the disorder.

    c. All sons of affected males will be normal.

    d. All daughters of affected males will be carriers (with each pregnancy).

    e. Heterozygous females transmit the gene to half their sons, who will be affected, and to half their daughters, who will be carriers.

    f. Transmission is horizontal among males in the same generation; in addition, a generation will be skipped, and second-generation males will be affected.

  2. Examples: Duchenne muscular dystrophy, hemophilia, color blindness, and glucose-6-phosphate dehydrogenase deficiency (Kingston, 2002).

Mitochondrial Disorders

  1. The great majority of genetic diseases are caused by defects in the nuclear genome. However, a small but significant number of diseases are the result of mitochondrial mutations.

  2. Because of the unique properties of mitochondria, these diseases display characteristic modes of inheritance and a large degree of phenotypic variability (Jorde et al., 2005).

  3. The mitochondria, which produce adenosine triphosphate (ATP), have their own unique DNA. Mitochondrial DNA is maternally inherited and has a high mutation rate. A number of diseases are known to be caused by mutations in mitochondrial DNA.

  4. Organ systems with large ATP requirements and high thresholds tend to be the ones most seriously affected by mitochondrial diseases; for example, the central nervous system consumes 20% of the ATP the body produces and is often affected by mtDNA mutations.

  5. Mitochondrial mutations are also involved in some common human diseases, for example, a form of deafness (Jorde et al., 2005).

CHROMOSOMAL DEFECTS
Abnormal Number

A. **Polyploidy:** more than two sets of homologous chromosomes, showing multiples of the haploid number.
B. **Nonmultiples** are designated by the suffix "-somy"; monosomy is one less than the diploid number (45), and trisomy is one more than the diploid (47).
C. **Causes.**
   1. Nondisjunction: failure of paired chromosomes to separate during cell division.
   2. Chromosome lag: failure of a chromosome to travel to the appropriate daughter cell.
   3. Anaphase lag: chromosome lag during the third state of division of a cell nucleus in meiosis and mitosis.
D. **Mosaicism:** nondisjunction of an anaphase lag that occurs during mitosis after fertilization, resulting in two different cell lines in the same person (Jones, 2005).

Abnormal Structure

A. **Deletion:** loss of a chromosomal segment.
B. **Duplication:** any duplication of a region of DNA that contains a gene. It is a process that can result in free mutation.
C. **Translocation:** occurrence of a chromosomal segment at an abnormal site, either on another chromosome or in the wrong position on the same chromosome (i.e., an inversion).
D. **Inversion:** occurs when a segment of the chromosome breaks off and reattaches in the reverse direction.
E. **Nonreciprocal translocation:** a one-way transfer of a chromosomal segment to another chromosome.
F. **Polygenic defects:** type of inheritance in which a trait is dependent on many different gene pairs with cumulative effects.
G. **Environmental influences.** Inadequate nutritional intake, certain drugs, irradiation, and viruses are examples that could alter the genetic makeup of an offspring while in vitro. Multifactorial: genes plus environment.
H. **Basic generalizations.**
   1. Loss of an entire autosome is usually incompatible with life.
   2. One X chromosome is necessary for life and development.
   3. If the male-determining Y chromosome is missing, life and development may continue but will follow female pathways.
   4. Extra entire chromosomes, the translocation of extra chromatin material, and the insertion of extra chromatin material are often compatible with life and development.
   5. Multiple congenital structural defects are present when gross aberrations are present (Blackburn, 2007).
I. **Incidence.**
   1. Autosomal aberrations: 5:1000 births.
   2. Sex chromosome aberrations: 2:1000 births.
   3. Spontaneous abortions: 60% are associated with chromosomal aberration (Jorde et al., 2005).

PRENATAL DIAGNOSIS

Recent technologic advances and marked progress in the understanding of the etiology and pathogenesis of many common disorders have allowed many families a prenatal diagnosis.

Indications and Advantages of Prenatal Diagnosis

A. **Indications.**
   1. Advanced maternal age.
   2. Prior child with a chromosomal disorder.
   3. Family history of neural tube defects.

4. Previous child with multiple malformations.
5. Carriers of X-linked diseases.
6. Carriers of chromosome translocation.
7. Couples at risk of having a child with a specific inborn error of metabolism (previous child or by carrier testing).
8. Ultrasonographic identification of major malformation, polyhydramnios, and/or intra-uterine growth restriction (Jorde et al., 2005).

B. **Advantages.**
1. Knowledge that the fetus is unaffected.
2. Time to explore options and prepare for an affected newborn infant.
3. Opportunity electively to choose either to avoid starting a pregnancy or to abort an affected fetus.
4. Opportunity for the physician to plan delivery, management, and care of the infant when the disease is diagnosed in the fetus (Jorde et al., 2005).

Prenatal Tests

Triple and Quad Screen Tests

A. **Screening test.** Performed at 15 to 20 weeks. The triple screen is a group of three tests that are used to screen pregnant woman in the second trimester of pregnancy. The quad screen adds a fourth test to the group. The test helps evaluate the risk that a fetus has certain abnormalities, including trisomy 21, and neural tube defects. Each test performed measures a different substance found in the blood: alpha-fetoprotein (AFP), human chorionic gonadotropin (hCG), unconjugated estriol (uE3), and with the quad test, inhibin A. The newest marker, inhibin A, increases both the sensitivity and specificity of the screen. These tests have been established as a triple or quad screen because the power lies in their use together. A mathematical calculation involving the levels of these three or four substances and considerations of maternal age, weight, race, and diabetic status are used to determine a numeric risk for trisomy 21 and other selected chromosomal anomalies (i.e., trisomy 18). This risk is compared with an established cutoff. If the risk is higher than the cutoff value, then it is considered positive or increased.
1. **Alpha-fetoprotein (AFP)** is a protein produced by fetal tissue. During development, AFP levels in fetal blood and amniotic fluid rise until about 12 weeks, then levels gradually fall until birth. Some AFP crosses the placenta and appears in the maternal blood.
2. **Human chorionic gonadotropin (hCG)** is a hormone produced by the placenta. Levels rise in maternal blood for the first trimester of pregnancy and then fall to less than 10% by the end of pregnancy.
3. **Unconjugated estriol (uE3)** is a form of estrogen that is produced by the fetus through metabolism. This process involves the liver, adrenals, and the placenta. Some of the unconjugated estriol crosses the placenta and can be measured in the mother's blood. Levels rise around the 8th week and continue to increase until shortly before delivery.
4. **Inhibin A** is a hormone also produced by the placenta. Inhibin is a dimer (has two parts) and is sometimes referred to as DIA or dimeric inhibin A. Levels in maternal blood decrease slightly from 14 to 17 weeks of gestation and then rise again.

B. **Preparation.** Explain to client that this is a screening test, not a diagnostic test. Explain that an abnormal result does not indicate an abnormality but will indicate the possible need for a diagnostic test to rule out abnormalities.

C. **Trisomy 21:** the levels of AFP and unconjugated estriol tend to be low and hCG and inhibin A levels high.

D. **Trisomy 18:** the levels of unconjugated estriol and hCG levels are low and AFP levels are variable.

E. **Open neural tube defects:** where there is an opening in the infant's spine, head, or abdominal wall that allows higher than usual amounts of AFP to pass to the mother's blood.

F. **Shortfalls of this test.**
1. The test result is very dependent on the accurate determination of the gestational age of the fetus. If the gestational age of the fetus has not been accurately determined, the results may be falsely high or low.

2. In multiple gestation pregnancies, calculation of the risk of trisomy 21 or trisomy 18 is difficult. For twin pregnancies, a "pseudo-risk" can be calculated comparing results to normal results in other twin pregnancies. For higher gestation pregnancies, risk cannot be calculated from these tests.

3. Evaluation of the risk of open neural tube defects in twin pregnancies can be determined, although it is not as effective as in singleton pregnancies.

G. **Results and further testing:** A multiple marker test or triple screen is used to determine if a fetus is at an increased risk of having certain congenital abnormalities. The test has a high rate of false positives; as few as 10% of women with abnormal results go on to have babies with congenital defects. The purpose of the test is to determine if further testing (such as ultrasound or amniocentesis) is warranted.

Ultrasonography

A. **Preparation for ultrasonography.** Explain to the client that a transducer coated with ultrasonic gel will be placed on her abdomen, with high-frequency sound waves used to display sectional planes of the uterine contents on a monitor. Explain that ultrasonography cannot detect all anomalies and cannot guarantee fetal outcome.

B. **Initial assessment** recommended by 16 to 20 weeks for the verification and evaluation of gestational age.

C. **Ultrasonography:** to detect abnormalities of fetus, placenta, amniotic fluid, and uterus; to monitor changes in anatomy and growth with serial ultrasonography.

D. **Diagnostic capability:** only as good as the person's training—not just contingent on the equipment.

E. **No known harmful effects.**

F. **Critical to safety of amniocentesis:** chorionic villus sampling and percutaneous blood sampling.

G. **Anatomic landmarks commonly observed:** fetal spine, kidneys, bladder, stomach, three-vessel cord, cord insertion, four-chambered heart, face, upper lip, biparietal diameter, head circumference, abdominal circumference, femur length, transcerebellar diameter, placenta, amount of amniotic fluid, uterus, and adnexa.

H. **Detectable anomalies:** many, including those indicative of various syndromes. Examples: anencephaly, atrial septal defect, cardiac anomalies, choroid plexus cyst, cleft lip, craniosynostosis, cystic hygroma, cystic kidneys, encephalocele, gastroschisis, hydrocephalus, microcephaly, myelomeningocele, omphalocele, skeletal dysplasia (Jorde et al., 2005).

Amniocentesis ("Amnio")

A. **Removal of 10 to 30 ml of amniotic fluid** through a needle placed into the woman's abdomen, for the purpose of chromosomal analysis and other biochemical tests as indicated.

B. **Preparation.** Review risks and benefits of the procedure, discuss options based on current information, and arrange to obtain results of amniocentesis. Explain that normal results of amniocentesis do not guarantee a good fetal outcome. Obtain written consent for this procedure. Obtain client's blood type before procedure. If she is Rh negative, obtain father's blood type.

C. **Usual timing of procedure:** 16 to 18 gestational weeks, but amniocentesis can be performed later in gestation and as early as 14 weeks.

D. **Indications.**
1. Woman of advanced maternal age (>35 years at the time of expected delivery).
2. Previous fetus with Down syndrome.
3. Previous fetus with neural tube defect.
4. Both parents known as heterozygous carriers of autosomal recessive chromosome.
5. Both parents known as carriers of sex-linked recessive disorder.
6. Client or partner with balanced chromosomal translocation of his or her chromosomes.
7. A woman with an abnormal triple or quad screen.

E. **Fluid analysis:** requires 2 to 3 weeks for cells to grow adequately for accurate analysis.

F. **Risks:** Overall risk to mother or fetus is 1%.
1. Spontaneous abortion: approximately 0.5% of cases.
2. Hemorrhage.
3. Infection.

4. Premature labor.
5. Rh sensitization from fetal bleeding into maternal circulation.
6. Trauma to fetus or placenta.

G. **Analysis.**
1. Fetal sex: determined through special staining techniques, karyotype, or amniotic fluid testosterone levels, providing risk information for X-linked disorder.
2. Alpha$_1$-fetoprotein: abnormally high or low levels raise concern (see earlier section on triple and quad screening, under Prenatal Tests).
3. Biochemical: metabolism disorders, including Tay-Sachs disease (a lipid disorder) and amino acid, carbohydrate, and mucopolysaccharide metabolism disorders, can be discovered by 20 weeks of gestation.
4. Chromosomes: abnormalities, including Down syndrome, other trisomies, and other chromosomal abnormalities, can be detected at 16 weeks of gestation by karyotyping.

H. **Postamniocentesis care.**
1. Assess fetal heart activity.
2. Cleanse insertion site and apply protective cover.
3. Instruct client to rest for 24 hours, to lift no more than 10 lb (approximately 4.5 kg), and to avoid straining.
4. Administer immune globulin (RhoGAM) if client is Rh negative and if father of fetus is either Rh positive or of unknown blood type. Do not give RhoGAM if Rh sensitization.
5. When results are available, explain their implications (Jenkins and Wapner, 2004).

Chorionic Villus Sampling

A. **Transvaginal or transabdominal sampling** of the chorionic villi. Obtain fetal cells for the purpose of chromosomal analysis and other biochemical tests. Chorionic villus sampling (CVS) cannot identify neural tube defects.

B. **Preparation:** Review risks and benefits of the procedure, discuss options, and arrange to obtain CVS results. Obtain written consent for this procedure.

C. **Timing of procedure:** usually 8 to 10 weeks of gestation.

D. **Indications.**
1. Client prefers to make decisions regarding pregnancy in the first trimester.
2. Severe oligohydramnios.

E. **Contraindications.**
1. Multiple gestation.
2. Uterine bleeding during this pregnancy.
3. Active genital herpes infection or other cervical infection.
4. Uterine fibroids.

F. **Fetal cell analysis:** requires 24 to 48 hours for initial results.

G. **Risks:** overall, 2% to 3%.
1. Infection.
2. Bleeding.
3. Cervical lacerations.
4. Miscarriage: 1% to 5%.

H. **Techniques of CVS.**
1. Vaginal CVS: Catheter is inserted through the vagina and cervix into the chorion outer tissue of the embryonic sac, and a tiny amount of the chorionic villi is aspirated by suction or cut with forceps.
2. Abdominal CVS: Needle is inserted through the abdomen into the chorion to obtain a sample of the chorionic villi.

I. **Post-CVS care.**
1. Same recommendations as for postamniocentesis care.
2. Nothing in the vagina (tampon, douche, intercourse) for 24 hours.
3. If transvaginal sample, instruct client to use sanitary napkins as needed for 24 to 48 hours.

Percutaneous Umbilical Blood Sampling

A. **Sampling:** removal of fetal blood through a needle placed into the woman's abdomen and into the umbilical vein.

B. **Preparation:** same as that recommended for CVS.
C. **Timing:** 18 weeks to term.
D. **Indications.**
   1. Client wants fast results to support her decision making regarding pregnancy.
   2. Abnormality is identified by ultrasonography late in pregnancy.
   3. Client has been exposed to infectious disease that could affect development of fetus.
   4. Blood incompatibility (Rh disease).
   5. Drug or chemical level in fetal blood needs to be assessed.
E. **Risks.**
   1. Same as amniocentesis: infection, bleeding, isoimmunization, miscarriage, trauma to the fetus—overall 1% to 5% risk factor.
   2. Perforation of uterine arteries, clotting in fetal cord.
   3. Premature delivery.
F. **Results:** fetal blood analysis takes 3 days.
G. **Postsampling care:** same as postamniocentesis care (Drugan et al., 2005).

POSTNATAL TESTING

A. **Chromosome analysis/karyotype:** an ordered display of an individual's chromosomes. This can be done on amniotic fluid prenatally. Chromosomes are analyzed by staining techniques that result in visibility of dark and light bands that are designated in a standardized way from the centromere.
B. **High-resolution banding/prometaphase banding:** Some disorders cannot be seen reliably on standard chromosome analysis and require special handling during processing. Prometaphase banding is used because the cell growth during culturing is adjusted to maximize the number of cells in prometaphase, where the chromosomes are much less condensed and therefore longer, rather than in metaphase, where the cell growth is stopped in standard chromosome studies. High-resolution banding can have from 550 to 800 bands and allows a much more detailed analysis.
C. **Fluorescence in situ hybridization (FISH)** is a technique called molecular cytogenetics that combines chromosome analysis with the use of fluorescence-tagged molecular markers (probes) that are applied after the chromosome preparation is produced. This method relies on the phenomenon of hybridization of complementary pieces of deoxyribonucleic acid (DNA). FISH is a powerful tool useful not only in diagnosing relatively common microdeletion or microduplication disorders but also for identifying the origin of extra chromosome material (Drugan et al., 2005).
D. **Polymerase chain reaction (PCR)** is a powerful technique in amplifying many copies of a segment of DNA so that it can be analyzed. PCR is useful in disorders with recurring muta-tion, for example, achondroplasia.
E. **Comparative Genomic Hybridization (CGH)** microarray testing: an advancement in cytoge-netic technology that is used for the detection of cytogenetic imbalances that are smaller than what can be detected through routine chromosome analysis. Testing will detect the loss (dele-tion) or gain (duplication) of chromosomal regions.

HUMAN GENOME PROJECT

A. **What is the Human Genome Project?**
   1. The Human Genome Project was an international 13-year effort formally begun in October 1990 to discover all the estimated 30,000 to 35,000 human genes and make them accessible for further biologic study.
   2. The project started in the mid-1980s and is the single most important coordinated medical research initiative in the history of biomedical research. It culminated in the completion of the full human genome sequence in April 2000 (www.genome.gov).
   3. The goals of the project were to map genes on chromosomes and to determine the sequence of the nucleotides that make up the human DNA, which is the basic genetic material. One of the top priorities was to generate complete sets of full-length chromosomal DNA

(cDNA) clones and sequences for both human and model organism genes. It is expected that genome research will produce a ream of new information about the genes involved in inherited disorders, birth defects, and common conditions influenced by genetic factors.

4. One insight already obvious is that even on a molecular level we are more than the sum of our 35,000 or so genes. However, surprisingly this new estimated number of genes is only one third of what was previously thought, although the numbers may be revised as more analyses are performed. This suggests to scientists that the genetic key to human complexity lies not in the number of genes but in how gene parts are used to build different products in a process called alternative splicing.

5. In December 1999, the first human chromosome, chromosome 22, was sequenced. This is the location of defects that can cause DiGeorge syndrome, chronic myeloid leukemia, and neurofibromatosis. It is also the final autosome in the human sequence as outlined by the NIH Human Genome Report in 2003 (Collins et al., 2003).

6. Though the outcome of the Human Genome Project itself is not ethically problematic, the use of the data generated presents major ethical questions that must be addressed. The future, then, presents the challenges of addressing the project's implications (Blackburn, 2007; Larsson, 2001).

B. **Ethical, legal, and social issues program.**

1. Study is now under way on the ethical, legal, and social issues related to increasingly rapid progress in the field of human genetics. Four areas were identified for initial emphasis: privacy of genetic information, safe and effective introduction of genetic information in the clinical setting, fairness in the use of genetic information, and professional and public education.

2. The program also emphasizes the importance of understanding the cultural, ethnic, social, and psychologic influences that must inform policy development and service delivery issues.

3. With time these issues must be addressed to ensure that the maximal benefit is gained from the project (Blackburn, 2007; Larsson, 2001).

GENETIC COUNSELING

A. **Definition:** a communication process that deals with the human problems associated with the occurrence, or the risk of occurrence, of genetic disorders in a family. This process involves collaboration of people from multiple disciplines (physician, sonographer, nurse, genetic counselor, social worker, neonatologist, and pediatric specialist, as indicated) and family support. Genetic counseling is a nondirective communication process that deals with the human problems associated with the occurrence, or the risk of occurrence, of a genetic disorder in a family.

B. **Principles of genetic counseling.**

1. Based on correct diagnosis and pattern of inheritance.
2. Nondirective.
3. Reinforcement of information previously presented.
4. Emphasis on communication with the primary care physician.

C. **Goal of genetic counseling** is to assist the family in comprehending the

1. Diagnosis,
2. Role of heredity,
3. Recurrence risks and options,
4. Possible courses of action, and
5. Methods of ongoing adjustment.

D. **Indications** (Blackburn, 2007; Drugan et al., 2005).

1. Previously affected child, parent, or grandparent.
   a. Congenital malformation.
   b. Sensory defect.
   c. Metabolic disorder.
   d. Mental retardation.

    e. Known or suspected chromosome abnormality.

    f. Neuromuscular disorder.

    g. Degenerative central nervous system (CNS) disease.

  2. Previously affected cousins.

    a. Muscular dystrophy.

    b. Hemophilia.

    c. Hydrocephalus.

  3. Consanguinity.

  4. Hazards of ionizing radiation.

  5. Recurrent miscarriages.

  6. Concern for teratogenic effect.

  7. Advanced maternal age.

  8. High or low MSAFP.

E. Methods of obtaining information needed.

  1. Questionnaire.

  2. Pedigree.

  3. Medical records.

  4. Physical examination.

  5. Laboratory tests.

  6. Carrier detection.

F. Provision of medical facts.

  1. Differential diagnosis.

  2. Risks to fetus and mother.

  3. Probable course of disorder.

  4. Recommended management for prenatal course.

  5. Type and timing of delivery.

  6. Neonatal, pediatric, and long-term-care requirements.

G. Explanation of hereditary factors that contribute to the disorder.

H. Discussion with parents regarding all alternatives.

  1. Home care of newborn infant.

  2. Institutionalization.

  3. Adoption.

  4. Appropriate method of termination for gestational age.

  5. Objective information regarding fetus and neonate status. Provide statistical risk factors as they relate to this individual fetus.

  6. Identification of the normal characteristics that can exist in the affected fetus. Point these out in pictures to promote awareness of the total condition of the fetus.

  7. Assistance to parents: understanding of causes, risks of recurrence, and limits of current treatments.

  8. Discussion of options available for dealing with risk of recurrence.

  9. Written information for parents and information regarding support groups.

  10. Explanation of recommended obstetric care, mode and timing of delivery, and neonatal care (Jones, 2005).

NEWBORN CARE

Diagnosis

A. Complete diagnosis: important in planning care. Consideration for the infant's overall problems, in addition to the defect, is essential.

B. Evaluation of infant with a birth defect. A birth defect is a structural or functional abnormality of the body that is present from birth. The effects of a birth defect may be either immediate or delayed until later in life.

C. Syndrome.

  1. Definition: a constellation of anomalies that cannot be explained otherwise and that result in similar patterns of expression.

  2. Examples: fetal alcohol syndrome, trisomy 21.

D. Sequence.
  1. Definition: a primary event or anomaly that sets a pattern of other events (anomalies). Designates a series of anomalies resulting from a cascade of events initiated from a single malformation.
  2. Example: Pierre Robin sequence. Lannelongue and Menard first described Pierre Robin syndrome in 1891 in a report on two patients with micrognathia, cleft palate, and retroglossoptosis. In 1926, Pierre Robin published the case of an infant with the complete syndrome. Until 1974, the triad was known as Pierre Robin syndrome; however, the term *syndrome* is now reserved for those errors of morphogenesis with simultaneous presence of multiple anomalies caused by a single etiology. The term *sequence* has been introduced to include any condition that includes a series of anomalies caused by a cascade of events initiated by a single malformation. The initial event, mandibular hypoplasia, occurs between the 7th and 11th week of gestation. This keeps the tongue high in the oral cavity, causing a cleft in the palate by preventing the closure of the palatal shelves. This explains the classic inverted U-shaped cleft and the absence of an associated cleft lip. Oligohydramnios could play a role in the etiology since the lack of amniotic fluid could cause deformation of the chin and subsequent impaction of the tongue between the palatal shelves (Collaboration for Craniofacial Development and Disorders, 2006).
E. Association.
  1. Is a nonrandom occurrence in two or more individuals of multiple anomalies not known to represent a sequence or syndrome.
  2. Example: Coloboma, Heart defect, Atresia choanae, Restricted growth and/or development, Genital anomalies and Ear anomalies (CHARGE) association
F. Malformation.
  1. Definition: an abnormality of morphogenesis due to intrinsic problems within the developing structures.
  2. Examples: neural tube defects, cleft lip and palate.
G. Deformation.
  1. Definition: an abnormality of morphogenesis owing to intrinsic problems within the developing structures.
  2. Examples: Pierre Robin sequence, uterine position defects, and oligohydramnios sequence.
H. Disruption.
  1. Definition: an abnormality of morphogenesis due to disruptive forces acting on the developing structure. Can be due to pressure on developing structures.
  2. Examples: amniotic bands, vascular accidents, and infections.
I. Genetic heterogeneity.
  1. Definition: different causes may produce similar characteristics.
  2. Examples: hydrocephalus, cleft lip, and cleft palate.

History

A. Family history.
  1. History of three generations.
  2. Defects in the family history related to the problem in the child.
  3. Medical records and/or photos of similarly affected relatives.
  4. History of consanguinity.
  5. Reproductive history, such as frequent spontaneous abortions.
  6. Pattern of inheritance of the problems.
B. Prenatal history.
  1. Length of gestation.
  2. Fetal activity level.
  3. Maternal exposures: infections, illness, high fevers, medications, x-ray examinations, known teratogens, alcohol, smoking, and use of street and prescription drugs.
  4. Obstetric factors: uterine malformations, complications of labor, and presenting fetal part.
  5. Neonatal factors: birth weight, length, head circumference, and Apgar scores.

Examination and Care

A. Physical examination.

1. General: asymmetry, problems of relationship, and inappropriate size and strength.
2. Face: configuration; centered features with normal spacing; round, triangular, flat, bird-like, elfin, coarse, or expressionless characteristics.
3. Head: size of anterior fontanelle, prominence of frontal bone, flattened or prominent occiput, abnormalities in shape (proportionally large or small).
4. Skin: intact, or presence of skin tags, open sinuses, tracts.
5. Hair: texture, hairline, presence of whorls.
6. Eyes: structure and color of iris, presence of colobomas, centering and spacing of epicanthal folds (hypotelorism or hypertelorism), ptosis, slanting, eyelash length.
7. Ears: protruding or prominent shape, location, low set, unilateral or bilateral defect, presence and/or degree of rotation.
8. Nose: beaked, bulbous, pinched, upturned, misshapen, two nares, flattened bridge, patency, centered on face.
9. Oral: intact palate, presence of smooth philtrum, natal teeth; shape and size of tongue, mouth, jaw (micrognathia).
10. Neck: short and/or webbed, redundant folds.
11. Chest: symmetric; presence of accessory nipples.
12. Abdomen: number of cord vessels, presence of abdominal wall defects and abdominal musculature, prune belly.
13. Genitourinary system (male): hypospadias—four degrees, dependent on placement of meatus; chordee; ambiguous genitalia; testes descended.
14. Anus: position, patency.
15. Spine: intact, scoliosis, lordosis, kyphosis.
16. Extremities: length, shape, absence of bones.
17. Hands and feet: broad, square, or spadelike shape, polydactyly, clinodactyly, syndactyly, abnormal creases in the palm of the hand (simian or Sydney creases), contractures, abnormally large or small size, overriding fingers, proximally placed thumb, rocker-bottom feet.

B. Causation of defect.

1. Identify the primary abnormality.
2. Recognize etiologic heterogeneity (a defect having more than one cause).
3. Determine category of congenital malformation, according to etiology.
   a. Malformation.
   b. Deformation.
   c. Disruption.
   d. Syndrome.
   e. Association.
   f. Sequence.
   g. Genetic heterogeneity.

C. Family care management for all genetic syndromes or disorders.

1. Provide grief counseling. Acknowledge short- and long-term grief; promote awareness that each of the parents may be in a different stage of the grief process, creating additional stress. Recommend that parents communicate their needs to each other and ask for support when needed.
2. Encourage genetic counseling.
3. Facilitate family use of support systems: social services; Aid to Families with Dependent Children; Women, Infants, and Children (WIC) program; March of Dimes; clergy; mental health services; support groups; Internet information.
4. Provide unconditional emotional support. Allow parents and siblings to verbalize feelings.
5. Identify normal aspects of neonate that can coexist with the syndrome or disorder.
6. Promote parent involvement in care; offer choices in care and interventions.
7. Discuss treatment options and their risks and benefits.

8. Provide literature.
9. Obtain legal and ethical counsel when parents prefer not to pursue medical interventions (Nelson, 2005).

Examples of Specific Disorders (for more specific disorders, see Chapter 35)

VATER Association

VATER is an acronym for *v*ertebral anomalies, *a*nal atresia, *t*racheo*e*sophageal fistula, and *r*adial and renal dysplasia.

A. **Etiology and precipitating factors: unknown.**
B. **Incidence: 1.6:10,000.**
C. **Clinical presentation. Three or more of the following defects are present:**
   1. Vertebral anomalies.
   2. Anal atresia with or without fistula.
   3. Tracheoesophageal fistula with esophageal atresia.
   4. Radial dysplasia, including thumb or radial hypoplasia, polydactyly, and syndactyly.
   5. Renal anomaly.
   6. Single umbilical artery.
D. **Complications and outcome.**
   1. Failure to thrive.
   2. Possibility of normal life after slow mental development during infancy.
E. **Care management.**
   1. Supportive: prognosis and management depend on the extent and severity of the anomalies.
   2. Surgery: surgical correction of anomalies.

VACTERL Association

VACTERL is an acronym for an association characterized by the sporadic, nonrandom association of specific abnormalities: *v*ertebral abnormalities, *a*nal atresia, *c*ardiac abnormalities, *t*racheo*e*sophageal fistula and/or esophageal atresia, *r*enal agenesis and dysplasia, and *l*imb defects.

A. **Etiology and precipitating factors.**
   1. Unknown.
   2. Injury between 4 and 6 weeks to a specific mesodermal area may produce simultaneous anomalies of the hindgut, lower vertebral column, lower urinary tract, and developing kidney.
   3. Abnormalities: average of 7 or 8 per patient.
B. **Incidence:** rare (about 250 reported cases worldwide).
C. **Clinical presentation** (Hockenberry, 2007; Jones, 2005).
   1. Vertebral anomalies.
   2. Anal atresia with or without fistula.
   3. Cardiac anomalies: commonly ventricular septal defects.
   4. Tracheoesophageal fistula with or without esophageal atresia.
   5. Radial dysplasia, including thumb or radial hypoplasia, polydactyly, and syndactyly.
   6. Renal anomaly.
   7. Single umbilical artery.
D. **Complications and outcome.**
   1. Failure to thrive.
   2. Normal life: minimal CNS anomalies with only occasional mental retardation.
E. **Care management** (Hockenberry, 2003).
   1. Supportive: prognosis and management depend on the extent and severity of the anomalies.
   2. Surgery: surgical correction of anomalies.

Common Trisomies

Trisomy 21 (Down Syndrome)

A. **Incidence and etiology**

1. Incidence by maternal age is as follows:
   a. 15 to 29 years, 1:1500
   b. 30 to 34 years, 1:800
   c. 35 to 39 years, 1:270
   d. 40 to 44 years, 1:100
   e. 45 years or older, 1:50
2. Accounts for 15% to 20% of cases of severe mental retardation.
3. Risk increases with maternal age.
4. 25% of Down syndrome infants receive an extra chromosome from their father.
5. Person has 47 chromosomes (3 of chromosome 21).
6. Extra chromosome fits into group G21,22. Extra chromosome results from nondisjunction during meiosis. May occur unrelated to maternal and appear as follows:
   a. Chromosomes: 46
   b. Translocation of chromosome 21.
   c. Familial transmission autosomal dominant.
   d. No abnormalities if chromosomes are balanced. There is one No. 21 and one No. 14 chromosome.
   e. Production of unbalanced gametes by balanced carriers: should consider prenatal diagnosis.
7. Some infants have mosaicism for trisomy 21 or translocation 14/21 or 21/22.
   a. Some have all the defects.
   b. Some have only a few.
   c. Some of this group may have normal intellectual ability.

B. Clinical presentation.
1. Size: small; 20% are premature.
2. Skull: short and round with a flat occiput.
3. Eyes: slant upward and outward.
4. Prominent epicanthal fold.
5. Flat face.
6. Brushfield's spots: iris may be speckled with a ring of round, grayish spots or flecks of gold in light-colored eyes.
7. Cheeks: red.
8. Palate: narrow and short.
9. Nose: short with a flat nasal bridge.
10. Tongue: protrudes; can become dry and wrinkled.
11. Skin loose around lateral and dorsal aspects of the neck.
12. Hands.
    a. Fingers: short
    b. Hands: square
    c. Single simian creases
13. Feet.
    a. Wide space between great toe and second toe.
    b. Deep crease that starts between the great toe and the second toe and curves
14. Muscular hypotonia.
15. Narrow acetabular angle.
16. Narrow iliac index.
17. Broadened iliac bones.
18. Delayed psychomotor development.
19. Cardiac ventricular septal defects or other congenital heart defects found in 50% of infants.
20. Duodenal atresia (Jones, 2005).

C. Complications and outcome.
1. Congestive heart failure due to congenital heart disease.
2. Upper respiratory tract infections.
3. Developmental delay: IQ ranges from 25 to 70.

Trisomy 18

A. **Etiology and precipitating factors.**
  1. Nondisjunction most frequent; also possible partial trisomy, translocation, or mosaicism.
  2. Advanced parental age.
B. **Incidence: 1:3500 births.**
C. **Clinical presentation.**
  Characteristics 1 to 7 appear in most cases:
  1. Weight: low birth weight in term infant.
  2. Ears: low set and/or abnormal shape.
  3. Micrognathia and microstomia.
  4. Mental retardation.
  5. Hands.
     a. Clenched hand with flexed fingers.
     b. Flexion contraction of the two middle digits.
     c. Unfolded thumb.
  6. Cardiac: usually ventricular septal defect with patent ductal arteriosus.
  7. Feet: rocker bottom.
  Characteristics 8 to 14 may also appear:
  8. Eyes: ptosis of one or both eyelids.
  9. Syndactyly.
  10. Head: abnormally prominent occiput.
  11. Genitourinary defects.
  12. Hernias, especially umbilical.
  13. Simian crease appears in 25%.
  14. Arches on seven or more fingers in 80% of cases.
D. **Complications and outcome.**
  1. Mortality rate: 30% die within 2 months of birth, usually of heart failure.
  2. Survival: 10% survive past the first year with severe developmental delay.
E. **Care management.**
  1. No treatment beyond supportive care.
  2. Gavage/gastric tube feedings as needed for poor feeding.
  3. Oxygen as needed for respiratory distress.
  4. Parental support.

Trisomy 13

Etiology: unknown; may be related to older maternal age.
A. **Incidence: 1:15,000 births.**
B. **Clinical presentation.**
  1. Psychomotor delay.
  2. Ears: malformed.
  3. Hands: flexion deformities of hand, fingers, and wrist: postaxial polydactyly.
  4. Cardiac: usually ventricular septal defect, patent ductus arteriosus, or rotational anomalies such as dextroposition.
  5. Feet: rocker bottom.
  6. Eyes: microphthalmos, colobomas of iris, cataracts.
  7. Nose: broad and flattened, cleft lip and palate (not always).
  8. Umbilicus: hernia, omphalocele.
  9. Genitalia:
     a. Female: bicornate or septate uterus.
     b. Male: cryptorchidism, small scrotum and anterior placement.
  10. Kidneys: polycystic.
  11. Skin: cutaneous hemangiomas, cutis aplasia.
  12. Brain: gross defects, grand mal seizures, myoclonic jerks.

13. Hematologic abnormalities, such as increased frequency of nuclear projections in neutrophils and/or persistence of embryonic and/or fetal type of hemoglobin.

C. Complications and outcome.
1. Mortality rate: 44% die within the first month.
2. Survival: 18% survive the first year.
3. Severe mental retardation.

D. Care management.
1. No treatment beyond supportive care.
2. Parental support.

REFERENCES

Allanson, J.E. and Cassidy S.B. (Eds.): *Management of genetic syndromes.* New York, 2005, Wiley-Liss.

Blackburn, S.T.: *Maternal, fetal & neonatal physiology. A clinical perspective* (3rd ed.). St. Louis, 2007, Saunders.

Collaboration for Craniofacial Development and Disorders, 2006. Retrieved February 2, 2009, from www. hopkinsmedicine.org/craniofacial/Gateway/PierreRobinSequence.

Collins, F.S., Green, E.D., Guttmacher, A.E., and Guyer, M.S.: A vision for the future of genomics research. *Nature, 422*(6934):835-848, 2003.

Drugan, A., Isada, N.B., and Evans, M.I.: Prenatal diagnosis in the molecular age—Indications, procedures, and laboratory techniques. In M.G. MacDonald, M. D. Mullett, and M.M.K. Seshia (Eds.): *Avery's neonatology: Pathophysiology & management of the newborn* (6th ed.). Philadelphia, 2005, Lippincott Williams & Wilkins, pp. 130-148.

Hockenberry, M.J.: *Wong's nursing care of infants and children* (8th ed.). St Louis, 2007, Mosby.

Jenkins, T.M. and Wapner, R.J.: Prenatal diagnosis of congenital disorders. In R.K. Creasy, R. Resnik, and J.D. Iams (Eds.): *Maternal-fetal medicine: Principles and practice* (5th ed.). Philadelphia, 2004, Saunders, pp. 235-280.

Jones, K.: *Smith's recognizable patterns of human malformation* (6th ed.). Philadelphia, 2005, Saunders.

Jorde, L.B., Carey, J.C., Bamshed, M.J., and White, R.L.: *Medical genetics* (3rd ed.). St Louis, 2005, Mosby.

Kingston, H.M.: *ABC of clinical genetics* (5th ed.). London, 2002, BMJ.

Larsson, A.: Neonatal screening for metabolic, endocrine, infectious and genetic disorders: Current and future directions. *Clinics in Perinatology, 28*(2):449-461, 2001.

March of Dimes Foundation, White Plains, New York, 2006. Retrieved February 2, 2009, from www. marchofdimes.com.

Nelson, R.M.: Ethical decisions in the neonatal-perinatal period. In H.W. Taeusch, R.B. Ballard, and C.A. Gleason (Eds.): *Avery's diseases of the newborn* (8th ed.). Philadelphia, 2005, Saunders, pp. 17-22.

Nussbaum, R.L., McInnes, R.R., and Willard, H.F.: *Thompson and Thompson genetics in medicine* (7th ed.). Philadelphia, 2007, Saunders.

Online Mendelian Inheritance in Man (OMIM). Retrieved February 2, 2009, from www.ncbi.nlm.nih.gov/omim.

21 Intrafacility and Interfacility Neonatal Transport

S. LOUISE BOWEN

OBJECTIVES

1. Discuss planning for an intrafacility transport of a critically ill neonate.
2. Identify important considerations in the selection of transport vehicles.
3. Discuss the important factors to be considered in selecting team composition.
4. Describe the process of neonatal transport from the referring call, to transport of the patient, to arrival at the receiving hospital.
5. List four methods to increase safety in the transport environment.
6. Discuss legal and ethical considerations relating to neonatal transport.

In the late 1950s and early 1960s, intensive care for newborn infants first became available. As the scope of care for critically ill infants expanded, so did the number of hospitals offering this service. Unfortunately, because of the uneven distribution of these services, many areas remained without available resources. In the early 1970s, the need to regionalize perinatal care was recognized by health care providers. In 1976 the National Foundation March of Dimes released the report "Toward Improving the Outcome of Pregnancy," which described regionalized care and identified criteria for level I, II, and III hospitals (Committee on Perinatal Health, 1976). The report also recommended the establishment of formal relationships between hospitals delivering different levels of care within a region so that every infant could receive appropriate care. The concept of regionalization led naturally to the need for the development of neonatal transport.

The United States Department of Health and Human Services reported that of the more than 4 million live births in the United States in 2005, 12.7% were premature (March of Dimes, 2005). This percentage of preterm births has continued to increase during the past 20 years. Advances in neonatology and technology have led to increased survival rates of these lower gestational age infants. These infants may be born outside a regional center and require transport to a neonatal intensive care unit. Infants with congenital anomalies or multisystem problems may also require transport to a regional neonatal intensive care center. The neonatal period is defined as the first 4 weeks of life and is the period of greatest mortality in childhood, with the highest risk occurring during the first 24 hours of life (March of Dimes, 2005). Intrafacility and interfacility transport of the critically ill neonate presents unique challenges. The goal is to transport these critically ill neonates in the most stable condition possible and to minimize adverse effects. The neonatal transport team must be knowledgeable about neonatal physiology and clinical requirements to provide optimal care and outcome. This chapter discusses various aspects of intrafacility and interfacility neonatal transport.

HISTORICAL ASPECTS

A. **1899:** When most infants were born at home, the first ambulance incubator was developed to transport premature infants from home to Chicago's Lying-In Hospital (Butterfield, 1993; Cone, 1985).

B. **1935:** The Chicago Board of Health operated a special ambulance with incubator, oxygen, and humidity and staffed with public health nurses (Chou and MacDonald, 1989).

C. **1948:** The New York City Department of Health, Maternity and Newborn Division established a well-organized transport service staffed with ambulance drivers, nurses, a pediatrician, and a transport clerk (Losty et al., 1950; Wallace et al., 1952).

D. **1966:** Dr. Sydney Segal published guidelines for neonatal transport (Segal, 1966) that were expanded in 1972 into a comprehensive transport manual (Segal, 1972).

E. **1970s:** The number of organized transport programs increased as a result of regionalization of perinatal care (Wood and Bose, 2005).

PHILOSOPHY OF NEONATAL TRANSPORT

A. **The neonatal transport team is an extension of the neonatal intensive care unit** (Walsh and Fanaroff, 2006).
   1. Interfacility neonatal transport is inherently different from typical emergency medical services (EMS) transport. Stabilization during interfacility transport is accomplished in the controlled setting of a medical facility, such as a hospital or medical clinic, in comparison with stabilization performed at the scene of an accident with limited support services. During interfacility transport, the patient is moved from a controlled setting, that is, referring hospital, to the transport environment before arriving in the controlled setting of the receiving center. Scene-response systems move a patient from an uncontrolled setting to the controlled setting of a medical facility. The focus of EMS is on immediate short-term stabilization to sustain the patient until arrival at the medical facility. Interfacility transport systems focus on providing intensive care services from the referral facility and throughout the transport; thus more time is spent in stabilization at the point of origin.
   2. The level of care should remain the same or increase during neonatal interfacility transport.

B. **Crew and patient safety must be the highest priority of a transport program** (American Academy of Pediatrics [AAP], 2007; Blumen, 2002; Levick, 2007).
   1. Crew and patient safety must be the highest priority for both ground and air neonatal transport programs. The focus of a transport safety program is accident prevention. However, when an accident does occur, a systematic approach should be used to minimize the impact. Every team member is responsible for a safe program. Crew members' attitudes, participation, education, and judgment are variables that influence the safety program. Unsafe behaviors or practices are unacceptable in the transport environment.

C. **The neonate is a member of a family unit** (Pillitteri, 2003).
   1. Parents and family of a critically ill neonate experience a mixture of emotions. Reactions of the parents may vary based on the condition of their infant and on their perception of the situation, past experiences, support systems, and coping mechanisms. The transport team plays a pivotal role assisting the family to cope with the crisis.

D. **Intrafacility and interfacility neonatal transport** should be planned and organized with appropriate transport staff and adequate equipment.

E. **Intrafacility and interfacility preparation, stabilization, and transport** should be performed as efficiently as possible using skilled staff and appropriate equipment. The continuum of care should not be interrupted during the transport process.

INTRAFACILITY NEONATAL TRANSPORT*

A. **Preparation.**
   1. Neonates may require intrafacility transport for diagnostic and invasive procedures. The same concepts used for interfacility transport apply to intrafacility transport to avoid adverse outcomes.
   2. Level of care must be maintained or increased.

B. **Staffing.**
   1. Staff must be knowledgeable in neonatal physiology and pathophysiology and have excellent assessment skills. They must have the combined expertise and skills to provide safe transport.

---

*Bowen, 2002.

2. The type and number of personnel required is determined by patient acuity level and equipment.
3. It is beneficial to have the bedside registered nurse as part of the staff because of patient knowledge. It may not be feasible with staffing shortages and patient care assignments.

C. **Effective communication** between staff of the neonatal intensive care unit, intrafacility transport team, and procedure department is critical.

D. **Equipment.**
   1. Type of equipment selected is based on patient acuity level.
   2. Anticipate potential complications.
   3. Maintenance of a neutral thermal environment during the procedure presents challenges. Prevention of hypothermia may require additional supplies.
      a. Radiant warming lights.
      b. Warm blankets.
      c. Hat.
      d. Crushable heat packs or thermal pad (do not place against fragile skin).
      e. Polyurethane wrap or bag.
   4. Monitoring devices should be compatible with the type of procedure performed.
   5. Equipment should have battery back-up capabilities. Plug in equipment to an electrical outlet to maintain the battery charge.

E. **Safety.**
   1. Use the most expeditious route between the unit and the procedure department.
   2. Anticipate and plan for potential problems, that is, elevator not functioning.
   3. Supplies and equipment should be packaged for safe transport.
   4. Staff remaining with patient during the procedure should be provided with protective clothing and monitoring devices depending on type of procedure.
   5. The neonate and monitoring equipment should be positioned for optimal visualization.
   6. Staff may be required to stay with the neonate during the procedure given that other health care providers may not have the expertise to manage a neonate.
   7. The neonate should be assessed frequently during the procedure.

INTERFACILITY NEONATAL TRANSPORT

Types of Transports (AAP, 2007)

A. **One-way transports.**
   1. One-way transport uses services of personnel, equipment, and vehicles dispatched by the referral hospital to the receiving center.
   2. Advantages of one-way transport.
      a. Time saving in patient arrival to the receiving center.
      b. Knowledge of the patient by referring staff.
   3. Disadvantages of one-way transport.
      a. Justification of the expense of maintaining experienced staff and equipment is difficult because of the small number of transports.
      b. May deplete the resources of local EMS or the referring hospital for the duration of the transport.
      c. Referring hospital and local EMS staff may not have appropriate equipment or training for transport of neonates. Studies have shown that there is an increased morbidity and mortality when neonates are transported by an untrained versus a trained neonatal team (Walsh and Fanaroff, 2006).

B. **Two-way transport.**
   1. Two-way transport uses the services of personnel, equipment, and vehicles dispatched by the receiving center.
   2. Advantages.
      a. More cost-effective use of expensive equipment.
      b. More experienced transport staff trained specifically in neonatal transport.
      c. Improved neonatal stabilization techniques.
      d. Provide equipment specifically for neonatal transport.

    3. Disadvantages.
       a. Time delay in moving patient from referring facility.
       b. Expense of maintaining transport program.
C. **Three-way transport.**
    1. The neonate is transported from the referring facility to the receiving facility by a transport team from a third facility or air medical company.
D. **Back/return transport** (Wood and Bose, 2005).
    1. Neonates are transferred back to the local or birth hospital when they no longer require the resources of the regional neonatal intensive care center. The family should be involved in the decision of transferring the infant.
       a. Parents should visit the local or birth hospital prior to the transfer.
    2. Advantages.
       a. More efficient use of beds at regional center.
       b. Improved relations between community hospitals and tertiary care center.
       c. Greater opportunity for parental involvement.
       d. Familiarity of primary physician with infant before discharge home.
       e. Decreased cost during convalescence.
    3. Disadvantages.
       a. Financial analysis of cost to keep infant at the regional facility versus cost of transport. Transfer of neonate back to referring hospital may depend on managed care or insurance contract.
       b. Potential need for transport back to higher-care facility if patient's condition deteriorates at community hospital.
       c. Parental anxiety and loss of continuity of care.
E. **Transfers out.**
    1. Neonates are transferred for a specialized procedure or treatment not available at the current facility, i.e., extracorporeal membrane oxygenation, surgical procedure.
    2. Neonate may be transported by a team from the receiving hospital, the referring hospital, or from a third facility or company.
    3. Receiving facility should consider back-transport after completion of the treatment or procedure.

SELECTION OF TRANSPORT VEHICLES

A. **General considerations** (AAP, 2007; James, 2002).
    1. Appropriate vehicle selection may be dictated by diagnosis, clinical condition of the patient, available resources at the referring hospital, location of referring hospital, distance and duration of transport, geographic characteristics (road conditions, traffic conditions, construction detours), size of team, vehicle availability, weather, cost of the transport, and reimbursement.
    2. Vehicles must be appropriately equipped, including power supplies, inverter, oxygen and air supply, suction, lighting, altitude pressurization where appropriate, means for securing incubators and all equipment, and room for adequate personnel.
    3. An integrated system using multiple modes of transportation allows maximum flexibility to meet patient needs in a cost-effective manner.
    4. Decisions regarding the appropriate vehicle for individual transport should be made by the medical control physician at the tertiary hospital, the transport team, and the referring physician in consideration of the impact on patient care and outcome, advantages and disadvantages of each vehicle, and cost.
    5. Vehicle design and equipment placement must allow for continuation of patient care throughout the transport.
    6. The vehicle must be equipped with appropriate locking devices and storage to secure the incubator and equipment.
B. **Specific vehicle considerations.**
    1. Ambulance (AAP, 2007; James, 2002).
       a. Advantages.

       (1) Lower transport costs.

       (2) Operate in weather conditions that restrict air transport.

       (3) Does not require a landing zone or runway.

       (4) Ability to carry equipment and personnel for two incubators in specially equipped ambulances.

       (5) Increased space and patient more accessible.

       (6) Ability to stop vehicle or divert to the closest hospital in an emergency.

    b. Disadvantages.

       (1) Long response times due to speed limitations, road conditions, traffic congestion, and geographic location.

       (2) Delay of admission to tertiary care center because of long-distance ground transport.

  2. Helicopters (AAP, 2007; Arndt, 2003).

    a. Advantages.

       (1) Speed in response to calls and in returning patient to the receiving center for distances up to 150 miles.

       (2) Decreased response time to the referring facility.

       (3) Use of one-way helicopter transport to increase team's response time to referring hospital.

       (4) Avoid traffic delays and ground obstacles.

    b. Disadvantages.

       (1) Increased noise and vibration levels.

       (2) Difficult to identify problems when they occur because of noise and vibration (pneumothorax, extubation).

       (3) High operational costs.

       (4) Space and weight limitations.

       (5) Increased downtime because of weather.

       (6) May require ground transportation depending on landing zone location.

       (7) Securing the same incubator in a helicopter and ambulance may not be possible because of different mounts and stretcher configurations. This must be evaluated prior to the transport.

  3. Fixed-wing aircraft (AAP, 2007).

    a. Advantages.

       (1) Primarily beneficial for long-distance transports, usually greater than 150 miles.

       (2) Although fixed-wing transportation is expensive, favorable cost comparison possible over long distances when staff time is taken into consideration.

    b. Disadvantages.

       (1) If no contractual agreements with aircraft vendors, possible inadequate equipment and unfamiliarity of team with the aircraft or with general vendor operation.

       (2) Requires coordination of ground transportation on both ends of the flight.

       (3) Space limitations.

       (4) Securing the same incubator in a fixed-wing aircraft and ambulance may not be possible because of different mounts and stretcher configurations. This must be evaluated before the transport.

       (5) Requires an airport for landing and takeoff.

       (6) Multiple patient movements from aircraft and ambulances.

TRANSPORT PERSONNEL

A. Composition of a neonatal transport team varies with federal, state, and local regulations, budget, availability, professional standards, patient population, mission, referral area, expectations and available resources at referral hospital, skill and educational level of team, acuity, and volume of transports. The team must possess the combined expertise to assess, plan, implement, and evaluate actual and potential complications during transport of a critically ill neonate (Commission on Accreditation of Medical Transport Systems [CAMTS], 2006; James,

2002; Woodward et al., 2002). The team may be staffed by using various combinations of personnel, with a minimum of two patient care providers trained in the management of critically ill neonates. These patient care providers are in addition to the ambulance drivers or pilots. At least one of the patient care providers should be a physician, registered nurse, or neonatal nurse practitioner. Team composition may remain constant or vary according to patient acuity (Woodward et al., 2002). When transporting two neonates in the same vehicle, specific patient care providers should be assigned to each infant. Cross-training staff within scope of practice and licensure increases efficiency of the team. Transport teams may be configured using a combination of the following personnel:

1. Physicians and neonatologists.
2. Fellows and residents.
3. Registered nurses.
4. Neonatal nurse practitioners.
5. Respiratory therapists.
6. Emergency medical technicians or paramedics.

B. **Roles for transport personnel**, including functions, responsibilities, qualifications, and competencies, must be clearly outlined in job descriptions.
   1. Transport personnel should function as a team.
   2. Cross-training personnel within scope of practice and licensure.
   3. The program should have a written policy specific to job performance for physical requirements and disqualifying mental conditions of team members.
      a. Weight and height requirements, especially in air transport.
      b. General physical condition.
      c. Notification to transport administration of use of prescription and over-the-counter medications (certain medications may delay mental function and reflexes).
   4. Staff should participate in neonatal transport with sufficient frequency to maintain expertise.

C. **Team composition considerations** (AAP, 2007; CAMTS, 2006).
   1. Physicians.
      a. Neonatologists should be utilized when their additional expertise is required.
      b. May limit resources in a busy neonatal practice.
      c. Residents provide less consistency as a result of rotations and lack of educational experience in neonatal intensive care.
      d. Fellows provide more consistency and increasing levels of expertise as they advance through their fellowship.
   2. Registered nurses.
      a. Requires advanced knowledge and experience in neonatal intensive care.
      b. May be the team leader.
      c. Educational requirements may include in-service programs, national certifications, the American Academy of Pediatrics/American Heart Association Neonatal Resuscitation Program, the American Academy of Pediatrics/American Heart Association Pediatric Advanced Life Support Course, Certified Flight Registered Nurse, Certified Transport Registered Nurse, and Board of Certification for Emergency Nursing.
   3. Neonatal nurse practitioners.
      a. Licensed in most states to perform diagnostic and therapeutic procedures.
      b. Highly skilled, in addition to their advanced knowledge of neonatal intensive care therapies.
      c. Increased cost in comparison to a registered nurse; however, this may obviate the need for resident/fellow/neonatologist presence.
   4. Respiratory therapists.
      a. Frequent team members because of the majority of neonates transported have a respiratory problem.
      b. Require advanced knowledge in neonatal intensive care.
      c. May assist with nursing functions as licensed by the state.
      d. Responsible for respiratory equipment, airway maintenance, and maintaining adequate oxygenation and ventilation during transport.

5. Emergency medical technicians and paramedics.
   a. Role varies, depending on experience and education in neonatal care.
   b. Functions may include nursing or respiratory therapy responsibilities.
6. Expertise required within the transport team (Arndt, 2003; James, 2002).
   a. Assessment.
      (1) History taking.
      (2) Physical examination and gestational age assessment.
      (3) Interpretation of laboratory and radiologic findings.
   b. Knowledge of neonatal physiology and pathophysiology.
   c. Excellent communication and public relations skills.
   d. Clinical experience and expertise.
   e. Physical examination and fitness criteria (physical agility and stamina).
   f. Knowledge of aviation physiology.
   g. Transport safety.
   h. Knowledge of transport environment and vehicles.
   i. Independence and flexibility.
   j. Procedures.
      (1) Bag-and-mask ventilation.
      (2) Endotracheal intubation.
      (3) Laryngeal mask airway insertion.
      (4) Arterial access (umbilical artery catheters, percutaneous artery catheters, arterial sampling).
      (5) Needle thoracostomy.
      (6) Thoracostomy tube insertion.
      (7) Venous access (umbilical venous catheters, peripheral intravenous [IV] lines).
      (8) Intraosseous insertion.
      (9) Administration of nitric oxide and nitrogen, as applicable.
      (10) Mobile extracorporeal membrane oxygenation, as applicable.
      (11) Administration of surfactant.
7. Justification for a neonatal team.
   a. Staffing: dedicated, unit based, on call.
   b. Use of personnel when there are no transports.
   c. Volume of transports.
   d. Review of other systems that could transport neonates. These systems should demonstrate appropriate clinical expertise and possess equipment to transport a critically ill neonate.
   e. Cost and reimbursement.
D. **Medical director** (AAP, 2007; Woodward et al., 2002). The role of the neonatal transport team medical director, including qualifications and responsibilities, must be clearly outlined in a job description.
   1. A neonatologist or a physician with acute care expertise or subspecialty training in neonatology.
   2. License to practice medicine in the transport program's state.
   3. Knowledgeable in transport medicine.
   4. Oversees medical aspects of the transport program.
   5. Involved in the quality management program.
   6. Involved in administrative aspects: selection of team members, orientation, education, program operation, policies, public relations, and outreach education.

TRANSPORT EQUIPMENT*

A. **Transport equipment and supplies must be checked regularly** to ensure that they are adequately stocked, functioning properly, and ready for immediate transport. Equipment should be scheduled for preventive maintenance program regularly.

---

*AAP, 2007.

B. Recommended equipment must be operable on battery power.
   1. Transport incubator.
   2. Cardiorespiratory monitor with pressure tracing and recorder.
   3. Pulse oximeter.
   4. Infant ventilator.
   5. Air–oxygen blender.
   6. End-tidal carbon dioxide monitor or adaptors.
   7. Airway humidification system.
   8. Invasive and noninvasive blood pressure monitors.
   9. Intravenous infusion safety pumps.
   10. Transilluminator.
   11. Point-of-care testing including portable blood gas analyzer and glucometer (state regulations vary regarding use and quality control checks in mobile intensive care environments).
   12. Defibrillator/pacer (minimum capacity, 2 watt-seconds).
   13. Liquid oxygen, oxygen tank in vehicle, or portable oxygen cylinders.
   14. Air tank in vehicle, portable air cylinders or air compressor.
   15. Inverter in vehicle. Equipment should have battery backup.
   16. Specialized equipment: nitric oxide, nitrogen, extracorporeal membrane oxygenation, and high-frequency ventilation during neonatal transport.
C. Supplies for neonatal transport (Box 21-1).
D. Fixed-wing transports.
   1. Ensure incubator fits through door of aircraft prior to the transport.
E. Evaluate type and grounding of electrical outlets in vehicles prior to the transport. Voltage and amperage differences may affect equipment.

NEONATAL TRANSPORT PROCESS*

A. Referral call. The initial transport request call may be taken by a dispatch center, transport team, neonatologist, or neonatal intensive care staff. The referring physician is responsible for

---

■ BOX 21-1
■ **SUPPLIES FOR NEONATAL TRANSPORT**

This supply list is designed for critical care interfacility neonatal transport.	Thoracentesis setups
Respiratory Equipment	Syringe, 60 ml
Laryngoscope handle with blades, sizes Miller 00, 0, and 1	Three-way stopcock
Spare laryngoscope bulbs and batteries	Angiocatheters, 20 and 22 gauge
ET tube stylet	Tubing T-connector
Anesthesia bag (not to exceed 750 ml) or self-inflating bag with oxygen reservoir	Antiseptic solution
Manometer	Heimlich valves/closed drainage system
Face mask (micropremie, premature, and term)	Chest tubes, sizes 8F, 10F, and 12F
ET tubes, sizes 2.0, 2.5, 3.0, 3.5, and 4.0	Oxygen hood
Suction catheter and glove sets, sizes 5F, 6F, 8F, and 10F	Laryngeal mask airway
Meconium aspirator	Bulb syringe
Blood gas kit	End-tidal carbon dioxide monitor/adapter
CPAP prongs	**IV Therapy Equipment**
Nasal cannula (premature, infant)	Bags of D_5W and $D_{10}W$
Ventilator circuit	IV pump tubing
	IV filters
	Platelet and blood infusion sets
	Umbilical catheters, sizes 3.5F and 5F
	IV extension tubing
	T-connectors, multiport connectors

---

*AAP, 2007; Jaimovich and Vidyasagar, 2002; Salyer, 2003.

■ BOX 21-1
■ **SUPPLIES FOR NEONATAL TRANSPORT—cont'd**

Sterile drapes
Syringes, sizes 1 to 60 ml
Needles, assorted sizes, 18 to 25 gauge; or
   needleless system
Three-way stopcock and stopcock plugs
Antiseptic wipes
Scalp vein needles, 23 and 25 gauge
IV catheters, 22, 24, and 26 gauge
Disposable razors
Medication additive labels
Tape measure
Tongue blades
Armboards, sizes premature and infant
Intraosseous needles
Assorted tape
Umbilical tape
Antiseptic solution
Size 4-0 silk suture with curved needle
Umbilical catheter and thoracotomy set,
   including:
   Two sterile drapes
   Iris forceps
   Needle holders
   Scissors
   Curved forceps
   Tongue tissue forceps
   Sterile gauze pads, 2×2
   Scalpel and blade
   Blunt-end adapters, 17, 18, and 20 gauge
Thermoregulation and Monitoring Equipment
   Hat
   Polyurethane wrap or bag
   Crushable heat packs and mattress
   Space blankets
   Thermometer
   Neonatal electrocardiogram electrodes
   Lead wires for heart monitor
   Capillary tubes
   Glucose level monitoring device
   Lancets
   Arterial transducer tubing
Miscellaneous
   Camera, film
   Parent information
   Blood culture bottles
   Scissors and hemostat
   Flashlight
   Gauze pads, 2×2
   Limb restraints
   Rubber bands
   Pacifiers (various sizes)
   Cotton balls
   Christmas tree adapters

Feeding tubes, sizes 5F and 8F
Salem sump tubes, sizes 10F and 12F
Dual-flow gastric tubes, sizes 10F and
   12F
Sterile glove packs (assorted sizes)
Sphygmomanometer with blood pressure
   cuffs, sizes premature, neonate, and
   infant
Neonatal stethoscope
Trash bag; needle disposal system
Personal protective equipment (goggles,
   gowns, masks, gloves)
Visceral pack: normal saline solution, sterile
   gauze, sterile operating room drape, or
   sterile plastic bag
Medications
Epinephrine 1:10,000
Sodium bicarbonate, 4.2%
Calcium gluconate 10%
Dopamine
Dobutamine
Isoproterenol (Isuprel)
Prostaglandin E_1 (Alprostadil)
Phenobarbital
Fosphenytoin
Diazepam (Valium)
Paralytic agent; pancuronium bromide
   (Pavulon); vecuronium (Norcuron)
Analgesics
Lidocaine (Xylocaine), 1%
Heparin (1000 U/ml)
Normal saline diluent, 0.9%
Sterile water diluent
Flush solution
Broad-spectrum antibiotics
Albumin 5% and/or normal saline solution
$D_{50}W$ (for making higher-glucose-concen-
   trated IV fluid)
Adenosine
Digoxin (Lanoxin)
Surfactant replacement therapy
Ophthalmic ointment
Vitamin K
Lorazepam (Ativan)
Sedative(s)
Milrinone
Reversals:
   Neostigmine (reverse neuromuscular
      blocking agents)
   Flumazenil (reverse benzodiazepine)
   Naloxone (reverse narcotic induced
      respiratory depression)

CPAP, Continuous positive airway pressure; D_5W and $D_{10}W$, 5% and 10% dextrose in water; *ET*, endotracheal; *IV*, intravenous.

selection of an appropriate receiving facility and contacting the receiving physician to request patient transfer. During the initial call, at a minimum information should be obtained to activate the appropriate team, select the mode of transport, and anticipate any special supplies or equipment that may be required during the transport. A neonatologist may provide consultation to the referring hospital as needed until the transport team arrives. Management given via phone must be accurately documented and preferably recorded. Transport computer electric medical record systems are available.

Information to be obtained during the referral call includes the following:

1. Time and date of referral call.
2. Patient name and gender.
3. Parent's name and demographic information.
4. Referring physician.
5. Referring institution, including city, state, and phone number.
6. Reason for transfer request/preliminary diagnosis.
7. Maternal prenatal, labor, and delivery history.
8. Date and time of birth.
9. Gestational age, birth weight, and current weight.
10. Apgar scores.
11. Current treatment and interventions.
12. Subsequent neonatal course.
    a. Significant findings of physical examination.
    b. Pertinent laboratory and radiographic data.
    c. Vital signs.
    d. Respiratory support.
    e. Fluid management. To prevent aspiration, the infant should receive nothing by mouth before transport.
    f. Other pertinent patient findings or medical management.
    g. Infection control issues.

B. **Selection and notification of team members.**
C. **Selection and dispatch of appropriate vehicle.**
D. **Selection of appropriate equipment and supplies.**
E. **Planning en route to referring hospital.**
   1. Team members will discuss provisional and differential diagnoses, proposed plan of care, and division of responsibilities.
   2. Referring hospital should be notified of time of team's dispatch, mode of transport, and estimated time of arrival to referring hospital.
   3. Emergency and anticipated medication dosages and intravenous fluid amounts are calculated on the basis of weight.
   4. Potential complications are anticipated.
   5. History and diagnostic study results to be obtained at referring hospital are identified.
F. **Stabilization at referral hospital.**
   1. Introduce transport team members to referring physicians, staff, and family members. Check identification band on infant. All patients should be transported with identification band on. Parents' religious, cultural, and ethnic preferences should be incorporated into care.
   2. Maintain latex-safe environment.
   3. Perform primary assessment of neonate to determine need for immediate interventions.
   4. Obtain further details of history and current management.
   5. Review previous radiographic images.
   6. Obtain vital signs and glucose screening results. Determine blood gas values if clinical situation warrants.
   7. Perform secondary assessment.
   8. Pain assessment using a validated pain-scoring tool should be completed as part of the initial assessment and reassessed during the transport Schechter et al., 2003).
      a. Recognition by the transport team that neonates feel pain.
      b. The neonate's response to pain becomes more defined with increased gestational age.

    c. Low birth weight and extremely low birth weight neonates display less organized and less vigorous response to pain.

    d. Transport team should observe for cues that the neonate is experiencing pain.

    e. The transport team should anticipate painful procedures to the neonate.

    f. The transport team should utilize nonpharmacologic techniques and or administer pain medication or sedation as ordered or by protocol.

    g. The neonate should be reassessed for effectiveness of therapy after treatment of pain.

9. Initiate monitoring systems as appropriate; may include cardiorespiratory, peripheral blood pressure, arterial blood pressure monitoring, end-tidal carbon dioxide, and pulse oximetry.

10. Consult with designated transport physician regarding management plan and anticipated complications en route, or follow transport protocols.

11. Attempt to achieve normal or optimal blood gas values, blood pressure, temperature, perfusion, serum glucose level, and acid–base balance according to the plan of care.

12. Begin switching to transport equipment, including ventilator and IV pumps, carefully monitoring changes in patient status.

13. Notify receiving unit of estimated time of arrival, current patient status, family's status, and equipment needs on admission.

14. Family support (Pillitteri, 2003). The transport team plays a pivotal role in recognizing the family in crisis, anticipating further crisis, intervening, and assisting the family through the transport process and admission to the receiving hospital.

    a. Identify members of the family unit, that is, parenting dynamics and extended family members. The family unit is often diverse. The "family" should be viewed as the object of care.

    b. If possible, allow the parents to remain in the room as their newborn is prepared for the transport.

    c. Update current patient status; discuss anticipated complications during transport and treatment plans. The parents should be involved in the plan of care.

    d. Assess the parents' understanding of the infant's condition, plans for traveling to the receiving center, and their needs for physical and emotional support.

    e. Provide information about the receiving center, including location, phone numbers, directions, attending physician, primary/admitting nurse, and visiting policy.

    f. Obtain written transport consents.

    g. Take a picture of the infant or provide a set of hand or footprints of the infant to leave with the parents. Initiate the process for bedside video if available at the receiving hospital.

    h. The family may request that special objects, such as toys, pictures, or religious and cultural objects, be transported with their infant. The team should attempt to support the request if it does not interfere with safe transport and it is within the hospital policy.

    i. Leave a bonding agent (i.e., cloth) with a parent to keep against the skin that will be given to the infant during visitation.

    j. Discuss feeding options. If the mother is planning to breast-feed, discuss storage and transport of milk to receiving hospital.

    k. The parents should be allowed to touch the infant prior to departure. This is helpful in bonding and in making the birth seem more real.

    l. Depending on the team's policy and mode of transport, one parent may be allowed to accompany the infant.

15. Obtain copies of prenatal, maternal, and neonatal medical records.
    The records should be secured during the transport in accordance with the Health Insurance Portability and Accountability Act.

16. Distribute transport evaluation form to referring hospital staff and/or parents.

G. Planning en route to receiving hospital.

1. Infant should be secured in incubator with a restraint device. Loose equipment must never be placed inside the incubator.

2. Continuously monitor temperature, pulse, respirations, blood pressure, oxygenation/ventilation, and pain status as indicated.
3. Documentation at regular intervals, as indicated by infant's condition.
   a. Vital signs, blood pressure, color, pain level.
   b. Readings of oxygenation and ventilation monitors and of respiratory support settings (including altitude if appropriate).
   c. Serum glucose screening.
   d. Important documentation times for status of infant, including arrival at referring hospital, departure from referring hospital, and time of transfer of care to receiving hospital staff.

H. Arrival to receiving facility.
1. Transport team should notify the parents/family.
2. Transport team provides report to hospital staff.
3. Follow-up may be provided to referring staff and physicians during the infant's hospitalization at the receiving center, maintaining patient confidentiality and following Health Insurance Portability and Accountability Act regulations.

I. Neonates should be transported using individualized developmental care techniques.
1. The sick premature infant experiences significant physiologic stress when incoming stimuli resulting from high noise levels, increased vibration, lighting, and handling exceed the immature nervous system's ability to respond. The infant responds with autonomic instability, hypoxia, and increased oxygen requirements. Incorporating developmental care techniques may decrease these maladaptive responses.
2. Ear protection should be provided for the neonate.
3. Shield the neonate's eyes from light or glare by placing an eye shield on the infant or covering the incubator with a flame-retardant incubator cover. The infant's eyes should be covered prior to use of lights in the vehicle. Limit use of overhead fluorescent lighting. Install and use dimmer switches in the vehicle. Indirect lighting should be directed away from the neonate to facilitate staff needs.
4. The neonate should be positioned in the incubator to support posture and movement and promote a calm, regulated behavioral state. Nesting or boundaries support the infant's position and conserve energy by containing movement. Positioning aids may be purchased or blanket rolls may be used.
5. Incubator portholes and doors should be closed with care. Objects should not strike the incubator.
6. A gel mattress may be used to decrease vibration and aid in positioning.
7. Decrease noise levels inside the vehicle by reducing speech levels, excluding radio or television use, and responding promptly to monitor alarms. An intercom system may be used for staff communication.
8. On ground transport, request that the ambulance driver avoid rough areas in road.

J. Special transport stabilization considerations.
1. Very low birth weight infant (VLBW) (Thigpen, 2002).
   a. Ventilation.
      (1) Susceptibility to barotrauma with high peak inspiratory pressures.
      (2) Administration of surfactant replacement therapy by the transport team may be considered for infants meeting specific clinical criteria or for long-distance transports. Ventilatory status must be closely monitored to prevent pulmonary air leaks because of changes in lung compliance after administration. Transport from the referring hospital may be delayed to stabilize the infant and monitor lung compliance changes prior to departure in the vehicle.
      (3) The VLBW infant may experience increased incidence of hypoxia and oxygen requirements because of the stresses of transport. Developmental care techniques should be incorporated into care. Sedation prior to transport may be required.
   b. Hypothermia.
      (1) May require supplemental warming devices in addition to the prewarmed transport incubator: crushable heat packs or mattresses; hats; polyurethane wrap or bags

especially designed for infants less than 28 weeks; increase environmental temperature, warm objects prior to placing in contact with neonate.
(2) Because of the fragility of the skin, extreme care must be taken to not place warming devices in direct contact with skin.
(3) Transport incubator door and portholes should be kept closed as much as possible.
(4) Cover the outside of the incubator with a flame-retardant incubator cover.
(5) In cold weather, preheat the vehicle prior to loading the incubator.
   c. Skin fragility.
(1) Minimal to gentle handling.
(2) Use monitoring devices designed for the VLBW infant.
(3) Minimize invasive procedures and placement of monitoring devices on skin.
(4) Maintain appropriate level of hydration. Intravenous fluid administration is calculated on increased insensible water loss with decreased gestational age. Glucose should be closely monitored.
(5) Application of a semipermeable polyurethane membrane or specific products designed for the VLBW infant may be placed on the skin to maintain integrity and decrease insensible water loss.
  2. Spinal immobilization (Jaimovich and Vidyasagar, 2002).
   a. Traumatic injuries to the neonatal spinal cord are rare.
   b. Injuries may occur because of a congenital defect, birth injury, fall, or nonaccidental trauma.
   c. The spinal column in the neonate is more susceptible to hyperextension injury as a result of increased elasticity.
   d. Spinal immobilization may be required. Immobilization device should fit into the incubator.
  3. Inhaled nitric oxide.
   a. Inhaled nitric oxide (iNO) may be initiated at the referring hospital or by the transport team. If initiated during transport, the treatment should continue for the duration of the transport.
   b. Requires continuous monitoring of all iNO delivery equipment.
   c. Follow Federal Aviation Administration for rotor-wing and fixed-wing transports. The pilot should be informed when iNO is taken on board the aircraft and when started.
   d. Ensure that a hand ventilation system is available.
  4. Ventilation and airway assist devices.
   a. Conventional ventilator.
   b. T-piece resuscitator (Neonatal Resuscitation Program, 2006).
   c. High-frequency jet ventilation (Jaimovich and Vidyasagar, 2002; Salyer, 2003).
   d. Heated humidified high-flow nasal cannula.
   e. Noninvasive positive-pressure ventilation.
   f. Continuous positive airway pressure (Murray and Stewart, 2008).

DOCUMENTATION

A. Necessity of documentation. Patient status and the care provided must be documented throughout the transport.
B. Logistical documentation.
  1. Time of transport call.
  2. Time of departure en route to referring hospital.
  3. Time of arrival at referring hospital.
  4. Time of departure from referring hospital.
  5. Time of arrival at receiving hospital.
  6. Transport delays.
  7. Names of transport staff.
  8. Mode of transport.
  9. Names of referring facility and physician.

C. Patient care documentation.
   1. Significant maternal history, including medical history before pregnancy and prenatal, labor, and delivery history.
   2. Date and time of birth.
   3. Gestational age.
   4. Birth weight.
   5. Delivery room resuscitation, including Apgar scores.
   6. Care provided before the team's arrival at the referring hospital, including laboratory and radiographic findings and medication administered.
   7. Patient status on arrival of the transport team to the referring hospital, including physical assessment, vital signs, and current patient management.
   8. Problem list, including current and resolved problems.
   9. Ongoing documentation of patient assessment, management, and consultations with designated transport physician.
   10. Patient status on arrival of the transport team to the receiving hospital, including assessment, vital signs, and monitor readings.

SAFETY*

A. Safety must be the highest priority in any transport program.
   1. The transport program should develop a comprehensive safety program for team members and patients. Training should consist of orientation to the vehicle, emergency and evacuation procedures, survival training, crew resource management, and quality management.
   2. Any passenger, that is, parent riding in the ambulance, should receive a safety briefing prior to the transport.
   3. During each transport, the team should review evacuation procedures for the crew and the neonate.
   4. Debriefing should be performed between crew members after each transport.
   5. Critical incident stress management (CISM) should be available for each crew member.
B. Uniforms.
   1. Team members should be appropriately attired to the environmental conditions when on transport.
      a. Flame- and heat-resistant uniforms.
      b. Garments such as jackets, gloves, socks, and underclothing should be made from fire-retardant or natural fibers.
      c. Protective footwear.
      d. Helmets should be worn during helicopter transports. Visors should be available to protect the eyes and face from projectile objects. Helmets may also be worn during fixed-wing and ground transport.
      e. Outer garments may be worn to protect against environmental conditions.
      f. Hearing protection should be worn by all crew who assist with patient loading and unloading while rotor blades are activated on the helicopter.
C. Flotation vests should be worn by all crew members who fly over water.
D. Survival and first-aid kit should be located on each vehicle.
E. All equipment and articles in the ambulance or aircraft must be secured.
   1. The incubator may be mounted on a cart or stretcher.
   2. The cart or stretcher must be locked into the vehicle.
   3. Majority of vehicles use longitudinal placement of the incubator rather than horizontal placement.
F. Restraint of all passengers, including the neonate, during transport.
   1. The neonate should be secured in the transport incubator with a restraint device. Owing to different gestational ages, the restraint device must adjust to fit various sizes and weights. The restraint must not constrict the thoracic cavity. A cushioned head pad should be placed in the incubator to provide protection to the neonate's head.
   2. All staff and/or passengers should have seat belts/shoulder harnesses fastened.

---

*AAP, 2007; ASTNA, 2006; CAMTS, 2006; James, 2002.

G. **Establish a written policy on the use of lights and sirens.**
   1. Follow state and local regulations.
   2. Use only for life-threatening emergencies.
H. **Communication equipment.**
   1. Communication devices are used between team members, dispatch and team, hospital and team, and team and medical control. All communication equipment must be maintained in full operating condition and in good repair.
   2. Types of communication devices:
      a. Head sets.
      b. Pagers.
      c. Cell phone.
      d. Satellite phone.
      e. Global system for mobile communication (GSM).
      f. Radio.
I. **Preaccident planning.**
   1. Ground and air transport programs must have a policy outlining the procedure to follow if the vehicle, staff, and patient are in an accident.
      a. Notification of transport and hospital administration, risk management, public relations.
      b. Provision for staff to receive care.
      c. Provision for patient care and completion of the transport. The patient may return to referring hospital for evaluation and treatment from the accident.
      d. Notification of transport team's emergency contact.
      e. Notification of the neonate's family.
      f. If appropriate, notification of other team members of the incident.
      g. If appropriate, lock-down of dispatch or transport office to limit the amount of personnel in the area.
      h. Assistance may be required to staff phones. Consider providing a separate phone number other than the team number to provide incident information and updates. A Web site may also be used to disseminate information.
   2. Staff must complete an emergency contact form that is updated annually or when there is a change of information. The form should include the following:
      a. Name of employee.
      b. Home address.
      c. Name, address, phone, cell, and pager numbers of emergency contact.
      d. Alternate emergency contact information.
      e. Information on children.
      f. General directions to crew member's home.
      g. Current photograph in uniform.
      h. Fingerprints.
      i. Name, address, and phone number to obtain dental records.
   3. Contact local or state agencies for critical incident stress debriefing for the team. Immediate- and long-term debriefing may be required.
   4. Staff should be aware of the benefits and services available prior to an incident.
J. **Infection control.** Infection control and adherence to universal precautions should be planned because of the confined space of transport vehicle.

DISASTER PREPARATION*

A. **The neonatal transport team may have to assist in evacuating a neonatal intensive care unit.**
B. **Nontraditional transport equipment may be required** because of the time limitation of having one infant in a transport incubator; size and weight of transport incubator may be prohibitive in certain aircraft.
C. **Established system of family notification of where the infant is being transported.**
D. **Established system of patient tracking, patient identification, and medical record transfer.**

---

*Orlando et al., 2007; Gershanik, 2006.

AIR TRANSPORT CONSIDERATIONS

A. **Altitude.**
  1. Anticipate increased oxygen requirement or ventilatory support at higher altitudes.
  2. Provide supplemental oxygen for staff above 10,000 feet if in a nonpressurized aircraft.
  3. Neonates are at increased risk in developing hypoxia as the partial pressure of alveolar oxygen decreases during ascent.
  4. Slow ascent and descent are recommended to prevent rapid reexpansion of gas, which increase the risk for pneumothorax and air embolism in the neonate.

B. **Dysbarism.**
  1. Increased atmospheric pressure results in expansion of gases.
  2. Anticipate expansion of "trapped" gases in body spaces (pulmonary air leaks, necrotizing enterocolitis, bowel obstruction).
     a. Gastrointestinal tract. Insert orogastric tube and empty stomach of air.
     b. Pulmonary air leaks. Consider needle thoracentesis or tube thoracotomy for decompression prior to the transport.
     c. Equalization of pressures in the eustachian tubes may be restricted in the neonate or in staff with upper respiratory or sinus problems. Providing a pacifier to the infant during descent, if appropriate, can maintain patency of the eustachian tubes.

C. **Effects of motion.**
  1. Staff should recognize and understand the stresses of transport and flight.
  2. Anticipate patient instability on ascent and descent.
  3. Staff should be able to differentiate monitor artifact from actual recordings.

D. **Noise and vibration.**
  1. Provide ear protection for staff and for the neonate (especially in rotor-wing aircraft).
  2. Provide routine hearing screens for staff.
  3. Minimize noise levels in patient compartment of vehicle.
  4. Anticipate patient instability.
  5. Use mattress and padding to minimize vibration in incubator.

E. **Evaluation for extubation and pulmonary air leaks:** possibly difficult during transport, especially in rotor-wing aircraft. Anticipate problems during transport on the basis of diagnosis and clinical presentation.

F. **Out-of-state and international transport.**
  1. The team should be knowledgeable regarding out-of-state and international transport regulations and issues.
     a. Language barriers.
     b. Time change issues.
     c. Landing permits and fees.
     d. Airport hours of operation.
     e. Fueling.
     f. Ground ambulance: availability, type, fees.
     g. Customs/immigration.
     h. Communication with regional neonatal intensive care center.

G. **Plan for crew hydration and nutrition on long-distance transports.**

H. **Transport configuration and on-loading/off-loading procedures should be predetermined, documented, and practiced prior to an actual patient transport.**

LEGAL AND ETHICAL CONSIDERATIONS

A. **Legal issues** (AAP, 2007; National Association of Neonatal Nurses, 1999).
  1. Determination of the level of responsibility of the receiving and referring staffs and institutions during the transport process has not been clearly defined and is open to legal interpretations.
     a. Referring institution's level of responsibility gradually decreases as the receiving physician and transport team assume increasing responsibility for the management and care of the infant.

      b. Transport team should be aware of national and state regulations regarding transport and professional standards: Federal Aviation Administration; National Health, Transportation and Safety Administration; Department of Transportation; Federal Communications Commission; Health Care Financing Agency; The Joint Commission; the Clinical Laboratories Improvement Act; Health Insurance Portability and Accountability Act; and the Consolidated Omnibus Budget Reconciliation Act.

      c. Receiving institution acquires increasing responsibility from the time of the transport call and the initial consultation until the time of admission to the receiving hospital.

  2. Parents or legal guardian must receive information regarding the infant's status, treatment options, the risks and benefits of transport, and the risk of not transferring.

      a. The transport program should have a policy on transporting a neonate in an emergency situation and the parent(s) are not able to provide consent.

  3. Responsibilities of transport team members should be clearly outlined in their job functions and should be compatible with practice acts.

  4. The transport nurse should be aware of federal and state regulations governing the transport and administration of controlled substances.

  5. The transport program may not be able to perform neonatal transport for a specific period owing to external and internal factors.

      a. The program may not be able to perform transports due to

         (1) weather, that is, hurricanes, tornadoes, and snowstorms;

         (2) transport accident; and

         (3) neonatal intensive care bed status.

      b. Develop a plan on how to communicate this information to referral centers.

      c. If team is operational, develop a plan for performing three-point transports. Team and facility will maintain relationship with the referring hospital.

      d. If team is not operational, develop a plan for contacting another neonatal transport service.

B. Ethical issues. Dilemmas regarding the transport of neonates should be addressed by administrative, medical, and transport staff and should include information on the following:

  1. Infants with expected poor outcomes, including those with genetic disorders, severely asphyxiated infants, extremely low birth weight infants, and those with lethal anomalies.

  2. Debriefing of the team may be required.

TOTAL QUALITY MANAGEMENT

The transport program should develop a quality management program to monitor, evaluate, and improve the service.

A. Quality indicators may include the following:

  1. Transport statistics (number of completed transports, referral hospitals, referral physicians).

  2. Equipment malfunction, failure, or supply.

  3. Transport delays.

  4. Stabilization times/use of lights or sirens.

  5. Crew and patient safety issues.

  6. Number of transports per team member.

  7. Procedures performed by crew on transport.

  8. Documentation of patient care and medications.

  9. Vehicle out-of-service time.

  10. Patient outcome.

  11. Appropriateness and timeliness of interventions and patient's response.

  12. Family and referring hospital customer satisfaction.

  13. Staff education and skills.

  14. Number of aborted and canceled transports.

B. Quality improvement may be attained through a number of mechanisms. A combination of these mechanisms is probably most effective.

1. Case review by the team, medical director, and transport director.
2. Use of peer review.
3. Regular staff meetings.
4. Case review with team members, which can be effectively accomplished by review of selected cases, including the following:
   a. Initial referral call.
   b. Transport logistics.
   c. Stabilization of the infant by the referring hospital as well as the transport team.
   d. Care provided during transport.
   e. Patient outcome.
C. **Peer review may be used to provide feedback to individuals.**
   1. Appropriateness of care provided.
   2. Clarity of treatment plan.
   3. Treatment plan rationale and outcome.
   4. Documentation.
D. **Issues identified through any of these mechanisms should be addressed with recommendations and plans for follow-up.**

REFERENCES

Air and Surface Transport Nurses Association: Position paper: Transport nurse safety in the transport environment. 2006. Retrieved January 14, 2008, from http://www.astna.org/PDF/ASTNASafetyPaper.pdf

American Academy of Pediatrics: *Guidelines for air and ground transport of neonatal and pediatric patients* (3rd ed.). Elk Grove Village, IL, 2007, American Academy of Pediatrics.

American Academy of Pediatrics/American Heart Association: *Textbook of neonatal resuscitation (NRP)* (5th ed.). Elk Grove Village, IL, 2006, American Academy of Pediatrics/American Heart Association.

Blumen, I.: *A safety review and risk assessment in air medical transport.* Salt Lake City, 2002, Air Medical Physician Association.

Bowen, S.L.: Transport of the mechanically ventilated neonate. *Respiratory Care Clinics*, 8:67-82, 2002.

Butterfield, L.J.: Historical perspectives of neonatal transport. *Pediatric Clinics of North America*, 40(2):221-239, 1993.

Chou, M. and MacDonald, M.G.: Landmarks in the development of patient transport systems. In M.G. MacDonald and M.K. Miller (Eds.): *Emergency transport of the perinatal patient.* Boston, 1989, Little, Brown.

Commission on Accreditation of Medical Transport Systems: *Accreditation standards of the commission on accreditation of medical transport systems.* Anderson, SC, 2006, Commission on Accreditation of Medical Transport Systems.

Committee on Perinatal Health: *Toward improving the outcome of pregnancy.* White Plains, NY, 1976, National Foundation of March of Dimes.

Cone, T.E.: *History of the care and feeding of the premature infant.* Boston, 1985, Little, Brown.

Gershanik, J.: Caring for and transporting very low birth weight infants during a disaster. *Pediatrics*, 117(5):5365-5368, 2006.

Jaimovich, D.G. and Vidyasagar, D.: *Handbook of pediatric and neonatal transport medicine* (2nd ed.). Philadelphia, 2002, Hanley & Belfus.

James, S.E.: *Standards for critical care and specialty ground transport.* Lexington, KY, 2002, Transport Nurses Association.

Levick, N.: Safety for pediatric ambulance transport webinar presentation. 2007. Retrieved February 27, 2007, from http://www.objectivesafety.net

Losty, M.S., Orlofsky, I., and Boles, T.: A transport service for premature babies. *American Journal of Nursing*, 50:10-12, 1950.

March of Dimes: Perinatal statistics. 2005. Retrieved January 14, 2008, from http://www.marchofdimes.com

Murray, P. and Stewart, M.: Use of nasal continuous positive airway pressure during retrieval of neonates with acute respiratory distress. *Pediatrics*, 121(4):54-75, 2008.

National Association of Neonatal Nurses: Position statement #3020: Transport of neonates across state lines. 1999. Retrieved January 14, 2008, from http://www.NANN.org

Orlando, S., Bernard, M., and Mathews, P.: Neonatal nursing care issues following a natural disaster: Lessons learned from the Katrina experience. *Journal of Perinatal and Neonatal Nursing*, 22(2):147-153, 2007.

Pillitteri, A.: *Maternal and child health nursing: Care of the childbearing and childrearing family* (4th ed.). Philadelphia, 2003, Lippincott Williams & Wilkins.

Salyer, J.W.: Transport of infants and children. In M. Czervinske and S. Barnhart (Eds.): *Perinatal and pediatric respiratory care* (2nd ed.) Philadelphia, 2003, Saunders, pp. 693-707.

Schechter, N.L., Berde, C.B., and Yaster, M. *Pain in infants, children and adolescents* (2nd ed.). Philadelphia, 2003, Lippincott Williams & Wilkins.

Segal, S.: Transfer of a premature or other high-risk newborn infant to a referral hospital. *Pediatric Clinics of North America*, 13(4):1195-1205, 1966.

Segal, S. (Ed.): *Manual for the transport of high-risk newborn infants.* Sherbrooke, Quebec, 1972, Canadian Pediatric Society.

Thigpen, J.: Developmental considerations for resuscitation of the VLBW infant. *Neonatal Network*, 21(4):21-26, 2002.

Wallace, H.M., Losty, M.A., and Baumgartner, L.: Report of two years' experience in the transportation of premature infants in New York City. *Pediatrics*, 22:439-447, 1952.

Walsh, M. and Fanaroff, A.: Epidemiology and perinatal services. In R. Martin, A.A. Fanaroff, and M.C. Walsh (Eds.): *Fanaroff and Martin's neonatal-perinatal medicine: Diseases of the fetus and infant* (8th ed.). Philadelphia, 2006, Mosby, pp. 25-34.

Wood, K.S. and Bose, C.: Neonatal transport. In M. MacDonald, M. Mullett, and M. Seshia (Eds.): *Avery's neonatology: Pathophysiology and management of the newborn* (6th ed.). Philadelphia, 2005, Lippincott Williams & Wilkins, pp. 40-53.

Woodward, G.A., Insoft, R.M., Pearson-Shaver, A.L., et al.: The state of pediatric interfacility transport: Consensus of the second national pediatric and neonatal interfacility transport medicine leadership conference. *Pediatric Emergency Care*, 18(1):38-43, 2002.

22 Care of the Extremely Low Birth Weight Infant

DIANNE SUSAN CHARSHA

OBJECTIVES

1. Discuss atraumatic care techniques for extremely low birth weight (ELBW) infants that eliminate or minimize the psychologic and physical distress experienced by infants and their families.
2. Identify principles of nursing management specific to the ELBW infant population and their families.

The ELBW infant challenges all assessment and management strategies and exemplifies the importance of holistic nursing care in the neonatal intensive care unit (NICU). Nursing skills must be finely honed and fully developed before they accept an ELBW infant assignment. The overriding approach must be one of extreme gentleness, with constant appreciation of the fragility of these infants. Every cell of the ELBW infant is immature and delicate, and demands special consideration. The purpose of this chapter is to describe a developmentally appropriate approach to nursing care of ELBW infants that emphasizes the special physiologic considerations pertinent to their care and management. Recent authors define ELBW infants as birth weight less than 1000 g, the definition adopted for this chapter (Blickstein et al., 2002; Msall and Tremont, 2002; Tommiska et al., 2003).

PRENATAL CONSIDERATIONS

A. **Whenever possible, ELBW infants** should be delivered in a tertiary care facility with a NICU. The best method of transportation for the infant is intrauterine, unless the mother cannot be stabilized or when labor is present or has progressed too far for transfer to be accomplished safely. Neonates born following maternal transport have better survival rates and decreased risk of long-term complications than those who were transferred after birth (American Academy of Pediatrics and American College of Obstetricians and Gynecologists, 2007).
   1. Neonatology consultation. Women who threaten to deliver an infant on the edge of viability should have a neonatal consultation. Consultations should be requested and performed as soon as possible to minimize parental stress. Consultations that occur when delivery is imminent are of little value. The goal of the consultation is to initiate a relationship with the mother and father that will build trust and facilitate decision making. Consultations are typically performed by neonatologists, as well as neonatal nurse practitioners.
   2. Parent participation in decision making. Understanding the parents' thoughts, wishes, and concerns will guide discussion and enable the family to participate in decision making. Collaborating with families on decision making ensures a family-centered approach. Parents must learn about the challenges and unknowns of ELBW infant delivery and resuscitation. Information should be provided in a nonbiased and factual manner. It is optimal to provide mortality and morbidity statistics specific to the institution that will be providing the neonatal care. In the best situation, parents should be given time to reflect

and talk with family, friends, and clergy. They should be encouraged to ask questions and should feel supported by the care team in the decisions they make.

DELIVERY ROOM MANAGEMENT

A. **Whenever possible, the neonatal team should prepare for the birth of an ELBW infant in advance.**

1. A neonatologist or neonatal nurse practitioner should attend the delivery, as well as a NICU nurse. Both should be skilled in the American Academy of Pediatrics/American Heart Association's Neonatal Resuscitation Program (NRP), and at least one should be skilled in intubation (NRP Steering Committee, 2006). Before the infant is born, the neonatal team should clearly define their roles with each other to avoid confusion in a stressful situation. If twins or other multiples are expected, one team should be assigned to each infant.

2. The usual resuscitation equipment must be available and its function verified. The warming table should be prewarmed, and warmed blankets available. The delivery room itself should be prewarmed whenever possible. It is optimal to place a portable warming pad under a warmed blanket on the delivery table. Consider placing the infant, neck down, in a reclosable polyethylene bag to minimize evaporative heat loss (Knobel et al., 2003; NRP Steering Committee, 2006). For centers that routinely deliver preterm infants of less than 32 weeks of gestation, blended oxygen and pulse oximetry should be available in the delivery room (NRP Steering Committee, 2006).

B. **At the time of delivery:**

1. As the infant is gently placed on the warming table, the clinician responsible for intubation should evaluate the infant's breathing, heart rate, and color. The NRP guidelines should be used to resuscitate if necessary. Blended oxygen should be administered during the resuscitation of the ELBW infant. A concentration between 21% and 100% oxygen should be administered to achieve optimal saturation levels between 85% and 95% (NRP Steering Committee, 2006). Research suggests that prophylactic surfactant is beneficial if given in the delivery room to ELBW infants after resuscitation even if they do not present with significant signs of respiratory distress (NRP Steering Committee, 2006). This clinician should also determine Apgar score at the appropriate times.

2. The second clinician should be responsible for thermoregulation by gently drying the infant and removing wet blankets or placing the infant in a reclosable polyethylene bag. If drying the infant, extreme care should be taken to avoid shearing the skin. The wet blankets around the infant should be removed so the infant remains as warm as possible.

3. As soon as possible, the infant's arms and legs should be gently flexed and supported with blanket rolls. If a small diaper is to be used, it should be slid under the buttocks rather than abruptly lifting the legs which may rapidly increase cerebral blood flow. In addition, studies suggest that maintaining an ELBW infant's head in a midline position to their torso for the first 96 hours of life decreases intracranial pressure (Carteaux et al., 2003; Cowen and Thoresen, 1985; Emery and Peabody, 1983). Midline position can be maintained in the supine or side-lying position.

4. Transfer the infant to the NICU as soon as possible in a warmed incubator equipped with the necessary gases and equipment. If the infant is intubated, the ventilator should be used rather than hand-bagging, which can deliver variable volume and pressure, to minimize risk of pneumothorax. The infant should be secured to the mattress with a blanket tucked under both sides to minimize bouncing and provide a sense of security. Care should be taken when moving the incubator over breaks in the floor, such as entry into an elevator or the change from tile to carpeting.

   a. Hospital transfer. Increased precautions must be taken to protect the ELBW infants transported in an ambulance or a fixed- or rotor-wing aircraft. Ensuring as smooth a ride as possible, promote body flexion by providing boundaries, minimize stimulus by placing cotton over the ears and applying a loose-fitting hat pulled down over the eyes and ears, which will contribute to a more developmentally supportive environment.

ADMISSION TO THE NICU

A. **Monitoring.**
   1. Hydrogel adhesive (water-based gel) cardiac leads or limb leads are optimal for use with the ELBW infant.
   2. Umbilical arterial catheters should be transduced with alarms.
   3. Skin temperature must also be monitored, whether the infant is admitted to a warming table or incubator.
   4. Oxygen saturation.
   5. Ventilator alarms (if the infant is mechanically ventilated).
B. **Thermoregulation.** ELBW infants are unable to thermoregulate themselves and require diligent attention to their temperature. Although research has not yet established an appropriate neutral thermal environment (NTE) for infants weighing less than 1000 g, caregivers must provide an adequate amount of heat to keep the ELBW infant warm. The NTE is achieved by providing the appropriate amount of warmth so the infant does not need to expend energy. ELBW infants lose a tremendous amount of heat and water through their thin skin, so interventions focused on their skin will contribute to maintaining an NTE.
   1. Bed type: incubators do decrease insensible water loss over radiant warmers, so providing care in an incubator may be preferred. Radiant warmers do have advantages but at present, not enough information exists to strongly recommend one bed type over the other (Flenady and Woodgate, 2003). Double-walled incubators decrease heat loss compared with single-walled incubators but the effects on outcome are minimal (Laroia et al., 2006). So if given a choice, a double-walled incubator should be selected for the smallest infants. Ultimately, a warmer bed that converts into a double-walled incubator provides the most flexibility for the care providers trying to meet the varying requirements of these tiny infants throughout their NICU stay.
   2. Probe: A temperature probe should be placed on a fleshy part of the abdomen, avoiding bony prominences and extremities. Apply a heat reflector backed with hydrogel adhesive if radiant heat or phototherapy is in use. Placing the probe on the left lateral side of the abdomen enables the infant to be repositioned on the back, front, and right side without moving the probe.
      a. Incubators and radiant warmers should be prewarmed with the linens.
      b. The temperature mode should be set to servocontrol, and the desired temperature set manually (36.2° C to 36.5° C).
   3. Other interventions to maintain NTE include:
      a. Addition of humidity to the microenvironment.
      b. Application of a semitransparent membrane on large skin surface areas.
      c. Application of plastic wrap across a radiant warmer.
      d. Application of a preservative-free, water-miscible, petrolatum-based topical ointment on the skin (Evidence Based Clinical Practice Guideline Development Team, 2007).
C. **Skin care.** The importance of excellent skin care in the ELBW infant population cannot be overstated. Their integumentary system does not provide a significant barrier against pathogens, infections, topical teratogens, and insensible water loss. Skin tears and shears easily because there is a minimal bond between the epidermis and dermis. Depending on gestational age, the stratum corneum may be as little as 1 or 2 cells thick (Rutter, 1996). The Neonatal Skin Care Guideline (Evidence Based Clinical Practice Guideline Development Team, 2007) provides an evidence-based approach to skin care. The guidelines were tested in a multicenter research utilization project that demonstrated improved skin conditions after guidelines were implemented (Lund et al., 2001).
   1. Vernix caseosa appears to provide a measure of antimicrobial activity (Yoshio et al., 2003), yet only the "larger" ELBW infants will have any.
   2. ELBW infants may need as many as 8 weeks for the stratum corneum to provide an effective barrier, and it may take 3 weeks for the skin pH to fall from 6.0 to 5.0 (Fox et al., 1998).
   3. Protect the skin with a piece of a pectin-based skin barrier that has a keyhole the size of the probe cut into it. Tape the probe to the skin barrier. These products should also be

used to protect the skin when taping endotracheal tubes and umbilical lines (Evidence Based Clinical Practice Guideline Development Team, 2007).

4. Avoid skin adhesives or solvents on the skin. Adhesives will create a stronger bond than that between the dermis and epidermis. Solvents will be absorbed into the skin, and are associated with liver and kidney toxicity (Evidence Based Clinical Practice Guideline Development Team, 2007).

5. Minimize the use of tape on the skin. In most cases, water-based gel adhesives are available to avoid skin trauma (Evidence Based Clinical Practice Guideline Development Team, 2007).

6. Clean the skin with sterile water. Soap is not necessary, and may alter the acidic protective nature of the skin and may be drying. If use of a cleanser is necessary, select a preservative-free neutral-pH product (Evidence Based Clinical Practice Guideline Development Team, 2007).

7. Remove antimicrobials (such as povidone-iodine) as soon as possible to minimize absorption (Evidence Based Clinical Practice Guideline Development Team, 2007).

8. Periodic application of a preservative-free, water-miscible, petrolatum-based emollient on the skin may help to protect dry skin (Evidence Based Clinical Practice Guideline Development Team, 2007). Routine application has been associated with increased nosocomial infections (Conner et al., 2003).

9. Cover wounds and cracks on skin with transparent adhesive dressings, hydrocolloid or pectin-based barrier, or nonadherent hydrogel dressing (Evidence Based Clinical Practice Guideline Development Team, 2007).
   a. Keeping clean wounds moist with transparent adhesive dressings, hydrocolloid or pectin-based barrier, or nonadherent hydrogel dressing can facilitate the healing process (Evidence Based Clinical Practice Guideline Development Team, 2007).
   b. Antifungal or antibacterial ointments can be used for infected areas.

10. Avoid using isopropyl alcohol on the skin, including the umbilical cord (Evidence Based Clinical Practice Guideline Development Team, 2007). Alcohol is drying to the skin, and is absorbed through the umbilical cord. The cord should be kept dry to enable it to fall off naturally.

PARAMETERS OF CLINICAL ASSESSMENT AND NURSING MANAGEMENT

A. **Respiratory support.**
   1. It is the rare ELBW infant who does not require respiratory support. Although some may require only blow-by oxygen or Oxyhood shortly after birth, ELBW infants may quickly tire and should be assessed closely for signs of respiratory failure.
   2. Continuous positive airway pressure (CPAP) provides alveolar distention and conserves surfactant, which decreases the work of breathing in ELBW infants with respiratory distress syndrome. Some centers choose to use bubble CPAP over ventilator-derived CPAP because of the theory that the bubbles produce vibrations, which is thought to enhance gas exchange (Morgan Stanley Children's Hospital of New York-Presbyterian, 2007). Care should be taken to ensure the correct device size because the skin of ELBW infants is extremely fragile. Both mask and nasal prongs have the potential to cause facial pressure ulcers, but the nasopharyngeal (NP) and endotracheal (ET) methods are more invasive. Place a feeding tube open to air to vent the stomach during CPAP administration (Kattwinkel et al., 2007).
      a. Permissive hypercarbia: tolerating $Paco_2$s in the 50s while maintaining a pH greater than 7.25 avoids providing excessive support, which increases the risk of trauma and added stress (Kattwinkel et al., 2007).
   3. Mechanical ventilation. Mechanical ventilation is indicated when the ELBW infant is not exchanging gases sufficiently, is acidotic, apneic, or bradycardic. When mechanical ventilation is required in the first few days of life in the ELBW infant, surfactant administration

is commonly indicated. Several different modes of mechanical ventilation are available (see Chapter 27.)

    a. Barotrauma and oxygen exposure that is associated with mechanical ventilation is responsible for the development of chronic lung disease.

B. Nursing management. Vigilant attention to all details is constantly necessary. Consistent nursing caregivers enable subtle changes to be recognized early.

  1. Minimize oxygen consumption.

    a. Conserve heat. Promote flexion and provide boundaries.

    b. Maintain blood pressure and hematocrit.

    c. Buffer metabolic acidosis as ordered.

    d. Handle minimally, reduce stimulus (light, noise), and provide cue-based, individualized care.

    e. Sedate with extreme caution. Midazolam is associated with adverse neurologic events such as death, grades III through IV intraventricular hemorrhage, and periventricular leukomalacia (Anand et al., 1999; Ng et al., 2003).

    f. Monitor for complications such as patent ductus arteriosus (PDA), and pneumothorax.

  2. Use supportive measures to decrease metabolic demands.

    a. Provide adequate fluid (start at approximately 100 ml/kg/day and adjust to maintain normal electrolyte levels) with at least 60 kcal/kg/day of caloric support and increase aggressively as tolerated to 110 to 140 kcal/kg/day (70 to 90 nonprotein calories) to promote growth (Gomella et al., 2004). Early parenteral nutrition with at least 1 to 1.5 g/kg/day amino acids is necessary to prevent negative nitrogen balance (Thureen and Hay, 2001). Enteral nutrition should be started early and advanced as tolerated.

    b. Accurately assess intake (including medications and flushes), output (including blood out), and daily weights.

    c. Monitor glucose.

    d. Monitor serum electrolytes and bilirubin levels.

    e. Monitor blood and urine cultures.

    f. Review differential and platelet counts.

    g. Provide antibiotic therapy when indicated.

  3. Maintain ventilatory support and supplemental oxygen.

    a. Maintain and protect patent airway.

    b. Monitor vital signs continuously.

    c. Monitor oxygen saturations (administering oxygen for saturations less than 85% but weaning for saturations greater than 95% [Kattwinkel et al., 2007]).

    d. Sample and monitor blood gases as clinically indicated.

    e. Maintain Pao_2 50 to 70 mm Hg.

    f. Wean ventilator settings as tolerated.

    g. Obtain x-rays, as clinically indicated.

    h. Administer surfactant replacement (should be considered in the first few days of life for oxygen requirements greater than 30% to 40%, mean airway pressure greater than 6 cm H_2O, and radiographic findings suggestive of respiratory distress syndrome).

  4. Assess airway patency, breathing patterns, and work of breathing (high risk of pulmonary hemorrhage and air leak).

  5. Assess changes in breathing following interventions (pulse oximetry, grunting, flaring, retracting).

  6. Assess changes in oxygenation and ventilation following interventions (pulse oximetry, blood gases).

  7. Ensure continuous and excellent fit of mechanical devices. All have a tendency to move or dislodge with patient movement.

  8. Maintain developmentally appropriate body positioning (support rounded shoulders and hips, flexed extremities, tucked head, hand to mouth).

  9. Regularly assess and reassess comfort and pain level with a standardized tool. Although sucrose appears to be safe in most preterm infants (repeated dosing should be used with caution) in the ELBW population (Johnston et al., 2002). Johnston and colleagues reported increased risk of poor neurobehavioral development and physiologic outcomes related to repeated use of sucrose in infants of less than 31 weeks of gestation. However, opioids should be considered for moderate and severely painful procedures (i.e., chest tube placement) (Anand, 2001).

C. **Cardiovascular support.** ELBW infants have approximately 90 to 105 ml/kg of circulating blood.
   1. Blood pressure. Blood pressures tend to be lower in ELBW infants, but should rise in the first 24 hours of life.
      a. Persistent low mean arterial pressure (MAP) has been associated with an increased risk of cerebral hemorrhage and ischemic lesions (Bada et al., 1990; Watkins et al., 1989).
      b. Blood pressures correlate directly with birth weights above 750 g.
      c. Mean arterial pressures should be monitored in conjunction with urine output and peripheral perfusion.
   2. PDA is a common congenital heart lesion. As pulmonary vascular resistance decreases and systemic vascular resistance increases, blood is shunted left to right through the PDA, which increases pulmonary blood flow.
      a. The incidence of PDA is inversely related to gestational age: as high as 80% in infants with birth weight less than 1000 g (Gomella et al., 2004).
      b. Incidence of PDA in the ELBW infant is increased because the lack of smooth muscle in the ductus prolongs patency.
      c. PDA often manifests at 3 to 7 days when respiratory distress improves and the pulmonary vascular resistance decreases. Classic signs (which may be subtle) include increased pulmonary vasculature, increased oxygen requirements, cardiomegaly, bounding peripheral pulses, widening pulse pressure, hyperactive precordium, and murmur.
      d. Patients are typically managed with conservative measures (fluid restrictions, diuretics, and positive end-expiratory pressure (PEEP), ibuprofen versus indomethacin (many more side effects [Donze et al., 2007]), or surgical management. Little and colleagues (2003) reported that medical closure of PDA failed more often when the infant was under 1000 g at birth.
      e. PDA causes increased pulmonary blood flow, which decreases systemic blood flow. Thus, ELBW infants with a PDA may be at an increased risk for necrotizing enterocolitis and renal failure.
   3. Blood transfusions. Blood removed for laboratory analysis far exceeds the ability of the ELBW infant to replace volume lost. Therefore, it is prudent to evaluate the need for every blood test performed along with the quantity of blood needed for each study.
      a. Low hematocrit level triggers the bone marrow to increase red blood cell production, but this is a weak stimulus in the ELBW infant.
      b. Packed red blood cell transfusions may be needed occasionally to raise the hematocrit level and improve oxygen-carrying capacity. It is optimal to divide units of blood to increase the number of aliquots that can be administered from each unit. Benefits of transfusion must be weighed against known risks.
      c. Erythropoietin has been shown to reduce the need for transfusion in ELBW infants, if started on days 3 to 5 of life (Maier et al., 2002).
   4. Nursing management. Vigilant attention to all details is constantly necessary. Consistent nursing caregivers enable subtle changes to be recognized early so that interventions can be made to decrease or minimize the severity of symptoms/complications. Nursing care includes diligent accounting for all blood removed, including estimates of bleeding episodes when present.
D. **Fluid and electrolyte balance.**
   1. The principles of nursing assessment and management include:
      a. Knowledge of daily requirements (start at approximately 100 mg/kg/day and adjust by 20 ml/kg for indicators of total body water status [electrolytes, weight, urine output]).
      b. Assessment of any unusual losses or gains.
      c. Prediction and measurement of ongoing losses or gains.

2. Basic elements of fluid and electrolyte balance.
   a. Body water is the major constituent of body tissue, approximately 85% in ELBW infants. Any large change in weight reflects water balance. A 20% weight loss in ELBW infants is expected, and beneficial. Most losses occur in the extracellular fluid (ECF) compartment.
   b. Electrolytes. In solution, they dissociate into ions (charged particles). Na^{2+} and K^{+} supplementation is usually needed in the parenteral nutrition formulation by day 3 to 4.
      (1) The chief cations are sodium (Na^{2+}, extracellular) and potassium (K^{+}, intracellular). Hydrogen (H^{+}) is also a cation.
      (2) The chief anions are chloride (Cl^{-}) and bicarbonate (HCO_3^{-}).
   c. pH. An alteration in pH always alters electrolyte balance. For example, hyperventilation increases the pH, and the kidneys respond by wasting bicarbonate to compensate for the elevated pH, and serum potassium is driven into the cells.
3. Body water is contained in two large compartments. The intracellular (55%) and extracellular (interstitial 40%, intravascular 5%) compartments freely exchange water.
   a. ELBW infants have severely decreased glomerular filtration rate, increased basal metabolic rate, and increased surface area in relation to body weight.
   b. Indicators of body water are weight, urine output, electrolyte balance, blood urea nitrogen, skin turgor, fontanelles, and cranial sutures. Parenteral nutrition fluid should be adjusted using these clinical and laboratory indicators with the goal of avoiding fluid overload or dehydration.
4. Fluid and electrolyte imbalances common in ELBW infants.
   a. Hypernatremia (greater than 148 mEq/l) due to excessive water losses from immature kidney function. This diagnosis should be suspected when there is increased urine output (>2 ml/kg/hour), and increasing serum sodium levels. Hypernatremia is treated by increasing fluid intake and trying to decrease sodium intake (parenteral nutrition, sodium bicarbonate, etc.).
   b. Hyponatremia (less than 133 mEq/l) due to excessive fluid administration or as a syndrome of inappropriate antidiuretic hormone (SIADH), in which a normal or excess ECF volume exists. The diagnosis should be suspected when there is sudden weight gain, no edema, increased urine osmolality, and decreased urine output. ELBW infants at risk of SIADH are those having intraventricular hemorrhage, birth asphyxia, pneumothorax, or positive-pressure ventilation. Treatment of SIADH is to restrict fluids if serum sodium is less than 120 mEq/l, and replace urinary sodium.
   c. Nonoliguric hyperkalemia (greater than 6 mEq/l) is a common problem in the ELBW infant population, resulting from movement of potassium from the intracellular space to the extracellular space. Although little research exists on the best treatment methods, Mildenberger and Versmold (2002) advocate administration of calcium, infusion of insulin and glucose, and correction of acidosis based on the best evidence available. Furosemide and sodium polystyrene sulfonate (Kayexalate) can be administered to excrete potassium (Gomella et al., 2004).
5. Transepidermal water loss (TEWL) is a measurable parameter, but is usually estimated.
   a. The Evaporimeter (ServoMed, Stockholm, Sweden) has been used in research (Vernon et al., 1990) as well as the Nova 9003 Dermal Phase Meter (NovaTech Corp, Portsmouth, NH) (Okah et al., 1995). Although expensive, the 9003 Dermal Phase Meter is easy to use and not affected by changes in the microenvironment.
   b. High humidity decreases TEWL and heat loss. Humidity also decreases fluid requirements, improves electrolyte balance, and increases urine output (Gaylord et al., 2001).
   c. ELBW infants can lose up to 200 ml/kg/day in combined TEWL and urine output (Simmons, 1998). The sum of evaporation and radiant water loss is inversely proportional to weight.
   d. 70% or higher humidity in the first week of life is needed to effect a difference (Evidence Based Clinical Practice Guideline Development Team, 2007).
   e. The use of double-walled incubators decreases TEWL (Laroia et al., 2006).

      f. The use of plastic wrap blankets that do not contact the skin surface or as-needed use of topical emollients may be used to decrease TEWL (Evidence Based Clinical Practice Guideline Development Team, 2007).

E. Hyperbilirubinemia. Most ELBW infants require treatment for elevated bilirubin levels. Their immature liver is not capable of processing the quantity of bilirubin produced during the initial weeks of life. In addition, they cannot eliminate bilirubin because they do not have the enteral intake or gut motility of term infants. The more immature the ELBW infant is, the easier his or her skin bruises and the more likely he or she is to experience intraventricular hemorrhages. Bruising and bleeds increase the problem of hyperbilirubinemia.

    Because hyperbilirubinemia is such a common problem of the ELBW infant, many institutions start phototherapy at birth. The new blue-green lamps with wavelengths of 420 to 475 nm produce less heat, which will conserve body water. If treatment is not initiated at birth, usually phototherapy is started when the bilirubin value approaches 50% of the birth weight (i.e., 3 mg/dl in a 600-g infant) (Subramanian et al., 2006). The goal is to keep bilirubin levels less than 10 to 12 mg/dl in the ELBW infant. Exchange transfusion is usually considered when values approach 12 mg/dl (Gomella et al., 2004).

F. Sepsis. Many ELBW infants are born infected or from an infected environment (Gomella et al., 2004). Infants with early-onset sepsis are more likely to die than uninfected infants (Stoll et al., 2002).

    1. Increased susceptibility to sepsis is due to
        a. Decreased antibody levels,
        b. Poor response to antigenic stimuli,
        c. Limited production of type-specific antibodies,
        d. Impaired circulating antibody,
        e. Depressed complement pathways,
        f. Decrease in neutrophil storage pool,
        g. Failure to increase stem cell proliferation during infection, and
        h. Altered neutrophil functions.
    2. Environmental risk factors include
        a. Prolonged length of stay,
        b. Multiple invasive procedures, and
        c. Frequent use of antibiotics.
    3. Reduce the risk of nosocomial bloodstream infections.
        a. Practice excellent handwashing skills.
        b. Use waterless hand disinfectants between patients after good handwashing.
        c. Optimize skin integrity and minimize skin punctures and invasive procedures.
        d. Use sterile technique when inserting invasive (venous or arterial) catheters.
        e. Use skin antimicrobials according to directions.
        f. Institute quality improvement measures to decrease the number of intravenous and central line days and improve nutrition.
        g. Standardize and minimize IV tubing connections.
        h. Prevent catheter hub contamination.
        i. Consider trophic feeds, preferably with breast milk (Edwards, 2002; Furman et al., 2003).

G. Nutrition. Nutritional management of ELBW infants is challenging.

    1. The goal of feeding is to provide nutrition that supports "postnatal growth that approximates the in utero growth of a normal fetus" (AAP, 1998).
        a. Nutrition must support the tremendous amount of physiologic growth that occurs toward the end of the second trimester and into the third trimester. Growth and development are vulnerable to nutritional deprivation.
        b. The ELBW infant gut is immature at birth and is at high risk of developing necrotizing enterocolitis.
        c. Parenteral nutrition (PN) should be initiated as soon as possible, at least within the first 24 hours of life (Evans and Thureen, 2001; Ziegler et al., 2002).
            (1) Early administration of amino acids with 1.5 g/kg/day to prevent catabolism (Thureen, Hay, 2001) and advancing to 4 g/kg/day appears to be necessary to meet the growth demands of the ELBW infant (Subramanian et al., 2006).

(2) Serum blood glucose must be followed closely for evidence of hyperglycemia. Titrating infusion rates down and/or decreasing dextrose content in the infusate may be necessary to prevent hyperglycemia.

(3) Continuous insulin infusion enables control of plasma glucose while continuing to provide nutrition to promote growth. Although not fully studied, insulin administration to promote ELBW infant growth is used with caution in many centers.

(4) Lipids provide essential fatty acids and long-chain polyunsaturated fatty acids. A 20% emulsion should be started at approximately 0.5 g/kg/day and advanced as tolerated to 2 g/kg/day while watching triglyceride levels to ensure that they remain less than 200 mg/dl (Gomella et al., 2004).

   d. Enteral nutrition.

(1) The preferred first feed is breast milk. Ziegler and colleagues (2002) recommend 1 to 2 ml per feed every 3 to 6 hours. Trophic feedings should be initiated as soon as the infant is physiologically stable and hopefully within the first few days of life. Once trophic feeds are tolerated with gastric residuals less than 0.5 ml, then advance feeds slowly 10 to 20 ml/kg/day. It is important to provide nonnutritive sucking opportunities during trophic/enteral feedings. Nonnutritive sucking is calming to the ELBW infant while it stimulates the release of digestive enzymes and develops the sucking behavior (Pinelli and Symington, 2005).

(2) ELBW infants have random, irregular motility, which causes gastric residuals. It often leads to a misdiagnosis of "feeding intolerance" when in fact it is a benign finding. The pattern reverts back to normal when feedings are started early (Berseth and Nordyke, 1993).

(3) Withholding feedings for prolonged periods leads to atrophy of the gut. Initiation of feedings that have been withheld for a prolonged period may actually be more unsafe in a gut that has atrophied as a result of starvation.

(4) Although the etiology of necrotizing enterocolitis (NEC) is unclear, it does not seem related to gastric residuals. Berseth et al. (2003) reported that NEC may be related to the rate at which feedings are incrementally increased. The incidence of NEC increased so drastically in their study group whose feeds were advanced from 30 to 40 ml/kg/day that they closed the study early.

(5) Breast milk will require fortification once enteral feedings reach 60 to 100 ml/kg/day. The goal of fortification is to add protein, calcium, phosphorus, and calories necessary to support growth and minimize protein malnutrition, osteopenia of prematurity, or rickets (Subramanian et al., 2006).

(6) The transition from gavage to breast/oral feedings must be attempted cautiously. Breathing compromise, oxygen desaturation, and bradycardia are likely to occur during oral feeds with a nasogastric (NG) tube in place (Shiao et al., 1995). Apnea appears to be an important factor that increases the length of time it takes a preterm infant to reach full oral feedings (Mandich et al., 1996).

H. Developmentally appropriate care. There is no more important subgroup of high-risk infants to integrate developmentally appropriate care into nursing than the ELBW infant. Ideally, developmentally appropriate care should be more of a philosophic approach to care than specific interventions. Developmentally appropriate care should be so well integrated into neonatal nursing that it becomes invisible and cannot be discerned from "regular" nursing care. Evidence exists that measures taken to minimize pain and stress may reduce the incidence of intraventricular hemorrhage and periventricular leukomalacia (McLendon et al., 2003).

  1. Stress. The most common sign of stress in the ELBW infant population is decreased activity and lack of "fight." They may become floppy and nonreactive.

    a. Protect from stress.

(1) Use gentle touch when handling the infant.

(2) Avoid swift changes in cerebral blood flow by gentle repositioning. Studies suggest that the head of the ELBW infant should be kept midline to the torso on a 30-degree elevation (Carteaux et al., 2003; Cowen and Thoresen, 1985; Emery and Peabody, 1983). Infants can be kept midline in a supine or side-lying position.

(3) Create a stress-free, womblike environment. Consider a heavy cover over the incubator to minimize light. When the infant gets older, approximately 32 weeks of

gestational age, some evidence exists that the circadian system becomes responsive to light and that low-intensity lighting can help regulate the developing clock (Rivkees and Hao, 2000).

    (4) Create a quiet environment.

    (5) Provide long periods of restful sleep.

    (6) Use an incubator or warming table that converts to incubator from the time of admission.

  b. Minimize stress.

    (1) Provide comfort measures after stressful events, continuing until the ELBW infant has recovered.

    (2) Use "facilitated tucking," a technique that brings flexed arms and legs to midline. Facilitated tucking mimics the fetal position, which is a universally comforting position. It is particularly useful following a stressful event, or one in which the infant is in an extended position.

    (3) Avoid clustering many stressful procedures together. Give the ELBW infant time and support to recover.

    (4) Enable hand-to-mouth positioning by flexing the arms and bringing the hands up to the mouth. This position also mimics the fetal position. In order to promote hand-to-mouth activities, avoid using hands as an intravenous (IV) site when possible.

    (5) Support position so shoulders and hips are rounded, and chin is tucked toward neck.

    (6) Use ventral support.

    (7) Use close boundaries, as in a nest (see Chapter 11).

    (8) Provide nonnutritive sucking and handholding.

    (9) Locate ELBW infant beds in quiet areas, away from telephones, sinks, and other noise producers.

  c. Learn ELBW infant cues.

    (1) Notice the emerging patterns of response from ELBW infants to caregiver's interventions.

    (2) Structure and time nursing interventions according to individual ELBW infant response.

  d. Involve family.

    (1) Teach family how ELBW infant cues are interpreted.

    (2) Consider skin-to-skin holding (kangaroo care) when appropriate.

I. Pain management. Untreated or inappropriately treated pain can have devastating effects on the ELBW infant. Unfortunately, we do not yet know all that causes pain in this population. Clinicians should proceed with caution, closely assessing ELBW infant response—and nonresponse—to all procedures and interventions.

  1. Procedures known to cause moderate or severe pain (such as chest tube insertion) should be treated with an opioid such as morphine or fentanyl.

  2. Procedures known to cause mild pain (i.e., heel stick) and those suspected of causing mild pain (i.e., endotracheal tube suctioning) should be treated using nonpharmacologic measures.

  3. Sucrose has been reported to be effective in decreasing pain responses when administered in single oral applications to preterm infants of between 26 and 34 weeks of gestation (Stevens et al., 2004). Not enough evidence exists regarding the safety of implementing sucrose interventions in ELBW infants to recommend its widespread use for repeated painful procedures in the NICU (Walden and Gibbins, 2008).

  4. Eutectic mixture of local anesthetic is not approved for use in infants of less than 37 weeks of gestation.

  5. ELBW infants treated with continuous opioid infusions for management of postoperative pain should be assessed at least every 3 to 4 hours for pain, using a valid and reliable pain scale developed specifically for preterm infants. The Premature Infant Pain Profile is such a pain scale (Ballantyne et al., 1999; Stevens et al., 1996).

    a. Infants on continuous opioid infusions may be oversedated, even at a low starting dose. All continuous doses must be titrated to achieve the desired effect. Titration occurs when the dose is decreased periodically throughout the 24-hour day when little or no pain is assessed to enable achievement of the right amount of opioid without overse-dating the ELBW infant.

b. The safety of sedatives in the ELBW infant population is not established, and should be avoided. Sedatives also blunt the infant's behavioral responses to pain without providing pain relief (Walden and Carrier, 2003).

c. Continuous infusions of opioids beyond 7 days will cause physical dependence. Depending on the dose and length of treatment, the dose should be reduced (weaned) on a regular schedule, while signs of withdrawal are closely assessed and treated if necessary.

d. Withdrawal symptoms should be treated with opioids rather than sedatives or anti-convulsants, which mask rather than treat the symptoms.

J. **Screening/Monitoring/Maintenance.** Routine health promotion and screening is an important part of the ELBW infant's care. The primary goal of health screening is to recognize and diag-nose potential significant health conditions and neurodevelopmental disabilities early. Early detection of health issues will promote more timely interventions, thereby optimizing the infant's health, growth, and development and avoiding or minimizing secondary complications.

1. Neuro Ultrasounds (NUS)—most intraventricular hemorrhage occurs within the first 3 to 4 days of life. Therefore, it's important to acquire the initial NUS by day 4 to 7 of life (Gomella et al., 2004). If signs of an intraventricular hemorrhage are present (neurologic changes, apnea/bradycardia, drop in hematocrit level, etc.) or if the ELBW infant is unsta-ble, it might be best to acquire the first NUS earlier to help the care team and parents decide what level of support is best to provide. If the initial NUS is normal, it is important to repeat an NUS at about 30 days of life to evaluate for periventricular leukomalacia.

2. Immunizations—following birth, ELBW infants starts to lose maternal antibodies that protect them from childhood diseases. At 60 days of age, the healthcare team should con-sider initiating the Centers for Disease Control and Prevention's (CDC) Recommended Immunization Schedule for Persons Aged 0-6 years (www.cdc.gov/vaccines/recs/acip). However, if the mother is positive for hepatitis B at delivery, then the hepatitis B vaccine and hepatitis B immune globulin (HBIG) should be given following birth.

3. Retinopathy of Prematurity Screening—the retina in ELBW infants is immature. Although the exact cause of retinopathy of prematurity is unclear, the greatest risk factor is prema-turity. These infants are frequently exposed to oxygen, light, and an NICU course that may be complex. An eye exam is indicated for ELBW infants once they reach 31 weeks of cor-rected age (Kattwinkel et al., 2007). The examining ophthalmologist will recommend follow-up screening based on the initial findings.

4. Hearing Screens—because the ELBW infant is commonly exposed to ototoxic drugs (ami-noglycosides, loop diuretics, etc.) and noise following birth, a hearing screen is recom-mended by 3 months of age or prior to discharge from the NICU (Kattwinkel et al., 2007). These infants should be screened using an auditory brainstem response (American Academy of Pediatrics Joint Committee on Infant Hearing, 2007).

K. **Palliative care** provides an integrated interdisciplinary approach by caregivers to support both the ELBW infant and the family through a difficult period (Carter and Bhatia, 2001). Palliative care is not limited to infants who are terminally ill or actively dying. Rather, it is a family-centered approach to care that should be offered to any family whose infant is admit-ted to the NICU. A program of palliative care may have several "levels" in which interventions change or escalate.

1. A supportive family-centered environment in which parents are encouraged to discuss concerns with health care providers is the first level of palliative care. Parents are active participants in their infant's plan of care. Clinicians spend time educating parents about their infant and condition.

2. Helping parents make decisions about resuscitation or withdrawing life support is another level of palliative care. When a model of palliative care is used as described above, deci-sions about life and death occur in a trusting relationship.

3. Infants with a lethal condition such as trisomy 13 who survive the initial neonatal period will require a higher level of palliative care. Parents may take home such an infant, but need help from community sources and respite care.

4. Infants who are actively dying require their care to be "redirected" to comfort care rather than treatment in the final level of palliative care. Clinicians caring for these patients and families must be sensitive to parents' wishes and cultural beliefs. They are intimately involved in creating the memory that parents and families will always have with them.

REFERENCES

American Academy of Pediatrics and American College of Obstetricians and Gynecologists: *Guidelines for perinatal care* (6th ed.). Elk Grove Village, IL, 2007, American Academy of Pediatrics and American College of Obstetricians and Gynecologists.

American Academy of Pediatrics Committee on Nutrition: *Pediatric nutrition handbook* (4th ed.). Elk Grove Village, IL, 1998, American Academy of Pediatrics.

American Academy of Pediatrics Joint Committee on Infant Hearing: Year 2007 position statement: Principles and guidelines for early hearing detection and intervention programs. *Pediatrics*, 120:898-921, 2007.

Anand, K.J.: Consensus statement for the prevention and management of pain in the newborn. *Archives of Pediatric and Adolescent Medicine*, 155(2):173-180, 2001.

Anand, K.J., Barton, B.A., McIntosh, N., et al.: Analgesia and sedation in preterm neonates who require ventilatory support: Results from the NOPAIN trial. *Archives of Pediatric and Adolescent Medicine*, 153(4):331-338, 1999.

Bada, H.S., Korones, S.B., Perry, E.H., et al.: Mean arterial blood pressure changes in premature infants and those at risk for intraventricular hemorrhage. *Journal of Pediatrics*, 117(4):607-614, 1990.

Ballantyne, M., Stevens, B., McAllister, M., et al.: Validation of the premature infant pain profile in the clinical setting. *Clinical Journal of Pain*, 15(4):297-303, 1999.

Berseth, C.L., Bisquera, J.A., and Page, V.U.: Prolonging small feeding volumes early in life decreases the incidence of necrotizing enterocolitis in very low birthweight infants. *Pediatrics*, 111(3):529-534, 2003.

Berseth, C.L. and Nordyke, C.: Enteral nutrients promote postnatal maturation of intestinal motor activity in preterm infants. *American Journal of Physiology*, 264(6 Part 1):G1046-G1051, 1993.

Blickstein, I., Jacques, D.L., and Keith, L.G.: The odds of delivering one, two or three extremely low birth weight (<1000 g) triplet infants: A study of 3288 sets. *Journal of Perinatal Medicine*, 30(5):359-363, 2002.

Carteaux, P., Cohen, H., Cleck, J., et al.: Evaluation and development of potentially better practices for the prevention of brain hemorrhage and ischemic brain injury in very low birth weight infants. *Pediatrics*, 111(4):e489-e496, 2003.

Carter, B.S. and Bhatia, J.: Comfort/palliative care guidelines for neonatal practice: Development and implementation in an academic medical center. *Journal of Perinatology*, 2(5):279-283, 2001.

Centers for Disease Control and Prevention: Recommended immunization schedule for persons aged 0-6 years—United States. 2008. Retrieved January 2008 from www.cdc.gov/vaccines/recs/acip

Conner, J.M., Roll, R.F., and Edwards, W.H.: Topical ointment for preventing infection in preterm infants.

Cochrane Database of Systematic Reviews 1998, Issue 3. Art. No.: CD001150. DOI:10.1002/14651858. CD001150.pub2, Revised 2003.

Cordero, L., Timan, C.J., Waters, H.H., and Sachs, L.A.: Mean arterial pressures during the first 24 hours of life in < or = 600-gram birth weight infants. *Journal of Perinatology*, 22(5):348-353, 2002.

Cowen, F. and Thoresen, M.: Changes in superior sagittal sinus blood velocities due to postural alteration and pressure on the head of the newborn infant. *Pediatrics*, 75:1038-1047, 1985.

Donze, A., Smith, J.R., and Bryowski, K.: Safety and efficacy of ibuprofen vs indomethacin for the treatment of patent ductus arteriosus in the preterm infant: Reviewing the evidence. *Neonatal Network*, 26(3):187-195, 2007.

Edwards, W.H.: Preventing nosocomial bloodstream infection in very low birth weight infants. *Seminars in Neonatology*, 7(4):325-333, 2002.

Emery, J. and Peabody, J.: Head position affects intracranial pressure in newborn infants. *Journal of Pediatrics*, 103:950-953, 1983.

Evans, R.A. and Thureen, P.: Early feeding strategies in preterm and critically ill neonates. *Neonatal Network*, 20(7):7-18, 2001.

Evidence Based Clinical Practice Guideline Development Team: *Evidence-based clinical practice guidelines: Neonatal skin care*. Washington, DC, 2001, AWHONN.

Flenady, V.J. and Woodgate, P.G.: Radiant warmers versus incubators for regulating body temperature in newborn infants. *Cochrane Database of Systematic Reviews* 1998, Issue 2. Art. No.: CD000435. DOI:10.1002/14651858. CD000435, Revised 2003.

Fox, C., Nelson, D., and Wareham, J.: The timing of skin acidification in very low birth weight infants. *Journal of Perinatology*, 18(4):272-275, 1998.

Furman, L., Taylor, G., Minich, N., et al.: The effect of maternal milk on neonatal morbidity of very low birth weight infants. *Archives of Pediatric and Adolescent Medicine*, 15(1):66-71, 2003.

Gaylord, M.S., Wright, K., Lorch, K., et al.: Improved fluid management utilizing humidified incubators in extremely low birth weight infants. *Journal of Perinatology*, 21(7):438-443, 2001.

Gomella, T.L., Cunningham, M.D., Eyal, F.G., et al.: *Neonatology: Management, procedures, on-call problems, diseases, and drugs*. New York, 2004, Lange Medical Books/McGraw-Hill.

Johnston, C.C., Filion, F., Snider, L., et al.: Routine sucrose analgesia during the first week of life in neonates younger than 31 weeks' postconceptual age. *Pediatrics*, 110(3):523-527, 2002.

Kattwinkel, J., Cook, L., Hurt, H., et al.: *Perinatal Continuing Education Program (PCEP): Specialized newborn care—Book 3*. Elk Grove Village, IL, 2007, AAP.

Knobel, R.B., Wimmer, J.E., Ahearn, C.J., et al.: *Placing infants <29 weeks' gestation in polyurethane bags after birth to reduce hypothermia.* Abstract, Southern Nursing Research Society, 17th Annual Conference, Orlando, FL, Conference Proceedings, February 13-15, 2003.

Laroia, N., Phelps, D.L., and Roy, J.: Double wall versus single wall incubator for reducing heat loss in very low birth weight infants in incubators. *Cochrane Database of Systematic Reviews* 2007, Issue 2. Art. No.: CD004215. DOI: 10.1002/14651858. CD004215.pub2, Revised 2006.

Little, D.C., Pratt, T.C., Blalock, S.E., et al.: Patent ductus arteriosus in micropreemies and full-term infants: The relative merits of surgical ligation versus indomethacin treatment. *Journal of Pediatric Surgery,* 38(3):492-496, 2003.

Lund, C.H., Osborne, J.W., Kuller, J., et al. Neonatal skin care: Clinical outcomes of the AWHONN/NANN evidence-based clinical practice guideline. *Journal of Obstetric, Gynecologic, and Neonatal Nursing,* 30(1):41-51, 2001.

McLendon, D., Check, J., Carteaux, P., et al.: Implementation of potentially better practices for the prevention of brain hemorrhage and ischemic brain injury in very low birth weight infants. *Pediatrics,* 111(4 Part 2):e497-e503, 2003.

Maier, R.F., Obladen, M., Müller-Hansen, I., et al.: Early treatment with erythropoietin beta ameliorates anemia and reduces transfusion requirements in infants with birth weights below 1000 g. *Journal of Pediatrics,* 141(1):8-15, 2002.

Mandich, M.B., Ritchie, S.K., and Mullett, M.: Transition times to oral feeding in premature infants with and without apnea. *Journal of Obstetric, Gynecologic, and Neonatal Nursing,* 25(9):771-776, 1996.

Mildenberger, E. and Versmold, H.T.: Pathogenesis and therapy of non-oliguric hyperkalemia of the premature infant. *European Journal of Pediatrics,* 161(8):415-422, 2002.

Morgan Stanley Children's Hospital of New York-Presbyterian: Bubble CPAP therapy: What every neonatologist should know. 2005. Retrieved December 2007, from www.childrensnyp.org/CPAP

Msall, M.E. and Tremont, M.R.: Measuring functional outcomes after prematurity: Developmental impact of very low birth weight and extremely low birth weight status on childhood disability. *Mental Retardation and Developmental Disabilities Research Reviews,* 8(4):258-272, 2002.

Ng, E., Taddio, A., and Ohlsson, A.: Intravenous midazolam infusion for sedation of infants in the neonatal intensive care unit. *Cochrane Database of Systematic Reviews* 2003, Issue 1. Art. No.:CD002052. DOI: 10.1002/14651858.CD002052, 2003.

NRP Steering Committee: *Textbook of neonatal resuscitation* (5th ed.). Elk Grove Village, IL, 2006, American Academy of Pediatrics and American Heart Association.

Okah, F.A., Wickett, R.R., Pickens, W.L., et al.: Surface electrical capacitance as a noninvasive bedside measure of epidermal barrier maturation in the newborn infant. *Pediatrics,* 96(4 Part 1):688-692, 1995.

Pinelli, J. and Symington, A.: Non-nutritive sucking for promoting physiologic stability and nutrition in preterm infants. *Cochrane Database of Systematic Reviews,* Issue 4. Art. No.: CD001071. DOI: 10.1002/14651858.CD001071.pub2, Revised 2005.

Rivkees, S.A. and Hao, H.: Developing circadian rhythmicity. *Seminars in Perinatology,* 24(4):232-242, 2000.

Rutter, N.: The immature skin. *European Journal of Pediatrics,* 155(Suppl 2):S18-S20, 1996.

Shiao, S.Y., Youngblut, J.M., Anderson, G.C., et al.: Nasogastric tube placement: Effects on breathing and sucking in very-low-birth-weight infants. *Nursing Research,* 44(2):82-88, 1995.

Simmons, C.F.: Fluid and electrolyte management. In J.P. Cloherty and A.R. Stark (Eds.): *Manual of neonatal care.* Philadelphia, 1998, Lippincott-Raven, pp. 87-100.

Stevens, B., Johnston, C., Petryshen, P., and Taddio, A.: Premature infant pain profile: Development and initial validation. *Clinical Journal of Pain,* 12(1):13-22, 1996.

Stevens, B., Yamada, J., and Ohlsson, A.: Sucrose for analgesia in newborn infants undergoing painful procedures. *Cochrane Database of Systematic Reviews* 1998, Issue 2. Art. No.:CD001069. DOI:10.1002/14651858.CD001069.pub2, Revised 2004.

Stoll, B., Hansen, N., Fanaroff, A.A., et al.: Changes in pathogens causing early-onset sepsis in very-low-birth-weight infants. *New England Journal of Medicine,* 347(4):280-281, 2002.

Subramanian, K.N.S., Barton, A.M., and Montazami, S.: Extremely low birth weight infant. 2006. Retrieved January 2008 from www.emedicine.com/ped/topic2784.htm

Thureen, P. and Hay, W.: Early aggressive nutrition in preterm infants. *Seminars in Neonatology,* 6:403-415, 2001.

Tommiska, V., Heinonen, K., Kero, P., et al.: A national two year follow up study of extremely low birthweight infants born in 1996-1997. *Archives of Disease in Childhood, Fetal Neonatal Edition,* 88(1):F29-F35, 2003.

Vernon, H.J., Lane, A.T., Wischerath, L.J., et al.: Semipermeable dressing and transepidermal water loss in premature infants. *Pediatrics,* 86(3):357-362, 1990.

Walden, M. and Gibbins, S.: *Pain assessment and management: Guidelines for practice* (2nd ed.). Glenview, IL, 2008, National Association of Neonatal Nurses.

Walden, M. and Carrier, C.T.: Sleeping beauties: The impact of sedation on neonatal development. *Journal of Obstetric, Gynecologic, and Neonatal Nursing,* 32(3):393-401, 2003.

Watkins, A.M.C., West, C.R., and Cooke, R.W.: Blood pressure and cerebral haemorrhage and ischaemia in very low birthweight infants. *Early Human Development,* 19(2):103-110, 1989.

Yoshio, H., Tollin, M., Gudmundsson, G.H., et al.: Antimicrobial polypeptides of human vernix caseosa and amniotic fluid: Implications for newborn innate defense. *Pediatric Research,* 53(2):211-216, 2003.

Ziegler, E.E., Thureen, P.J., and Carlson, S.J.: Aggressive nutrition of the very low birthweight infant. *Clinics in Perinatology,* 29(2):225-244, 2002.

23 Care of the Late Preterm Infant

BARBARA ELIZABETH PAPPAS and BRENDA WALKER

OBJECTIVES

1. Review fetal development for the last 6 weeks of gestation.
2. Discuss the health and developmental risks for late preterm infants.
3. Describe emerging standards of care for the late preterm infant.
4. Identify short- and long-term outcome concerns for late preterm infants.

The rate of premature births continues to rise despite advancing medical and nursing science. Neonates born between 34 and 36 weeks of gestation continue to account for 8.9% of all deliveries and more than 75% of the preterm population (Lee et al., 2006). Outcome data continues to be collected but mortality and morbidity risks are increased. The late preterm infant is at greater risk for medical problems, has a sevenfold increase risk of death, and consumes more health care dollars than full-term infants (Lee et al., 2006; Wang, 2006). A standard of care is just emerging for these infants. Often not ill enough to justify care in the neonatal intensive care unit, the late preterm neonate is often cared for in the normal newborn nursery where policies and care models are focused toward needs of the full-term neonate. Thorough assessment of risk and health status, interventions, and parent education for these neonates should be individualized (Campbell, 2006).

Definition: previously defined as near-term infant; gestational age of $34\frac{0}{7}$ to $36\frac{6}{7}$ weeks (Engle, 2006).

A. **Thermoregulation.**
   1. Anatomy and physiology:
      a. Decreased brown and subcutaneous fat.
      b. Decreased glycogen stores and ability to convert stored glycogen.
      c. Neuromuscular immaturity with decreased ability to flex extremities and decrease surface area.
      d. Increased susceptibility to large temperature gradient between neonate and environment, especially during transition.
   2. Risk factors:
      a. Temperature may decrease as much as 2° to 3° C in the first 30 minutes of life; risk for temperature instability continues beyond first day for life.
      b. Increased susceptibility to heat loss.
      c. Increased comorbidities with hypothermia such as hypoglycemia, respiratory distress, and respiratory and/or metabolic acidosis.
   3. Clinical management:
      a. More frequent and prolonged assessment; after stable, continue to assess at feedings and PRN.
      b. Warm and humidify oxygen and keep away from drafts to decrease convective losses.
      c. Encourage skin to skin holding.
      d. Provide additional layers of clothing, prewarmed hats, and blankets.
      e. May need additional support from incubator or radiant warmer—use servocontrol to maintain normal temperature.
      f. Utilize institutional protocol for weaning to open crib.

B. Respiratory issues.
1. Anatomy and physiology:
   a. Respiratory system is one of the last systems to mature.
   b. Normal lung fluid production and absorption for gestational age suggest difficulty with clearance of fluid, increased fluid retention, and delayed completion of transition.
   c. Surfactant production incomplete.
   d. Increased chest compliance, decreased muscle mass and muscle immaturity.
   e. Central nervous system immaturity and increased risk for apnea and bradycardia.
   f. Decreased airway stability due to larger head size and decreased neck stability.
   g. Higher percentage of fetal hemoglobin and risk for tissue and end-organ hypoxia.
2. Risk factors:
   a. Altered metabolic stability and increased risk for hypothermia, hypoglycemia, acidosis, and anemia.
   b. More likely to require mechanical ventilation if delivered by cesarean section without labor (Jain and Dudell, 2006).
3. Common conditions:
   a. Transient tachypnea of newborn.
   b. Respiratory distress syndrome.
   c. Meconium aspiration.
   d. Pneumonia.
   e. Pulmonary hypertension of the newborn.
   f. Apnea and bradycardia.
   g. Pneumothorax.
4. Clinical management (refer to Chapter 24):
   a. Supplemental respiratory support as needed.
   b. NPO if respiratory distress present.
C. Infection.
1. Anatomy and physiology:
   a. Immature immune system despite normal cell counts.
   b. Decreased transference of maternal antibodies.
   c. Impaired skin integrity.
   d. Increased exposure to microorganisms due to increased hospitalization and invasive tests and procedures.
2. Clinical management:
   a. Increased likelihood to be screened for infection and treated with antibiotics; initiate antibiotics within 1 hour of recognition of need (Wang, 2006).
   b. Identify if meets criteria for RSV prophylaxis.
D. Hyperbilirubinemia.
1. Anatomy and physiology:
   a. Immature liver function.
   b. Decreased gastric motility.
   c. Increased normal breakdown of RBCs.
   d. Hyperbilirubinemia levels generally peak by 5 to 7 days of life; increased risk for kernicterus (Askin et al., 2007).
2. Risk factors:
   a. Suboptimal feeding and risk for dehydration
   b. Presence of cephalohematoma, subgaleal hemorrhage, and ecchymosis.
3. Clinical management:
   a. Assess and ensure adequate feeding and hydration status.
   b. Assess for jaundice with each feeding and with routine physical assessment.
   c. Screen for hyperbilirubinemia using transcutaneous and/or serum levels when jaundiced and/or prior to discharge.
   d. Evaluate need for phototherapy and initiate per AAP Guidelines (see Figs. 23-1 and 23-2).

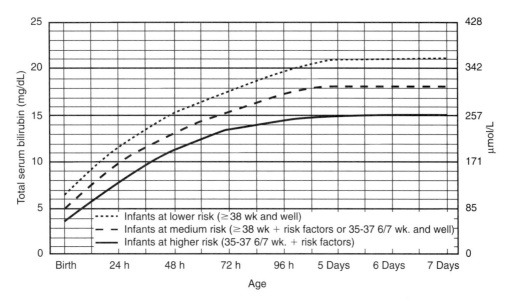

FIGURE 23-1 ■ Guidelines for phototherapy in hospitalized infants of 35 or more weeks of gestation. (From American Academy of Pediatrics: Management of hyperbilirubinemia in the newborn infant 35 or more weeks gestation. *Pediatrics, 114*[1]:297-316, 2004.)

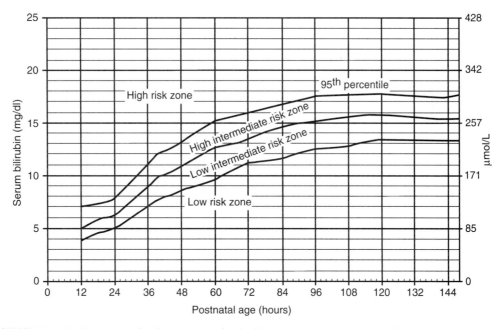

FIGURE 23-2 ■ Nomogram for designation of risk. (From American Academy of Pediatrics: Management of hyperbilirubinemia in the newborn infant 35 or more weeks gestation. *Pediatrics, 114*[1]:297-316, 2004.)

E. Hypoglycemia and feeding challenges.

   1. Anatomy and physiology:

   a. Increased risk for hypoglycemia due to low glucose stores, increased utilization, and inadequate nutritional intake.

   b. Immature oro-motor development, including rooting and sucking reflexes; coordination of suck, swallow, and breathe.

   c. Decreased gastric motility and absorption of nutrients.

   d. Difficulty maintaining tone in large and small muscle groups.

      (1) Poor latch and inadequate milk transfer.
      (2) Decreased suction and tongue tone.
      (3) Increased drooling and gulping.
      (4) Fatigue.
  e. Immature neurobehavioral development.
      (1) Immature brain development.
      (2) In-turning stage and focus on physiologic stability until approximately 34 to 35 weeks of gestation.
  f. Decreased ability to tolerate environment and stimulation and decreased ability to habituate.
      (1) Cues inconsistent, unsustained, and subtle.
  g. Fatigues easily; increased sleep and decreased awake time.
      (1) Disorganized and rapid change in behavior state.
  h. Health status affects ability to feed (e.g., respiratory distress, hypoglycemia, hypothermia) (McGrath and Braescu, 2004).
  i. Metabolic needs increased.
  j. Clinical problems related to feeding challenges:
      (1) Hypoglycemia.
      (2) Hypothermia.
      (3) Feeding residual.
      (4) Hyperbilirubinemia.
      (5) Excessive weight loss and/or dehydration.
      (6) Failure to establish or maintain breast milk volume and feeding.
      (7) Delay in discharge as much as 76% (Adamkin, 2006).
      (8) Failure to thrive.
  k. General feeding considerations:
      (1) Increased need for intravenous fluid support; assess for dehydration by monitoring for adequate intake.
      (2) Consider abdominal girth measurements, especially if low Apgar scores or feeding residuals.
      (3) Assess for feeding readiness based on cues; use cues to direct feeding method (e.g., bottle/breast vs. gavage feeding; cessation of nippling effort).
      (4) Feed early in awakening; delay care and stimulation that tire neonate.
      (5) May feed well first few feedings or days and then fatigue.
      (6) Bottle or breastfeeding should not be pushed if neonate is not awake or does not have sufficient energy; feeding relationship should be positive.
      (7) Provide external pacing if necessary.
      (8) Transition method from gavage to breast and/or bottle has not been defined by the evidence.
      (9) Decrease overall stimulation during feeding (e.g., noises, light).
     (10) Utilize nonnutritive sucking between feedings and 2 to 3 minutes prior to feeding.
     (11) Promote skin-to-skin care.
     (12) Avoid thermal stress.
     (13) May need transitional formula or fortified breast milk.
     (14) Consider consultation with feeding team or specialist.
     (15) If hospital stay 1 week or more, measure/plot length and head circumference.
  l. Breastfeeding management.
      (1) Support early lactogenesis.
      (2) Lactation support.
      (3) Initiate pumping after each feeding.
      (4) Thorough assessment of latch, suck–swallow–breath coordination.
      (5) Test weights may be helpful for some populations.
      (6) Establish a defined discharge plan to promote transition to full breastfeeding (Wright, 2004).
      (7) Follow up at discharge with lactation support.

     m. Bottle feeding.
        (1) Low-flow bottle nipple.
        (2) May need supplementation with gavage feeding.
        (3) Swaddle with hands to midline in tucked position.
        (4) Hold close in crook of arm for feeding.
     n. Nonsupportive feeding interventions.
        (1) Manipulation of nipple into or in mouth (e.g., twisting, turning, pushing, pulling nipple).
        (2) Nipple with enlarged hole.
        (3) "Preemie" nipple (McGrath and Braescu, 2004).
        (4) Interpretation of "gulping" as hunger.
        (5) Pushing neonate to continue.
        (6) Adding medication or vitamins to feeding.

F. Developmental.
  1. Anatomy and physiology:
     a. Incomplete development of the central nervous system.
     b. Despite development of some sensory systems, continues to be vulnerable to stimulation as a result of illness and/or difficulty with habituation; may be sensitive especially with multiple stimuli.
     c. Ability to focus on visual stimuli limited.
     d. State system stability emerging as demonstrated by limited awake time, lack of smooth transition from sleep to awake, and rapid movement between sleep and awake states.
     e. Decreased stability of subsystems with illness and transition to extrauterine life.
  2. Clinical management.
     a. Apply developmentally supportive care practices (i.e., developmental tools, facilitated tucking, skin-to-skin care, imposed rest during care).
     b. Offer cue-based, individualized care teaching parents cues and supportive measures.
     c. Offer singular stimulation observing cues for tolerance before adding stimulation (i.e., offer voice or face separately).
     d. Transition to increased lighting; promote dimmed light when alert, quiet
     e. Support day–night cycling of light and stimulation.

G. Miscellaneous—Drug toxicity.
  1. Anatomy and physiology.
     a. Immaturity of gastric motility and acidity; decreased bile acid secretion and protein binding may alter drug absorption, metabolism, and elimination.
     b. Altered water, fat, and tissue distribution may alter absorption, distribution, metabolism, and elimination of drugs.
     c. Increased risk for dehydration (Raju et al., 2006; Ward, 2006).
  2. Clinical management.
     a. Follow therapeutic values of medications closely.

H. Discharge criteria.
  1. Normoglycemic.
  2. Temperature stability.
  3. Stable or decreasing bilirubin.
  4. Feeding to sustain growth.
  5. Feeding plan in place and parent(s) educated on plan.
  6. Consider neuroimaging and ophthalmic examination.
  7. RSV prophylaxis considered.
  8. Scheduled home care and follow-up appointments (i.e., lactation support, weight checks, home treatment for hyperbilirubinemia).

I. Parent education.
  1. When and how often to see primary healthcare provider (i.e., respiratory distress, jaundice, feeding, weight checks).
  2. Temperature assessment and maintenance at home; avoid overdressing and underdressing.

3. Feeding plan (e.g., minimum number or volume of feeding per day).
4. Assessment for jaundice and dehydration.
5. Offer instruction in infant CPR.
6. Education on RSV prophylaxis and prevention.
7. Behavior expectations—amount of sleep–awake time to expect, cues.
8. Car seat—findings of pulse oximetry testing, information on car bed or car seat for neonates less than 5 to 7 pounds depending on individual needs.
9. Hip ultrasound at 6 weeks if breech at birth.
10. Information on infection control, SIDS.
11. Information on early intervention services.

J. Long-term outcome.
1. Increased risk for SIDS by as much as 50% (Darnall et al., 2006).
2. Increased risk for at least one hospital readmission within the first 6 to 12 months of life, especially if never admitted to NICU (Cuevas et al., 2005; Jain and Cheng, 2006).
3. Potential for growth and developmental delay (Chyi et al., 2008).

REFERENCES

Adamkin, D.H.: Feeding problems in the late preterm infant. *Clinics in Perinatology, 33*(4):831-837, 2006.

American Academy of Pediatrics: Management of hyperbilirubinemia in the newborn infant 35 or more weeks gestation. *Pediatrics, 114*(1):297-316, 2004.

Askin, D.F., Bakewell-Sachs, S., Medoff-Cooper, B., Rosenberg, S., and Santa-Donato, A.: *Late preterm assessment guide.* Washington, DC, 2007, Association of Women's Health, Obstetric and Neonatal Nurses.

Campbell, M.A.: Development of a clinical pathway for near-term and convalescing premature infants in a level II nursery. *Advances in Neonatal Care, 6*(3):150-164, 2006.

Chyi, L.J., Lee, H.C., Hintz, S.R., Gould, J.B., and Sutcliffe, T.L.: School outcomes of late preterm infants: Special needs and challenges for infants born at 32 to 36 weeks gestation. *Journal of Pediatrics, 153*(1):5-6, 2008.

Cuevas, K.D., Silver, D.R., Brooten, D., Youngblut, J.M., and Bobo, C.M.: The cost of prematurity: Hospital charges at birth and frequency of rehospitalizations and acute care visits over the first year of life. *American Journal of Nursing, 105*(7):56-65, 2005.

Darnall, R.A., Ariagno, R.L., and Kinney, H.C.: The late preterm infant and the control of breathing, sleep, and brainstem development: A review. *Clinics in Perinatology, 33*(4):883-914, 2006.

Escobar, G.J., Clark, R.H., and Greene, J.D.: Short-term outcomes of infants born at 35 and 36 weeks gestation: We need to ask more questions. *Seminars of Perinatology, 30*:28-33, 2006.

Engle, W.A.: A recommendation for the definition of "late preterm ("near-term") and the birth weight-gestational age classification system. *Seminars in Perinatology, 30*:2-7, 2006.

Jain, S. and Cheng, J.: Emergency department visits and rehospitalizations in late preterm infants. *Clinics in Perinatology, 33*(4):935-945, 2006.

Jain, L. and Dudell, G.G.: Respiratory transition in infants delivered by cesarean section. *Seminars in Perinatology, 30*:296-304, 2006.

Lee, Y.M., Cleary-Goldman, J., and D'Alton, M.E.: The impact of multiple gestations on late preterm (near-term) births. *Clinics in Perinatology, 33*(4):777-792, 2006.

McGrath, J.M. and Braescu, A.V.B.: State of science: Feeding readiness in the preterm infant. *Journal of Perinatal and Neonatal Nursing, 18*(4):353-368, 2004.

Raju, T.N.K., Higgins, R.D., Stark, A.R., and Leveno, K.J.: Optimizing care and outcome for late-preterm (near term) infants: A summary of the workshop sponsored by the National Institute of Child Health and Human Development. *Pediatrics, 118*:1207-1214, 2006.

Wang, M.L., Dorer, D.J., Fleming, M.P., and Catlin, E.A.: Clinical outcomes of near-term infants. *Pediatrics, 114*(2):372-376, 2004.

Ward, R.M.: Drug disposition in the late preterm ("near-term") newborn. *Seminars in Perinatology, 30*:48-51, 2006.

Wright, N.E.: Breastfeeding the borderline (near-term) preterm infant. *Breastfeeding Review, 12*(3):17-24, 2004.

24 Respiratory Distress

DEBBIE FRASER ASKIN

OBJECTIVES

1. Describe the anatomic and biochemical events associated with lung development.
2. Discuss the physiology of respiration.
3. Describe common respiratory disorders seen in the newborn infant.
4. Discuss common findings in respiratory distress syndrome (RDS), meconium aspiration syndrome, pneumonia, pulmonary hypertension, and bronchopulmonary dysplasia.
5. Describe nonpulmonary causes of respiratory distress.
6. Identify treatment strategies for common respiratory problems.
7. Formulate a plan of care for infants with respiratory disorders.

The most common group of life-threatening diseases in newborns is respiratory in origin. This is evidenced by the number of infants admitted to the neonatal intensive care unit (NICU) in respiratory distress. Respiratory distress syndrome, retained lung fluid syndromes, aspiration syndromes, air leaks, and congenital pneumonia account for approximately 90% of all respiratory distress in newborns. Pulmonary disease, however, is not the cause of all respiratory distress in newborn infants. Congenital malformations, metabolic abnormalities, central nervous system (CNS) disorders, and congenital heart disease may also present with respiratory distress. This chapter discusses common respiratory problems of the newborn infant, along with pathophysiology, clinical presentation, differential diagnosis, and management.

LUNG DEVELOPMENT

A. **Anatomic events.** Five stages of lung development have been identified and are described as follows (Larsen, 2001; Moore and Persaud, 2003):
   1. Embryonic development (weeks 1 to 5). The endoderm-derived embryonic foregut provides a single lung bud that begins to divide ventrocaudally through the mesenchyme surrounding the foregut. The pulmonary vein develops and extends to join the lung bud. The trachea develops at the end of the embryonic period. There are three divisions on the right side and two on the left side that will eventually become the lobes of the lungs.
   2. Pseudoglandular period (weeks 5 to 17). All conducting airways are formed. Cartilage appears; main bronchi are formed; demarcation of major lobes occurs; formation of new bronchi are complete; capillary bed is formed with connecting bronchial blood supply; no connection made with terminal air sacs. The lung at this time undergoes 14 more generations of branching and the formation of the terminal bronchioles. The lung resembles an exocrine organ because of surrounding loose mesenchymal tissues, hence the name *pseudoglandular*.
   3. Canalicular period (weeks 17 to 24). Formation of gas-exchanging acinar units (i.e., respiratory units). The appearance of glycogen-rich cuboidal cells and inclusions for surface-active material storage are seen; capillaries invade terminal airway walls; type II alveolar epithelial cells appear. Airway changes from glandular to tubular and increases in length and diameter. Vascular system proliferates and the capillaries are now closer to the epithelium-conducting airways. Respiratory bronchioles that will participate in gas exchange can be differentiated.
   4. Terminal sac period (weeks 24 to 37). Between weeks 24 and 26 alveolar sacs are formed; air–blood surface area is limited for gas exchange; and type II cells are unable to release

surfactant in sufficient quantity to maintain air breathing. Capillary loops increase; type II cells cluster at alveolar ducts, become numerous and mature; more budding occurs from alveolar ducts; and lung size increases rapidly because there is an exponential increase in surface area for gas exchange.

5. Alveolar period (week 37 to 8-10 years). This phase is characterized by continued alveolar proliferation and development.

B. **Biochemical events.**

1. Surface-active phospholipids line terminal air spaces and maintain alveolar stability by reducing surface tension.

2. Surfactant is a mixture of at least six phospholipids and four apoproteins.

   a. Dipalmitoylphosphatidylcholine (DPPC) is the major surface-active lipid component of surfactant. DPPC reduces the surface tension at the air–water interface in the alveolus almost to zero (Jobe and Ikegami, 2001).

   b. Surfactant includes cholesterol, proteins, complex carbohydrates, and glycolipids.

   c. Phospholipids are responsible for the surface-active properties of surfactant. Surfactant proteins have recently been found to have important properties.

   d. The two groups of surfactant proteins: the hydrophilic surfactant proteins A and D (SP-A and SP-D) and the hydrophobic surfactant proteins B and C (SP-B and SP-C). SP-B and SP-C are known to enhance the surface tension–lowering properties of surfactant and facilitate its absorption and spread.

      (1) SP-A with SP-B forms the tubular myelin lattice network. SP-A probably also has a role in the recycling of surfactant. SP-A activates alveolar macrophages and thus has a role in host defenses. SP-A is the most abundant of the surfactant proteins.

      (2) SP-B is important in the formation of tubular myelin, enhances the uptake of phospholipids by the type II cell, and is also important in the recycling of surfactant.

      (3) SP-C may have a role in surfactant dispersal and recycling, enhancing the rate of absorption and spreading of surfactant.

      (4) SP-D may also have a role in host defense mechanisms (Jobe and Ikegami, 2001; Moise and Hansen, 2003).

   e. Surfactant reduces surface-tension forces in the alveoli that are capable of producing collapse at expiration (Jobe and Ikegami, 2001).

      (1) Surfactant is produced in the type II pneumocyte beginning at 24 to 28 weeks of gestation and continuing to term (Shapiro, 1988). Type II pneumocytes synthesize, store, secrete, and recycle surfactant (Blackburn, 2007; Moise and Hansen, 2003).

      (2) When the lungs are inflated, receptors in type II cells mobilize intracellular calcium, which causes the release of the contents of lamellar bodies into the air space. After secretion, surfactant may be taken back into type II cells with a turnover time of 10 hours (Moise and Hansen, 2003).

3. The changing pattern of phospholipids in amniotic fluid can be used to assess surfactant production and maturation of pathways.

   a. Material from the fetal lung contributes to amniotic fluid.

   b. Concentrations of various phospholipids can be measured and will assist in determining lung maturity.

4. Sphingomyelin concentration remains stable, with a small peak at 28 to 30 weeks.

5. Lecithin and phosphatidylinositol concentrations remain low until 26 to 30 weeks, when an increase begins. A peak occurs at 36 weeks.

6. Phosphatidylglycerol (PG) appears at 30 weeks, peaks at 35 to 36 weeks, and increases as the phosphatidylinositol level falls.

   a. When PG is present, the risk that RDS will develop in the infant is less than 1%.

   b. PG is measured as absent or present.

   c. Blood and meconium do not affect test results.

7. The lecithin/sphingomyelin (L/S) ratio has been used to assess fetal lung maturity.

   a. An L/S ratio greater than 2:1 is considered to indicate fetal lung maturity.

   b. An infant of a diabetic mother may develop RDS even with a mature L/S ratio (presence of PG ensures lung maturity).

     c. Chronic fetal stress (e.g., maternal hypertension, retroplacental bleeding, maternal drug use, smoking) will tend to accelerate surfactant production, resulting in a mature L/S ratio in premature infants.

  8. Fetal lung maturity (FLM).

     a. Measures ratio of surfactant to albumin.

     b. Sample should be free of blood and meconium.

     c. Less than 50 = immaturity; 50 to 70 = borderline maturity; greater than 70 = mature lungs.

C. Role of antenatal steroids.

  1. Antenatal corticosteroids and glucocorticoids (e.g., betamethasone or dexamethasone) affect lung maturation and present a strategy for preventing RDS. Betamethasone appears to significantly decrease neonatal death and morbidity (National Institutes of Health [NIH] Consensus, 2000; Roberts and Dalziel, 2008). Steroids accelerate the normal pattern of lung growth by increasing the rate of glycogen depletion and glycerophospholipid biosynthesis. This leads to thinning of the intraalveolar septa and increases the size of the alveoli. The number of surfactant-producing type II pneumocytes increases as do the number of lamellar bodies inside the cells. This leads to increased synthesis of surfactant phospholipids. Steroids may also increase the amount of fibroblast pneumocyte factor, which increases surfactant production (Blackburn, 2007).

     a. Treatment with steroids is recommended for:

       (1) Maternal risk of preterm delivery between 24 and 34$\frac{6}{7}$ weeks of gestation (Roberts and Dalziel, 2008).

       (2) Treatment with corticosteroids less than 24 hours prior to delivery is still associated with a decrease in mortality, RDS, and intraventricular hemorrhage (IVH). It should be given unless immediate delivery expected.

     b. Administration of corticosteroids in premature rupture of the membranes is not associated with a higher risk of chorioamnionitis (Ghidini et al., 1997). The recommendation from the NIH consensus statement is the use and efficacy of a single course of antenatal corticosteroid (NIH Consensus, 2000).

     c. Two doses of betamethasone 12 mg should be given intramuscularly (IM) 24 hours apart, or four doses of dexamethasone 6 mg should be given IM every 12 hours in patients at risk for preterm delivery between 24 and 34$\frac{6}{7}$ weeks of gestation with intact membranes or between 24 and 32 weeks of gestation for patients with ruptured membranes. Repeated courses of glucocorticoids should not be routinely used (American Academy of Pediatrics and American College of Obstetricians and Gynecologists [AAP/ACOG], 2002).

  2. Infants exposed to chronic stress in utero are usually small for gestational age and have more mature lungs (they also have small thymuses and large adrenal glands, suggesting high glucocorticoid levels in utero).

PHYSIOLOGY OF RESPIRATION

Refer to Chapters 4 and 26.

RESPIRATORY DISORDERS

Respiratory Distress Syndrome

A. Definition.

  1. Developmental disorder starting at or soon after birth and occurring most frequently in infants with immature lungs.

  2. Increasing respiratory difficulty in the first 3 to 6 hours, leading to hypoxia and hypoventilation.

  3. Progressive atelectasis.

B. Incidence.

  1. Approximately 20,000 to 30,000 infants per year affected in the United States (Whitsett et al., 2005).

2. The incidence of RDS is inversely related to gestational age, affecting 10% of all premature infants, the majority of these born at less than 28 weeks of gestation (ALA, 2008).

C. **Etiology.**
1. Surfactant deficiency.
2. Pulmonary hypoperfusion.
3. Anatomic immaturity.
4. Precipitating factors associated with incidence and/or severity of RDS.
   a. Prematurity.
   b. Cesarean delivery without labor.
   c. Maternal diabetes, especially if infant was born at less than 38 weeks of gestation.
   d. Acute antepartum hemorrhage.
   e. Second twin.
      (1) May be due to greater risk of asphyxia.
      (2) First twin usually smaller, suggesting chronic stress leading to early lung maturation.
   f. Asphyxia at birth.
   g. Male/female ratio of 2:1.

D. **Pathophysiology.**
1. Production of surfactant is inadequate, occurring when the utilization of surfactant exceeds the rate of production. This leads to diffuse alveolar atelectasis, pulmonary edema, and cell injury (Hagedorn et al., 2006). Progressive worsening of these three factors will contribute to a loss of functional residual capacity, alteration in ventilation perfusion ratio, and uneven distribution of ventilation (Whitsett et al., 2005).
2. Serum proteins, which inhibit surfactant function, leak into the alveoli. The increased water content, immature mechanisms for clearance of lung liquid, lack of alveolar–capillary apposition, and decreased surface area for gas exchange, typical of the immature lung, also contribute to the disease (Liley and Stark, 1998).
3. Histologic findings are the presence of hyaline membranes and an eosinophilic material derived from injury to epithelial cells. The alveolar spaces are generally collapsed, with pulmonary edema, hemorrhage, and hemorrhagic edema noted (Whitsett et al., 2005).

E. **Clinical presentation.**
1. Almost exclusively in premature infants.
   a. May appear to be a normally grown, healthy premature infant with good Apgar scores at birth.
   b. Distress begins at or soon after birth.
2. Increasing respiratory difficulty related to progressive atelectasis. Symptoms are progressive.
   a. Tachypnea (>60 breaths per minute) is usually the first sign; color is maintained.
   b. Audible expiratory grunt.
      (1) Heard during first few hours.
      (2) Caused by forcing of air past a partially closed glottis.
      (3) Used to maintain positive end-expiratory pressure (PEEP) at the alveolar level in an attempt to prevent alveolar collapse.
      (4) More pronounced with severe disease.
   c. The chest wall in an infant is very compliant. When an infant breathes spontaneously, pleural pressure decreases during inspiration. When there is parenchymal disease, the chest wall produces greater negative pressure and the more compliant chest wall caves inward with a moderate decrease in pleural pressure, which results in retractions. Retractions are seen at the xiphoid and intercostal markings of the infant's chest and reflect a decrease in lung volume (McClure et al., 2005).
   d. Nasal flaring.
   e. Cyanosis due to increasing hypoxemia.
3. Oxygen requirements increase to maintain arterial Po_2 at 50 to 70 mm Hg because of decreased lung compliance secondary to decreased surfactant. Additional physical effort is needed to keep terminal airways open, resulting in increased work of breathing.
4. Paradoxic seesaw respirations may be seen.

5. If signs and symptoms are unattended, infant becomes obtunded and flaccid.
   a. Pallor may obscure severe central cyanosis.
   b. Poor capillary filling time (>3 to 4 seconds).
   c. Progressive edema, usually seen in the face, palms, and soles.
6. Oliguria is common in the first 48 hours.
7. Breath sounds diminish and lung auscultation is usually described as "poor air entry" despite vigorous effort on the infant's part.
8. Crackles become audible as the disease progresses.
9. Cardiac murmurs are generally not heard until after 24 hours of age.
10. Tachycardia (heart rate >160 beats per minute [bpm]) is common and even more prevalent if acidosis and hypoxemia are present.

F. **Diagnosis.**
1. Signs and symptoms as previously described.
2. Hypoxemia (defined as arterial Po_2 level <50 mm Hg in room air) as a result of ventilation–perfusion mismatch and right-to-left intrapulmonary shunting, responding to supplemental inspired oxygen; respiratory failure secondary to alveolar hypoventilation (Pco_2 >50; pH ≤7.25).
3. Chest x-ray reveals low lung volumes, hazy lung fields, and a fine reticulogranular pattern of density with air bronchograms. Occasionally the disease may appear worse in one lung than the other (Moise and Hansen, 2003).
4. Diagnostic studies.
   a. Chest x-ray examination.
   b. Arterial blood gas (ABG) measurements.
   c. Blood cultures, complete blood cell count. Pneumonia caused by group B streptococcus has similar radiographic features; therefore infection must be considered.
   d. Blood glucose level. Increased work of breathing results in increased glucose consumption.

G. **Differential diagnosis.**
1. Pneumonia. Similar signs, symptoms, and radiologic features can be found in neonates with pneumonia and those with RDS.
2. Transient tachypnea of the newborn (TTN) can present with the same signs and symptoms, but these infants usually require ≤40% Fio_2, improve quicker, and have larger lung volumes on chest x-ray (CXR).
3. Pulmonary edema. A primary cardiac disorder with pulmonary edema (caused by patent ductus arteriosus [PDA]) can mimic RDS.

H. **Complications.**
1. Pulmonary.
   a. Air leaks.
   b. Pulmonary edema.
   c. Bronchopulmonary dysplasia (BPD).
2. Cardiovascular.
   a. PDA.
   b. Systemic hypotension.
3. Renal.
   a. Oliguria.
      (1) Most likely to follow hypoxia, hypotension, or shock ("prerenal" renal failure).
   b. Immature renal function with decreased glomerular filtration in very low birth weight infants.
   c. Natural diuresis will occur at approximately 48 to 72 hours of age, as infant's condition improves.
4. Metabolic.
   a. Acidosis. Atelectasis with increased work of breathing will lead to hypoxemia and acidemia, resulting in vasoconstriction of the pulmonary vasculature. This then limits alveolar capillary blood flow, which further impedes the production of surfactant and compounds the problem (Hagedorn et al., 2006).
   b. Hyponatremia or hypernatremia.

      c. Hypocalcemia.

      d. Hypoglycemia.

  5. Hematologic.

      a. Anemia—may be iatrogenic due to blood loss required for diagnostic testing. Hematocrit should be near normal to ensure adequate oxygen-carrying capacity.

  6. Neurologic.

      a. Seizures: may result from hypoglycemia or an IVH.

      b. Ventilator manipulations, rapid fluid infusions, shock, and acidosis are all factors causing changes in cerebral blood flow that may precipitate an IVH (Paige and Moe, 2006).

  7. Other.

      a. Secondary nosocomial infections.

      b. Retinopathy of prematurity (ROP).

      c. Dislodged endotracheal tubes.

      d. Thrombus formation. Complication of umbilical catheters needed to monitor respiratory status.

I. Management. RDS is a disease that is self-limited and transient. Adequate surfactant can be produced by the premature infant within 48 to 72 hours.

  1. Goal of treatment is supportive until disease resolves and to prevent further lung injury (Moise and Hansen, 2003).

  2. Surfactant replacement therapy.

      a. Benefits include the following (Engle and the Committee on Fetus and Newborn, 2008; Kattwinkel, 1998; Moise and Hansen, 2003):

         (1) Reduced morbidity and mortality rates.

         (2) Improved compliance and decreased resistance in surfactant-poor acini, thereby reducing the pressure needed to inflate the lungs and decreasing work of breathing.

         (3) Improved ventilation in low-volume lung units, which increases the Pao_2, decreases the right-to-left intrapulmonary shunt, and improves overall oxygenation of the infant.

      b. Surfactants approved by U.S. Food and Drug Administration (FDA) for treatment of RDS:

         (1) Natural surfactants: beractant (Survanta), poractant alfa (Curosurf), and calfactant (Infasurf). Composed of minced bovine, porcine, or calf lung with added lipids.

         (2) A synthetic form of surfactant (Exosurf) was approved but is no longer being manufactured.

      c. Two treatment methods are related to timing.

         (1) Prophylaxis. Treatment soon after birth: infants born at less than 27 to 30 weeks of gestation; dose given via endotracheal tube after initial resuscitation. Additional doses may be given if necessary. Prophylactic use of surfactant has been shown to decrease the incidence and severity of RDS and to reduce the risk of air leak, BPD, and death (Engle and the Committee on Fetus and Newborn, 2008; Soll, 2000).

         (2) Rescue. Treatment of infants with progressive oxygen requirements (usually ≥40% Fio_2) in the first day of life; multiple doses can be given. The goal of intervention is to avoid progressive alveolar atelectasis leading to respiratory failure requiring intermittent positive pressure ventilation (IPPV) (Egberts et al., 1993; Kattwinkel et al., 1993; Kendig et al., 1991).

         (3) Beractant (Survanta): Dose is 4 ml/kg given through an in-line catheter or a 5F orogastric catheter threaded through the endotracheal tube with the tip extended just beyond the end of the endotracheal tube, above the carina. Repeated doses can be given every 6 hours during the first 48 hours of life (Hagedorn et al., 2006).

         (4) Poractant alfa (Curosurf): Initial dose is 2.5 ml/kg given in 2 aliquots via an in-line catheter or a 5F orogastric catheter threaded through the endotracheal tube. Two subsequent doses of 1.25 ml/kg can be administered at 12-hour intervals if needed (Hagedorn et al., 2006).

         (5) Calfactant (Infrasurf): Dose is 3 ml/kg divided in 2 aliquots, every 12 hours for a total of three doses. After each aliquot, the infant is repositioned in either the right

or left side dependent positions to enhance distribution in the lungs (Hagedorn et al., 2006).

3. Provide warm, humidified oxygen to maintain normal Pao_2.
4. Provide continuous positive airway pressure (CPAP) via nasal prongs or endotracheal tube if indicated.
5. Use assisted ventilation for profound hypoxemia (Pao_2 <50 mm Hg) and/or hypercapnia ($Paco_2$ >60 mm Hg).
6. Monitor oxygenation by pulse oximetry and/or transcutaneous monitoring.
7. Monitor pulmonary status with chest x-ray examination, as clinically indicated.
8. Other measures.
   a. Stabilize temperature.
   b. Provide adequate fluid and electrolyte intake. Monitor intake and output, serum BUN, and creatinine.
   c. Restore acid–base balance by administration of sodium acetate and/or sodium bicarbonate ($NaHCO_3$) for severe metabolic acidosis.
   d. Monitor arterial/capillary blood gases, electrolytes, calcium, bilirubin, and glucose.
   e. Monitor blood pressure for hypotension. Give volume replacement and pharmacotherapeutic agents (e.g., dopamine or dobutamine) as indicated.
   f. Maintain hematocrit.
   g. Administer antibiotics for associated pneumonia/rule out sepsis.

J. **Prevention of RDS.**
   1. Maternal glucocorticoid administration prenatally.
   2. Use of L/S ratio, fetal lung maturity, and PG determination for timing labor induction or elective cesarean delivery.
   3. Perinatal management to avoid situations leading to pulmonary circulation compromise in the fetus or newborn infant.
      a. Obstetric.
         (1) Maternal hypotension.
         (2) Oversedation.
         (3) Maternal hypoxia.
         (4) Fetal distress without prompt delivery.
      b. Neonatal.
         (1) Delayed resuscitation.
         (2) Uncorrected hypoxia or acidosis.
         (3) Hypothermia, hypoglycemia, and hypovolemia.

K. **Outcome.**
   1. Infants with chronic lung disease improve slowly and progressively if they can be kept infection free. May have episodes of bronchiolitis and pneumonia (especially pneumonia caused by respiratory syncytial virus [RSV]); long-term sequelae are related to specific complications (e.g., BPD, IVH, ROP).
   2. Infants who weigh greater than 1500 g who have mild to moderate RDS have the same developmental outcome as infants of the same gestational age without RDS. The infants with the most severe developmental outcomes are those who weigh less than 1500 g and who have had an IVH (Hagedorn et al., 2006).
   3. Cerebral palsy (CP)—the most prevalent major impairment encountered in premature infants. Premature infants less than 3.3 pounds are 20 to 80 times more likely to develop CP than term infants (March of Dimes, 2007). Respiratory distress has only a modest association with CP, with an odds ratio ranging from 1.3 to 2.1. Infants with pneumothorax and respiratory distress increase their incidence of CP. Infants who develop chronic lung disease have an increased incidence of CP, with an odds ratio of 2.4 to 5.8. Infants who have been treated with dexamethasone to decrease the risk of chronic lung disease (CLD) increase their risk of CP (Stark et al., 2001).
   4. Factors associated with poorer neurodevelopmental outcome include BPD, steroid use for BPD, Grade 3 or 4 IVH, necrotizing enterocolitis, and male sex (Hagedorn et al., 2006).

Pneumonia

A. Definition. Infection of the fetal or newborn lung; may be intrauterine or neonatal.

    1. Intrauterine infection.

        a. Passage of infecting agent by infection of fetal membranes.

        b. Transplacental transmission.

        c. Aspiration of meconium or infected amniotic fluid during delivery.

    2. Neonatal infection.

        a. Acquired during nursery stay.

        b. Pathogens are generally different from those acquired in utero.

        c. Results by passage from other infants, equipment, or caretakers.

B. Incidence.

    1. Neonatal pneumonia occurs 1% in the term infant and 10% in the preterm infant (Carey and Trotter, 2000). The incidence varies by institution and according to causative agent.

    2. Bacterial pneumonia incidence is comparable with that of sepsis.

C. Etiology.

    1. Risk of infection greatest in premature infants because of immature immune system and lack of protective maternal antibodies. Pneumonia can occur by several routes: transplacental, amniotic fluid, at delivery, and nosocomially (Moise and Hansen, 2003).

    2. Immature ciliary system in the tracheobronchial tree, leading to suboptimal removal of inflammatory debris, mucus, and pathogens. The number of pulmonary macrophages are insufficient for bacterial clearance (Orlando, 1997).

    3. Multiple agents cause neonatal pneumonia (Box 24-1).

■ BOX 24-1
■ **COMMON ORGANISMS ASSOCIATED WITH NEONATAL PNEUMONIA**

TRANSPLACENTAL	**AMNIOTIC FLUID**
Rubella	Cytomegalovirus
Cytomegalovirus	Herpes simplex virus
Herpes simplex virus	Enteroviruses
Adenovirus	Genital mycoplasma
Mumps virus	*Listeria monocytogenes*
Toxoplasma gondii	*Chlamydia trachomatis*
L. monocytogenes	*Mycobacterium tuberculosis*
M. tuberculosis	Group B streptococcus (GBS)
Treponema pallidum	*Escherichia coli*
	Haemophilus influenzae (nontypeable)
	Ureaplasma urealyticum
AT DELIVERY	**NOSOCOMIAL**
GBS	*Staphylococcus aureus*
E. coli	*Staphylococcus epidermidis*
S. aureus	GBS
Klebsiella spp.	*Klebsiella* spp.
Other streptococci	*Enterobacter* spp.
H. influenzae (nontypeable)	*Pseudomonas* spp.
Candida spp.	Influenza viruses
C. trachomatis	Respiratory syncytial virus
U. urealyticum	Enteroviruses

From Weisman, L.E. and Hansen, T.N. (Eds.): *Contemporary diagnosis and management of neonatal respiratory diseases* (3rd ed.). Newtown, PA, 2003, Handbooks in Health Care (division of AMM Co.), p. 142.

D. Pathophysiology.
1. Congenital pneumonia.
   a. Infant may be born critically ill or stillborn to a mother with a history of chorioamnionitis. Evidence of pulmonary inflammation is found in 15% to 38% of stillborn infants at autopsy (Speer and Weisman, 2003). Other factors linked to congenital pneumonia include excessive obstetric manipulation, prolonged labor with intact membranes, and maternal urinary tract infection (Orlando, 1997).
   b. Prolonged rupture of membranes (>24 hours); ascending organisms may infect amniotic fluid. If mother is in active labor, contamination occurs more rapidly.
   c. Infective organisms may cross the placenta and enter the fetal circulation, causing septicemia that may present as pneumonia.
   d. Infants usually show signs of generalized illness from birth, but signs of illness may be delayed hours to days if the infective fluid is aspirated during delivery.
2. Neonatal pneumonia.
   a. Infection occurs days to weeks after birth.
   b. Pathogenic organism is acquired from hospital personnel, parents, or other infected infants.
   c. Both bacterial and viral pathogens are associated with neonatal pneumonia. The most common bacterial organisms include group B streptococcus, *Escherichia coli, Klebsiella, Pseudomonas, Proteus, Staphylococcus epidermidis,* group A streptococci, *Listeria, Enterobacter, Staphylococcus aureus, Mycoplasma,* and *Ureaplasma.* Viral infections such as herpes, cytomegalovirus (CMV), varicella zoster, RSV, enterovirus, adenovirus, and parainfluenza virus are also seen (Carey and Trotter, 2000; Whitsett et al., 2005).

E. Clinical presentation.
1. Labor greater than 24 hours.
   a. Prolonged rupture of membranes (>24 hours).
   b. Maternal fever/chorioamnionitis.
   c. Foul-smelling or purulent amniotic fluid.
   d. Fetal tachycardia.
   e. Decreased fetal heart rate variability.
2. Signs and symptoms.
   a. Often indistinguishable from other forms of respiratory distress and sepsis.
   b. Tachypnea, grunting, retractions, cyanosis, hypoxemia, hypercapnia, and hypoglycemia.
   c. With severe involvement, shock-like syndrome, usually in the first 24 hours of life, with recurrent apnea followed by cardiovascular collapse, profound hypoxemia, and persistent pulmonary hypertension. These signs represent a poor prognosis.
3. Physical examination.
   a. Physical signs are variable.
   b. Diminished breath sounds may be present over one or more areas.
   c. In addition, localized dullness, harshness, or rales may be audible.
   d. Radiologic findings can mimic those seen with RDS. In addition, pleural effusions may be seen on chest x-ray with group B streptococci (GBS) pneumonia.

F. Diagnostic evaluation.
1. History of any previously mentioned contributing factors is suggestive.
2. Infant may require resuscitation in the delivery room.
3. Chest x-ray findings are variable.
   a. Unilateral or bilateral alveolar infiltrates.
   b. Diffuse interstitial pattern.
   c. Pleural effusions.
4. Blood culture because septicemia may present as pneumonia.
5. A complete blood cell count may show neutropenia/leukopenia or may have an abnormal ratio of immature to total neutrophils.
6. Polymerase chain reaction (PCR) can be used to detect herpes viruses.

7. ABG values should be obtained because metabolic acidosis may be severe.
8. Tracheal aspirate culture should be obtained, especially if the infant has an endotracheal tube in place.
9. Cerebrospinal cultures should be obtained when infant is stable, because meningitis often accompanies pneumonia.

G. **Differential diagnosis.**
   1. RDS.
   2. Sepsis/meningitis.
   3. TTN.
   4. Meconium aspiration.
   5. Lung hypoplasia.
   6. Pulmonary hemorrhage.
   7. Congenital heart disease.

H. **Complications.**
   1. Cardiopulmonary complications similar to those of RDS.
   2. Systematic inflammatory response syndrome (SIRS).
   3. Disseminated intravascular coagulation (DIC).
   4. Persistent pulmonary hypertension.
   5. Meningitis.

I. **Management.**
   1. Antibiotic therapy (see Chapter 32).
   2. Maintain normal temperature.
   3. Monitor glucose levels.
   4. Monitor blood pressure and treat hypotension.
   5. Use oxygen with or without assisted ventilation to maintain normal ABG values.
   6. Correct respiratory and metabolic acidosis.
   7. Provide adequate fluid and electrolyte intake.
   8. Monitor for evidence of DIC.
   9. High-frequency ventilation, nitric oxide, and extracorporeal membrane oxygenation have been used for patients who are critically ill with pneumonia, with variable outcomes.
   10. Provide support for the family.

Retained Lung Fluid Syndromes—Transient Tachypnea of the Newborn (TTN)

A. **Definition.** Delayed clearance of the fetal lung fluid—TTN.

B. **Incidence**
   1. TTN occurs at a rate of 11 per 1000 live births (Whitsett et al., 2005).

C. **Clinical presentation.**
   1. Term and near-term infants.
   2. In first few hours, tachypnea results in respiratory rates of 60 to 120 breaths per minute; grunting and retractions may also be present.
   3. Minimal cyanosis may require fractional inspired oxygen of 0.30 to 0.40.
   4. Duration may be 1 to 5 days.

D. **Etiology.**
   1. Delay in removal of lung fluid.
   2. Excessive amount of lung fluid.

E. **Pathophysiology.**
   1. Fetal lung fluid has a higher chloride concentration than plasma, interstitial fluid, or amniotic fluid. During labor, active transport of chloride stops and the fluid is reabsorbed via a protein gradient and removed by the lymphatic system. Two thirds of the lung fluid are removed before birth. Infants born without labor or prematurely may not have the time to reabsorb the fetal lung fluid (Speer and Hansen, 2003).
   2. Infants at highest risk for retained fetal lung fluid include the following:
      a. Birth near or at term.

       b. Cesarean delivery without labor.

       c. Breech delivery.

       d. Second twin.

       e. Maternal asthma.

       f. Precipitous delivery.

       g. Delayed cord clamping (results in a transfusion of blood, which may transiently elevate the central venous pressure).

       h. Macrosomia.

       i. Male sex.

       j. Maternal sedation.

   3. TTN may originate from reduced lung compliance because of delayed reabsorption of lung fluid at the time of birth and/or the distention of interstitial spaces by fluid, leading to alveolar air trapping and decreased lung compliance (Whitsett et al., 2005).

   4. Delayed clearance of lung fluid by pulmonary lymphatic system. The retained fetal lung fluid accumulates in the peribronchiolar lymphatics and bronchovascular spaces and interferes with forces promoting bronchiolar patency, and results in bronchiolar collapse with air trapping or hyperinflation. Hypoxemia results from continued perfusion of poorly ventilated alveoli, and hypercarbia results from mechanical interference with alveolar ventilation. Decreased lung compliance results in tachypnea and increased work of breathing (Whitsett et al., 2005).

F. Diagnosis.

   1. Early signs and symptoms may be difficult to distinguish from those of other respiratory problems; however, they are usually milder.

   2. Chest x-ray examination reveals diffuse haziness and streakiness in both lung fields, with clearing at the periphery. Fluid may be present in the interlobar fissures, and mild hyperinflation may be present.

   3. Diagnosis is frequently one of exclusion.

G. Differential diagnosis.

   1. RDS.

   2. Pneumonia/sepsis.

H. Management.

   1. Because diagnosis is not conclusive, other disorders should be ruled out.

   2. Supportive management.

       a. Oxygen with or without CPAP.

       b. Temperature regulation.

       c. Adequate fluid intake.

       d. Maintain ABGs within normal levels.

       e. Maintain blood glucose at normal levels.

   3. If respiratory rate is greater than 60 breaths per minute, delay feedings to avoid possible aspiration.

   4. If history indicates risk of infection, broad-spectrum antibiotics (e.g., ampicillin and gentamicin) should be administered until culture results are negative.

I. Outcome.

   1. Self-limited.

   2. Oxygen requirement and tachypnea decrease steadily over several days. Infant may remain mildly tachypneic beyond the need for oxygen.

   3. Some infants with TTN have high pulmonary artery pressures documented by echocardiography. If hypoxemia and tachypnea persist, a further complication may be persistent pulmonary hypertension of the newborn.

Persistent Pulmonary Hypertension of the Newborn

A. Definition. Persistent pulmonary hypertension of the newborn (PPHN) is caused by right-to-left shunting through the fetal shunts at the atrial and ductal levels. It is secondary to persistent elevation of pulmonary vascular resistance (PVR) and pulmonary artery pressure (Wood, 2003). Seventy-seven percent of infants are diagnosed in the first 24 hours of life, 93% diagnosed by 48 hours of life, and 97% of the infants by 72 hours of life (Hagedorn et al., 2006). Incidence is 1.9 per 1000 live births (Walsh-Sukys et al., 2000).

B. **Pathophysiology.**
   1. After delivery, adequate oxygenation depends on lung inflation, closure of fetal shunts, decreased PVR, and increased pulmonary blood flow.
   2. Over the first 12 to 24 hours of life, PVR falls by 80% of its total decline.
   3. When PVR remains high, adaptation from fetal to neonatal circulation is impaired.
   4. Neonatal pulmonary vessels have greater vasoactive properties than adult pulmonary vessels and respond to hypoxia and acidosis with vasoconstriction. Numerous factors increase and decrease PVR.
   5. Development of increased vascular smooth muscle contributes to vasospasm. Development of pulmonary artery musculature occurs late in gestation, making PPHN generally a condition of the term and postterm infant.
   6. High PVR and pulmonary hypertension impede pulmonary blood flow, which promotes hypoxemia, acidemia, and lactic acidosis.
   7. Once vasoconstriction is induced, it can persist even when the precipitating cause is removed (Kinsella and Abman, 1995; Morin and Stenmark, 1995; Steinhorn et al., 1995).
   8. Studies have described low plasma arginine and nitric oxide metabolites in infants with PPHN, suggesting that a genetic link of the urea cycle may contribute to this process of PPHN (Pearson et al., 2001).

C. **Etiology.**
   1. Maladaptation. The pulmonary vascular bed is structurally normal, but PVR remains high. Maladaptation generally results from active vasoconstriction, which may be transient or persistent.
      a. Hypoxia/asphyxia. This is the most common precipitating factor in PPHN. It is correlated with abnormal muscularization and remodeling of small pulmonary arteries. Acute asphyxia may induce persistent pulmonary vasospasm.
      b. Pulmonary parenchymal disease (RDS, meconium aspiration, pneumonia, other aspiration syndromes) can cause pulmonary vasospasm and may be associated with vascular remodeling.
      c. Bacterial sepsis. The underlying mechanism may be endotoxin-mediated myocardial depression or pulmonary vasospasm associated with high levels of thromboxanes and leukotrienes.
      d. Prenatal pulmonary hypertension.
         (1) Fetal systemic hypertension.
         (2) Premature closure of ductus arteriosus (associated with maternal use of aspirin, prostaglandin inhibitors, phenytoin [Dilantin], lithium, or indomethacin).
      e. Any condition preventing normal circulatory transition at delivery (CNS depression, delayed resuscitation, hypothermia).
      f. Hypothermia and hypoglycemia contributing to acidosis, which will potentiate pulmonary vasoconstriction.
      g. Hyperviscosity/polycythemia. This may lead to a functional obstruction of the pulmonary vascular bed.
   2. Maldevelopment: abnormal pulmonary vessels. Musculature is hypertrophied and extends into normally nonmuscularized arteries. The excessive muscularization affects lumen size, which increases vascular resistance. Causes of maldevelopment include the following:
      a. Intrauterine asphyxia: increases systemic arterial blood pressure in the fetus and diverts more blood to the lung, resulting in pulmonary vessel development.
      b. Fetal ductal closure: forces cardiac output from the right ventricle through the lungs, resulting in maldevelopment.
      c. Congenital heart disease: abnormal pulmonary vessels resulting from various defects.
   3. Underdevelopment: decreased number of pulmonary vessels. Blood is shunted because there are too few vessels for blood to flow through the lungs. There is a decreased cross-

sectional area available for gas exchange. Severity depends on the timing of the interruption of lung development in utero: reduced numbers of bronchial generations if early (<16 weeks) and decreased number of alveoli if later in gestation. Contributing conditions include the following:

  a. Pulmonary hypoplasia (i.e., Potter sequence).
  b. Space-occupying lesions or lung masses (e.g., diaphragmatic hernia, cystic adenomatoid malformation) that prevent normal development of lung tissue and the capillary bed.
  c. Congenital heart disease. Pulmonary atresia or tricuspid atresia may lead to decreased blood flow and vascular underdevelopment (Van Marter, 1998; Wearden and Hansen, 2003).

D. Clinical presentation.
  1. Near-term, term, or postterm infants.
  2. History of hypoxia or asphyxia at birth.
      a. Low Apgar scores.
      b. Infant usually slow to breathe or difficult to ventilate.
      c. Meconium-stained fluid, nuchal cord, abruptio placentae or any acute blood loss, and maternal sedation.
  3. Respiratory abnormalities.
      a. Symptoms seen before 12 hours of age.
      b. Tachypnea.
      c. Retractions if airway is obstructed (e.g., because of aspiration).
      d. Cyanosis out of proportion to degree of distress (may not see cyanosis with Pao_2 <50 mm Hg); cyanosis of sudden onset that often is intractable.
      e. Low Pao_2 despite high oxygen concentration administration because of right-to-left shunting. Differences are seen between preductal and postductal oxygenation.
      f. Chest x-ray may be normal unless aspiration or pneumonia present (will see infiltrates in these cases).
  4. Cardiovascular abnormalities.
      a. Blood pressure is usually lower than normal.
      b. Electrocardiogram will show a right axis deviation.
      c. Systolic murmur is frequently heard, usually from a PDA, foramen ovale, or tricuspid insufficiency. Single loud second heart sound (S_2), resulting from high pulmonary pressures, may be heard.
      d. Echocardiogram shows dilated right side of the heart and evidence of pulmonary hypertension.
      e. Congestive heart failure has been reported occasionally.
  5. Metabolic abnormalities.
      a. Hypoglycemia.
      b. Hypocalcemia.
      c. Metabolic acidosis.
      d. Decreased urine output or coagulopathy caused by kidney and liver damage from asphyxia may occur.

E. Diagnosis.
  1. PPHN will be suspected on the basis of history and clinical course.
  2. Shunt study. Because of the right-to-left shunting at the level of the ductus arteriosus, there will be a preductal and a postductal Pao_2 difference. Difference in Pao_2 of 10 mm Hg or greater documents ductal shunting.
  3. Hyperoxia test. A right-to-left shunt is demonstrated if Po_2 does not increase in 100% oxygen. Cause may be either PPHN or congenital heart disease.
  4. An echocardiogram will rule out structural heart disease, evaluate myocardial function, measure pulmonary artery pressures, and diagnose right-to-left shunting at the level of the PDA or foramen ovale.
  5. Chest x-ray may or may not be helpful, but should be taken to rule out other lung pathology.

6. Electrolytes, calcium, and glucose levels and complete blood cell count should be obtained.
7. An ABG measurement is done to determine degree of acidosis and hypoxemia.

F. **Differential diagnosis.**
   1. Congenital heart disease.
   2. Pulmonary disease.
      a. Severe disease may mimic PPHN.
      b. Disease may coexist with PPHN.

G. **Complications.**
   1. Pulmonary.
      a. Air leaks. Related to high mean airway pressures used in ventilator management.
      b. BPD.
   2. Cardiovascular.
      a. Systemic hypotension.
      b. Congestive heart failure.
   3. Renal.
      a. Decreased urine output related to asphyxia and hypotension.
      b. Acute tubular necrosis caused by asphyxia.
      c. Hematuria, proteinuria.
   4. Metabolic.
      a. Hypoglycemia, hypocalcemia.
      b. Metabolic acidosis.
   5. Hematologic.
      a. Thrombocytopenia.
      b. DIC: depends on precipitating cause of PPHN.
      c. Hemorrhage (e.g., gastrointestinal, pulmonary).
   6. Neurologic.
      a. CNS irritability.
      b. Seizures.
   7. Iatrogenic.
      a. Thrombus formation or complications of invasive monitoring equipment.
      b. Dislodged endotracheal tube.
   8. Other.
      a. Edema due to third spacing.
      b. Side effects of pharmacologic agents used for treatment.

H. **Management.**
   1. Main goal is to correct hypoxia and acidosis (major contributing factors) and promote pulmonary vascular dilation, as well as support extrapulmonary systems.
   2. Management will depend on the cause of PPHN.
   3. Supportive care.
      a. Monitor vital signs.
      b. Temperature stabilization.
      c. Adequate IV fluid infusion.
      d. Monitor electrolytes, glucose, calcium, complete blood cell count, ABGs.
      e. Correction of metabolic abnormalities.
      f. Blood cultures and antibiotics.
   4. Specialized monitoring.
      a. Umbilical catheters.
         (1) Arterial: blood gas access, arterial pressure monitoring.
         (2) Venous: central pressure monitoring, infusion of vasopressors.
      b. Right radial arterial line: monitor preductal blood gases.
      c. Transcutaneous monitoring and pulse oximetry. Preductal and postductal applications can be helpful.
   5. Oxygen: most potent pulmonary vasodilator.
   6. Ventilation.
      a. Conventional mechanical ventilation (CMV).

    b. High-frequency ventilation (HFV), high-frequency oscillatory ventilation (HFOV), or high-frequency jet ventilation (HFJV). Used when CMV fails or when excessive barotrauma is a concern.

      (1) Hyperoxygenation.

        (a) Goal is to keep Pao_2 at greater than 90 mm Hg.

        (b) Danger of ROP is minimal because most infants are born at or near term.

      (2) Hyperventilation to keep $Paco_2$ values in the low normal range. Hyperventilation may aid in reducing acidosis and pulmonary artery pressure caused by the vasodilatory effect of alkalosis.

    c. Inhaled nitric oxide (iNO).

      (1) iNO is a selective pulmonary vasodilator.

        (a) Potent and short acting, with a half-life of 3 to 5 seconds.

        (b) Combines with hemoglobin and becomes inactivated.

        (c) Inactivation results in formation of methemoglobin; levels need to be monitored during treatment.

      (2) Exact dosage has not been determined. Current evidence supports using starting doses of 20 ppm in term newborn infants with PPHN (Finer and Barrington, 2006; Kinsella and Abman, 2003; Moise and Gomez, 2003).

      (3) iNO withdrawal (weaning) needs to be systematic; in some infants abrupt discontinuation may result in rebound increased PVR (Kinsella and Abman, 2003).

      (4) Infants with severe parenchymal lung disease/underinflation and PPHN respond better to iNO when it is combined with HFOV.

    d. Surfactant replacement: especially for etiology based on significant parenchymal disease (Hagedorn et al., 2006).

    e. Extracorporeal membrane oxygenation (ECMO) may be used when conventional therapies are unsuccessful.

7. Minimal stimulation and handling.

    a. Infants will show marked fluctuation (generally decreases) in their Pao_2 if handled or manipulated.

    b. The pulmonary arteries are very reactive to changes in Pao_2; therefore, any action that causes a decrease in Pao_2 (e.g., suctioning, blood sampling, vital signs, ventilator changes) will cause further vasoconstriction.

    c. Suction only as needed to maintain a patent airway.

    d. Sedatives and analgesics are used for procedures and treatments.

    e. The bedside nurse must be a strong advocate for these patients and keep noise and environmental stimuli to a minimum.

8. Pharmacologic support.

    a. Muscle relaxants.

      (1) Used when infant's own respirations interfere with assisted ventilation.

      (2) Paralysis prevents resisting the ventilator, reduces pulmonary vascular resistance, and reduces the risk of air leaks and BPD. It should be used with caution because it can decrease venous return and compromise ventilation (Whitsett et al., 2005).

      (3) Pancuronium bromide (Pavulon). Dosage: 0.04 to 0.15 mg/kg every 1 to 2 hours, or as needed for paralysis (Young and Mangum, 2008).

      (4) Vecuronium. Dosage: 0.03 to 0.15 mg/kg IV every 1 to 2 hours or as needed (Young and Mangum, 2008).

    b. Vasopressors.

      (1) Goal is to keep the systemic pressure above pulmonary pressure to decrease right-to-left shunting.

      (2) Dopamine is the drug of choice. Dopamine is an endogenous catecholamine with a short half-life and must be given by constant infusion. Dosage: 2 to 20 mcg/kg/minute of continuous IV infusion. Begin at lowest dose and titrate by monitoring effects (i.e., blood pressure, urine output, capillary refill, perfusion, and heart rate (Hagedorn et al., 2006; Young and Mangum, 2008).

      (3) Dobutamine is a synthetic catecholamine with primary β_1 effects to support blood pressure in patients with shock and hypotension related to myocardial ischemia,

pulmonary hypertension, and cardiomyopathy. Dosage: 10 mcg/kg/minute by continuous infusion; titrate by monitoring effects (i.e., blood pressure, urine output, capillary refill, perfusion, and heart rate (Hagedorn et al., 2006; Young and Mangum, 2008).

    (4) Nitroprusside increases cardiac output by decreasing left ventricular preload and afterload, acting on the arterial and venous smooth muscle. Dosage: 0.4 to 5 mcg/kg/minute. Closely follow thiocyanate and cyanide levels (Hagedorn et al., 2006).

    (5) Epinephrine is an adrenergic agonist that increases systemic blood pressure, improves cardiac contractility, and elevates heart rate. Dosage: 0.05 to 1 mcg/kg/minute given as a continuous infusion (Zenk et al., 2003).

  c. Pulmonary vasodilators.

    (1) iNO (previously described).

    (2) Sildenafil may be as effective as iNO in improving pulmonary vasodilation (Hagedorn et al., 2006). It has been suggested as adjunctive therapy to facilitate weaning of iNO. A Cochrane review of this therapy suggests the need for additional research before widespread adoption (Shah and Ohlsson, 2007).

    (3) Milrinone improves oxygenation without decreasing systemic blood pressure. Dosage: 0.5 mcg/kg/minute (Lulic-Botica et al., 2005).

  d. Analgesics and sedatives.

    (1) Fentanyl citrate. In addition to analgesic effect, fentanyl produces a sedative effect. Dosage: 1 to 5 mcg/kg per dose by IV slow push. Repeat as required (usually every 2 to 4 hours). Frequently used as a constant infusion at 1 to 5 mcg/kg/hour. Tolerance may develop rapidly, requiring weaning to prevent significant withdrawal symptoms (Gardner et al., 2006; Young and Mangum, 2008).

    (2) Morphine sulfate. Dosage: 0.05 to 0.2 mg/kg per dose IV. Repeat as required, usually every 4 hours. For continuous infusion, usual dose is 10 to 15 mcg/kg/hour. Tolerance may develop with prolonged use, requiring slow weaning to prevent significant withdrawal symptoms (Gardner et al., 2006; Young and Mangum, 2008).

I. Outcome.

  1. PPHN survival rate is dependent on the center and the underlying disease process.

  2. Residual chronic lung disease is common, although recently low-dose iNO has reduced the need for ECMO and has reduced the occurrence of chronic lung disease in neonates with hypoxemic respiratory failure (Clark et al., 2000).

  3. Sensorineural hearing loss is higher among children treated for PPHN.

  4. Incidence of abnormal neurologic outcome is 12% to 25% (Wearden and Hansen, 2003).

Meconium Aspiration Syndrome

A. Definition and etiology of meconium aspiration syndrome (MAS).

  1. Meconium is a mixture of epithelial cells and bile salts found in the fetal intestinal tract.

  2. With intrauterine stress or asphyxia, peristalsis is stimulated and relaxation of the anal sphincter occurs, releasing meconium into the amniotic fluid.

  3. Aspiration may occur whenever meconium passes into the amniotic fluid, but the risk increases when repeated episodes of severe asphyxia lead to gasping respirations in utero.

B. Incidence. Meconium-stained amniotic fluid (MSAF) is present in approximately 13% of all newborns delivered. Of these, 5% to 12% develop MAS (Wiswell, 2001).

C. Pathophysiology.

  1. Complete or partial airway obstruction can occur.

  2. Atelectasis or ball-valve air trapping leads to hyperinflation.

  3. A chemical pneumonitis develops (probably caused by bile salts). Hemorrhagic pulmonary edema in the alveoli interferes with surfactant production and increases surface tension (Wiswell, 2001).

  4. Meconium decreases the levels of surfactant proteins, SP-A and SP-B, and large number of phospholipids (Gelfand et al., 2004).

5. The hypoxia associated with meconium aspiration increases pulmonary vascular resistance.

D. Clinical presentation/diagnosis.

1. MAS is a disease of term or postterm infants. MAS is rarely seen in infants born at less than 36 weeks of gestation.
2. Asphyxia and the results of chronic hypoxia may predispose these infants to PPHN.
3. Vigorous resuscitation is frequently needed in the delivery room because of central depression.
4. Respiratory distress signs are nonspecific and may include tachypnea, nasal flaring, and retractions.
5. Respiratory distress may range from mild and transient to severe and prolonged.
6. If there has been prolonged placental insufficiency, infants may appear to be wasted, with hanging skinfolds (usually around knees, buttocks, and axillae).
7. Nail beds and skin are usually stained a yellow-green.
8. The chest may appear to be hyperinflated or barrel shaped.
9. Chest x-ray shows hyperexpanded lucent areas mixed with areas of atelectasis throughout lung fields.
10. Expiration phase of respirations may be prolonged.
11. Coarse crackles are common on auscultation.
12. No specific laboratory data are useful for diagnosis of MAS.
13. ABGs will show the following:
    a. Respiratory and metabolic acidosis in severe cases.
    b. Low Pao_2 even with 100% oxygen administration.

E. Complications.

1. Pulmonary.
    a. Air leaks (pneumothorax and pneumomediastinum) due to ball-valve phenomenon leading to overinflation and air trapping and high ventilator pressures.
    b. Pneumonia.
    c. PPHN.
    d. BPD.
2. Metabolic.
    a. Acidosis.
    b. Hypoglycemia.
    c. Hypocalcemia.
3. Neurologic: will depend on degree of asphyxia.

F. Management and prevention.

1. Delivery room management.
    a. If the infant is depressed with no respiratory effort, muscle tone and/or has a heart rate less than 100, direct suctioning of the trachea soon after delivery is indicated, before respirations are established. While administering free-flow oxygen, clear the mouth and posterior pharynx with a suction catheter to facilitate visualization of the glottis. Tracheal suctioning with an endotracheal tube is recommended. Using a meconium aspirator, suction as you slowly withdraw the endotracheal tube. This procedure should be repeated, if necessary (American Academy of Pediatrics [AAP], 2006).
2. Respiratory care.
    a. ABGs to determine degree of respiratory compromise and type of therapy needed.
    b. Oxygen and/or assisted ventilation.
       (1) Use same parameters for therapy as with RDS. May want to use a lower level of positive end expiration pressure (PEEP) to avoid inadvertent PEEP and a higher respiratory rate to induce alkalosis and prevent PPHN.
       (2) May choose HFV.
       (3) iNO if PPHN develops.
    c. Improved oxygenation and reduced pulmonary morbidity has been demonstrated in infants given surfactant within 6 hours after birth (Johnson et al., 2003). The use of surfactant in infants with MAS has also decreased the need for ECMO (Lotze et al., 1998; Wiswell, 2001). Although surfactant therapy seems to be effective in the manage-

ment of MAS, this treatment strategy has not been approved by any regulatory agencies (Wiswell, 2001).

   d. For infants with MAS requiring ventilation, the use of sedatives and paralytics may be necessary.

G. Outcome.

   1. The prognosis for infants with mild cases of MAS is generally excellent unless complications such as seizures, PPHN, or severe asphyxia occur during the course of the disease.

   2. In more severe cases, neurologic sequelae are common and death may occur despite vigorous, maximal support.

Bronchopulmonary Dysplasia

A. Definition.

   1. In 1967 Northway, Rosan, and Porter originally described the four stages of BPD based on the time that the change occurred (from birth to 30 days of life) and on the type of alveolar and bronchial damage and repair that occurred.

   2. A more clinically useful definition now is a 36-week postmenstrual-age infant with an O_2 requirement, an abnormal chest x-ray, and abnormal physical examination findings (Barrington and Finer, 1998; Farrell and Fiascone, 1997).

   3. A new proposed definition is an infant less than 32 weeks of gestation who has reached 36 weeks of postmenstrual age, was treated with oxygen greater than 28 days, and requires oxygen or positive pressure at 36 weeks of postmenstrual age (see Table 24-1). This definition also established criteria for mild, moderate, and severe BPD (Jobe and Bancalari, 2001).

B. Incidence.

   1. Statistics vary because of the difference in diagnostic criteria and practices in individual centers.

   2. Recent literature has provided estimates of BPD in low birth weight infants (<1250 g) ranging from 7.4% (Sahni et al., 2005) to 35% (Walsh et al., 2004) and up to 77% in extremely low birth weight infants <1000 g (Ehrenkranz et al., 2005).

C. Etiology.

   1. The etiology of BPD is multifactorial, resulting from acute lung injury, arrested lung development, as well as abnormal repair processes that occur in the lung.

■ TABLE 24-1
■ ■ **Definition of Bronchopulmonary Dysplasia: Diagnostic Criteria**

Gestational Age	<32 Weeks	≥32 Weeks
Time point of assessment	36 weeks' PMA or discharge to home, whichever comes first	>28 days but <56 days of postnasal age or discharge to home, whichever comes first
	Treatment with oxygen >21% for at least 28 days **plus**	
Mild BPD	Breathing room air at 36 weeks' PMA or discharge, whichever comes first	Breathing room air by 56 days' postnatal age or discharge, whichever comes first
Moderate BPD	Need* for <30% oxygen at 36 weeks' PMA or discharge, whichever comes first	Need* for <30% oxygen at 56 days' postnatal age or discharge, whichever comes first
Severe BPD	Need* for ≥30% oxygen and/or positive pressure (PPV or NCPAP) at 36 weeks' PMA or discharge, whichever comes first	Need* for ≥30% oxygen and/or positive pressure (PPV or NCPAP) at 56 days' postnatal age or discharge, whichever comes first

BPD, Bronchopulmonary dysplasia; *NCPAP*, nasal continuous positive airway pressure; *PMA*, postmenstrual age; *PPV*, positive-pressure ventilation.
*A physiologic test confirming that the oxygen requirement at the assessment time point remains to be defined. This assessment may include a pulse oximetry saturation range.
From Jobe, A.H. and Bancalari, E.: Bronchopulmonary dysplasia. *American Journal of Respiratory and Critical Care Medicine*, *163*(7):1723-1729, 2001.

    a. Prior to delivery, chorioamnionitis triggers an inflammatory response that is thought to alter the development of alveoli and lung vasculature in the immature fetus (Jobe, 2003; Speer, 2006).

    b. Oxygen toxicity can be a cause of BPD (Chess et al., 2006).

        (1) High inspired oxygen concentrations cause the production of reactive oxygen species (ROS) and the release of chemotactic factors that attract neutrophils to the lung, initiating the inflammatory cycle (Weinberger et al., 2002). An ongoing inflammatory process in the lung ensues that causes and continues parenchymal damage (Barrington and Finer, 1998; Farrell and Fiascone, 1997).

        (2) Inflammatory mediators and proteolytic enzymes are released. The preterm infant has lower levels of antiproteases such as α_1-protease (α_1-antitrypsin) and the antioxidant enzymes dismutase and glutathione. These together make the premature pulmonary system especially vulnerable to oxygen toxicity (Gitto et al., 2002; Higgins et al., 2007).

        (3) When ROS injure epithelial and endothelial cells, pulmonary edema and activation of inflammatory cells results (Weinberger et al., 2002).

        (4) Pulmonary edema results in a leak of proteins into the alveoli, which inactivates surfactant, exacerbating the surfactant deficiency of prematurity (Gitto et al., 2002).

        (5) Tissue damage from ROS results in proliferation of alveolar Type II cells and eventually tissue fibrosis (Weinberger et al., 2002)

2. There are three pathways of injury that occur in the clinical evolution of BPD.

    a. Structural injury to the airway and alveoli in conjunction with inhibition of maturational processes.

    b. Stimulation of elastic tissue production and the accelerated fibrosis.

    c. Activation of an intense inflammatory response, which contributes to ongoing airway damage (Adams and Cooper, 2003).

3. Assisted ventilation with positive pressure results in lung damage (barotrauma and volutrauma), which contributes to BPD development.

    a. Intubation interrupts normal pulmonary function (mucociliary function is damaged; dead space is increased, leading to increased pressure needs).

    b. Correlation exists between the severity of the initial pulmonary process and BPD (Barrington and Finer, 1998).

    c. Barotrauma is related to the intensity and amount of time exposed to elements of positive-pressure ventilation (peak inspiratory pressure [PIP], inspiratory time, and PEEP). Repeated distention of distal airways during mechanical ventilation of infants with poor alveolar compliance results in ischemia. Because of the immaturity of the pulmonary system, the alveolar capillary unit is further disrupted by mechanical ventilation, leading to pulmonary edema. Many factors contribute to barotrauma, such as the structure of the tracheobronchial tree and the physiologic effects of surfactant deficiency. Changes in the method of ventilation are being evaluated in order to prevent barotrauma (Davis and Rosenfeld, 2005).

    d. Ventilation using volumes that are too low results in cycles of alveolar collapse (atelectrauma), which is as damaging as overventilation (Jobe and Ikegami, 2004).

4. Increased shunting (left to right) via a PDA has been described as a possible cause of BPD. Improved lung compliance may follow PDA ligation in infants with RDS.

5. Excessive fluid intake in the first 4 days of life contributes to the development of BPD (Adams et al., 2004).

6. Colonization by *Ureaplasma urealyticum, Chlamydia,* or cytomegalovirus (CMV) has been associated with higher incidence of BPD (Adams and Cooper, 2003; Benstein et al., 2003; Davis and Rosenfeld, 2005; Jobe and Bancalari, 2001).

7. Gestational age plays an important role in the development of BPD.

    a. Damage to the developing lung is more likely in infants weighing less than 1500 g.

    b. Damage may occur with less exposure to the previously noted factors in the infant <1250 g.

8. Nutritional deficits contribute to the risk for developing BPD.

    a. Adequate caloric and protein intake is required for cell growth and division.

    b. Vitamin A is essential for differentiation, integrity, and repair of respiratory epithelial cells (Van Marter, 2006; Young, 2007). Vitamin A supplementation in neonates has been shown to reduce the production of proinflammatory cytokines (Bessler et al., 2007).

    c. Poor nutrition may impair macrophages and neutrophil and lymphocyte function (Biniwale and Ehrenkranz, 2006).

D. Pathophysiology. All levels of the tracheobronchial tree are involved.

  1. Large airways.

    a. Submucosal glandular hypertrophy.

    b. Increased bronchial smooth muscle.

    c. Bronchial mucosa replaced by metaplastic squamous epithelium.

    d. Submucosal fibrosis.

    e. Inflammatory infiltrates.

    f. Granulation tissue.

    g. Loss of cilia.

    h. Tracheomalacia or bronchomalacia frequently develops.

  2. Small airways.

    a. Bronchiolar smooth muscle hypertrophy.

    b. Focal mucosal squamous metaplasia.

    c. Chronic inflammation.

    d. Peribronchial edema.

    e. Peribronchiolar fibrosis.

    f. Necrosis with intraluminal debris.

    g. Luminal narrowing.

    h. Excessive production of mucus.

  3. Alveoli.

    a. Decreased number of alveoli.

    b. Enlarged alveoli.

    c. Alveolar septal destruction, which leads to emphysematous blebs.

  4. Pulmonary vascular bed.

    a. Muscular hypertrophy of the medial layer of pulmonary arterioles leads to increased pulmonary pressures.

    b. Fibrosis.

    c. Endothelial cell hyperplasia, which leads to a decreased cross-sectional area.

  5. Asthma (Ng et al., 2000).

E. Clinical presentation.

  1. Predisposing risk factors.

    a. Oxygen, intubation, and assisted ventilation.

    b. Gestational age <32 weeks.

    c. Nutritional deficiencies.

    d. Underlying lung disease.

    e. Air leaks.

    f. Infection.

    g. Patent ductus arteriosus.

  2. Increase in ventilatory requirements or inability to be weaned from ventilator.

  3. Hypoxia, hypercapnia, and respiratory acidosis.

  4. Audible crackles and wheezing.

  5. Retractions.

  6. Increased secretions.

  7. Bronchospasm.

  8. Electrocardiogram showing right ventricular hypertrophy and right axis deviation.

  9. Chest x-ray showing hyperinflation, infiltrates, blebs, and cardiomegaly.

  10. Fluid intolerance, evidenced by increase in weight, edema, and decrease in urine output, despite no change in fluid intake.

F. Diagnosis.

  1. Diagnosis of exclusion.

2. Chest x-ray findings (see Chapter 14).
3. Clinical signs (e.g., tachypnea, hypercapnia, hypoxia, rales) help make diagnosis.

G. Complications.
  1. Intermittent bronchospasm.
  2. Inability to be weaned from ventilator and/or oxygen supplementation.
  3. Recurrent infections.
      a. Pneumonia.
      b. Upper respiratory tract infections.
      c. Otitis media.
  4. Congestive heart failure from cor pulmonale.
  5. BPD "spells."
      a. Infant becomes irritable, agitated, and dusky; has increased respiratory effort, hypoxia, and hypercapnia.
      b. Cause is unknown but may be bronchospasm or increased pulmonary vascular resistance.
  6. Gastroesophageal reflux.
  7. Developmental delays.

H. Prevention.
  1. Administration of antenatal steroids reduces the incidence of RDS and the need for mechanical ventilation (Roberts and Dalziel, 2008).
  2. Surfactant rescue therapy decreases mortality rates, and prophylaxis may decrease the incidence of BPD slightly.
  3. Routine use of steroids (e.g., dexamethasone) for prevention of treatment of chronic lung disease in preterm infants is not recommended (AAP Committee on Fetus and Newborn and CPS Fetus and Newborn Committee, 2002).
  4. Gentle ventilation, permissive hypercapnia, and early extubation have all been suggested as ways to decrease BPD. Early use of surfactant combined with extubation to NCPAP results in a lower rate of BPD than in infants receiving surfactant later (Stevens et al., 2007).
  5. Synchronized intermittent mandatory ventilation (SIMV) is associated with less severe BPD because the incidence of pulmonary air leaks decreases.
  6. HFV: Animal data suggest that high-frequency ventilation results in lower rates of BPD, but newborn studies have shown mixed results (Henderson-Smart et al., 2003).
  7. Aggressive nutrition is needed to promote lung growth, maturation, and repair, and protect the damaged lung from infection (Biniwale and Ehrenkranz, 2006; Davis and Rosenfeld, 2005).

I. Management.
  1. Minimize length of exposure to mechanical ventilation.
  2. Continue respiratory support as needed.
      a. Continue assisted ventilation.
          (1) Weaning should be slow, to allow time for the infant to compensate.
          (2) Use synchronized modes of ventilation with the minimal amount of pressure and volume needed to deliver adequate tidal volumes, but always assess each infant individually.
      b. After extubation, oxygen is needed to prevent hypoxia and avoid cor pulmonale.
          (1) Oxygen inhalation alleviates airway constriction seen in infants with BPD.
          (2) Maintain Pao_2 at greater than 55 mm Hg and pH at greater than 7.25.
          (3) Supplemental oxygen may enhance overall growth of the infant.
      c. Weaning can usually be accomplished by use of pulse oximetry and occasional monitoring of blood gas.
  3. Diuretics are used to control fluid retention leading to pulmonary edema. Furosemide (Lasix) is used most often. Benefits include decreased airway resistance, increased airway compliance, and a decrease in total body water, extracellular water, and interstitial water. Metabolic alkalosis may result in compensatory hypoventilation. Calcium wasting may lead to nephrocalcinosis, cholelithiasis, and osteopenia (Zenk et al., 2003). Chlorothiazide (Diuril) has been used with results similar to those seen with furosemide. Follow serum

electrolyte values to monitor for hyponatremia, hypokalemia, and metabolic alkalosis (Zenk et al., 2003).

4. Bronchodilators.

   a. Systemic bronchodilator: theophylline (aminophylline). Use varies with individual centers; levels must be monitored. Can cause tachycardia and gastrointestinal (GI) irritation.

5. Fluid restriction may help reduce pulmonary edema and right-sided heart failure.

6. Cardiac evaluation for complications.

   a. Cor pulmonale (right ventricular hypertrophy) due to prolonged pulmonary hypertension.

   b. Electrocardiography and echocardiography should be performed periodically to evaluate the progression/development of right ventricular hypertrophy.

7. Optimal nutrition. Provide increased calories to compensate for increased work of breathing and fluid restriction. Infant may need 150 to 180 kcal/kg/day. Growth failure is common (Reynolds and Thureen, 2007).

8. Monitor for osteopenia beginning at 6 weeks and follow every 2 to 3 weeks (Rusk, 1998). BPD infants are at high risk because of their gestational age, often protracted respiratory course, and medications (e.g., diuretics).

9. Chest physiotherapy and suctioning may be helpful in loosening and removing bronchial secretions. Caregivers must use caution so as not to precipitate a BPD "spell" or cause a rib fracture.

10. Use of steroids.

   a. Early administration of systemic dexamethasone in preterm neonates who are mechanically ventilated may reduce the incidence of chronic lung disease and extubation failure, but can cause complications (AAP Committee on Fetus and Newborn and CPS Fetus and Newborn Committee, 2002; Stark et al., 2001).

   b. Complications include impairment of growth, possible increase in neurodevelopmental abnormalities, hypertension, myocardial hypertrophy, gastrointestinal hemorrhage and perforation, gastric ulcerations, nosocomial sepsis, hyperglycemia, and transient adrenal suppression (AAP/ACOG, 2002; Parad and Berger, 1998; Stark et al., 2001).

   c. Have not been found to have a substantial impact on long-term outcomes such as duration of supplemental oxygen requirement, length of hospital stay, or mortality (Parad and Berger, 1998).

   d. Early treatment of inhaled corticosteroids to very low birth weight infants has no discernible benefits in the prevention and treatment of chronic lung disease (AAP Committee on Fetus and Newborn and CPS Fetus and Newborn Committee, 2002).

11. RSV: BPD infants are at high risk for RSV outbreaks and account for many readmissions, with 25% of BPD infants needing assisted ventilation. Treatment modalities include the following:

   a. Benefits of RSV prophylaxis:

      (1) RespiGam (RSV IGIV): decreases the severity of RSV infection, decreases hospitalizations, and reduces the incidence of concurrent otitis media (Impact-RSV Study Group, 1998; Welliver, 1998).

      (2) Palivizumab (Synagis): humanized monoclonal antibody against RSV. Unlike RSV-IGIV, palivizumab is not a human blood product and therefore is not associated with the risk of bloodborne pathogens (AAP/ACOG, 2002). Monthly administration of Synagis results in a 45% to 55% decrease in hospital admissions for RSV (Meissner et al., 2003). For high-risk infants, palivizumab is preferred over RSV-IGIV for most high-risk children because of its ease of administration, safety, and effectiveness (American Academy of Pediatrics Committee on Infectious Diseases and Committee on Fetus and Newborn, 2003).

   b. AAP recommendations include the following:

      (1) Prophylaxis to infants who are less than 2 years of age with chronic lung disease requiring medical therapy within 6 months before the anticipated start of the RSV season, infants born at 29 to 32 weeks of gestation (prophylaxis up to 6 months of

age), and infants born at 28 weeks of gestation and younger (prophylaxis until 12 months of age)

   (2) Infants with severe CLD may benefit from prophylaxis during a second RSV season if they continue to require medical therapy.

   c. Palivizumab dose is 15 mg/kg, intramuscular route, given monthly during RSV season, with the first dose to be given before the start of the season (Meissner et al., 2003).

J. Outcome.

   1. Mortality rate:

   a. The prognosis for infants with BPD is dependent on the severity of the disease and the infant's overall health status

   b. After discharge, mortality rate is less than 10%.

   (1) Death is usually not caused by respiratory failure.

   (2) Complications such as cor pulmonale or infection are the usual causes of death.

   2. Some infants will be discharged home with oxygen supplementation.

   3. Pulmonary function:

   a. Long-term follow-up of BPD infants suggests that there is progressive normalization of lung mechanics and to some extent lung volumes; however, abnormalities of the small airways persist (Bhandari and Panitch, 2006).

   b. By 3 years of age, pulmonary compliance is near normal; however, airway resistance may be 30% higher than that of controls (Adams and Cooper, 2003).

   4. Neurologic and developmental sequelae.

   a. Infants with BPD demonstrate deficits compared with VLBW and term children in intelligence; reading, mathematics, and gross motor skills; and special education services (Short et al., 2003).

   b. Sensorineural hearing loss. Incidence of 0.7% to 2% in very low birth weight infants. Conductive hearing loss has an incidence of 14% to 42%.

   c. Factors that increase the risk of poor neurodevelopmental outcomes in infants with BPD include moderate to severe intraventricular hemorrhage and low socioeconomic and parent education levels (Bregman and Farrell, 1992).

PULMONARY AIR LEAKS (PNEUMOMEDIASTINUM, PNEUMOTHORAX, PNEUMOPERICARDIUM, PULMONARY INTERSTITIAL EMPHYSEMA)

A. Definition. Alveolar overdistention and rupture. May occur spontaneously or as a secondary cause, usually when assisted ventilation is used.

B. Incidence. In infants receiving CPAP, bag-and-mask ventilation, or mechanical ventilation, the incidence ranges from 2% to 10% (Hagedorn et al., 2006).

C. Pathophysiology.

   1. Generally iatrogenic, resulting from the use of excessive airway pressure during resuscitation or with assisted ventilation.

   2. Can occur spontaneously if there is uneven air distribution at birth.

   a. Some areas are expanded, whereas others remain collapsed.

   b. Infant will generate pressure to expand unopened areas, leading to greater pressure in already expanded areas, which results in the air leak.

   3. Frequently, underlying lung disease is present.

   a. Obstructive: such as ball-valve trapping of air, seen with MAS.

   b. Poor lung compliance: such as seen with RDS.

   4. Overdistention of alveoli leads to rupture, with gas moving into nonventilated tissues. Air travels via vascular sheaths to the lining of the lung. Interstitial air can dissect around blood vessels or along lymphatics, becoming pulmonary interstitial emphysema (PIE). Air can move from the lining to the mediastinum, resulting in pneumomediastinum, through to the thoracic cavity and visceral pleura, resulting in a pneumothorax. When the air moves along the great vessels to the pericardium, a pneumopericardium results. If air dissects

down from the mediastinum through the sheaths of the great vessels, pneumoperitoneum results.

D. **Clinical presentation and diagnosis** (see Chapter 14 for x-ray findings).

   1. Pneumothorax.

     a. Sudden deterioration if air leak is large.

     b. Decreased breath sounds on the affected side, hypotension, skin mottling, and shift of the mediastinum (detected by shift of the point of maximal cardiac impulse on auscultation) to the unaffected side.

     c. Obtain chest x-ray.

     d. Transillumination (translucent glow when fiberoptic light is placed against the skin) of the chest wall may confirm presence of pneumothorax, without having to wait for a chest x-ray.

     e. If the air leak is small, may be asymptomatic.

   2. Pneumomediastinum.

     a. Should be anticipated with MAS.

     b. Signs include increased anteroposterior diameter of chest and indistinct heart sounds.

     c. Chest x-ray may show "sail sign," indicating elevation of the thymus surrounded by air.

   3. Pneumopericardium.

     a. Immediate presentation with hypotension, muffled heart sound, and bradycardia from cardiac tamponade.

     b. Life-threatening.

     c. Chest x-ray will show air encircling the heart, halo appearance.

   4. PIE.

     a. Difficult to interpret.

     b. Limited to infants with poor lung compliance who are receiving CPAP or positive-pressure ventilation.

     c. Chest x-ray shows microcystic areas throughout one or both lungs; may show hyperinflated lungs and flattened diaphragm.

     d. May progress to pneumomediastinum and/or pneumothorax.

     e. Hypoxia and hypercapnia commonly present.

E. **Management.**

   1. Pneumothorax.

     a. If asymptomatic, will often resolve without treatment.

     b. Symptomatic (tension) pneumothorax requires emergency removal of air. Associated with hypoxia, hypotension, and cardiopulmonary arrest.

       (1) Thoracentesis (needle aspiration to remove air) may be necessary, until a chest tube can be placed, if infant's condition has acutely deteriorated or until adequate pain, pharmacologic support can be administered.

       (2) Thoracostomy tube is placed in the anterior chest and connected to underwater seal drainage system, with continuous negative pressure of 10 to 15 cm H_2O, and left in place until air ceases to bubble from the chest tube for at least 24 hours and pneumothorax is resolved by chest x-ray examination. The chest tube is then placed to the water seal for 24 hours, and the infant is observed for reaccumulation of air. The chest tube is removed 12 to 24 hours after the tube has been placed to water drainage if the infant remains free of symptoms.

       (3) In asymptomatic infants or nonventilated infants, administration of supplemental oxygen may aid the absorption of the air in the pneumothorax by the pleural capillaries. Because of the toxic effects of oxygen, this treatment is not recommended for preterm infants.

   2. Pneumomediastinum.

     a. Usually not treated.

     b. If associated with pneumothorax (common occurrence), supplemental oxygen may help resolve condition, as described previously.

3. Pneumopericardium. Emergency treatment is required by placement of a long catheter or chest tube into the pericardial sac with constant application of gentle negative pressure.
4. PIE.
   a. If unilateral and persistent, intubation of mainstem bronchus supplying opposite lung may show improvement in condition.
   b. If bilateral, supportive treatment is given (e.g., oxygen, ventilation, fluids).
   c. Minimize positive inspiratory pressure and shorten inspiratory time.
   d. High-frequency ventilation.
   e. Place affected side in dependent position.
F. **Outcome.**
   1. Outcome depends on underlying lung pathology.
   2. Mortality rate is high with pneumopericardium, bilateral pneumothoraces, and bilateral PIE.
   3. In survivors of bilateral PIE, the risk of chronic lung disease is high.

PULMONARY HYPOPLASIA

A. **Definition.** Defective or inhibited growth of the lungs, either unilateral or bilateral. Developmental disorder that results in decreased numbers of alveoli, bronchioles, and arterioles.
B. **Pathophysiology.**
   1. Conditions that compress the lungs or limit lung growth (e.g., diaphragmatic hernia, cystic adenomatoid malformation) are one cause of pulmonary hypoplasia.
   2. Conditions that result in oligohydramnios (e.g., renal disorders, amniotic fluid leakage) are associated with pulmonary hypoplasia caused by thoracic compression.
   3. Associated congenital malformations, such as renal dysgenesis (Potter syndrome), phrenic nerve absence, and vertebral and chromosomal anomalies, should be considered.
C. **Diagnosis.**
   1. Often very difficult to diagnose.
   2. Any of the above conditions are suggestive of pulmonary hypoplasia.
   3. Usually present with severe respiratory distress.
   4. Higher than usual pressures needed for ventilation; pneumothorax common.
   5. Hypercapnia difficult or impossible to treat early in disease course.
   6. Chest x-ray will usually show decreased volume of the thorax.
   7. Symptoms of PPHN possible.
D. **Management.** Treatment is supportive and directed at respiratory failure.
   1. Assisted ventilation/HFV.
   2. Treatment of PPHN.
   3. iNO (nitric oxide).
   4. ECMO.
E. **Outcome.**
   1. Degree and etiology of hypoplasia determines outcome.
   2. Mortality rate is high.
   3. Management is difficult, but infant can function adequately if treatment and support can be continued until lung growth occurs, although this outcome is rare.

PULMONARY HEMORRHAGE

A. **Definition.**
   1. Localized areas of bleeding into alveoli (generally found at autopsy); also known as hemorrhagic pulmonary edema.
   2. Can be a massive generalized bleeding event.
B. **Etiology and pathophysiology.**
   1. Usually occurs as a complication of other disorders such as prematurity, erythroblastosis, intracranial hemorrhage, asphyxia, aspiration, heart disease, sepsis, hypothermia, PDA, and surfactant replacement.

2. May be due to trauma from improper suctioning technique.
3. Usually due to large increase in capillary hydrostatic pressure; results in capillary rupture and fluid transudation from other capillaries (Welty and Hansen, 2003).

C. **Clinical presentation.**
 1. May present with sudden, severe respiratory distress.
 2. Bright red blood or frothy pink secretions may be suctioned from the trachea.

D. **Management.**
 1. Use of assisted ventilation is necessary to maintain gas exchange and PEEP.
 2. Transfusion of packed red blood cells if large hemorrhage with decreased hematocrit/hemoglobin.
 3. Identify any clotting abnormalities and treat.
 4. Assess for and treat PDA.
 5. Treat other underlying diseases.

E. **Outcome.**
 1. If bleeding is massive, death will occur quickly despite vigorous management.
 2. If hemorrhage is small or isolated, infant will recover and outcome will be dependent on underlying disease.

OTHER CAUSES OF RESPIRATORY DISTRESS

A. **Upper airway disorders.**
 1. Choanal atresia:
    a. Incidence is 2 to 4 in 10,000 births with female/male ratio of 2:1.
    b. Bone or membrane protrudes into nasal passages, causing blockage or narrowing.
    c. If condition is bilateral, gasping respirations and cyanosis occur immediately after birth because neonates are obligate nose breathers. Many infants have associated anomalies (Treacher Collins syndrome, tracheoesophageal fistula, palatal abnormalities, CHARGE association [Coloboma, Heart disease, choanal Atresia, Restricted growth and development, Genital hypoplasia, and Ear anomalies]), congenital heart disease.
    d. Signs of distress are intermittent when condition is unilateral.
    e. Failure to pass a catheter through the nasal passages to the posterior oropharynx will make the diagnosis.
    f. Initially treat by placing infant in prone position with a large oral airway taped securely in place (an endotracheal tube can be used if placement of an oral airway is difficult).
    g. Surgical correction of the problem is necessary and consists of perforation of the obstruction and serial dilation by use of obturators.
 2. Micrognathia.
    a. Defined as mandibular undergrowth.
    b. Occurs with certain syndromes and sequences such as Pierre Robin syndrome, trisomy 18, trisomy 22, and cri-du-chat syndrome (deletion of the short arm of chromosome 5).
    c. Airway distress may be alleviated by prone positioning.
    d. Use of an oral airway or endotracheal tube will provide an open airway.
    e. If an endotracheal tube is in place, humidification will be needed to prevent the drying of secretions.
    f. Tracheostomy may be necessary.
    g. Generally mandibular growth "catches up" by 6 to 12 months of age.
 3. Cystic hygroma.
    a. Form of cystic lymphangioma, with benign water cysts occurring most frequently in the neck (80%); can also be found in the groin, axilla, and mediastinum.
    b. Usually seen at birth.
    c. Mass will occupy the submandibular region and may compromise the airway in 25% of cases.
    d. Symptoms depend on the size and location.

  e. Treatment is related to complications.

   (1) If infant is free of symptoms, surgical excision is performed between 4 and 12 months of age.

   (2) Excision must be performed at an earlier age if the airway is compromised or if infections are recurrent.

   (3) Multiple excisions are usually performed to prevent damage to nerves and vascular structures.

 4. Obstruction of larynx or trachea.

  a. Stridor is a major symptom and usually requires no specific treatment, but mechanical causes must be ruled out.

  b. Direct laryngoscopy will reveal structural abnormalities such as polyps, webs, and granulomas.

  c. Hemangiomas of the larynx or trachea may cause obstruction.

  d. Extrinsic compression of the upper airway occurs with thyroglossal duct cyst, cervical neuroblastoma, vascular ring, and double aortic arch.

  e. Laryngotracheomalacia results from collapse of the larynx and cervical trachea, which produces stridor; condition is usually self-limiting and resolves by 6 to 12 months of age, when the tracheal diameter increases and the cartilage matures.

 5. Tracheoesophageal fistula (refer to Chapter 29).

B. Thoracic disorders.

 1. Cystic adenomatoid malformation (CAM).

  a. Primary pulmonary tissue dysplasia with failure of terminal bronchioles to canalize, which leads to intrapulmonary mass consisting of multiple small cysts.

  b. Three types.

   (1) Type I CAM is the most common, occurring in 70% of cases. It presents as a single or multiple large (3 to 10 cm) cysts that communicate with the bronchi; 11% are associated with anomalies; survival rate of 90%.

   (2) Type II CAM is found in 18% of cases. It is composed of multiple medium-size, evenly distributed cysts that resemble terminal bronchioles (0.5 to 2.0 cm); 50% of these infants have other anomalies, and only 56% survive. Most common associated anomalies are sirenomelia, renal agenesis, and extralobar pulmonary sequestration.

   (3) Type III CAM is found in 10% of cases. It is a large bulky lesion composed of evenly distributed small (<0.2 cm in size) cysts. This type resembles the early canalicular stage of fetal lung development and may be the result of an insult at the time of lung bud branching. Only 60% of these infants survive (Johnson and Cooper, 2003).

  c. Respiratory distress may be seen at birth, or the malformation may cause no symptoms.

  d. May be confused with diaphragmatic hernia or pulmonary sequestration on x-ray.

  e. Treatment of choice is surgical excision of the involved lobe.

 2. Bronchogenic cyst.

  a. Mucus-producing cyst.

  b. May cause tracheal, bronchial, or esophageal obstruction.

  c. Distress usually not severe.

  d. Treatment is surgical excision.

 3. Congenital lobar emphysema.

  a. Overdistention of one or more lobes of the lung (upper lobes generally affected; 10% in right middle lobe).

  b. Inability of the lung to deflate properly, possibly because of a defect in bronchial cartilage.

  c. Possibility of severe respiratory distress within hours of birth but usually delayed for weeks or months.

  d. Chest x-ray examination is diagnostic (refer to Chapter 14).

  e. Treatment of choice: surgical resection.

4. Chondrodystrophies.
   a. Group of disorders of bone growth, resulting in short stature.
   b. Possible respiratory distress because of small thoracic cavities.
   c. Treatment: based on degree of distress.
5. Neuromuscular disorders.
   a. Conditions resulting in hypotonia, such as spinal muscular atrophy and myotonic dystrophy, result in varying degrees of respiratory distress.
   b. Management will depend on degree of distress.

C. **CNS disorders.**
   1. Seizures.
   2. Hypoxic-ischemic injury.
   3. Intracranial hemorrhages.
   4. Drugs.
   5. Meningitis.

D. **Cardiovascular and hematologic disorders.**
   1. Congenital heart disease.
   2. Anemia.
   3. Polycythemia.
   4. Shock.
   5. Sepsis.
   6. Respiratory distress, varying from mild to severe.
   7. Treatment in relation to underlying cause.

E. **Diaphragmatic disorders** (see also Chapter 14).
   1. Diaphragmatic hernia.
   2. Diaphragmatic paralysis.
   3. Diaphragmatic eventration.

F. **Renal disorders.**
   1. Pulmonary hypoplasia results from renal agenesis or renal dysgenesis.
   2. Conditions are usually untreatable, and death will occur within hours or days.

REFERENCES

Adams, J.M. and Cooper, T.R.: Bronchopulmonary dysplasia. In L.E. Weisman and T.N. Hansen (Eds.): *Contemporary diagnosis and management of neonatal respiratory diseases* (3rd ed.). Newtown, PA, 2003, Handbooks in Health Care, pp. 163-178.

Adams, E.W., Harrison, M.C., Counsell, S.J., et al.: Increased lung water and tissue damage in bronchopulmonary dysplasia. *Journal of Pediatrics, 145*(4):503-507, 2004.

American Academy of Pediatrics Committee on Fetus and Newborn and Canadian Pediatric Society Fetus and Newborn Committee: Postnatal Corticosteroids to treat or prevent chronic lung disease in preterm infants. *Pediatrics, 109*(2):330-338, 2002.

American Academy of Pediatrics Committee on Infectious Diseases and Committee on Fetus and Newborn: Revised indications for the use of palivizumab and respiratory syncytial virus immune globulin intravenous for the prevention of respiratory syncytial virus infections. *Pediatrics, 112*(6 Pt 1):1442-1446, 2003.

American Academy of Pediatrics: Initial steps in resuscitation. In J. Kattwinkel (Ed.): *Textbook of neonatal resuscitation* (5th ed.). Elk Grove Village, IL, 2006, American Academy of Pediatrics, pp. 21–2-26.

American Academy of Pediatrics and the American College of Obstetricians and Gynecologists: *Guidelines for perinatal care* (5th ed.). Elk Grove Village, IL, 2002, AAP/ACOG, pp. 125-306.

American Lung Association: *American Lung Association Fact Sheet: Respiratory distress syndrome and bronchopulmonary dysplasia.* American Lung Association, 2008. Retrieved November 14, 2008, from www. lungusa.org

Barrington, K.J. and Finer, N.N.: Treatment of bronchopulmonary dysplasia: A review. *Clinics in Perinatology, 25*(1):177-202, 1998.

Benstein, B.D., Crouse, D.T., Shanklin, D.R., and Ourth, D.D.: Ureaplasma in lung. 2. Association with bronchopulmonary dysplasia in premature newborns. *Experimental and Molecular Pathology, 75*(2):171-177, 2003.

Bessler, H., Wyshelesky, G., Osovsky, M., Prober, V., Sirota, L.: A comparison of the effect of vitamin A on cytokine secretion by mononuclear cells of preterm newborns and adults. *Neonatology, 91*(3):196-202, 2007.

Biniwale, M.A. and Ehrenkranz, R.A.: The role of nutrition in the prevention and management of bronchopulmonary dysplasia. *Seminars in Perinatology, 30*(4):200-208, 2006.

Bhandari, A., and Panitch, H.B.: 2006. Pulmonary outcomes in bronchopulmonary dysplasia. *Seminars in Perinatology, 30*(4):219-226, 2006.

Blackburn, S.T.: *Maternal, fetal, and neonatal physiology: A clinical perspective* (3rd ed). St. Louis, 2007, Saunders.

Bregman, J. and Farrell, E.E.: Neurodevelopmental outcome in infants with bronchopulmonary dysplasia. *Clinics in Perinatology, 19*(3):673-694, 1992.

Carey, B.E. and Trotter, C.: Neonatal pneumonia. *Neonatal Network, 19*(4):44-50, 2000.

Clark, R.H., Kueser, T.J., Walker, M.W., et al.: Low-dose nitric oxide therapy for persistent pulmonary hypertension of the newborn: Clinical Inhaled Nitric Oxide Research Group. *New England Journal of Medicine, 342*(7):469-474, 2000.

Chess, P.R., D'Angio, C.T., Pryhuber, G.S., and Maniscalco, W.M.: Pathogenesis of bronchopulmonary dysplasia. *Seminars in Perinatology, 30*(4):171-178, 2006.

Davis, J.M. and Rosenfeld, W.: Bronchopulmonary dysplasia. In M.G. MacDonald, M.D. Mullett, and M.M.K. Seshia (Eds.): *Avery's neonatology: Pathophysiology and management of the newborn* (5th ed.). Philadelphia, 2005, Lippincott, pp. 578-599.

Egberts, J., de Winter, J.P., Sedin, G., et al.: Comparison of prophylaxis and rescue treatment with Curosurf in neonates less than 30 weeks' gestation: A randomized trial. *Pediatrics, 92*(6):768-774, 1993.

Ehrenkranz, R.A., Walsh, M.C., Vohr, B.R., et al. for the National Institutes of Child Health and Human Development Neonatal Research Network: Validation of the National Institutes of Health consensus definition of bronchopulmonary dysplasia. *Pediatrics, 116*(6):1353-1360, 2005.

Engle, W.A., and the Committee on Fetus and Newborn: Surfactant-replacement therapy for respiratory distress in the preterm and term neonate. *Pediatrics, 121*(2):419-426, 2008.

Farrell, P.A. and Fiascone, J.M.: Bronchopulmonary dysplasia in the 1990s: A review for the pediatrician. *Pediatrics, 27*:129-172, 1997.

Finer, N.N. and Barrington, K.J.: Nitric oxide for respiratory failure in infants born at or near term. *Cochrane Database of Systematic Reviews, 18*(4):CD000399, 2006.

Gardner, S.L., Hagedorn, M.I., and Dickey, L.A.: Pain and pain relief. In G.B. Merenstein and S.L. Gardner (Eds.): *Handbook of neonatal intensive care* (6th ed.). St. Louis, 2006, Mosby, pp. 223-272.

Gelfand, S., Fanaroff, J., and Walsh, M.: Controversies in the treatment of meconium aspiration syndrome. *Clinics in Perinatology, 31*(3):445-452, 2004.

Ghidini, A., Salafia, C.M., Miniar, V.K., et al.: Repeated courses of steroids in preterm membrane rupture do not increase the risk of histologic chorioamnionitis. *American Journal of Perinatology, 14*(6):309-313, 1997.

Gitto, E., Reiter, R.J., Karbownik, M., et al.: Causes of oxidative stress in the pre- and perinatal period. *Biology of the Neonate, 81*(3):146-157, 2002.

Hagedorn, M.I.E., Gardner, S.L., Dickey, L.A., and Abman, S.H.: Respiratory diseases. In G.B. Merenstein and S.L. Gardner (Eds.): *Handbook of neonatal intensive care* (6th ed.). St. Louis, 2006, Mosby, pp. 595-698.

Henderson-Smart, D.J., Bhuta, T., Cools, F., and Offringa, M.: Elective high frequency oscillatory ventilation versus conventional ventilation for acute pulmonary dysfunction in preterm infants. *Cochrane Database of Systematic Reviews, 4*:CD000104, 2003.

Higgins, R.D., Bancalari, E., Willinger, M., and Raju, T.N.: Executive summary of the workshop on oxygen in neonatal therapies: Controversies and opportunities for research. *Pediatrics, 119*(4):790-796, 2007.

Impact-RSV Study Group: Palivizumab, a humanized respiratory syncytial virus monoclonal antibody, reduces hospitalization from respiratory syncytial virus infection in high-risk infants. *Pediatrics, 102*(3 Part 1):531-537, 1998.

Jobe, A.: Antenatal factors and the development of bronchopulmonary dysplasia. *Seminars in Neonatology, 8*(1):9-17, 2003.

Jobe, A.H. and Bancalari, E.: Bronchopulmonary dysplasia. *American Journal of Respiratory Care Medicine, 163*(7):1723-1729, 2001.

Jobe, A.H and Ikegami, M.: Pathophysiology of respiratory distress syndrome and surfactant metabolism. In R.A. Polin, W.W. Fox, and S.H. Abman (Eds.): *Fetal and neonatal physiology* (3rd ed.). Philadelphia, 2004, Saunders, pp. 1055-1068.

Jobe, A.H. and Ikegami, M.: Biology of surfactant. *Clinics in Perinatology, 28*(3):655-669, 2001.

Johnson, K.E. and Cooper, T.R.: Congenital diseases affecting the lung parenchyma. In L.E. Weisman and T.N. Hansen (Eds.): *Contemporary diagnosis and management of neonatal respiratory diseases* (3rd ed.), Newton, PA, 2003, Handbooks in Health Care, pp. 186-200.

Johnson, K.E., Cooper, T.R., and Hansen, T.N.: Meconium aspiration syndrome. In L.E. Weisman and T.N. Hansen (Eds.): *Contemporary diagnosis and management of neonatal respiratory diseases* (3rd ed.). Newtown, PA, 2003, Handbooks in Health Care, pp. 135-141.

Kattwinkel, J.: Surfactant: Evolving issues. *Clinics in Perinatology, 25*(1):17-32, 1998.

Kattwinkel, J., Bloom, B.T., Delmore, P., et al.: Prophylactic administration of calf lung surfactant is more effective than early treatment of respiratory distress syndrome in neonates 29 through 32 weeks' gestation. *Pediatrics, 9*(1/2):90-98, 1993.

Kendig, J.W., Notter, R.N., Cox, C., et al.: A comparison of surfactant as immediate prophylaxis and as rescue therapy in newborns of less than 30 weeks' gestation. *New England Journal of Medicine, 324*(13):865-871, 1991.

Kinsella, J.P. and Abman, S.H.: Recent developments in the pathophysiology and treatment of persistent pulmonary hypertension of the newborn. *Journal of Pediatrics, 12*(6):853-864, 1995.

Kinsella, J.P. and Abman, S.H.: Special ventilatory techniques and modalities III. In J.P. Goldsmith and E.H. Karotkin (Eds.): *Assisted ventilation of the neonate.* Philadelphia, 2003, Saunders, pp. 235-248.

Larsen, W.J.: Embryonic foldings. In *Human embryology* (3rd ed.). New York, 2001, Churchill Livingstone, pp. 134-155.

Liley, H.G. and Stark, A.R.: Respiratory distress syndrome: Hyaline membrane disease. J.P. Cloherty and A.R. Stark (Eds.): *Manual of neonatal care.* Philadelphia, 1998, Lippincott-Raven, pp. 329-335.

Lotze, A., Mitchell, B.R., Bulas, D.I., et al.: Multicenter study of surfactant (beractant) use in the treatment of term infants with severe respiratory failure. *Journal of Pediatrics*, 132(1):40-47, 1998.

Lulic-Botica, M., Biglin, K., Aranda, J.V.: Drug formulary for the newborn. Appendix A-1. In S.J. Yaffe and J.V. Aranda (Eds.): *Neonatal and pediatric pharmacology. Therapeutic principles in practice* (3rd ed.). Philadelphia, 2005, Lippincott Williams & Wilkins, pp. 861-888.

March of Dimes, 2007: *Cerebral palsy*. Retrieved February 5, 2009, from www.marchofdimes.com.

McClure, P.C., Patel, M.R., and Le, T.T.: *Hyaline membrane disease*. EMedicine, 2005. Retrieved November 14, 2008, from www.emedicine.com/radio/topic350.htm

Meissner, H.C., Long, S.S., and the American Academy of Pediatrics Committee on Infectious Diseases and Committee on Fetus and Newborn: Revised indications for the use of palivizumab and respiratory syncytial virus immune globulin intravenous for the prevention of respiratory syncytial virus infections. *Pediatrics*, 112(6 Pt 1):1447-1452, 2003.

Moise, A.A. and Gomez, M.R.: Nonventilatory management of respiratory failure. In L.E. Weisman and T.N. Hansen (Eds.): *Contemporary diagnosis and management of neonatal respiratory diseases*. Newtown, PA, 2003, Handbooks in Health Care, pp. 286-291.

Moise, A.A. and Hansen, T.N.: Acute, acquired parenchymal lung disease. In L.E. Weisman and T.N. Hansen (Eds.): *Contemporary diagnosis and management of neonatal respiratory diseases* (3rd ed.). Newtown, PA, 2003, Handbooks in Health Care, pp. 90-107.

Moore, K.L. and Persaud, T.V.N.: The respiratory system. In *Before we are born: Essentials of embryology and birth defects* (6th ed.). Philadelphia, 2003, Saunders, pp. 190-199.

Morin, F.C., III and Stenmark, K.R.: Persistent pulmonary hypertension of the newborn. *American Journal of Respiratory and Critical Care Medicine*, 151(6):2010-2032, 1995.

National Institutes of Health: Antenatal corticosteroids revisited: Repeat courses. *NIH Consensus Statement 2000. August 17-18*:17(2)1-18, 2000.

Ng, D.K., Lau, W.Y., and Lee, S.L.: Pulmonary sequelae in long-term survivors of bronchopulmonary dysplasia. *Pediatrics International*, 42(6):603-607, 2000.

Northway, W.H., Rosan, R.C., and Porter, D.Y.: Pulmonary disease following respiratory therapy of hyaline membrane disease. *New England Journal of Medicine*, 276(7):357-368, 1967.

Orlando, S.: Pathophysiology of acute respiratory distress. In D.F. Askin (Ed.): *Acute respiratory care of the neonate*. Petaluma, CA, 1997, NICU Ink Books, pp. 37-41.

Paige, P.L. and Moe P.C.: Neurologic disorders. In G.B. Merenstein and S.L. Gardner (Eds.): *Handbook of neonatal intensive care* (6th ed.). St. Louis, 2006, Mosby, pp. 773-811.

Parad, R.B. and Berger, T.M.: Chronic lung disease. In J.P. Cloherty and A.R. Stark (Eds.): *Manual of neonatal care*. Philadelphia, 1998, Lippincott-Raven, pp. 378-387.

Pearson, D.L., Dawling, S., Walsh, W.F., et al.: Neonatal pulmonary hypertension: Urea-cycle intermediates, nitric oxide production, and carbamoyl-phosphate synthetase function. *New England Journal of Medicine*, 344(24):1832-1838, 2001.

Reynolds, R.M. and Thureen, P.J.: Special circumstances: Trophic feeds, necrotizing enterocolitis and bronchopulmonary dysplasia. *Seminars in Fetal and Neonatal Medicine*, 12(1):64-70, 2007.

Roberts, D. and Dalziel, S.R.: Antenatal corticosteroids for accelerating fetal lung maturation for women at risk of preterm birth. *Cochrane Database of Systematic Reviews*, 4:CD004454, 2008.

Rusk, C.: Rickets screening in the preterm infant. *Neonatal Network*, 17(1):55-57, 1998.

Sahni, R., Ammari, A., Suri, M.S., et al.: Is the new definition of bronchopulmonary dysplasia more useful? *Journal of Perinatology*, 25(1):41-46, 2005.

Shah, P.S. and Ohlsson, A.: Sildenafil for pulmonary hypertension in neonates. *Cochrane Database of Systematic Reviews*, 18(3):CD005494, 2007.

Shapiro, D.L.: The development of surfactant therapy and the various types of replacement surfactants. *Seminars in Perinatology*, 12(3):174-179, 1988.

Short, E.J., Klein, N.K., Lewis, B.A., et al.: Cognitive and academic consequences of bronchopulmonary dysplasia and very low birth weight: 8-year-old outcomes. *Pediatrics*, 112(5):e359, 2003.

Soll, R.F.: Prophylactic natural surfactant extract for preventing morbidity and mortality in preterm infants. *Cochrane Database of Systematic Reviews*, 2: CD000511, 2000.

Speer, M.E. and Hansen, T.N.: Transient tachypnea of the newborn. In L.E. Weisman and T.N. Hansen (Eds.): *Contemporary diagnosis and management of neonatal respiratory diseases* (3rd ed.). Newtown, PA, 2003, Handbooks in Health Care, pp. 108-113.

Speer, M.E. and Weisman, L.E.: Pneumonia. In L.E. Weisman and T.N. Hansen (Eds.): *Contemporary diagnosis and management of neonatal respiratory diseases* (3rd ed.). Newtown, PA, 2003, Handbooks in Health Care, pp. 140-144.

Speer, C.P.: Inflammation and bronchopulmonary dysplasia: A continuing story. *Seminars in Fetal and Neonatal Medicine*, 11(5):354-362, 2006.

Stark, A.R., Carlo, W.A., Tyson, J.E., et al.: Adverse effects of early dexamethasone treatment in extremely-low-birth-weight-infants: National Institute of Child Health and Human Development Neonatal Research Network. *New England Journal of Medicine*, 344(2):95-101, 2001.

Steinhorn, R.H., Millard, S.L., and Morin, F.C.: Persistent pulmonary hypertension of the newborn. *Clinics in Perinatology*, 22(2):405-428, 1995.

Stevens, T.P., Harrington, E.W., Blennow, M., and Soll, R.F.: Early surfactant administration with brief ventilation vs. selective surfactant and continued mechanical ventilation for preterm infants with or at risk for respiratory distress syndrome. *Cochrane Database of Systematic Reviews*, 17(4):CD003063, 2007.

Van Marter, L.J.: Persistent pulmonary hypertension of the newborn. In J.P. Cloherty and A.R. Stark (Eds.): *Manual of neonatal care*. Philadelphia, 1998, Lippincott-Raven, pp. 364-369.

Van Marter, L.J.: Progress in discovery and evaluation of treatments to prevent bronchopulmonary dysplasia. *Biology of the Neonate*, *89*(4):303-312, 2006.

Walsh-Sukys, M.C., Tyson, J.E., Wright, L.L., et al.: Persistent pulmonary hypertension of the newborn in the era before nitric oxide: Practice variation and outcomes. *Pediatrics*, *105*(1):14-20, 2000.

Walsh, M.C., Yao, Q., Gettner, P., et al.: Impact of a physiologic definition on bronchopulmonary dysplasia rates. *Pediatrics*, *114*(5):1305-1311, 2004.

Wearden, M.E. and Hansen, T.N.: Persistent pulmonary hypertension of the newborn. In L.E. Weisman and T.N. Hansen (Eds.): *Contemporary diagnosis and management of neonatal respiratory diseases* (3rd ed.). Newtown, PA, 2003, Handbooks in Health Care, pp. 113-124.

Weinberger, B., Laskin, D.L., Heck, D.E., Laskin, J.D.: Oxygen toxicity in premature infants. *Toxicology and Applied Pharmacology*, *181*(1):60-67, 2002.

Welliver, R.C.: Respiratory syncytial virus immunoglobulin and monoclonal antibodies in the prevention and treatment of respiratory syncytial virus infection. *Seminars in Perinatology*, *22*(1):87-95, 1998.

Welty, S.E. and Hansen, T.N.: Pulmonary hemorrhage. In L.E. Weisman and T.N. Hansen (Eds.): *Contemporary diagnosis and management of neonatal respiratory diseases* (3rd ed.). Newtown, PA, 2003, Handbooks in Health Care, pp. 130-135.

Whitsett, J.A., Rice, W.R., Warner, B.B., Wert S.E., and Pryhuber, G.S: Acute respiratory disorders. In M.G. MacDonald, M.D. Mullett, M.M.K. Seshia (Eds.): *Avery's neonatology: Pathophysiology and management of the newborn* (5th ed.). Philadelphia, 2005, Lippincott, pp. 553-577.

Wiswell, T.E.: Expanded uses of surfactant therapy. *Clinics in Perinatology*, *28*(3):695-711, 2001.

Wood, B.R.: Physiologic principles. In J.P. Goldsmith and E.H. Karotkin (Eds.): *Assisted ventilation of the neonate*. Philadelphia, 2003, Saunders, pp. 15-40.

Young, T.E. and Mangum, O.B.: *Neofax: A manual of drugs used in neonatal care* (21st ed.). Raleigh, NC, 2008, Acorn.

Young, T.E.: Nutritional support and bronchopulmonary dysplasia. *Journal of Perinatology*, *27*(Suppl. 1):S75-S78, 2007.

Zenk, K., Sills, J., and Koeppel, R.: *Neonatal medications and nutrition*. Santa Rosa, CA, 2003, NICU Ink.

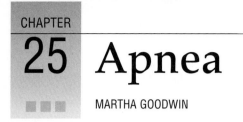

25 Apnea

MARTHA GOODWIN

OBJECTIVES

1. Define types of apnea seen in the newborn infant.

2. Identify three causes of apnea.

3. Describe the pathogenesis of apnea in the premature infant.

4. Describe the evaluation process for the infant with apnea.

5. Discuss management techniques for controlling apnea.

6. Discuss the current status of home monitoring.

Apnea represents one of the most frequently encountered respiratory problems in the premature infant. It is not known why some infants are affected and others are not, although certain factors have a good predictive value. Apnea in the term infant is not ever a normal finding and must always be investigated. In the preterm infant, apnea that presents in the first 24 hours has historically been perceived as pathologic, whereas that occurring later has most often been attributed to immaturity. The mechanism of action is not fully understood but can be characterized as an immature respiratory system faced with demands it is ill equipped to handle. This chapter will provide a comprehensive review of apnea of the premature infant, including causes, evaluation, treatment, and long-term home follow-up.

DEFINITIONS OF APNEA

A. Periodic breathing.

1. Definition: recurrent sequences of pauses in respiration lasting 5 to 10 seconds followed by 10 to 15 seconds of rapid respiration.

2. Seen in less than 2% of well term infants and in 30% to 95% of healthy preterm infants more than 24 hours of age.

3. Not accompanied by cyanosis or changes in heart rate.

4. Episodes of periodic breathing in the preterm infant decrease significantly by 39 to 41 weeks of postmenstrual age (Miller et al., 2006).

5. Studies do not support a link between periodic breathing and significant apnea or sudden infant death syndrome (SIDS) (American Academy of Pediatrics [AAP] Committee on Fetus and Newborn, 2003; Miller and Martin, 2003).

B. Apnea.

1. Definition: cessation of respiration for at least 20 seconds, or less if complicated by cyanosis, pallor, hypotonia, or bradycardia.

2. Most apnea occurs in the healthy preterm infant without organic disease. Up to 80% of infants weighing less than 1000 g and 25% weighing less than 2500 g at birth will have apnea during their neonatal course (Miller and Martin, 2003).

TYPES OF APNEA

A. Primary apnea.

1. Definition: initial cessation of respiratory movements after a period of rapid respiratory effort as a result of asphyxia during the delivery process.

2. Exposure to stimulation and/or oxygen will usually induce spontaneous respiratory effort.

B. **Secondary apnea.**
   1. Definition: apnea occurring after a period of deep, gasping respirations and fall in blood pressure and heart rate, brought about by prolonged asphyxia during the delivery process. The gasping becomes slower and weaker and then ceases.
   2. Infant will not respond to stimulation and will require more vigorous resuscitation.
   3. For each minute in secondary apnea before resuscitation, there is a 2-minute delay before gasping is reestablished and another 2 minutes before the onset of regular respirations.
   4. It is not usually possible to distinguish primary from secondary apnea at birth (Kattwinkel, 2006).

C. **Central apnea.**
   1. Definition: absence of airflow and respiratory effort.
   2. Cause of central apnea in the preterm infant is not fully understood.
   3. Contributing factors are thought to include the following:
      a. Chest wall afferent neuromuscular signals and chest wall instability.
      b. Diaphragmatic fatigue.
      c. Immature, paradoxic response of neonate to hypoxia and hypercapnia.
      d. Altered levels of local neurotransmitters in the brain stem region of the central nervous system (CNS).
   4. Fifteen percent of apnea episodes are central in origin.
   5. Closure of upper airway occurs in about half of cases of central apnea (Hanson and Corbet, 2005).

D. **Obstructive apnea.**
   1. Definition: absence of airflow with continued respiratory effort, associated with blockage of airway at the level of pharynx and/or larynx (Miller et al., 2006).
   2. Hyperextension or flexion of the neck may induce obstruction of the airway.
   3. May be caused by obstruction of airflow at the mouth or nose as a result of anatomic abnormalities such as macroglossia (Beckwith–Wiedemann syndrome, congenital hypothyroidism) or micrognathia (Pierre Robin syndrome).
   4. Up to 30% of apnea episodes are obstructive in origin.

E. **Mixed apnea.**
   1. Definition: a combination of central and obstructive apnea, obstruction usually at the level of the pharynx.
   2. Fifty to sixty percent of neonatal apnea episodes are mixed.

F. **Idiopathic apnea, or apnea of prematurity.**
   1. Diagnosis after exclusion of pathologic processes in the premature infant.
   2. Not necessarily associated with the presence of periodic breathing.
   3. Recurrent apnea seen in preterm infants who show no other abnormalities.
   4. Onset within the first week of life, usually at 24 to 48 hours. If not present within the first week of life, will usually not appear unless later illness develops.
   5. More likely to be obstructive than central in the first 2 days of life.
   6. Episodes of apnea cease by term in 95% of infants: may persist longer in infants born at less than 28 weeks of gestational age (Stokowski, 2005).

PATHOGENESIS OF APNEA IN THE PREMATURE INFANT

A. **Immature central respiratory center.**
   1. Decreased afferent traffic occurs as a result of
      a. Poor CNS myelinization,
      b. Decreased number of synapses, and
      c. Decreased dendritic arborization.
   2. Decreased amounts of neurotransmitters have been measured in infants with apnea and may play an important role in respiratory control (Kattwinkel, 1977).
   3. Fluctuating respiratory center output has been implicated (Martin and Abu-Shaweesh, 2005).

B. Chemoreceptors.

1. Located in the medulla (central) and the carotid and aortic bodies (peripheral), chemoreceptors relay information to the respiratory center in the brain regarding pH, Po_2, and Pco_2 via the vagus and glossopharyngeal nerves.

   a. Hypoxemia is sensed in the carotid and aortic bodies and results in an increase in alveolar ventilation. Premature infants with apnea do not respond to hypoxemia as effectively as infants who do not have apnea (Khan et al., 2005).

   b. Hypercapnia is sensed centrally. The normal response to an increased arterial Pco_2 is an increase in minute ventilation. Neonates can increase ventilation by only 3 or 4 times the baseline values, in comparison with the 10- to 20-fold increase that adults can obtain. Premature infants exhibit a blunted response to elevated Pco_2, resulting in ongoing hypoventilation and hypercapnia. This diminished response predisposes them to apnea (Khan et al., 2005).

2. Biphasic response of the premature infant to hypoxia.

   a. During the first minute of hypoxia, a brief increase in respiratory effort occurs. It is followed in the next 2 to 3 minutes by a decrease in respiratory rate and by periodic breathing, respiratory depression, and apnea. Initial stimulation of the peripheral chemoreceptors is followed by overriding depression of the respiratory centers as a result of hypoxia (Miller et al., 2006).

   b. At 7 to 18 days of postnatal age, an infant can maintain the adult response to hypoxia of sustained hyperventilation.

3. Depressed response to hypercapnia. The premature infant exhibits decreased sensitivity to increased levels of carbon dioxide, requiring higher levels of carbon dioxide to stimulate respirations (Cohen and Katz-Salamon, 2005).

C. Thermal afferents.

1. Apnea is increased in an environment that may be too warm for the infant (Stokowski, 2005).

2. Thermal receptors in the trigeminal area of the face produce an apneic response to stimulation by a cold or hot gas mixture.

D. Mechanoreceptors.

1. Stretch receptors alter the timing of respiration at various lung volumes.

   a. Head's paradoxic reflex: a gasp followed by apnea after abrupt lung inflation.

   b. Hering–Breuer reflex.

      (1) Vagally mediated, it acts to inhibit inspiration and/or prolong expiration.

      (2) Lung inflation initiates inhibitory impulses that terminate inspiration and prolong expiratory time.

      (3) Mechanoreceptors are very active in the neonate but rarely seen in the adult.

2. Pharyngeal collapse and airway obstruction are produced by negative pharyngeal pressure generated during inspiration.

3. Intercostal phrenic inhibitory reflex, an inward movement of the ribcage during inspiration, prematurely ends inspiration (Martin and Abu-Shaweesh, 2005).

E. Protective reflexes.

1. Stimulation of the posterior portion of the pharynx with suctioning, endotracheal or gavage tube placement, or gastroesophageal reflux can stimulate apnea.

2. Pulmonary irritant receptors can produce an apneic response to direct bronchial stimulation.

3. Laryngeal taste receptors can produce an apneic response to various chemical stimuli (Kattwinkel, 1977).

F. Sleep state.

1. Eighty percent of the neonate's day is spent in sleep.

2. Respiratory depression occurs predominantly in rapid eye movement (REM) or transitional sleep (Darnall et al., 2006).

   a. May be influenced by central mechanisms at the level of the brainstem.

      (1) May be due to a defect in a sleep-related feedback loop or respiratory command.

      (2) Variability of respiratory rhythmicity is seen in active sleep (Hanson and Corbet, 2005).

b. May be related to paradoxic respirations in which chest wall movements are out of phase, resulting in ribcage collapse with abdominal expansion during inspiration. This would lead to a decrease in lung volume and functional residual capacity.

c. May be related to decreased skeletal muscle tone of the tongue and pharynx during sleep, which could lead to increased resistance and obstruction in the upper airway (Bhat et al., 2006).

CAUSES OF APNEA

A. **Prematurity.**
B. **Hypoxia.**
C. **Respiratory disorders.**
   1. Respiratory distress syndrome.
   2. Pneumonia.
   3. Aspiration.
   4. Acidosis.
   5. Airway obstruction.
   6. Pneumothorax.
   7. Atelectasis.
   8. Pulmonary hemorrhage.
   9. Postextubation status.
  10. Congenital anomalies of the upper airway.
D. **Cardiovascular disorders.**
   1. Hypotension.
   2. Arrhythmias.
   3. Congestive heart failure.
   4. Patent ductus arteriosus.
E. **Infection.**
   1. Sepsis.
   2. Pneumonia.
   3. Meningitis.
   4. Viral infections.
   5. Necrotizing enterocolitis.
F. **CNS disorders.**
   1. Congenital malformations.
   2. Seizures.
   3. Asphyxia.
   4. Intracranial hemorrhage.
   5. Kernicterus.
   6. Tumors.
G. **Drugs.**
   1. Maternal drugs.
     a. Narcotics.
     b. Analgesics.
     c. Anesthesia.
     d. β-Blocker antihypertensive agents.
     e. Magnesium sulfate.
   2. Neonatal drugs.
     a. Anticonvulsants: phenobarbital, pentobarbital.
     b. Cardiovascular drugs: prostaglandin E_1.
     c. Narcotics/analgesics.
       (1) Fentanyl.
       (2) Morphine.
       (3) Midazolam hydrochloride.
       (4) Lorazepam.

H. Metabolic disorders.
   1. Hypocalcemia.
   2. Hypoglycemia.
   3. Hypomagnesemia.
   4. Hyponatremia.
   5. Acidosis.
   6. Hyperammonemia.
I. Hematopoietic disorders.
   1. Polycythemia.
   2. Anemia.
J. Reflex stimulation.
   1. Posterior pharyngeal stimulation.
   2. Gastroesophageal reflux—controversial, recent studies do not support a link. Some studies have shown apnea precedes reflux when the two are linked (Finer et al., 2006; Nimavat et al., 2007).
K. Environmental factors.
   1. Rapid warming.
   2. Hypothermia.
   3. Hyperthermia.
   4. Elevated environmental temperature.
   5. Feeding.
   6. Stooling.
   7. Painful stimuli.

EVALUATION FOR APNEA

A. History.
   1. Perinatal risk factors.
      a. Maternal bleeding, drugs, fever, hypertension, prolonged rupture of membranes, polyhydramnios, chorioamnionitis, decreased fetal movements, abnormal fetal presentation.
      b. Fetal hypoxia, trauma.
   2. Neonatal risk factors.
      a. Prematurity.
      b. Cardiorespiratory disease.
      c. Metabolic abnormalities.
      d. Temperature instability.
      e. Infection.
      f. Environmental causes.
      g. CNS disorders.
B. Physical examination. A complete physical and neurologic examination should be performed. Observe for congenital malformations, especially those involving the airway. Observe for signs of respiratory distress and heart disease. Abnormal behavior, tone, or posturing may be associated with a neurologic focus. An abdominal examination should be performed, which may reveal symptoms related to obstruction, infection, necrotizing enterocolitis, or congestive heart failure.
C. Documentation of apnea episodes. A record of apneic episodes should be maintained as part of the infant's record. This allows the caregiver to determine a pattern, if any, to the apnea. It may also provide information about precipitating events or specific events associated with the apnea. Information documented should include the following:
   1. Duration of apnea episode.
   2. Time of apnea episode and any relation to feeding, activity, stooling, sleep, or procedures.
   3. Infant's position: prone or supine, with head of bed elevated or flat.
   4. Associated bradycardia/heart rate.
   5. Associated color change and/or oxygen desaturation.

6. Type of stimulation required to resolve the episode:
   a. None, self-resolved.
   b. Gentle tactile stimulation.
   c. Vigorous tactile stimulation.
   d. Oxygen.
   e. Bag–mask ventilation.
D. **Laboratory evaluation.**
   1. Basic evaluation to look for infection, respiratory deterioration, and metabolic problems.
      a. Complete blood cell count, with differential cell and platelet counts.
      b. Blood gas.
      c. Serum glucose, electrolytes, calcium, magnesium.
      d. Blood culture, lumbar puncture for evaluation of cerebrospinal fluid, and urine culture.
   2. Extensive laboratory evaluation for less common causes of apnea.
      a. Toxicology screen.
      b. Urine collection for detection of amino acids and organic acids.
      c. Serum ammonia.
      d. State screen and expanded neonatal screen for metabolic disease.
E. **Other.**
   1. Echocardiogram or electrocardiogram: may detect cardiac abnormality or conduction disorders.
   2. Electroencephalogram: may confirm suspected seizures.
   3. Chest x-ray: may demonstrate respiratory or cardiac abnormalities.
   4. Cranial ultrasound, computed tomography, or magnetic resonance imaging: may demonstrate structural abnormalities or hemorrhages.
   5. Barium swallow and pH study: to evaluate pharyngeal structure and function or gastroesophageal reflux.
   6. Pneumogram.
      a. Measures chest wall movement, heart rate, oxygen saturation, and nasal airflow by thermistor or carbon dioxide probe; measures esophageal pH.
      b. No predictive value for SIDS; recording monitors are as effective at detecting apnea over a prolonged period (AAP Committee on Fetus and Newborn, 2003).

MANAGEMENT TECHNIQUES

A. **Treat underlying cause if determined.**
B. **Provide needed medical or surgical intervention.**
C. **Maintain environmental temperature at the low end of the neutral thermal zone.**
D. **Avoid triggering reflexes:**
   1. Vigorous catheter suctioning.
   2. Hot or cold to the face.
   3. Sudden gastric distention.
E. **Maintain infant in the prone position whenever possible.** Prone positioning is associated with higher oxygen saturation, shorter gastric emptying time, and decreased incidence of regurgitation and aspiration. Supine positioning has been associated with an increase in apnea and severity of apneic episode. Elevation of the head of the bed by 15 degrees reduces hypoxemic events in preterm infants. Babies should be placed supine at 36 weeks of postmenstrual age (Bhat et al., 2006).
F. **Maintain the neck in a neutral position, not flexed or hyperextended. Use of a neck roll is recommended.**
G. **Avoid vigorous manual ventilation to prevent intermittent hyperoxia, hypocapnia, and blunting of the CO_2 response.**
H. **Attempt to control apnea by avoiding painful stimuli, loud noises, extremely vigorous tactile stimulation, or potent odors.** No evidence supports effectiveness of kinesthetic

stimulation in reduction of apnea (Henderson-Smart and Osborn, 2002). A recent small study showed reduction in apnea with use of pleasant olfactory stimulation; further research is needed (Marlier et al., 2005).

I. Consider providing continuous positive airway pressure.

    1. Increases end-expiratory lung volumes and splints the upper airway and weak chest wall, thereby improving compliance and oxygenation and decreasing respiratory muscle work so that diaphragmatic movements are less tiring and more effective.

    2. Complicates gavage feedings and may increase risk of aspiration. Increases risk of air leak.

J. Pharmacologic therapy.

    1. Methylxanthine (aminophylline, theophylline, caffeine), administered orally or intravenously. Used to treat apnea of prematurity after pathologic causes have been eliminated.

        a. Mechanisms of action include the following:

            (1) Stimulation of central respiratory chemoreceptors.

            (2) Increased ventilatory response to carbon dioxide.

            (3) Increased oxygenation.

            (4) Increased minute ventilation (theophylline).

            (5) Stabilization of oscillations in breathing (theophylline).

            (6) Improved diaphragmatic contractility.

            (7) Relaxation of bronchial smooth muscle (theophylline).

            (8) CNS excitation.

            (9) Increased respiratory drive.

            (10) Increased respiratory muscle activity.

            (11) Increased skeletal muscle activity.

        b. Pharmacokinetics.

            (1) Half-life of aminophylline and theophylline is approximately 30 hours.

            (2) Half-life of caffeine is approximately 100 hours.

            (3) Both theophylline and caffeine are rapidly absorbed intravenously. Oral absorption of caffeine is rapid, and oral absorption of theophylline is variable.

            (4) Metabolism of caffeine and theophylline takes place in the liver. This is slower in the neonate than in the adult.

            (5) Theophylline is metabolized to caffeine by a metabolic pathway unique to the preterm infant.

            (6) Serum concentrations must be checked to avoid toxic levels (Lopes and Aranda, 2005).

        c. Dosage:

            (1) Aminophylline.

                (a) Route: intravenous (IV).

                (b) Loading dose: 5 mg/kg.

                (c) Maintenance dose: 1 to 2 mg/kg every 8 to 12 hours.

                (d) Therapeutic level: 5 to 15 mcg/ml.

            (2) Theophylline.

                (a) Route: by mouth.

                (b) Loading dose: 5 mg/kg.

                (c) Maintenance dose: 1 to 2 mg/kg every 8 to 12 hours.

                (d) Therapeutic level: 5 to 15 mcg/ml.

            (3) Caffeine.

                (a) Route: IV or by mouth.

                (b) Loading dose: 10 mg/kg, caffeine base; 20 mg/kg, caffeine citrate.

                (c) Maintenance dose: 2.5 mg/kg, caffeine base; 5 mg/kg, caffeine citrate; every 24 hours.

                (d) Avoid use of caffeine benzoate preparation, which can displace bilirubin from albumin-binding sites.

                (e) Therapeutic level: 5 to 20 mcg/ml.

                (f) Higher doses and therapeutic levels have been studied, with no reported adverse effects but not in common use (Steer et al., 2004).

    d. Side effects.

        (1) Caffeine: tachycardia, cardiac dysrhythmias, increased wakefulness, increased active sleep, gastrointestinal distention, gastrointestinal bleeding, and diuresis with sodium loss.

        (2) Theophylline: tachycardia, cardiac dysrhythmias, seizures, jitteriness, feeding intolerance, gastroesophageal reflux, dehydration, hyperglycemia, and hypotension.

    e. Caffeine versus theophylline.

        (1) Theophylline is a more potent vasodilator.

        (2) Theophylline causes a more rapid and sustained tachycardia.

        (3) Caffeine diffuses more rapidly in the CNS.

        (4) Caffeine is given only once a day.

        (5) Caffeine has a wider therapeutic index.

        (6) Caffeine may be effective in apnea not responsive to theophylline and vice versa.

        (7) Caffeine has a longer half-life, resulting in smaller changes in its plasma concentration.

        (8) On the basis of its higher therapeutic ratio, more reliable enteral absorption, and longer half-life, caffeine is recommended over theophylline for treatment of apnea of prematurity (Lopes and Aranda, 2005).

  2. Doxapram.

    a. Potent respiratory stimulant for apnea refractory to methylxanthine therapy.

    b. Mechanism of action thought to be stimulation of the peripheral chemoreceptors at low doses (0.5 mg/kg/hour) and of the CNS at higher doses.

    c. Increases minute ventilation, tidal volume, and mean inspiratory flow and decreases Pco_2 (Dani et al., 2006).

    d. Pharmacokinetics.

        (1) Half-life is approximately 10 hours in the first few days of life and 8 hours at 10 days of age.

        (2) Steady-state levels are reached within 24 hours.

    e. Dosage.

        (1) Route: IV.

        (2) Dosage range: 0.25 to 2.5 mg/kg/hour, administered by continuous infusion.

        (3) Controversy exists over therapeutic and toxic plasma levels. Guidelines include the following:

            (a) Therapeutic level: less than 5 mg/l.

            (b) Toxic level: 5 mg/l. Levels greater than 3.5 mg/l may produce side effects.

    f. Side effects.

        (1) Jitteriness, irritability, vomiting, seizures, abdominal distention, increased gastric residuals, hyperglycemia, and glycosuria.

        (2) Hypertension, tachycardia, and increased cardiac output.

        (3) Increased work of breathing resulting from respiratory stimulation, consequent increased oxygen consumption and carbon dioxide production, and increased tidal volume and respiratory rate.

        (4) Increased risk of intraventricular hemorrhage if used in the first few days of life.

    g. Contraindication: use in newborn infant not routinely recommended because preparation contains benzyl alcohol.

        (1) Benzyl alcohol is associated with "gasping syndrome," characterized by metabolic acidosis, renal failure, liver failure, and cardiovascular collapse.

        (2) Cumulative doses might be toxic for the liver, kidney, or brain.

        (3) Insufficient data exist on clinical benefit and long-term effects (Lopes and Aranda, 2005).

K. Assisted ventilation. Used for apnea resistant to other methods of therapy.

HOME MONITORING

A. Effectiveness of home monitoring. The American Academy of Pediatrics states that cardiorespiratory monitoring is effective in preventing death from apnea for certain selected infants but is clearly inappropriate for others, with the primary objective being to serve the best interest of the infant based on the infant's history (Task Force on Sudden Infant Death Syndrome, 2005).

B. Indications for home monitoring.
1. Premature infant with symptoms of idiopathic apnea of prematurity who is otherwise ready for hospital discharge.
2. A survivor of an apparent life-threatening event defined as apnea, cyanosis, altered muscle tone, choking, or gagging.
3. Sibling death due to SIDS.
4. Tracheostomy, mechanically supported ventilation.
5. A sleep apnea syndrome caused by a neurologic disorder, periodic breathing, upper-airway abnormality, or idiopathic syndromes.
6. Other conditions of ill or high-risk infants, as determined on an individual basis.

C. Home monitoring is not indicated in prevention of SIDS in symptom-free, healthy infants.

D. Monitoring technology.
1. Transthoracic impedance combined with electrocardiography is current standard.
   a. Electrodes are placed on infant's chest or inside an adjustable belt worn around the chest.
   b. A small electric current passes between the electrodes. The impedance to this current is measured as the chest wall diameter changes. The monitor senses this change and equates it with respiration.
   c. Electrocardiograph reads cardiac activity.
   d. High and low limits for respirations and heart rate are set by the clinician.
   e. Monitor is compact and portable, weighing less than 5 pounds. A battery pack is available for use outside the home.
2. Technical problems include artifact from signal interference, false alarms caused by shallow breathing, and the monitor's inability to detect obstructive apnea. Incorrect placement of leads can result in false alarms as well.
3. Advances in technology allow recording of home monitor events for evaluation by the clinician.
   a. Recording of events allows monitoring of compliance.
   b. True events can be distinguished from false alarms.
   c. Fewer rehospitalizations are needed.
   d. Recording is as sensitive as a pneumogram for evaluating whether monitoring can be discontinued.
   e. Fewer monitor days are needed for infants without events.

E. Follow-up care.
1. Multidisciplinary team includes physician, nurse, social worker, case manager, and equipment company representatives.
2. Family and other caretakers of the infant are trained in cardiopulmonary resuscitation before hospital discharge. Thorough education in use of the monitor is also provided before discharge.
3. Care includes close telephone contact—within 24 hours after discharge and every week to 2 weeks afterward as needed.
4. Visiting nurse makes home visit within the first week and then as needed.
5. A team member is available 24 hours a day for answering questions and solving problems. Equipment company representative is available as needed for problems and information.
6. Home follow-up does not replace clinic visits.
7. In 80% of infants apnea of prematurity will cease between 40 and 44 weeks of postmenstrual age; in asymptomatic infants home monitoring can be stopped at 45 weeks of postmenstrual age (AAP Committee on Fetus and Newborn, 2003).

REFERENCES

American Academy of Pediatrics, Committee on Fetus and Newborn: Apnea, sudden infant death syndrome, and home monitoring. *Pediatrics, 111*:914-917, 2003.

Bhat, R., Hannam, S., Pressler, R., Rafferty, G., Peacock, J. and Greehough, A.: Effect of prone and supine position on sleep, apneas and arousal in preterm infants. *Pediatrics, 118*:101-107, 2006.

Cohen, G. and Katz-Salamon, M.: Development of chemoreceptor responses in infants. *Respiratory Physiology and Neurobiology, 149*:233-242, 2005.

Dani, C., Bertini, G., Pezzati, M., Pratesi, S., Filippi, L., Tronchin, M., and Rubaltelli, F.: Brain hemodynamic effects of doxapram in preterm infants. *Biology of the Neonate, 89*:69-74, 2006.

Darnall, R.A., Ariagno, R.L., and Kinnery, H.C.: The late preterm infant and the control of breathing, sleep and brainstem development: a review. *Clinics in Perinatology, 33*(4):883-914, 2006.

Finer, N., Higgins, R., Kattwinkel, J., and Martin, R.: Summary proceedings from the apnea-of-prematurity group. *Pediatrics, 117*:S47-S51, 2006.

Hanson, T.N. and Corbet, A.: Control of breathing. In H.W. Tausch, R.A. Ballard, and C.A. Gelason (Eds.): *Avery's diseases of the newborn* (8th ed.). Philadelphia, 2005, Saunders, pp. 616-633.

Henderson-Smart, D.J. and Osborn, D.A.: Kinesthetic stimulation for preventing apnea in preterm infants. *Cochrane Database of Systematic Reviews, 92*(2): CD000373, 2002.

Kattwinkel, J.: Neonatal apnea: Pathogenesis and therapy. *Journal of Pediatrics, 90*(3):342-347, 1977.

Kattwinkel, J.: *Textbook of neonatal resuscitation* (5th ed.). Elk Grove Village, IL, 2006, American Academy of Pediatrics and American Heart Association.

Khan, A., Qurashi, M., Kwiatkowski, K., Cates, D., and Rigatto, H.: Measurement of the CO_2 apneic threshold in newborn infants: Possible relevance for periodic breathing and apnea. *Journal of Applied Physiology, 98*:1171-1176, 2005.

Lopes, J. and Aranda, J.: Pharmacologic treatment of neonatal apnea. In S. Yaffe and J. Aranda (Eds.): *Neonatal and pediatric pharmacology: Therapeutic principles in practice* (3rd ed.). Philadelphia, 2005, Lippincott, Williams, & Wilkins, pp. 218-229.

Marlier, L., Gaugler, C., and Messer, J.: Olfactory stimulation prevents apnea in premature newborns. *Pediatrics, 115*:83-88, 2005.

Martin, R. and Abu-Shaweesh, J.: Control of breathing and neonatal apnea. *Biology of the Neonate, 87*:288-295, 2005.

Miller, M. and Martin, R.: Pathophysiology of apnea of prematurity. In R. Polin and W. Fox (Eds.): *Fetal and neonatal physiology* (3rd ed.). Philadelphia, 2003, Saunders, pp.1129-1140.

Miller, M.J., Fanaroff, A.A., and Martin, R.: Respiratory disorders in preterm and term infants. In R. Martin, A.A. Fanaroff, and M.C. Walsh (Eds.): *Fanaroff and Martin's neonatal-perinatal medicine: Diseases of the fetus and infant* (8th ed.). Philadelphia, 2006, Mosby, 1122-1146.

Nimavat, D., Sherman, M., Santin, R., and Porat, R.: Apnea of prematurity. Article on Emedicine, 2007. Retrieved January 28, 2008, from www.emedicine.com/ped/topic1157/htm

Steer, P., Shearman, A., Charles, B., et al.: High dose caffeine citrate for extubation of preterm infants: A randomised controlled trial. *Archives of Disease in Childhood Fetal and Neonatal Edition, 89*:F499-F503, 2004.

Stokowski, L.: A primer of apnea of prematurity. *Advances in Neonatal Care, 5*(3):155-170, 2005.

Task Force on Sudden Infant Death Syndrome: The changing concept of sudden infant death syndrome: diagnostic coding shifts, controversies regarding the sleeping environment, and new variables to consider in reducing risk. *Pediatrics, 116*:1245-1255, 2005.

26 Assisted Ventilation

DEBBIE FRASER ASKIN and WILLIAM DIEHL-JONES

OBJECTIVES

1. Identify the concepts of FRC, Vᴛ, VC, and TLC and describe their importance in the physiology of ventilation.
2. Describe the concepts of elastic recoil, compliance, resistance, and gas trapping and their importance in ventilating the lungs of the newborn infant.
3. Explain the relationship of fetal hemoglobin, pH, and temperature to the oxyhemoglobin dissociation curve.
4. List potential causes of respiratory and metabolic acid–base disturbance in the newborn infant. Identify ranges of pH, PaO_2, $PaCO_2$, HCO_3^-, and base excess/deficit in various respiratory disease states in the newborn infant.
5. Identify treatment modalities for neonates in respiratory distress.
6. Describe various types of mechanical ventilation devices available for the neonate.
7. List nursing interventions required to care for ventilated infants, based on the theories of mechanical ventilation.
8. Differentiate among the three types of high-frequency ventilation: jet, oscillatory, and high-frequency flow interrupter.
9. Identify the nursing interventions required for high-frequency ventilation that differ from those required for conventional ventilation.
10. Identify changes in patient status that indicate potential complications with assisted ventilation.
11. Describe various medications used to enhance lung status in the ventilated patient.

■
■ ■ Caring for an infant requiring assisted ventilation is a challenge. It is necessary for the nurse to understand the normal pulmonary physiology as well as the pathophysiology of pulmonary diseases in the neonate. An understanding of the basic mechanical principles of various ventilators is important to providing optimal care for a neonate. New ventilation techniques are being developed rapidly, and the choices for ventilating the neonate are greater now than ever before. The focus of this chapter is to provide the basic knowledge needed to care for the infant requiring oxygen therapy or mechanical ventilation.

PHYSIOLOGY

A. **Definitions** (Blackburn, 2007).
   1. Tidal volume (Vᴛ): the amount of air that moves into or out of the lungs with each single breath at rest (4 to 6 ml/kg).
   2. Vital capacity (VC): the volume of air maximally inspired and maximally expired (40 ml/kg).
   3. Functional residual capacity (FRC): the volume of gas that remains in the lungs after a normal expiration (30 ml/kg).
   4. Total lung capacity (TLC): the amount of air contained in the lung after a maximal inspiration (63 ml/kg).
   5. Physiologic dead space: anatomic plus alveolar dead space (Wood, 2003).
      a. Anatomic dead space: the volume of gas within the area of the pulmonary conducting airways that cannot engage in gas exchange.
      b. Alveolar dead space: the volume of inspired gas that reaches the alveoli but does not participate in gas exchange because of inadequate perfusion to those alveoli.

6. Mechanical dead space: gas that fills the ventilator circuit for availability in inspiration, as well as exhaled gas. Minimal dead space is desirable. Excessive dead space can cause increased retention of carbon dioxide.

B. **Concepts.**

1. Elastic recoil: the natural tendency for a stretched object to return to the original resting volume. With inhalation, alveoli stretch to a certain point, and during exhalation the alveoli return to their original size in an infant with normal lungs.

2. Lung compliance: the change in volume that occurs with a change in pressure (elasticity of the lung). It also refers to the relationship between a given change in volume and the pressure required to produce that change. An infant with severe hyaline membrane disease will have decreased compliance (because of lack of surfactant) requiring increased pressure to overcome the resistance generated by the surface tension in the alveoli. The major force contributing to elastic recoil of the lung is surface tension at the air–liquid interface in distal bronchioles and alveoli. The amount of distal airway pressure needed to counteract the tendency of the alveoli and bronchioles to collapse is demonstrated by the Laplace relationship: the relationship between pressure, surface tension, and the radius of a structure. The pressure needed to stabilize an alveolus is directly proportional to twice the surface tension and inversely proportional to the radius of that alveolus.

3. Lung resistance: the result of friction between moving parts. Airway resistance is determined by the flow rate, viscosity, and density of the respiratory gases as well as the length and diameter of the airways (Wood, 2003). An increase in airway resistance increases the time needed for air to reach the alveoli. High rates of airflow increase airway resistance by creating turbulence. Resistance to gas in a 2.5-mm endotracheal tube (ETT) is higher than in a 3.5-mm ETT because of the narrow lumen of the smaller tube. It takes greater pressure to force air through a small tube. Anatomic sources of resistance in the newborn infant include nasal passages, the glottis, the trachea, and the main bronchi. During intubation, the ETT is also a source of resistance.

4. Gas trapping: more gas entering the lung than leaving the lung. A partially occluded ETT can cause gas trapping. Debris from meconium can allow gas into the lung but may occlude the airway during exhalation (known as a ball-valve effect).

5. Inadvertent positive end-expiratory pressure (PEEP): a result of gas trapping in which volume and pressure increase in the distal airways through end expiration. Providing oxygen by nasal cannula can result in inadvertent PEEP in the small premature infant.

6. Ventilation–perfusion ratio ($\dot{V}_A/\dot{Q}_C$) (Fig. 26-1). Matching pulmonary ventilation and perfusion is necessary for efficient gas exchange. The relationship between ventilation and perfusion is expressed as a ratio and describes the relationship between alveolar ventilation and capillary perfusion of the lungs. A 1:1 ratio indicates that the alveoli are in perfect contact with the pulmonary capillaries, allowing exchange of O_2 and CO_2. A $\dot{V}_A/\dot{Q}_C$ ratio of zero indicates a shunt whereby no ventilation occurs during passage of blood through the lungs. Abnormalities of the $\dot{V}_A/\dot{Q}_C$ ratio may be due to
   a. too little ventilation with normal blood flow,
   b. too little blood flow with normal ventilation, or a
   c. combination of the above.

7. Mean airway pressure (MAP): mean or average pressure transmitted to the airways throughout an entire respiratory cycle (Hagedorn et al., 2006). MAP is dependent on the ventilator rate, gas flow through the ventilator circuit, peak inspiratory pressure (PIP), PEEP, and inspiratory time. Increasing MAP can greatly influence the management of respiratory distress in decreasing atelectasis and true intrapulmonary shunting and is a useful tool in determining oxygenation.

8. Permissive hypercapnia: ventilation strategy that allows carbon dioxide levels to remain elevated providing the pH does not fall below 7.25. This strategy is designed to minimize barotrauma by avoiding the use of mechanical ventilation or by using minimal ventilatory rates and pressures.

C. **Oxygen transport.**

1. The amount of oxygen that can be delivered to the tissues is dependent on cardiac output and the oxygen content of the blood.

V_A/Q Relationships

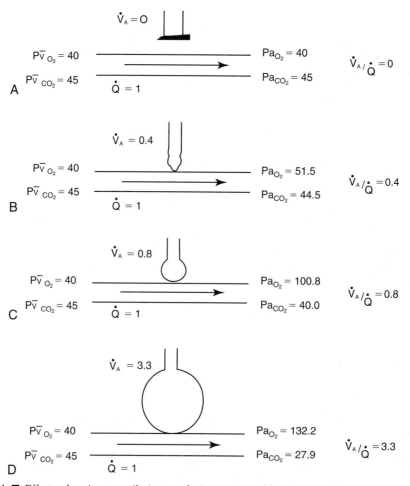

FIGURE 26-1 ■ Effects of various ventilation–perfusion ratios on blood gas tensions. **A,** Direct venoarterial shunting ($\dot{V}_A/\dot{Q} = 0$). Venous gas tensions are unaltered, and arterial blood has the same tension as venous blood. **B,** Alveolus with a low $\dot{V}_A/\dot{Q}$ ratio. Only partial oxygenation and CO_2 removal take place in this alveolus because of underventilation in relation to perfusion. **C,** Normal alveolus. **D,** Underperfused alveolus with high $\dot{V}_A/\dot{Q}$ ratio. Note that although the oxygen tension is 32 mm greater than alveolus (**C**), this results in only a slightly higher saturation and O_2 content. (From Thibeault, D.W. and Gregory, G.A.: *Neonatal pulmonary care.* Norwalk, CT, 1986, Appleton Century-Crofts.)

2. Oxygen is transported to tissue cells bound reversibly to hemoglobin and dissolved in plasma O_2. The amount of O_2 that is dissolved in the plasma is small (0.3 ml of O_2 dissolved in 100 ml of plasma per 100 mm Hg of O_2) compared with the amount that is bound to hemoglobin (1.34 ml of O_2 per gram of 100% saturated hemoglobin).
3. The amount of oxygen carried in the blood by hemoglobin depends on the hemoglobin concentration and the percent saturation of the hemoglobin. Adequate saturation is affected by the amount of hemoglobin available. Hemoglobin is almost fully saturated at a P_{O_2} of 80 to 100 mm Hg.
4. The binding of oxygen to hemoglobin varies with the Pao2. The relationship is nonlinear and gives rise to an S-shaped curve—the oxyhemoglobin dissociation curve. The amount of oxygen that combines with hemoglobin at a given Po2 depends on the position of the hemoglobin–oxygen dissociation curve (Fig. 26-2). Factors that determine the position of the dissociation curve are:
   a. Concentration of 2,3-diphosphoglycerate and the proportion of hemoglobin A (adult) to hemoglobin F (fetal).

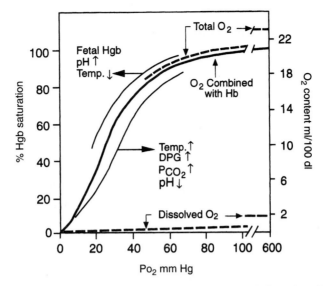

FIGURE 26-2 ■ Hemoglobin–oxygen dissociation curve. Nonlinear or S-shaped oxyhemoglobin curve and the linear or straight-line dissolved O_2 relationships between the O_2 saturation (Sao_2) and the Po_2. Total blood O_2 content is shown with division into a portion combined with hemoglobin and a portion physically dissolved at various levels of Po_2. Also shown are the major factors that change the O_2 affinity for hemoglobin and thus shift the oxyhemoglobin dissociation curve either to the left or to the right. *DPG*, 2,3-diphosphoglycerate. (Modified from West, J.B.: *Respiratory physiology: The essentials* [2nd ed.]. Baltimore, 1979, Williams & Wilkins, pp. 71, 73.)

      b. Temperature.

      c. Pco_2.

      d. pH.

   5. With decreased affinity (shift to the right), hemoglobin releases O_2 more easily to the tissues.

   6. With increased affinity (shift to the left), oxygen is unloaded less rapidly and efficiently in the peripheral tissues.

D. Control of breathing (Hagedorn et al., 2006). Control of ventilation (Box 26-1) is affected by both neurologic and chemical factors. The neurologic factors include central nervous system (CNS) maturity, sleep state, and reflexes. The chemoreflexes include responses to hypoxemia, hyperoxia, and hypercapnia.

E. Hypoxia. Delivery of O_2 to tissues is inadequate. Causes include the following:

   1. Heart failure.

   2. Anemia. Hemoglobin available to transport oxygen is reduced although completely saturated. Pao_2 levels are usually normal.

   3. Abnormal hemoglobin. O_2 is not released to the tissues.

      a. Methemoglobin.

      b. Bart hemoglobin.

   4. Cardiogenic or hypovolemic shock.

F. Hypoxemia. O_2 content of arterial blood is low because of extrapulmonary or intrapulmonary shunts. The blood has bypassed adequately ventilated alveoli.

   1. Intrapulmonary shunt.

      a. Ventilation–perfusion mismatch caused by lung diseases such as atelectasis, respiratory distress syndrome, or pneumonia.

      b. Can occur whenever alveoli are inadequately ventilated (hypoventilation).

   2. Extrapulmonary shunt.

      a. Cyanotic congenital heart disease. Abnormal heart structure causes blood to bypass the lungs for oxygenation.

      b. Pulmonary artery hypertension. Blood shunts from the right side of the heart to the left side via a patent foramen ovale or ductus arteriosus, or both, causing blood to bypass the lungs.

■ BOX 26-1
■ **FACTORS AFFECTING CONTROL OF VENTILATION IN THE SPONTANEOUSLY BREATHING NEONATE**

A. Neurologic Factors

1. "Maturity" of the CNS.
   a. Degree of myelination, which largely determines speed of impulse transmission and response time to stimuli affecting ventilation.
   b. Degree of arborization, or dendritic interconnections (synapses) between neurons, allowing summation of excitatory potentials coming in from other parts of the CNS, and largely setting the neuronal depolarization threshold and response level of the respiratory center.
2. Sleep state (i.e., REM sleep vs. quiet or non-REM sleep).
   a. REM sleep is generally associated with irregular respirations (both in depth and frequency), distortion, and paradoxic motion of the ribcage during inspiration, inhibition of Hering–Breuer and glottic closure reflexes, and blunted response to CO_2 changes.
   b. Quiet sleep is generally associated with regular respirations, a more stable ribcage, and a directly proportional relationship between Pco_2 and degree of ventilation.
3. Reflex responses.
   a. Hering–Breuer reflex, whereby inspiratory duration is limited in response to lung inflation sensed by stretch receptors located in major airways. Not present in adult humans, this reflex is very active during quiet sleep of newborn babies but absent or very weak during REM sleep.
   b. Head reflex, whereby inspiratory effort is further increased in response to rapid lung inflation. Thought to produce the frequently observed "biphasic sighs" of newborn infants that may be crucial for promoting and maintaining lung inflation (and therefore breathing regularity) after birth.
   c. Intercostal–phrenic reflex, whereby inspiration is inhibited by proprioception (position-sensing) receptors in intercostal muscles responding to distortion of the lower ribcage during REM sleep.
   d. Trigeminal–cutaneous reflex, whereby tidal volume increases and respiratory rate decreases in response to facial stimulation.
   e. Glottic closure reflex, whereby the glottis is narrowed through reflex contraction of the laryngeal adductor muscles during respiration, "breaking" exhalation and increasing subglottic pressure (as with expiratory "grunting").

B. Chemical Drive Factors (Chemoreflexes)

1. Response to hypoxemia (falling Pao_2) or to decrease in O_2 concentration breathed (mediated by peripheral chemoreceptors in carotid and aortic bodies):
   a. Initially there is increase in depth of breathing (tidal volume), but subsequently (if hypoxia persists or worsens), there is depression of respiratory drive, reduction in depth and rate of respiration, and eventual failure of arousal.
   b. For the first week of life, at least, these responses are dependent on environmental temperature (i.e., keeping the baby warm).
   c. Hypoxia is associated with an increase in periodic breathing and apnea.
2. Response to hyperoxia (increase in Fio_2) breathing causes a transient respiratory depression, stronger in term than in preterm infants.
3. Response to hypercapnia (rising $Paco_2$ or $[H^+]$) or to increase in CO_2 concentration breathed (mediated by central chemoreceptors in the medulla):
   a. Increase in ventilation is directly proportional to inspired CO_2 concentration (or, more accurately stated, to alveolar CO_2 tension), as is the case in adults.
   b. Response to CO_2 is in large part dependent on sleep state: in quiet sleep, a rising $Paco_2$ causes increase in depth and rate of breathing, whereas during REM sleep the response is irregular and reduced in depth and rate. The degree of reduction closely parallels the amount of ribcage deformity occurring during REM sleep.
   c. Ventilatory response to CO_2 in newborn infants is markedly depressed during behavioral activity, such as feeding, and easily depressed by sedatives and anesthesia.

CNS, Central nervous system; *REM*, rapid eye movement.
From Goldsmith, J.P. and Karotkin, E.H.: *Assisted ventilation of the neonate* (3rd ed.). Philadelphia, 1996, W.B. Saunders, p. 26.

(1) Comparison of the Pao_2 or O_2 saturation of preductal and postductal blood can help determine whether a right-to-left shunt is present.

(2) In the presence of shunting, preductal blood obtained from the right radial artery has a greater than 5% difference in saturation from postductal blood obtained from the umbilical artery or posterior tibial artery.

TREATMENT MODALITIES

A. **Blow-by oxygen.** Free flow of O_2 from a bag and mask or flow of O_2 through O_2 tubing near the infant's face may be useful for short-term O_2 delivery to an infant who is breathing but needs an O_2-enriched atmosphere for oxygenation (i.e., in the delivery room following a trial of room air, during caregiving activities, during placement of an intravenous (IV) line, during weighing). There is no way to determine the exact content of O_2 delivered to the infant. O_2 content depends on O_2 concentration, flow rate, the distance of the O_2 source from the infant, and the ventilatory efforts of the infant.

B. **Oxygen hood.** Warm, humidified oxygen is provided at a measured concentration via a plastic hood placed over the infant's head.

  1. Indications are respiratory distress, hypoxemia, and cyanosis.
  2. Disadvantages are the possibility of temperature instability, loss of O_2 when hood is removed, the possibility that the oxygen tubing will become disconnected from the hood, and difficulty in positioning and comforting the infant.
  3. O_2 concentration must be measured with an appropriately calibrated oxygen analyzer.
  4. Pulse oximeter should be used to monitor O_2 saturation.
  5. Adequate gas flow is required to avoid CO_2 accumulation within the hood.
  6. Hood size should be appropriate to the size of the infant.
  7. A blender system should be used to provide a fixed oxygen concentration to the hood.

C. **Nasal cannula. Humidified O_2 is delivered at a set flow rate via a cannula, with the flow directed into the nares. The exact concentration of oxygen delivered by nasal cannula cannot be measured.**

  1. Conventional nasal cannula. O_2 is delivered through the cannula and is regulated by the flow (measured in liters). Low-flow meters are capable of delivering amounts as small as 0.02 l/minute. The concentration of oxygen used may be 100% or may be regulated with the use of a blender system.
  2. High-flow nasal cannula (HFNC). Flow is >1.5 to 2 l/minute, with oxygen blended to a known concentration. High flow rates result in the delivery of various levels of continuous positive airway pressure (CPAP) depending on the type of cannula, size of the infant, and the flow rate used (Courtney and Barrington, 2007). Adequate humidification is essential with the use of high flow to prevent drying and damage to the nasal passages. HFNC may be comparable to NCPAP in level of respiratory support supplied (Saslow et al., 2006).
  3. A blender should be used to adjust the concentration of oxygen being delivered by cannula although the amount of oxygen entering the infant's lungs cannot be accurately determined because of the entrainment of room air around the cannula.
  4. Indications. A nasal cannula is used when there is a need for prolonged oxygen therapy as in chronic lung disease, transfer or transport, and increased mobility of the infant for feedings or for other developmental activities.
  5. Complications. Pressure-related tissue damage may occur because of improper or infrequent changing, O_2 concentration may vary, hypoxemia may result from a displaced cannula, and the cannula may be occluded by nasal secretions (may cause significant respiratory distress). Flow through the cannula may result in drying of the nasal mucosa, predisposing the infant to tissue damage and thickened nasal secretions.

D. **CPAP.**

  1. Mask CPAP: delivery of positive pressure (5 to 8 cm H_2O pressure) with variable amounts of O_2 via face mask. Requires appropriate-sized mask and tight seal around the nose and mouth.

    a. Indications: atelectasis, apnea, respiratory distress, and pulmonary edema.

    b. Advantages: short-term use to assist with alveolar expansion and to inhibit alveolar collapse (atelectasis); intubation not required.

    c. Complications: pulmonary hyperexpansion potentially leading to air leaks (i.e., pneumothorax, pneumomediastinum), aspiration of stomach contents, and ineffective ventilation leading to increasing respiratory difficulty.

2. Nasal CPAP: generally started at 5 to 7 cm H_2O pressure and titrated up to 10 cm H_2O pressure (Morley and Davis, 2004) delivered by prongs that fit into the nares, in addition to a measured concentration of oxygen.

    a. Indications: atelectasis, apnea, mild to moderate respiratory distress, and pulmonary edema.

    b. Advantage: intubation not required.

    c. Complications: ineffective ventilation, pneumothorax, variable pressure delivery when infant's mouth is open, molding of the head from securing straps, erosion of the septum from poorly fitting prongs, nasal obstruction as a result of increased secretions, agitation, dislodging of prongs by an active infant, and gastric distention and perforation.

3. Nasopharyngeal CPAP: delivered by ETT or long nasal prongs, passed through the nares and positioned with the tip of the tube in the oropharynx.

    a. Indications: atelectasis, apnea, respiratory distress, pulmonary edema, and to assist in weaning from mechanical ventilation.

    b. Advantage: stable placement of tube, which an infant is less likely to dislodge than with nasal CPAP.

    c. Disadvantages: need for a skilled provider to place the tube, possible damage to the nasal septum and oropharynx, more invasive than other forms of CPAP, variable pressure delivery when infant's mouth is open, and gastric distention.

4. Endotracheal CPAP: delivered via an ETT placed into the trachea.

    a. Indications: atelectasis, apnea, respiratory distress, pulmonary edema, improved pulmonary suctioning, upper airway obstruction, and CNS disorders.

    b. Advantage: constant delivery of O_2 and pressure.

    c. Disadvantage: skilled provider required for intubation. Intubation is an invasive procedure exposing the neonate to potential infection and tissue damage during intubation as a result of the presence of a tube in the trachea. Breathing through an ETT increases airway resistance and may result in increased work of breathing.

    d. Complications: malpositioned or dislodged tube, trauma resulting from intubation, port of entry for pathogens, hypoventilation, mucous plugging, possible airway injury (subglottic stenosis, laryngomalacia, tracheomalacia) with prolonged use, and increased risk of pulmonary air leaks.

5. Mechanical ventilation: respiratory support of infant using mechanical assistance.

    a. Gas exchange mechanisms in spontaneous and conventional mechanical ventilation.

        (1) Convection (bulk flow) in large airways goes to approximately the eighth bronchial generation. Gas moves along a negative pressure gradient from the upper airways to the alveoli.

        (2) Molecular diffusion occurs in terminal airways and alveoli. This is the exchange of gases in adjacent spaces.

        (3) The status of alveolar ventilation is determined as follows: Alveolar ventilation = respiratory rate × (tidal volume delivered − anatomic dead-space volume).

    b. Indications: respiratory failure (hypoxemia, hypercapnia, and/or acidemia), pulmonary insufficiency, need for surfactant administration, severe apnea and bradycardia episodes, cardiovascular support, CNS disease, and surgery.

    c. Advantages: consistent delivery of assisted ventilation and oxygen therapy, decreases the work of breathing, and stabilizes the airway.

    d. Disadvantages: intubation by skilled provider, x-ray examination to confirm placement, possible intermittent x-ray examinations to verify placement or lung status, continuous monitoring of vital signs and oxygen saturation. Exposes the neonate to potential volutrauma/barotrauma of the lung tissue.

e. Complications: tube malposition or dislodgment, underventilation or overventilation, tracheobronchial injury, pulmonary air leaks, infection, intracranial hemorrhage, bronchopulmonary dysplasia, and retinopathy of prematurity.

Types of Assisted Ventilation

A. Positive-pressure devices.

1. Bag-and-mask ventilation. Positive pressure and O_2 are delivered via face mask applied with an adequate seal around the mouth and nose. Maximal pressure relief valves should be present to prevent administration of excessive pressure. A manometer should measure pressure delivered to the patient. Device does not require intubation and can be very effective for short-term use, including initial resuscitation.

2. T-Piece Resuscitator (NeoPUff, Fischer & Paykel Healthcare Corp, Auckland, NZ). Levels of positive pressure and PEEP are preset. Breaths are delivered by occluding the PEEP cap on the T-piece. A gas source is required to operate the T-piece resuscitator. Has the advantage of controlling the amount of pressure applied with each breath, thus eliminating variable pressure delivery inherent in bag-and-mask ventilation (Hussey et al., 2004).

3. Pressure-cycled ventilator. Inspiratory phase ends when a preset pressure is reached within the ventilator circuit, regardless of the volume of gas delivered during inspiration.

4. Time-cycled, pressure-limited, continuous-flow ventilator. A predetermined pressure of gas is administered; the duration of inspiration and expiration can be adjusted. Ventilator also allows for the infant's spontaneous respiratory efforts, facilitating a gradual reduction of support. The operator determines the rate, PIP, PEEP, inspiratory time, and flow.

5. Volume-cycled ventilator. Inspiration ends when a preset volume of gas is delivered, regardless of the pressure reached within the ventilator circuit. The pressure used to deliver the breath will vary inversely with the infant's lung compliance and respiratory effort. An increase in ventilation is achieved by increasing V_T or rate; oxygenation is improved by increasing PEEP, Fio_2, or V_T (Carlo, 2007).

6. Pressure-support ventilator (PSV): PSV supports breaths initiated by the infant by delivering a mechanical breath to a preset volume. PSV uses a variable inspiratory time to allow the infant greater control and synchrony with the ventilator. PSV is flow cycled such that when inspiratory flow decreases by a certain percentage, inspiration ends. PSV ventilators usually have a maximum inspiratory time (T_i) that is preset. PSV is often used as a weaning mode of ventilation (Spitzer, 2005).

Ventilator Modes

A. Intermittent mandatory ventilation. "Breaths" are delivered at a predetermined rate, regardless of where the patient is in the respiratory cycle. The ventilator continues to deliver fresh gas, which allows spontaneous respirations as well. It is possible to stack a ventilator breath on top of a spontaneous breath during either inspiration or expiration. This may lead to air trapping, air leaks, CNS dysfunction, and irregularity of blood pressure and cerebral blood flow.

B. Patient-triggered ventilation (PTV). Mechanical breaths are delivered in response to a signal derived from the patient and detected as a spontaneous respiratory effort. The signal may be derived from a sensor that detects airflow, airway pressure, chest wall movement, or esophageal pressure (Carlo, 2007). The goal of patient-triggered ventilation is to avoid asynchrony of breathing by the patient and breaths given by the ventilator. Asynchrony may lead to air trapping, air leaks, CNS dysfunction, and irregularity of blood pressure and cerebral blood flow. Patient-triggered ventilation has been shown to improve gas exchange, decrease the need and duration of ventilation, reduce the incidence of air leaks, and provide ventilation that better matches the infant's own efforts (Baumer, 2000; Beresford et al., 2000; Cole and Fiascone, 2000; Greenough et al., 2004; Herrera et al., 2002).

1. Synchronized intermittent mandatory ventilation.

a. Preset number of ventilator breaths is synchronized with the onset of spontaneous breaths. When the infant initiates a breath, the ventilator supports that breath according to the preset PIP and inspiratory time.

    b. Unassisted breaths occur between ventilator breaths, with continuous flow of gas from the ventilatory circuit.

    c. Partial asynchrony may occur if inspiratory times are different, in that the patient may attempt to terminate the inspiratory effort while the ventilator continues to be in the inspiratory phase.

  2. Assist/control mode of ventilation (A/C).

    a. A synchronized breath is delivered each time a spontaneous patient breath meeting the threshold criteria is detected, or back-up mechanical breaths are delivered at a preset regular rate if the patient does not exhibit spontaneous respiratory effort (i.e., if the patient has apnea).

    b. A detection system signals the start of inspiratory effort, which allows for synchronous initiation of inspiration.

    c. Asynchronous expiratory-phase breaths may still occur.

  3. Volume-targeted ventilation.

    a. Volume-targeted ventilation (VG) can be used in conjunction with synchronized intermittent mandatory ventilation or Assist/Control modes in patient-triggered ventilation.

    b. A V_T is set by the operator based on the infant's weight and disease condition.

    c. The benefits of VG include lower peak inspiratory pressures; enhanced spontaneous respiratory effort (Herrera et al., 2002).

NURSING CARE OF THE PATIENT REQUIRING RESPIRATORY SUPPORT OR CONVENTIONAL MECHANICAL VENTILATION

A. Care of O_2 delivery devices.

  1. Oxygen hood. Warm, humidified (to prevent heat loss) O_2, delivered via head hood, is usually blended to select the appropriate amount needed. The percentage of O_2 in the hood must be monitored by a properly calibrated O_2 analyzer placed in the hood near the infant's nose. Ensure a hood of correct size for each infant. To prevent buildup of CO_2, do not block openings in the hood and ensure an adequate flow of 5 to 7 l/minute. Clean and change per unit protocol.

  2. Nasal cannula. Remove and clean secretions every 4 to 6 hours as needed. Inspect surrounding tissue for pressure-related injury. If sudden onset of respiratory distress occurs, inspect cannula for secretions and suction nasopharynx for mucus. Change cannula according to unit protocol. Some infants receiving oxygen by nasal cannula benefit from the administration of saline drops to moisten the mucosa. These should be administered according to unit protocol.

  3. Nasopharyngeal or nasal prong CPAP. Ensure that CPAP device is of the correct size to decrease the incidence of pressure necrosis of the nares. Nasal CPAP units come in a variety of sizes and should be short and wide, with thin walls to allow for maximal airflow. They should be soft and flexible and should be easy to secure and maintain. Humidification of 90% to 100% should be provided in the CPAP system to prevent drying out of the mucous membranes and subsequent formation of thick secretions. Evaluate the need for suctioning every 2 to 4 hours. Inspect surrounding tissue for pressure-related injury. Secure the device to a stockinette cap or with soft straps provided by some manufacturers. Lightweight tubing is helpful for ease in securing the device and in keeping the unit in the nose. The infant can be positioned supine, on either side, or prone, generally with the head of the bed at approximately a 30-degree angle. Observe for abdominal distention resulting from excessive air entering the stomach from the CPAP device. Consider aspirating every few hours from an orogastric tube or leaving it open to continuously vent gas from the stomach. Feeding is not contraindicated during delivery of CPAP. The clinical condition must be evaluated before institution of feedings. During CPAP delivery, feedings must be administered via orogastric tube either intermittently or by continuous drip. Change prongs according to unit protocol, generally every 2 or 3 days.

  4. ETT. After correct placement has been determined, note the depth of the tube at the gum or lip and post at the bedside. This is important for future reference in case the tube slips, reintubation is needed, or to determine suction catheter length. Secure the ETT with tape or other method. Each institution generally develops a method that works well for the staff and patients. Observe for evidence of slipping or tape loosening and secure again when necessary to prevent accidental extubation. Position the infant supine, on either side, or in the prone position, with the head in a neutral position. Be aware that the tube moves with the chin and can move several centimeters with flexion or extension of the head. Signs of extubation include sudden deterioration in clinical status, abdominal distention, crying, decreased chest wall movement, breath sounds in the abdomen, agitation, cyanosis, or bradycardia. Notify the physician or neonatal nurse practitioner if extubation is a concern and prepare for reintubation as soon as possible. Intubation equipment should be readily available. A bag and mask with pressure manometer or a T-piece resuscitator should also be available at each bedside and should be tested during each shift. Suction the ETT when necessary. Complications of an ETT include palatal grooves (consider a palate protector, which can be made by a pediatric dentist or is commercially available), nasal erosion, subglottic stenosis, tracheoesophageal perforation during insertion of the tube, aspiration, infection, and tracheal granuloma.

5. Tracheostomy tube. Daily changing of the dressing and weekly changing of the tube are usually adequate. Inspect the site for signs of tissue pressure and/or necrosis. Suctioning is necessary to keep the airway clear of secretions. Family members need to be included in this procedure, thus facilitating discharge.

B. Suctioning the airway.
1. Nontracheal tubes.
   a. Suctioning of the mouth, nose, and tubes should be performed on an as-needed basis. The presence of a foreign body in the mouth or nose will cause an increase in secretions.
   b. Suctioning can coincide with the cleaning or changing of the tubes or with routine caregiving.
2. Endotracheal tubes.
   a. The amount of secretions will be disease related. Infants with resolving respiratory distress syndrome, patent ductus arteriosus (PDA), bronchopulmonary dysplasia, and pneumonia are more likely to require suctioning because of an increased production of mucus. Patients with early-stage respiratory distress syndrome and those with most types of congenital heart disease will not have much mucus and will require less suctioning. Suctioning is done on an as-needed basis, never on a routine schedule (Hagedorn et al., 2006). Criteria for suctioning include evidence of secretions (audible or visible), changes in vital signs, agitation or restlessness, and changes in oxygenation or ventilation.
   b. Protocols for suctioning vary from one institution to another. Administering manual breaths with the ventilator or hand ventilating for 30 to 60 seconds before and after suctioning may be necessary to maintain lung volumes during the procedure.
   c. In-line suction devices allow suctioning while ventilation continues and are associated with a decreased risk of infection, smaller changes in cerebral blood flow, and other hemodynamic changes (Kalyn et al., 2003; Ruof and Fahwenstich, 2000).
   d. Do not advance the suction catheter farther than the distance of the ETT, and do not suction too vigorously.
   e. Vacuum pressure range should be 60 to 100 mm Hg (Hagedorn et al., 2006). A 5F or 6F suction catheter for a 2.5 to 3.5 ETT, or an 8F suction catheter for a 4 to 4.5 ETT, is usually appropriate.
   f. Complications of suctioning include hypoxemia, bradycardia, barotrauma, changes in blood pressure, alterations in cerebral blood flow, intraventricular hemorrhage, tracheal damage, atelectasis, infection, and pneumothorax.

C. Initiating mechanical ventilation. The goal of mechanical ventilation is to assist in providing adequate tissue oxygenation and eliminating CO_2.
1. Establish an airway. Endotracheal intubation should be performed by a skilled provider (see Chapter 15).

2. Ventilator selection. The ventilator selected for use is based on the patient's condition and disease process, the patient's response to previous ventilatory support, and staff experience and comfort with the device. Patient-triggered or synchronized ventilation is now the preferred method of mechanically ventilating neonates in most NICUs. There are a number of devices and ventilator modalities that allow the operator to control the peak inspiratory pressure or volume delivered to the neonate as well as the rate, PEEP, flow, and inspiratory time.

3. Parameters to be set and/or monitored during mechanical ventilation.

   a. Rate of intermittent mandatory ventilation. Infants without respiratory failure have a resting respiratory rate of approximately 40/minute, whereas infants with respiratory failure may have a respiratory rate of 0/minute to more than 100/minute. A beginning ventilator rate of 30 to 40/minute for an infant with respiratory failure should be adequate. For infants without respiratory failure, a rate of 20 to 30/minute should be adequate. The ventilator rate will affect the ability to blow off CO_2. The rate is adjusted to maintain the arterial tension of CO_2 in the range of 40 to 50 mm Hg and to avoid excessive respiratory effort, which would exhaust the infant. A rate greater than 40/minute may shorten the expiratory phase of ventilation and cause air trapping.

   b. PIP. PIP is the primary factor used for determining tidal volume and affecting Pao_2 (Spitzer, 2005). Determining the appropriate PIP requires careful and skilled assessment. The complications of excessive PIP include air leaks, decreased venous return, intraventricular hemorrhage, and decreased cardiac output. Factors such as weight, gestational age, disease process, lung compliance, and airway resistance must be considered. Auscultation of breath sounds to assess aeration and compliance is necessary. Experimenting with an anesthesia bag to find the best rate and pressure may be useful and allows the clinician to determine the infant's ventilation needs. Visual inspection of chest wall movement, in conjunction with the use of a pressure gauge connected to the anesthesia bag, may guide your assessment. A beginning PIP of 20 cm H_2O is appropriate for most preterm infants. The lowest PIP that will provide adequate ventilation is ideal, with the goals of preventing barotrauma and volutrauma and decreasing the incidence of air leaks and chronic lung disease (Donn and Sinha, 2002; Halliday, 2004). Certain conditions may warrant use of high PIP, including poor compliance, atelectasis, or pulmonary hypertension. Before connecting the patient to the ventilator, ensure that the inspiratory pressure is correct. Recheck after the connection has been made, and adjust as necessary.

   c. Vt. Vt is the primary factor affecting both oxygenation and ventilation. When using volume-targeted ventilation, the operator determines the desired volume to be delivered with each breath rather than setting the PIP. Based on averaging a series of breaths, the ventilator determines the PIP needed to deliver the desired volume of gas. An upper limit for the PIP should be set by the operator to prevent the delivery of excessive pressure.

      An increase in ventilation is achieved by increasing the volume of gas to be delivered (Vt) or the rate. Increased oxygenation is achieved by increasing the Fio_2, the PEEP, or the Vt (Carlo, 2007). Determination of tidal volume is based on the infant's weight, with a beginning Vt of 4 to 5 ml/kg being most common.

   d. PEEP. This measure aids in maintaining functional residual capacity, stabilizing and recruiting atelectatic areas for gas exchange, improving compliance, and improving ventilation–perfusion matching in the lung (Hagedorn et al., 2006). PEEP is important in assisted ventilation for infants with surfactant deficiency because of the likelihood of alveolar collapse. Physiologic PEEP is estimated at 2 cm H_2O. Levels lower than 2 cm H_2O are not generally recommended. In most instances, medium levels, about 4 to 7 cm H_2O, are recommended. Levels greater than 8 cm H_2O are associated with pulmonary air leaks and reduction of cardiac output.

   e. Inspiratory/expiratory (I/E) ratio: ratio of time spent in inspiration to time spent in expiration. Determining this time should be based on the underlying reason for ventilation. A physiologic I/E ratio in a nondisease state is equal to 1:2 or 1:3, meaning a short inspiratory time with a longer expiratory time. Prolonged expiratory time is

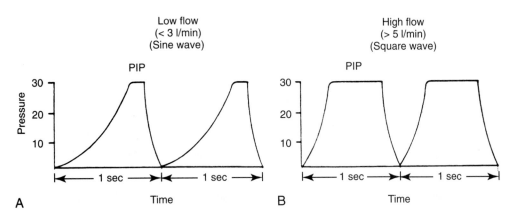

FIGURE 26-3 ■ Comparison of ventilator waveforms. **A,** Relative sine wave. **B,** Relative square wave. (From Goldsmith, J.P. and Karotkin, E.H. [Eds.]: *Assisted ventilation of the neonate* [3rd ed.]. Philadelphia, 1996, Saunders, p. 169.)

useful during weaning, when oxygenation is not as problematic. The I/E ratio will affect the Pao_2 and $Paco_2$. Changes affect mean airway pressure and oxygenation.

    f. Flow rate: flow of gas (measured in liters per minute) through the patient's circuit. The flow rate determines the ability of the ventilator to deliver the desired amount of PIP, waveform, I/E ratio, and respiratory rate. A flow rate of at least twice the infant's minute ventilation ensures that the ventilator can reach the desired pressure. Flow rates of 5 to 10 l/minute are usually adequate (Spitzer, 2005). With low flow rates (<3 l/min), inspiratory pressure gradually builds to a peak just before expiration, closely resembling a sine waveform (normal breaths are shaped like a sine waveform). There may be less barotrauma to the airways with a sine waveform. High flows of 4 to 10 l/minute or higher are necessary with square waveform ventilation or when high rates are used. A square waveform pattern moves the ventilator breath rapidly from the resting or expiratory pressure level to the PIP. Because the PIP is reached sooner than with a sine waveform, the PIP is held for a longer period (Fig. 26-3). This may be advantageous with atelectatic areas of the lung. It may also contribute to barotrauma.

    g. MAP: average distending pressure throughout a complete respiratory cycle. It is the major determinant of oxygenation. MAP, most affected by changes in PEEP, PIP, and I/E ratio. Increases in oxygenation are directly related to increases in MAP, and increased barotrauma to the lungs can result with high MAP. Close attention to the MAP during ventilation is essential, especially once the underlying disease begins to resolve.

  4. For effects of different ventilator changes, see Box 26-2.

HIGH-FREQUENCY VENTILATION

High-frequency ventilation (HFV) is any of several forms of mechanical ventilation that use small tidal volumes at rates of at least 150 breaths per minute (Truog and Golombek, 2005) to ventilate patients with severe respiratory failure. The advantage of HFV over conventional mechanical ventilation is the ability to deliver adequate minute volumes with lower proximal airway pressures.

A. Gas-exchange mechanisms in HFV. The tidal volumes used may be less than or equal to anatomic dead-space volume. According to gas-exchange theories for conventional ventilation, alveolar ventilation during HFV should be zero.

B. Theories of gas exchange during HFV.

  1. Augmented (facilitated) diffusion: Gas molecules diffuse higher in the airways.

  2. Coaxial diffusion: Fresh gases travel down the center of the airway, and CO_2 elimination occurs along the periphery of the airway (Fig. 26-4).

■ BOX 26-2
■ **SPECIFIC EFFECTS OF DIFFERENT VENTILATOR CHANGES**

Increasing PIP
1. Increases VT and Ve
2. Adds little to MAP unless combined with a reversal of I/E ratio or prolongation of IT
3. Affects maximum dilation of alveoli already open, contributing to barotrauma
4. Opens alveoli with high critical opening pressures

Reversing I/E Ratio (for Lengthening IT while Respiratory Rate is Kept Constant)
1. Has little effect on VT or Ve beyond the minimum IT needed to deliver VT or reach desired PIP level (or both)
2. Can contribute on more than one-to-one basis to MAP, depending on original PIP and degree of reversal of I/E ratio
3. Allows expansion of atelectatic alveoli at lower PIP
4. May cause inadvertent PEEP, overinflation of alveoli, and reduction of pulmonary blood flow

Increasing Background CPAP or PEEP
1. Decreases VT and Ve unless significant atelectasis is overcome
2. Adds to MAP on a one-to-one basis
3. Holds open alveoli and terminal airways on end-expiration, thus raising closing volume and aiding in equal distribution of ventilation
4. Reduces likelihood of inadvertent PEEP

CPAP, Continuous positive airway pressure; *I/E*, inspiratory/expiratory; *IT*, inspiratory time; *MAP*, mean airway pressure; *PEEP*, positive end-expiratory pressure; *PIP*, peak inspiratory pressure; *VT*, tidal volume; *Ve*, expired volume per unit time.
From Goldsmith, J.P. and Karotkin, E.H. (Eds.): *Assisted ventilation of the neonate* (3rd ed.). Philadelphia, 1996, Saunders, p. 62.

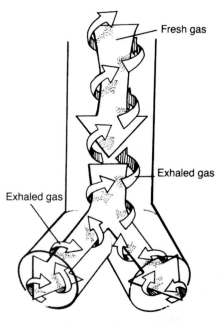

Fresh gas

Exhaled gas

Exhaled gas

FIGURE 26-4 ■ Coaxial diffusion.

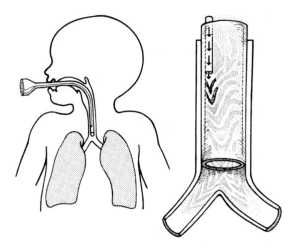

FIGURE 26-5 ■ Entrainment during high-frequency jet ventilation. Gas molecules near the jet orifice are "entrained," or dragged along with the jet pulse, whereby additional volume is delivered to the patient without substantially increasing static airway pressure. (From Harris, T.R.: Physiologic principles. In J.P. Goldsmith and E.H. Karotkin [Eds.]: *Assisted ventilation of the neonate* [2nd ed.]. Philadelphia, 1988, Saunders.)

3. Entrainment: Gas molecules from higher in the airway are pulled into the area of low pressure created behind a high-velocity gas entry point, such as a jet cannula port (Fig. 26-5).

4. Interregional gas mixing ("pendelluft"): Because of the different time constants of the respiratory units, gases in the periphery of the lung may move between alveolar units to provide better matching of ventilation and perfusion.

C. **Effectiveness of gas exchange.** All forms of HFV produce gas exchange with lower PIPs, theoretically reducing the risk of barotrauma.

D. **Types of high-frequency ventilators.**

1. High-frequency jet ventilation (HFJV): Bunnell Life Pulse Jet Ventilator (Bunnell Inc., Salt Lake City, Utah).

   a. A jet injector or narrow-bore cannula that delivers short, rapid, high-velocity pulses from a pressurized gas source directly into the trachea via a small cannula. Requires the use of a triple-lumen ETT adapter ("jet nozzle") that attaches to a standard ETT.

   b. Servocontrolled driving pressure: continuously adjusts the pressure of the gas supply to the jet cannula to maintain desired peak airway pressure. Solenoid valve: opens and closes gas supply to the jet cannula.

   c. Humidification system: built in-line.

   d. Proximal airway pressures: monitored and continuously displayed; used in servo-control of pressure delivery.

   e. Conventional ventilator: used in tandem to provide gas for entrainment, PEEP, and background ventilation (sighs).

   f. Exhalation: passive.

   g. Ventilation (CO_2 removal) is primarily determined by the amplitude or size of the breath.

   h. Oxygenation is related to mean airway pressure, a complex interrelationship between jet PIP and frequency and the rate, PEEP and inspiration time provided by conventional breaths (Keszler, 2005).

   i. Indications for use: effective with disorders in which CO_2 elimination is the major problem. CO_2 elimination is achieved at lower peak and mean airway pressures than with high-frequency oscillatory ventilation (HFOV). Severe atelectatic disorders such as respiratory distress syndrome may also benefit from HFJV (Keszler, 2005) as do obstructive disorders such as meconium aspiration syndrome (Keszler and Durand, 2001) and restrictive lung diseases and air leaks (Mammel, 2003).

j. Parameters to be set and/or monitored:
  (1) PIP: set on both the jet and the conventional ventilator.
   (a) Jet PIP is usually initially set at the same PIP required during conventional ventilation, and the conventional ventilator PIP is lowered by 2 to 5 cm H_2O.
   (b) A higher conventional PIP may cause interruption of the jet.
  (2) Servocontrolled pressure: internal adjustment of driving pressure by the ventilator as patient compliance and pressure settings change.
   (a) Lower servopressure reflects worsening lung disease, airway obstruction, pneumothorax, or kinked ventilator tubing.
   (b) Higher servopressure indicates improved lung compliance or a leak in the patient/system.
  (3) PEEP: set on conventional ventilator; displayed on jet ventilator. Value displayed may be lower than value set, because of where and how it is measured. The PEEP provided by the conventional ventilator assists in lung recruitment when atelectasis is a problem.
  (4) Jet valve on time: percentage of time that the jet valve is open; similar to inspiratory time, usually 0.02 second.
  (5) Rate set on jet and conventional ventilators:
   (a) The jet rate is usually 400 to 500 breaths per minute; Bunnell default setting of 420/minute appears to be most effective for this ventilator.
   (b) The rate for conventional intermittent mandatory ventilation is usually set between 5 and 20 breaths per minute to provide background ventilation (sigh breaths), which helps to prevent atelectasis.
  (6) Fio_2: set on jet and conventional ventilators.
k. Weaning from HFJV is usually accomplished as the acute phase of the illness resolves. Air leaks should be resolved for 1 or 2 days before switching back to conventional mechanical ventilation. Weaning is accomplished by decreasing the PIP and reducing the HFJV rate to 250 to 350 breaths per minute. Support from conventional mechanical ventilation is increased using small tidal volume breaths.
l. Patient assessment and care.
  (1) Patient will require an ETT adapter that is attached to the standard ETT (Fig. 26-6).
  (2) Suctioning may be performed with HFJV on or off.
   (a) Placing jet ventilator on stand-by mode during suctioning may prevent airway damage caused by the shearing force of opposing positive and negative pressures.
   (b) Suctioning with the jet ventilator on may help decrease respiratory decompensation during the procedure in some patients.
   (c) If suctioning is performed with the jet ventilator running, suction must be applied as the catheter is inserted, as well as when withdrawn, to prevent overpressurization of the circuit and alveolar rupture.
  (3) Humidification of gases is important with HFJV in preventing obstruction of the ETT.
   (a) Jet port should be irrigated with 0.5 ml normal saline solution or air every 3 to 4 hours.
   (b) Main port of ETT is suctioned as usual.
  (4) Tubing to the conventional ventilator must never be kinked because overpressurization of the circuit and alveolar rupture may occur if expiratory gas cannot escape.
  (5) Vibration of the chest wall is an indicator of lung compliance, airway patency, and effectiveness of ventilator settings.
   (a) Chest wall vibration must be assessed after head position changes to ensure that the jet port of the ETT has not been occluded by the tracheal wall.
   (b) Sudden decrease in chest wall vibration may indicate a plugged ETT or a pneumothorax.
  (6) Vibration may interfere with electrical monitoring of heart rate and respiratory rate.

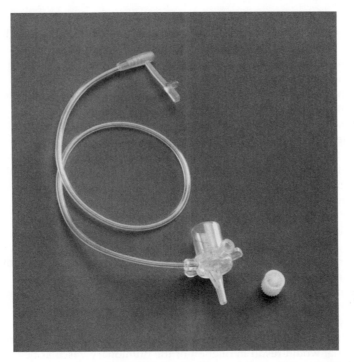

FIGURE 26-6 ■ LifePort endotracheal tube adapter. (Courtesy Bunnell, Inc., Salt Lake City, Utah.)

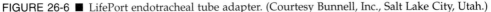

(a) Use pulse from arterial line or pulse oximeter to monitor heart rate if necessary.
(b) Respiratory rate cannot be monitored.
(7) Jet ventilation is more efficient at CO_2 elimination than at oxygenation.
(a) Increasing the background ventilation rate may improve oxygenation.
(b) Pressure difference between PIP and PEEP is the major determinant of ventilation.
(c) MAP is the major determinant of oxygenation.
(8) Patients are generally weaned to a low PIP and then switched back to conventional ventilation before extubation.
m. Complications and problems:
(1) Airway obstruction, which may be indicated by decreased chest wall vibration, increased Pco_2, and decreased servopressure.
(2) Necrotizing tracheobronchitis (inflammatory injury to tracheal mucosa).
(3) Microatelectasis and poor oxygenation, possible after prolonged HFJV; necessitates return to conventional ventilation.
(4) Air trapping occurs at very high rates or with excessive jet valve on-times.
n. A Cochrane Review of jet ventilation in newborns has demonstrated a reduction in chronic lung disease at 36 weeks of gestation in infants electively ventilated with the jet (Bhuta and Henderson-Smart, 2000).
2. High-frequency oscillatory ventilation. In the United States the majority of HFOVs is provided by SensorMedics 3100 (Sensor Medics Inc., Yorba Linda, Calif). In Canada and the United Kingdom the Dräger Babylog (Dräger Medical, Lübeck, Germany) HFOV is more commonly used.
a. Piston, or vibrating diaphragm, moves a small volume of gas toward and then away from the patient.
b. The amount of gas moved is referred to as the amplitude.
c. Oscillators deliver very little bulk gas. A continuous flow of fresh gas flows past the source that powers the oscillations, producing bias gas flow in a resulting push–pull

fashion and thereby eliminating CO_2 buildup and delivering O_2. A low-pass filter allows gas to exit the system while maintaining vibration of gas in the airway (Carlo, 2007).

    d. Mean airway pressure is governed by the rate of gas flow into the circuit and the resistance to flow out of the circuit (Durand and Asselin, 2004).

    e. Amplitude is determined by the driving pressure or stroke volume of the piston or vibrating diaphragm.

    f. Proximal airway pressure is monitored by the ventilator, but clinical relevance is questionable because it probably does not reflect alveolar pressure.

    g. HFOV allows for the use of higher MAP with less barotrauma, in comparison with conventional mechanical ventilation and ventilation with small tidal volumes.

    h. Exhalation is active, assisted by the oscillating device.

    i. Oxygenation is determined by MAP. Ventilation (CO_2 removal) is governed by amplitude or MAP.

    j. Indications for use are as follows:

        (1) Severe lung disease that is unresponsive to conventional ventilation.

        (2) Pulmonary air leaks, pulmonary interstitial emphysema, pneumothorax, and bronchopleural fistula.

        (3) Pulmonary hypoplasia and diaphragmatic hernia: treated with limited success. HFV can be used to stabilize the condition of these patients.

        (4) Persistent pulmonary hypertension and meconium aspiration syndrome: treated with mixed results. The improved CO_2 exchange may lead to a respiratory alkalosis that would result in dilation of the pulmonary vascular bed.

        (5) Failure of conventional mechanical ventilation.

    k. Parameters to be set or monitored:

        (1) MAP: affects oxygenation.

        (2) Amplitude or stroke volume: size of pressure wave produced by oscillator (another way to describe volume delivered).

        (3) Fio_2: set on the ventilator as with conventional ventilation.

        (4) Frequency: 180 to 900 "breaths" per minute (3 to 15 Hz where 1 Hz = 60 breaths).

    l. Patient care and assessment:

        (1) No special ETT is required.

        (2) Suctioning procedure is performed as usual. Infants on high-frequency ventilation often benefit from the use of an in-line suctioning device to minimize postsuctioning atelectasis.

        (3) Chest wall vibration is assessed, rather than breath sounds, to determine the effectiveness of ventilator settings and lung compliance changes. Breath sounds are not audible during HFOV.

        (4) Vibration may interfere with electrical monitoring of heart rate and respiratory rate.

            (a) Use pulse from arterial line or pulse oximeter for heart rate monitoring if necessary.

            (b) Respiratory rate cannot be monitored.

            (c) Sighs help reduce microatelectasis and improve oxygenation.

        (5) Complications and problems are:

            (a) Microatelectasis, poor oxygenation.

            (b) Increased incidence of intraventricular hemorrhage in the collaborative trial of HFV using oscillators for treatment of respiratory distress syndrome in preterm infants (HIFI Study Group, 1989; Moriette et al., 2001). Recent studies have failed to demonstrate an increased risk.

    m. Studies evaluating the use of HFO ventilation have demonstrated mixed results depending on the volume strategy used. Bhuta and colleagues (2000) completed a Cochrane Review of HFOV for term or near-term infants and found no data to support the routine use of HFOV. A Cochrane Review comparing HFOV to conventional ventilation for preterm infants found that elective HFOV resulted in a reduction in chronic lung disease at term. Results were inconsistent across studies and some short-term neurologic morbidity was found, but this did not reach statistical significance (Henderson-Smart et al., 2001). Other benefits include decreased need for surfactant replacement (Moriette et al., 2001) and decreased days on oxygen and ventilation (Rimensberger et al., 2000).

NURSING CARE DURING THERAPY

A. Physical assessment.

1. Observation. One of the most valuable tools in assessing an infant's respiratory status is observation. Does the infant appear to be comfortable while breathing, or does the infant show signs and symptoms of distress by grunting, flaring, and retracting? The Silverman–Andersen score is a screening tool that uses five signs or symptoms to assess respiratory distress in the newborn infant (Fig. 26-7). Assess the skin color of the infant. It should be uniformly pink. Skin color that is blue, dusky, or pale needs to be evaluated further. A dramatic change in skin color needs to be investigated immediately to rule out a pneumothorax versus a mechanical obstruction. Observe the infant's respiratory rate. Is it within the normal range (40 to 60 breaths per minute)? When observing the respiratory rate, consider variables such as environment, temperature, and the infant's state of activity or inactivity, which can increase or decrease the respiratory rate. Observe whether the chest rises symmetrically; if asymmetric, suspect a possible pneumothorax, diaphragmatic hernia, or phrenic nerve palsy. With accidental extubation, chest movement may not be observable or may be decreased from previous observations.

2. Auscultation. Listen to the breath sounds carefully to determine differences in the upper and lower lung fields and differences in the left and right lung fields. Is aeration equal bilaterally? Are fine coarse crackles evident? Are other abnormal sounds audible? A finding in a ventilated infant may be louder breath sounds on the right; if so, suspect that the ETT may have slipped into the right bronchus or that a pneumothorax may have occurred, necessitating evaluation. Rule out other noises and their points of origin. Bowel sounds heard in the chest are an indication of a diaphragmatic hernia. In the patient receiving HFV, chest wall vibration is an indicator of lung compliance, airway patency, and effectiveness of ventilator settings. Chest wall vibration must be assessed after repositioning. Sudden decrease in chest wall vibration may indicate a plugged ETT or a pneumothorax.

SILVERMAN-ANDERSEN RETRACTION SCORE

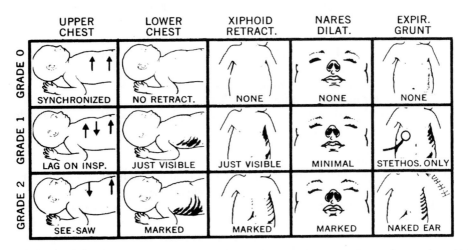

FIGURE 26-7 ■ Silverman–Andersen scale to assess respiratory distress in the newborn infant. (Adapted from Silverman, W.A. and Andersen D.H.: A controlled clinical trial of effects of water mist on obstructive respiratory signs, death rate, and necropsy findings among premature infants. *Pediatrics,* 17[1]:1-10, 1956.)

3. ETT observation. Fogging or condensation in the ETT is a sign that the infant is intubated. The condensation occurs on exhalation and is visible in the ETT. Observation of the tube position more than 1 cm from its desired location may indicate extubation or placement in the right mainstem bronchus.
4. Signs of extubation:
   a. Audible crying.
   b. Absent or decreased breath sounds.
   c. Cyanosis.
   d. Bradycardia.
   e. Hypoxemia.
   f. Agitation, restlessness.
   g. Increased abdominal distention.
B. **Equipment function.** All ventilators used for conventional mechanical ventilation should have been approved by the U.S. Food and Drug Administration and should display rate (intermittent mandatory ventilation), peak inspiratory pressure, PEEP, tidal volume (where applicable), inspiratory time, I/E ratio, mean airway pressure, and O_2 concentration. Ventilators must be plugged into an electrical outlet that provides emergency power in the event of a power failure.
   1. All mechanical ventilators should have:
      a. Alarms activated to alert caregivers to ventilator malfunction or disconnection,
      b. Preset pressure-relief valves to ensure against administration of excessive PIP and PEEP,
      c. Frequently scheduled inspections by licensed respiratory therapists,
      d. Ventilator tubing changed routinely per unit policy,
      e. O_2 concentration analyzed routinely and documented in the patient record, and
      f. Routine cleaning between patient use.
   2. The following equipment, to be located in the immediate area of all infants requiring mechanical ventilation, should be checked for proper functioning and replaced as needed:
      a. Laryngoscope with blade.
         (1) Size 0 for infants weighing less than 3 kg.
         (2) Size 1 for infants weighing more than 3 kg.
      b. Sterile ETTs.
         (1) Size 2.5 for infants weighing less than 1000 g.
         (2) Size 3 for infants weighing 1000 to 2000 g.
         (3) Size 3.5 for infants weighing 2000 to 3000 g.
         (4) Size 3.5 or 4 for infants weighing more than 3000 g.
      c. Sterile stylet (plastic coated).
      d. Magill forceps (nasal intubation).
      e. Suction tubing and catheters (suction control gauge set at 60 to 100 mm Hg).
      f. Sterile orogastric tubes.
         (1) Size 5F or 6F for infants weighing less than 1 kg.
         (2) Size 8F for infants weighing more than 1 kg.
      g. Anesthesia bag with manometer and mask or T-piece resuscitator, capable of delivering blended O_2, and O_2 source.
      h. Tape, scissors.
C. **Noninvasive monitoring.**
   1. All infants receiving O_2 therapy should be considered as potential candidates for mechanical ventilation and should be monitored with the following:
      a. Heart rate monitor: audible beat-to-beat capability and alarm device for bradycardia (<100 beats per minute [bpm]) or tachycardia (>180 bpm); should provide a visual display of electrocardiogram and actual heart rate.
      b. Respiratory monitor: visual display of respiratory wave pattern and actual respiratory rate; should include alarm device for apnea and tachypnea. Respiratory rate trend mode is preferred.

    c. Blood pressure monitoring: peripheral (cuff) blood pressure or arterial blood pressure monitoring, performed on a scheduled interval, and documented on the permanent record.

    d. O_2 analyzer: continuous monitoring of O_2 content of the gas delivered to the patient, with mandatory alarm device for O_2 concentration greater than or less than the desired range.

    e. Pulse oximetry: continuous monitoring for critically ill infants; intermittent checks with documentation of peripheral O_2 saturations indicated for infants not critically ill.

    f. Additional requirements for all infants requiring mechanical ventilation, based on clinical condition:

       (1) Arterial access (usually via umbilical artery catheter) for:

          (a) Blood gas sampling.

          (b) Blood pressure monitoring.

       (2) Transcutaneous Po_2 and Pco_2 monitoring as indicated by clinical status.

2. Pulse oximetry.

    a. Pulse oximetry is a noninvasive and continuous method of measuring hemoglobin O_2 saturation. With the use of red and infrared light, the saturation of hemoglobin bound to O_2 is determined and displayed by a digital readout on the monitoring device. The main advantage of pulse oximetry is the short response time in determining O_2 saturation in a neonate. It also reduces the number of invasive blood gas measurements necessary for a particular infant. It can be used in various settings outside the NICU (e.g., in neonatal transport, delivery room care, and surgery). The alarm device will alert attendants if O_2 saturations are at less or greater than the desired range. **Pulse oximetry does not eliminate the need for blood gas analysis because clinical signs of ventilation and acid–base balance must still be evaluated.**

    b. An accurate reading is dependent on several factors, a primary factor being the perfusion status of the infant. The accuracy of pulse oximetry decreases with low perfusion states. Phototherapy, motion artifact, dyes (ink from footprints), and vasoconstricting drugs (dopamine) can affect saturation readouts. Recent research has shown that the incidence of severe retinopathy of prematurity in low birth weight infants can be reduced by lowering the oxygen saturation alarm limits and implementing oxygen targeting guidelines and educational programs (Chow et al., 2003; VanderVeen et al., 2006).

3. End-tidal CO_2 monitoring.

    a. Measures CO_2 tension through gas analysis during respiration.

    b. Most accurate when infants have normal lung function and a normal ventilation to perfusion ($\dot{V}A/\dot{Q}A$) ratio.

    c. Markedly less accurate in infants with severe lung disease (large alveolar–arterial gradient) and cannot be relied on for accuracy.

    d. May be useful in premature infants with mild to moderate lung disease and in infants with normal lung function.

    e. Transcutaneous CO_2 monitoring is more accurate in the infant with severe lung disease.

D. **Blood gas measurement.** Blood gas measurement is the standard method for monitoring oxygenation, ventilation, and acid–base balance in the ill neonate. Different methods are available for obtaining the blood sample, with umbilical arterial catheterization being the most common. Other methods for sampling include the use of indwelling peripheral arterial catheters, intermittent arterial puncture, and capillary sampling. Arterial samples are preferred over capillary samples (heel stick) because arterial samples are more reliable in obtaining an accurate Pao_2 value. Capillary samples are useful for measuring Pco_2 and pH in infants with chronic lung disease. All these methods are invasive, with potential for complications (see Chapter 15).

MEDICATIONS USED DURING VENTILATION THERAPY

A. **Surfactant:** A deficiency of surfactant in the lungs of premature infants results in impaired gas exchange and increased work of breathing. Administration of exogenous surfactants is routine in preterm infants with evidence of respiratory distress syndrome. Surfactant therapy may also be indicated for more mature infants with meconium aspiration or pulmonary hypertension (American Academy of Pediatrics, 2008). Exogenous surfactant may be in a natural form taken from the lungs of pigs or calves (Beractant [Survanta], Bovine Lung Exogenous Surfactant, Curosurf, Infasurf. Exogenous surfactant is a liquid preparation administered directly into the endotracheal tube.

1. Dose: depends on the product used; approximately 4 or 5 ml/kg/dose.
2. Administration: Ensure that the endotracheal tube is in proper position prior to beginning surfactant administration. Follow the manufacturer's recommendations regarding positioning for administration.
3. Monitor: continuous cardiac, respiratory, and oxygen saturation monitoring during and after administration, frequent vital signs and blood pressure, and ongoing assessment of air entry and chest excursion.
4. Considerations: infants may become hypoxic, bradycardic, or distressed during surfactant administration. Rapid changes in lung compliance may occur during and immediately following dosing. Changes in lung compliance increase the risk of pulmonary hemorrhage in infants with a PDA.
5. Endotracheal suctioning is delayed for at least 1 to 2 hours after dosing to avoid removing the drug.
6. Results: Cochrane Review of natural surfactant use in preterm infants found an improvement in respiratory status, a decreased risk of pneumothorax, a decrease in pulmonary interstitial emphysema, a decreased risk of bronchopulmonary dysplasia, and a decreased mortality (Soll, 2000).

B. **Bronchodilators.**
1. Methylxanthines: Theophylline and caffeine citrate are routinely used to stimulate respirations in preterm neonates (see Chapter 24). In addition to improving respiratory drive, methylxanthines also increase the contractility of the diaphragm and enhance chemoreceptor sensitivity to carbon dioxide. Both drugs have been shown to reduce the number of apneic spells and the need for mechanical ventilation in premature neonates. These drugs also improve renal and pulmonary blood flow, causing mild diuresis and bronchodilation, and increased heart rate and cardiac output (Lopes and Aranda, 2005).
   a. Theophylline (aminophylline).
      (1) Dose: loading dose, 5 to 6 mg/kg; maintenance dose, 2 to 4 mg/kg/dose every 8 to 12 hours (Lopes and Aranda, 2005).
      (2) Monitor: trough level obtained 30 minutes before dose, 72 hours after therapy is initiated; therapeutic range: apnea, 5 to 15 mg/l (Lopes and Aranda, 2005).
      (3) Aminophylline is approximately 80% theophylline.
      (4) Considerations: holding dose if heart rate exceeds 180 bpm.
      (5) Adverse effects: gastrointestinal upset, tachycardia, diuresis, poor weight gain, hyperreflexia, jitteriness, and reduced sleep.
   b. Caffeine: preferred by many clinicians over theophylline because it is given once daily and has fewer adverse effects. Caffeine does not have as great a bronchodilator or diuretic effect as theophylline.
      (1) Dose: loading dose, 20 mg/kg; maintenance 5 mg/kg every 24 hours beginning 24 hours after loading dose (Zenk, 2003).
      (2) Serum drug concentrations are not routinely monitored.
      (3) Adverse effects: usually well tolerated. Tachycardia, jitteriness, and mild glycosuria may occur at higher serum concentrations.

C. **Diuretics.**
1. Furosemide (Lasix): affects chloride transport in the loop of Henle, causes loss of chloride, sodium, potassium, and calcium. Diuresis may decrease pulmonary blood flow, decrease vascular resistance, and increase pulmonary compliance.
   a. Dose: 1 to 2 mg/kg/dose IV or by mouth (Guignard, 2005); a higher oral dose may be required because of reduced bioavailability. Interval: premature infant, every 24 hours; term, every 12 hours; full-term greater than 1 month, every 6 to 8 hours. Long-term therapy: consider a dose every other day.

      b. Monitor: accurate intake and output; specific gravity to evaluate response; frequent electrolyte values to monitor losses and replacement.

      c. Considerations: ototoxic, with transient and permanent hearing losses reported; renal calculi reported with long-term use.

  2. Spironolactone (Aldactone): exerts inhibitory effect of aldosterone on the tubules, with resultant increase in sodium losses and sparing of potassium.

      a. Dose: 1 to 3 mg/kg/dose by mouth every 24 hours (Guignard, 2005).

      b. Monitor: accurate intake and output; specific gravity to evaluate response; electrolyte values after 48 to 72 hours to detect hyperkalemia.

      c. Considerations: may cause rash, vomiting, and diarrhea. Use with caution in infant with impaired renal function.

  3. Hydrochlorothiazide with spironolactone (Aldactazide): Thiazides inhibit sodium reabsorption in the distal nephron, resulting in increased excretion of sodium chloride. The spironolactone is an aldosterone antagonist that helps to prevent potassium excretion and hypokalemia.

      a. Dose: 1 to 3 mg/kg/day given as a single daily dose or divided every 12 hours (Guignard, 2005).

      b. Monitor: accurate intake and output when first starting spironolactone, signs of dehydration, serum electrolytes.

      c. Considerations: may cause hyperglycemia or altered glucose tolerance; hypokalemia may result despite the potassium sparing effect of spironolactone.

D. Corticosteroids.

  1. Dexamethasone (Decadron): a long-acting antiinflammatory medication used in the treatment of chronic lung disease and tracheal edema before and after extubation. Studies have documented an increased risk of adverse neurodevelopmental outcomes in infants receiving systemic steroid therapy. These findings have resulted in the following recommendations developed by the American Academy of Pediatrics and the Canadian Paediatric Society (AAP and CPS, 2006):

      a. Routine use of corticosteroids for the prevention or treatment of chronic lung disease in low birth weight (LBW) infants is not recommended.

      b. The use of corticosteroids outside of randomized controlled trials should be limited to exceptional clinical circumstances.

      c. Monitoring of long-term neurodevelopmental outcomes of infants in systemic steroid clinical trials is strongly encouraged.

      d. Clinical trials investigating alternative antiinflammatory corticosteroids are needed before further recommendations can be made.

      e. Further recommendations suggest that dexamethasone use be restricted to ventilator-dependent infants unlikely to survive without corticosteroids (Grier and Halliday, 2005), that informed parental consent be obtained (Halliday, 2000), and that the lowest dose and shortest course possible be prescribed (Grier and Halliday, 2005).

  2. Monitor serum and urine glucose, blood pressure, and gastric aspirates for blood. Echocardiogram is indicated if treatment continues longer than 7 days.

  3. Considerations: adverse effects—hyperglycemia, glycosuria, hypertension, cardiac effects, sodium and water retention, poor weight gain, hypokalemia, hypocalcemia, and increased risk of sepsis.

E. Paralytic agents.

  1. Pancuronium (Pavulon): pharmacologic relaxation/paralysis of the skeletal muscle to promote improved mechanical ventilation with improved oxygenation/ventilation, decreased barotrauma, decreased fluctuations in cerebral blood flow.

      a. Dose: 0.1 to 0.15 mg/kg/dose IV push. Interval: every 1 to 4 hours as needed for paralysis (Lieh-Lai and Sarnaik, 2005).

      b. Monitor: vital signs including blood pressure continuously.

      c. Considerations: mandatory use of mechanical ventilation, adequate pulmonary toilet mandatory because no swallow or gag reflex is present, eye lubricant necessary. Signs of toxicity: tachycardia, hypertension, or hypotension.

2. Vecuronium (Norcuron): similar to pancuronium, but shorter acting. Dose: 0.1 mg/kg/dose IV push every 1 to 2 hours as needed for paralysis (Lieh-Lai and Sarnaik, 2005).

F. **Pain control/sedation (see Chapter 16).**

G. **Inhaled nitric oxide (iNO):** Endogenous nitric oxide is released from the endothelium and is responsible for vascular smooth muscle relaxation. iNO is used to promote relaxation of the pulmonary smooth muscle to facilitate perfusion of the lung and gas exchange. iNO has been approved by the FDA for the treatment of near-term and term infants with persistent pulmonary hypertension of the newborn (Hagedorn et al., 2006). Use of iNO in preterm infants remains experimental.

1. Dose: initial 20 parts per million (ppm); after 4 hours reduce dose to 6 ppm. iNO is then weaned by 20% in a stepwise fashion to a dose of 1 ppm before discontinuation (Zenk, 2003).

2. Duration of therapy: usually less than 5 days.

3. Monitor: vital signs including blood pressure continuously, complete blood count (CBC), methemoglobin levels, and environmental levels of NO.

4. Considerations: may cause methemoglobinemia, decreased platelet aggregation.

5. Term and near-term infants—significant reduction in the need for ECMO (Field, 2002; Finer, 2000). Cochrane Review concluded that enough evidence exists to recommend iNO for this population of infants with hypoxic respiratory failure who do not have diaphragmatic hernia (Finer and Barrington, 2007). A randomized controlled trial of iNO in preterm infants found a decrease in the incidence of death or CLD from 64% to 49% in premature infants (<34 weeks of gestation) receiving iNO at 10 ppm on day 1 of life followed by 5 ppm for 6 days (Schreiber et al., 2003). A meta-analysis of iNO in preterm infants concluded that when used as rescue therapy for very ill preterm infants undergoing ventilation, iNO may increase severe intracranial hemorrhage but that early routine use of inhaled nitric oxide for mildly sick, preterm infants decreases the risk of serious brain injury and may improve rates of survival without bronchopulmonary dysplasia (Barrington and Finer, 2007).

WEANING FROM CONVENTIONAL VENTILATION

A. **Indications.**
1. Clinical status of infant consistent with beginning resolution of pulmonary condition.
2. Ventilation becomes easier with less support and may result in hypocapnia.
3. Less inspiratory pressure is required to achieve desired V_T.

B. **Techniques.**
1. Physical assessment of respiratory status: breath sounds, aeration, chest wall excursion, and spontaneous respiratory rate. Physical assessment of cardiovascular status: color, perfusion, heart rate, pulses, blood pressure, and presence or absence of murmur. Physical assessment of neurologic status: presence of spontaneous respirations, tone, irritability, and reflexes.
2. Radiographic evaluation: useful in documenting improved lung status and absence of pathologic changes.
3. Laboratory analysis: fluid, electrolyte, and hematologic stability.
4. Blood gas analysis: primary information for weaning an infant from conventional mechanical ventilation. If all other assessments indicate improvement, blood gas analysis provides information about the appropriate ventilator settings to adjust. To decrease the Pao_2, alter the Fio_2 or the MAP: reduce PIP, inspiratory/expiratory time (I/t) ratio, or PEEP. To increase $Paco_2$, decrease ventilation: decrease rate or tidal volume. During weaning it is important to try to decrease the most injurious parameters first. O_2 toxic effects from free O_2 radicals damage lung tissue, and O_2 is associated with retinopathy of prematurity. Therefore it is important to keep O_2 use at a minimum. PIP, PEEP, I/t ratio, and rate are all associated with barotrauma, so weaning should be achieved as soon as possible.

C. **Extubation from mechanical ventilation.** When low ventilator parameters have been achieved (intermittent mandatory ventilation, 10 to 20/min; PIP, 14 to 18; V_T 3.5 to 5 ml/kg; Fio_2, 0.21

to 0.30), the infant should be evaluated for extubation. Some infants may need a transition to nasal CPAP, nasal prong, cannula, or O_2 hood.

Nursing Care During Weaning Process

A. **Airway management, equipment function, and monitoring of the infant do not change during the weaning process.**
B. **Frequent assessment of the infant's vital signs, blood pressure, O_2 saturation, and neurologic status is essential.** Documentation of this assessment will facilitate appropriate changes in ventilator support.
C. **Be alert for decompensation of respiratory or cardiovascular status during this time, and notify the appropriate personnel when necessary.**
D. **Preparation for extubation.**
   1. Equipment for reintubation available at the bedside.
   2. Suction of ETT and oropharynx.
   3. Postextubation equipment ready for use.
   4. Blood gas determination after extubation.
   5. X-ray examination of chest to rule out atelectasis if decompensation occurs.
   6. Frequent physical assessment every 1 to 2 hours after extubation for 24 hours.
   7. Frequent position changes; suctioning as needed.
   8. Explanation of the plan and process to the family before extubation.

INTERPRETATION OF BLOOD GAS VALUES

The purpose of obtaining blood gas values is to determine whether the patient has adequate ventilation and perfusion. Blood gas values also facilitate analysis of oxygenation and acid–base status. Oxygenation is determined by the Pao_2 value. The Pao_2 is the amount of O_2 dissolved in the serum—3% of the total O_2 content. The remainder of the body's O_2 is bound to hemoglobin. Acceptable arterial blood gas values are illustrated in Table 26-1. Capillary Pao_2 reliability is uncertain. The value is lower than with an arterial specimen. Acid–base balance is indicated by the pH and the base deficit or excess. Ventilation is measured by Pco_2.

A. **Acidosis and alkalosis.** Changes in the pH from the normal range indicate a change in the acid–base status of the infant. An elevated pH, greater than 7.45, is alkalosis, which is caused by excess base or decreased acid level in the blood. A decreased pH, less than 7.35, is acidosis, which is caused by decreased base or increased acid level in the blood.
   1. Respiratory acidosis ($Paco_2 > 45$; $pH < 7.35$), caused by the accumulation of CO_2, the respiratory acid, results from hypoventilation.
   2. Respiratory alkalosis ($Paco_2 < 35$; $pH > 7.45$), caused by the decrease of CO_2, results from hyperventilation.
   3. Metabolic alkalosis ($HCO_3^- > 26$, base excess $> +2$; $pH > 7.45$) is caused by a failure to excrete HCO_3^-, which is controlled by kidney function.
   4. Metabolic acidosis ($HCO_3^- < 22$, base deficit > -2 and < 7.35) is caused by failure to retain HCO_3^- or by an increase in blood acid, which is controlled by the kidney.
   5. For causes of acidosis and alkalosis, see Table 26-2.
B. **Disorders of acid–base balance (see Chapter 8).**

■ TABLE 26-1
■ ■ **Normal Arterial Blood Gas Values**

pH	7.35 to 7.45
$Paco_2$	35 to 45 mm Hg
Pao_2	50 to 80 mm Hg
HCO_3^-	22 to 26 mEq/L
Base excess	−2 to +2

■ TABLE 26-2
■ ■ **Causes of Acidosis and Alkalosis**

Cause	Mechanism
Respiratory Acidosis ($\uparrow$Paco$_2$, $\downarrow$pH)	
CNS depression	Maternal narcotics during labor, asphyxia, intracranial hemorrhage, neuromuscular disorder, CNS dysmaturity (apnea of prematurity)
Decreased ventilation–perfusion ratio	Obstructed airway, meconium aspiration, choanal atresia
Decreased lung compliance	Respiratory distress syndrome, pulmonary insufficiency, diaphragmatic hernia
Injury to the thorax	Phrenic nerve paralysis, pneumothorax
Metabolic Acidosis ($\downarrow$HCO$_3^-$, pH, and base deficit [negative value])	
Decreased tissue perfusion	Increased lactic acid production
Sepsis, congestive heart failure	
Renal failure	Increased organic acids
Renal tubular acidosis	Renal loss of base
Diarrhea	Gastrointestinal loss of base
Respiratory Alkalosis ($\downarrow$Paco$_2$, $\uparrow$pH)	
Iatrogenic	Excessive mechanical ventilation
Hypoxemia	Increase in alveolar ventilation
CNS irritation (pain)	
Metabolic Alkalosis ($\uparrow$HCO$_3^-$, pH and base excess [positive value])	
Gastric suction	Loss of acid
Vomiting	Loss of acid
Diuretic therapy	Renal losses of H$^+$ ion
Iatrogenic	Administration of HCO$_3^-$ (base added)

CNS, Central nervous system.

C. **Interpreting a blood gas value.**
   1. Evaluate the pH. Is there an acidosis or an alkalosis?
   2. Evaluate the Paco$_2$. If it is not normal, does it contribute to the acid–base status? Or is it a compensating factor?
   3. Evaluate the HCO$_3^-$ and the base excess or deficit. If they are not normal, do they contribute to the acid–base status? Or are they compensating factors?
   4. Evaluate the Pao$_2$. Is there hypoxia or hyperoxia?
   5. From this information, you can attempt to identify the specific cause of the abnormal acid–base status and treat as indicated.

REFERENCES

American Academy of Pediatrics and Canadian Paediatric Society: Postnatal corticosteroids to treat or prevent chronic lung disease in preterm infants. *Pediatrics*, *109*(2):330-338, Reaffirmed 2006.

American Academy of Pediatrics Committee on Fetus and Newborn: Surfactant-replacement therapy for respiratory distress in the preterm and term neonate. *Pediatrics*, *121*(2):419-432, 2008.

Barrington, K.J. and Finer, N.N.: Inhaled nitric oxide for preterm infants: A systematic review. *Pediatrics*, *120*(5):1088-1099, 2007.

Baumer, J.H.: International randomized controlled trial of patient triggered ventilation in neonatal respiratory distress syndrome. *Archives of Disease in Childhood*, *82*:F5-F10, 2000.

Beresford, M.W., Shaw, N.J., and Manning, D.: Randomized controlled trial of patient triggered and conventional fast rate ventilation in neonatal respiratory distress syndrome. *Archives of Disease in Childhood*, *82*:F14-F18, 2000.

Bhuta, T., Clark, R.H., and Henderson-Smart, D.J.: Rescue high frequency oscillatory ventilation vs conventional mechanical ventilation for infants with severe pulmonary dysfunction born at or near term (Cochrane Review). *Cochrane Database of Systematic Reviews*, 2:CD000438, 2000.

Bhuta, T. and Henderson-Smart, D.J.: Elective high frequency jet ventilation versus conventional ventilation for respiratory distress syndrome in preterm infants (Cochrane Review). *Cochrane Database of Systematic Reviews*, 2:CD000328, 2000.

Blackburn, S.T.: *Maternal, fetal, and neonatal physiology: A clinical perspective* (3rd ed.). St. Louis, 2007, Saunders.

Carlo, W.A.: Emerging technologies for the management of respiratory disorders. In C. Kenner and J. Lott (Eds.): *Comprehensive neonatal care: An interdisciplinary approach* (4th ed.). St. Louis, 2007, Saunders, pp. 18-31.

Chow, L.C., Wright, K.W., Sola, A., and the CSMC Oxygen Administration Study Group: Can changes in clinical practice decrease the incidence of severe retinopathy of prematurity in very low birth weight infants? *Pediatrics*, 111(2):339-345, 2003.

Cole, C. and Fiascone, J.: Strategies for prevention of neonatal chronic lung disease. *Seminars in Perinatology*, 24(6):445-462, 2000.

Courtney, S.E. and Barrington, K.J.: Continuous positive pressure and noninvasive ventilation. *Clinics in Perinatology*, 34(1):73-92, 2007.

Donn, S.M. and Sinha, S.K.: Newer techniques of mechanical ventilation: An overview. *Seminars in Neonatology*, 7:401-407, 2002.

Durand, D.J. and Asselin, J.M.: High-frequency ventilation. In R.A. Polin, W.W. Fox, and S.H. Abman (Eds.): *Fetal and neonatal physiology* (3rd ed.). Philadelphia, 2004, Saunders, pp. 979-984.

Field, D.: Alternative strategies for the management of respiratory failure in the newborn—Clinical realities. *Seminars in Neonatology*, 7(5):429-436, 2002.

Finer, N.N.: Inhaled nitric oxide in term and near-term infants: Neurodevelopmental follow-up of the neonatal inhaled nitric oxide study group (NINOS). *Journal of Pediatrics*, 136(5):611-617, 2000.

Finer, N.N. and Barrington, K.J.: Nitric oxide for respiratory failure in infants born at or near term (Cochrane Review). *Cochrane Database of Systematic Reviews*, 3: CD000509, July 18, 2007.

Greenough, A., Milner, A., and Dimitriou, G.: Synchronized mechanical ventilation for respiratory support in newborn infants (Cochrane Review). *Cochrane Database of Systematic Reviews*, 4: CD000456, 2004.

Grier, D.G. and Halliday, H.L.: Management of bronchopulmonary dysplasia in infants: Guidelines for corticosteroid use. *Drugs*, 65(1):15-29, 2005.

Guignard, J.P.: Diuretics. In S.J. Yaffe and J.V. Aranda (Eds.): *Neonatal and pediatric pharmacology*. Philadelphia, 2005, Lippincott Williams & Wilkins, pp. 595-611.

Hagedorn, M.I., Gardner, S.L., Dickey, L.A., and Abman, S.: Respiratory diseases. In G.B. Merenstein and S.L. Gardner (Eds.): *Handbook of neonatal intensive care* (6th ed.). St. Louis, 2006, Mosby, pp. 595-698.

Halliday, H.L.: Perinatal corticosteroid treatment—helpful or harmful. *Archives of Perinatal Medicine*, 6:7-9, 2000.

Halliday, H.L.: What interventions facilitate weaning from the ventilator? A review of the evidence from systematic reviews. *Paediatric Respiratory Reviews*, 5(Suppl A):S347-S352, 2004.

Henderson-Smart, D.J., Bhuta, T., Cools, F., and Offringe, M.: Elective high frequency oscillatory ventilation vs conventional ventilation for acute pulmonary dysfunction in preterm infants (Cochrane Review). *Cochrane Database of Systematic Reviews, 3:* CD000104, 2001.

Herrera, C.M., Gerhardt, T., Claure, N., et al.: Effects of volume-guaranteed synchronized intermittent mandatory ventilation in preterm infants recovering from respiratory failure. *Pediatrics*, 110(3):529-533, 2002.

HIFI Study Group: High-frequency oscillatory ventilation compared with conventional mechanical ventilation in the treatment of respiratory failure in preterm infants. *New England Journal of Medicine*, 320(2):88-93, 1989.

Hussey, S.G., Ryan, C.A., and Murphy, B.P.: Comparison of three manual ventilation devices using an intubated mannequin. *Archives of Disease in Childhood Fetal and Neonatal Edition*, 89:F490-F493, 2004.

Kalyn, A., Blatz, S., Feuerstake, S., Paes, B., and Bautista, C.: Closed suctioning of intubated neonates maintains better physiologic stability: A randomized trial. *Journal of Perinatology*, 23(3):218-222, 2003.

Keszler, M.: High-frequency jet ventilation. In A.R. Spitzer (Ed.): *Intensive care of the fetus and neonate* (2nd ed.). Philadelphia, 2005, Saunders, pp. 655-669.

Keszler, M. and Durand, D.J.: Neonatal high-frequency ventilation. Past, present, and future. *Clinics in Perinatology*, 28(3):579-607, 2001.

Lieh-Lai, M. and Sarnaik, A.P.: Therapeutic application in pediatric intensive care. In S.J. Yaffe and J.V. Aranda (Eds.): *Neonatal and pediatric pharmacology*. Philadelphia, 2005, Lippincott Williams & Wilkins, pp. 261-277.

Lopes, J.M. and Aranda, J.V.: Pharmacologic treatment of neonatal apnea. In S.J. Yaffe and J.V. Aranda (Eds.): *Neonatal and pediatric pharmacology*. Philadelphia, 2005, Lippincott Williams & Wilkins, pp. 217-229.

Mammel, M.C.: High-frequency ventilation. In J.P. Goldsmith and E.H. Karotkin (Eds.): *Assisted ventilation of the neonate* (4th ed.). Philadelphia, 2003, Saunders, pp.183-201.

Moriette, G., Paris-Llado, J., Walti, H., et al.: Prospective randomized multi-center comparison of high-frequency oscillatory ventilation and conventional ventilation in preterm infants of less than 30 weeks with RDS. *Pediatrics*, 107(2):363-372, 2001.

Morley, C. and Davis, P.: Continuous positive airway pressure: Current controversies. *Current Opinion in Pediatrics*, 16(2):141-145, 2004.

Rimensberger, P., Beghetti, M., Hanquinet, S., et al.: First intention high-frequency oscillation with early lung volume optimization improves pulmonary outcome in VLBW infants with RDS. *Pediatrics*, 105(6):1202-1208, 2000.

Ruof, H. and Fahwenstich, H.: Closed versus open ET suctioning in ventilated preterm infants. *Pediatric Research*, 47:430A, 2000.

Saslow, J.G., Aghai, Z.H., Nakhla, T.A., et al.: Work of breathing using high-flow nasal cannula in preterm infants. *Journal of Perinatology*, *26*(8):476-480, 2006.

Schreiber, M.D., Gin-Mestan, K., Marks, J.D., Hou, D., Lee, G., and Srisuparp, P.: Inhaled nitric oxide in premature infants with respiratory distress syndrome. *New England Journal of Medicine*, *349*(22):2099-2107, 2003.

Soll, R.F.: Prophylactic natural surfactant extract for preventing morbidity and mortality in preterm infants (Cochrane Review). *Cochrane Database of Systematic Reviews*, *2*:CD000511, 2000.

Spitzer, A.R.: Positive pressure ventilation: The use of mechanical ventilation in the treatment of neonatal lung disease—general principles. In A.R. Spitzer (Ed.): *Intensive care of the fetus and newborn*. Philadelphia, 2005, Saunders, pp. 623-654.

Truog, W.E. and Golombek, S.G.: Principles of management of respiratory problems. In M.G. MacDonald, M.D. Mullett, and M.M.K. Seshia (Eds.): *Avery's neonatology: Pathophysiology and management of the newborn* (6th ed.). Philadelphia, 2005, Lippincott Williams & Wilkins, pp. 553-577.

VanderVeen, D.K., Mansfield, T.A., and Eichenwald, E.C.: Lower oxygen saturation alarm limits decrease the severity of retinopathy of prematurity. *Journal of AAPOS*, *10*(5):445-448, 2006.

Wood, B.: Physiologic principles. In J.P. Goldsmith and E.H. Karotkin (Eds.): *Assisted ventilation of the neonate* (4th ed.). Philadelphia, 2003, Saunders, pp. 15-40.

Zenk, K.: *Neonatal medications and nutrition: A comprehensive guide* (3rd ed.). Santa Rosa, CA, 2003, NICU Ink.

27 Extracorporeal Membrane Oxygenation

CAROLYN HOUSKA LUND

OBJECTIVES

1. Discuss the history of neonatal ECMO and related survival statistics.
2. Discuss indications and contraindications for ECMO.
3. Discuss the criteria used to determine an infant's need for ECMO.
4. Review the technical and mechanical aspects of the ECMO procedure.
5. Review the physiology of extracorporeal circulation.
6. Discuss the general care given to infants undergoing the ECMO procedure and the support provided to their families.
7. Review follow-up and outcome of ECMO survivors.

■■ Extracorporeal membrane oxygenation (ECMO) is the use of a modified heart–lung machine for days or weeks to support life and allow treatment and recovery during severe cardiac or pulmonary failure (Bartlett et al., 2000). Despite recent advances in ventilatory management, respiratory failure remains the most frequent cause of neonatal death. ECMO is used as a "rescue" therapy for the 2% to 5% of critically ill infants who do not respond to maximal ventilatory, pharmacologic, and surgical treatments.

ECMO: A HISTORICAL PERSPECTIVE

A. **John Gibbon (1937) invented the first heart–lung machine** and was the first physician to use the technology to perform cardiac surgery successfully. This prototype required direct exposure of the blood to oxygen and a roller pump.
B. **Development of a membrane lung by Clowes (1956)** allowed for separation of the blood and gas phases and dramatically reduced complications (thrombocytopenia, hemolysis, organ failure) of the direct exposure of blood to oxygen.
C. **Development of silicone rubber by Kammermeyer (1957)** made the membrane lung feasible for long-term support.
D. **Kolobow (1969 to 1970) demonstrated the safe use of extracorporeal support for up to 7 days in lambs,** using a coiled silicone membrane lung.
E. **Prolonged ECMO support for moribund neonates in respiratory failure was attempted from 1965 to 1971.** Bartlett began extensive clinical studies and reported improvements in survival and morbidity rates (Bartlett, 1986; Bartlett and Gazzaniga, 1978; Bartlett et al., 1982, 1985).
F. **First survivor was successfully treated in 1975.**
   1. Survival rate of 55% in 1981 (Bartlett et al., 1982).
   2. Survival rate of 100% in 1985 (Bartlett et al., 1985).
G. **Bartlett's success prompted randomized, prospective clinical trials at ECMO centers.**
   1. O'Rourke et al. (1989), in a prospective clinical trial, demonstrated that the overall survival rate of ECMO-treated infants was 99%, in comparison with 60% of infants treated with conventional mechanical therapy.

2. The UK Neonatal ECMO Trial Group (1996) found that the mortality in infants who were randomized to ECMO support was 29%, compared with 61% for the control infants who received maximal conventional therapy.

H. **Extracorporeal Life Support Organization (ELSO) International Registry Report (July 2008) lists a total of 22,429 infants treated since 1975, with an overall survival rate of 76%.**

1. A total of 92 ECMO centers reported. Survival by diagnosis was as follows: meconium aspiration syndrome 94%, persistent pulmonary hypertension of the newborn/persistent fetal circulation 78%, respiratory distress syndrome/hyaline membrane disease 84%, pneumonia 59%, sepsis 75%, air-leak syndrome 74%, congenital diaphragmatic hernia (CDH) 51%, and other diagnoses 63%.

2. After a peak of ECMO cases during the years 1989 to 1995 (927 to 1181 cases per year), the number of ECMO cases for neonates has decreased (472 to 571 cases per year) for the years 2003 to 2008, while the survival rate has declined to 63% to 68%. This decline in both cases and survival reflects a change in the kinds of neonates who require ECMO support, having failed the more sophisticated ventilator management, surfactant, and use of inhaled nitric oxide that is currently standard practice (Ford, 2006).

CRITERIA FOR USE OF ECMO

A. **Neonatal ECMO patient criteria** (Van Meurs et al., 2005).
1. Gestational age greater than 34 weeks.
2. Birth weight greater than 2000 g; SGA infants should not be excluded.
3. Significant coagulopathy or uncontrolled bleeding should be corrected prior to initiating ECMO, if possible.
4. Intracranial hemorrhage grade 2 or less.
5. Mechanical ventilation for less than 10 to 14 days is a relative contraindication.
6. Reversible lung injury.
7. No lethal malformations.
8. No major cardiac malformations (except in infants requiring stabilization and life support before or after surgery).

B. **Acute and reversible respiratory or cardiac pathology.**
1. Respiratory distress syndrome.
2. Meconium aspiration syndrome.
3. Persistent pulmonary hypertension of the newborn.
4. Congenital diaphragmatic hernia.
5. Sepsis.
6. Life support before or after cardiac surgery.
7. Acute respiratory distress syndrome.

C. **Cranial and cardiac ultrasonography findings** ruling out severe intracranial hemorrhage and cyanotic congenital heart disease.

D. **Objective criteria for final selection predictive of greater than 80% mortality rate** (Box 27-1). To achieve specificity, each ECMO center must determine its own mortality indicators and criteria. Criteria may differ in different disease states, such as septic shock, CDH, or severe air leak caused by barotrauma.

E. **Pre-ECMO stabilization, including optimal ventilatory management and trial of high-frequency ventilation, volume support, vasopressors, vasodilator medications, surfactant, and nitric oxide if indicated.** These should be used at a center where ECMO can be initiated quickly if the infant does not respond adequately.

VENOARTERIAL PERFUSION

A. **Technique for venoarterial perfusion (VA).**
1. Deoxygenated blood is drained from the right side of the heart through a cannula placed in the right atrium via the right internal jugular vein.
2. Venous cannula must be a size that is capable of delivering total cardiac output (120 to 150 ml/kg/minute) to the membrane lung; cannulas of largest possible internal diameter (8F to 14F) are inserted.

■ BOX 27-1
■ **NEONATAL ECMO PATIENT QUALIFYING CRITERIA**

Alveolar-Arterial Difference in Partial Pressure of Oxygen: 600 to 624 mm Hg for 4 to 12 Hours at Sea Level

$$AaDo_2 = \frac{Atmospheric\ pressure - 47 - (Paco_2 + Pao_2)}{Fio_2}$$

Note: 47 is the partial pressure of water vapor.
Oxygenation Index: 25 to 60 for 30 Minutes to 6 Hours

$$OI = \frac{MAP \times Fio_2 \times 100}{Pao_2}$$

where MAP is mean airway pressure.
Pao$_2$: 35 to 50 mm Hg for 2 to 12 Hours
Acute Deterioration
   Pao$_2$ ≤30 to 40 mm Hg
   pH ≤7.25 for 2 hours
   Intractable hypotension

From Rosenberg, E. and Seguin, J.: Selection criteria for use of ECLS in neonates. In J. Zwischenberger and R.H. Bartlett (Eds.): *ECMO: Extracorporeal cardiopulmonary support in critical care.* Ann Arbor, 1995, Extracorporeal Life Support Organization.

3. Oxygenated blood is returned through a cannula placed into the ascending aorta via the right common carotid artery (Bartlett, 2005).

B. Advantages.
   1. Technique provides both respiratory and cardiac support by decompressing pulmonary circulation, decreases pulmonary artery and pulmonary capillary filtration pressure, and supports circulation by augmenting the pumping action of the heart.
   2. Positive-pressure ventilation can be reduced to minimal parameters: peak inspiratory pressure, 15 to 20 cm H$_2$O; positive end-expiratory pressure, 5 to 10 cm H$_2$O; respiratory rate, 10 to 20/min; and fractional concentration of oxygen in inspired gas (Fio$_2$), 21%.

C. Disadvantages.
   1. Emboli (air or particulate) could be infused directly into the arterial circulation.
   2. Ligation of carotid artery may affect cerebral perfusion.

VENOVENOUS PERFUSION

A. Technique for venovenous (VV) perfusion.
   1. Double-lumen cannula is used (size 12F, 14F, or 15F). Deoxygenated blood is drained from the venous limb, positioned in the right atrium.
   2. Blood is returned through the arterial limb, also located in the right atrium, with side holes positioned at the tricuspid valve.
   3. Blood flow is directed across the valve, into the right ventricle, and through the pulmonary circulation. It returns to the left atrium before entering the systemic circulation via the aorta.

B. Advantages (Fortenberry et al., 2005).
   1. No ligation of the carotid artery is necessary.
   2. Oxygenated blood flows through pulmonary circulation, which may help reverse pulmonary hypertension.
   3. Oxygenated blood is provided to the coronary arteries.
   4. Emboli (air or particulate) are less likely to result in severe compromise to the infant because blood is not returned directly to the arterial circulation.

C. Disadvantages.
1. VV perfusion can be used only with adequate cardiac function because systemic flow is dependent on cardiac output. In the event of cardiac "stun," or decreased function, emergent conversion to VA ECMO may be needed.
2. Recirculation of oxygenated blood can occur. Oxygenated blood returned to the right atrium may be emptied again into the venous side of the double-lumen cannula, rather than across the tricuspid valve.
3. Use of somewhat higher ventilatory support may be required because lower flow rates are achieved with the smaller lumens of the double-lumen cannula.
4. Vasopressor therapy may need to be continued to support blood pressure and ECMO flow.

CIRCUIT COMPONENTS AND ADDITIONAL DEVICES

A. Cannulas (Fig. 27-1).
1. Cannulas are surgically placed in large blood vessels to remove deoxygenated venous blood and return oxygenated blood to the circulation.
2. Before insertion of the cannulas, the infant is paralyzed and given opiates to prevent respiratory movement and air embolism, and systemic heparin is given to prevent clotting of the cannulas and the circuit; this is because when circulating blood comes into contact with artificial surfaces, coagulation is activated (Annich and Miskulin, 2005).
3. In VA ECMO, the venous cannula tip is positioned in the right atrium to drain blood flow from the inferior vena cava and the superior vena cava. The arterial cannula tip reaches just to the aortic arch.
4. In VV ECMO, the double-lumen cannula is positioned in the right atrium, with the arterial side directed toward the tricuspid valve.

B. ECMO circuit.
1. The ECMO circuit consists of polyvinyl chloride tubing, Luer lock connectors, stopcocks, infusion sites, and usually a silicone bladder.

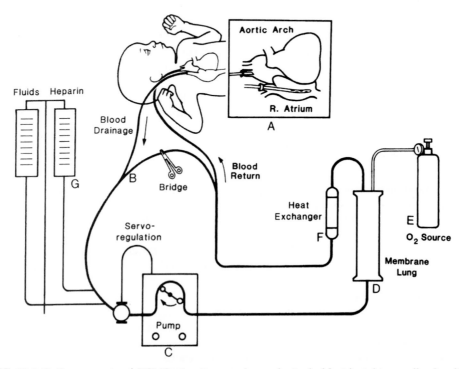

FIGURE 27-1 ■ Components of ECMO circuit: cannulas, polyvinyl chloride tubing, roller head pump, membrane oxygenator (lung), gas source, heat exchanger, and infusion pumps.

2. Some manufacturers have developed surface bonding materials for circuit tubing and cannulas, in an effort to minimize the activation of complement, platelets and inflammatory mediators, and are thought to be less thrombogenic (Hansell, 2005).
3. Blood circulates throughout all components of the ECMO circuit; parenteral fluids, medications, and blood products are administered into the venous side of the circuit (before the membrane oxygenator).
4. Only platelets are infused on the arterial side of the circuit, or into the patient directly, to prevent adherence to the membrane oxygenator.
5. Precautions and guidelines for placing medications and blood products into the circuit are the same as those for safely administering medications and blood products directly to patients.

C. **Servo-regulation of venous return: bladder reservoir, pressure monitoring.**
1. Collapsible silicone bladder distends with returning venous blood.
2. Inadequate flow (decreased venous return) into the ECMO circuit causes the bladder to collapse, which triggers a microswitch and an audible alarm and stops the roller head pump.
3. When the bladder reexpands, the microswitch engages the pump and normal pump operation continues.
4. Adequate venous return is critical for maintaining cardiorespiratory support; therefore the cause of decreased return must be recognized and corrected immediately.
5. Servomechanism regulation of ECMO flow can also be achieved by transducers placed in the circuits. Premembrane (venous) pressure and postmembrane (arterial) pressure may be monitored continuously to signal extracorporeal flow problems before collapse of the silicone bladder. This allows for early detection and timely intervention.
   a. Fall in premembrane pressure indicates decreased venous return.
   b. Rise in postmembrane pressure indicates malfunction of membrane oxygenator or heat exchanger.
6. Other devices have been recently introduced to regulate venous flow, including a thin-walled section of tubing encased in rigid housing that is mounted vertically in the circuit, and does not have the clotting issues associated with the conventional silicone bladder (Hansell, 2005).

D. **Pumps.**
1. Roller head pumps and centrifugal pumps are both used to provide ECMO support.
2. Roller head pumps compress and displace the blood in the PVC tubing placed in the pump raceway.
   a. Blood is pushed forward, creating gentle suction in the venous cannula and assisting left ventricular function when VA bypass is used.
   b. Digital display indicates circuit flow in cubic centimeters per minute.
   c. Electrically powered; must be hand cranked or attached to battery pack if power failure occurs.
3. Centrifugal pumps generate flow by means of a spinning motor.
   a. Negative pressure pulls blood into the pump, and directs it out at the top of the vortex.

E. **Gas exchange devices.**
1. Silicone membrane oxygenator is made of a solid silicone polymer membrane envelope with a plastic space screen that is wrapped spirally around a spool; encased in a silicone rubber sleeve.
   a. Maximizes gas exchange across the membrane.
   b. Only oxygenator currently approved by FDA for long-term use.
2. Hollow-fiber oxygenator contains microporous tubes with tiny holes through which gas exchange takes place (Hansell, 2005).
   a. Potential advantage during priming; can have bioactive coating.

F. **Heat exchanger.**
1. Located after the oxygenator, or incorporated into the oxygenator.
2. Rewarms blood before returning it to the infant's circulation.
3. Heat loss occurs from cooling effect of ventilating gases inside the oxygenator and circuit exposure to ambient air temperature.

G. **Bubble detector.**
   1. Placed beyond heat exchanger to detect air in blood flowing through arterial side of pump as the blood is returned to the patient.
   2. In some systems, when air is detected, the roller head pump is shut off and flow to the patient ceases.
   3. Critical importance in veno-arterial ECMO.
H. **Activated clotting time (ACT) monitoring.**
   1. ACT is the most practical bedside method to measure anticoagulation in the ECMO patient (Annich and Miskulin, 2005).
   2. Initial bolus of heparin during cannulation (usually 100 units/kg).
   3. Infusion pump for continuous infusion of heparin solution at 25 to 100 units/kg/hour into ECMO circuit.
   4. Titration of heparin solution to keep ACT within the desired range (usually 180 to 220 seconds).
   5. For control of heparin administration, no heparin added to any other medications or fluids (an exception may be the fluids being infused into umbilical or peripheral arterial lines).
   6. Factors that influence heparin requirements: thrombocytopenia, abnormal clotting studies, urinary output, and infusions of blood products that contain clotting factors.
I. **Blood gas monitoring.**
   1. Mixed venous oxygen saturation (Svo_2), monitored continuously, is the optimal parameter to assess tissue oxygen delivery. It can be measured through fiberoptic catheters or by using optical reflectance technology. Correlation with co-oximeter values measured by a blood gas machine is required.
   2. Arterial blood gas measurements obtained beyond the membrane oxygenator in the ECMO circuit reflect the function of the membrane lung.
   3. Patient blood gas values and noninvasive oxygen saturation monitoring are used to assess the recovery of lung function and the infant's acid–base balance.

PHYSIOLOGY OF EXTRACORPOREAL CIRCULATION

The physiology of extracorporeal circulation has been discussed by Bartlett (2005) and Ford (2006).
A. **Blood flow.**
   1. VA bypass is instituted by draining venous blood into the ECMO circuit; a like amount of oxygenated blood is returned to the arterial circulation.
   2. As bypass flow increases, flow through the pulmonary artery decreases faster than bypass flow and reduces total flow in the systemic circulation, causing peripheral and pulmonary hypotension.
   3. Blood volume replacement is required for optimal tissue perfusion.
   4. ECMO perfusion is nonpulsatile (pulse contour decreases as flow rate increases); kidneys interpret this as inadequate flow and promote the release of renin and aldosterone, which causes sodium retention, extracellular fluid expansion, and a decreased total body potassium concentration.
   5. Total patient flow is the sum of ECMO flow and pulmonary blood flow; adequate flow is reached when oxygen delivery and tissue perfusion result in normoxia, normal pH, normal $S\bar{v}o_2$, and normal organ function.
   6. Total gas exchange and support are achieved at a flow rate of 120 to 150 ml/kg/minute.
B. **Gas exchange.**
   1. The membrane lung has two compartments divided by a semipermeable membrane: ventilating gas is on one side and blood is on the other.
   2. Oxygen diffuses into the blood because of a pressure gradient between the elevated oxygen pressure in the gas compartment and the low oxygen pressure in the venous blood.
   3. Carbon dioxide diffuses from the blood compartment to the gas compartment as a result of a pressure gradient between venous carbon dioxide pressure and the ventilating gas. The carbon dioxide transfer rate is 6 times greater than that of oxygen transfer. The ventilating gas mixture is usually enriched with carbon dioxide to prevent hypocapnia.

C. Blood–surface interface.
1. During ECMO, up to 80% of the cardiac output is exposed to a large artificial surface each minute.
2. Clot formation is prevented by systemic heparinization; platelet destruction is minimized by preexposure of the circuit to albumin.
3. Platelets show the greatest effect of exposure to a foreign surface, as evidenced by decreased platelet count (thrombocytopenia) and function.
4. Hemolysis is monitored regularly by measuring plasma free hemoglobin levels. It is usually not significantly altered by ECMO flow, although increases may indicate problems with red blood cell destruction in the membrane oxygenator or small-lumen cannula.
5. All types of white blood cells decrease in concentration, and phagocytic activity is significantly decreased.
6. After cessation of ECMO, platelets and white blood cell counts return to normal.

CARE OF THE INFANT DURING ECMO

Remenapp et al. (2005), Sheehan (1999), and Nugent and Matranga (1997) have discussed the responsibilities of the ECMO specialist and the bedside nurse in the care of the infant during ECMO.

A. Cannulation.
1. Cannulation requires the initiation of systemic anesthesia and analgesia; the operating room staff is in attendance.
2. See Table 27-1 for nursing responsibilities and interventions.
3. ECMO specialist responsibilities:
   a. Maintain and monitor ECMO circuit.
   b. Assess physiologic stability.
   c. Maintain physiologic parameters such as blood gas values, blood pressure, platelet count, Svo_2 and arterial oxygen saturation (Sao_2) and ACT.
   d. Assist nurse in the general care of the infant.
   e. Be prepared for circuit emergencies.
B. During ECMO "run."
1. Bypass is gradually instituted until approximately 80% (120 to 150 ml/kg/minute) of cardiac output is diverted through the ECMO circuit.
2. At maximal flow, blood gas values should normalize and Svo_2 is maintained at greater than 70%.
3. Svo_2 is an excellent indicator of adequate flow during VA ECMO because it is a measure of tissue perfusion and efficiency of extracorporeal circulation in meeting metabolic demands.
4. Oxygenation during VV ECMO is assessed by infant's arterial blood gas values and continuous oxygen saturation monitoring via pulse oximetry. Svo_2 is not an accurate reflection of deoxygenated blood because of recirculation; Svo_2 is used as a trending parameter during VV ECMO.
5. Ventilator settings are reduced to a minimum; vasopressor therapy and chemical paralysis are usually discontinued; enteral feedings are generally withheld because of concern about hypoxic injury to the gastrointestinal tract, which has never been exposed to nutrients; and blood loss is quantified and replaced.
6. Emergencies during ECMO (DeBerry et al., 2005):
   a. Circuit emergencies.
      (1) Air embolism.
      (2) Tubing rupture.
      (3) Oxygenator malfunction.
      (4) Accidental decannulation.
      (5) Power failure.
      (6) Gas source failure.
   b. Responsibilities of the nurse during a circuit emergency:
      (1) Notification of physician.
      (2) Ventilation.

■ TABLE 27-1
■ ■ **Nursing Responsibilities and Interventions for ECMO**

Responsibility	Intervention
Before Cannulation	
Obtain and document baseline physiologic data.	Record weight, length, and head circumference.
	Draw blood samples for CBC, electrolytes, calcium, glucose, BUN, creatinine, PT/PTT, platelet count and function, arterial blood gas values.
	Record vital signs: heart rate; respiratory rate; systolic, diastolic, and mean blood pressure; and temperature.
Ensure adequate supply of blood products for replacement.	Draw, type, and cross-match samples for two units of packed red blood cells and fresh frozen plasma.
	Keep one unit of packed cells and fresh frozen plasma always available in the blood bank.
Maintain prescribed pulmonary support.	Maintain ventilator parameters.
	Administer muscle relaxants if indicated.
Assemble and prepare equipment.	Prepare infusion pumps to maintain arterial lines and infusion of parenteral fluids and medications into the ECMO circuit.
	Place the infant on a radiant warmer with the head positioned at the foot of the bed to provide thermoregulation and access for cannulation.
	Attach infant to physiologic monitoring devices to monitor heart rate, intraarterial blood pressure, transcutaneous oxygen, and other parameters.
	Insert urinary catheter and nasogastric tube; place to gravity drainage.
	Remove IV lines just prior to heparinization (optional).
	Prepare loading dose of heparin (50 to 100 units/kg).
	Prepare heparin solution for continuous infusion (100 units/ml 5% dextrose in water).
	Prepare paralyzing drug (pancuronium bromide, 0.1 mg/kg, or succinylcholine, 1 to 4 mg/kg).
	Assist in insertion of arterial line (umbilical or peripheral).
	Administer prophylactic antibiotics.
During Cannulation	
Monitor cardiopulmonary status during procedure.	Monitor heart rate and intraarterial blood pressure continuously.
	Obtain blood gas values after paralysis and during cannulation, as indicated by the infant's response to the procedure.
Be prepared to administer cardiopulmonary support.	Have medications and blood products available to correct hypovolemia, bradycardia, acidosis, and cardiac arrest.
Administer medications.	Give loading dose of heparin systemically when vessels are dissected free and are ready to be cannulated.
	Give paralyzing drug systemically just before cannulation of internal jugular vein if infant has not been previously paralyzed. Give analgesia for anesthetic effect.
Reduce ventilator parameters to minimal settings.	Once adequate bypass is achieved, reduce PIP to 16 to 20 cm H_2O, PEEP to 4 cm H_2O, ventilator rate to 10 to 20 breaths per minute, and Fio_2 to 21% to 30%. Patients undergoing VV bypass may require greater respiratory support.
During ECMO Run	
Monitor and document physiologic parameters.	Record hourly: heart rate, blood pressure (systolic, diastolic, mean), respirations, temperature, oxygen saturation, ACT, ECMO flow.
	Measure hourly accurate intake and output of all body fluids (urine, gastric contents, blood); test all stools for occult blood.
	Assess hourly: color, breath sounds, heart tones, murmurs, cardiac rhythm, arterial pressure waveform, peripheral perfusion.

■ TABLE 27-1
■ ■ **Nursing Responsibilities and Interventions for ECMO—cont'd**

Responsibility	Intervention
	Assess hourly: level of consciousness, reflexes, tone, and movement of extremities; assess neurologic examination, including fontanelle tension, pupil size, and reaction every 8 to 12 hours.
	Record ventilator parameters hourly.
	Assess weight and head circumference daily.
Monitor and document biochemical parameters.	Draw samples for arterial blood gas values from umbilical or peripheral line as indicated.
	All other blood specimens are drawn from ECMO circuit by ECMO specialist: electrolytes, calcium, platelets, Chemstrip blood tests, hematocrit every 4 to 8 hours, CBC, PT/PTT, BUN, creatinine, total and direct bilirubin, plasma hemoglobin, fibrinogen, fibrin split products, and blood culture as indicated.
Administer medications.	Remove air bubbles and double-check dosages before infusion.
	Administer no medications intramuscularly or by venipuncture.
	Place all medications and fluids into the venous side of the ECMO circuit.
	Prepare and administer the arterial line (umbilical or peripheral) infusion.
	Administer parenteral alimentation.
Provide pulmonary support.	Perform endotracheal suctioning according to individual assessment and need.
	Maintain patent airway; be alert to extubation or plugging.
	Obtain daily chest films and tracheal aspirate cultures as indicated.
	Maintain ventilator parameters.
Prevent bleeding.	Avoid all of the following: rectal probes, injections, venipunctures, heel sticks.
	Avoid invasive procedures. Do not change nasogastric tube, urinary catheters, or endotracheal tube unless absolutely necessary; use premeasured endotracheal tube suction technique.
	Observe for blood in urine, stools, and endotracheal or nasogastric tubes.
Maintain excellent infection control.	Change all fluids and tubing daily.
	Change dressings daily and as needed.
	Maintain closed system for urinary catheter drainage.
	Maintain strict aseptic and handwashing techniques.
	Use universal barrier precautions.
Provide physical care.	Keep skin dry, clean, and free of pressure points.
	Give mouth care as needed.
	Provide range of motion as indicated.
	Turn side to side every 1 to 2 hours.
Provide pain management, sedation, stress reduction.	Minimize noise level.
	Cluster patient care to maximize sleep period.
	Administer analgesia: fentanyl or morphine as continuous IV drip.
	Manage iatrogenic physical dependency by following dose reduction regimen.
Be alert to complications and emergencies.	See text.

ACT, Activated clotting time; *BUN*, blood urea nitrogen; *CBC*, complete blood cell count; *Fio$_2$*, fractional concentration of oxygen in inspired gas; *PEEP*, positive end-expiratory pressure; *PIP*, peak inspiratory pressure; *PT/PTT*, prothrombin time/partial thromboplastin time; *VV*, venovenous.

Adapted from Nugent, J. and Matranga, G.: Extracorporeal membrane oxygenation. In D.F. Askin (Ed.): *Acute respiratory care of the newborn* (2nd ed.). Petaluma, CA, 1997, NICU Ink, pp. 341-368.

        (3) Anticoagulation.

        (4) Chemical resuscitation.

        (5) Blood loss replacement.

    c. Responsibilities of the ECMO specialist during a circuit emergency:

        (1) Clamp catheters.

        (2) Open bridge.

        (3) Remove gas source.

        (4) Repair circuit.

C. ECMO patient complications (DeBerry et al., 2005).

1. Electrolyte/glucose/fluid imbalance. Sodium requirements decrease; potassium requirements increase because of the action of aldosterone. Calcium replacement may be needed if citrate-phosphate-dextrose anticoagulated blood is used. Hyperglycemia may necessitate a decrease in the glucose concentration of IV fluids.

2. CNS deterioration: cerebral edema, intracranial hemorrhage, and seizures. Deterioration results from initial hypoxia, acidosis, hypercapnia, or vessel ligation.

3. Generalized edema. The extracellular space is enlarged by the distribution of crystalloid solution and the action of aldosterone and antidiuretic hormone. The use of diuretics or hemofiltration may be necessary if edema causes brain or lung dysfunction.

4. Renal failure. Acute tubular necrosis results from pre-ECMO hypotension and hypoxia. Indicators of renal failure are abnormal blood urea nitrogen and creatinine values. Low-dose dopamine therapy and/or hemodialysis may be necessary.

5. Hemorrhage due to thrombocytopenia, coagulopathy.

6. Decreased venous return and/or hypovolemia due to inadequate circulating blood volume, pneumothorax, and/or partial venous catheter occlusion or malposition.

7. Hypertension due to overinfusion of blood products, renal ischemia, and excretion of renin-angiotensin.

8. Patent ductus arteriosus. Left-to-right shunting may cause increased blood flow to the lung, necessitating high pump flows without the expected increase in Pao_2. Ligation may be necessary.

9. Cardiac "stun." Transient loss of ventricular contractility (1 to 3 days) is manifested by hypotension, decrease in aortic pulse pressure, poor peripheral perfusion, and decreased Pao_2. It is possibly due to mismatch between afterload and ventricular contractility during ECMO.

10. Mechanical complications. These include incorrect catheter placement, oxygenator failure, power failure, air entrainment, and accidental decannulation.

D. Weaning/decannulation.

1. Signs of improvement and indicators that the infant is ready to be weaned are as follows:

    a. Improvement of lung fields on chest x-ray examination.

    b. Clinical findings: improved breath sounds, rising Pao_2 on fixed ECMO flow, improvement in lung compliance.

2. Once improvement has been ascertained, flow rate is decreased slowly in 10- to 20-ml increments until ECMO support is no longer needed to maintain adequate gas exchange at low ventilator settings (Bartlett, 2005).

3. When flow rate is 50 to 100 ml/kg/minute, a state of "idling" is achieved, the infant remains at this lowest possible flow rate for 4 to 8 hours.

4. If improvement in lung function remains stable, cannulas are clamped, heparin is infused directly into the infant, and the circuit is recirculated via a bridge. If blood gas values deteriorate, the cannulas are unclamped and ECMO support is resumed.

5. In VV ECMO the cannulas are not clamped during the "trial off" procedure; gas flow to the membrane oxygenator is discontinued. Low flow rates are maintained, and patient response is assessed by measurement of blood gases.

6. Decannulation proceeds if blood gas values remain satisfactory.

7. Before decannulation, the infant undergoes chemical paralysis and ventilator parameters are increased to compensate for loss of spontaneous respiratory function.

8. After adequate anesthesia and analgesia has been administered, the cannulas are removed. Both the internal jugular vein and the carotid artery are ligated. In some ECMO centers, carotid reconstruction is attempted (Cheung et al., 1997; Levy et al., 1995). The efficacy of this procedure is debatable because of clot formation at the site of reconstruction.

9. After decannulation, the infant is weaned as tolerated from the ventilator and routine NICU care is resumed.

POST-ECMO CARE

A. **Lung recovery is achieved through weaning of the infant from assisted ventilation.** Occasionally the use of steroids and/or diuretics is necessary to improve recovery.

B. **Assessment of neurologic recovery involves clinical evaluation and CT scan.** It may be difficult to assess neurologic status during opiate use or while the infant is recovering from significant illness, so assessment may be deferred until the infant is ready for discharge.

C. **Weaning from opiate analgesics and sedatives involves a gradual reduction of doses and careful monitoring for withdrawal symptoms.** Infants receiving ECMO therapy require opiate infusions or scheduled dosing of opiates and sedatives throughout their course of ECMO to prevent excessive movement, which can dislodge the cannulas (Arnold et al., 1990; Caron and Maguire, 1990; Franck and Vilardi, 1995).

D. **Establishing oral feedings may be difficult.** Prolonged respiratory compromise, the effect of opiates on state control, alterations in swallowing caused by neck dissection during cannula placement, and gastroesophageal reflux, particularly in infants with CDH, are some of the causes of feeding problems in the post-ECMO infant. Feeding difficulties are generally more common in infants with CDH than in those with other diagnoses such as meconium aspiration syndrome or persistent pulmonary hypertension of the newborn.

PARENTAL SUPPORT

A. **The ECMO candidate's parents are in crisis.** They are aware that ECMO is a method of last resort with no guarantee of positive result, and the technology is overwhelming.

B. **Parents need concise, accurate information** about their child's condition and the required procedures.

C. **Parent-to-parent support, using parents of "ECMO graduates,"** is efficacious and a positive experience.

D. **Parents should have access to their infant.** The ECMO candidates have an increasingly bright outcome, and every effort should be made to encourage involvement and bonding.

FOLLOW-UP AND OUTCOME

The follow-up and outcome of ECMO have been discussed by Bernbaum et al. (1995), Boggs and LaPrade-Wolf (1992), Boykin et al. (2003), Glass et al. (1989, 1995), Glass and Brown (2005), Hofkosh et al. (1991), and Kanto (1994).

A. **Critical scrutiny of survivors is essential to assess the value and safety of ECMO.** Survivors should be evaluated at 4 to 6 months, and then yearly until school age. The following are assessed:
   1. Growth and development.
   2. Cardiorespiratory development.
   3. Cerebrovascular status.
   4. Neurologic and psychologic functioning.

B. **Medical morbidity includes poor somatic growth, feeding problems, chronic lung disease, and rehospitalizations.** Predictors include diagnosis of CDH, lower birth weight, and age at initiation of ECMO.

C. **Rate of bilateral hearing loss requiring amplification is approximately 5%.** By 5 years of age, the majority of ECMO-treated neonates are functioning in normal range for IQ, although lower than control children who were not ill in the neonatal period (Glass et al., 1995). Risk for developmental disability is similar to pre-ECMO mortality risk, whether they receive CPR, degree of prematurity, and neuroimaging abnormality (Glass and Brown, 2005).

D. **School-age ECMO survivors are twice as likely as other children to have neuropsychologic deficits and are at risk of having academic problems.** Predictors include lower birth weight, abnormal findings on neurologic imaging, chronic lung disease, and failure to thrive. However, even children who do not have these risk factors can have neuropsychologic testing to predict the need for special education services.

E. **Psychologic morbidity, including behavioral problems, is also reported and may be due to altered parenting styles and family stress.** Early trauma from severe illness may set the stage for problems in parent–child interactions.

REFERENCES

Annich, G. and Miskulin, J.: Coagulation, anticoagulation, and the interaction of blood and artificial surfaces. In K. Van Meurs, K.P. Lally, G. Peek, and J.B. Zwischenberger (Eds.): *ECMO: Extracorporeal cardiopulmonary support in critical care* (3rd ed.). Ann Arbor, 2005, Extracorporeal Life Support Organization, pp. 29-58.

Arnold, J., Truog, R., Orav, E.J., et al.: Tolerance and dependence in neonates sedated with fentanyl during extracorporeal membrane oxygenation. *Anesthesiology*, 73(6):1136-1140, 1990.

Bartlett, R.: Physiology of ECLS. In K. Van Meurs, K. Lally, G. Peek, and J. Zwischenberger (Eds.): *ECMO: Extracorporeal cardiopulmonary support in critical care* (3rd ed.). Ann Arbor, 2005, Extracorporeal Life Support Organization, pp. 5-27.

Bartlett, R.: Respiratory support: Extracorporeal membrane oxygenation in newborn respiratory failure. In K. Welch, et al. (Eds.): *Pediatric surgery*. Chicago, 1986, Year Book Medical Publishers, pp. 74-77.

Bartlett, R., Andrews, A.F., Toomasian, J.M., et al.: Extra-corporeal membrane oxygenation for newborn respiratory failure: Forty-five cases. *Surgery,* 92(2):425-433, 1982.

Bartlett, R. and Gazzaniga, A.: Extracorporeal circulation for cardiopulmonary failure. *Current Problems in Surgery*, 12(5):1-96, 1978.

Bartlett, R., Roloff, D.W., Cornell, R.G., et al.: Extracorporeal circulation in neonatal respiratory failure: A prospective randomized study. *Pediatrics*, 76(2):479-487, 1985.

Bartlett, R., Roloff, D.W., Custer, J.R., et al: Extracorporeal life support: The University of Michigan experience. *Journal of the American Medical Association*, 28(7):904-908, 2000.

Bernbaum, J., Schwartz, I.P., Gerdes, M., et al.: Survivors of extracorporeal membrane oxygenation at 1 year of age: The relationship of primary diagnosis with health and neurodevelopmental sequelae. *Pediatrics*, 96(5 Pt 1):907-913, 1995.

Boggs, K. and LaPrade-Wolf, P.: Beyond survival: Strategies for establishing a follow-up program for infants with extracorporeal membrane oxygenation. *Neonatal Network*, 11(1):7-13, 1992

Boykin, A., Quivers, E., Wagenhoffer, K., et al.: Cardiopulmonary outcome of neonatal extracorporeal membrane oxygenation at ages 10-15 years. *Critical Care Medicine*, 31(9):2380-2384, 2003.

Caron, E. and Maguire, D.: Current management of pain, sedation and narcotic physical dependency of the infant on ECMO. *Journal of Perinatal and Neonatal Nursing*, 4(10):63-74, 1990.

Cheung, P.Y., Vickar D.B., Hallgren R.A., et al.: Carotid artery reconstruction in neonates receiving extracorporeal membrane oxygenation: A 4-year follow-up study. Western Canadian ECMO Follow-up Group. *Journal of Pediatric Surgery*, 32(4):560-564, 1997.

DeBerry, B., Lynch, J., Chung, D., and Zwischenberger, J.: Emergencies during ECLS and their management. In K. Van Meurs, K.P. Lally, G. Peek, and J.B. Zwischenberger (Eds.): *ECMO: Extracorporeal cardiopulmonary support in critical care* (3rd ed.). Ann Arbor, 2005, Extracorporeal Life Support Organization, pp. 133-156.

Ford, J.: Neonatal ECMO: Current controversies and trends. *Neonatal Network*, 25(4):229-238, 2006.

Fortenberry, J., Pettignano, R., and Dykes, F.: Principles and practice of venovenous ECMO. In K. Van Meurs, K.P. Lally, G. Peek, and J.B. Zwischenberger (Eds.): *ECMO: Extracorporeal cardiopulmonary support in critical care* (3rd ed.). Ann Arbor, 2005, Extracorporeal Life Support Organization, pp. 85-105.

Franck, L. and Vilardi, J.: Assessment and management of opioid withdrawal in ill neonates. *Neonatal Network*, 14(2):39-48, 1995.

Glass, P. and Brown, J.: Outcome and follow-up of neonates treated with ECMO. In K. Van Meurs, K.P. Lally, G. Peek, and J.B. Zwischenberger (Eds.): *ECMO: Extracorporeal cardiopulmonary support in critical care* (3rd ed.). Ann Arbor, 2005, Extracorporeal Life Support Organization, pp. 319-328.

Glass, P., Miller, M., and Short, B.: Morbidity for survivors of extracorporeal membrane oxygenation: Neurodevelopmental outcome at 1 year of age. *Pediatrics*, 83(1):72-78, 1989.

Glass, P., Wagner, A., Papero, P., et al.: Neurodevelopmental status at age five years of neonates treated with extracorporeal membrane oxygenation. *Journal of Pediatrics*, 127(3):447-457, 1995.

Hansell, D.: ECLS equipment and devices. In K. Van Meurs, K.P. Lally, G. Peek, and J.B. Zwischenberger (Eds.): *ECMO: Extracorporeal cardiopulmonary support in critical care* (3rd ed.). Ann Arbor, 2005, Extracorporeal Life Support Organization, pp. 107-119.

Hofkosh, D., Thompson, A., Nozza, R., et al.: Ten years of extracorporeal membrane oxygenation:

Neurodevelopmental outcome. *Pediatrics, 87*(4):549-555, 1991.

Kanto, W.P.: A decade of experience with neonatal extracorporeal membrane oxygenation. *Journal of Pediatrics, 124*(3):335-347, 1994.

Levy, M.S., Share, J.C., Fauza, D.O., et al: Fate of the reconstructed carotid artery after extracorporeal membrane oxygenation. *Journal of Pediatric Surgery, 30*(7):1046-1049, 1995.

Neonatal ECMO Registry Report, January. Ann Arbor, 2008, Extracorporeal Life Support Organization.

Nugent, J. and Matranga, G.: Extracorporeal membrane oxygenation. In D.F. Askin (Ed.): *Acute respiratory care of the newborn* (2nd ed.). Petaluma, CA, 1997, NICU Ink, pp. 341-368.

O'Rourke, P., et al.: Extracorporeal membrane oxygenation and conventional medical therapy in neonates with persistent pulmonary hypertension of the newborn: A prospective randomized study. *Pediatrics, 84*(6):957-963, 1989.

Remenapp, R., WinklerPrins, A., and Mossberg, I.: Nursing care of the patient on ECMO. In K. Van Meurs, K.P. Lally, G. Peek, and J.B. Zwischenberger (Eds.): *ECMO: Extracorporeal cardiopulmonary support in critical care* (3rd ed.). Ann Arbor, 2005, Extracorporeal Life Support Organization, pp. 595-607.

Sheehan, A.: Bedside nursing care and ECMO specialist responsibilities. In K. Van Meurs (Ed.): *ECMO specialist training manual* (2nd ed.). Ann Arbor, 1999, Extracorporeal Life Support Organization, pp. 199-206.

UK Neonatal ECMO Trial Group: UK collaborative randomized trial of neonatal extracorporeal membrane oxygenation. *Lancet, 348*(9020):75-82, 1996.

Van Meurs, K.P., Hintz, S.R., and Sheehan, A.M.: ECMO for neonatal respiratory failure. In K. Van Meurs, K.P. Lally, G. Peek, and J. Zwischenberger (Eds.): *ECMO: Extracorporeal cardiopulmonary support in critical care* (3rd ed.). Ann Arbor, 2005, Extracorporeal Life Support Organization, pp. 273-295.

28 Cardiovascular Disorders

SHARYL L. SADOWSKI

OBJECTIVES

1. Describe how to differentiate between cyanosis that is cardiac in origin and that which is pulmonary in origin.
2. Name the major classifications of congenital heart disease; list two anomalies in each.
3. Discuss the link between congenital heart disease and genetics, including use of available tests.
4. Define and describe the anatomy, clinical manifestations, and the possible medical and/or surgical treatment of tetralogy of Fallot (TOF), coarctation of the aorta, patent ductus arteriosus (PDA), ventricular septal defect (VSD), atrial septal defect (ASD), and hypoplastic left heart syndrome (HLHS).
5. Describe the basic medical rationale for care of the newborn infant with a suspected or identified cardiac defect.
6. Describe basic surgical rationale for treatment of major cardiovascular defects.
7. List signs and symptoms of congenital heart abnormalities in the newborn infant.
8. Discuss available diagnostic modalities and the congenital cardiac defects they are used to diagnose.
9. List the signs and symptoms of PDA and the current medical, transcatheter, and surgical interventions.
10. Discuss the treatment modalities used in congestive heart failure, including the risks and benefits to the neonate.
11. Define the three classifications of shock, and list one cause under each category.
12. Discuss the major complications and sequelae of open-heart surgery and list two factors that contribute to the sequelae.

■ ■ Until the 20th century, there was limited clinical interest in congenital heart disease. In the majority of cases, the cardiac anomaly was incompatible with life; in the others, no treatment existed either to remedy the condition or to relieve its symptoms. Today, with advances in treatment of congenital heart defects (CHDs), the survival and quality of life of infants with congenital heart disease have markedly improved. There are a million adults now living with complex CHD that required surgery in the neonatal period (Wernovsky, 2005).

Advances in fetal echocardiography have resulted in a significant increase in the prenatal diagnosis of many CHDs, allowing for extensive parental counseling, thus providing time for parents to make decisions about treatment prior to birth (Dorfman et al., 2008; Kaplan et al., 2005). In addition, advancements in echocardiography, angiography, and interventional catheterization, coupled with a more complete understanding of newborn physiology, have led to improvements in diagnostic capabilities with decreased risk. In addition, newer surgical techniques that may limit time spent in deep hypothermia with circulatory arrest or on continuous cardiopulmonary bypass (CPB) permits the total correction of many forms of CHDs in the neonatal period (Zannini and Borini, 2007). In some cases, early intervention is essential to prevent long-term morbidity or early death (Ades and Wernovsky, 2005).

Whereas these advances have allowed for correction of many CHDs with dramatic decreases in mortality, long-term outcomes have been identified as neurodevelopmental morbidities. Multiple clinical trials reported in the literature substantiate earlier findings of neurodevelopmental impairments in patients following neonatal surgery (Gaynor and Wernovsky, 2005). Although overall intelligence has been spared, only 21% of school-age patients function at age-appropriate levels, 37% have moderate disabilities, and 6% have severe disabilities. The disabilities were identified as motor and cognitive impairments, including speech and language delays, gross and fine motor deficiencies, and visual–motor delays.

Many studies have linked these outcomes with the deep hypothermic cardiac arrest and continuous cardiopulmonary bypass that is used during open-heart surgery. In the past few years, pediatric heart surgeons have begun to perform some of these procedures using minimally invasive techniques, and on "beating" hearts, circumventing the need for circulatory arrest. It remains to be seen if this approach will improve the adverse neurodevelopmental outcomes presently linked to open-heart surgery in the neonatal period.

CARDIOVASCULAR EMBRYOLOGY AND ANATOMY
Cardiac Development
Fetal cardiac development occurs rapidly from day 18 to the 12th week of fetal life (Collins-Nakai and McLaughlin, 2002).

A. **Cardiac tube.**
   1. Heart development is first identified at 18 to 19 days of fetal life with formation of a heart tube (Table 28-1; Fig. 28-1, *A*).
   2. The heart tube elongates and develops dilatations and contractions that will later form the ventricles, bulbus cordis, and outflow tracts (Fig. 28-1, *B*).
   3. The pairs of aortic arches develop from the cephalic, extracardial portion of the heart tube. The caudal end will form the early ventricle (Fig. 28-1, *C*).
   4. Abnormal development during this time will include corrected transposition and dextrocardia (Collins-Nakai and McLaughlin, 2002).

B. **Cardiac septation:** begins in the middle of the fourth week and is complete by the end of the fifth week of fetal life (Fig. 28-1, *D*).
   1. Atrial septum and foramen ovale are formed from two septa and endocardial cushions.
      a. Atrial septum primum is formed by unidirectional growth from the top of the atrium toward the endocardial cushions, resulting in formation of the septum.
      b. A second septum (septum secundum) appears to the right of the septum primum and grows to overlap the ostium secundum. Thus the flapped opening, the foramen ovale, is created (Fig. 28-2).
   2. Ventricular septation results from fusion of the endocardial cushions and dilation and fusion of the ventricles (Fig. 28-3).

■ TABLE 28-1
■ ■ **Timeline for Fetal Heart Development**

Age (Days)	Cardiovascular Morphogenesis
18	Angiogenic tissue appears
19 to 20	Endothelial heart tubes appear
21	Fusion of endothelial heart tubes
23 to 25	Differentiation of atria, ventricle, and bulbus cordis; heart begins to beat
25	Fusion of atria, dorsal mesocardium regresses, formation of bulboventricular loop
26 to 27	Circulation is established
32	Appearance of septum primum
33	Intraventricular septum begins to form
35	Foramen secundum present
36 to 37	Fusion of atrial endocardial cushions
43	Ridges form in the bulbus cordis
46	Closure of ventricular septum, formation of coronary arteries
47	Septum secundum appears

Data from Collins-Nakai, R. and McLaughlin, P.: How congenital heart disease originates in life. *Cardiology Clinics*, *20*(3):367-383, 2002; Park, M.K.: *Pediatric cardiology for practitioners* (5th ed.). Philadelphia, 2008, Mosby; Theorell, C.: Cardiovascular assessment of the newborn. *Newborn and Infant Nursing Reviews*, *2*(2):111-127, 2002.

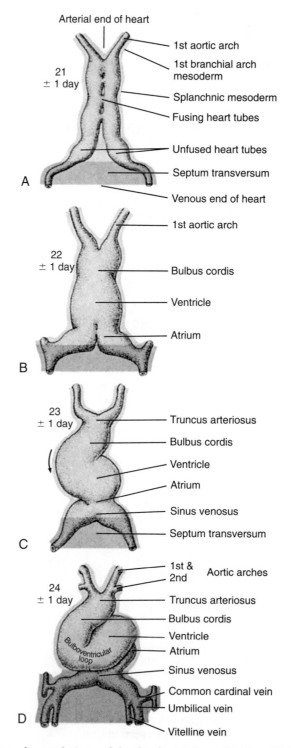

FIGURE 28-1 ■ Sketches of ventral views of the developing heart (at 20 to 25 days), showing fusion of endocardial heart tubes to form a single heart tube. Bending of the heart tube to form a bulboventricular loop is also illustrated. (Adapted from Moore, K.L. and Persaud, T.V.N.: *The developing human: Clinically oriented embryology* [8th ed.]. Philadelphia, 2008, Saunders.)

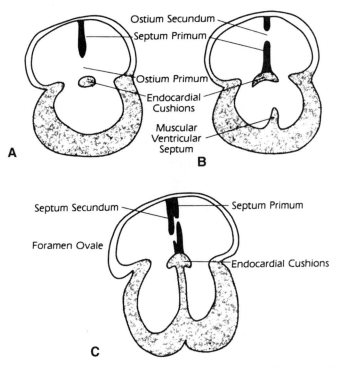

FIGURE 28-2 ■ Atrial septation. **A,** Septum primum begins to form, extending toward endocardial cushion (note ostium primum). **B,** Ostium primum is closed and perforation (called ostium secundum) forms in the septum primum. **C,** Septum secundum forms, creating the foramen ovale. (From Hazinski, M.F.: Congenital heart disease in the neonate. *Neonatal Network, 21*[3]:31-42, 1983.)

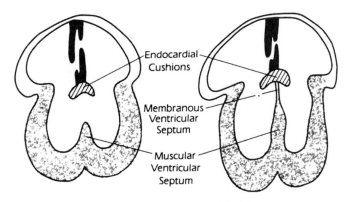

FIGURE 28-3 ■ Ventricular septation (with muscular and membranous septum). (From Hazinski, M.F.: Congenital heart disease in the neonate. *Neonatal Network, 21*[3]:31-42, 1983.)

3. Tissue of endocardial cushion forms the atrioventricular valves (Fig. 28-4).
   a. Tricuspid valve: between right atrium and ventricle.
   b. Mitral valve: between left atrium and ventricle.
4. Abnormal development during cardiac septation can lead to the following:
   a. VSD, ASD, and endocardial cushion defect (atrioventricular canal).
   b. Absence, deformation, stenosis, or atresia of the tricuspid and/or mitral valves.

Great Vessel Development

A. Single vessel (truncus arteriosus) extends from the ventricles until the fourth week of fetal life. It will then separate into the aorta and the pulmonary artery (Fig. 28-5).

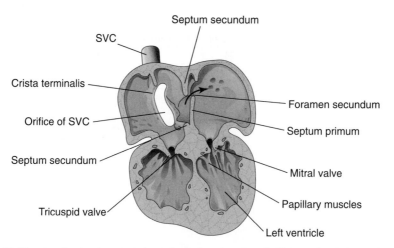

FIGURE 28-4 ■ The developing heart at about 8 weeks, showing the heart after it is partitioned into four chambers. Arrow indicates flow of well-oxygenated blood from right to left atrium. (From Moore, K.L. and Persaud, T.V.N.: *The developing human: Clinically oriented embryology* (8th ed.). Philadelphia, 2008, Saunders.)

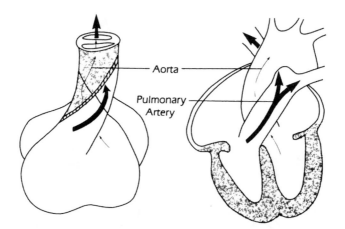

FIGURE 28-5 ■ Closing of the truncus arteriosus and division into the pulmonary artery and aorta. (From Hazinski, M.F.: Congenital heart disease in the neonate. *Neonatal Network, 21*[3]:31-42, 1983.)

1. The semilunar valves (aortic and pulmonic valves) develop from three ridges of tissue at the opening to the aorta and pulmonary trunk.

B. **Development of aorta and aortic branches** (Table 28-2). The truncus arteriosus connects with the aortic sac, which in turn connects with the paired aortic branches. A series of six paired aortic arches then form in succession (Fig. 28-6).
   1. The third arches become part of the common carotid arteries.
   2. The right fourth arch becomes the proximal portion of the right subclavian artery.
   3. The left fourth arch becomes the aortic arch segment between the left common carotid artery and left subclavian artery.
   4. The left sixth arch becomes part of the left pulmonary artery and the ductus arteriosus.
   5. The right sixth arch forms the right pulmonary artery.
   6. Abnormalities include interrupted aortic arch and coarctation of the aorta.

C. **Developmental abnormalities of truncal septation include** (Collins-Nakai and McLaughlin, 2002):
   1. Truncus arteriosus.
   2. TOF.
   3. Pulmonary and/or aortic valve atresia or stenosis.

■ TABLE 28-2
■ ■ **Development of Aorta and Aortic Branches**

Embryonic Vessel	Results In
Truncus arteriosus	Aorta and pulmonary artery
First pair of aortic arches	Pieces remain as stapedial arteries
Second pair of aortic arches	Pieces remain as stapedial arteries
Third pair of aortic arches	Common carotid arteries and proximal portion of internal carotid arteries
Fourth pair of aortic arches	
Right	Proximal portion of the right subclavian artery
Left	Aortic arch segment between left common carotid and left subclavian artery
Fifth pair of aortic arches	Regresses totally
Sixth pair of aortic arches	
Left	Proximal portion of the left pulmonary artery and ductus arteriosus
Right	Proximal portion of the right pulmonary artery

Data from Collins-Nakai, R. and McLaughlin, P.: How congenital heart disease originates in life. *Cardiology Clinics, 20*(3):367-383, 2002; Park, M.K.: *Pediatric cardiology for practitioners* (5th ed.). Philadelphia, 2008, Mosby; Theorell, C.: Cardiovascular assessment of the newborn. *Newborn and Infant Nursing Reviews, 2*(2):111-127, 2002.

4. Transposition of the great vessels (dextroposition).
5. Double-outlet right ventricle.

Circulatory Development

A. **Heart contractions begin around 21 days**; the atrium and ventricle muscle layers are continuous. Contractions result in a rhythmic peristalsis.
B. **Electrical conduction system** is functional around 10 weeks, with normal sinus rhythm seen by 16 weeks (Blackburn, 2007).
C. **Establishment of fetal circulation:** With completion of atrial and ventricular septation, development of valves between chambers and outflow tracks, and separation of the truncus arteriosus into the great vessels, fetal circulation is established.
D. **Fetal circulation is anatomically and physiologically different from adult circulation**, and adaptation after birth is necessary (Blackburn, 2007). For a full discussion of fetal circulation and cardiopulmonary adaptation at birth, see Chapter 4.

Cardiovascular Physiology

A. **Normal circulation** (see Fig. 4-2).
   1. Oxygen-poor blood enters the right atrium and passes through the tricuspid valve into the right ventricle, where it is pumped through the pulmonary artery to the lungs.
   2. As the blood flows through the lungs, it gives up carbon dioxide and gains oxygen.
   3. Oxygen-rich blood returns from the lungs through the pulmonary veins. It enters the left atrium and then passes through the mitral valve into the left ventricle, which pumps it through the aortic valve and into the aorta.
   4. The aorta then delivers oxygenated blood to all body organs and tissues.
B. **Cardiac depolarization:**
   1. Results from the electrical discharge across the myocardial cell (total net movement of ions across the cell wall) and is measured by the electrocardiograph (ECG).
   2. Shortening of muscle fibers (contraction) usually follows cardiac depolarization. Strength of cardiac (ventricular) contraction is measured by blood pressure or arterial pulse palpation.
   3. Cardiac electrical activity does not ensure adequate cardiac function.
      a. Congenital defects or surgical injury to the conduction system may result in arrhythmias or heart block.

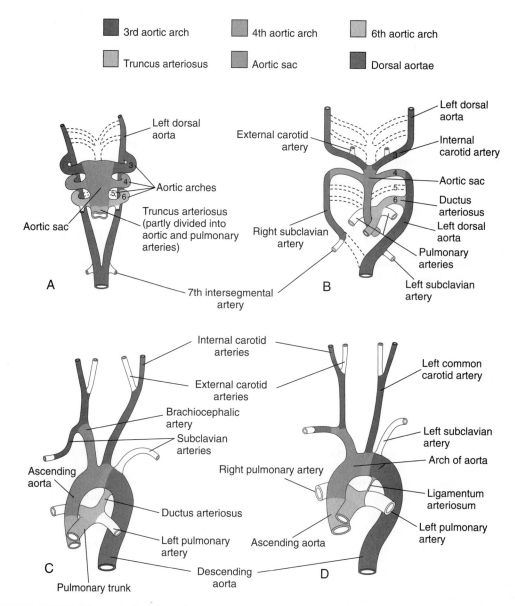

FIGURE 28-6 ■ Schematic drawings illustrating arterial changes that result during transformation of the truncus arteriosus, aortic sac, aortic arches, and dorsal aortas into the adult arterial pattern. **A**, Aortic arches at 6 weeks. **B**, Aortic arches at 7 weeks. **C**, Arterial arrangement at 8 weeks. **D**, Sketch of arterial vessels of 6-month-old infant. (From Moore, K.L. and Persaud, T.V.N.: *The developing human: Clinically oriented embryology* [8th ed.]. Philadelphia, 2008, Saunders.)

    b. Electrolyte disturbance (i.e., altered fluid composition surrounding the cells) can affect electrical activity.
        (1) Hypokalemia and hyperkalemia.
        (2) Hypocalcemia and hypercalcemia.
        (3) Hypoxia.
        (4) Acidosis.
C. Cardiac output.
    1. Cardiac output is the volume of blood ejected by the heart in 1 minute. Approximations vary from 120 to 200 ml/kg/minute.

2. Cardiac output = stroke volume × heart rate (in liters per minute).
   a. As heart rate fluctuates, so will cardiac output.
      (1) Normal term newborn heart rate is 120 to 160 beats per minute (bpm), although it may range from 70 to 180 bpm on an individual basis (Gardner and Johnson, 2006).
      (2) Significant or persistent bradycardia will result in a drop in the neonate's cardiac output.
   b. Tachycardia seems to be an effective mechanism for improving cardiac output as long as the tachycardia does not compromise diastolic filling time and decrease coronary artery perfusion.
3. Stroke volume is relatively fixed at 1.5 ml/kg and is affected by three factors: preload, contractility, and afterload.
   a. Preload: the volume of blood in the ventricles before contraction.
      (1) Clinically, preload is a measurement of pressure, rather than volume, in the ventricles before contraction.
      (2) Increasing the volume in the ventricles, consequently lengthening the myocardial fibers before contraction, should result in improved stroke volume (Frank–Starling law). The newborn infant is capable of increasing stroke volume provided there is no increase in systemic vascular resistance or rapid rise in aortic pressure. Given the neonate's smaller contractile mass, less compliant myocardium, and normal maximization of myocardial fiber length, volume infusions are likely to increase aortic pressure and afterload, resulting in a decline in stroke volume (Wernovsky et al., 2005).
   b. Contractility: speed of ventricular contraction.
      (1) Cardiac cycle consists of ventricular contraction (systole), followed by ventricular relaxation (diastole). As contraction time decreases, relaxation time (diastole) increases, with an increase in ventricular filling volume (preload) before contraction.
      (2) Ventricular contractility cannot be directly measured. Measurements of cardiac shortening fractions and ejection fraction provide an indirect assessment of contractility.
      (3) Contractility in neonates is influenced by the following:
         (a) Exogenous catecholamine (dopamine/dobutamine) use, which increases blood pressure and cardiac output.
         (b) Factors that decrease contractility:
            (i) Acidosis, which impairs myocardial response to catecholamines.
            (ii) Hypoxia.
            (iii) Electrolyte disturbances.
            (iv) Hypoglycemia.
   c. Afterload: the resistance to blood leaving the ventricle.
      (1) Dependent on systemic vascular resistance (SVR) and pulmonary vascular resistance (PVR); if SVR or PVR increases, afterload increases.
      (2) The neonate's myocardium is very sensitive to increased afterload; with small increases in afterload, stroke volume can fall significantly.
      (3) Afterload can be reduced by intravenous (IV) infusion of vasodilators (e.g., nitroglycerin, amrinone, and nitroprusside). Dobutamine can be used to decrease PVR (Young and Mangum, 2008).
4. Concepts of blood flow.
   a. Flow is directly proportional to pressure/resistance.
   b. Blood flow will always take the path of least resistance.
   c. If heart action (pressure) remains unchanged but vasoconstriction or dilation or obstruction to flow (resistance) changes, flow will change (i.e., cardiac output will vary).
   d. PVR starts to fall by almost 80% after delivery resulting in a dramatic increase in pulmonary blood flow and subsequent increase in systolic blood pressure (Blackburn, 2007). This normal decline is influenced by prematurity, low birth weight, and hypoxia episodes.

CONGENITAL HEART DEFECTS

Occurrence

A. **Incidence:** 6 to 8:1000 live births (<1%) (Wechsler and Wernovsky, 2004). According to Glickstein (2007), the incidence in premature infants is 12.5:1000 live births excluding isolated ASD and PDA.
   1. 85% of cases are due to multifactorial causes.
   2. 10% to 12% are due to chromosomal factors.
   3. 1% to 2% are due to genetic factors.
   4. 1% to 2% are due to exposure to maternal or environmental teratogens (Lott, 2007).
B. **Genetic factors:** Chromosomal abnormalities: overall incidence of CHD in patients with a chromosome aberration is 30%. Isolated cardiac defects result from multiple genes and their interaction with factors in the environment. Advances in technology have identified genetic factors for many of these defects.
   1. Incidence of CHD varies with chromosomal abnormality. Syndromes with an entire extra chromosome or syndromes with a missing chromosome are detected with normal chromosomal studies (Beck and Hudgins, 2003):
      a. Trisomy 21: 40% to 50%.
      b. Trisomy 18: 90% to 100%.
      c. Trisomy 13: 90%.
      d. Turner syndrome: 25% to 45% (45,X0 karyotype or mosaic 46,XX).
   2. Syndromes requiring fluorescence in situ hybridization (FISH) analysis include those with mosaicism and those with deletions in a chromosome.
      a. Chromosome deletion syndromes 18, 13, 5, and 4: 25% to 50%.
      b. Mosaic Turner's syndrome: X and Y chromosome. FISH probe needed to rule out Y chromosome (Bishara and Clericuzio, 2008).
   3. Microdeletions that are detected through FISH:
      a. 22q11 deletion syndrome: 80% to 85%.
      b. Williams syndrome: 50% to 70% (deletion of elastin gene at 7q11.23).
      c. Alagille syndrome: 90% (JAGI deletion on 20p12).
      d. Noonan syndrome: >50% (12q24.1, PTPN11 gene).
      e. DiGeorge deletion: 50% (22q11.2).
   4. Single-mutant-gene syndromes: 1% to 2% of all cardiovascular abnormalities in newborn infants. Both autosomal dominant and recessive syndromes have been associated with CHD. According to Bishara and Clericuzio (2008), the tests for these syndromes include gene mutation analysis via array comparative genomic hybridization (aCGH). This type of testing can detect smaller imbalances in the genome, allowing for detection of mutations, insertions, deletions, and imprinting abnormalities.
      a. Holt–Oram syndrome: >85% to 95% (TBX5 gene found at 12q24.1).
      b. X-linked situs inversus Xq25, ZIC3 gene.
      c. Kartagener syndrome (Fleiner, 2006): 100% (DNAI1 on 9p21-p13, DNAH5 on 5p15-p14).
      d. Beckwith–Wiedemann syndrome: 10% to 35%, imprinting defects of KIP2/LIT1 and paternal IGF2 genes at 11p15.5 (Jonas and Demmer, 2007).
   5. Multifactorial: approximately 90% due to genetic predisposition coupled with a causative factor.
      a. Cornelia de Lange: approximately 30%.
      b. VACTERL (*V*ertebral anomalies, *A*nal atresia/stenosis, *C*ardiac defects: 50%, *T*racheo-*E*sophageal fistula, *R*adial defects, *L*imb anomalies) (Wechsler and Wernovsky, 2004).
      c. CHARGE (*C*oloboma, *H*eart defects: 50% to 70%, choanal *A*tresia, *R*estriction of growth and development, *G*enital anomalies, *E*ar anomalies) (Wechsler and Wernovsky, 2004).
   6. Genetic Counseling is done to evaluate cause and recurrence risk. The risk of having another child with a cardiac lesion is 3% to 4% if the cause is unknown (Beck and Hudgins, 2003). However, this risk may be as much as 13% higher in specific syndromes.

   a. DiGeorge syndrome: parents should be offered FISH deletion studies.
      (1) 7% of parents carry the deletion.
      (2) Recurrence risk is up to 50% (Bishara and Clericuzio, 2008).
      (3) Prenatal diagnosis in future pregnancies via CVS or amniocentesis, with FISH requested specifically.
   b. Trisomies 13, 18, and 21 all carry recurrence risk of 1%, and prenatal diagnosis in future pregnancies is done using CVS or amniocentesis. The recurrence risk for trisomy 21 increases after maternal age 40.
C. **Environmental factors and teratogens** can include fetal exposure to drug, chemical, infectious, or physical agents; maternal disease or altered metabolic state with the period of greatest risk at 14 to 50 days of fetal life (Lott, 2007).
   1. Cardiac teratogenesis is associated with maternal ingestion of the following:
      a. Thalidomide: dramatically illustrated the extraordinarily deleterious effects of prescribed drug on a developing fetus.
      b. Anticonvulsants: 2% to 3% of infants exposed to anticonvulsants will have associated congenital cardiac defects such as pulmonary stenosis, coarctation of the aorta, and PDA. Glickstein (2007) reports the following defects with use of specific anticonvulsants in pregnancy:
         (1) Phenytoin (fetal hydantoin syndrome): VSD, d-transposition of the great vessels (d-TGV), TOF, HLHS, pulmonary atresia, ASD, aortic stenosis, and pulmonic stenosis.
         (2) Carbamazepine (Tegretol): VSD, TOF.
         (3) Valproic acid: VSD, coarctation of the aorta, interrupted aortic arch, TOF, HLHS, aortic stenosis, ASD, pulmonary atresia.
         (4) Trimethadione (fetal trimethadione syndrome): VSD, TGV, TOF, HLHS, double-outlet right ventricle, pulmonary atresia, ASD, aortic stenosis, pulmonic stenosis.
         (5) Pentobarbital: no confirmed specific embryopathy but may potentiate the effects of other drugs taken concurrently.
      c. Anticoagulants.
         (1) Warfarin (Coumadin): abortion or fetal embryopathic development in weeks 6 to 9 of gestation. Cardiac malformations have been identified, but no consistent cardiac defect has been noted.
         (2) Heparin: because of its larger molecular weight, does not cross the placenta.
      d. Antineoplastic medications.
         (1) Aminopterin: cardiac manifestations include dextroposition but are not as prominent as other defects resulting from drug ingestion.
         (2) In general, the disorders for which antineoplastic agents are used are serious enough to preclude pregnancy (Glickstein, 2007).
      e. Lithium: approximately 10% of infants exposed will have defects such as Ebstein anomaly, ASD, and tricuspid atresia.
      f. Retinoic acid: aortic arch abnormalities, other congenital heart malformations.
      g. Isotretinoin.
      h. Alcohol: fetal alcohol syndrome (FAS) is accompanied by a variety of cardiac lesions (e.g., VSD with or without subpulmonic and subaortic stenosis, ASD, coarctation of the aorta, TOF.
      i. Amphetamine: 5% to 10% will have congenital cardiac defects such as VSD, PDA, ASD, and TGV (Knight and Washington, 2006).
   2. Exposure to environmental hazards such as radiation, heat, and gases may produce teratogenic effects, but there are no specific associated cardiac malformations.
D. **Maternal disease and viral infections** (Box 28-1).
   1. Women with diabetes mellitus, especially insulin-dependent, have a 5 times greater risk of their children being born with cardiac anomalies than the general population of pregnant women have. Disorders include hypertrophy of the septum and myocardium, VSD, double-outlet right ventricle, TGV, truncus arteriosus, and coarctation of the aorta.
   2. Maternal lupus erythematosus may be linked to complete congenital heart block and dilated cardiomyopathy.

■ BOX 28-1
■ CLASSIFICATION OF MATERNAL DISEASES AFFECTING THE FETAL CARDIOVASCULAR SYSTEM

Category I: Maternal Diseases That Directly Affect the Fetal Cardiovascular System (Excluding Teratogenic Effects)
Pheochromocytoma
Hyperthyroidism
Diabetes mellitus
Collagen vascular disease (e.g., Ro antibody)
Rubella
Cytomegalovirus
Enterovirus infection
Toxoplasmosis
Listeriosis
Maternal group B streptococcal colonization with fetal invasion
Syphilis
Inherited metabolic diseases

Category II: Maternal Diseases That May Indirectly Affect the Fetal Cardiovascular System as a Result of Abnormalities of Uteroplacental Function
Neoplastic diseases
Diabetes mellitus
Maternal cardiac disease
Anemia (including the hemoglobinopathies)
Hypertensive disorders
Collagen vascular disease (e.g., lupus anticoagulant and systemic lupus erythematosus)
Renal disease (associated with hypertension)
Asthma
Cholestatic jaundice of pregnancy
Cytomegalovirus
Bacterial infections

From Katz, V. and Bowes, W.: Maternal diseases affecting the fetal cardiovascular system. In W. Long (Ed.): *Fetal and neonatal cardiology.* Philadelphia, 1990, Saunders, p. 135.

3. Rubella and cytomegalovirus produce clinically significant heart disease (Knight and Washington, 2006). Disorders seen are PDA, pulmonary stenosis and branch pulmonary artery stenosis, VSD, and ASD.

4. Maternal obesity has been recently linked to congenital heart disease (Glickstein, 2007).

RISK ASSESSMENT AND APPROACH TO DIAGNOSIS OF CARDIAC DISEASE

Sex Preferences Associated with Cardiac Lesions

A. Males.
   1. Coarctation of the aorta.
   2. Aortic stenosis.
   3. TGV.
   4. HLHS.
B. Females.
   1. ASD.
   2. PDA.

History (Knight and Washington, 2006)

A. **Gestational age.**
   1. Preterm. Infants born prematurely are much more likely to have pulmonary problems resulting in cyanosis than to have congestive heart failure (CHF), but they do have a higher incidence of:
      a. PDA.
      b. Left-to-right shunts (e.g., VSD or atrioventricular canal).
   2. Term. The majority of infants with CHF are term infants.
B. **Maternal history** (see Box 28-1).
   1. Infants of mothers with uncontrolled diabetes have an increased risk of
      a. TGV,
      b. VSD,
      c. Cardiomyopathy, or
      d. Complex congenital heart disease.
   2. Lupus may cause congenital heart block and cardiomyopathy.
   3. Viral and bacterial illnesses may directly and indirectly affect the fetal cardiovascular system.
   4. Seizures or coagulation disorders can be linked to congenital heart defects because the medications used may be teratogens.
   5. Maternal congenital heart disease can lead to an increased risk of same defect in infant.
   6. Maternal age greater than 35 years increases risk.
   7. Alcohol consumption: increase in cardiac defects seen with FAS.
C. **Familial.**
   Incidence of congenital heart defects increases by 3- to 4-fold when a first-order relative (parent or sibling) has CHD (Park, 2008). Risk increases by 10-fold if two first-order relatives have congenital heart disease (Table 28-3).
D. **Perinatal history.**
   1. Intrauterine growth pattern and birth weight.
   2. Prenatal diagnosis with ultrasound.
   3. Mode of delivery.
      a. Vaginal delivery most common for CHD, and initial Apgar scores are usually good.
      b. History of cesarean section and poor Apgar scores more indicative of asphyxia and respiratory distress.

Clinical Presentation

A. **Cyanosis** (in the first week may be sole evidence of a heart lesion).
   1. With cardiovascular problems, cyanosis is unexpected or gradual in onset.
   2. Cyanosis observation.
      a. Dependent on hemoglobin levels; at least 5 g of desaturated hemoglobin/dl is necessary before cyanosis becomes apparent.
      b. Will be influenced by presence of anemia or polycythemia and the levels of 2,3-diphosphoglycerate.
   3. Differentiation between central and peripheral cyanosis.
      a. Peripheral or acrocyanosis results from sluggish movement of blood through the extremities and increased tissue oxygen extraction.
         (1) Persists from birth and can last several days.
         (2) Does not involve mucous membranes.
         (3) May be caused by peripheral vasomotor instability.
      b. Central cyanosis results from desaturated blood leaving the heart.
         (1) Seen as bluish discoloration of tongue and mucous membranes, reflecting arterial desaturation.
         (2) Central cyanosis may present difficulties in making a differential diagnosis between respiratory and cardiac origin.

■ TABLE 28-3
■ ■ Familial Recurrence Risks

Cardiac Anomaly	Family Member with Congenital Heart Defect	Risk (%)
PDA—patent ductus arteriosus	Mother	3.5 to 4
	Father	2.5
	Sibling	3
VSD—ventricular septal defect	Mother	6
	Father	2
	Sibling	3
ASD—atrial septal defect	Mother	4 to 4.5
	Father	1.5
	Sibling	2.5
AVC—atrioventricular canal	Mother	14
	Father	1
	Sibling	2
Tetralogy of Fallot	Mother	6 to 10
	Father	1.5
	Sibling	2.5
Aortic stenosis	Mother	13 to 18
	Father	3
	Sibling	2
Pulmonary stenosis	Mother	4 to 6.5
	Father	2
	Sibling	2
Coarctation of the aorta	Mother	4
	Father	2
	Sibling	2
Other defects (TGA, tricuspid atresia, truncus arteriosus, HLHS)	Sibling	1.4 (average)

HLHS, Hypoplastic left heart syndrome; *TGA*, transposition of the great arteries.
Data from Park, M.K.: *Pediatric cardiology for practitioners* (5th ed.). Philadelphia, 2008, Mosby; Theorell, C.: Cardiovascular assessment of the newborn. *Newborn and Infant Nursing Reviews, 2*(2):111-127, 2002.

B. **Respiratory pattern.**
  1. Useful in the differentiation of cyanosis.
  2. Tachypnea (respiratory rate >60) without dyspnea is an important, often subtle, clue to cardiac anomalies. In the absence of cyanosis, it may indicate a left-to-right shunt lesion. Tachypnea is significant if coupled with feeding difficulty. It is suggestive of CHF if the infant must stop feeding to catch its breath.
  3. Hyperpnea (increased respiratory depth) is observed in congenital heart lesions resulting in diminished pulmonary blood flow.
  4. Crying may exacerbate cyanosis in neonates with CHD because of increased oxygen consumption by the tissues.
C. **Heart sounds.**
  1. First heart sound (S_1) represents closure of the mitral and tricuspid valves at the onset of ventricular systole.
    a. Best heard at the fourth intercostal space in the left midclavicular line (mitral) and at the fourth intercostal space at the sternal borders (tricuspid).
    b. S_1 is accentuated with the following:
      (1) Increased cardiac output.
      (2) Increased flow across atrioventricular valves.
      (3) Specific conditions such as the following:
        (a) PDA.
        (b) VSD with increased mitral flow.

      (c) Total anomalous pulmonary venous return (TAPVR).

      (d) Arteriovenous malformation.

      (e) TOF.

      (f) Anemia.

      (g) Fever.

  c. Conditions decreasing S_1 include the following:

    (1) Decreased atrioventricular conduction.

    (2) CHF.

    (3) Myocarditis.

2. Second heart sound (S_2) occurs at the end of ventricular systole from closure of aortic and pulmonic valves.

  a. Heard best at upper left sternal border.

  b. Split S_2 is a normal occurrence, reflecting closure of aortic valve before the pulmonic valve.

    (1) Increases on inspiration.

    (2) Single S_2 is often heard in the first 2 days of life because of increased PVR.

    (3) Splitting of S_2 is influenced by:

      (a) Abnormalities of aortic or pulmonic valves.

      (b) Conditions altering PVR or SVR.

  c. Conditions widening the S_2 are influenced by the following:

    (1) ASD.

    (2) TAPVR.

    (3) TOF.

    (4) Pulmonary stenosis.

    (5) Ebstein anomaly.

  d. Absent S_2 splits occur in the following:

    (1) Pulmonary atresia and severe pulmonary stenosis.

    (2) Aortic stenosis/atresia.

    (3) Persistent pulmonary hypertension.

    (4) L-TGV.

    (5) Truncus arteriosus.

3. Third heart sound (S_3) is due to increased flow across the atrioventricular (AV) valves from rapid, passive ventricular filling from the atria.

  a. Follows S_2 and is a low-pitched, broad sound.

  b. Prominent in situations of increased atrioventricular flow and increased ventricular filling (Lott, 2007).

    (1) Left-to-right shunts (e.g., ASD, VSD, PDA).

    (2) Anemia.

    (3) Mitral valve insufficiency.

4. Fourth heart sound (S_4) occurs at the final phase of ventricular filling and active atrial contraction during late diastole.

  a. Occurs just before S_1 and is low pitched.

  b. Rarely heard in the newborn infant.

  c. Always pathologic and indicates decreased ventricular compliance.

5. Ejection clicks are heard as snapping sounds just after the first heart sound in the first 24 hours of life.

  a. Abnormal (except during first 24 hours of life) and indicate cardiac disease.

  b. Audible for short duration after S_1.

  c. Associated with dilation of the great vessels or deformity of aortic or pulmonic valve.

  d. Other conditions associated with ejection clicks include the following:

    (1) Aortic valve stenosis.

    (2) Truncus arteriosus.

    (3) TOF (severe).

    (4) Pulmonary valve stenosis.

    (5) HLHS.

    (6) Coarctation of the aorta.

6. Murmurs.

    a. Murmurs are audible vibrations resulting from turbulence of blood flow and may be due to

        (1) Abnormal valves,

        (2) Septal defects,

        (3) Regurgitated flow through incompetent valves, or

        (4) High blood flow across normal structures.

    b. Physiologic murmurs have been noted in 50% of neonates in the first 48 hours of life (Theorell, 2002). Generally, these murmurs are due to

        (1) Transient left-to-right flow via the ductus arteriosus,

        (2) Increased flow over the pulmonary valve associated with a fall in PVR, or

        (3) Mild bilateral peripheral pulmonary arterial stenosis because of size and pressure differences between the main pulmonary trunk and the left and right pulmonary arterial branches.

    c. Absence of murmur does not indicate absence of significant cardiac disease.

    d. Evaluation of murmurs includes the following:

        (1) Intensity of sound.

           (a) Murmurs are graded I through VI. Grade III or less generally present no hemodynamic problems (Lott, 2007).

              (i)   Grade I: barely audible, only after careful auscultation.

              (ii) Grade II: soft, easily audible on auscultation.

              (iii) Grade III: moderately loud, not associated with a thrill.

              (iv) Grade IV: loud murmur associated with a thrill.

              (v) Grade V: very loud. May be heard with stethoscope just touching the chest wall.

              (vi) Grade VI: extremely loud. Can be heard with stethoscope off the chest wall.

           (b) Presence of a thrill on palpation is associated with a loud murmur of at least grade 4.

        (2) Timing within cardiac cycle.

           (a) Systolic: heard during ventricular systole (i.e., between S_1 and S_2) or if feeling the pulse during auscultation, at the upstroke of the pulse.

              (i)   Identified as early, mid-, or late systolic.

              (ii) Pansystolic (holosystolic): heard throughout systole. Heard in mitral or tricuspid insufficiency and VSD.

              (iii) Ejection murmurs: turbulence of blood flow leaving the heart; noted in aortic or pulmonic valve stenosis, TOF, ASD, and TAPVR. The majority of innocent murmurs are systolic ejection murmurs (Lott, 2007).

           (b) Diastolic: heard during period of ventricular filling (i.e., between S_2 and S_1) and are usually indicative of a cardiac disorder.

              (i)   Early: results from aortic or pulmonic valve insufficiency.

              (ii) Mid: increased blood flow across normal mitral or tricuspid valve.

              (iii) Late: associated with stenotic mitral or tricuspid valve.

           (c) Continuous: audible throughout cardiac cycle but can be louder in systole or diastole (e.g., PDA).

        (3) Quality and pitch.

           (a) Pitch: reflects frequency of vibrations.

              (i)   High-pitched sound from turbulent blood flow from a high-pressure area to a low-pressure area. Generally reflects valve insufficiency on the left side of the heart, whereas a low-pitched sound reflects right-sided valve insufficiency.

              (ii) Low-pitched sound is from a low-pressure difference in turbulent blood flow reflecting right-sided valve insufficiency.

           (b) Quality is described as

              (i)   Harsh,

              (ii) Blowing, or

              (iii) Musical.

(4) Location: in terms of maximal intensity described by anatomic location on chest wall.

(5) Radiation if present.

D. Peripheral pulses (Knight and Washington, 2006).

1. Pulses should be synchronous with equal intensity.

2. Upper- and lower-extremity pulses should be palpated simultaneously and differences documented.

3. Discrepancies (e.g., pulses that are greater in upper than in lower extremities) raise the possibility of an abnormal aortic arch.

4. Right brachial artery pulse should be compared with pulses in lower extremities because the right subclavian is always preductal.

5. Pulse volume graded from 0 to 4.
   a. 0 = absent.
   b. 1+ = weak.
   c. 2+ = weak to average.
   d. 3+ = strong.
   e. 4+ = bounding.

6. Weak pulses indicate low cardiac output, as seen in
   a. Left heart outflow obstructive lesions,
   b. Myocardial failure, or
   c. Shock.

7. Bounding pulses indicate aortic runoff.
   a. PDA.
   b. Aortic insufficiency.
   c. Systemic to pulmonary shunts.

8. Visible precordial impulse persisting after the first 12 hours of life occurs in defects with volume overload and is suggestive of left-to-right shunt (Wechsler and Wernovsky, 2004).

E. Blood pressure.

1. Normal values are dependent on birth weight and gestational age. The mean arterial pressure (MAP) is reported as being the same as the gestational age of the infant (Seri and Evans, 2001).
   a. Healthy term infant: average systolic pressure is 56 to 77 mm Hg; average diastolic pressure is 33 to 50 mm Hg. MAP is 42 to 60 mm Hg (Sansoucie and Cavaliere, 2007).
   b. Premature infant's blood pressure varies with size and gestational age; the lower limit of the MAP is similar numerically to the gestational age for infants of 26 to 32 weeks of gestation. For neonates weighing less than 800 g, the MAP may be lower than the gestational age (Swinford et al., 2006).

2. Blood pressure values may also be affected by postnatal age, body temperature, infant's behavioral state, and cuff size.

3. Cuff width should be 25% greater than the width of the extremity. If the width is too narrow, the blood pressure will have a false high reading. If the cuff width is too wide, the blood pressure will have a false low reading (Swinford et al., 2006).

4. Compare upper- and lower-extremity pressures. Systolic blood pressure of the upper extremities 20 mm Hg above that of lower extremities is suggestive of the following:
   a. Coarctation of the aorta. PDA may mask these pressure differences.
   b. Aortic arch abnormalities.
      (1) In addition, blood pressure differences between the upper extremities are seen with aortic arch abnormalities.
      (2) To evaluate, simultaneously measure blood pressure in both arms and one leg. Either leg can be evaluated because the blood supply to both legs comes from the descending aorta below the level of the defect.

5. In a term infant, neonatal hypertension is defined as a systolic blood pressure greater than 90 mm Hg and a diastolic pressure greater than 60 mm Hg.
   a. In a premature infant, systolic pressure greater than 80 mm Hg and diastolic pressure greater than 50 mm Hg indicates hypertension.

    b. Structural and/or functional renal abnormalities are the most common causes of hypertension.

F. Congestive heart failure.

1. CHF is defined as inadequate delivery of oxygen by the heart (Lott, 2007) and is typically associated with congenital heart lesions. The timing of CHF appearance may assist in the diagnosis of the lesion (Knight and Washington, 2006).
2. Structural heart defects leading to a presentation of CHF symptoms:
    a. At birth:
    (1) HLHS.
    (2) Severe tricuspid or pulmonary regurgitation.
    (3) Large systemic arteriovenous fistula.
    b. First week of life:
    (1) TGA.
    (2) Premature infant with large PDA.
    (3) TAPVR below the diaphragm.
    c. 1 to 4 weeks of life:
    (1) Critical aortic or pulmonary stenosis.
    (2) Coarctation of the aorta.
3. Noncardiac causes.
    a. Birth asphyxia resulting in transient myocardial ischemia.
    b. Metabolic, including hypoglycemia and hypocalcemia.
    c. Severe anemia.
    d. Overhydration.
    e. Neonatal sepsis.
4. Primary myocardial disease.
    a. Myocarditis.
    b. Transient myocardial ischemia.
    c. Cardiomyopathy (seen in infants of diabetic mothers).
5. Disturbances in the heart rate.
    a. Supraventricular tachycardia.
    b. Atrial flutter or fibrillation.
    c. Congenital heart block.
6. Late-onset CHF may result from bronchopulmonary dysplasia or other pulmonary stressors (see Chapter 24).
7. Clinical presentation.
    a. Depends on the cause of the CHF and the age of the patient.
    (1) Newborns. CHF interferes with breathing and feeding, crying or stooling. Poor perfusion is the hallmark sign, with pale, cyanotic, or gray coloring, poor capillary refill, and diaphoresis. These newborns may take as long as 45 to 60 minutes to finish a feeding that should only take 10 to 15 minutes.
    b. Physical examination (Fleiner, 2006).
    (1) Respiratory rate greater than 60, tachypnea from interstitial pulmonary edema.
    (2) Heart rate. Tachycardia from compensation for decreased cardiac output; may have a gallop rhythm.
    (3) Four-limb blood pressure may yield a higher blood pressure in the right arm than in either leg, indicating an aortic obstruction.
    (4) Central or peripheral cyanosis may be a clue to poor perfusion.
    (5) Decreased peripheral pulses and mottling of extremities from redistribution of blood flow to vital tissues.
    (6) Precordium may be hyperactive.
    (7) Hepatomegaly.

Diagnostic Adjuncts

A. Arterial blood gas values are used primarily to help differentiate lung disease vs. heart disease as the cause of cyanosis.

1. Paco$_2$: generally normal in CHD and elevated in pulmonary parenchymal disease.
2. Hyperoxygen test: should be performed on all neonates with suspected CHD.
   a. Sample arterial Po$_2$ with infant breathing room air if tolerated. Have the patient breathe 100% oxygen for at least 10 minutes and repeat the arterial Po$_2$. Measurements should be at both pre- and postductal sites (Wechsler and Wernovsky, 2004).
      (1) Umbilical artery sample may detect right-to-left shunts via PDA. The lowered Pao$_2$ is usually a reflection of lung disease and not of primary heart disease.
      (2) Administration of oxygen to infants with cardiac disease resulting in high pulmonary blood flow and CHF will improve oxygen levels (i.e., increased Pao$_2$) through decreased PVR and increased pulmonary blood flow.
      (3) Most accurate assessment of cardiac vs. pulmonary disease can be made if the right radial or temporal (preductal) and umbilical artery samples (postductal) are taken simultaneously.
      (4) Monitoring of preductal and postductal transcutaneous oxygen pressure or pulse oximetry provides a noninvasive evaluation for cardiac versus pulmonary disease.
   b. Preductal Pao$_2$ will rise to greater than 100 mm Hg with pulmonary disease, whereas an increase to less than 100 mm Hg is consistent with cardiac disease. The response of arterial Po$_2$ in the hyperoxia test should be interpreted in view of the clinical picture (Hagedorn et al., 2006).

B. **Pulse oximetry is noninvasive and inexpensive.**
   1. The combination of pulse oximetry and clinical examination has a sensitivity of 76.9% and specificity of 99.9% in detecting CHD (Thangaratinam et al., 2007).

C. **Chest x-ray examination is used to** (Knight and Washington, 2006; Lott, 2007)
   1. Rule out pulmonary parenchymal disease,
   2. Identify increased pulmonary vascular markings, as seen in lesions with left-to-right shunting,
   3. Evaluate aortic arch, and
   4. Evaluate cardiac size, shape, and position (Wechsler and Wernovsky, 2004).
      a. Cardiomegaly: defined as cardiac/thoracic ratio greater than 0.6.
      b. See Chapter 14 for chest x-ray findings in heart disease.

D. **Electrocardiography.**
   1. Reflects abnormal hemodynamic burdens placed on the heart.
   2. Used to determine severity of disease by assessing the degree of atrial or ventricular hypertrophy. Right ventricular predominance is normal shortly after birth. (In utero the right ventricle does most of the cardiac work.)
   3. Changes in ST segments or T waves may suggest myocardial ischemia.
      a. Tall, peaked P waves are common in right-sided heart failure.
      b. Wide, notched P waves are seen with left-sided heart failure.
   4. ECG is the major diagnostic tool for evaluating arrhythmias and the impact of electrolyte imbalances (e.g., potassium and calcium) on electrical conductivity.
   5. Normal ECG values in term neonates (Flanagan et al., 2005; Knight and Washington, 2006):
      a. Heart rate: 120 to 160 bpm in first week.
      b. Normal sinus rhythm: P wave precedes QRS complex.
      c. P wave: duration 0.04 to 0.08 second.
      d. PR interval: 0.09 to 0.12 second. Prolonged interval is seen in first-degree heart block and is usually benign.
      e. Rightward deviation of the QRS complex with a maximum of −180° and duration of 0.03 to 0.07 second. Prolonged complex indicates interventricular conduction delay.
      f. Occasional Q waves in V1.
      g. Premature infants have higher resting heart rates with greater variation. Duration of P wave is shorter. PR and QRS intervals are decreased (0.10 and 0.04 second, respectively).

E. **Echocardiography** (Rychik and Cohen, 2005):
   1. Provides rapid, noninvasive, and relatively painless evaluation of cardiovascular anatomy and function by use of ultrasonic sound waves. Used to estimate pressures, measure

gradients, and evaluate cardiac function. Echocardiography is important in the overall assessment of disorders of the cardiac system that are unique to the neonate. The soft tissue and fluids that comprise the heart provide clear windows for cardiac imaging using echocardiography. Although advances in technology and decrease in size of transducers have increased the sensitivity of echocardiography, it does have some limitations.

a. There are three types of echocardiograms.
  (1) Transthoracic echo: most common.
  (2) Transesophageal echo: small transducer is placed in the esophagus in neonates weighing ≥2.5 kg. Used to visualize structures in the posterior chest such as the pulmonary veins. It is also used to guide interventional procedures.
  (3) Fetal echo: conducted on the pregnant mother to examine the fetal heart and major blood vessels for structural defects, and arrhythmias prior to birth. A family history of CHD, fetal abnormalities detected during routine obstetric ultrasound, abnormal amniocentesis, abnormal fetal heart rhythm, maternal insulin-dependent diabetes mellitus, and exposure to known teratogens are all indications for a fetal echocardiogram (Kaplan et al., 2005).

b. M-mode (single-dimension) echocardiography permits evaluation of anatomic relationships of heart and vessels, including relative sizes of each. It is also used to evaluate the motion of the cardiac valves and detect pericardial fluid. Most commonly used to determine ventricular function.

c. Two-dimensional (real-time) echocardiography has greater versatility, providing more specific information regarding anatomic relationships. This mode is used to diagnose PDA, or ventricular dysfunction in premature infants.

d. Color-flow Doppler echocardiography shows
  (1) Patterns of blood flow (i.e., right-to-left vs. left-to-right shunting),
  (2) Location of restrictions and/or regurgitation, and
  (3) Direction of motion, i.e., warm colors indicate movement toward the transducer and cool, away from the transducer.

e. Continuous-wave Doppler echocardiography shows the quantity of flow across an obstruction, giving an estimate of pressure gradients, which is beneficial in aortic, pulmonary, and mitral stenosis (Kipps and Silverman, 2005). It is used to detect the direction of shunting, to estimate cardiac output, and to assess ventricular diastolic function.

f. Contrast echocardiography is accomplished by rapid injection of sterile contrast solution, saline or dextrose in water solution in a vein while conducting an ultrasonographic examination. It allows for greater evaluation of flow patterns throughout the heart and identifies the presence of shunts.

g. 3-D echocardiography provides a great number of cross-sectional images. The newest technique in pediatric echocardiography is real-time 3-D, which enhances the ability to identify spatial relationships and can record a large amount of image data using limited examination times.

F. Magnetic resonance imaging (Knight and Washington, 2006):
  1. Three-dimensional, providing high-resolution images of the heart and great vessels. Used in conjunction with echocardiograms and cardiac catheterization to evaluate pulmonary arteries and veins, and systemic veins.

G. Cardiac catheterization (Kanter and Hellenbrand, 2005):
  1. The focus of this invasive procedure has changed over the past 10 to 15 years from a diagnostic modality to an interventional procedure. However, noninterventional cardiac catheterization remains an important tool in presurgical hemodynamic evaluation, and reevaluation of previously repaired defects and biopsies of transplanted hearts to detect rejection.
    a. Measures pulmonary artery pressure, detects pulmonary artery stenosis.
    b. May be used in palliative treatment (e.g., in the use of balloon atrial septostomy to treat TGV).
    c. Radiofrequency perforation of atrial septum and atretic valves.
    d. Balloon valvuloplasty.

   e. Acyanotic heart lesions; catheterization can be delayed until the full effect of medical management of CHF is seen.
   f. Treatment modalities during catheterization include coil placement to close the ductus arteriosus, placement of stents following balloon dilation of stenotic heart valves or narrow vessels, and implantation of devices to close ASDs and VSDs, as well as post cardiac transplant biopsy.
2. Procedure: advancement of a catheter through the umbilical, subclavian, femoral, or right internal jugular vessels and into the heart.
   a. If balloon septostomy is anticipated, a large vessel will be needed.
   b. Pressure measurements are made of all chambers and outlet tracts.
3. Concomitant angiography (injection of contrast medium): often performed to achieve maximal cardiac information.
4. Interventional techniques have replaced conventional surgery for many lesions.
   a. Objective is improvement or preservation of cardiac function and improvement in quality and quantity of life.
   b. Common procedures.
      (1) Dilation of valvular lesions (mitral stenosis).
      (2) Balloon valvuloplasty for critical aortic or pulmonary valve stenosis.
      (3) Dilation of coarctation of the aorta.
      (4) Dilation of pulmonary artery stenosis.
      (5) Balloon atrial septostomy.
      (6) Transcatheter defect occlusion for PDA.
      (7) Catheter-delivered devices for ASD closure and certain muscular VSD closures.
5. Complications.
   a. Mortality risk is related to the defect, severity of symptoms, and the patient's condition.
   b. High sodium content of contrast medium contributes to myocardial depression and exerts an osmotic effect, temporarily increasing intravascular volume.
   c. Hemorrhage with catheter insertion or removal may lead to
      (1) Hypotension,
      (2) Shock, and
      (3) Cardiac tamponade if bleeding is in the pericardial sac.
   d. Dysrhythmias are not uncommon (e.g., premature atrial and ventricular beats, heart block, and tachycardia), because of catheter manipulation.
   e. In infants younger than 4 months of age, the rate of nonfatal serious complications is 12%.
   f. Need for increased awareness of a possible link between diagnostic procedures using ionizing radiation and increase in biomarkers of genetic damage for carcinogenesis (Andreassi et al., 2006).

H. Laboratory data.
1. Complete blood cell count with differential cell count.
   a. Rules out anemia or polycythemia as cause of CHF.
   b. Decreased number of neutrophils and presence of left shift: possible indication of sepsis. Group β-hemolytic streptococci can mimic HLHS.
2. Blood glucose concentration. Used to evaluate hypoglycemia as potential cause of cardiomyopathy.
3. Electrolytes (especially potassium and calcium). Both potassium and calcium are major cations in electrical conductivity. Alterations can adversely affect cardiac contractility.

DEFECTS WITH INCREASED PULMONARY BLOOD FLOW

Patent ductus arteriosus: failure of the ductus arteriosus to close within 72 hours after birth.
A. **Incidence** (fourth most common lesion).
   1. Isolated PDA in term gestations: 1:2000 live births.
   2. In preterm gestations:
      a. Incidence is inversely related to gestational age and weight.
      b. Appears in 45% of infants weighing less than 1750 g at birth.

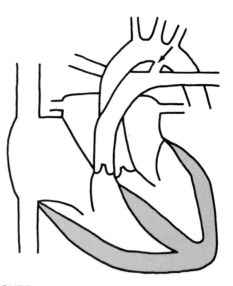

FIGURE 28-7 ■ Patent ductus arteriosus (PDA).

    c. Is apparent in 80% of infants weighing less than 1200 g at birth.

    d. Symptomatic PDA with CHF in 31% of premature infants with a birthweight (BW) of 500 to 1500 g (Knight and Washington, 2006; Lott, 2007).

  3. Occurs 3 times more commonly in females than in males.

B. Anatomy: persistent patency of the ductus arteriosus after birth (Fig. 28-7).

  1. In utero patency of this structure is functional, diverting blood to the placenta for gas exchange. About 90% of right ventricular outflow is through the ductus arteriosus.

  2. Persistent patency is influenced by several factors.

    a. Improvement in oxygenation causes the pulmonary vascular resistance to drop rapidly. Although increased oxygen tension is a potent stimulant of smooth muscle contraction, which should decrease patency, premature infants have an immature response to oxygen; thus the PDA remains open.

    b. Lack of ductal smooth muscle (e.g., in premature infants) prolongs patency.

    c. Prostaglandins inhibit closure of ductus.

C. Hemodynamics.

  1. As PVR falls and SVR rises, a left-to-right shunt via the PDA results in blood flow from the aorta into the pulmonary artery, increasing pulmonary blood flow. The increased pulmonary artery pressure and increased left ventricular pressure and volume lead to bilateral CHF.

  2. Because left-to-right flow is dependent on a drop in PVR, infants with pulmonary disease (e.g., respiratory distress syndrome) will show symptoms when lung disease improves. Before this time, PVR greater than SVR leads to a right-to-left shunt via the patent ductus (commonly referred to as persistent pulmonary hypertension of the neonate).

D. Clinical manifestations.

  1. Presents at 4 to 7 days of life with inability to wean from the ventilator or has a need for increased ventilatory and oxygen support. May present with apneic and/or bradycardic spells if not on a ventilator.

    a. Increased pulmonary vasculature and cardiomegaly.

    b. Bounding peripheral pulses and hyperactive precordium.

    c. Widening pulse pressure (>20 mm Hg).

    d. Low diastolic blood pressure.

    e. Unexplained metabolic acidosis.

  2. Continuous murmur may be present at the upper left sternal border but may be "silent" in 10% to 20% of the preterm infants despite hemodynamically significant shunt.

3. Radiographic findings consist of normal size or mild cardiomegaly (cardiothoracic ratio >0.60), pulmonary edema, and increased pulmonary vascularity. These "typical" signs may be absent if the infant is receiving positive-pressure ventilation.

4. Echocardiography is the gold standard for diagnosis. Two-dimensional echocardiography will provide anatomic information about the diameter, length, and shape of the ductus. Doppler flow will provide information on the ductal shunt magnitude and patterns (Dice and Bhatia, 2007).

5. B-type natriuretic peptide levels may be useful. Some studies have reported specificity of 73% and sensitivity of 93% using a cutoff value of 70 pg/ml (Dice and Bhatia, 2007).

E. **Management.**

1. Dependent on whether shunt is hemodynamically significant. In premature infants the PDA may prolong ventilator use beyond the dictates of the initial lung disease.

2. Hemodynamically significant ductus arteriosus includes the following:
    a. Heart rate greater than 170 bpm.
    b. Respiratory rate greater than 70 per minute.
    c. Hepatomegaly greater than 3 cm below costal margin.
    d. Bounding pulses.

3. Conservative measures are generally employed initially, which may minimize exposure to pharmacologic agents. However, delaying treatment may decrease response to nonsteroidal anti-inflammatory drugs.
    a. Fluid restriction.
    b. Diuretics: if employed with fluid restriction, may lead to electrolyte imbalance, dehydration, and caloric deprivation.
    c. Positive end-expiratory pressure: useful in reducing left-to-right shunt via PDA.

4. Medical management using a nonsteroidal anti-inflammatory agent that inhibits COX-1 and/or COX-2. Treatment choices are indomethacin and ibuprofen lysine, both manufactured by Ovation Pharmaceuticals, Inc. The cost of either drug is approximately $1800 for three doses, and the need for surgical intervention increases the treatment cost by approximately 77% (Turck et al., 2007). Ductal recurrence rate may approach 30% (Markham, 2006).
    a. Ibuprofen lysine gained FDA approval in 2006 for treatment of clinically significant PDA in neonates with birth weight 500 to 1500 g and GA ≤32 weeks at time medication is given (Overmeire, 2007). Inhibits both COX-1 and COX-2 enzymes but has less COX-1 inhibition than indomethacin.
        (1) Initial dose 10 mg/kg IV followed by two doses of 5 mg/kg at 24 and 48 hours after the first dose.
        (2) Significantly lower incidence of oliguria as compared to indomethacin (Hermes-DeSantis and Aranda, 2007).
        (3) Does not decrease cerebral blood flow (Corff and Sekar, 2007).
        (4) Does not reduce mesenteric blood flow (Capparelli, 2007).
        (5) According to Aranda and Thomas (2005), ibuprofen lysine is equally safe and effective as indomethacin, with maintenance of cerebral, mesenteric, and renal blood flow favoring ibuprofen lysine.
        (6) Monitor serum creatinine, BUN, platelet count, and urine output during treatment course.
    b. Indomethacin management includes the following:
        (1) As a prostaglandin inhibitor, indomethacin can constrict and close the PDA in some premature infants.
        (2) Initial dosage is 0.2 mg/kg IV, followed by 2 doses 0.1 mg/kg IV every 12 to 24 hours, for a total of three doses (Corff, 2007). An alternative long-course treatment is associated with an increased risk of NEC and is no longer recommended (Herrera et al., 2008).
        (3) Prophylactic treatment in the ELBW premature neonate in the first 24 hours after birth showed a decrease in IVH when compared to placebo (Markham, 2006).

(4) Complications related to indomethacin being a stronger COX-1 inhibitor are as follows:

(a) Transient oliguria and decreased renal blood flow.

(b) Increased incidence of gastrointestinal bleeding.

(c) Inhibition of platelet aggregation for 7 to 9 days, with potential for intracerebral hemorrhage.

(5) Contraindications are (Corff, 2007):

(a) Renal failure (blood urea nitrogen [BUN] concentration >30 mg/dl, serum creatinine concentration >1.8 mg/dl, urine output <0.5 ml/kg/hour).

(b) Active bleeding.

(c) Suspected NEC.

(d) Thrombocytopenia.

(e) Sepsis: suspected or proven.

5. Surgical management: ligation of the PDA.

   a. Standard approach is surgical ligation via posterolateral thoracotomy incision risk.

   b. New techniques include placement of a stainless-steel spring coil or Amplatzer PDA occlusion device via interventional cardiac catheterization with complete occlusion rates of approximately 90% 24 hours after the procedure and 98% at 6 months. Minimally invasive video-assisted thoracoscopic surgery allows for PDA closure using two titanium clips that are placed using a trocar (Dutta and Albanese, 2006).

F. Prognosis. Surgical mortality is less than 1%. If the defect is asymptomatic or medically or surgically ligated, prognosis is excellent.

Ventricular Septal Defect

A. Incidence. At 1:3000 live births, VSDs are the most common of all CHDs.

B. Anatomy. Abnormal opening in the septum between the right and left ventricle. Sizes range from pinhole to almost complete absence of the ventricular septum (Fig. 28-8).

C. Hemodynamics.

1. The degree of hypertrophy of ventricles and the pressure relationships are dependent on the size of the defect. A small defect allows pressure differences between ventricles.

2. PVR less than SVR results in a left-to-right shunt, producing increased pulmonary blood flow and leading to decreased pulmonary compliance and pulmonary edema.

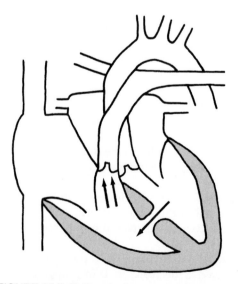

FIGURE 28-8 ■ Ventricular septal defect (VSD).

3. Excessive pulmonary artery blood flow eventually results in pulmonary artery hypertrophy and stenosis.

4. High pulmonary artery pressure can delay maturation of pulmonary arterioles.

D. **Clinical manifestations.**

1. Size dependent.

2. Small VSD.

   a. Asymptomatic.

   b. High-pitched pansystolic murmur along the left sternal border 4 to 10 days after birth.

3. Moderate VSD: asymptomatic except for murmur, fatigue with feeding, and recurrent respiratory infections.

4. Large VSD.

   a. Present at 1 to 2 months of age with CHF, hepatomegaly, recurrent pulmonary infections, and increased precordial activity.

   b. Loud, blowing pansystolic murmur at the left lower sternal border.

   c. Chest x-ray examination: cardiomegaly and increased pulmonary vascular markings.

   d. Two-dimensional echocardiography is capable of identifying 90% of VSDs. Doppler and/or color flow mapping increases the accuracy of diagnosis of VSD. Color flow is extremely useful in identifying multiple VSDs and the direction of blood flow across the VSD.

E. **Management.**

1. 50% to 75% of small defects will close spontaneously; 20% of large defects become smaller or close.

2. Plasma B-type natriuretic peptide is useful in the diagnosis of CHF in pediatrics (Maghsood and Das, 2007). With mild CHF, treatment consists of digoxin and diuretics.

3. Surgery is indicated if patient has failure to thrive or intractable CHF.

   a. Palliative: surgical banding of pulmonary artery to reduce pulmonary blood flow, decrease CHF, and prevent pulmonary vascular resistance.

   b. Surgical: repair by suturing defect or patching defect through a median sternotomy. The defect is approached via the right atrium and tricuspid valve through ventriculotomy. Indicated when closure is necessary in the first 6 to 12 months of life. If the infant is less than 2000 g, it may be necessary to perform pulmonary artery banding to decrease blood flow to the lungs. Surgical closure is then done when the infant is greater than 2000 g. Newer approaches include a combination of surgery and intraoperative device placement in multiple and complex muscular VSDs (Zannini and Borini, 2007).

   c. Transcatheter devices such as the clamshell, double-umbrella, and buttoned devices may be used.

F. **Prognosis: excellent.** Mortality rate is less than 5% in infants. Complications from surgical closure may include right bundle-branch block, third-degree heart block, and aortic and/or tricuspid insufficiency. Earlier surgical repair, rather than palliative banding with delayed repair, is associated with better results. If VSD remains open with a large left-to-right shunt after 9 months of age, complications may result in pulmonary vascular disease (Knight and Washington, 2006).

Atrial Septal Defect

A. **Incidence:** 1:5000 live births, 7% to 10% of all cardiac defects. Female to male ratio 2:1.

B. **Anatomy:** defect in formation of septum, resulting in a communication between right and left atria. Defect may be an ostium primum defect, an ostium secundum defect (most common), or a partial endocardial cushion defect (Fig. 28-9). By definition, a patent foramen ovale is generally excluded, although symptoms can be the same.

C. **Hemodynamics.**

1. Immediately after birth, right ventricular pressure is greater than left ventricle pressure, so there is no shunt or only a small right-to-left shunt.

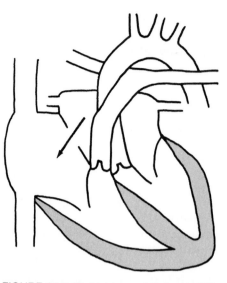

FIGURE 28-9 ■ Atrial septal defect (ASD).

2. As PVR decreases, left-to-right shunt develops with concomitant right ventricular volume overload and hypertrophy.
D. **Clinical manifestations.**
1. The isolated defect is generally asymptomatic and unrecognized. If ASD is diagnosed in infancy, greater than 50% of the patients will be symptomatic.
2. CHF from left-to-right shunt with mitral valve insufficiency.
3. Failure to thrive.
4. Recurrent respiratory infections.
5. Systolic murmur at the second intercostal space at the left sternal border, persistent split S_2 if shunt is large, diastolic murmur heard at the left lower sternal border.
6. Chest x-ray examination: increased pulmonary vascular markings with enlarged right atrium and ventricle (Knight and Washington, 2006).
E. **Management.**
1. If defect is small, clinical follow-up is indicated; the defect may close spontaneously.
2. ASD with CHF: medical treatment of CHF and delay surgical repair.
3. ASD with intractable CHF or if defect is very large or lacks significant borders for positioning of closure device: early surgical repair (i.e., suturing or patching of defect).
4. Surgical repair is done by placement of a patch using the patient's own pericardium, a bovine pericardium, Gore-Tex, or Dacron. All surgical repairs are done with the patient on cardiopulmonary bypass. Complications include residual shunting, arrhythmias, and embolization of the device (American Heart Association, 2008).
5. Transcatheter closure devices are only appropriate for small ostium secundum ASDs. Owing to the size of the occlusion devices, the patient needs to weigh a minimum of 8 kg. Implantation of the device is guided by transesophageal echocardiography. One side of the device is placed on the left side of the septum and the other on the right, which forms a sandwich over the defect. This acts as a framework for normal tissue to grow over the defect. The FDA requires follow-up at 1, 3, 6, and 12 months following the procedure. They also require follow-up to 5 years if there is any adverse effect during placement of the device (Moake and Ramaciotti, 2005).
F. **Prognosis.**
1. Spontaneous closure occurs in up to 20% of ASDs during the first year of life.
2. If left unrepaired, lifetime mortality risk is 25% (Moake and Ramaciotti, 2005).
3. Perioperative mortality rate is less than 1%, with good long-term results in survivors. Survival at 5 years of age is 97% and at 10 years, 90%.

Endocardial Cushion Defect (Atrioventricular Canal)

A. **Incidence:** 1:9000 live births. Most common heart defect found in Down syndrome.

B. **Anatomy.**
1. Endocardial cushions form the lower portion of the atrial septum, the upper portion of the ventricular septum, and septal portions of the mitral and tricuspid valves.
2. A wide range of defects is possible, from simple cleft of the mitral and/or tricuspid valves to complete absence of the lower atrial and upper ventricular septa with common atrioventricular valve (i.e., atrioventricular canal) (Fig. 28-10).

C. **Hemodynamics.**
1. With PVR less than SVR, blood dependently shunts left to right via the ASD and the VSD.
2. Higher pressure of the left ventricle creates obligatory left-to-right shunting via the atrioventricular valve (atrioventricular valve regurgitation). Blood flows from the left ventricle to the mitral portion of the atrioventricular valve to the left atrium to the ASD, and to the right atrium.

D. **Clinical manifestations.**
1. Isolated ostium primum atrial defect: rarely identified in the neonatal period.
2. Isolated ventricular defect: see clinical features of VSD, p. 557.
3. Complete atrioventricular canal.
   a. Atrioventricular valve regurgitation controls age at presentation.
      (1) Severe: seen at 1 to 2 weeks of age with CHF.
      (2) Valves competent: seen in first or second month of life.
   b. Respiratory distress.
   c. Active precordium, with a thrill at the left lower sternal border.
   d. Variable murmurs; usually loud pansystolic murmur at the lower left sternal border, radiating to left back.
   e. Recurrent respiratory infections.
   f. Chest x-ray examination: cardiomegaly, bilateral atrial and ventricular hypertrophy, increased pulmonary markings.

E. **Management.**
1. Objective: avoid development of pulmonary vascular obstructive disease.
2. Medical management: prevent or control CHF with digoxin and diuretics.
3. Palliative pulmonary artery banding to decrease pulmonary overload. Does not influence obligatory shunting of the atrioventricular valve.

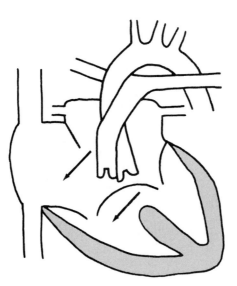

FIGURE 28-10 ■ Atrioventricular canal (AVC).

4. Primary repair with closure of atrial and ventricular septal defects and mitral and tricuspid valve reconstruction (Zannini and Borini, 2007). If complete AV canal, surgery is done before 6 months of age, if partial, surgery is done between 6 and 12 months.

F. **Prognosis.**
   1. Prognosis is dependent on details of anatomic form and on the presence of significant associated noncardiac anomalies and significant pulmonary obstructive vascular disease.
   2. Best results are seen with ostium primum defect or common atrium; long-term prognosis is good.
   3. Outlook for complete atrioventricular canal without operation is poor.
   4. Mortality rate for surgical repair is under 5%. A 10% to 20% incidence in repeat surgery is noted for left AV residual regurgitation (Zannini and Borini, 2007).

OBSTRUCTIVE DEFECTS WITH PULMONARY VENOUS CONGESTION
Coarctation of the Aorta

A. **Incidence:** 3% to 5% of congenital heart lesions (Killian, 2006).
   1. Most common congenital heart defect presenting in week 2 of life.
   2. Male dominance: 2:1.
   3. 30% of those with Turner syndrome will have this defect.
B. **Anatomy:** constriction of aorta at the junction or the transverse aortic arch or the vicinity of the ductus arteriosus (Fig. 28-11).
   1. Most common site is below the origin of the left subclavian artery.
   2. Preductal coarctation is associated with hypoplasia of the aortic arch. Defects such as VSD, PDA, and transposition of the great arteries (TGA) will be found in 40%.
   3. Up to 60% of infants with coarctation will have a bicuspid aortic valve.
C. **Hemodynamics.**
   1. Isolated coarctation: obstruction to left ventricular outflow, leading to increased left ventricular, left atrial, and pulmonary venous pressures. Pulmonary venous congestion develops.
   2. Coarctation with VSD: elevated left ventricular pressure, shunting blood left to right via VSD and causing pulmonary overload.
   3. Preductal coarctation: dependent on PDA for distal aorta and lower-body blood flow.
D. **Clinical manifestations.**
   1. CHF as a result of pressure overload on the left ventricle.
      a. If severe, will result in cardiovascular collapse after ductus closes.

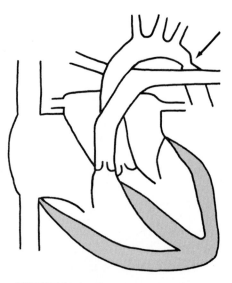

FIGURE 28-11 ■ Coarctation of aorta.

2. Decreased or absent pulses in the lower extremities.
3. Lower extremities cool to touch.
4. Higher blood pressure (>15 mm Hg) in upper extremities is the most consistent factor in critical coarctation. If blood pressures are lower in the upper extremities, the following applies:
    a. Decreased blood pressure in left arm, indicative of left subclavian artery as site of coarctation.
    b. Decreased blood pressure in right arm: right subclavian artery arises below coarctation (rare).
    c. Pulses that "wax and wane": related to increase or decrease in PDA blood flow.
5. Heart sounds.
    a. Postductal: no murmur or short systolic ejection click in axilla or back.
    b. Preductal with VSD: harsh pansystolic murmur at the left lower sternal border.
    c. Gallop rhythm possible.
6. Systolic thrill heard at the suprasternal notch.
7. Chest x-ray examination: enlarged heart with left ventricular hypertrophy and increased pulmonary vascular markings.
8. Echocardiography may be useful in detecting coarctation of the aorta when PDA is present by measuring the isthmus diameter (Lu et al., 2006).
9. Magnetic resonance imaging (MRI) to determine the location of the coarct and whether it affects any other vessels (Mayo Clinic Staff, 2006).
10. Cardiac catheterization is diagnostic and usually performed prior to surgical management to evaluate for other anomalies.

E. **Management.**
1. Aggressive medical management of CHF.
2. Prostaglandin E_1 (PGE_1) to dilate ductus arteriosus (preductal lesion).
    a. Dose: 0.05 to 0.1 mcg/kg/min IV infusion, titrate dose.
    b. Response: Ductus arteriosus will reopen 30 to 120 minutes after infusion starts.
    c. Adverse effects: apnea, fever, hypotension.
3. Palliative balloon angioplasty in critically ill neonate, followed by surgery.
4. Isolated postductal coarctation: control of CHF first, then delayed surgical correction.
5. Surgical correction: two common repairs.
    a. Either resection of abnormal segment and reanastomosis.
    b. Or subclavian patch across area of obstruction.
    c. With associated anomalies, variable approaches according to type of defect.

F. **Prognosis.**
1. Outcome is dependent on complexity of coarctation, with mortality rates at 1 month ranging from zero for simple coarctation to 10%; can be higher for complex coarctation associated with VSD or other left-sided obstruction (Reade et al., 2006).
2. Long-term prognosis after coarctation repair is determined by the presence of residual or recurrent coarctation, persistence of pulmonary hypertension, and residual cardiovascular lesions (Knight and Washington, 2006).
    a. Incidence of recurrence of 5% to 25% after resection and end-to-end anastomosis has been reported after repair in infancy.
    b. Overall surgical mortality is 2% to 10% in infancy; however, earlier detection and use of PGE_1 has reduced mortality.
    c. The most common complication is hypertension.

Aortic Stenosis

A. **Incidence:** 1:24,000 live births, accounts for 5% to 6% of all cardiac anomalies.
1. Four times more likely in males.
B. **Anatomy:** may be subvalvular, valvular, or supravalvular, with valvular stenosis being the most common form. The myocardium of the left ventricle is hypertrophied (Fig. 28-12).
1. Valvular stenosis usually has a bicuspid aortic valve.
2. Supravalvular stenosis is the least common and is seen with Williams syndrome.

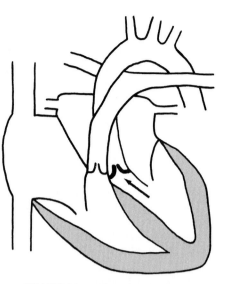

FIGURE 28-12 ■ Aortic stenosis.

C. **Hemodynamics:** Obstruction to left ventricular outflow leads to increased left ventricular pressures and hypertrophy. If aortic stenosis is severe in utero, blood flow through the ventricle is decreased, resulting in left ventricular hypoplasia and left-sided heart syndrome.

D. **Clinical manifestations.**
   1. Usually asymptomatic at birth (Knight and Washington, 2006).
   2. Acrocyanosis.
   3. Heart sounds include a grade II to IV/VI harsh systolic murmur in upper right sternal border, radiating to the neck and lower left sternal border.
   4. Suprasternal notch thrill may be present.
   5. CHF symptoms may be delayed by weeks but progress rapidly after onset.
   6. Chest x-ray examination shows cardiomegaly with normal pulmonary vascular markings.
   7. If critical aortic stenosis is present, sudden deterioration is likely.

E. **Management.**
   1. Medical management is usually not successful.
   2. Initially, CHF is treated with fluid restriction, diuretics, digoxin, acidosis management, and antibiotic prophylaxis.
   3. If stenosis is critical, use PGE_1 to prevent hypoxia.
   4. The treatment of choice in neonates is balloon valvuloplasty. Early mortality rate is 11%. However, 25% will develop significant aortic insufficiency (Killian, 2006). Multiple procedures are common in childhood (Wechsler and Wernovsky, 2004).
   5. Surgery is reserved for patients who fail balloon valvuloplasty and involves aortic valvotomy or valve replacement. The number of aortic valvotomies have declined substantially since balloon valvuloplasty has gained favor (Weber and Seib, 2006).

F. **Prognosis.**
   1. Success rate of balloon valvuloplasty is very high.
   2. Aortic stenosis accounts for 1% of all sudden death in children with heart disease.

OBSTRUCTIVE DEFECTS WITH DECREASED PULMONARY BLOOD FLOW

Tetralogy of Fallot

A. **Incidence:** 1:5000 live births. Most common cyanotic heart lesion, accounting for 10% of all defects.

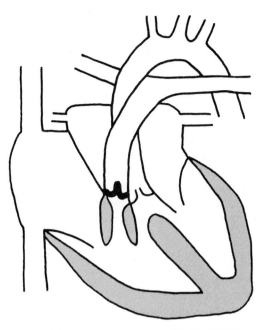

FIGURE 28-13 ■ Tetralogy of Fallot (TOF).

B. **Anatomy:** classified as a combination of four defects, although numbers 3 and 4, below, are consequences of numbers 1 and 2, below (Fig. 28-13).
   1. Pulmonary stenosis: obstruction of outflow tract.
   2. VSD.
   3. Aorta overriding VSD.
   4. Right ventricular hypertrophy.
C. **Hemodynamics.**
   1. Dependent primarily on degree of pulmonary stenosis and to a lesser extent on VSD size.
   2. In severe pulmonary stenosis, blood flow passes from right to left via the VSD, with resulting hypoxia and cyanosis.
   3. In mild pulmonary stenosis, blood flows from left to right via the VSD, with CHF resulting.
   4. In mild to moderate pulmonary stenosis, blood flow via the VSD may be minimal as long as PVR and SVR are balanced. With crying, right-to-left shunting occurs.
D. **Clinical manifestations.**
   1. Presentation is a function of the degree of pulmonary stenosis.
   2. Severe obstruction presents in the first days of life with severe cyanosis, hypoxia, and dyspnea.
   3. Milder pulmonary obstruction presents in the first days of life with mild cyanosis.
   4. Harsh grades II to IV/VI, systolic murmur with thrill present at mid- to upper left sternal border.
   5. Chest x-ray examination shows normal-sized boot-shaped heart with normal or decreased pulmonary vascular markings.
   6. Traditional "TET spells" (paroxysmal dyspnea and severe cyanosis) are common in infants and can occur in neonates.
E. **Management.**
   1. Medical (Knight and Washington, 2006).
      a. Propranolol is the drug of choice for treating hypercyanotic infants.
      b. PGE₁ is used to maintain patency of the ductus arteriosus until the infant can be taken to surgery in severe TOF.

2. Corrective surgery involves closure of the VSD with a patch and eliminating the pulmo-nary stenosis by resection. The pulmonary outflow tract may be enlarged by a patch. This procedure is done while the infant is on cardiopulmonary bypass.
   a. Surgical correction is now preferred before 6 months of age (Wechsler and Wernovsky, 2004).
   b. If the neonate has severe pulmonary stenosis or atresia, a Blalock–Taussig procedure is generally performed, with full correction at a later time (Ahmad et al., 2007).
3. Prognosis.
   a. Prognosis without surgery is very poor. Mortality rate in infancy is less than 10% (Knight and Washington, 2006).
   b. Complications/residual effects include arrhythmias, decreased or absent pulses in affected arm, inadequate shunt, and CHF resulting from large shunt.
   c. Postoperative mortality is less than 5% for uncomplicated TOF. This rate increases with the more severe forms of TOF (Zannini and Borini, 2007).

Pulmonary Stenosis

A. **Incidence:** 1 : 14,000 live births, 5% to 8% of all congenital heart defects.
B. **Anatomy:** narrowed opening either in pulmonary valve as a consequence of pulmonary valve cusp fusions (Fig. 28-14) or above or below the valve because of tissue hypertrophy.
C. **Hemodynamics.**
   1. In utero, right ventricular hypoplasia can develop, depending on the degree of pulmonary valve stenosis and subsequent decrease in right ventricular blood flow.
   2. After birth, the combination of right ventricular hypoplasia and severe pulmonary valve stenosis redirects blood flow from right to left at the atrial level via the foramen ovale. Pulmonary blood becomes dependent on a left-to-right flow via the PDA.
   3. In mild stenosis, the pulmonary blood flow is not excessively restricted and is PDA inde-pendent. As PVR decreases, atrial right-to-left shunt will decrease, improving systemic hypoxia.
D. **Clinical manifestations.**
   1. Mild pulmonary stenosis: loud systolic murmur at left upper sternal border is the only finding.
   2. Moderately severe stenosis.
      a. Murmur is less prominent. Murmur of tricuspid insufficiency may be noted.
      b. Cyanosis is present and increases with PDA closure.
      c. Generally, hepatomegaly is present.

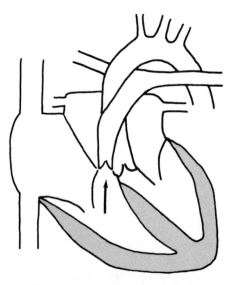

FIGURE 28-14 ■ Pulmonary stenosis (PS).

3. Chest x-ray examination: mild cardiomegaly with bulging right heart border and decreased pulmonary vascular markings.
4. Two-dimensional echocardiography used to make anatomic and physiologic diagnosis (Wechsler and Wernovsky, 2004).

E. **Management.**
   1. Cyanotic neonate.
      a. Initial management: oxygen, bicarbonate, and PGE_1.
      b. Nonsurgical treatment with transcatheter balloon valvuloplasty.
         (1) Few complications; effective.
         (2) Treatment of choice for most lesions.
      c. Surgical valvotomy or tissue excision is reserved for specific cases or when valvuloplasty fails and patient is symptomatic.
   2. Noncyanotic neonate: conservative management includes catheterization at 6 to 12 months if stenosis is severe, with subsequent surgery if right ventricular pressure exceeds systemic.

F. **Prognosis:** Excellent. Operative mortality rate for valvuloplasty is less than 3%.

Pulmonary Atresia

A. **Incidence:** 1:14,000 live births, accounting for less than 1% of cardiac defects.
B. **Anatomy:** complete obstruction of the pulmonic valve, resulting in a hypoplastic right ventricle and tricuspid valve (Fig. 28-15). In the presence of a VSD the right ventricle may be of adequate size.
C. **Hemodynamics.**
   1. Venous blood returning to the right atrium goes across the foramen ovale into the left atrium, into the left ventricle, and out the aorta.
   2. Blood flow to the lungs is derived entirely from a left-to-right shunt at the ductus arteriosus, which is generally small and tortuous. As the PDA closes, severe hypoxemia ensues.
   3. Regurgitant blood flow occurs at the tricuspid valve.
D. **Clinical manifestations.**
   1. Mild cyanosis at birth, progressing to intense cyanosis by 24 hours.
   2. Tachypnea.
   3. Heart sounds.

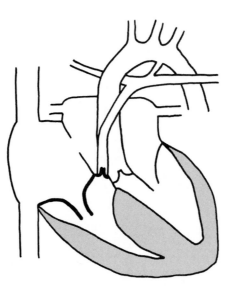

FIGURE 28-15 ■ Pulmonary atresia.

    a. PDA murmur is present.

    b. Soft systolic murmur is heard at the upper left sternal border, and harsh systolic murmur at the lower right and upper left sternal border if tricuspid insufficiency is present.

  4. Chest x-ray examination shows increased heart size with decreased pulmonary markings; right atrial hypertrophy is seen in 70%.

  5. Two-dimensional echocardiography with Doppler and color flow mapping is used to determine absence of blood flow across the pulmonary valve and is standard for diagnosis (Khairy et al., 2007).

E. Management.

  1. Initial treatment is use of oxygen and bicarbonate for metabolic acidosis and PGE_1 to maintain patency of the ductus arteriosus.

  2. Cardiac catheterization is done with balloon atrial septostomy in infants with pulmonary atresia.

  3. Mild right ventricle hypertrophy: surgical valvotomy may be effective.

  4. With severe hyperplasia of right ventricle and tricuspid valve, usually a Blalock–Taussig shunt to provide systemic-to-pulmonary shunting in the neonatal period that may be converted at 3 to 6 months to a bidirectional Glenn procedure. These infants will later require definitive repair via completion of the Fontan, resulting in communication between the right atrium and pulmonary artery. Closure of ASD or VSD is done at this time (Jones et al., 2006).

F. Prognosis.

  1. Without surgery, the mortality rate is 100%. If reconstruction of the right ventricular outflow tract is needed, the mortality rate is 25%.

  2. Long-term complications are arrhythmias, CHF, and sudden death.

  3. Reported survival rates range from 65% to 75%, depending on anatomy of defect, size of right ventricle, and operative procedure (Charpie, 2007).

Tricuspid Atresia

A. Incidence: 1:18,000 live births.

B. Anatomy: agenesis of the tricuspid valve development with associated patent foramen ovale or ASD (Fig. 28-16).

  1. VSD is often associated with the hypoplastic right ventricle.

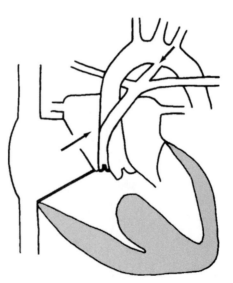

FIGURE 28-16 ■ Tricuspid atresia. Arrows identify shunting through the patent foramen ovale and the patent ductus arteriosus.

2. Pulmonary atresia or stenosis typically present.
3. Transposition of the great vessels occurs in 30% of the cases.

C. **Hemodynamics.**
1. Systemic venous blood is shunted from the right atrium across the foramen ovale or ASD into the left atrium. With an isolated defect, the pulmonary blood flow is supplied by the left ventricular outflow via the PDA.
2. In the presence of a VSD, some of the blood entering the left ventricle shunts across into the hypoplastic right ventricle and out the pulmonary artery—or out the aorta in the case of coexisting transposition. If severe pulmonary stenosis or atresia is present, blood does not flow through the VSD (see also item C.1, above.)

D. **Clinical manifestations.**
1. Cyanosis usually presents soon after birth with an isolated defect or coexisting VSD and pulmonary outflow tract obstruction. Increasing cyanosis occurs with closure of the ductus.
2. Dyspnea; tachypnea may be present.
3. CHF ensues with large VSD and absent pulmonary stenosis usually within the first month of life.
4. Murmur is absent unless associated with pulmonary stenosis, VSD, or PDA.
5. Chest x-ray examination shows variable heart size, depending on the degree of pulmonary stenosis; size is generally nondiagnostic.
6. Cardiac catheterization to perform a balloon septostomy to improve intraatrial mixing of blood.

E. **Management.**
1. Primary treatment: oxygen, bicarbonate, and PGE_1 for severe hypoxia.
2. Palliative treatment.
   a. Systemic–pulmonary artery shunt including Blalock–Taussig procedure.
   b. Large VSD with no pulmonary stenosis: pulmonary artery banding is performed to control CHF.
3. Reparative surgery.
   a. Right atrium is connected to either the right ventricular outflow track or the pulmonary artery (Fontan or modified Fontan), so that the right atrium forces blood into the lungs. Closure of the ASD and VSD is done at this time if they are present.
   b. Modified Fontan procedure separates oxygenated and unoxygenated blood inside the heart but does not restore normal hemodynamics or anatomy.

F. **Prognosis:** Survival is 82% at 1 year, 72% at 5 years, and 61% at 20 years. Complications include heart failure, persistent shunts, and dysrhythmias (Wald et al., 2007).

MIXED DEFECTS
Transposition of the Great Vessels

A. **Incidence:** 1:5000 live births; male predominance, 2:1. Most common cardiac cause of cyanosis in neonates (DeBord et al., 2007).
B. **Anatomy:** positions of the great arteries are reversed (i.e., the pulmonary artery arises from the left ventricle and the aorta from the right ventricle). Without other intracardiac defects (e.g., VSD, ASD), an independent, parallel circuit exists (Fig. 28-17). In dextroposition (D presentation), the aorta is situated to the left of the pulmonary artery.
C. **Hemodynamics.**
1. Oxygenated blood returns from the lungs to enter the left atrium and ventricle, then recirculates to the lungs by way of the pulmonary artery.
2. Unoxygenated blood returns to the right atrium and ventricle and is returned through the aorta to the body.
3. Mixing of oxygenated and unoxygenated blood occurs at the ductus arteriosus (as long as patency exists) or through any existing septal defects (ASD, VSD).
   a. Mixing is required for survival.
   b. Shunting occurs from left to right through septal defects or the PDA, ameliorating the degree of cyanosis and hypoxia.

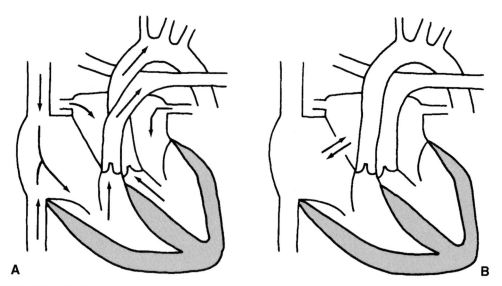

FIGURE 28-17 ■ Transposition of great vessels (TGV). **A,** Normal anatomy. **B,** Appearance of heart with TGV.

D. Clinical manifestations.
1. Cyanosis is present within the first 24 hours of life and becomes progressively more intense.
2. Prominent murmurs are uncommon; VSD (if present) will have a loud murmur.
3. Chest x-ray findings are usually normal; the heart may have an "egg on a string" appearance. Pulmonary vasculature may be increased or decreased.
4. Echocardiography is the standard diagnostic test (Westmoreland, 1999).

E. Management: TGA is a cardiac emergency.
1. Correction of metabolic acidosis.
2. PGE_1 to maintain patency of the PDA until palliative surgery can be performed (Chamberlin and Lozynski, 2006).
3. Palliation of choice: catheter-introduced balloon atrial septostomy.
   a. Balloon catheter is inserted into the femoral or umbilical vein; it is advanced across the foramen ovale into the left atrium. The balloon is inflated and pulled across the atrium, creating an ASD.
   b. Procedure rapidly improves systemic and pulmonary circulation admixing, thus increasing Pao_2 (30s) and saturation (70s).
4. Blade septostomy: if balloon septostomy is unsuccessful, surgical excision of the posterior aspect of the septum is done during cardiac catheterization (Knight and Washington, 2006; Lott, 2007) technique, and a hole is excised in the atrial septum.
5. Pulmonary artery banding: to prevent pulmonary vascular disease, to decrease CHF, or to exercise the left ventricle before surgery by increasing the ventricular workload.
6. Corrective surgery.
   a. Arterial switch operation (Jatene procedure) is the treatment of choice: detaches aorta, coronary arteries, and pulmonary artery, reattaching to correct ventricles. Procedure is generally performed within the first 2 weeks of life and provides both anatomic and physiologic correction.
   b. Mustard or Senning procedure: creates a baffle at the atrium to divert systemic venous blood into the left ventricle and pulmonary artery and pulmonary venous blood into the right ventricle and aorta.
   c. Rastelli procedure: intraventricular repair combined with placement of an extracardiac shunt from the right ventricle to the pulmonary artery. Used for TGV with large VSD and extensive left ventricular outflow tract obstruction.

F. **Prognosis.**
1. Changes in medical operative management make short-term data potentially misleading and long-term data out of date.
2. Without surgery, 90% will die within the first year.
3. Survival outcomes are >98% at 4 years, if arterial switch is performed (Freed et al., 2006).
4. Complications are myocardial ischemia and aortic and/or pulmonary stenosis.
5. The incidence of neurologic and developmental complications is relatively high after neonatal arterial switch. These complications include gross motor deficits, fine motor deficits, sensory dysfunction, and speech and language difficulties (Freed et al., 2006).

Truncus Arteriosus

A. **Incidence:** 1:33,000 live births, 1% to 2% of cardiac defects.
B. **Anatomy:** a single great artery arises from both ventricles, overriding a VSD (Fig. 28-18).
1. Type I: most common, short pulmonary artery arising from the base of the common trunk, then divides into the right and left arteries.
2. Type II: right and left pulmonary arteries arise from the posterior surface of the common trunk.
3. Type III: right and left pulmonary arteries have separate origins in the lateral walls of the common trunk (Jones et al., 2006).
C. **Hemodynamics.**
1. Both ventricles pump blood into the common trunk supplying the systemic and pulmonary circulation. As PVR drops, preferential shunting to the pulmonary circulation occurs, increasing blood flow to the lungs and workload of the left ventricle.
2. If pulmonary arteries are stenotic or hypoplastic, blood flow to the lungs is restricted.
D. **Clinical manifestations.**
1. CHF with bounding pulses and widened pulse pressure.
2. Intermittent cyanosis: severe cyanosis with pulmonary artery stenosis.
3. Heart sounds: harsh systolic murmur at the mid- to lower-left sternal border and systolic ejection click with single S_2.
4. Chest x-ray examination: cardiomegaly with increased pulmonary vascular markings. (Exception: if pulmonary artery stenosis exists, decreased pulmonary markings are seen.)
5. Echocardiography with cross-section, and Doppler flow and color mapping is the standard diagnostic test and is used to identify the number of truncal valve leaflets, presence of pulmonary stenosis, and to assess the aortic arch (Wernovsky and Gruber, 2005).

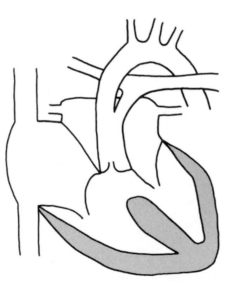

FIGURE 28-18 ■ Truncus arteriosus.

E. Management.
1. Medical management is temporary and is directed toward treating CHF.
   a. Diuretics, digoxin, and angiotensin-converting enzyme (ACE) inhibitors are used to control pulmonary overload and decrease systemic resistance, which leads to a decrease in pulmonary vascular resistance.
2. Surgical repair at 6 to 8 weeks is the treatment of choice.
   a. Homograft between the right ventricle and the pulmonary artery.
   b. VSD closure using a patch.
   c. Separation of the pulmonary arteries from the truncus (Wechsler and Wernovsky, 2004).
3. Homografts are preferred to synthetic because they are more flexible, easier to use during surgery, and less prone to obstruction.

F. Prognosis.
1. Mortality rate ranges from 70% to 95% in the first year of life if unrepaired (Wechsler and Wernovsky, 2004).
2. Postsurgical mortality is <10% and survival is >80% at the 10- to 20-year follow-up.

Total Anomalous Pulmonary Venous Return

A. Incidence: 1:17,000 live births, 1% of all cardiac defects.
B. Anatomy: Pulmonary veins drain into the right atrium either directly or indirectly via a systemic venous channel (Fig. 28-19).
1. Presence of a patent foramen ovale or true ASD is required for survival.
2. Varying degrees of pulmonary venous obstruction occur.
3. Three types of TAPVR occur.
   a. Supracardiac. Pulmonary veins attach above the diaphragm, often to the superior vena cava (common form).
   b. Cardiac. Pulmonary veins attach directly to the coronary sinus and drain into the right atrium.

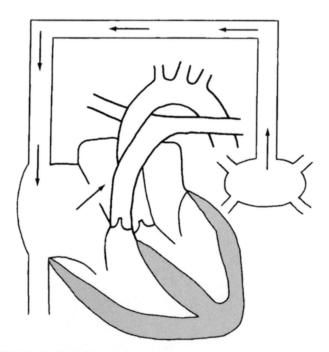

FIGURE 28-19 ■ Total anomalous pulmonary venous connection (TAPVR).

    c. Infracardiac. Pulmonary veins attach below the diaphragm into the portal venous system, draining into the inferior vena cava (most severe form).

C. Hemodynamics.

1. Oxygenated blood from the lungs drains into the right atrium, mixing with the systemic venous return. Part of this flow passes into the left atrium via the patent foramen ovale or ASD, into the left ventricle, and out the aorta. With the normal decrease in PVR, pulmonary blood flow will increase.

2. If obstruction to pulmonary venous return exists, the resulting increase in PVR leads to pulmonary edema and diversion of blood from the pulmonary artery to the aorta via the PDA. Closure of the PDA then increases right-to-left atrial shunting.

D. Clinical manifestations.

1. Nonobstructed.
    a. CHF.
    b. Mild cyanosis.
    c. Heart sounds: systolic murmur at the upper left sternal border, diastolic rumble at the lower left sternal border. Wide split S_2 may be present but is generally nonspecific.
    d. Chest x-ray examination: right ventricle dilation, increased pulmonary vascular markings, and "snowman" appearance after 4 months of age.
    e. Echocardiography will demonstrate a right ventricular dilation (Stein, 2007).

2. Obstructed.
    a. Profound cyanosis present.
    b. Respiratory distress, may not respond to mechanical ventilation. This form may require emergent surgical repair (Wechsler and Wernovsky, 2004).
    c. ECG will show right ventricular hypertrophy with a right-axis deviation.
    d. Chest x-ray examination: normal size, with pulmonary edema.

3. Echocardiography with color flow mapping reveals an extra cavity behind the left atrium, a right-to-left shunt across the atrial septum and the anomalous return as the blood enters the atrium, superior vena cava, or coronary sinus. It may be difficult to visualize the pulmonary veins (Knight and Washington, 2006).

E. Management: Surgical treatment of obstructed TAPVR is an emergency.

1. Medical management of nonobstructed TAPVR is only a temporary measure and is aimed at preventing or treating CHF.

2. Cardiac catheterization may be omitted to speed time to operation, with surgery based on echocardiography.

3. Anomalous veins are detached and transplanted to the left atrium; the ASD is repaired.

F. Prognosis.

1. Mortality rate for infants with TAPVR who undergo surgery is 2% to 20% in infancy (Stein, 2007); the highest mortality is in the infracardiac type.

2. Long-term prognosis is excellent because TAPVR is closer to a surgically "curable" condition, approximately 90%, than are most congenital cardiac lesions.

Hypoplastic Left Heart Syndrome

A. Incidence: 2 to 2.6 : 10,000 live births; 1% to 4% of all cardiac defects; 28% have chromosomal abnormalities. HLHS is the most common cardiac cause of death in the first week of life (Killian, 2006).

B. Anatomy.

1. Hypoplastic left ventricle, aortic arch, and ascending aorta.

2. Atretic or hypoplastic mitral and aortic valves (Fig. 28-20).

C. Hemodynamics.

1. Obstruction of blood flow through the left side of the heart due to hypoplastic aorta and ventricle leads to pulmonary venous congestion and edema.

2. Blood supply to the descending aorta and to the aortic arch and coronary arteries (retrograde flow) is dependent on the PDA.

3. Coarctation of the aorta is present in 75% of patients.

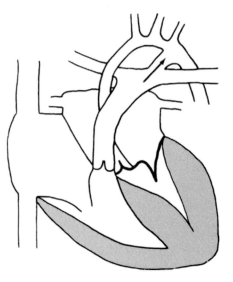

FIGURE 28-20 ■ Hypoplastic left heart syndrome.

D. Clinical manifestations.

1. Asymptomatic at birth.
2. Tachypnea and dyspnea with increasing pulmonary blood flow.
3. CHF: usually presents at 24 to 48 hours of life.
4. Cyanosis: rarely permanent despite mixing of systemic and pulmonary circulations.
5. Rapid deterioration as PDA closes (Wechsler and Wernovsky, 2004).
    a. Severe mottling.
    b. Gray pallor of skin.
    c. Markedly diminished pulses.
    d. Cardiovascular collapse and shock.
    e. Systolic murmur present in two thirds.
6. Chest x-ray examination: cardiomegaly with increased pulmonary blood flow and pulmonary edema.
7. Prenatal diagnosis by fetal echocardiography at 18 to 22 weeks. Fetal interventions to prevent development of the syndrome are being studied, including balloon dilation and stent placement in areas of restriction. However, results are variable (Connor and Thiagarajan, 2008). Postnatal diagnosis with echocardiography to determine size of interatrial communication, AV valve function, and ascending aorta size (Connor and Thiagarajan, 2008). Echocardiography should include Doppler and color-flow mapping (Khairy et al., 2007).

E. Management.

1. Treatment options include comfort care, a multistaged surgical approach, or cardiac transplantation.
2. Initial management.
    a. PGE_1 to maintain ductus arteriosus patency and systemic circulation.
    b. Use of inhaled O_2 and nitrogen combination for an inspired FIO_2 of less than 21% to maintain an oxygen saturation of 70% to 85%. Nitrogen therapy creates pulmonary hypoxia and vasoconstriction, which may maximize right-to-left shunting and systemic blood flow, with a resulting increase in systemic oxygen saturation (Green et al., 2002).
    c. Transcatheter balloon atrial septostomy to decompress the left atrium.
3. Staged surgical repair "Norwood" procedure has an overall mortality rate of 25% to 40% (Bleiweis and Saidi, 2006).
    a. First (Norwood) stage can be performed on infants with BW as low as 1.5 kg and has a greater than or equal to 35% mortality, with 12-month survival around 61% (Khairy et al., 2007).

(1) Division of the main pulmonary artery and ligation of the ductus arteriosus.

(2) Gore-Tex shunt is placed to maintain pulmonary blood flow and prevent CHF.

(3) Atrial septectomy to ensure pulmonary venous return to the right atrium.

(4) Connection of the right pulmonary artery and the aorta using an aortic allograft.

(5) Newer Sano procedure for first stage includes placement of a conduit between the right ventricle and pulmonary artery has improved survival to second stage repair (Bleiweis and Saidi, 2006).

(6) "Hybrid" approach: involves placement of a stent in the ductus arteriosus along with pulmonary artery banding. This is done in a special suite that has catheterization and surgery capabilities. Complications include narrowing of the ductus, which requires balloon dilation, and increased pulmonary blood flow (Killian, 2006).

    b. Second stage: bidirectional Glenn procedure (anastomosis of the superior vena cava to the right pulmonary artery) done before 6 months of age to reduce volume overload to the right ventricle. Mortality rate for this stage is less than 9.5%.

    c. Third stage, or modified Fontan procedure, with a mortality rate of 10% (Khairy et al., 2007).

(1) Involves completion of Fontan procedure between 12 and 24 months of age to connect the inferior vena cava to the pulmonary artery and close the atrial communication.

(2) Completion of stages 2 and 3 separates the pulmonary from the systemic circulation.

    d. Disadvantages.

(1) Two or three open surgeries in the first 2 years of life.

(2) Single right ventricle supplies the systemic circulation.

    e. Contraindication: significant tricuspid valve or pulmonic valve dysplasia associated with functional disturbances.

  4. Cardiac transplantation.

    a. Provides a structurally and physiologically normal heart in one operation.

    b. 25% of infants die while waiting for a donor heart (Bleiweis and Saidi, 2006).

    c. Complications include the following:

(1) Increased susceptibility to infections as a result of immunosuppression.

(2) Allograft rejection, with acute rejection as the leading cause of death in the first year after transplant.

(3) Systemic hypertension: usually seen only in the first year after transplantation.

(4) Recurrent or residual coarctation: managed with angioplasty or surgical repair.

(5) Abnormal neurologic findings in as many as 19%, including seizures.

  5. Prognosis.

    a. Comparison of staged repair versus heart transplantation outcomes requires evaluation of numbers of surviving children who completed procedures and numbers of those "lost" through death awaiting procedure or death between stages of the procedure.

    b. According to Web sites that list survival data, survival following transplant has improved and varies from 79% to 89% at 1 year, not including deaths while awaiting a transplant, which can approach 40%. Recent advancements in ABO-incompatible transplant and use of ventricular assist devices have increased survival rates (American Heart Association, 2007). Centers in Germany have reported survival rates of 82%, 80%, and 78% at 1, 5, and 10 years, respectively (Minami et al., 2005).

    c. Overall, 1-year survival after completion of the staged procedure is 60% to 75% (Bleiweis and Saidi, 2006).

CONGESTIVE HEART FAILURE

Etiology

A. CHF is a set of clinical signs and symptoms that reflect the heart's inability to deliver adequate oxygen to meet the metabolic requirements of the body.

■ TABLE 28-4
■ ■ **Causes of Congestive Heart Failure and Time of Onset**

Age at Onset of Symptoms	Underlying Cause
At birth	Hypoplastic left heart syndrome (HLHS) Severe tricuspid or pulmonary regurgitation Systemic arteriovenous fistula
In first week of life	Patent ductus arteriosus (PDA) in premature infants Transposition of the great vessels (TGV) Total anomalous pulmonary venous return (TAPVR) with pulmonary venous obstruction
1 to 4 weeks after birth	Coarctation of the aorta Critical aortic or pulmonary stenosis All other lesions listed above

Data from Park, M.K.: *Pediatric cardiology for practitioners* (5th ed.). Philadelphia, 2008, Mosby.

1. Cardiac output is unable to meet the body's metabolic requirements.
2. Right and/or left ventricular end-diastolic pressures are elevated, impeding systemic and/or pulmonary venous returns.
B. **Although structural heart defects are the most common cause of CHF** in neonates, other causes such as birth asphyxia, severe anemia, dysrhythmias, and sepsis should be considered.
    1. Timing of detection is often helpful in predicting causes because the diseases causing CHF characteristically show up at certain ages. Table 28-4 indicates conditions associated with CHF and their time of onset.
    2. CHF in utero that is detected at birth may be due to the following (Sharma et al., 2003):
        a. Profound anemia: erythroblastosis fetalis or twin-to-twin transfusion.
        b. Arrhythmia: supraventricular tachycardia or congenital heart block.
        c. Intrauterine infection with myocarditis.
        d. Arteriovenous malformations.
        e. Absent pulmonary valve.
        f. Premature ductus arteriosus closure: maternal use of prostaglandin inhibitor (e.g., aspirin, ibuprofen).
        g. Volume overload: twin-to-twin or mother-to-infant transfusion.

Clinical Manifestations

A. **Common signs.**
    1. Tachypnea (60 to 100 respirations per minute at rest) is the first clinical sign of pulmonary edema.
    2. Tachycardia (160 to 180 bpm at rest) from compensation for decreased cardiac output.
    3. Arrhythmias.
    4. Cardiomegaly on x-ray.
        a. Dilational or hypertrophic cardiomyopathy.
        b. Diminished or engorged pulmonary vasculature.
    5. Hepatomegaly (3 to 5 cm below coastal margin): one of the most useful signs.
    6. Pulmonary fine rales and coarse rales (rhonchi).
    7. Fatigue or difficulty with feeding leading to failure to thrive (Fleiner, 2006).
B. **Less common signs.**
    1. Peripheral edema: usually not obvious unless CHF is present for some time.
    2. Diaphoresis.
    3. Gallop rhythm.
    4. Altered pulses (variable, depending on underlying cause).

5. May have mottling of the extremities from redistribution of blood flow to vital tissues.
6. ECG indicating the following:
    a. Hypertrophy of one or more chambers.
    b. Abnormal mean QRS axis.
    c. Rhythm disturbances.
7. Grading the severity of CHF is difficult and not standardized. Several tools have been reported in the literature but lack testing to suggest reliability.

Management of Congestive Heart Failure

A. **General measures** (appropriate for any heart disease).
    1. Use semi-Fowler or prone position to achieve maximal diaphragmatic excursion and lung expansion.
    2. Decrease oxygen consumption.
        a. Maintain neutral thermal environment.
        b. Minimize stimulation (e.g., heel sticks, radial sticks).
        c. Provide sedation with morphine or fentanyl for agitated infant.
        d. Consider assisted ventilation to reduce work of breathing and decrease pulmonary edema if present.
    3. Provide supplemental oxygen. The amount is dictated by the Pao$_2$ and the presence of CHD with admixing of arterial and venous blood.
    4. Correct acidosis and any metabolic derangements (e.g., hypoglycemia or hypocalcemia).
B. **Specific measures.**
    1. Fluid and nutritional support.
        a. During acute phase, volume intake is reduced, generally to two thirds of maintenance levels.
        b. Use of glucose polymers (Polycose) or medium-chain triglycerides (MCT oil) enhances caloric content without significant volume increase.
        c. IV infusions of up to 50% fat emulsions can also be used to increase caloric intake with minimal intake volume.
    2. Pharmacologic therapy.
        a. Digoxin therapy (Table 28-5).
            (1) Achieve maximal cardiac output; use in patients with left-to-right shunt is controversial (Sharma et al., 2003).
            (2) Digitalize patient and observe for bradycardia (discontinue if heart rate <100 bpm).
                (a) Arrhythmias or heart block.
                (b) Hypokalemia.
                (c) Toxic effects: increased in premature infants because of a longer serum half-life (61 to 170 hours) for digoxin than in term or older infants (18 to 45 hours) (Takemoto et al., 2003).
        b. Diuretic therapy.
            (1) Used to eliminate excess intravascular fluid.
            (2) Furosemide (Lasix), 1 to 2 mg/kg every 12 hours IV, or 1 to 3 mg/kg every 12 hours by mouth.
                (a) In severe CHF the IV route is preferable for its rapid onset of action.
                (b) Hypokalemia and hypochloremia are side effects that can result in metabolic alkalosis.
                (c) May cause hypocalcemia, with urinary loss of calcium leading to nephrocalcinosis.
                (d) Use is contraindicated in renal failure.
            (3) Chlorothiazide (Diuril), 20 to 40 mg/kg/day in two oral doses (Hay et al., 2003).
                (a) Administered when less acute oral diuresis is required.
                (b) Does not produce the profound potassium losses seen with furosemide; may reduce urinary calcium losses seen with furosemide.

■ TABLE 28-5
■ ■ **Pressure Values from Cardiac Catheterization**

Pressure	Normal Neonatal Values
Systemic arterial pressure	60 to 90/20 to 60 mm Hg (birth to 5 days of age)
Right atrial pressure	3 mm Hg
Right ventricular pressure	30/3 mm Hg
Pulmonary artery occlusion pressure/pulmonary wedge pressure	6 to 10 mm Hg
Left atrial pressure	8 mm Hg
Left ventricular pressure	100/6 mm Hg

  (4) Spironolactone (Aldactone), 1 to 3 mg/kg/day by mouth.
   (a) Potassium sparing; must monitor for hyperkalemia.
 c. Inotropic agents.
  (1) May be necessary in severe CHF or cardiogenic shock.
  (2) Most commonly used are dopamine, dobutamine, and isoproterenol.
 d. Nesiritide has shown promise in pediatric patients older than 1 month who have low cardiac output and those with CHF who have not responded to traditional therapy (Mahle et al., 2005). Further investigation is needed.
C. Cardiology consultation to rule out or establish presence of congenital heart lesion. Cardiac catheterization, angiocardiography, and surgery may be indicated.

POSTOPERATIVE CARDIAC MANAGEMENT

Noninvasive Monitoring

A. Electrocardiography.
 1. Continuous display of a limb lead, which shows P wave and QRS complex should be monitored (Wernovsky and Gruber, 2005).
  a. Tachycardia.
  b. Bradycardia.
  c. Fibrillation.
  d. Asystole.
 2. Lead II: assessment of amplitude, axis, and presence and absence of P waves.
 3. Lead V_5 changes: septal or lateral wall ischemia.
B. Blood pressure: manual.
 1. Cuff can be used to occlude an arterial catheter leak.
 2. Measurement of upper and lower extremities after repair of coarctation of the aorta gives pressure gradient across repair site.
 3. Avoid extremity for blood pressure measurement when an artery has been used for surgical repair (e.g., subclavian patch for coarctation of the aorta, Blalock–Taussig shunt).
C. Pulse oximetry.
 1. Decreasing oxygen saturations may indicate
  a. Decreased cardiac output,
  b. Increasing intracardiac shunting, or
  c. Increased intrapulmonary shunting.
 2. Continuous monitoring is useful in pulmonary hypertension. Small decrease in saturation may be the first sign of increased pulmonary artery pressure with onset of right-to-left shunting.
D. Urinary output.
 1. Hourly output rate of 1 to 2 ml/kg/hour is a good clinical indicator of renal perfusion (Spence, 2007).

    a. Invalid in first 2 hours postoperatively after diuretic administration.

    b. Urinary retention can be induced by analgesics.

    c. A sudden decrease in urine output may indicate renal failure.

  2. Oliguria may persist for up to 48 hours following cardiopulmonary bypass.

  3. It is common to see increased urine output secondary to osmotic diuresis in the initial postoperative period, followed by decreased urine output after 6 to 8 hours (Pike and Falco, 2002).

  4. Indwelling catheter is generally not required in those with uncomplicated procedures, stable vital signs, and good peripheral perfusion.

Invasive Monitoring

For pressure values from cardiac catheterization, see Table 28-5.

A. Arterial pressure.

  1. Mandatory for timely vasoactive medication adjustments.

  2. Arterial tracing provides information for analysis of waveform and calculation of pulse pressure.

  3. Pronounced phasic variations during mechanical ventilation may indicate hypovolemia or heart failure (Wernovsky and Gruber, 2005).

B. Right-sided cardiac pressures.

  1. In patients with normal cardiac anatomy: right atrial pressure = right ventricular end-diastolic pressure = central venous pressure.

  2. Increasing values seen with (Artman et al., 2002)

    a. Right ventricular overload,

    b. Poor ventricular function,

    c. Elevated pulmonary artery pressure, resulting from reactive pulmonary hypertension,

    d. Tricuspid regurgitation,

    e. Cardiac tamponade, or

    f. Residual shunting.

  3. Particularly useful for evaluating the following:

    a. Right-sided cardiac lesions.

      (1) Pulmonic stenosis.

      (2) TOF.

    b. Those lesions requiring high right atrial pressures, such as in the Fontan procedure.

  4. Right-sided line may be used to give vasoactive and inotropic medications, and to provide parenteral nutrition.

    a. May be left in place for up to two weeks (Wernovsky and Gruber, 2005).

C. Pulmonary artery pressure.

  1. Surgical placement using a pursestring structure or transthoracic placement of a pulmonary artery catheter into the right ventricular outflow tract is indicated for those neonates at risk for pulmonary hypertension (Artman et al., 2002; Hill et al., 2002).

  2. Measurements guide the medical management of pulmonary hypertension and are most frequently used in conditions in which postoperative pulmonary hypertension is anticipated, as in endocardial cushion repair, TAPVR, and mitral stenosis (Wernovsky and Gruber, 2005). Incidence of severe pulmonary hypertension following pediatric cardiac surgery found to be 2%.

  3. Mixed venous oxygen saturation ($S\overline{v}o_2$) monitoring can be obtained from pulmonary artery catheters with continuous oximetry capabilities.

    a. $S\overline{v}o_2$ reflects a balance between oxygen delivery and consumption.

    b. Alterations are seen in

      (1) Anemia,

      (2) Shock, and

      (3) Left-to-right or right-to-left shunts.

    c. Change in $S\overline{v}o_2$ generally precedes detectable hemodynamic changes by several minutes.

D. Left-sided cardiac pressures are monitored using a left atrial line.
   1. In patients with normal cardiac anatomy: left ventricular end-diastolic pressure = left atrial pressure = pulmonary artery occlusion pressure = pulmonary artery wedge pressure.
   2. Used to monitor systemic ventricular function and pulmonary shunting (Wernovsky and Gruber, 2005).
   3. Useful in patients with mitral valve dysfunction, as seen in postendocardial cushion repair.
   4. Requires meticulous line care because the risk of air or particulate embolization is high.
   5. Usually removed 1 to 2 days postoperation.
E. Epicardial pacing wires.
   1. Usually attached to right atrium and/or right ventricle.
   2. Provides temporary back-up pacing for up to 10 days (Dubin and Van Hare, 2002).
   3. Access to dual-chamber pacing is most important after surgical repairs near the cardiac conduction system. For example:
      a. VSD.
      b. Transposition of the great arteries.
      c. Truncus arteriosus.
      d. Endocardial cushion defects.

Hemodynamic Management

Neonates experience wide swings in physiologic responses, namely, heart rate, temperature, glucose metabolism, and systemic and pulmonary vascular resistance.
A. Bradycardia.
   1. Common result of intraoperative cooling; proportional to degree of hypothermia.
   2. After extensive atrial surgery, such as arterial switch procedure, TAPVR repair.
   3. After injury to sinoatrial node.
   4. With conducting problems:
      a. Sinoatrial block.
      b. Sinus asystole.
      c. Atrioventricular block is of most concern in the postoperative period (Wernovsky and Gruber, 2005).
   5. As a consequence of edema around conduction system (generally resolves in 3 to 4 days).
B. Tachycardia: Observed as a consequence of or in response to the following (Dubin and Van Hare, 2002):
   1. Pain.
   2. Anxiety/agitation.
   3. Fever.
   4. Hypovolemia.
   5. Junctional conduction disturbance.

POSTOPERATIVE DISTURBANCES

Heart Failure

Etiology

A. Most common postoperative event resulting from decreased neonatal cardiac reserve, limited by
   1. Decreased myofilament numbers;
   2. Decreased ventricular compliance;
   3. Greater oxygen consumption, cardiac output, and resting heart rate in the neonate; and
   4. Nearly maximal neonatal cardiac performance in the absence of stress.
B. Causes (Wernovsky and Gruber, 2005):
   1. Cardiopulmonary bypass adversely affects myocardial performance.
      a. Peak effect is 6 to 18 hours postoperatively.

2. Residual anatomic lesions.
   a. Transesophageal echocardiography in the operating room has minimized the incidence.
3. Pulmonary artery hypertensive crisis.
   a. Life-threatening right heart failure may be caused by an acute increase in pulmonary artery pressure.
4. Arrhythmias.

C. **Preload or diastolic filling:**
1. Hypovolemia.
   a. Inadequate volume replacement.
   b. Inadequate mechanical hemostasis.
   c. Impaired clotting.
2. Iatrogenic volume overload.
3. Left ventricular dysfunction.
4. Cardiac compression.

D. **Afterload** (Wernovsky and Gruber, 2005):
1. In the postoperative period, the neonatal heart is extremely sensitive to increased afterload.
2. Evidenced by peripheral vasoconstriction.
   a. Vasodilators are used to enhance the reduction of ventricular afterload.

E. **Contractility:**
1. Decreased peripheral perfusion.
2. Decreased urine output.
3. Treat with inotropic medications.

F. **Inadequate systemic venous return:**
1. Excessive positive end-expiratory pressure.
2. Tension pneumothorax.
3. Atrial baffle obstruction.
4. Postpericardial effusions.

G. **Increased pulmonary vascular resistance.**

H. **Decreased cardiac contractility**, resulting from the following:
1. Accidental discontinuation of vasoactive drugs.
2. Electrolyte disturbances.
3. Hypoglycemia.
4. Surgical manipulation or damage.

Recognition of Low Cardiac Output

A. **Frequently seen with changes in preload, afterload, and contractility** in the postoperative period, identified by impaired multiorgan system perfusion and elevated filling pressures (Mahle et al., 2005).

B. **Factors that influence the severity of low cardiac output:**
1. Age less than 1 month.
2. Weight less than 2.5 kg (Wernovsky et al., 2005).
3. Preoperative condition.
4. Type of defect.

C. **Observation: "just not doing well."**
1. Noninteractive or becoming less interactive with environment.
2. Lack of/or decreasing vigor of cry.
3. Awake but "floppy."

D. **Color:**
1. Violet color of mucosa.
2. Gray skin or mottling of skin.

E. **Extremities:**
1. Cool to touch.
2. Lack of or decrease in pedal pulses.
3. Capillary refill time longer than 3 seconds.

4. Edema: often seen postoperatively as third spacing, but also indicative of fluid overload (Spence, 2007).

F. **Oliguria (urine output <0.5 to 1 ml/kg/hour).**
   1. Transient acute renal failure may occur in 5% of neonates who require cardiopulmonary bypass during cardiac surgery (Wernovsky and Gruber, 2005).

G. **Tachycardia.**
   1. Gallop rhythm.
   2. Distant heart sounds: possible indication of pericardial effusions.

H. **Low arterial blood pressure.**

I. **Respiratory distress.**
   1. Retractions, tachypnea, grunting, and/or stridor in infant after extubation.
   2. Rales: often heard after bypass procedure.

J. **Weight gain disproportionate to caloric intake.**
   1. May be early indicator of fluid retention.

K. **X-ray findings.**
   1. Excessive cardiac size or enlargement of specific chamber.
   2. Large cardiac silhouette or "bag of waters" appearance may indicate pericardial effusions.
   3. Increased fluffy densities; these are not seen if elevated positive end-expiratory pressure is used in ventilation.

L. **Metabolic derangement.**
   1. Metabolic acidosis, generally resulting from low bicarbonate levels and lactic acid buildup that results from diminished tissue perfusion.
   2. Low sodium value, in part due to excessive free water.

Management of Low Cardiac Output

A. **Use blood for volume replacement.**
   1. Maintain hemoglobin greater than 12 g/dl for noncyanotic lesions and greater than 15 g/dl for cyanotic lesions (Cuadrado, 2002).

B. **Volume challenge is appropriate in light of cardiopulmonary bypass third spacing.**
   1. Close monitoring required.
   2. Strict intake and output.
   3. Neonates are easily fluid overloaded when given excessive fluids (Spence, 2007).

C. **Provide correction of metabolic disorders.**
   1. Hypocalcemia, hyponatremia, and hypoglycemia.
   2. Acid–base balances.
      a. Acidosis may result from poor tissue perfusion, prolonged hypovolemia, or impaired renal function (Spence, 2007). Correction depends on the underlying cause.

D. **Reduce right ventricular afterload.**
   1. Hyperventilation.
   2. Pulmonary vasodilating agents.
      a. PGE_1.
      b. Nitroglycerin.
      c. Nitroprusside is a mixed vasodilator frequently used with dopamine or dobutamine (Park, 2008).
      d. Inhaled nitric oxide.
   3. Provide sedation and analgesia (Cuadrado, 2002).

E. **Treat rate or rhythm disturbance.**
   1. Increased heart rate.
      a. Rate of 200 to 210 bpm is tolerated well, with acceptable myocardial work and oxygen consumption.
      b. Cardioversion can be used for supraventricular tachycardia, atrial flutter/fibrillation, and ventricular tachycardia (Hay et al., 2003).
   2. Atrial or atrioventricular pacing is often necessary.

F. **Consider pharmaceutical agents.**
   1. Isoproterenol (Isuprel): acts to decrease pulmonary and systemic vascular resistance (decreases afterload).

2. Nitroprusside or nitroglycerin: a venodilator that reduces afterload.
3. Milrinone: increases heart rate and contractility with some vasodilatory properties. Does not affect platelet function (Young and Mangum, 2008).
4. Nesiritide is a venous and arterial dilator with diuretic properties. In recent studies, has shown to be well-tolerated and improves diuresis; however, more studies are needed (Mahle et al., 2005).
5. Volume replacement: often necessary because of vasodilation (maintain preload). Central venous pressure is useful in determining volume needs.
6. Vasopressors (i.e., dopamine >10 µg/kg/min, or dobutamine). Potential for increasing PVR. Careful monitoring of effects is necessary.

G. Monitor blood pressure.

Bleeding

A. Provide sedation. Avoid agitation, prevent hypertension and pressure at active and potential bleeding sites, which may aggravate or disrupt clot formation.

B. Assess and treat coagulopathy (Miller and Spitzer, 2002).
1. Coagulation factors are 30% to 40% lower in neonates with congenital heart defects than in neonates without defects (Pike and Falco, 2002).
2. Use fresh whole blood less than 48 hours old for volume and clotting.
   a. Maintain hematocrit greater than 40% to 45% (Artman et al., 2002).
3. Use cryoprecipitate for fibrinogen (aids clotting).
4. Evaluate platelets: count is low and function is inadequate because of "bypass" and deep hypothermia.
   a. Give platelet infusion.
   b. Give desmopressin (DDAVP), 0.3 mcg/kg, to increase levels of von Willebrand factor (vWF), which stimulates platelets to aggregate.

Pulmonary Hypertension/Pulmonary Vasospasm (see Chapter 24)

A. Avoid hypoxemia and acidosis.
1. Hypoxia increases PVR and acidosis.
2. Neonates at risk for postoperative pulmonary hypertension need to be identified on return from the recovery room (Wernovsky and Gruber, 2005).
   a. Large VSD.
   b. Complete AV canal.
   c. Truncus arteriosus.
   d. Total anomalous venous return.
   e. D-transposition of the great arteries.

Maintenance of Fluid and Electrolyte Balance (see Chapter 8)

A. Hypoglycemia, hypokalemia, and hypocalcemia are potential problems.
1. All result in decreased myocardial function.
2. Potential for seizures is present.
   a. Poor cardiac output to the brain may cause seizures.
   b. Cardiopulmonary bypass and circulatory arrest also predispose an infant to seizures.

B. Avoid acidosis.
1. Metabolic acidosis is common in tissue hypoxia and suboptimal perfusion from lowered cardiac output.
2. Respiratory acidosis may be caused by poor pulmonary compliance, decreased respiratory drive, pulmonary disease, or inadequate mechanical ventilation.

C. Avoid fluid overload.
1. Meticulous monitoring of intake and output.

Shock

Etiology

A. Shock is a complex state of inadequate circulating blood volume, resulting in insufficient perfusion, oxygenation, and nutrients to the tissues (Kourembanas, 2004). Several varieties of shock are recognized.

B. **Hypovolemic shock** may be caused by (Karlsen and Tani, 2003):
   1. Blood loss from placental abnormalities (e.g., umbilical cord rupture, abruptio placentae, placenta previa, and twin-to-twin transfusion syndrome).
   2. Acute blood loss postnatally (such as intracranial or pulmonary hemorrhage).
   3. Acute or chronic blood loss postsurgically.
   4. Plasma and fluid losses.
      a. Skin integrity losses (e.g., myelomeningocele, gastroschisis).
      b. Pleural effusions (e.g., erythroblastosis fetalis or nonimmune hydrops).
      c. Body water loss from persistent vomiting/continuous gastric suctioning, diarrhea, or evaporative skin losses.
      d. Capillary leak syndrome resulting in third spacing.
C. **Cardiogenic shock** may be caused by (Karlsen, 2006):
   1. Myocardial failure due to severe hypoxemia, hypoglycemia, hypocalcemia, or acidosis.
   2. Congenital heart lesions.
   3. Cardiac arrhythmias.
      a. Sustained supraventricular tachycardia.
      b. Complete atrioventricular block (third degree).
   4. Restriction of cardiac function by
      a. Tamponade,
      b. Tension pneumothorax, or
      c. Excessive levels of ventilatory distending pressures.
   5. Myocarditis: often associated with sepsis.
D. **Distributive shock** (septic shock):
   1. Results from impaired peripheral arterial resistance usually caused by sepsis (i.e., release of bacterial toxins). The toxins cause capillary leak, which then leads to hypovolemic shock (Karlsen, 2006).
   2. Typically is associated with gram-negative organisms; however, gram-positive organisms may be the causative agent.

Clinical Indicators

A. **Signs of shock are frequently nonspecific.** (Cardiogenic shock may be indistinguishable from CHF.)
B. **Cardiopulmonary status changes.**
   1. Tachycardia at rest.
   2. Bradycardia.
   3. Tachypnea, increased work of breathing, dyspnea.
   4. Poor peripheral perfusion.
      a. Pallor (especially with acute blood loss).
      b. Capillary refill time longer than 3 seconds.
      c. Mottling.
      d. Weak, thready pulses.
      e. Cool extremities.
   5. Hypotension (blood pressure may be normal in early stages).
   6. Hypotonia, lethargy that may progress to a comatose state.
C. **Decreased urinary output.**
D. **Metabolic disturbances.**
   1. Metabolic acidosis.
   2. Hypoglycemia.
   3. Hypothermia.
E. **Evidence of coagulation defects.**
   1. Oozing from IV sites, suture lines, etc.
   2. Coagulopathy: abnormal PT, PTT, fibrinogen.
F. **Indicators of blood volume** (or effective blood volume):
   1. Change in hemoglobin and hematocrit values.
   2. Response to fluid challenge of 10 ml of saline solution per kilogram of body weight, while blood pressure and urine output are monitored.

3. Positive Betke–Kleihauer test result indicates fetal-to-maternal transfusion in utero. This test examines the maternal blood for the presence of fetal erythrocytes.

G. Indicators of cardiac function.

1. See Cardiopulmonary Status Changes, point B, above.
2. Echocardiogram establishes anatomic defects and/or specific myocardial function abnormalities.
3. Central venous pressure is generally elevated, except during hypovolemic shock.

H. Indicators of septic shock.

1. Clinical signs of sepsis or positive culture results.
2. Normal blood pressure in the face of prominent hypoperfusion.
3. Edema or sclerema from capillary protein and fluid leakage.
4. Oliguria, proteinuria.
5. Persistent pulmonary hypertension of the neonate (common).

Management of Shock

A. Depends largely on prevailing pathogenesis. A large proportion of the care is supportive.

B. Supportive care.

1. Maintain oxygenation and ventilation as dictated by arterial blood gas values.
   a. Give ventilatory support if concurrent pulmonary disease exists.
   b. Provide neutral thermal environment to decrease oxygen consumption.
   c. Decrease external stress (i.e., handling, peripheral blood sampling).
   d. Consider sedatives, analgesics, and neuromuscular blockade to decrease stress.
2. Promptly treat acidosis to avoid adverse effects on myocardial contractility. Sodium bicarbonate is often necessary.
3. Maintain fluid and electrolyte balance.

C. Specific therapies.

1. Increase blood volume and erythrocyte mass.
   a. Maintain blood pressure and maximize oxygen content.
   b. Treatment of acute blood loss may require large volume transfusion.
   c. Monitoring arterial blood pressure is essential; monitoring of central venous pressure ideally should be included.
   d. Caution: In cardiogenic shock, added volume may increase the myocardial workload.
2. Treat the infectious process in septic shock.
   a. Antibiotic therapy should be initiated.
   b. Consider use of granulocyte colony-stimulating factor, giving 5 to 10 mcg/kg/day for 3 to 5 days for infants who are in septic shock and have an absolute neutrophil count less than $1000/mm^3$ (Takemoto et al., 2003).
3. Maximize cardiac output.
   a. Inotropic agents such as epinephrine are useful in cardiogenic shock to increase cardiac output and support circulation. Start early in septic shock if evidence of oliguria, hypotension, or acidosis exists. Monitor for hypertension and edema (Takemoto et al., 2003). Norepinephrine may prove useful in dopamine-resistant shock (Carcillo and Fields, 2002). According to Takemoto and colleagues (2003), the usual dose is 0.5 mcg/kg/minute.
   b. Isoproterenol (Isuprel): increases heart rate and contractility (β_1-adrenergic effects). Simultaneous effects produce bronchodilation and smooth muscle relaxation (β_2-effects). Usual dose is 0.05 to 2 mcg/kg/minute. Observe for ventricular arrhythmias and tachycardia.
   c. Dopamine: increases cardiac contractility and cardiac output, affecting preload, contractility, and afterload, all three components of cardiovascular function (Evans and Seri, 2005). Effects are dose dependent. At low doses (1 to 3 mcg/kg/min, IV), selective vasodilation of the renal, mesenteric, cerebral, and coronary vascular beds occur, with little effect on heart rate or blood pressure. With moderate doses (5 to 10 mcg/kg/min), increased blood pressure and improved tissue perfusion can be observed. Beneficial effects are dependent largely on adequate blood volume. Correct hypovolemia before the dopamine infusion. At higher doses (>10 mcg/kg/min, IV), vasoconstriction occurs,

and includes vasoconstriction of the pulmonary vasculature, increased right ventricular afterload, reduction in pulmonary blood flow, right-to-left shunting through fetal structures, increased blood pressure, and increased hypoxemia. Tachycardia, dysrhythmias, and ectopic beats can occur as a consequence of dopamine infusion.

 d. Dobutamine (Dobutrex): increases cardiac contractility and heart rate while exerting limited effects on vasculature. Cardiac output increases, depending on myocardial catecholamine stores. Dose is 5 to 15 mcg/kg/minute as a continuous IV infusion (Kourembanas, 2004).

 e. Milrinone has proven beneficial in pediatric patients who continue to have increased vascular resistance after cardiac output is corrected to a low normal state (Wechsler and Wernovsky, 2004). Milrinone should be given for more than 72 hours (Young and Mangum, 2008). In term neonates, a loading dose of 75 mcg/kg IV is given over 60 minutes, followed by an infusion of 0.5 to 0.75 mcg/kg/min. In preterm neonates of <30 weeks of gestational age, loading dose is 0.75 mcg/kg/min for 3 hours, followed by 0.2 mcg/kg/min IV infusion.

 f. Corticosteroids have been used in premature infants to treat hypotension when volume expanders and standard modalities have failed. Recent studies have shown that steroids do improve blood pressure in this population; however, this has not been found in term neonates (Langer et al., 2006). It is unclear if corticosteroid use in preterm neonates is safe and effective.

 g. Digitalis should be considered and used selectively, especially in the face of hypoxia or toxic myocardiopathy.

 4. Correct any tension pneumothorax or cardiac tamponade.

D. Treatment goals.

 1. Reduce morbidity.

 2. Normalization of hemodynamic status.

 3. Halt progression of the shock state.

Pain Control and Sedation (see Chapter 16)

A. Pain assessment is the fifth vital sign; however, assessment of pain in newborn infants remains a major challenge for healthcare providers. Of even greater concern is assessment of pain in critically ill neonates. These infants have marginal organ system reserves, which leads to lack of adequate compensatory mechanisms (Wernovsky et al., 2005).

B. Postoperative pain management.

 1. Patients recovering from cardiac surgery are highly sensitive to stressful interventions and procedures and require analgesia and anesthesia to suppress responses to painful stimuli (Wernovsky et al., 2005).

  a. Intermittent or continuous neuromuscular blockade.

  b. Fentanyl infusion (2 to 4 mcg/kg/hour).

  c. Extending anesthesia beyond the immediate postoperative period may decrease hemodynamic variations, with improved outcomes.

  d. Minimize handling.

 2. Spinal anesthesia blockade (SAB) combined with general anesthesia.

 3. Nonpharmacologic measures.

  a. Comfort measures, such as swaddling, facilitated tucking, nonnutritive sucking, have proven beneficial.

  b. Environmental measures such as decreased lighting and noise levels are effective in reducing noxious stimuli.

Developmental Care (see Chapter 11)

A. Measures taken to facilitate developmentally appropriate care.

 1. Decrease noise and lighting.

 2. Decrease hands-on care; cluster tasks.

 3. Nonnutritive sucking.

4. Use positional devices and facilitated tucking.
5. Administer analgesics and sedatives.
6. Involve the family (Ward and Lugo, 2005).

Long-term Outcomes

A. There are more than a million adults now living with complex congenital heart disease who required surgery in the first month of life (Wernovsky et al., 2005).
B. Mortality has decreased dramatically over the last decade; however, mortality remains higher in low-birth-weight infants with the same defects (Wernovsky et al., 2005).
C. **Neurodevelopmental outcomes.**
   1. Adverse outcomes are well-documented in the literature.
      a. Infancy.
         (1) Feeding issues are present in 50%.
         (2) Delay in milestones by several months.
   2. Damage to central nervous system secondary to stroke remains at 1% to 5% after cardiac surgery (Wernovsky et al., 2005).
B. **Factors associated with poor outcomes.**
   1. Preoperative factors (Freed et al., 2006; Gaynor and Wernovsky, 2005).
      a. Gestational age (inversely related).
      b. Type of defect; increased risk of aneurysms with coarctation of the aorta (Padula and Ades, 2006).
      c. Seizures, acidosis.
      d. Age at time of repair.
   2. Operative factors.
      a. Type of circulatory support during surgery.
         (1) Deep hypothermic circulatory arrest.
            (a) Period of cerebral ischemia followed by reperfusion.
         (2) Continuous cardiopulmonary bypass.
      b. Hemodilution.
      c. Degree of cooling.
   3. Postoperative (Wernovsky, 2007).
      a. Seizures within 48 hours of surgery.
         (1) Linked to increase in cerebral palsy and neurodevelopmental delays.
         (2) Hypoxemia, low cardiac output; cardiac arrest.
         (3) Ventilator days (Dorfman et al., 2008).
         (4) CHF.

Parental Support and Education (see Chapter 17)

General Information

Whether made prenatally or postnatally, the diagnosis of a congenital heart defect or disease is stress-inducing for parents and other family members. Although this is well known, the psychological impact of prenatal diagnosis of congenital heart disease has not been well studied (Brosig et al., 2007). Having the diagnosis made prenatally does not lessen the stress experienced after birth. It is imperative that families be given support, accurate education, and skills to care for their newborn. This may be facilitated by a family-centered approach to care (McGrath and Kolwaite, 2006).

REFERENCES

Ades, A.A. and Wernovsky, G.: Management considerations and outcomes of low-birth weight infants who have congenital heart disease. *NeoReviews*, 6(7):e332-e338, 2005.

Ahmad, U.A., Fatimi, S.H., Naqvi, I., et al.: Modified Blalock-Taussig shunt: Immediate and short-term follow-up results. *Heart Lung Circulation*, doi:10.1016/j.hlc, 2007.

American Heart Association: Blood-incompatible infant heart transplants safe, may save more lives. *AHA News.* 2007. Retrieved January 18, 2008, from www. americanheart.org

American Heart Association: Surgical management of atrial septal defect. *AHA News.* 2008. Retrieved January 26, 2008, from www.americanheart.org

Andreassi, M.G., Ait-Ali, L., Botto, N., Manfredi, et al.: Cardiac catheterization and long-term chromosomal damage in children with congenital heart disease. *European Heart Journal,* 27:2703-2704, 2006.

Aranda, J.V. and Thomas, R.: Pharmacology review: Pharmacokinetic considerations with intravenous ibuprofen lysine. *NeoReviews,* 12(3):e516-e523, 2005.

Artman, M., Mahony, L., and Teitel, D.F.: *Neonatal cardiology.* New York, 2002, McGraw-Hill, pp. 196-199, 231-243.

Beck, A.E. and Hudgins, L.: Congenital cardiac malformations in the neonate: Isolated or syndromic? *NeoReviews,* 4(4):e105-e110, 2003.

Bishara, N. and Clericuzio, C.L.: Common dysmorphic syndromes in the NICU. *NeoReviews,* 3(1):e29-e38, 2008.

Blackburn, S.T.: Cardiovascular system. In S.T. Blackburn (Ed.): *Maternal, fetal, and neonatal physiology: A clinical perspective* (3rd ed.). St. Louis, 2007, Saunders, pp. 267-314.

Bleiweis, M.S. and Saidi, A.: Advances in neonatal cardiac surgery: Historical perspectives and current status. *NeoReviews,* 7(9):e463-e473, 2006.

Brosig, C.L., Whitstone, B.N., Frommelt, M.A., et al.: Psychological distress in parents of children with severe congenital heart disease: The impact of prenatal versus postnatal diagnosis. *Journal of Perinatology,* 27(11):687-692, 2007.

Capparelli, E.V.: Pharmacologic, pharmacodynamic, and pharmacokinetic considerations with intravenous ibuprofen lysine. *The Journal of Pediatric Pharmacology and Therapeutics,* 12(3):158-170, 2007.

Carcillo, J.A. and Fields, A.I.: Clinical practice parameters for hemodynamic support of pediatric and neonatal patients in septic shock. *Critical Care Medicine,* 30(6):1365-1378, 2002.

Chamberlin, M. and Lozynski, J.: To go against nature: Manipulating the neonatal ductus arteriosus with prostaglandin. *Newborn and Infant Nursing Reviews,* 6(3):158-164, 2006.

Charpie, J.R.: Pulmonary atresia with intact ventricular septum. *eMedicine.* 2007. Retrieved January 24, 2008, from www.emedicine.com/PED/topic2526.htm

Collins-Nakai, R. and McLaughlin, P.: How congenital heart disease originates in life. *Cardiology Clinics,* 20(3):367-383, 2002.

Connor, J.A. and Thiagarajan, R.: Hypoplastic left heart syndrome. *Neonatal Intensive Care,* 21(1):40-43, 2008.

Corff, K.E.: *Clinical considerations in the management of PDA in premature infants.* Symposia presented at 2007 National Association of Neonatal Nurses Conference, 2007.

Corff, K.E. and Sekar, K.C.: Clinical considerations for the pharmacologic management of patent ductus arteriosus with cyclooxygenase inhibitors in premature infants. *The Journal of Pediatric Pharmacology and Therapeutics,* 12(3):147-157, 2007.

Cuadrado, A.R.: Management of postoperative low cardiac output syndrome. *Critical Care Nursing Quarterly,* 25(3):63-71, 2002.

DeBord, S., Cherry, C., and Hickey, C.: The arterial switch procedure for transposition of the great arteries. *AORN Journal,* 86(2):211-226, 2007.

Dice, J.E. and Bhatia, J.: Patent ductus arteriosus: An overview. *The Journal of Pediatric Pharmacology and Therapeutics,* 12(3):138-146, 2007.

Dorfman, A.T., Marino, B.S., Wernovsky, G., et al.: Critical heart disease in the neonate: Presentation and outcome at a tertiary care center. *Pediatric Critical Care Medicine,* 9(3):1-10, 2008.

Dubin, A.M. and Van Hare, G.: Postoperative arrhythmias. In B.A. Reitz and D.D. Yuh (Eds.): *Congenital cardiac surgery.* New York, 2002, McGraw-Hill, pp. 203-215.

Dutta, S. and Albanese, C.T.: Minimal access surgery in the neonate. *NeoReviews,* 7(8):e400-e409, 2006.

Evans, N. and Seri, I.: Cardiovascular compromise in the newborn infant. In H.W. Taeusch, R.A. Ballard, and C.A. Gleason (Eds.): *Avery's diseases of the newborn.* Philadelphia, 2005, Saunders, pp. 398-437.

Flanagan, M.F., Yeager, S.B., and Weindling, S.N.: Cardiac disease. In M.G. MacDonald, M.M.K. Seshia, and M.D. Mullett (Eds.): *Avery's neonatology: Pathophysiology & management of the newborn* (6th ed.). Philadelphia, 2005, Lippincott Williams & Wilkins, pp. 633-709.

Fleiner, S.: Recognition and stabilization of neonates with congenital heart disease. *Newborn and Infant Nursing Reviews,* 6(3):137-150, 2006.

Freed, D.H., Robertson, C.M., Sauve, R.S., et al.: Intermediate-term outcomes of the arterial switch operation for transposition of great arteries in neonates: Alive but well? *Journal of Thoracic and Cardiovascular Surgery,* 132(4):845-852, 2006.

Gardner, S.L. and Johnson, J.L.: Initial nursery care. In G.B. Merenstein and S.L. Gardner (Eds.): *Handbook of neonatal intensive care* (6th ed.). St. Louis, 2006, Mosby, pp. 79-121.

Gaynor, J.W. and Wernovsky, G.: Long-term neurologic outcomes in children with congenital heart disease. In H.W. Taeusch, R.A. Ballard, and C.A. Gleason (Eds.): *Avery's diseases of the newborn.* Philadelphia, 2005, Saunders, pp. 896-901.

Glickstein, J.S.: Cardiology. In R.A. Polin and A.R. Spitzer (Eds.): *Fetal and neonatal secrets.* Philadelphia, 2007, Mosby, pp. 80-114.

Green, A., Pye, S., and Yetman, A.: The physiologic basis for and nursing considerations in the use of subatmospheric concentrations of oxygen in HLHS. *Advances in Neonatal Care,* 2(4):177-186, 2002.

Hagedorn, M.I.E., Gardner, S.L., Dickey, L.A., and Abman, S.H.: Respiratory diseases. In G.B. Merenstein and S.L. Gardner (Eds.): *Handbook of neonatal intensive care* (6th ed.). St. Louis, 2006, Mosby, pp. 595-698.

Hay, W.W., Hayward, A.R., Levin, M.J., and Sondheimer, J.M.: Cardiovascular diseases. In S. Reinhardt, H. Lebowitz, and L.A. Sheinis (Eds.): *Current pediatric diagnosis and treatment* (16th ed.). New York, 2003, McGraw-Hill.

Hermes-DeSantis, E.R. and Aranda, J.V.: Clinical experience with intravenous ibuprofen lysine in the pharmacologic closure of patent ductus arteriosus. *The Journal of Pediatric Pharmacology and Therapeutics*, 12(3):171-182, 2007.

Herrera, C., Holberton, J., and Davis, P.: Prolonged versus short course of indomethacin for the treatment of patent ductus arteriosus in preterm infants. *Cochrane Database of Systematic Reviews*, 1: CD003480, 2008.

Hill, L.L., Lammers, C.R., and Boltz, M.G.: Pediatric cardiac anesthesia. In B.A. Reitz and D.D. Yuh (Eds.): *Congenital cardiac surgery*. New York, 2002, McGraw-Hill, pp. 81-85.

Jonas, J.M. and Demmer, L.A.: Genetic syndromes determined by alterations in genomic imprinting pathways. *NeoReviews*, 8(20):e120-e126, 2007.

Jones, K.J., Willis, M., and Uzark, K.: The blues of congenital heart disease. *Newborn and Infant Nursing Reviews*, 6(3):117-127, 2006.

Kanter, J.P. and Hellenbrand, W.E.: Recent advances in non-interventional pediatric cardiac catheterization. *Current Opinion in Cardiology*, 20:75-79, 2005.

Kaplan, J.H., Ades, A.M., and Rychik, J.: Effect of prenatal diagnosis on outcome in patient with congenital heart disease. *NeoReviews*, 6(7):e326-e331, 2005.

Karlsen, K.A.: Transporting newborns the S.T.A.B.L.E. way. A manual for community hospital caregivers: Pre-transport stabilization of sick newborns. In *The S.T.A.B.L.E. program instructor manual*. Park City, UT, 2006, S.T.A.B.L.E. Program, pp. 130-149.

Karlsen, K.A. and Tani, L.Y.: *S.T.A.B.L.E. cardiac module*. Park City, UT, 2003, S.T.A.B.L.E. Program.

Khairy, P., Poirier, N., and Mercier, L.: Univentricular heart. *Circulation*, 115:800-812, 2007.

Killian, K.: Left sided obstructive congenital heart defects. *Newborn and Infant Nursing Reviews*, 6(3):128-136, 2006.

Kipps, A. and Silverman, N.H.: Historical perspectives: The introduction of ultrasonography in neonatal cardiac diagnosis. *NeoReviews*, 6(7):e315-e325, 2005.

Knight, S.E. and Washington, R.L.: Cardiovascular diseases and surgical interventions. In G.B. Merenstein and S.L. Gardner (Eds.): *Handbook of neonatal intensive care* (6th ed.). St. Louis, 2006, Mosby, pp. 699-735.

Kourembanas, S.: Shock. In J.P. Cloherty, E.C. Eichenwald, and Stark, A.R. (Eds.): *Manual of neonatal care* (5th ed.). Philadelphia, 2004, Lippincott Williams & Wilkins, pp. 181-184.

Langer, M., Modi, B.P., and Agus, M.: Adrenal insufficiency in the critically ill neonate and child. *Current Opinion in Pediatrics*, 18:448-453, 2006.

Lott, J.L.: Cardiovascular system. In C. Kenner and J.W. Lott (Eds.): *Comprehensive neonatal care: An interdisciplinary approach* (4th ed.). St. Louis, 2007, Saunders, pp. 32-64.

Lu, C., Wang, J., Chang, C., Lin, M., Wu, E., Lue, H., et al.: Noninvasive diagnosis of aortic coarctation in neonates with patent ductus arteriosus. *Journal of Pediatrics*, 148:217-221, 2006.

Maghsood, S. and Das, B.: Index of suspicion in the nursery. *NeoReviews*, 8(3):e133-e135, 2007.

Mahle, W.T., Cuadrado, A.R., Kirshbom, P.M., Kanter, K.R., and Simsic, J.M.: Nesiritide in infants with congestive heart failure. *Pediatric Critical Care Medicine*, 6(5):543-546, 2005.

Markham, M.: Patent ductus arteriosus in the premature infant: A clinical dilemma. *Newborn and Infant Nursing Reviews*, 6(3):151-157, 2006.

Mayo Clinic Staff: *Coarctation of the aorta*. 2006. Retrieved February 8, 2008, from www.mayoclinica.com

McGrath, J.M. and Kolwaite, A.: Families and chronicity of diagnosis with congenital heart defects. *Newborn and Infant Nursing Reviews*, 6(3):175-178, 2006.

Miller, B.E. and Spitzer, K.K.: Anesthetic and perfusion issues in contemporary pediatric cardiac surgery. *Critical Care Nursing Quarterly*, 25(3):48-62, 2002.

Minami, K., Knyphausen, E., Niino, T., et al.: Long-term results of pediatric heart transplantation. *Annals of Thoracic and Cardiovascular Surgery*, 11(6):386-390, 2005.

Moake, L. and Ramaciotti, C.: Atrial septal defect treatment options. *AACN Clinical Issues*, 16(2):252-266, 2005.

Overmeire, B.V.: Common clinical and practical questions on the use of intravenous ibuprofen lysine for the treatment of patent ductus arteriosus. *The Journal of Pediatric Pharmacology and Therapeutics*, 12(3):194-206, 2007.

Padula, M.A. and Ades, A.M.: Neurodevelopmental implications of congenital heart disease. *NeoReviews*, 7(7):e363-e369, 2006.

Park, M.K.: *Pediatric cardiology for practitioners* (5th ed.). St. Louis, 2008, Mosby.

Pike, N.A. and Falco, D.A.: Postoperative care of the neonate/infant after cardiac surgery. In B.A. Reitz and D.D. Yuh (Eds.): *Congenital cardiac surgery*. New York, 2002, McGraw-Hill, pp. 193-202.

Reade, C., Maziarz, D.M., and Koutlas, T.C.: Coarctation of the aorta and interrupted aortic arch: Surgical perspectives. *eMedicine*. 2006. Retrieved February 1, 2008, from www.emedicine.com/Ped/topic2824.htm

Rychik, J. and Cohen, M.S.: Echocardiography in the neonatal intensive care unit. In H.W. Taeusch, R.A. Ballard, and C.A. Gleason (Eds.): *Avery's diseases of the newborn* (8th ed.). Philadelphia, 2005, Saunders, pp. 802-811.

Sansoucie, D.A. and Cavaliere, T.A.: Newborn and infant assessment. In C. Kenner and J.W. Lott (Eds.): *Comprehensive neonatal care: An interdisciplinary approach* (4th ed.). St. Louis, 2007, Saunders, pp. 677-718.

Seri, I. and Evans, J.: Controversies in the diagnosis and management of hypotension in the newborn infant. *Current Opinion in Pediatrics*, 13(2):116-123, 2001.

Sharma, M., Nair, M., Jatana, S.K., and Shahi, B.N.: Congestive heart failure in infants and children. *Medical Journal of Armed Forces of India*, 59:228-233, 2003.

Spence, K.: Surgical considerations in the newborn and infant. In C. Kenner and J.W. Lott (Eds.): *Comprehensive neonatal care: An interdisciplinary approach* (4th ed.). St. Louis, 2007, Saunders, pp. 385-391.

Stein, P.: Total anomalous pulmonary venous connection. *AORN Journal*, 85(3):509-520, 2007.

Subhedar, N.V., Duffy, K., and Ibrahim, H.: Corticosteroids for treating hypotension in preterm infants. *Cochrane Database of Systematic Reviews, 1*: CD003662, 2007.

Swinford, R.D., Bonilla-Felix, M., Cerda, R.D., and Portman, R.J.: Neonatal nephrology. In G.B. Merenstein and S.L. Gardner (Eds.): *Handbook of neonatal intensive care* (6th ed.). St. Louis, 2006, Mosby, pp. 736-772.

Takemoto, C.K., Hodding, J.H., and Kraus, D.M.: *Pediatric dosage handbook: Including neonatal dosing drug administration and extemporaneous preparations* (6th ed.). Cleveland, 2003, Lexi-Comp.

Thangaratinam, S., Daniels, J., Ewer, A.K., Zamara, J., and Khan, K.S.: Accuracy of pulse oximetry in screening for congenital heart disease in asymptomatic newborns: A systematic review. *Archives of Diseases in Childhood 92*(3):f176-180, 2007.

Theorell, C.: Cardiovascular assessment of the newborn. *Newborn and Infant Nursing Reviews, 2*(2):111-127, 2002.

Turck, C.J., Marsh, W., Stevenson, J.G., York, J.M., Miller, H., and Patel, S.: Pharmacoeconomics of surgical interventions vs. cyclooxygenase inhibitors for the treatment of patent ductus arteriosus. *The Journal of Pediatric Pharmacology and Therapeutics*, 12(3):183-193, 2007.

Wald, R.M., Tham, E.B., McCrindle, B.W., et al.: Outcome after prenatal diagnosis of tricuspid atresia: A multicenter experience. *American Heart Journal* 153(5):772-778, 2007.

Ward, R.M. and Lugo, R.A.: Pharmacologic principles and practices. In H.W. Taeusch, R.A. Ballard, and C.A. Gleason (Eds.): *Avery's diseases of the newborn* (8th ed.). Philadelphia, 2005, Saunders, pp. 427-437.

Weber, H.S. and Seib, P.M.: Aortic stenosis, valvar. *eMedicine.* 2006. Retrieved February 8, 2008, from www.emedicine.com/PED/topic2491.htm

Wechsler, S.B. and Wernovsky, G.: Cardiac disorders. In J.P. Cloherty, E.C. Eichenwald, and A.R. Stark (Eds.): *Manual of neonatal care* (5th ed.). Philadelphia, 2004, Lippincott Williams & Wilkins, pp. 407-460.

Wernovsky, G., Ades, A.M., and Spray, T.L.: Management of congenital heart disease in the low-birth-weight infant. In H.W. Taeusch, R.A. Ballard, and C.A. Gleason (Eds.): *Avery's diseases of the newborn* (8th ed.). Philadelphia, 2005, Saunders, pp. 888-895.

Wernovsky, G. and Gruber, P.J.: Common congenital heart disease: Presentation, management, and outcomes. In H.W. Taeusch, R.A. Ballard, and C.A. Gleason (Eds.): *Avery's diseases of the newborn* (8th ed.). Philadelphia, 2005, Saunders, pp. 827-871.

Westmoreland, D.: Critical congenital cardiac defects in the newborn. *Journal of Perinatal and Neonatal Nursing*, 12(4):67-87, 1999.

Young, T.E. and Mangum, B.: *Neofax* (21st ed.). Montvale, NJ, 2008, Thomson Healthcare.

Zannini, L. and Borini, I.: State of the art cardiac surgery in patients with congenital heart disease. *Journal of Cardiovascular Medicine*, 8:3-6, 2007.

29 Gastrointestinal Disorders

WANDA T. BRADSHAW

OBJECTIVES

1. Discuss normal and abnormal abdominal assessment findings.
2. Discuss common laboratory and diagnostic tests used to evaluate the gastrointestinal system.
3. Differentiate between omphalocele and gastroschisis.
4. Identify four common associations in infants with intestinal obstruction.
5. Identify the clinical presentation of a neonate with tracheoesophageal fistula.
6. Describe radiographic findings in an infant with duodenal atresia.
7. Identify one gastrointestinal disorder that is considered a surgical emergency.
8. Identify the gastrointestinal presentation of infants with cystic fibrosis.
9. Describe the defect in Hirschsprung disease.
10. Identify the three mechanisms involved in the pathogenesis of necrotizing enterocolitis.
11. Describe the clinical presentation of an infant with biliary atresia.
12. Identify at least three management strategies for the infant with cholestasis.
13. Identify at least three management strategies for the infant with gastroesophageal reflux.
14. Identify the triad of anomalies occurring in prune-belly syndrome.
15. Describe the symptoms of diaphragmatic hernia.
16. Differentiate between unconjugated and conjugated bilirubin.
17. Compare and contrast physiologic and nonphysiologic jaundice.
18. Describe management of an infant receiving phototherapy.
19. Define "hydrops."

■■ Unique embryologic features of the gastrointestinal (GI) tract, such as the obliteration and recanalization of the GI tract, midgut herniation into the umbilical cord, and rotation of the intestines, make the GI tract prone to a variety of congenital anomalies. Anomalies may affect any part of the GI tract, from the mouth to the anus. Atresias, stenoses, and functional obstructions account for the vast majority of congenital defects. As for acquired defects, necrotizing enterocolitis is the most common serious GI illness in neonates. This chapter will review the more common GI anomalies, and a variety of multisystem disorders that have significant GI involvement such as prune-belly syndrome, congenital diaphragmatic hernia, hyperbilirubinemia, and hydrops.

GASTROINTESTINAL EMBRYONIC DEVELOPMENT

A. **Week 3.** Tubular intestine begins to form; omphalomesenteric (yolk stalk) duct forms; mesentery is forming; major digestive (salivary, liver, pancreas, gall bladder) and endocrine (thyroid) gland formation is initiated.
B. **Week 4.** Intestine is present; esophagus and trachea separate and are distinct; stomach becomes obvious; liver is present.
C. **Week 5.** Esophagus, stomach, proximal duodenum present; intestine elongates into a loop and begins to rotate.

D. **Week 6.** Stomach rotates into adult position; distal duodenum, jejunum, ileum, cecum, ascending colon, and proximal two-thirds of transverse colon present; rapidly developing midgut herniates into umbilical cord.

E. **Week 7.** Rapid endothelial proliferation results in temporary duodenal occlusion; intestinal loops herniate into umbilical cord, lengthen, and rotate; and urorectal septum fuses with cloacal membrane, separating rectum from the developing urinary bladder.

F. **Week 8.** Small intestine recanalizes; intestinal villi develop; diaphragm complete.

G. **Weeks 9 and 10.** Intestines begin to reenter abdominal cavity and continue counterclockwise rotation around the axis of the superior mesenteric artery.

H. **Week 12.** Muscular layers of intestine are present; active transport of amino acids begins; pancreatic islet cells appear; bile appears; lactase appears.

I. **Week 16.** Meconium is present; swallowing is observed.

J. **Week 24.** Ganglion cells are detected in the rectum.

K. **Week 26.** Random peristalsis begins.

L. **Weeks 34 to 36.** Sucking and swallowing become coordinated.

M. **Weeks 36 to 38.** Maturity of GI system completed.

N. **Weeks 5 to 40.** Intestine elongates approximately 100-fold (small intestine is 6 times the length of the colon).

FUNCTIONS OF THE GASTROINTESTINAL TRACT

A. **Absorption and digestion of nutrients.**
B. **Elimination of waste products.**
C. **Maintenance of fluid and electrolyte balance.**
D. **Protection of host from toxins and pathogens.**

ASSESSMENT OF THE GASTROINTESTINAL SYSTEM

A. **History.**
1. Family: presence of GI disease.
2. Presence of genetic syndrome: Major syndromes associated with GI defects include (Jones, 2006) the following:
   a. Apert syndrome: pyloric stenosis, tracheoesophageal fistula/esophageal atresia (TEF/EA), congenital diaphragmatic hernia (CDH).
   b. Beckwith–Wiedemann syndrome: umbilical defects, diastasis recti, posterior diaphragmatic eventration, pancreatic hyperplasia resulting in hypoglycemia.
   c. Fetal hydantoin syndrome: umbilical hernia, duodenal atresia.
   d. Meckel–Gruber syndrome: liver defects (bile duct proliferation, fibrosis, cysts), single umbilical artery, patent urachus, omphalocele, intestinal malrotation, imperforate anus.
   e. Sirenomelia: imperforate anus, anal agenesis.
   f. Trisomy 13: umbilical defects, intestinal malrotation, CDH.
   g. Trisomy 18: umbilical defects, pyloric stenosis, intestinal malrotation, TEF/EA, CDH, single umbilical artery.
   h. Trisomy 21: Hirschsprung, pyloric stenosis, duodenal atresia, intestinal malrotation.
   i. VATERR association (*v*ertebral defects, imperforate *a*nus, *t*racheo*e*sophageal fistula and/or esophageal atresia, and *r*adial and *r*enal dysplasia). Additional: single umbilical artery.
   j. VACTERL association (*v*ertebral defects, *a*nal atresia, *c*ardiac abnormalities, *t*racheo*e*sophageal fistula and/or esophageal atresia, *r*enal agenesis or dysplasia, and *l*imb defects).
3. History of present illness.
   a. Fetal ultrasonography.
      (1) Abdomen can be seen by 10 weeks of gestation, stomach by 13 weeks.
      (2) Abdomen can be assessed for intactness of abdominal wall, umbilical cord insertion, stomach as fluid-filled chamber, bowel dilation, or indication of obstruction.

(3) Polyhydramnios (>2000 ml) may indicate interference with fetal swallowing or intestinal obstruction.

(4) Oligohydramnios (<500 ml) may indicate renal agenesis or dysgenesis.

b. Birth weight, weight loss/gain, reflux, vomiting, timing of passage of first meconium stool, diarrhea, constipation, abdominal distention or tenderness, jaundice (Seidel et al., 2006).

B. Abdominal assessment (Goodwin, 2003; Seidel et al., 2006).

1. Inspection.

  a. Size, shape, and color.

    (1) Should be rounded, soft, symmetric, pink.

    (2) Distended: intestinal obstruction, infection, organomegaly, ascites.

    (3) Scaphoid: associated with congenital diaphragmatic hernia.

    (4) Asymmetric: mass, organomegaly, intestinal obstruction.

  b. Muscular development.

    (1) Flat, flabby, lumpy: prune-belly syndrome.

    (2) Gap between rectus muscles: diastasis recti.

    (3) Externalization of abdominal contents: omphalocele, gastroschisis, bladder exstrophy.

    (4) Hernias: protrusions of an organ or tissue through an abnormal opening. Common in three areas:

      (a) Umbilical: common in African Americans, low birth weight males, trisomy 21, hypothyroidism, and mucopolysaccharidosis.

      (b) Inguinal.

        (i) More common in males, especially very low birth weight.

        (ii) Frequently bilateral.

        (iii) May not be evident until second or third month of life.

        (iv) Usually readily reducible.

      (c) Femoral.

        (i) Rare but more common in females.

        (ii) Located just below inguinal ligament on anterior aspect of thigh.

  c. Umbilicus/umbilical cord.

    (1) Normally pearly white.

    (2) Green or yellow staining suggests in utero meconium passage.

    (3) Wet, foul-smelling cord, or periumbilical redness: omphalitis.

    (4) Persistent clear drainage: patent urachus.

    (5) Ileal fluid drainage: omphalomesenteric duct.

    (6) Serous or serosanguineous drainage: granuloma.

    (7) Abnormally thick: single herniated loop of intestine.

    (8) Thick, gelatinous: large for gestational age.

    (9) Thin, small: intrauterine growth restriction.

    (10) Normally three vessels: two ventrally situated arteries, one dorsally situated vein.

    (11) Usually dries and spontaneously detaches in 10 to 14 days.

  d. Bowel loops.

    (1) Normally not visible.

    (2) Presence: obstruction.

  e. Movements.

    (1) Should move in synchrony with respirations.

    (2) Movements not in synchrony may represent respiratory distress, peritoneal irritation, or central nervous system (CNS) disease.

    (3) Peristalsis: not normally seen.

      (a) May be seen in premature infants with thin abdominal walls.

      (b) Presence: associated with hypertrophic pyloric stenosis.

  f. Veins.

    (1) Superficial veins become more prominent with abdominal distention.

    (2) Dilated veins: venous obstruction.

  g. Perineum: inspected for patency of anus and presence of fistulas.

2. Auscultation.
   a. Done before palpation (to avoid altering sounds).
   b. Bowel sounds.
      (1) Become audible within 15 to 30 minutes after birth (Thigpen and Kenner, 2003).
      (2) Should have a metallic clicking quality.
      (3) Hyperactive or hypoactive does not necessarily represent pathologic change. Other historical or clinical findings should be taken into consideration when interpreting bowel sounds.
      (4) Increased sounds.
         (a) Malrotation.
         (b) Hirschsprung disease.
         (c) Diarrhea.
      (5) Decreased or absent sounds.
         (a) Ileus.
         (b) Starvation.
   c. Vascular sounds: bruit, similar to murmur. Caused by turbulent blood flow through an artery, especially if heard despite position change of infant. Bruits may indicate partial vascular obstruction.
   d. Friction rub: peritoneal inflammation, splenic involvement, hepatic tumor, abscess.
3. Percussion.
   a. Provides information regarding size and location of organs, presence of masses, fluids, gases. Not a significantly useful tool in the newborn infant.
   b. Two main sounds to listen for:
      (1) Tympanic: low pitched, heard over gas-filled structures (stomach).
      (2) Dullness: high pitched, short, heard over dense or solid organs (liver, spleen).
4. Palpation.
   a. Performed to assess:
      (1) Abdominal tone.
      (2) Organ position.
         (a) Liver should be 1 to 2 cm below right costal margin, midclavicular line.
         (b) Spleen rarely palpable. Tip should not be more than 1 cm below left costal margin.
         (c) Kidneys are about 4 to 5 cm in length. Right kidney is easier to palpate and is lower than left.
      (3) Organomegaly.
      (4) Masses.
      (5) Pulsations.
      (6) Fluid.
   b. Technique: start in lower quadrants and progress to upper quadrants using a bimanual approach. Place one hand under infant's back; using free hand start with light palpation, then progress to deep palpation.
   c. Hints to relax infant.
      (1) Use warm hands.
      (2) Flex legs.
      (3) Use gentle circular motion.
      (4) Slowly increase depth of palpation.
      (5) Palpate any known areas of tenderness last.
C. **Diagnostic tests.**
   1. Gastric tests.
      a. Gastric aspirate. Measure pH of gastric contents.
      b. Apt test.
         (1) Differentiates swallowed maternal blood from fetal blood. Fetal hemoglobin remains pink; adult hemoglobin turns yellow-brown.
         (2) Can be done on gastric fluid or stool.

2. Stool examination.
   a. Examined for color, consistency, odor, blood, mucus, pus, tissue fragments, bacteria, and parasites.
   b. Color may be influenced by diet, dyes, drugs, pathology.
      (1) Green: indomethacin, meconium.
      (2) Greenish black: iron, meconium.
      (3) Black: iron, swallowed blood, blood from high GI tract lesion.
      (4) Pale: biliary atresia.
      (5) White: antacids, barium.
      (6) Red: bright red indicates blood from low GI tract lesion; currant jelly indicates intussusception.
   c. Odor.
      (1) Sweet, yeasty, or acidic in odor suggests carbohydrate malabsorption typical of osmotic diarrhea of viral enteritis.
      (2) Purulent odor suggests colitis.
   d. pH less than 5 in infants suggests carbohydrate malabsorption.
   e. Guaiac.
      (1) Detects occult blood.
3. pH probe test: 24-hour pH probe study to diagnose GI reflux. Detects acid reflux only; does not detect nonacid (milk) or gas reflux.
4. Radiologic studies.
   a. Plain radiograph (see Chapter 14).
      (1) Bowel gas pattern (Thigpen and Kenner, 2003).
         (a) At birth, GI tract is fluid filled and gasless.
         (b) Within 30 minutes, gas should be in stomach.
         (c) By 3 to 4 hours, gas should be in small intestine.
         (d) After 6 to 8 hours, gas should be in entire intestine.
      (2) Absence of gas below pylorus: possible indication of obstruction.
   b. Upper GI series: done to assess structure and function of esophagus, pyloric stenosis, malrotation.
      (1) Contrast material such as barium or a water-soluble product is administered via a nasogastric tube and observed by fluoroscopy.
      (2) Water-soluble products are preferred in cases of suspected perforation.
   c. Lower GI series: may be used to detect presence of malrotation, Hirschsprung disease, meconium ileus, and meconium plug syndrome. May be therapeutic in meconium ileus and meconium plug syndrome.
5. Ultrasonography: may be used to diagnose suspected cases of pyloric stenosis, duplications, gastroesophageal reflux, or biliary atresia.
6. Scintigraphy (nuclear scan): used to evaluate gastric emptying, aspiration with swallowing, reflux with aspiration, and liver excretory function. Radionuclide tagged formula is fed to the infant and recorded by a gamma camera.
7. Endoscopy: used to directly visualize the upper or lower GI mucosa. Endoscopic retrograde cholangiopancreatography (ERCP) visualizes the biliary pancreatic ducts.
8. Fecal fat: used to diagnosis malabsorption syndromes. Fecal fat content greater than 6 g/24 hours is associated with malabsorption syndrome.
9. Culture: helpful in differentiating bloody diarrhea caused by infection vs. hypoxic insult to intestine.

D. **Laboratory tests** (Table 29-1) (Kee, 2005).
   1. Albumin.
      a. Synthesized in the liver; it is the most abundant plasma protein.
      b. Decreased levels occur in hepatocellular injury; usually a late finding.
   2. Alkaline phosphatase (ALP).
      a. ALP is derived from the epithelium of the intrahepatic bile ducts and excreted into the bile. It is also found in the bone, kidney, and small intestine.
      b. Elevated levels occur in obstructive liver disease (e.g., biliary atresia) and hepatitis, as well as in bone disease.

■ TABLE 29-1
■ ■ **Laboratory Tests Used to Evaluate the Gastrointestinal System**

Test	Preterm	Term	Reference
Alanine aminotransferase (ALT) (units/l)	—	10 to 33	1
Aspartate aminotransferase (AST) (units/l)		24 to 81	1
Alkaline phosphatase (ALP) (units/l)	207 ± 60 to 320 ± 142	164 ± 68	1
Albumin	—	2.8 to 4.4 g/dl	2
Bile acids	⅙ of adult value	½ of adult value	3
Bilirubin, total (mg/dl)			1
Cord	<2.8	<2.8	
24 hours	1 to 6	2 to 6	
48 hours	6 to 8	6 to 7	
3 to 5 days	10 to 12	4 to 6	
≥1 month	<1.5	<1.5	
Bilirubin, direct (mg/dl)	<0.5	<0.5	
Ammonia (μg/dl)	—	90 to 150	1
Gamma-glutamyl-transferase (GGT) (units/l)	—	14 to 131	1
5'-nucleotidase (5′N, 5′NT) (units/l)	—	5 to 10	4
Prothrombin (PT) (seconds)	—	13 to 18	2

Adapted from Blackburn, S.T.: *Maternal, fetal, and neonatal physiology: A clinical perspective* (3rd ed.). St. Louis, 2003, Saunders; Martin, R.J., Fanaroff, A.A., and Walsh, M.C. (Eds.): *Fanaroff and Martin's neonatal-perinatal medicine: Diseases of the fetus and infant* (8th ed.). Philadelphia, 2006, Mosby; Malarkey, L.M. and McMorrow, M.E.: *Saunders nursing guide to laboratory and diagnostic tests.* St. Louis, 2005, Saunders; Simone, S.: Gastrointestinal critical care problems. In M.C. Curley and P.A. Moloney-Harmon (Eds.): *Critical care nursing of infants and children* (2nd ed.). Philadelphia, 2001, Saunders, pp. 765-804.

3. Aminotransferase activity.
   a. Alanine aminotransferase (ALT) catabolizes the reversible transfer of the α-amino group of aspartic acid to the α-keto group of α-ketoglutaric acid, leading to the formation of pyruvic acid.
   b. Aspartate aminotransferase (AST) catabolizes the reversible transfer of the α-amino group of aspartic acid to the α-keto group of α-ketoglutaric acid, leading to the formation of oxaloacetic acid.
   c. ALT and AST are the most sensitive tests of hepatocyte necrosis. ALT is more specific than AST because it is not found in high concentrations in other tissues.
   d. High elevations occur in hepatocellular injury. Slight elevations occur in cholestasis. Serum ALT >300 units coupled with jaundice signals a liver disorder and not a hemolytic disorder.
   e. ALT-to-AST ratio is often performed to help differentiate types of liver disease.
4. Ammonia.
   a. Produced from the deamination of amino acids during protein metabolism and is a by-product of colonic bacteria protein breakdown. Liver is responsible for metabolizing ammonia.
   b. Elevated in liver failure.
   c. Elevations occur in acute or chronic liver disease.
5. Bilirubin.
   a. By-product of heme breakdown.
   b. Increased indirect bilirubin occurs when liver function is reduced (prematurity, injury) or when there is an excessive load of unconjugated bilirubin (hemolysis).
   c. Increased direct bilirubin occurs when the liver cannot excrete conjugated bilirubin into the bile ducts or biliary tract (biliary atresia, cholestasis).
6. Prothrombin time (PT).
   a. Measures the time required for prothrombin (factor II) to be converted to thrombin.

    b. In cases of obstructive liver disease in which bile acids do not reach the intestine, fat-soluble vitamins are not absorbed (required for coagulation factors).

    c. Prolonged PT occurs in patients with hepatocellular injury and biliary obstruction.

  7. Serum bile acids.

    a. In the absence of abnormalities of the ileum, normal serum values reflect functioning of the enterohepatic circulation.

    b. Elevations occur in acute and chronic liver disease.

ABDOMINAL WALL DEFECTS

A. Omphalocele (exomphalos) (Farrell and Elias, 2007; Kalousek and Oligny, 2007; Magnuson et al., 2006; Oligny, 2007).

  1. Definition: central defect with herniation of the abdominal viscera into the umbilical cord covered by a thin, avascular membranous sac composed of amnion and peritoneum with a small amount of Wharton jelly. Umbilical arteries and veins insert into the apex of the defect (Fig. 29-1).

  2. Etiology: multifactorial, including environmental, chromosomal (recessive and dominant forms), and folding abnormality of the germ disc, with failure to close the ventral abdominal wall.

  3. Incidence: 2.5 per 10,000 live births.

  4. Associated conditions: a large number will have associated anomalies or be part of a syndrome.

    a. Prematurity; small for gestational age.

    b. Cardiac defects (50%).

    c. Intestinal malrotation and/or atresia.

    d. Pentalogy of Cantrell: upper abdominal omphalocele above the umbilical cord, diaphragmatic hernia, sternal cleft, pericardial defect, ectopia cardiac defect.

    e. Neurologic anomalies, neural tube (40%).

    f. Genitourinary anomalies.

    g. Skeletal anomalies.

    h. Chromosomal anomalies (50% to 65%). Common anomalies include trisomy 13, 18, and 21, with 18 being the most frequent. Frequent in infants with Beckwith–Wiedemann syndrome (chromosome 11).

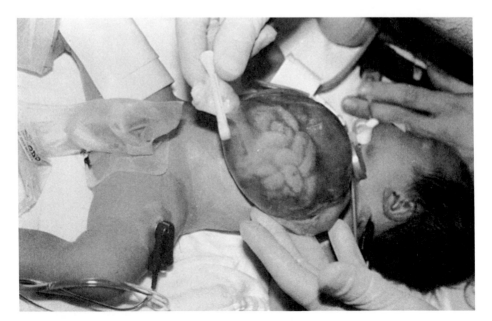

FIGURE 29-1. ■ Omphalocele.

5. Diagnosis.
   a. Maternal serum markers: elevated serum α-fetoprotein to detect open defects.
   b. High-resolution prenatal ultrasound.
   c. Amniocentesis: chromosome analysis for associated defects; amniotic fluid α-fetoprotein and acetylcholinesterase levels to evaluate for defects associated with abnormal values.
   d. Inspection at birth.
      (1) Small defect: contains few loops of intestine, slightly enlarged umbilical ring. Any umbilical cord that is unusually fat should be inspected carefully before clamping to prevent intestinal trauma.
      (2) Large defect: may contain intestines, stomach, liver, spleen, bladder, uterus and ovaries, testicle; deficient upper musculature of umbilical ring.
      (3) The thin, avascular membranous sac may rupture before or at time of delivery; must be differentiated from gastroschisis because of the high rate of associated anomalies with omphalocele.
6. Prognosis.
   a. Mortality rate is related to size of defect and severity of associated anomalies.

B. **Gastroschisis** (Farrell and Elias, 2007; Magnuson et al., 2006; Oligny, 2007).
   1. Definition: herniation of abdominal contents through an abdominal wall defect lateral to the umbilical ring; umbilical ring and cord are normal; right sided predominance (Fig. 29-2). See Table 29-2 for a comparison of omphalocele and gastroschisis.
   2. Etiology: unclear; theories include rupture of umbilical stalk, right periumbilical ischemia due to atrophy or persistence of the right umbilical vein, or a vascular accident of the right omphalomesenteric artery.
   3. Incidence: overall 1 per 10,000 live births, with 7 per 10,000 in women <20 years old, low socioeconomic status, and exposure to vasoconstrictors (decongestants, NSAIDs, cocaine).
   4. Associated conditions.
      a. Prematurity.
      b. Intestinal malrotation (100%) and atresia (5% to 25%).
      c. Other anomalies are uncommon.
   5. Diagnosis.
      a. Maternal serum markers: elevated serum α-fetoprotein to detect open defects.
      b. Prenatal ultrasonography, including a high-resolution method.

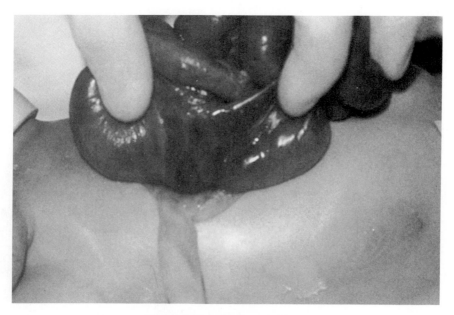

FIGURE 29-2. ■ Gastroschisis.

■ TABLE 29-2
■ ■ **Comparison of Omphalocele and Gastroschisis**

	Omphalocele	**Gastroschisis**
Incidence	1 : 5000 to 1 : 6000	1 : 30,000 to 1 : 50,000
Covering	Present, may be ruptured	None
Site	Umbilical	Paraumbilical, usually to the right
Fascial defect	Small or large	Small
Herniated organs	Intestines; stomach, liver, spleen sometimes	Intestines; rarely liver
Appearance of herniated bowel	Normal, unless sac is ruptured	Often edematous, matted
Associated anomalies	45% to 55%	10% to 15%
IUGR	Less common	Common

IUGR, Intrauterine growth restriction.

    c. Amniocentesis: chromosome analysis for associated defects; amniotic fluid α-fetoprotein and acetylcholinesterase levels to evaluate for defects associated with abnormal values.
    d. Inspection at birth.
       (1) Eviscerated abdominal organs without a thin, avascular membranous sac to protect the viscera.
       (2) Usually includes small and large intestines and rarely the liver.
       (3) Intestine may be thickened, edematous, and inflamed as a result of amniotic fluid exposure.
       (4) Fascial defect is smaller than with omphalocele.
       (5) Umbilical cord is intact.
       (6) Must be differentiated from ruptured omphalocele because of the high rate of associated anomalies with omphalocele.
  6. Prognosis.
    a. Mortality rate is related to size of defect and severity of associated anomalies.
    b. Morbidity almost entirely related to intestinal dysfunction (impaired absorption, reduced enzymes, dysmotility) as a result of in utero injury to eviscerated, unprotected bowel.
C. Care of the neonate with an abdominal wall defect (omphalocele and gastroschisis) (Magnuson et al., 2006).
  1. No research has demonstrated the efficacy of delivering infants with omphalocele or gastroschisis early.
  2. Goals.
    a. Prevent hypothermia and hypovolemia (heat and evaporative fluid loss).
       (1) At the time of delivery, if there is exposed viscera, place infant in a sterile bowel bag from the feet to the axilla. Secure drawstring around torso at axilla. The bowel bag maintains a sterile environment for, and allows visualization of, the exposed viscera. If bowel bag is not available, cover the exposed defect and viscera with warm, sterile normal saline dressings. Then cover the dressing with plastic. Gauze dressings require rehydration to prevent drying, adherence to viscera, and tissue trauma when removed. Such dressings may contribute to hypothermia as the gauze cools over time.
       (2) Begin IV fluid as soon as possible. Add TrophAmine and electrolytes as needed. IV fluid may need to be increased to approximately 150 ml/kg/day because of increased fluid loss through exposed bowel. Ideally, IV infusions should not be started in the lower extremities owing to postoperatively increased intraabdominal pressure and venous stasis.

    b. Gastric decompression.

        (1) NPO. Insert Replogle tube (Sherwood Medical, Norfolk, NE) and place to continuous low suction. Bowel distention restricts normal intestinal blood flow and makes primary surgical repair more difficult.

    c. Maintain perfusion to the viscera; prevent vascular compromise from torqued viscera.

        (1) Position infant side lying or support viscera with a small roll.

    d. Prevent infection.

        (1) Maintain sterile environment. Minimize handling of viscera, wear sterile gloves.

        (2) Administer antibiotics.

  3. Laboratory studies: complete blood count (CBC) with manual differential; electrolytes; acid–base and blood gas; clotting studies; and blood type and cross-match.

  4. Assess for associated anomalies, syndromes, or malformations.

  5. Most newborn infants with abdominal wall defects require surgical repair. The types of repair include the following:

    a. Primary repair: All contents are returned to the abdominal cavity, and the fascia and skin are closed. The infant may require prolonged respiratory support because of increased intraabdominal pressure. Preferred repair, but not possible in all cases.

    b. Staged repair: Not all the organs are returned to the abdominal cavity during the primary surgery. The viscera remaining outside the cavity are placed in an extra-abdominal prosthetic compartment (typically a mesh-reinforced, Silastic-covered Marlex sac [silo]). The sac is either sutured to the edge of the defect or secured underneath the fascia, allowing gradual reduction of the intestines on a daily basis. The silo must be supported at a 90-degree angle to the infant to promote reduction by gravity and prevent vascular compromise. This technique is employed with infants with large defects and for those who cannot tolerate primary repair. A variation of this technique is the insertion of a spring-loaded silo over the exposed viscera under the fascia performed in the delivery room or in the NICU with subsequent closure on an elective basis. This latter technique is gaining in popularity and has been associated with fewer complications, fewer ventilator days, and shorter hospital stays (Wu et al., 2003).

        (1) Reduction minimizes the stress on the respiratory and vascular systems by allowing these systems to adjust slowly to the increased pressure of the organs as they are slowly returned to the abdominal cavity.

        (2) Reduction can usually be accomplished during a period of 10 days or less, after which infection becomes a major consideration.

        (3) Assess perfusion of herniated contents frequently through the silo. Compromise of mesenteric vasculature can occur within the silo.

        (4) The abdominal wall is closed after the reduction is completed.

    c. Skin flap closure. Only the skin is pulled over the exposed organs. This method is not a long-term solution and is used when the fascia cannot be initially repaired.

        (1) Definitive repair done at 6 to 12 months of age.

    d. Closure by porcine small intestinal submucosal graft using Surgisis ES (Cook, West Lafayette, IN), a biomaterial (collagen, proteins, and bio molecules). The graft is sewn to the fascia. Complete epithelialization and vascularization over the graft occurs, closing the abdomen (Gabriela and Gollinb, 2006).

    e. Nonsurgical repair. The defect is painted with an escharotic agent such as silver nitrate, or silver sulfadiazine and allowed to air dry and epithelialize.

        (1) This uncommon procedure is used only if the defect is large, if the infant cannot tolerate surgery or has uncorrectable congenital anomalies, or if the reduction fails.

        (2) Systemic side effects are associated with most of the escharotic agents. The health care team should be aware of such effects and assess the infant for them.

  6. Postoperative care.

    a. Pain management (see Chapter 16).

    b. Prevent infection: dressing changes are performed with aseptic technique; administer antibiotics.

    c. Oxygen saturation, urine output, and blood pressure are monitored continuously. Other parameters to watch closely include fluid-and-electrolyte balance, pH, and clotting times.

d. Observe for complications: respiratory distress, sepsis, intestinal obstruction, skin necrosis over repaired defect, and venous stasis distal to the repair.

e. When staged reduction is employed, the silo must be supported to prevent tilting or torsion of the enclosed viscera. Sterile gauze may be wrapped around the base of the silo for this purpose.

f. Gastric suction is required postoperatively until the gastric output is minimal. Gastric losses should be replaced with physiologic IV solutions. To prevent dehydration, measure gastric suction drainage every 4 hours and replace this volume over the ensuing 4 hours with physiologic IV fluid.

g. Total parenteral nutrition is provided until the infant can tolerate feedings.

h. Bowel sounds are assessed to determine readiness to feed. A prolonged ileus is a common complication in gastroschisis, but relatively uncommon in omphalocele.

i. Feeding is begun very slowly when gastric output is minimal and bowel sounds are active.

   (1) Low osmolality feeding, such as half-strength formula, breast milk, or mineral–electrolyte solution (Pedialyte) is usually preferred. Feedings are frequently stopped and started because of reduced intestinal function.

   (2) Soy-based and elemental formulas are used for infants who exhibit signs of feeding intolerance or malabsorption.

j. Support parents through the often long recovery process (see Chapter 17).

OBSTRUCTIONS OF THE GASTROINTESTINAL TRACT

A. **General considerations** (Adamson and Hebra, 2004).

   1. Obstructions may be either mechanical (in which there is a specific point of obstruction) or functional (usually related to motility) in nature and can be found anywhere from the esophagus to the anus.

   2. Obstruction occurs because of an intrinsic or extrinsic blockage (Table 29-3).

   3. Common associations in infants with intestinal obstruction.

      a. History of polyhydramnios.

         (1) Occurs more often in proximal obstructions.

         (2) 15% to 20% of polyhydramnios is associated with fetal GI obstructions.

■ TABLE 29-3
■ ■ **Causes of Intestinal Obstruction in the Newborn Infant**

Mechanical		Functional
Congenital	**Acquired**	**Functional**
INTRINSIC	Necrotizing enterocolitis	Hirschsprung disease
Atresias	Intussusception	Meconium plug syndrome
Stenoses	Peritoneal adhesions	Ileus
Meconium ileus		Peritonitis
Anorectal malformations		
Enteric duplications		
EXTRINSIC		Intestinal pseudo-obstruction syndrome
Volvulus		
Peritoneal bands		
Annular pancreas		
Cysts and tumors		
Incarcerated hernias		

From Taeusch, H.W., Ballard, R.A., and Gleason, C.A.: *Avery's diseases of the newborn* (8th ed.). Philadelphia, 2005, Saunders.

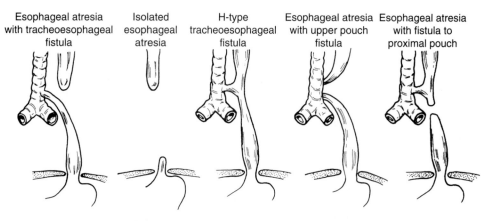

FIGURE 29-3. ■ Esophageal malformations.

    b. Failure to pass meconium within 24 to 48 hours: 95% of term infants pass meconium by 24 hours (Anderson et al., 2006).

    c. Abdominal distention: occurs more often in distal obstructions and tracheoesophageal fistula.

    d. Bilious vomiting: occurs when obstruction is distal to the ampulla of Vater, located in the duodenum.

  4. General preoperative management.

    a. NPO.

    b. Gastric decompression with Replogle tube to low intermittent suction. To prevent dehydration, measure amount every 4 hours and consider replacement with physiologic IV fluid.

    c. Correct fluid, electrolyte and acid–base status (see Chapter 8).

    d. Maintenance IV therapy (may include TPN).

    e. Antibiotics.

B. Esophageal atresia (EA) and tracheoesophageal fistula (TEF).

  1. Definitions: EA, an interruption in the esophagus; TEF, an abnormal communication between the esophagus and trachea. EA and TEF may occur as separate defects or, more commonly, in association with each other.

    a. Types of TEFs (Fig. 29-3) (Roaten et al., 2006).

      (1) Esophageal atresia (blind proximal pouch) with distal esophageal communication with the trachea (85%).

      (2) Isolated esophageal atresia (blind proximal pouch), no esophageal–tracheal communication (8%).

      (3) H-type: Communication between normal esophagus and normal trachea (5%).

      (4) Esophageal atresia (blind proximal pouch) with proximal or proximal and distal communication with trachea (2%).

  2. Etiology: hedgehog signaling abnormality leading to incomplete elongation and separation of esophagus and trachea during the fourth week of gestation (Lees et al., 2005).

  3. Incidence: approximately 1 per 1000 to 2500 live births (Askins and Gilbert-Barness, 2007).

  4. Associated anomalies (Wert, 2004).

    a. Low birth weight is associated with other malformations and poor outcome.

    b. Cardiac defects: primarily atrial septal defects and ventricular septal defects.

    c. GI anomalies: pyloric stenosis, duodenal obstruction, and imperforate anus.

    d. EA/TEF are components of both VATERR and VACTERL associations. Infants with EA/TEF should have a cardiac, renal, and skeletal evaluation.

    e. Esophageal abnormalities are also seen in the CHARGE (Colobomata, *H*eart disease, choanal *A*tresia, mental *R*etardation, *G*enital hypoplasia, and *E*ar anomalies with deafness) association.

5. Diagnosis (Magnuson et al., 2006).
   a. Fetal ultrasound showing small or absent stomach.
   b. History of polyhydramnios.
   c. Clinical presentation.
      (1) Dependent on the type of tracheoesophageal anomaly.
      (2) Accumulation of oral secretions in mouth, drooling.
      (3) Coughing, choking, respiratory distress, or cyanosis.
      (4) Inability to pass gastric tube. Passage terminates in proximal esophageal pouch at approximately 10 cm. On radiographic examination gastric tube appears coiled in the proximal esophageal pouch. In addition, air in the GI tract indicates the presence of a TEF. A gasless abdomen indicates an isolated EA (see Chapter 14).
      (5) Abdominal distention if fistula between distal esophagus and trachea.
      (6) Recurrent pneumonia (especially with communication between normal esophagus and normal trachea [H-type]).
      (7) Use of contrast studies is not recommended because of the risk of aspiration and subsequent chemical pneumonitis.
6. Prognosis: survival rate excellent for healthy term infants. Prognosis is dependent on birth weight, presence of other congenital anomalies, especially cardiac, and preoperative condition. Highest mortality occurs in infants less than 1500 g and those associated with cardiac or chromosomal abnormalities.
7. Preoperative care (Magnuson et al., 2006).
   a. See section A, "General Considerations," p. 599.
   b. Manage airway; prevent aspiration-induced lung injury.
      (1) EA/TEF: elevate head of bed 30 to 45 degrees to avoid reflux and aspiration of gastric secretions.
      (2) EA without TEF: normal positioning.
      (3) Evacuate EA pouch using a Replogle tube to low continuous suction. Replogle is the desired tube because evacuation holes are near the distal end. Assess and maintain patency of tube. If tube appears clogged, move tube slightly as it may have adhered to the esophageal mucosa or inject air only (to prevent aspiration) into the pigtail.
      (4) Use comfort measures to prevent crying, which leads to increased swallowed air, abdominal distention, and increased risk of gastric content reflux into the trachea.
      (5) Medications: gastric acid blockade and antibiotics.
      (6) For lung disease requiring ventilation, use low mean airway pressures or use high-frequency oscillation to minimize shunting of tidal volume from the trachea to the stomach.
   c. Perform complete evaluation for associated anomalies.
8. Surgical repair.
   a. Primary repair.
      (1) EA: end-to-end anastomosis of the esophagus.
      (2) TEF: ligation of the TEF.
   b. Staged repair is used with infants who are very premature, who have pneumonia or other coexisting life-threatening problems, or in whom the gap between the two esophageal segments is great (more than four vertebral bodies, with both segments in a neutral position).
      (1) Initial surgery: ligation of TEF, placement of gastrostomy tube for gastric decompression, minimize risk of aspiration of gastric contents, and provide route for enteral feedings.
      (2) Continue suction of proximal esophageal pouch until final surgery.
      (3) Final surgery is usually delayed for 6 to 12 months.
   c. When end-to-end anastomosis is impossible because the gap between the esophageal pouches is too great or a previous repair has failed, the upper segment may be elongated surgically.

9. Postoperative care (Magnuson et al., 2006).
   a. Provide pain management (see Chapter 16).
   b. Prevent aspiration: continue elevation of head of bed and gastric acid blockade.
   c. Prevent infection: administer antibiotics.
   d. Protect anastomosis site
      (1) Ventilate using low mean airway pressure.
      (2) Suction length of endotracheal tube (ETT) only. Prevent suction catheter extrusion beyond the ETT.
      (3) Do not extubate until certain that reintubation will not be necessary.
      (4) If accidental extubation occurs, do not bag–mask ventilate; only experienced personnel should reintubate if needed.
      (5) Suction posterior pharynx using a premeasured catheter to limit the distance.
      (6) If the orogastric/nasogastric tube placed during surgery is dislodged, do not attempt to reinsert.
   e. Monitor: extrathoracic drain, gastric drainage. Note amount, color, and consistency.
   f. Gastrostomy tube care.
   g. Nutrition.
      (1) TPN is used until sufficient enteral intake is established.
      (2) Enteral nutrition is initiated when the anastomosis site has healed. Confirmation may be obtained by esophagram.
10. Postoperative complications.
   a. Aspiration.
   b. Infection, pneumonia.
   c. Anastomosis site complications.
      (1) Leak: delays feeding, may result in infection.
      (2) Stricture: suspect in infants exhibiting dysphagia, inability to handle secretions, or respiratory distress after the immediate postoperative period. Strictures require long-term periodic dilation.
   d. Dysmotility of lower esophageal segment. Most often a problem with long gap atresia and when oral intake is delayed for a prolonged period of time.
   e. Recurrent fistula, usually resulting from a leak.
   f. Unilateral diaphragmatic paralysis.
   g. Tracheomalacia. This complication is occasionally severe enough to require a tracheostomy. Caused by deformation and softening of tracheal cartilages from compression of posterior trachea by enlarged proximal esophageal pouch.
   h. TEF cough. Characterized by stridor, brassy cough, and bronchospastic airway symptoms.
   i. Gastroesophageal reflux (common).
C. **Pyloric stenosis** (Evers, 2006).
   1. Definition: obstruction of pylorus caused by hypertrophy of the pyloric musculature.
   2. Etiology: unknown but higher incidence in infants whose mother had increased gastrin secretion in the third trimester of pregnancy or infants who received prostaglandin E administration. The pyloric muscle demonstrates both hypertrophy and hyperplasia.
   3. Incidence: overall 3 per 1000 live births.
      a. Predominance: males 5 per 1000 live births; females 1 per 1000 live births.
      b. Prevalence: more common in infants who are Caucasian, full term, and have trisomy 21.
      c. Occurs in approximately 20% of males and 10% of females who had affected mothers.
   4. Associated conditions: uncommon. Three major malformations associated with pyloric stenosis are Apert syndrome, trisomy 18, and trisomy 21 (Jones, 2006).
   5. Diagnosis.
      a. Presence of signs and symptoms usually between 3 weeks to 5 months of age.
      b. Clinical presentation.
         (1) Nonbilious vomiting that becomes projectile over time.
         (2) Visible peristaltic waves in epigastrium.

        (3) Palpable pyloric "olive" in right upper quadrant (70% to 90%).
        (4) Dehydration, electrolyte imbalances, acid–base disturbance (hypochloremia, hypokalemia, metabolic alkalosis).
        (5) Chronic weight loss, malnutrition, and failure to thrive (late sign).
    c. Ultrasound (almost exclusively).
    d. Upper GI tract contrast study.
6. Prognosis: excellent. Generally, complete recovery with no residual effects; some continued vomiting possible in the first few days after surgery, followed by quick resolution.
7. Preoperative care (Evers, 2006):
    a. See section A, "General Considerations," p. 599.
    b. Prevent aspiration-induced lung injury: use gastric decompression.
8. Medical repair (Evers, 2006):
    a. Pyloric stenosis may resolve spontaneously before 1 year of life. Infant requires medical and nutritional support. Procedure is associated with slow improvement and higher mortality.
9. Surgical repair (Evers, 2006):
    a. Pyloromyotomy: pyloric muscles are split/separated either by laparotomy or laparoscopic techniques.
10. Postoperative care (Evers, 2006):
    a. Pain management (see Chapter 16).
    b. Routine wound care.
    c. Nutrition: initially NPO for a few hours, then rapid progression of enteral feeds leading to full volume and discharge 24 hours after surgery.
    d. Prevention of perforation of the mucosa at the pyloromyotomy site by avoiding placement of a gastric tube postoperatively.

D. **Duodenal atresia and stenosis** (Magnuson et al., 2006; Ross, 2004).
    1. Definition: congenital obstruction of the duodenum. The defect usually occurs distal to the ampulla of Vater. The obstruction can be partial or complete and is further stratified as intrinsic or extrinsic. Duodenal atresia exhibits 3 forms: a membranous web causes obstruction in Type I and is associated with common bile duct anomalies; a fibrous atretic cord connects two segments of duodenum in Type II; while Type III exhibits discontinuous segments of the duodenum.
    2. Etiology: During early gestation, the duodenal epithelium proliferates rapidly and completely obliterates the bowel lumen. Obstruction is thought to be a failure of recanalization during weeks 8 to 10 of fetal life. With extrinsic obstruction, anomalies outside the duodenum affect patency. These anomalies include malrotation with Ladd's bands, annular pancreas, and supraduodenal portal vein.
    3. Incidence: approximately 1 per 7000 live births.
    4. Associated conditions.
        a. Trisomy 21 syndrome (approximately 30%).
        b. Congenital heart disease (approximately 30%).
        c. Intestinal malrotation (approximately 20%).
        d. Tracheoesophageal abnormalities (10% to 20%).
        e. Anorectal defects (10% to 20%).
    5. Diagnosis.
        a. Fetal ultrasound showing classic double bubble echogenicity.
        b. History of polyhydramnios.
        c. Clinical presentation.
            (1) Abdominal distention.
            (2) Absence of stools.
            (3) Bilious vomiting within the first 24 hours; nonbilious vomiting does not rule out duodenal atresia or obstruction.
            (4) Jaundice.
        d. Plain radiograph showing double bubble pattern (see Chapter 14).
    6. Prognosis: excellent. Long-term outcome is primarily dependent on associated anomalies and malformations.

7. Preoperative care.
   a. See section A, "General Considerations," p. 599.
   b. Place Replogle tube to low intermittent suction. To prevent dehydration gastric losses should be replaced with physiologic IV solutions.
   c. Perform complete evaluation for associated anomalies.
8. Surgical repair.
   a. For intrinsic lesions surgery is performed to excise the atretic or stenosed portions and perform primary reanastomoses. For extrinsic etiology, surgery removes or redirects the tissue causing duodenal blockage.
9. Postoperative care.
   a. Pain management (see Chapter 16).
   b. Prevent infection.
      (1) Routine wound care.
      (2) Continue antibiotics.
   c. Gastric decompression is required postoperatively until gastric output is minimal. Gastric losses should be replaced with physiologic IV solutions to prevent dehydration.
   d. Gastrostomy tube care if placed (rare).
   e. Nutrition: initially NPO for 3 to 10 days. Initiate enteral feeding and progress slowly as tolerated. Expect possible intolerance due to delayed gastric emptying and microcolon distal to repair site. Continue TPN until adequate enteral nutrition is established.
E. **Jejunal or ileal atresia** (Hartman et al., 2005; Magnuson et al., 2006).
   1. Definition: congenital obstruction of the jejunum, ileum, or both. Type I: membranous web; Type II: segments connected by fibrous cord; Type IIIa: segments separated by V-shaped mesenteric defect; Type IIIb: apple-peel defect, with distal small bowel corkscrewing around the ileocecal artery; Type IV: multiple atresias (Fig. 29-4).

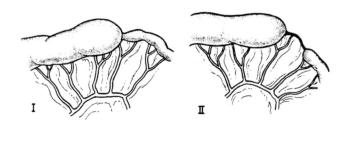

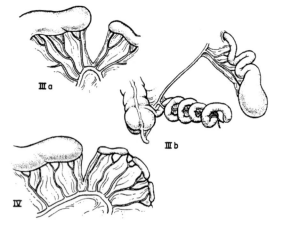

FIGURE 29-4. ■ Types of jejunal atresia. Type I—mucosal atresia with intact muscularis. Type II—atretic ends are separated by a fibrous band. Type IIIa—atretic ends are separated by a V-shaped gap defect. Type IIIb—apple-peel deformity of the distal atretic segment with retrograde blood supply from the ileocolic or right colic artery. Type IV—multiple atresias (string-of-sausage effect). (From Rowe, M.I., O'Neill, J.A., Grosfeld, J.L., et al.: *Essentials of pediatric surgery.* St. Louis, 1995, Mosby, p. 511.)

2. Etiology: two proposed etiologies: failure of recanalization during weeks 8 to 10 of fetal life or, second, and most supported hypothesis is a mesenteric vascular insult with subsequent necrosis and resorption of the affected segment or segments.

3. Incidence: 1 per 1000 live births. Males and females are equally affected. Anatomic distribution: jejunal (50%), ileum (50%).

4. Associated conditions.
   a. Intestinal malrotation (10% to 18%).
   b. Meconium peritonitis (12%).
   c. Meconium ileus (10%).

5. Diagnosis.
   a. Fetal ultrasound showing distended intestinal loops.
   b. History of polyhydramnios.
   c. Clinical presentation.
      (1) Abdominal distention. The lower the obstruction, the greater the distention.
      (2) Absence of stools.
      (3) Bilious vomiting within the first 24 to 48 hours.
      (4) Jaundice.
   d. Radiologic studies.
      (1) Plain radiograph showing dilated bowel loops and multiple air-fluid levels (see Chapter 14). With proximal jejunal atresia, classic triple bubble is noted. With in utero bowel perforation, peritoneal calcifications may be visible.
      (2) Barium enema reveals a microcolon.

6. Prognosis: generally good, with return to normal bowel function within 10 days. Mortality is usually related to short bowel syndrome and complex defects (Types IIIb and IV). Morbidity includes ileus, peritonitis, and prolonged intestinal dysfunction.

7. Preoperative care.
   a. See section A, "General Considerations," p. 599.
   b. Place Replogle tube to low intermittent suction. Gastric losses should be replaced with physiologic IV solutions to prevent dehydration.
   c. Perform complete evaluation for associated anomalies.

8. Surgical repair.
   a. Dependent on location of atresia and amount of intestinal involvement.
   b. Atretic intestinal portion is often resected proximally to the point of normal bowel dimensions and then connected to the distal segment using an end-to-oblique-side anastomosis.
   c. Occasionally, exteriorization of the proximal and even distal ends may be necessary with reanastomosis later.

9. Postoperative care.
   a. Pain management (see Chapter 16).
   b. Prevent infection.
      (1) Routine wound care.
      (2) Continue antibiotics.
   c. Gastric decompression until gastric output is minimal. Gastric losses should be replaced with physiologic IV solutions to prevent dehydration.
   d. Nutrition: initially NPO until motility returns. Initiate enteral feeding (often with elemental formula or maternal breast milk) and progress slowly as tolerated. Expect possible intolerance due to delayed gastric emptying and microcolon distal to repair site. Continue TPN until adequate enteral nutrition is established.

F. **Malrotation** (Louie, 2007).
   1. Definition: an assortment of intestinal anomalies of rotation and retroperitoneal fixation.
   2. Etiology: hedgehog signaling abnormality leading to failure of the intestines to rotate and fixate appropriately during weeks 6 to 10 of gestation (Lees et al., 2005). Intestines may twist on themselves (midgut volvulus), occluding the intestinal lumen, or may twist around the superior mesenteric artery, occluding intestinal blood supply. Ischemia and bowel necrosis follows.

3. Incidence: 1 per 5000 live births. The incidence of malrotation without significant symptoms is much higher than cases with clinically significant symptoms. More males affected than females.

4. Associated anomalies.
   a. Intestinal atresia.
   b. Diaphragmatic hernia.
   c. Duodenal obstruction due to peritoneal (Ladd) bands encircling the duodenum.
   d. Omphalocele.
   e. Gastroschisis.

5. Diagnosis.
   a. Presence of symptoms.
      (1) 80% of patients who become symptomatic do so within the first month of life, with the majority presenting within the first week. Approximately 90% of clinical symptoms appear in children in the first year of life.
      (2) Acute presentation.
         (i) Bilious vomiting, suggestive of malrotation with volvulus formation; needs immediate attention.
         (ii) Abdominal distention.
         (iii) Abdominal pain.
         (iv) Signs of shock and sepsis.
         (v) Rectal bleeding.
      (3) Less acute presentation.
         (i) Intermittent bilious vomiting.
         (ii) Abdominal tenderness.
         (iii) Failure to thrive.
   b. Radiologic examination.
      (1) Upper GI is the gold standard.
      (2) Plain radiographs. May appear normal in 20% of cases.
      (3) Ultrasound.
      (4) Classic early studies show distended stomach and proximal duodenum and scanty gas distributed throughout remainder of bowel. An airless abdomen is an ominous sign.

6. Prognosis: excellent if uncomplicated by infarction or associated anomalies. Mortality increases with intestinal necrosis, prematurity, or other abnormalities. Amount of intestinal resection is an important predicting factor in outcome. Major postoperative complication is short bowel syndrome.

7. Preoperative care.
   a. See section A, "General Considerations," p. 599.
   b. Perform complete evaluation for associated anomalies.

8. Surgical repair.
   a. Surgery is emergent and cannot be delayed. Degree of surgery is dependent on pathology and amount of intestinal involvement.
   b. Volvulus is detorsed, Ladd's bands are divided, incidental appendectomy, and nonrotational return of bowel to the abdomen with the small bowel to the right and large bowel to the left.

9. Postoperative care.
   a. Pain management (see Chapter 16).
   b. Prevent infection.
      (1) Routine wound care.
      (2) Continue antibiotics.
   c. Gastric decompression until gastric output is minimal. Gastric losses should be replaced with physiologic IV solutions to prevent dehydration.
   d. Nutrition: initially NPO until motility returns. Initiate enteral feeding (often with elemental formula or maternal breast milk) and progress slowly as tolerated. Expect possible intolerance due to delayed gastric emptying and microcolon distal to repair site. Continue TPN until adequate enteral nutrition is established.

G. Meconium ileus (Neff, 2005; Winfield and Beierle, 2006).

1. Definition: mechanical obstruction of the distal ileum due to intraluminal accumulation of thick, inspissated meconium. Although meconium ileus has been reported in a few patients without cystic fibrosis (CF), it is the predominant cause of meconium ileus in infants.

   a. Types of meconium ileus.

      (1) Simple meconium ileus.

         (a) More common.

         (b) Distal segment of the small bowel is obstructed with thick, tar-like, tenacious meconium and the proximal segment of the small bowel is dilated.

         (c) Clinical presentation is usually within 48 hours.

      (2) Complicated meconium ileus.

         (a) Volvulus.

         (b) Intestinal necrosis and perforation.

         (c) Meconium peritonitis or pseudocyst formation.

         (d) Clinical presentation is usually within 24 hours.

2. Etiology: exact cause unknown. Two implicating factors are hyposecretion of pancreatic enzymes, which may play a part in some but not all meconium ileus (as a result, meconium contains an abnormal amount of proteins and glycoproteins, making the meconium thick and viscid); or abnormal viscid secretions from the mucous glands of the small intestine.

3. Incidence: exact incidence unknown. Cystic fibrosis occurs in 1 in 2000 live births of white infants; 10% to 15% of children with cystic fibrosis have meconium ileus.

4. Associated conditions.

   a. Cystic fibrosis.

   b. Hepatobiliary disease.

5. Diagnosis.

   a. Abdominal distention at birth.

   b. Bilious vomiting.

   c. Failure to pass meconium within 12 to 24 hours.

   d. Palpable, rubbery loops of bowel. Small grapelike pellets of meconium may be palpated distally.

   e. Complicated form has earlier presentation, and these infants appear sicker, with signs of sepsis and respiratory distress.

   f. Family history of cystic fibrosis (CF). Definitive diagnosis of CF based on sweat chloride iontophoresis (sodium and chloride concentrations >60 mEq/L), or chromosome analysis (defect located on chromosome 7).

   g. Radiologic studies.

      (1) Plain radiograph shows soap bubble or ground glass appearance of distal intestine created by the mixture of air and meconium; distended bowel loops without air–fluid levels; scattered calcifications due to intrauterine intestinal perforations may be seen in complicated form.

      (2) Contrast radiograph may show microcolon.

6. Prognosis: dependent on number and degree of organs affected by CF as well as associated anomalies.

7. Pre–nonsurgical procedure and preoperatively.

   a. See section A, "General Considerations," p. 599.

   b. Perform complete evaluation for associated conditions; volvulus, atresia, perforation, and peritonitis must be ruled out.

   c. Evaluation by pediatric surgeon who remains in attendance during nonsurgical procedure.

   d. Patient should be prepared for surgery should complications occur during nonsurgical procedure.

8. Nonsurgical procedure.

   a. A hypertonic contrast water-soluble enema may be successful in dislodging the meconium by drawing fluid into the intestine and allowing for normal intestinal activity.

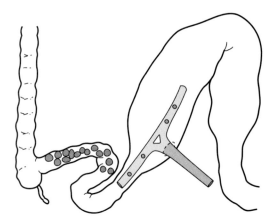

FIGURE 29-5. ■ T-tube. (From Mak, G.Z., Harberg, F.J., Hiatt, P., Deaton, A., Calhoon, R., and Brandt, M.: T-tube ileostomy for meconium ileus: Four decades of experience. *Journal of Pediatric Surgery, 35*[2]:349-352, 2000.)

    Successful in up to 60% of patients. Usually meconium pellets are passed quickly, followed by liquid meconium for 24 hours after the procedure. A second enema may be required.

9. Surgical repair: uncomplicated meconium ileus.
   a. Used when nonsurgical procedure has failed.
   b. A T-tube (Fig. 29-5) is inserted into the ileum, which is irrigated postoperatively with *N*-acetylcysteine pancreatic enzymes.
10. Surgical repair: complicated meconium ileus.
    a. Always requires surgical intervention.
    b. Compromised intestine is resected.
    c. If the bowel is viable, end-to-end anastomosis is performed.
    d. In extreme cases in which bowel necrosis has occurred, all compromised intestine is resected and an ostomy is placed at the proximal and/or distal segments.
11. Postprocedural care.
    a. Fluids at one-and-one-half times maintenance. Hypovolemic shock can occur secondary to rapid fluid shift resulting from hypertonic solution used for enema. Careful monitoring of urine output, urine specific gravity or osmolality, blood urea nitrogen, creatinine, and serum osmolality.
    b. Physical assessment. Intestinal perforation may occur up to 48 hours after administration of enema. Risk of intestinal perforation increases with successive attempts at nonoperative techniques.
12. Postprocedural management and postoperative care.
    a. Pain management (see Chapter 16).
    b. Prevent infection: administer antibiotics; chest physiotherapy, aerosolized mucolytic agents (acetylcysteine sodium [Mucomyst]), and supplemental humidity to prevent atelectasis and pneumonia, which infants with cystic fibrosis are prone to develop.
    c. NPO; gastric decompression until normal bowel function is restored (approximately 3 to 7 days).
    d. Irrigation of distal stoma or T-tube with *N*-acetylcysteine or pancreatic enzymes around postoperative day 3.
    e. Nutrition.
       (1) TPN is used until sufficient enteral intake is established.
       (2) Enteral nutrition is initiated when the surgical site has healed.
       (3) Begin feedings with elemental formula or breast milk, supplemented with pancreatic enzymes.
    f. Parental education.
       (1) Genetic counseling.
       (2) Pulmonary hygiene, infection prevention, nutritional supplements.

      g. Observe for postoperative complications.

        (1) Volvulus.

        (2) Gangrene.

        (3) Perforation.

H. Meconium plug syndrome (Winfield and Beierle, 2006).

  1. Definition: a mechanical obstruction, usually of the distal segment of the colon and the rectum, that occurs from thick, inspissated meconium in the absence of an abnormality of ganglion cells or enzymatic deficiency. Because the meconium plug is formed primarily by mucous and intestinal secretions, the plug appears yellowish white and is gelatinous.

  2. Etiology: unclear; results from diminished colonic motility and meconium clearance. More common with:

    a. Maternal diabetes, probably because of increased fetal glycogen production leading to decreased bowel motility.

    b. Neonatal hypermagnesemia: usually occurs after mother has been treated with magnesium sulfate for pregnancy-induced hypertension or preterm labor; the decreased bowel motility is secondary to myoneural depression.

    c. Prematurity.

    d. Hypotonia in infant with CNS disease.

    e. Sepsis.

  3. Incidence: 1 in 100 newborns; 75% of newborns are able to expel the plug spontaneously, avoiding the complication of intestinal obstruction.

  4. Associated conditions.

    a. Hirschsprung.

    b. Cystic fibrosis.

  5. Diagnosis.

    a. Clinical presentation.

      (1) Abdominal distention. Multiple dilated loops of bowel.

      (2) Failure to pass meconium by 48 hours of life.

      (3) Hyperactive bowel sounds.

      (4) Bilious vomiting (late sign).

    b. Plain radiograph showing multiple distended loops of bowel (see Chapter 14).

    c. Water-soluble contrast enema often outlines an intraluminal plug. Such an enema will commonly dislodge the plug, and no further interventions will be required.

  6. Prognosis: generally excellent if no associated conditions exist.

  7. Pre–nonsurgical procedure and preoperatively.

    a. See section A, "General Considerations," p. 599.

    b. Medications: generally not required.

    c. Perform complete evaluation for associated conditions; volvulus, atresia, perforation, and peritonitis must be ruled out.

  8. Interventions.

    a. Rectal examination may expel plug in some circumstances.

    b. Enemas of warm saline, meglumine diatrizoate, or acetylcysteine.

      (1) Meglumine diatrizoate is hyperosmolar, drawing fluid into the bowel from interstitial space. Careful assessment and management of fluid status are important.

    c. Surgery rarely necessary.

I. Hirschsprung disease (HD) (congenital megacolon, aganglionic megacolon) (Dasgupta, 2008; Kessman, 2006).

  1. Definition: congenital absence of parasympathetic innervation to the colon. The affected intestine is unable to relax, resulting in a functional obstruction.

    a. Length of bowel involvement is dependent on the time during which migration of neuroblasts ceased.

    b. Agangliosis commonly involves rectum or rectosigmoid portion of colon only.

    c. Agangliosis may extend to proximal colon. Total colon agangliosis is rare.

  2. Etiology: failure of ganglion cells to migrate cephalocaudally before week 12 of gestation resulting in partial or complete agangliosis of the submucosal and mesenteric plexuses of the colon. Eight genomes have been associated with HD. The lack of intestinal ganglion cells prevents the inhibitory relaxation normally regulated by parasympathetic nerves. The affected segment is unable to relax, and functional obstruction ensues. The normally innervated proximal colon becomes hypertrophied from its attempts to overcome the functional obstruction.

3. Incidence: 1 in 5000 live births. Males are affected 4 times more often than females. More than one third of affected patients have a relative with Hirschsprung disease (HD).

4. Associated conditions: not common but may include colonic atresia or imperforate anus; 3% to 10% of children with trisomy 21 have HD. Congenital deafness and ocular neuropathies are found in a small number of affected infants. The oral, facial, and cranial ganglia arise from the same craniocervical neural crest as the ganglionic plexus of the bowel.

5. Diagnosis.
    a. Clinical presentation.
        (1) Early symptom: failure to pass meconium within 24 to 48 hours after birth.
        (2) Bilious vomiting.
        (3) Progressive abdominal distention.
        (4) Poor feeding with failure to thrive.
        (5) Late symptom: inability to stool normally. Abnormal stooling since birth is a common symptom of HD. As the obstruction continues, enterocolitis may develop, with fever, abdominal distention, and diarrhea. The infant usually has symptoms in the first several weeks and then has diarrhea, abdominal distention, and/or vomiting. In advanced cases, urinary obstruction may occur secondary to mechanical compression of the ureters and bladder.
    b. Radiologic examination.
        (1) Plain radiograph demonstrating proximal bowel dilation with an absence of air in the rectum is suggestive.
        (2) Contrast studies showing a nondistensible rectal ampulla, with a dilated bowel above and a transition zone (an area between the normal and abnormal aganglionic intestine having a conical tapering appearance) is suggestive.
        (3) Retained barium in the rectum for more than 24 hours after the procedure is suggestive.
    c. Anal manometry is useful in very-short-segment agangliosis or in patients who have normal findings on contrast studies.
    d. Confirmation: rectal biopsy demonstrating absence of ganglion cells. Punch or suction biopsy may be done in the nursery. Full-thickness biopsy under general anesthesia is rarely needed. Increased acetylcholinesterase content in rectal tissue is identified by histochemical staining.
    e. Under current development is a test for a serum protein marker in which initial trials were 100% sensitive and specific for the disease (Wang, 2007).

6. Prognosis: excellent. Mortality rate increases when diagnosis is delayed and enterocolitis occurs as a result of bowel wall distention and ischemia followed by bacterial translocation into circulation, resulting in sepsis. Enterocolitis is the leading cause of death. Approximately 10% of patients with HD will have subsequent elimination problems, such as constipation and delayed toilet training.

7. Preoperative care.
    a. See section A, "General Considerations," p. 599.
    b. Perform complete evaluation for associated conditions; volvulus, atresia, perforation, and peritonitis must be ruled out.
    c. Rectal irrigation is routinely performed to allow repeated emptying of colon and prevent enterocolitis.

8. Surgical repair. Goal: bring the normal ganglionated bowel down to the anus. The transanal procedure eliminates an abdominal incision and results in a primary pull through repair.

9. Postoperative care.
    a. Pain management (see Chapter 16).
    b. NPO; gastric decompression with replacement of losses with physiologic IV fluid.

  c. Nutrition.
   (1) TPN is used until sufficient enteral intake is established.
   (2) Enteral nutrition is initiated when the anastomosis site has healed.
  d. Careful monitoring of fluid and electrolyte balance.
  e. Close observation for shock and recurrent enterocolitis.
  f. Routine ostomy care if applicable. Complications include ostomy prolapse, intestinal obstruction, skin dehiscence and excoriation, and stomal ulceration and bleeding.
  g. Routine rectal irrigations with normal saline to decrease risk of postoperative enterocolitis.
  h. If frequent and liquid stools cause perineal irritation, loperamide may be administered to reduce stool frequency and kaolin–pectin suspension can solidify stools.
  i. Special diets may be necessary to improve stool consistency.
  j. Genetic counseling should be offered to the infant's family.
  k. A regimen of anal dilation begins approximately 2 weeks postoperatively in primary pull-through patients.
 10. Complications.
  a. Fecal incontinence.
  b. Persistent constipation.
  c. Anastomotic leakage with subsequent stricture formation.
  d. Rectal stenosis.
J. Imperforate anus (anorectal agenesis) (Hartman et al., 2005; Roaten et al., 2006).
 1. Definition: a broad spectrum of anorectal malformations characterized by a stenotic or atretic anal canal. A fistula between the rectum and the perineum, vagina in females or urethra in males, may also occur.
 Classified dependent on level of defect (i.e., above [high] or below [low] a line drawn from the symphysis pubis to the coccyx [pubococcygeal line]).
  a. High imperforate anus (IA).
   (1) More common and generally more complex.
   (2) Male predominance.
   (3) Rectourinary and rectovaginal fistulas are common associations. Infants with a fistula are at risk for hyperchloremic acidosis as a result of colonic absorption of urine.
   (4) High IA with sacral anomaly can be associated with lack of innervation of the bowel and/or bladder, resulting in incontinence.
  b. Low imperforate anus.
   (1) Male/female ratio closer to 1:1.
   (2) Perineal fistula is common.
 2. Etiology: failure of differentiation of the urogenital sinus and cloaca during embryologic development (Blackburn, 2007). The failure to differentiate is a hedgehog signaling abnormality (Lees et al., 2005).
 3. Incidence: 1 in 5000 live births.
 4. Common associations: anomalies, including vertebral, genitourinary, cardiovascular, and GI malformations, in 20% to 75% of infants. Specific anomalies include cryptorchidism, congenital heart defects, esophageal atresia, spinal dysraphism.
 5. Diagnosis.
  a. Physical examination. An infant with anal stenosis or imperforate anal membrane may have a normal-appearing rectum, with the condition detected only after the absence of stooling is noted.
  b. Radiologic examination.
   (1) Plain and contrast radiographs. An inverted lateral radiograph may be obtained to determine the level of the air-filled rectal pouch in relation to the pubococcygeal line.
   (2) Ultrasonography.
 6. Prognosis: level of defect significantly influences outcome regarding fecal continence (Fig. 29-6).

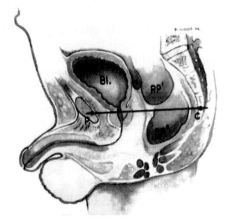

FIGURE 29-6. ■ Imperforate anus. Rectal pouch 1 (RP[1]) sits above the pubococcygeal line (PC) and would be classified as a "high type" anomaly. Rectal pouch 2 (RP[2]) sits below the PC line and represents a "low type" anomaly. The level of the rectal pouch is crucial in decisions of management. *Bl,* Bladder. (From Ross, A.J.: Intestinal obstruction in the newborn. *Pediatrics in Review, 15*[9]:338-347, 1994.)

Outcome is generally excellent with low imperforate anus although there is an association with constipation. High imperforate anus is associated with bowel incontinence.

    7. Preoperative care.
        a. See section A, "General Considerations," p. 599.
    8. Surgical repair.
        a. Surgical intervention is always necessary, with the procedure dependent on the level of the anorectal pouch. High and intermediate pouches are treated with a colostomy and a definitive pull-through procedure performed after the infant is approximately 8 months of age and weighs 18 pounds. A low pouch can usually be repaired by anoplasty with good results.
    9. Postoperative care.
        a. Pain management (see Chapter 16).
        b. NPO; gastric decompression continued until normal bowel function is restored.
        c. Nutrition.
            (1) TPN is used until sufficient enteral intake is established.
            (2) Enteral nutrition is initiated when the anastomosis site has healed.
        d. Routine ostomy care if applicable. Complications include ostomy prolapse, intestinal obstruction, skin dehiscence and excoriation, and stomal ulceration and bleeding.
        e. Anal dilation for approximately 2 weeks postoperatively in infants with anoplasty to prevent anal stenosis.

NECROTIZING ENTEROCOLITIS*

A. General considerations.
    1. Definition: an acquired disease that affects the GI system, particularly that of premature infants. It is characterized by inflammation of the bowel wall followed by areas of necrosis, most commonly in the terminal ileum and proximal colon, but may affect any or all of both small and large intestine.
    2. Etiology: unknown, thought to be multifactorial. Three mechanisms have been suggested including
        a. Intestinal ischemia (asphyxia/hypoxemia; redistribution of blood flow [hypotension, hypovolemia, polycythemia, patent ductus arteriosus, severe stress, hypothermia, umbilical catheter, blood transfusion, exchange transfusion]).

*Caplan, 2006; Louie, 2007; Sharma et al., 2006.

b. Bacterial colonization of the initially sterile intestinal tract. The occurrence of necrotizing enterocolitis (NEC) in clusters suggests a role for microorganism involvement. Organisms commonly associated with NEC include *Klebsiella, Escherichia coli, Clostridia* species.

c. Enteral feedings. Majority of NEC cases preceded by enteral feeding (90% to 95%). Increased occurrence when hyperosmolar formulae and medications (aminophylline, vitamin E) are administered enterally, and when feeding volume increases exceed 20 ml/kg/day. Mechanism is unclear; formula may provide a substrate for bacterial proliferation; feeding and medications may increase intestinal oxygen demand during absorption, resulting in tissue hypoxia; fluid shifts into the intestine, resulting in decreased GI blood flow and intestinal ischemia. Breast milk may have a protective effect against development of NEC. Protective ingredients include secretory immunoglobulin (IgA), lactobacilli, which is an antistaphylococcal agent, complement components, lysozymes, lactoferrins, macrophages, and lymphocytes. However, NEC can occur in infants who have received breast milk.

d. Prevention.
  (1) Emphasis is on minimizing the factors contributing to NEC.
  (2) Prevent/correct acid–base imbalance, hypoxemia, hypovolemia, hypotension.
  (3) Correct hyperviscosity.
  (4) Cautious initiation of enteral feedings in small premature infants and in infants who have had perinatal asphyxia.
  (5) Careful monitoring of feeding tolerance.
  (6) Oral administration of immunoglobulins and bifidobacterium may be beneficial (Barclay, 2007).

3. Focal intestinal perforation.
  a. Can occur in the absence of NEC.
  b. Factors distinguishing focal perforation from NEC:
    (1) Less hemodynamic instability.
    (2) Less metabolic acidosis.
    (3) Improved survival rate.
    (4) Use of umbilical artery catheters and indomethacin more common.
    (5) Pathologic finding of coagulation necrosis found in NEC is absent in focal intestinal perforations.

4. Incidence: up to 10% of all admissions to the NICU; approximately 90% of cases occur in preterm infants. Occurs sporadically and in clusters. Occurs within first week of life to several weeks after birth.
  a. Factors contributing to the preterm infant's susceptibility to NEC:
    (1) Decreased immunologic factors in the intestinal tract.
    (2) Increased gastric pH.
    (3) Immature intestinal barrier.
    (4) Decreased intestinal motility.

5. Associated conditions.
  a. Prematurity.
  b. Patent ductus arteriosus.
  c. Infection.

6. Diagnosis.
  a. Physical examination.
    (1) Positive abdominal signs: distention, visible bowel loops, diminishing peristalsis, tenderness, discoloration.
  b. Clinical presentation.
    (1) Gastric residuals.
    (2) Lethargy.
    (3) Apnea and bradycardia.
    (4) Blood in stools: occult or frank blood.
    (5) Temperature instability.
    (6) Diminished urinary output.

(7) Hypoperfusion.

(8) Hypotension due to third-space fluid loss from the intravascular space into the extracellular (third-space) compartment.

(9) Bilious vomiting.

c. Radiologic examination (plain film).

(1) Diffuse gaseous distention of intestines is an early but nonspecific sign.

(2) Asymmetric bowel gas pattern and a relative lack of gas in a certain area with dilation in another area.

(3) Persistently dilated loop of bowel usually represents advanced disease.

(4) Pneumatosis intestinalis (air within the wall of the intestine) is pathognomonic of NEC (see Chapter 14).

(5) Air in the portal venous system (see Chapter 14).

(6) Pneumoperitoneum: represents intestinal perforation (see Chapter 14). Absence of free air does not rule out intestinal perforation.

d. Laboratory studies.

(1) Abnormal CBC: leukocytosis or leukopenia, thrombocytopenia.

(2) Abnormal blood chemistry: metabolic acidosis, electrolyte imbalances.

(3) Abnormal blood gases: hypoxemia, hypercapnia.

(4) Abnormal clotting studies: disseminated intravascular coagulation (DIC).

(5) Presence of blood in stools.

(6) Carbohydrate malabsorption; may be an early sign of NEC.

7. Prognosis: survival rate varies between institutions and also depends on amount of bowel involvement and resection.

B. **Care of the infant with NEC.**

1. Medical management.

a. See section A, "General Considerations," p. 612.

b. Medications: antibiotics (both penicillin-based beta lactam and an aminoglycoside), 3 to 14 days, depending on clinical status.

c. Frequent CBCs and electrolytes to evaluate infant for thrombocytopenia and electrolyte imbalances.

d. Serial plain radiographs (usually every 6 to 8 hours).

e. Respiratory and ventilatory support as needed.

f. Circulatory support as needed to prevent hypotension. Fresh-frozen plasma, vasopressors should be considered.

g. Platelet transfusions for thrombocytopenia.

h. Fresh-frozen plasma for DIC; consider use of vitamin K.

i. Careful monitoring of intake and output. Third-spacing of fluids is common and may lead to hypovolemia and hypotension.

j. Frequent serial abdominal girth measurements.

k. Frequent blood glucose measurements.

2. Surgical management.

a. Preoperative care: continue medical management.

b. Surgery is used if medical management is not possible or fails. Indications for surgery include:

(1) Absolute indication.

(a) Pneumoperitoneum.

(2) Relative indications.

(a) Intestinal gangrene.

(b) Progressive clinical deterioration.

(c) Portal venous gas.

(d) Persistent fixed dilated loop of bowel.

(e) Abdominal wall edema or erythema.

(f) Progressive pneumatosis.

(g) Progressive acidosis.

(h) Progressive thrombocytopenia.

(i) Leukopenia or leukocytosis.

c. Surgical repair.
  (1) Principles of surgery for NEC are to decompress the bowel, resect necrotic bowel, and divert the proximal fecal stream. Actual procedures performed are dependent on condition and age of infant and amount of bowel necrosis.
  (2) In an infant who has isolated necrosis with remaining bowel appearing viable and no intestinal perforation, resection of necrotic bowel and primary anastomosis is appropriate.
  (3) When there is less than 25% viable bowel, options include simple closure of abdomen (always fatal), resection of all necrotic bowel and creation of stomas (frequently results in short bowel syndrome), and proximal diversion without bowel resection (may allow healing of part of bowel). Subsequent operations are usually required to resect gangrenous bowel, but there may be enough remaining bowel for survival.
  (4) Placement of peritoneal drains without surgery has been very successful for the initial management of extremely low birth weight infants with perforated NEC (Nguyen and Lund, 2007). Further surgery may not be required.
d. Postoperative care.
  (1) Pain management (see Chapter 16).
  (2) NPO; gastric decompression continued until normal bowel function is restored.
  (3) Nutrition.
    (a) TPN is used until sufficient enteral intake is established.
    (b) Enteral nutrition is initiated when the operative site has healed. Initiate enteral feeding (often with elemental formula or maternal breast milk) and progress slowly as tolerated.
  (4) Routine ostomy care if applicable. Complications include ostomy prolapse, intestinal obstruction, skin dehiscence and excoriation, and stomal ulceration and bleeding.
  (5) Maintenance of fluid and electrolyte balance.
  (6) Medications: continue antibiotics.
  (7) Observation of stomas for color and drainage.
  (8) Observe for complications.
    (a) Strictures occur in approximately a third of infants with resection. Signs of strictures include bloody stools, failure to thrive, feeding abnormalities, and diarrhea.
    (b) Enteric fistulas and short bowel syndrome (malabsorption and diarrhea).
    (c) Recurrent NEC is not common but can occur.

SHORT BOWEL SYNDROME*

A. **General considerations.**
  1. Definition: syndrome of chronic malabsorption and malnutrition as a result of bowel shortening. Pathophysiology depends on length of intestine, segment of remaining intestine, and whether or not the ileocecal valve is intact. Following bowel resection, the remaining bowel has the ability to adapt to increase its digestive and absorptive capabilities. Villi and crypts elongate and epithelial hyperplasia occurs. Adaptive process is greater in the ileum than in the jejunum. Adaptation occurs over 1 to 2 years. Consequences of short bowel syndrome (SBS) are related to malabsorption due to decreased surface area and loss of specific functions of resected segments.
  2. Etiology.
    a. Surgery requiring extensive resection of bowel.
      (1) NEC (most common, as high as 50%).
      (2) Jejunal or ileal atresia.
      (3) Midgut volvulus.
      (4) Extensive Hirschsprung disease.
      (5) Omphalocele or gastroschisis.

---

*Goulet and Sauvat, 2006; Misiakos et al., 2007.

3. Incidence: 2 per million per year.
4. Associated conditions.
   a. GI tract defects: atresia, malrotation, gastroschisis, omphalocele, Hirschsprung disease.
5. Diagnosis.
   a. Substantial small intestine is removed during surgery.
   b. Clinical presentation: in general, infants experience malabsorption and diarrhea; specific problems are dependent on length of small bowel remaining, presence of ileocecal valve, and site of intestinal loss.
6. Prognosis.
   a. Both the length of intestine and site of intestinal loss influence survival of infants receiving enteral nutrition. Increasing length alone permits longer contact between the product of digestion and the mucosa. If enteral feeding is inadequate, TPN is required. Long-term TPN carries the risk of cholestasis and hepatic damage. Cholelithiasis may occur, owing to depletion of bile acids, resulting in a cholesterol–bile salt ratio abnormality.
   b. Loss of stomach is well tolerated if vitamin B_{12} is periodically given parenterally to prevent anemia.
   c. Jejunum is the primary site of digestion and absorption; however, these functions can be performed in other areas of the intestine after adaptation occurs. Infants with loss of jejunum tend to do much better than those whose ileum is removed. Loss of jejunum can result in nutritional deficiencies, steatorrhea, and cholestasis.
   d. Ileum is responsible for absorption of fat-soluble vitamins, vitamin B_{12}, and bile salts. Loss of ileum has significant metabolic and nutritional consequences.
   e. Ileocecal valve delays intestinal transit time and prevents overgrowth of colonic bacteria in the small intestine. Loss of ileocecal valve results in small bowel colonization with colonic bacteria and less time for digestion and absorption of nutrients in the small intestine.
   f. Loss of the colon may result in hypovolemia, dehydration, and electrolyte disturbances.
   g. Overall survival has improved with new therapies.
   h. With an intact ileocecal valve, infants with as little as 15 cm of small bowel can survive.
   i. Without an intact ileocecal valve, infants require approximately 30 to 45 cm of small bowel for survival.
B. **Care of the infant with short bowel syndrome.**
   1. Medical management.
      a. Stabilize fluid and electrolytes.
      b. Nutrition.
         (1) TPN is used until sufficient enteral intake is established. Cyclic administration of TPN is often used. Careful monitoring for associated complications is required.
         (2) Initiate enteral feeding (often with elemental formula or maternal breast milk) and progress very slowly as tolerated.
      c. Medications:
         (1) Gastric acid blockade (50% have a temporary increase in gastric acid postoperatively).
         (2) Cholestyramine for steatorrhea.
         (3) Antiperistaltic agents for persistent diarrhea. Somatostatin is used to suppress intestinal hormones, decrease gastric and pancreatic secretions, and decrease GI motility. Octreotide is a somatostatin mimetic.
         (4) Trimethoprim-sulfamethoxazole, metronidazole, or other nonabsorbable antibiotics for bacterial overgrowth.
         (5) Vitamin B_{12} is required if the stomach or ileum is lost.
         (6) Vitamins A, D, E, and K are required if the ileum is lost.
      d. Provision of nonnutritive sucking.
      e. Prevention of skin breakdown due to diarrhea.
   2. Surgical management.
      a. Any of a variety of surgical procedures to increase intestinal surface area or decrease intestinal motility.

b. Small bowel transplant. Successful for only a small number of infants; reserved for infants in whom medical and other surgical management has been unsuccessful or who have life-threatening complications of TPN. Contraindications: profound neurologic disabilities, life-threatening and other noncorrectable illnesses not directly related to the digestive system, severe congenital or acquired immunologic deficiencies, and insufficient vascular patency to guarantee easy central venous access for up to 6 months following transplant.

BILIARY ATRESIA*

A. General considerations.
   1. Definition: obstruction of bile flow in the bile duct system. Two types:
      a. Intrahepatic. An embryonic form with failure of ductal formation. Associated with other congenital anomalies.
      b. Extrahepatic. Perinatal fibro-obliteration of ducts which has three forms: Type I with atresia of the common bile duct with patent proximal ducts; Type II with atresia of the common hepatic duct with patent proximal ducts; and Type III with atresia of the right and left hepatic ducts at the porta hepatic.
      c. With both intra and extrahepatic forms of biliary atresia (BA), bile fails to exit the liver resulting in hepatic fibrosis and cirrhosis with progressive liver failure and portal hypertension. With liver failure, liver functions diminish (clotting factors, albumin, drug biotransformation, phagocytosis of foreign substances and bacteria, and excretion of waste material and toxins). Deficiencies of fat-soluble vitamins and vitamin K occur as a result of alterations in fat digestion and absorption.
   2. Etiology: exact mechanism unknown. Suggested theories: alteration in embryologic development, immune or autoimmune response, and association with viral infections. Research points to a genetic causation in some cases.
   3. Incidence: 1 in 8,000 to 18,000 live births, with a slight preponderance in females; 20% intrahepatic and 80% extrahepatic.
   4. Associated anomalies: occurrence in 10% to 15% of infants; including cardiovascular disorders, polysplenia or asplenia with or without situs inversus, preduodenal or absent portal vein, malrotation, and intestinal atresias.
   5. Diagnosis.
      a. Clinical presentation.
         (1) Normal appearance at birth, with gradual manifestation during first month of life.
         (2) Jaundice: usually becomes apparent between second and sixth week of life. Skin is not yellow but rather of green-bronze color because of conjugated hyperbilirubinemia, which is always pathologic.
         (3) Acholic stools (meconium is normal in color). Dark urine.
         (4) Portal hypertension. Seen in advanced liver disease when high pressure exists between portal vein and inferior vena cava.
            (a) Engorged veins: periumbilical, esophageal, and rectal.
            (b) Ascites: result of low albumin levels and increased hydrostatic pressure in abdominal vessels.
      b. Physical examination.
         (1) Abdominal distention.
         (2) Distended, tortuous abdominal veins.
         (3) Hepatosplenomegaly. Liver is hard.
      c. Radiologic examination.
         (1) Ultrasound.
         (2) Hepatobiliary scintigraphy (HIDA scan).
         (3) Operative cholangiography.
         (4) Endoscopic retrograde cholangiopancreatography (ERCP). Recent development of a new side-view instrument makes ERCP now possible in infants.

---

*Shih et al., 2005; Winfield and Beierle, 2006; Wong et al., 2006.

    d. Laboratory studies.

      (1) Elevated serum levels of aminotransferase, alkaline phosphatase, gamma-glutam-yltranspeptidase, and 5′-nucleotidase and hyaluronic acid (Ukarapol et al., 2007).

      (2) Late findings: abnormal clotting studies, hypoalbuminemia.

    e. Other.

      (1) Liver biopsy.

6. Prognosis.

    a. Without surgical treatment, most infants will die by 2 years of age.

    b. Less than 20% of patients who have a portoenterostomy survive to adulthood without a liver transplant.

    c. Survival is improved for patients who initially undergo a portoenterostomy, followed by a liver transplant (LT) (Diem et al., 2003).

B. Care of the infant with biliary atresia.

1. Preoperative care.

    a. Evaluation for additional anomalies.

2. Surgical procedures.

    a. Intrahepatic form requires LT. Lack of intrahepatic ducts precludes any drainage procedures.

    b. Extrahepatic form. Goal: reestablishment of bile drainage. Treatment is dependent on the type.

      (1) Resection of atretic segments and end-to-end anastomosis: possible in only a few cases.

      (2) Hepatoportoenterostomy (Kasai procedure). Intestinal conduit is created between the liver surface and small intestine. Typically performed by laparotomy, recently performed using robotic laparoscopic technique (Meehan et al., 2007). This is most successful when performed by 2 months of age. The conduit is sometimes exteriorized temporarily to allow assessment of bile flow. Complications include the following:

        (a) Cholangitis: Most common complication; results from bile stasis and bacterial contamination of the intestinal conduit. Presents with fever, leukocytosis, increased serum bilirubin, and nonspecific signs of infection.

        (b) Cessation of bile flow.

        (c) Portal hypertension.

      (3) Liver transplant.

3. Postoperative care.

    a. Pain management (see Chapter 16).

    b. NPO; gastric decompression.

    c. Medications.

      (1) Antibiotics to decrease risk of cholangitis.

      (2) Fat-soluble vitamins (A, D, E, K).

      (3) Choleretic agents such as ursodiol (Actigall) may be given to increase bile flow.

      (4) Steroids are commonly given for a month, then tapered. Used for their choleretic effect and to decrease scarring at the site of anastomosis.

    d. Nutrition.

      (1) TPN is used until sufficient enteral intake is established.

      (2) Enteral nutrition is initiated when the operative site has healed. Initiate enteral feeding containing medium-chain triglycerides and progress as tolerated.

    e. Assessment of bile flow and replacement as appropriate (if exteriorized).

    f. Monitor for hemorrhage secondary to portal hypertension and bleeding tendencies.

CHOLESTASIS*

A. General considerations.

1. Definition: marked impairment in bile flow.

---

*Shih et al., 2005; Steinbach et al., 2008; Suchy, 2004; Wong et al., 2006.

2. Etiology: the main determinant of bile flow is the enterohepatic circulation, with the rate-limiting step being secretion of bile by the hepatocyte. The neonatal liver is prone to cholestasis because its bile acid pool size is diminished and hepatic uptake and excretion mechanisms are immature. In addition, new research points to a genetic causation in some cases. Causes of cholestasis by anatomic location:
   a. Extrahepatic bile duct: biliary atresia, choledochal cyst, choledocholithiasis, and bile duct perforation.
   b. Intrahepatic bile duct: syndromic paucity of bile ducts (Alagille syndrome [70% with abnormal chromosome 20p12]), nonsyndromic paucity of bile ducts, bile duct dysgenesis, cystic fibrosis, Langerhans cell histiocytosis, and hyper-IgM syndrome.
   c. Hepatocyte: bacterial and viral infection, progressive familial intrahepatic cholestasis syndrome, inborn errors of metabolism, neonatal hemachromatosis, and total parenteral nutrition-associated cholestasis (TPNAC).
3. Incidence: overall incidence is 1 in 2500. Incidence of cholestasis associated with TPN varies from 7% to 50%. Frequency increases with younger gestational age and longer duration of TPN. Most cases occur within 2 to 10 weeks after starting TPN; 90% of infants develop cholestasis within 13 weeks.
4. Associated conditions: see etiology above.
5. Diagnosis: there is no one test for cholestasis. Once it is established that the infant has conjugated hyperbilirubinemia, the diagnostic evaluation should be individualized.
   a. History.
   b. Clinical presentation.
      (1) Normal appearance at birth, with gradual manifestation during first month of life.
      (2) Jaundice; usually becomes apparent between second and sixth week of life. Skin is not yellow but rather of green-bronze color due to conjugated hyperbilirubinemia.
      (3) Acholic stools, malabsorption of fat (steatorrhea) and lipid-soluble vitamins, mineral and trace mineral deficiency, growth failure. Dark urine.
      (4) Hepatomegaly due to hepatocellular damage. Portal hypertension if cholestasis is prolonged and liver failure occurs.
      (5) Pruritus, xanthomas due to retention of bile acids and cholesterol.
   c. Radiologic examination.
      (1) Ultrasound.
      (2) Hepatobiliary scintigraphy (HIDA scan).
      (3) Percutaneous or endoscopic cholangiography.
      (4) Endoscopic retrograde cholangiopancreatography (ERCP).
      (5) Radiographs of long bones and skull for congenital infections.
   d. Laboratory studies.
      (1) Urinalysis.
      (2) Bacterial cultures of blood and urine.
      (3) Serology for vital hepatitides, human immunodeficiency virus (HIV), and toxoplasmosis, other [congenital syphilis and viruses], rubella, cytomegalovirus, herpes simplex (TORCH).
      (4) Bilirubin fractionation: Direct bilirubin greater than 2 mg/dl. Direct to total bilirubin ratio greater than 15%.
      (5) Liver enzymes: Elevated aminotransferase concentrations (hepatocellular damage). Elevated alkaline phosphatase, 5'-nucleotidase or γ-glutamyl transpeptidase (GGTP) (biliary injury or obstruction).
      (6) Assessment of synthetic liver function: serum albumin, glucose, ammonia, cholesterol, prothrombin time.
      (7) Test for inborn errors of metabolism.
      (8) Sweat chloride iontophoresis.
   e. Other.
      (1) Ophthalmologic examination.
      (2) Liver biopsy.
6. Prognosis: related to underlying cause.

B. **Management of the infant with cholestasis: management is specific to the etiology.** No specific therapy reverses cholestasis or prevents its progression. In cases of outflow obstruction, eliminate the obstruction (see Biliary Atresia, p. 617). Chromosomal abnormalities cannot be reversed but may be palliated. With an infectious etiology, treat underlying infection. For TPNAC, minimize TPN concentration and duration and provide enteral nutrition if possible. Goals of therapy are to improve nutritional status, maximize growth, and minimize discomfort.

1. TPN management.
   a. Decrease parenteral protein to 1 to 2 g/kg/day.
   b. Decrease parenteral dextrose concentration to 10%.
   c. Eliminate hepatic trace elements.
2. Enteral feeding management.
   a. Increase enteral feedings as tolerated. Caloric intake should be 125% to 150% of recommended dietary additives.
   b. Administer formulas with medium-chain triglycerides (e.g., Pregestimil, Alimentum).
   c. Encourage breastfeeding as long as infant grows appropriately.
3. Medications.
   a. Supplemental fat-soluble vitamins. TPGS-tocopherol (Liqui-E or Nutr-E-Sol) is the preferred vitamin E preparation, to be given with a multivitamin supplement (e.g., Poly-Vi-Sol) and vitamin K. These preparations should all be mixed together for administration.
   b. Cholestyramine to increase fecal excretion of bile acids. The decrease in bile acids returning to the liver stimulates the production of new bile acids from cholesterol, resulting in the reduction of toxic bile acids in the liver and a decrease in cholesterol. May help decrease pruritus.
   c. Ursodeoxycholic acid for pruritus and to increase intestinal excretion of bile acids (San Luis and Btaiche, 2007).
   d. Phenobarbital to decrease bile acid pool size.

GASTROESOPHAGEAL REFLUX*

A. **General considerations.**
   1. Definition: Gastroesophageal reflux (GER) is the retrograde movement of gastric contents into the esophagus and above. With gastroesophageal reflux disease (GERD), there are symptoms of disease resulting from GER events. GERD has not been well defined in neonates. Regurgitation is a movement of gastric contents into the mouth. Regurgitation may be a sign of GER, but GER can occur without regurgitation.
      a. Spectrum of GER.
         (1) Reflux episodes occur to some extent in all individuals, especially after meals.
         (2) Reflux is considered physiologic as long as the individual continues to thrive and has no complications.
         (3) Complications generally do not occur as long as the frequency and duration of reflux are in the normal range.
         (4) Infants who have regurgitation as their only sign of reflux are considered to have physiologic GER and are referred to as "happy spitters."
         (5) Pathologic GER usually manifests as malnutrition, respiratory disorders, or esophagitis.
   2. Etiology. Mechanisms for reflux in infants includes a transient relaxation of the lower esophageal segment (LES), delay in esophageal clearance of contents, air entry into stomach during swallowing, excessive swallowing, delayed gastric emptying, and decreased esophageal motility. A complete understanding of the pathophysiology of GER remains unclear.

---

*Bhat et al., 2007; Blackburn, 2007; Moukarzel et al., 2007; Sondheimer, 2006; U.S. Department of Health and Human Services (USDHHS), 2006; Winfield and Beierle, 2006.

3. Incidence: varied; 40% to 50% of infants regurgitate more than once a day. GER with symptoms has been noted in 3% to 10% of premature infants less than 1500 g.
4. Associated conditions.
   a. Prematurity.
   b. Birth asphyxia with neurodevelopmental delay. Infants treated with extracorporeal membrane oxygenation (ECMO) are at risk for GER because of the acute status requiring ECMO.
   c. GI tract anomalies/conditions: esophageal atresia/tracheoesophageal fistula, esophagitis, hiatal hernia, pyloric stenosis, gastroschisis/omphalocele, duodenal atresia, malrotation.
   d. Diaphragmatic hernia/paralysis.
   e. Chronic lung disease.
   f. Medications: xanthines, betamimetics, prostaglandin E_1, dopamine.
5. Diagnosis.
   a. Clinical presentation.
      (1) Feeding difficulties.
         (a) Regurgitation; most common presentation in infants.
         (b) Gagging.
         (c) Feeding refusal.
         (d) Aspiration.
         (e) Failure to thrive.
      (2) Fussiness, irritability, colic-like behavior, back arching with feeding.
      (3) Respiratory difficulty.
         (a) Apnea.
            (i) Protective airway reflexes may respond to refluxed pharyngeal material, causing laryngospasm and obstructive apnea.
            (ii) Reflux-related apnea most commonly occurs after a meal, with the infant supine or seated. The infant may not cough, choke, or gag prior to the apneic episode.
         (b) Stridor.
   b. Radiologic examination.
      (1) Fluoroscopy or upper GI series (30% false positive).
      (2) Scintigraphy.
   c. Other studies.
      (1) Esophageal pH probe. Detects acid reflux only; does not detect nonacid (milk) or gas reflux.
      (2) Intraesophageal electrical impedance (pH independent).
      (3) Esophageal manometry.
      (4) Endoscopy.
6. Prognosis. Resolves in almost all infants by 12 to 18 months of age; 10% to 15% require prolonged medical management; 10% to 15% also require surgery. Success after fundoplication varies. Prognosis depends on complications: respiratory (worsening of chronic lung disease; bronchospasm and pneumonia), esophageal (esophagitis [occurs in 61% to 83% of infants with clinically significant reflux], bleeding, strictures), and hematologic (anemia from chronic bleeding).
B. **Management of the infant with GER.**
   1. Conservative measures.
      a. Interventions to minimize simple regurgitation.
         (1) Thicken feedings with rice cereal. Thickening increases viscosity. It also increases caloric density, thus reducing the volume needed to supply adequate calories.
         (2) Feed slowly.
         (3) Frequent burping.
         (4) Small frequent feedings.
         (5) Position infant at a 45- to 60-degree angle during feeding.
         (6) Avoid pressure on abdomen during feeding.

      (7) Avoid jiggling or bouncing the infant during feeding and for at least an hour afterwards.

  b. Minimize/eliminate provoking and aggravating factors.

      (1) Provoking factors: frequent suctioning, chest physical therapy.

      (2) Aggravating factors: xanthine and betamimetic agents (increase LES relaxation).

  c. Position.

      (1) Upright for 30 minutes after feeding (infant held upright by caregiver) (USDHHS, 2006). Upright position in a car seat can make reflux worse as typically the infant's lower body slides forward, increasing intraabdominal pressure and possibly compromising the airway by a chin-on-chest position.

      (2) Supine position (Bhat et al., 2007; USDHHS, 2006). Preterm delivery and GER do not exempt an infant from supine position recommendations (American Academy of Pediatrics [AAP], 2000). This policy was not changed at a subsequent review and revision of the policy (AAP, 2005).

      (3) The surface on which the infant is placed for sleep should be firm and without soft bedding or gas-trapping objects (AAP, 2005).

2. Pharmacologic measures.

  a. Prokinetics. Used to increase gastric motility. Commonly used agents include bethanechol, metoclopramide, and erythromycin.

  b. H_2 antagonists or proton pump inhibitors. Reduce gastric acid when complications such as esophagitis occur. Commonly used agents include ranitidine, famotidine, and omeprazole.

  c. Acid-neutralizing agents (e.g., calcium- and aluminum-containing antacids). Facilitate healing of esophagitis but are infrequently given to neonates because of the side effect of constipation.

3. Surgical measures: initiated when conservative and medical management has failed and the infant has developed or is anticipated to develop sequelae and complications. Frequently performed using laparoscopic technique.

  a. Nissen fundoplication (Fig. 29-7). Stomach fundus is wrapped 360 degrees around the LES. Is the procedure most commonly performed.

  b. Variations of Nissen technique including the Thal procedure (270-degree); the Mutaf gastric tube cardioplasty; posterior 180-degree procedure; anterior 180-degree procedure; and recently an anterior 90-degree procedure.

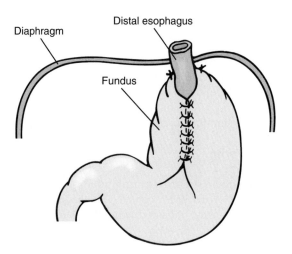

FIGURE 29-7. ■ Nissen fundoplication for repair of hiatal hernia. Fundus of stomach is wrapped around distal esophagus and sutured to itself. (From Lewis, S.M., Heitkemper, M.M., Dirksen, S.R., O'Brien, P.G., and Bucher, L.: *Medical-surgical nursing: Assessment and management of clinical problems* [7th ed.]. St. Louis, 2007, Mosby.)

MULTISYSTEM DISORDERS WITH GASTROINTESTINAL INVOLVEMENT*

A. Eagle–Barrett syndrome (prune-belly syndrome).

1. Definition: triad of congenital anomalies consisting of absence of abdominal musculature, genitourinary tract abnormalities, and cryptorchidism (undescended testes). Most common genitourinary defects are as follows:
   a. Megaloureter.
   b. Cystic renal dysplasia.
   c. Urethral obstruction.
   d. Megacystitis.

2. Etiology: unclear, but may be the result of a generalized developmental defect of abdominal parietes and mesenchyma. The condition is rarely familial, and no cytogenic abnormality has been discovered.

3. Incidence: 1 in 30,000 to 40,000 live births. Approximately 97% of affected infants are male. With familial cases, the incidence of affected males decreases to 72%. The incidence is also higher in twin gestations and African American infants.

4. Associated conditions.
   a. Pulmonary conditions: hypoplasia.
   b. GI tract anomalies (30%): malrotation, volvulus, atresia or stenosis, imperforate anus, persistent cloaca.
   c. Cardiac anomalies (10%): patent ductus arteriosus, atrial and ventricular septal defects, tetralogy of Fallot.
   d. Genitourinary conditions: patent urachus, posterior urethral valves.
   e. Musculoskeletal anomalies: limb abnormalities (clubfoot and other positional deformations), scoliosis, congenital hip dysplasia, contractures.

5. Diagnosis.
   a. Prenatal ultrasonography including high resolution method. May show a dilated renal pelvis (>5 mm at 16 to 18 weeks of gestation), dilated ureters, and bladder distention.
   b. History of oligohydramnios: suggestive of renal pathologic changes.
   c. Inspection at birth: shapeless, flat abdomen with wrinkled skin; respiratory distress, compression deformities.
   d. Physical examination: Potter's facies and skeletal deformities; bell-shaped chest, respiratory distress, cardiac murmur; wrinkled abdomen with visible bowel loops and possible margins of liver and spleen, enlarged kidneys, distended bladder (4 cm from symphysis by percussion), urinary drainage via the umbilicus; bilateral cryptorchidism, pseudohermaphroditism in females.

6. Radiologic examination.
   a. Ultrasound: kidneys, ureters, bladder, urethra.
   b. Voiding cystourethrogram: controversial. Evaluates urethra, bladder, vesicoureteral reflux, ureteral stenosis, and detects patent urachus.
   c. CT scan.
   d. Nuclear scan: technetium Tc 99m dimethylsuccinic acid (DMSA) renal scan.

7. Other: karyotyping if sex is indeterminate.

8. Prognosis: directly related to degree of urinary tract dysfunction, especially renal. Approximately 20% of infants die during the first month of life from renal dysplasia or hypoplasia. Renal failure develops in childhood in approximately 30% of those who survive infancy. Treatment required includes dialysis or transplant. Long-term considerations includes difficulty voiding and the need for nephrostomy or uretostomy; constipation is common; long-term antibiotic therapy may be necessary to prevent infection.

B. Management of the infant with Eagle–Barrett syndrome.

1. Medical management.
   a. Respiratory: support as needed; alert for pulmonary air leak.

---

*Levine et al., 2007; Siebert and Kapur, 2007; Woods and Brandon, 2007.

    b. Correct fluid, electrolyte, and acid–base status. Sodium reabsorption is diminished or deficient; hyponatremia may rapidly result. BUN and serum creatinine: rising values may indicate renal insufficiency.

    c. Nutrition. Low protein intake reduces renal workload.

    d. Antibiotics to prevent urinary tract infection due to urinary stasis and reflux, and invasive procedures.

  2. Surgical procedures.

    a. Prenatal: shunting to preserve renal function by preventing bladder distention. Procedures include vesicoamniotic shunting, open fetal surgery, and fetoscopic surgery.

    b. Postnatal: urinary diversion is essential to sustain renal function. Procedures include urethrotomy for urethral obstruction; cutaneous vesicostomy with the bladder brought to the abdominal surface; repair of posterior urethral valves; closure of patent urachus, although many spontaneously close; orchiopexy to prevent testicular malignancy; and abdominal wall reconstruction.

C. Congenital diaphragmatic hernia (Hayakawa et al., 2007; Holder et al., 2007; Migliazza et al., 2007).

  1. Definition: herniation of abdominal organs into the thoracic cavity through a defect in the diaphragm. About 85% occur on the left. Approximately 95% occur posteriorly (Bochdalek type) while 5% occur anteriorly (Morgagni type). The defect can vary from a small slit to the complete absence of the diaphragm on the affected side. Severity is related to timing and degree of prenatal herniation. Early herniation through a large defect is associated with bilateral pulmonary hypoplasia, pulmonary hypertension, and intrapulmonary shunt (V/Q mismatch). A right-to-left shunt occurs through the ductus arteriosus and/or foramen ovale, further compromising pulmonary blood flow and sending deoxygenated blood to the body.

  2. Etiology: unknown. May occur as isolated defect or part of a syndrome. Numerous genetic abnormalities are associated with CDH.

  3. Incidence: 1 in 3000 live births.

  4. Associated conditions.

    a. Chromosomal abnormalities: most common are trisomies 13, 18, 21, and 45X.

    b. Associated anomalies are reported to be greater than 40% and include CNS, cardio-vascular, skeletal, GI, and genitourinary defects. Intestinal malrotation is common.

  5. Diagnosis.

    a. Prenatal ultrasonography, including the high-resolution method.

    b. History of polyhydramnios.

    c. Clinical presentation.

      (1) Respiratory distress and cyanosis at birth or shortly after birth typically followed by worsening presentation. Condition worsens rather than improves with bag–mask ventilation as intestines distend with air and further compromise lung function.

      (2) Hypoperfusion and decreased oxygen saturation due to right-to-left shunting through the ductus arteriosus, foramen ovale, and intrapulmonary shunts.

    d. Physical examination.

      (1) Diminished breath sounds: decreased on ipsilateral side due to lung compression by abdominal organs; decreased on contralateral side due to mediastinal shift.

      (2) Heart tones may be shifted from their normal point of maximal intensity.

      (3) Barrel chest.

      (4) Scaphoid abdomen.

    e. Radiologic examination.

      (1) Plain radiograph showing displaced gastric bubble and a bowel gas pattern in the thorax (see Chapter 14). A radiograph taken immediately after birth may not demonstrate bowel gas in the intestines while later radiographs demonstrate it clearly.

    f. Laboratory tests: blood gas analysis demonstrating hypoxemia, hypercapnia, and combined metabolic and respiratory acidosis.

6. Prognosis: survival varies depending on the size of the defect and amount of herniated viscera, early intervention especially at a tertiary care center, pulmonary hypertension, and associated conditions. Despite current interventions, survival is approximately 50% (Colvin et al., 2005). Although some institutions report higher survival rates, the reported survival rates do not include infants who expired prior to arrival at the respective institution. Structured follow-up care is required for infants with long-term sequelae (AAP, 2008).

D. **Management of the infant with congenital diaphragmatic hernia.**
   1. Prenatal treatment: the gravid mother must be transferred to a facility capable of management of the infant postpartum including neonatal intensive care, inhaled nitric oxide, ECMO, pediatric surgery, and genetic evaluation.
   2. Preoperative care: CDH is no longer considered a surgical emergency. Concerns immediately after birth include pulmonary hypoplasia and pulmonary hypertension. In addition, not rushing to surgery allows stabilization of the infant and evaluation for associated conditions that may preclude ECMO or surgery.
      a. Respiratory.
         (1) Intubate and support as needed. Avoid bag–mask ventilation to prevent GI distention. Remain alert for pulmonary air leak. Immediate treatment must be prompt and aggressive. Primary considerations are as follows:
            (a) Establishment of adequate perfusion. Use of inotropes to increase systemic blood pressure and decreased right-to-left shunting.
            (b) Correction of acid–base imbalances and provision of adequate oxygenation.
            (c) May require high-frequency ventilation, administration of inhaled nitric oxide (iNO). Prophylactic surfactant treatment at birth has no benefit in both preterm and term infants (Lally et al., 2004; Van Meurs, 2004) because surfactant maturation is unaffected in infants with CDH (Boucherat et al., 2007). Hyperventilation and hyperalkalinization to force alkalinization are no longer recommended because they cause ventilation-induced lung injury, complicate electrolyte management, and decrease cerebral blood flow.
      b. ECMO is instituted if ventilation does not effectively stabilize the pulmonary status. ECMO may be used preoperatively to stabilize the patient for surgery, intraoperatively, and/or postoperatively to rest the lungs.
      c. NPO with continuous gastric decompression.
      d. Complete examination for other anomalies.
   3. Surgical procedures.
      a. Prenatal surgery.
         (1) Procedures to occlude the trachea have been used in fetuses but have not proven beneficial (Cortes et al., 2005).
         (2) In utero repair of CDH does not improve survival over conventional postpartum care.
      b. Postnatal surgery.
         (1) Primary closure of the diaphragmatic defect is usually possible. With large defects or a totally absent diaphragm, a synthetic patch can be used to close the diaphragmatic defect.
      c. Postoperative care.
         (1) Pain management (see Chapter 16).
         (2) Continue preoperative care.
            (a) Respiratory support with oxygenation, ventilation, iNO, ECMO.
            (b) NPO with continuous gastric decompression until peristalsis is normal.
            (c) Inotropes: decrease right-to-left shunting.
            (d) If placed during surgery, a chest tube for drainage should be placed on water seal (without suction) to prevent acute mediastinal shift.

E. **Hyperbilirubinemia** (AAP, 2004; Deshpande and Ramer, 2006; Frank and Frank, 2006; Hansen, 2007; Wong et al., 2006).
   1. Definitions.
      a. Hyperbilirubinemia: an elevated total serum bilirubin (TSB) level. Abnormal values differ by gestational age, days of life, concomitant illness or conditions. A recognizable

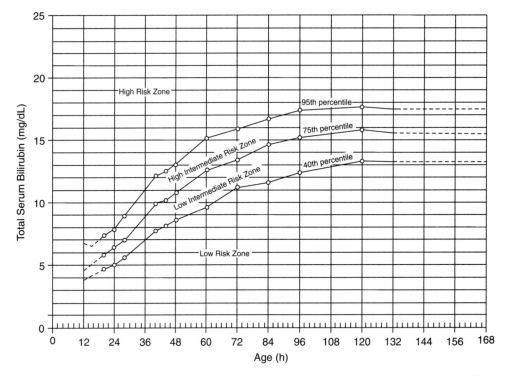

FIGURE 29-8. ■ Risk designation of term and near-term well newborns based on their hour-specific serum bilirubin values. The high-risk zone is designated by the 95th percentile track. The intermediate-risk zone is subdivided to upper- and lower-risk zones by the 75th percentile track. The low-risk zone has been electively and statistically defined by the 40th percentile track. (Dotted extensions are based on <300 total serum bilirubin [TSB] values/epoch.) (From Bhutani, V.K., Johnson, L., and Sivieri, E.M.: Predictive ability of a predischarge hour-specific serum bilirubin for subsequent significant hyperbilirubinemia in healthy term and near-term newborns. *Pediatrics, 103*[1]:6-14, 1999.)

    sign is jaundice. TSB is the combination of conjugated and unconjugated serum bilirubin levels (see Figure 29-8).

  b. Jaundice (icterus): the yellowish coloration of the skin and sclera caused by the presence of bilirubin in elevated concentrations. Jaundice appears cephalad to caudal and regresses in the reverse order.

  c. Conjugated: direct serum hyperbilirubinemia.

  d. Unconjugated: indirect hyperbilirubinemia.

  e. Acute bilirubin encephalopathy: acute bilirubin toxicity manifested by a direct correlation between lethargy and unconjugated serum bilirubin concentration, and abnormal brainstem auditory evoked response. Brain MRIs show focal changes. If not reversed the process progresses to permanent neurologic impairment or death. Survivors demonstrate cerebral palsy and sensorineural hearing loss. Autopsy also reveals renal, intestinal, and pancreatic cell involvement. Calculation of a risk index score (Fig. 29-9).

    (1) Phase 1: poor sucking, hypotonia, depressed sensorium.

    (2) Phase 2: fever, retrocollis, hypertonia, opisthotonos, high-pitched cry.

    (3) Phase 3: shrill cry, hearing and visual derangements, no feeding, athetosis, apnea, seizures, deep stupor to coma, death.

  f. Kernicterus: for consistency the AAP recommends this definition: irreversible, chronic sequelae of bilirubin toxicity (AAP, 2004).

    (1) During the first year of life, characteristic findings are hypotonia, active deep tendon reflexes, persistent tonic neck reflex, and delayed acquisition of motor skills.

VARIABLE	SCORE
Exclusive breast-feeding	6
Family history of jaundice in a newborn	6
Bruising noted	4
Asian race	4
Cephalohematoma noted	3
Maternal age ≥25 years	3
Male sex	1
Black race	−2
Gestational age, weeks	2 (40-GA)

*Risk index score is calculated as the sum of all characteristics that apply to the patient, except that points for gestational age (GA) are assigned based on twice the difference of GA from 40 weeks. For example, a 37-week bottle-fed Asian male newborn whose mother was 30 years old would receive a score of 14: 6 (2×[40−37])+4 (Asian)+1 (male)+3 (mother ≥25y).

FIGURE 29-9. ■ Risk index for predicting total serum bilirubin (TSB) greater than or equal to 428 mcmol/ L (25 mg/dl) in newborns who do not have early jaundice. (From Newman, T.B., Xiong, B., Gonzales, V.M., and Escobar, G.J.: Prediction and prevention of extreme neonatal hyperbilirubinemia in a mature health maintenance organization. *Archives of Pediatric and Adolescent Medicine, 154*[11]:1144-1147, 2000.)

(2) Characteristics of fully developed encephalopathy include hearing loss, choreoathetoid cerebral palsy, and gaze abnormalities, especially upward gaze. Intellectual deficits are common but usually not severe.

(3) Treatment: None.

2. Etiology.
   a. Bilirubin metabolism (Fig. 29-10).
      (1) Synthesis: bilirubin is primarily the metabolic end product of erythrocyte (RBC) breakdown. One gram of heme produces 34 mg of bilirubin; normal neonates produce 8 to 10 mg/kg/day.
      (2) Transport: heme reversibly binds to albumin (1 g of albumin can bind with approximately 8 mg of bilirubin) and is transported via the bloodstream to the liver as an unconjugated, fat-soluble product with a propensity for fatty tissues such as subcutaneous and brain tissue.
      (3) Metabolism: glucuronyl transferase converts bilirubin and glucuronic acid into water soluble glucuronide.
      (4) Excretion: glucuronide is excreted into bile, enters the intestine where bacteria convert it to urobilinogen. Urobilinogen is converted to stercobilin and excreted in feces, giving feces a brownish color.
      (5) Enterohepatic reabsorption of bilirubin: In the small intestine, the high concentration of β-glucuronidase in newborn infants can convert conjugated bilirubin into the unconjugated form, which is easily absorbed from the small intestine into the portal circulation. In fetal life, this permits bilirubin to be transported across the placenta for maternal excretion. Increased amounts of bilirubin in the amniotic fluid may indicate hemolytic disease or fetal intestinal obstruction below the bile ducts.
   b. Nonpathologic unconjugated hyperbilirubinemia: a result of an elevated hematocrit level at birth, increased RBC destruction (neonatal RBCs have a 70- to 90-day life span), reduced hepatic uptake of unconjugated bilirubin, and enterohepatic reabsorption of bilirubin. TSB levels generally peak on day 3 of life in full-term infants and on days 5 to 6 in preterm infants. Factors that may further accentuate this normal process include:
      (1) Hemolysis.
         (a) ABO/Rh incompatibilities.
         (b) Bacterial and viral infection (especially TORCH infections).
         (c) Inherited disorders of RBC metabolism.
            (i) RBC membrane defects: spherocytosis, elliptocytosis.
            (ii) RBC enzyme defects: glucose-6-phosphate dehydrogenase deficiency (G6PD) and pyruvate kinase deficiency.

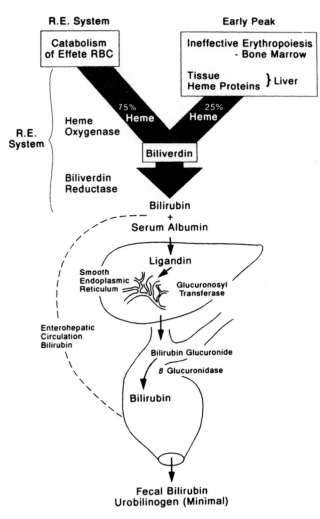

FIGURE 29-10. ■ Neonatal bile pigment metabolism. *RE,* Reticuloendothelial; *RBC,* red blood cells. (From Maisels, M.J.: Jaundice. In G.B. Avery, M.A. Fletcher, and M.G. MacDonald [Eds.]: *Neonatology: Pathophysiology and management of the newborn* [5th ed.]. Philadelphia, 1999, Lippincott Williams & Wilkins, p. 767.)

    (d) Inherited disorders of bilirubin metabolism: Crigler-Najjar types I and II, Gilbert disease.

    (e) Medications that cause hemolysis or compete with albumin for binding sites, and free fatty acids from emulsified fats (Intralipid®).

(2) Extravasation of blood.

    (a) Cephalohematoma or bruising.

    (b) Pulmonary, cerebral, or retroperitoneal hemorrhage.

    (c) Swallowed blood.

(3) Increased enterohepatic circulation.

    (a) Delayed feeding.

    (b) Intestinal obstructions.

(4) Decreased hepatic function and perfusion.

    (a) Metabolic derangements: hypoxia, acidosis, hypothermia, hypoglycemia, starvation.

    (b) Infection.

(5) Endocrine disorders.

    (a) Hypothyroidism.

    (b) Hypopituitarism.

(6) Inborn errors of metabolism (with both unconjugated and conjugated hyperbilirubinemia).
(a) Galactosemia.
(b) α_1-Antitrypsin deficiency.
(c) Tyrosinosis.
(d) Hypermethioninemia.
(e) Cystic fibrosis.
(7) Globin synthesis defect: α-thalassemia.
c. Pathologic unconjugated hyperbilirubinemia (for blood incompatibilities, see Chapter 31): when the nonpathologic unconjugated hyperbilirubinemia processes are exaggerated and when available albumin binding sites are saturated, unconjugated bilirubin circulates as free bilirubin and can cross the blood-brain barrier (BBB). This BBB breach is accentuated with meningitis.
(1) Unconjugated hyperbilirubinemia is pathologic when (Frank & Frank, 2006)
(a) Jaundice appears in the first 24 hours of life,
(b) TSB level increases by more than 5 mg/dl per day,
(c) TSB level exceeds 12.9 mg/dl in a term infant or 15 mg/dl in a preterm infant,
(d) TSB level is in the 95th percentile for age in hours or is "jumping the tracks" (Fig. 29-8), or
(e) Jaundice lasts for more than 1 week in a term infant or 2 weeks in a preterm infant.
d. Conjugated hyperbilirubinemia.
(1) Hepatic cell injury: TPN, infection (TORCH and viral hepatitis, and systemic bacterial), medications, metabolic derangements and inborn errors in metabolism.
(2) Biliary obstruction: see Biliary Atresia, p. 617.
(3) Excessive bilirubin load.
(4) Maternal–fetal blood group incompatibility: ABO, Rh (see Chapter 31).
e. Breastfeeding jaundice: onset 2 to 4 days of life; related to low enteral intake. Self-limiting as milk supply increases.
f. Breast milk jaundice: onset 4 to 7 days of life; exaggerated physiologic jaundice related to substances in maternal breast milk that cause glucuronyl transferase inhibition. Occurs in 10% to 30% of breastfed newborns; TSB levels may reach 12 to 20 mg/dL and persist for up to 2 months.
3. Incidence: dependent on etiology.
a. Influenced by the following:
(1) Ethnicity (higher in infants of Chinese, Japanese, Korean, Native American, and Greek descent).
(2) Elevated hematocrit level (delayed cord clamping, maternal diabetes).
(3) Extravasated blood (bruising, cephalohematoma, intracranial hemorrhage, swallowed blood).
(4) Maternal medications: oxytocin and bupivacaine. Mechanism is unclear but may involve hemolysis.
(5) Hepatic dysfunction: prematurity, asphyxia.
(6) Feeding: early enteral feeds promote peristalsis and passage of bilirubin-containing stool, and introduce bacteria into the gut (contributes to the conversion of bilirubin to urobilin, a substance that cannot be reabsorbed).
b. Nonpathologic unconjugated hyperbilirubinemia (physiologic jaundice): jaundice develops in more than 60% of term newborn infants and 80% of preterm infants; it is visible when the serum bilirubin concentration is greater than 6 to 7 mg/dl.
c. Conjugated hyperbilirubinemia: dependent on etiology.
d. Breastfeeding jaundice: 1 in 10 breastfed infants.
e. Breast milk jaundice: 1 in 200 breastfed infants.
4. Associated conditions.
a. Prematurity.
b. Infection.

5. Diagnosis.
   a. Nonpathologic unconjugated hyperbilirubinemia.
      (1) Clinical presentation: onset of jaundice around day 2 to 3 of life. No hepatosplenomegaly.
      (2) Laboratory tests: transcutaneous bilirubin (TcB) meter helps establish a risk assessment but does not determine exact TSB levels. Usefulness in preterm infants, infants receiving phototherapy, and infants with TSB values above 15 mg/dL requires further study. Definitive bilirubin levels are obtained only by analysis of TSB levels.
   b. Pathologic unconjugated hyperbilirubinemia.
      (1) See nonpathologic unconjugated hyperbilirubinemia.
      (2) Clinical presentation: jaundice within 24 hours of birth. Signs of acute bilirubin encephalopathy.
      (3) Laboratory tests: TSB increase of 5 mg/dL or more in a 24-hour period or above the 95th percentile for age (hours).
   c. Conjugated hyperbilirubinemia.
      (1) See Biliary Atresia.
   d. Breastfeeding jaundice: Peaks around day 3 as enteral intake increases, then resolves.
   e. Breast milk jaundice: Prolonged appearance, no signs of bilirubin encephalopathy.
6. Prognosis: dependent on etiology and early detection and treatment, when necessary.

F. **Care of the infant with hyperbilirubinemia.**
   1. **Management of nonpathologic unconjugated hyperbilirubinemia.**
      a. Frequent enteral feeding including promotion and support of breastfeeding.
      b. Establish protocols to identify hyperbilirubinemia and measure bilirubin levels. Interpret results by infant's age—gestationally and hours of life. Follow-up care postdischarge is required for all infants discharged before 48 hours of age.
      c. At discharge, provide caretakers with verbal and written information about hyperbilirubinemia, need for follow-up monitoring, and how monitoring will be accomplished.
   2. **Management of pathologic unconjugated hyperbilirubinemia.**
      a. Goal: prevent bilirubin toxic effects. Recognize that all infants are at risk. Risk is increased with decreasing gestational age, infants less than 38 weeks of gestation who are breastfeeding, and in the ill neonate.
      b. Guidelines for treating hyperbilirubinemia in healthy term infants are listed in Table 29-4. Management of hyperbilirubinemia in low-birth-weight infants is determined by clinical status, age, weight, and history (Table 29-5).
      c. Jaundice before 24 hours of age and rising TSB levels exceeding 5 mg/dL per day requires investigation.
      d. Phototherapy: converts bilirubin to a water-soluble product. Effectiveness influenced by the following:
         (1) Energy output of phototherapy unit. Bulbs require changing as energy output decreases. Light irradiance meters are used to determine bulb output.
         (2) Spectrum of light: special blue light labeled F20T12/BB (General Electric, Westinghouse, Sylvania) or TL52/20W (Phillips, Eindhoven, The Netherlands) at 450 nm is most effective. Disadvantage: distortion of infant's color. White lamps, high-intensity gallium nitride light-emitting diodes, and fiberoptic blankets are effective alternatives.
         (3) Amount of infant's body surface area exposed to light. Turn infant frequently to allow all areas of the skin to be exposed.
         (4) Distance between light and infant. Follow equipment manufacturer's recommendations. Monitor infant's temperature. Fluorescent lights should be at a distance of 10 cm from the infant, who is placed naked in a bassinet. When bank lights are used, lamps should be covered with a clear acrylic shield to protect the infant from ultraviolet light.
      e. Monitor fluid and electrolytes. Phototherapy increases insensible water loss and stooling. The AAP (2004) recommends milk-based enteral feeding that inhibits enterohepatic reabsorption of bilirubin.

■ TABLE 29-4
■ ■ **Management of Hyperbilirubinemia in Healthy Term Neonate***

			TSB Level, mg/dl (μmol/l)	
Age (hours)	Consider Phototherapy*	Phototherapy	Exchange Transfusion If Intensive Phototherapy Fails†	Exchange Transfusion and Intensive Phototherapy
≤24‡	C	C	C	C
25 to 48	≥12 (170)	≥15 (260)	≥20 (340)	≥25 (430)
49 to 72	≥15 (260)	≥18 (310)	≥25 (430)	≥30 (510)
>72	≥17 (290)	≥20 (340)	≥25 (430)	≥30 (510)

TSB, Total serum bilirubin.
*Phototherapy at these TSB levels is a clinical option, meaning that the intervention is available and may be used on the basis of individual clinical judgment.
†Intensive phototherapy should produce a decline of TSB of 1 to 2 mg/dl within 4 to 6 hours and the TSB level should continue to fall and remain below the threshold level for exchange transfusion. If this does not occur, it is considered a failure of phototherapy.
‡Term infants who are clinically jaundiced at ≤24 hours of age are not considered healthy and require further evaluation.
From American Academy of Pediatrics Provisional Committee for Quality Improvement and Subcommittee on Hyperbilirubinemia: Practice parameter: Management of hyperbilirubinemia in the healthy term newborn. *Pediatrics, 94*(4 Pt 1):558-565, 1994.

■ TABLE 29-5
■ ■ **Management of Hyperbilirubinemia in the Low-Birth-Weight Infant**

	Total Serum Bilirubin Level, mg/dl			
	Healthy		Sick	
Gestational Age	Phototherapy	Exchange Transfusion	Phototherapy	Exchange Transfusion
Premature				
<1000 g	5 to 7	Variable	4 to 6	Variable
1001 to 1500 g	7 to 10	Variable	6 to 8	Variable
1501 to 2000 g	10 to 12	Variable	8 to 10	Variable
2001 to 2500 g	12 to 15	Variable	10 to 12	Variable

From Martin, R.J., Fanaroff, A.A., and Walsh, M.C.: *Fanaroff and Martin's neonatal-perinatal medicine: Diseases of the fetus and infant* (8th ed.). Philadelphia, 2006, Mosby.

    f. Monitor TSB during and after therapy. A rebound of 1 to 2 mg/dL can be expected.
    g. Side effects: bronze skin if conjugated bilirubin is elevated; lethargy; skin rashes; risk of eye damage if eye patches are not secure; abdominal distention; hypocalcemia; lactose intolerance; and thrombocytopenia.
    h. Home phototherapy: an option that decreases hospitalization time for an otherwise healthy infant.
    i. Intensive phototherapy uses multiple phototherapy units above and below the completely naked infant. In addition, aluminum foil or a white cloth on the bassinet side is employed to reflect light onto the infant. All facilities providing care to infants should be capable of providing intensive phototherapy.
    j. Exchange transfusion.
        (1) Used when intensive phototherapy has been unsuccessful in controlling TSB, and at any time signs of acute bilirubin encephalopathy are present regardless of TSB level; used more often in hemolytic conditions.
        (2) Hemolyzed and antibody-coated RBCs are removed over approximately 2 hours in small aliquots (3 to 5 ml/kg in preterm infants, 10 ml/kg in term infants) and

replaced with donor blood. Double volume exchange (160 ml/kg) will reduce the TSB by 50%. Expect a rebound TSB of 60% to 70% of the preexchange transfusion level.

(3) Intravenous γ-globin (0.5 to 1 mg/kg over 2 hours) if phototherapy fails to control bilirubin levels or the TSB is approaching exchange transfusion level decreases isoimmune hemolysis.

(4) The administration of albumin prior to the exchange transfusion is not recommended.

(5) Stabilize infant prior to procedure: treat hypoglycemia, acid–base derangements, hypotension, and temperature abnormalities.

(6) Cytomegalovirus (CMV)-negative blood less than 48 hours old should be used to minimize problems with elevated potassium that occurs in older blood.

(7) Procedure.

    (a) Exchange transfusion is performed only by trained personnel in a neonatal intensive care unit with monitoring and resuscitation capabilities.

    (b) Secure infant on radiant warmer bed. Ensure oxygen, suction, and resuscitation equipment are immediately available. Observe neonate with a cardiorespiratory monitor and assess vital signs frequently.

    (c) Ideally, an umbilical artery catheter (UAC) and umbilical venous catheter (UVC) are placed (see Chapter 15 for procedure). A UVC may be inserted for several days to 2 weeks after delivery.

    (d) Laboratory studies.

        (i) On initial blood removed: CBC, bilirubin and calcium levels, and blood cultures.

        (ii) During procedure: calcium level (if signs of hypocalcemia present).

        (iii) On final aliquot removed: CBC, bilirubin, and calcium.

    (e) Accurate recording of blood volumes exchanged is essential during the procedure.

    (f) Observe for hypocalcemia. Anticoagulant citrates (acid–citrate–dextrose and citrate–phosphate–dextrose negative [CPD–] adenosine) bind to calcium. Symptoms of hypocalcemia include irritability, tachycardia, and prolonged QT interval.

    (g) Calcium gluconate is used to treat hypocalcemia. Normal dose is 1 to 2 ml/kg (100 to 200 mg/kg) per dose of 10% calcium solution.

    (h) Evaluate medications. Medications whose levels are known to decrease significantly during an exchange transfusion should be administered after the exchange: ampicillin, gentamicin, digoxin, phenobarbital, vancomycin.

(8) Complications.

    (a) Electrolyte and substrate abnormalities: hyperkalemia, hypocalcemia, hypomagnesemia, hypoglycemia, hyperglycemia.

    (b) Clotting abnormalities: thrombocytopenia, embolization, thrombosis.

    (c) Respiratory and cardiovascular events: apnea, bradycardia, cardiac dysrhythmias and arrest, cyanosis, vasospasm, heart failure, acidosis.

    (d) NEC and infection.

(9) Postexchange care.

    (a) Continue phototherapy.

    (b) Laboratory studies: TSB every 4 hours. Rebound usually occurs within 1 hour after the exchange.

    (c) Monitor blood glucose levels frequently. Dextrose in the blood preservative is equivalent to 300 mg of glucose per liter of blood. Rebound hypoglycemia can occur following an insulin response to the glucose.

    (d) Monitor for complications.

  3. Management of conjugated hyperbilirubinemia.

    a. Management is related to etiology (see Etiology: Unconjugated hyperbilirubinemia, p. 629).

   b. Eliminate or reduce causative factors; treat the remainder as appropriate (see Biliary Atresia, p. 617, and Cholestasis, p. 618).
   c. Evaluate liver function; evaluate for infection, including urinalysis and urine culture; check newborn screen for thyroid deficiency and galactosemia. Evaluate for G6PD disease.
4. **Management of breastfeeding jaundice.**
   a. Increase enteral intake by breastfeeding 8 to 12 times per day. The AAP does not encourage the interruption of breastfeeding (2004).
   b. No supplementation with water or glucose water in term, nondehydrated infants.
   c. Systematic assessment for hyperbilirubinemia risk including maternal blood typing and neonatal direct antibody testing for incompatibility.
   d. Establish protocols for jaundice assessment and follow-up, including when the nurse can obtain a transcutaneous and serum bilirubin level. TcB or TSB if jaundiced before 24 hours of age; follow-up required.
5. **Management of breast milk jaundice.**
   a. Obtain total and direct serum bilirubin to evaluate for cholestasis if jaundice is present at or beyond 3 weeks of age. Ensure normal thyroid and galactosemia screen.
6. **Alternative therapies.**
   a. Binding agents: agar and activated charcoal bind bilirubin in the gut and decrease the enterohepatic circulation.
   b. Phenobarbital: increases hepatic ligandin concentration and induces the CYP450 enzymatic system.
   c. Metalloporphyrins: inhibit heme oxygenase, the enzyme that catalyzes the conversion of heme to biliverdin, thereby decreasing bilirubin production. Tin mesoporphyrin and tin protoporphyrin are the two metalloporphyrins most commonly used; however, their use is not approved by the FDA and is still investigational.
G. Hydrops (Abrams et al., 2007; Gruslin and Moore, 2006; Hamdan, 2007; Trainor and Tubman, 2006; Wolf and Moore, 2006).
   1. Definition: a prenatal form of heart failure almost always caused by fetal anemia; characterized by generalized subcutaneous edema and fluid in 2 compartmental spaces.
   2. Etiology: an imbalance of interstitial fluid production and lymphatic return.
      a. Immune hydrops (IH), also known as alloimmune or isoimmune hydrops: fetal RBCs enter maternal circulation, inducing maternal antibodies that cross the placenta and attack and destroy fetal RBCs. Seen in Rh and ABO disease.
      b. Nonimmune hydrops (NIH): disease or anomalies interfere with fetal fluid management. Most conditions associated with hydrops cause edema through either anemia with hypoxia and subsequent capillary leak or through cardiovascular anomalies with heart failure and subsequent tissue hypoxia, vascular permeability, and decreased lymphatic flow.
         (1) Cardiovascular (most frequent cause).
            (a) Dysrhythmias: supraventricular tachycardia, atrial flutter, complete heart block.
            (b) Cardiac malformation: left and right outflow tract obstructions; hypoplastic left heart syndrome and endocardial cushion defects are the most common.
            (c) Myocarditis.
         (2) Chromosomal: aneuploidy including trisomies 13, 18, 21, triploidy, and 45X (Turner's syndrome); achondroplasia.
         (3) Infection: TORCH, parvovirus B19, and congenital hepatitis.
         (4) Hematologic.
            (a) α-Thalassemia.
            (b) Glucose-6-phosphate dehydrogenase deficiency.
            (c) Chronic fetal–maternal or twin-to-twin transfusion.
            (d) Hemorrhage, including fetomaternal hemorrhage.
            (e) Bone marrow failure.

(5) Renal.
  (a) Nephrosis.
  (b) Renal vein thrombosis.
  (c) Renal hypoplasia.
  (d) Urinary obstruction.
(6) Pulmonary.
  (a) Pulmonary hypoplasia.
  (b) Cystic adenomatoid malformations.
  (c) Pulmonary lymphangiectasis.
  (d) Congenital diaphragmatic hernia.
(7) Gastrointestinal.
  (a) In utero volvulus.
  (b) Meconium peritonitis.
  (c) Prune-belly syndrome.
(8) Maternal.
  (a) Toxemia.
  (b) Diabetes.
  (c) Systemic lupus erythematosus.
(9) Placenta and cord (uncommon).
  (a) Chorioangioma.
  (b) Umbilical vein thrombosis.
  (c) Arteriovenous malformation.
(10) Idiopathic: approximately 25% of cases have no identifiable cause. Incidence of idiopathic NIH is dependent on the thoroughness of the diagnostic workup of the populations studied.

3.   Incidence: exact figure unknown, as some fetuses die or hydrops resolves in utero. Current estimates range from 1 in 600 to 1 in 4000 live births. Males affected more than females (X-linked genetic disorder).
  a.   IH: incidence has significantly decreased to approximately 10% to 20% of hydrops cases with the wide use of anti-D prophylaxis using Rh immunoglobulin for Rh-negative mothers at 28 weeks of gestation (following suspected fetomaternal hemorrhage) and postpartum (following the delivery of an Rh-positive infant). In addition, in utero fetal transfusion has lessened the incidence.
  b.   NIH: approximately 80% to 90% of hydrops cases.
4.   Associated conditions.
  a.   Chromosomal abnormalities.
  b.   Congenital malformations: heart defects especially outflow tract obstruction (both left and right).
  c.   Prematurity.
  d.   Inborn errors of metabolism.
5.   Diagnosis.
  a.   Prenatal.
    (1) Polyhydramnios.
    (2) High-resolution ultrasound and fetal echocardiography: hepatosplenomegaly, cardiomegaly, cardiac defects, pleural effusion, pericardial effusion, ascites, generalized edema.
    (3) Fetal blood sampling via cordocentesis.
    (4) Amniocentesis: chromosome analysis for associated defects, bilirubin level.
    (5) Serologic testing for isoimmunization and infection (TORCH; PCR for parvovirus B19).
    (6) Kleihauer–Betke test for fetomaternal hemorrhage.
  b.   Postnatal.
    (1) Clinical presentation.
      (a) Physical examination: generalized edema; respiratory distress; cardiovascular abnormalities including dysrhythmia, murmur, diminished perfusion; abdominal findings, including hepatosplenomegaly, distention.

(2) Radiologic examination: skeletal radiographs, ultrasound.

(3) Laboratory studies.

(a) Hematology: CBC to evaluate anemia, thrombocytopenia, reticulocytosis; hemoglobin electrophoresis.

(b) Other: serum albumin, metabolic panel, chemistries, karyotype if not already done.

6. Prognosis. Immune hydrops is associated with a survival rate of approximately 75%. Prognosis in NIH is very poor and is related to the underlying cause. Multiple anomalies and chromosomal abnormalities carry an extremely high mortality. Neurologic outcomes in survivors is concerning.

H. Care of the infant with hydrops.

1. Prenatal: depends on etiology. The gravid mother must be transferred to a facility capable of management of the infant postpartum, including neonatal intensive care, ventilatory and inotropic support, and genetic evaluation.

   a. Intrauterine transfusion to ameliorate anemia.

   b. Amniocentesis to determine karyotype, follow bilirubin level, and reduce uterine volume to prevent premature delivery.

   c. Thoracentesis or thoracoamniotic shunt placement.

   d. Maternal medication administration to control fetal dysrhythmias.

   e. Fetal medication administration.

   f. Delivery.

2. Postnatal.

   a. Resuscitation is frequently required including intubation, bilateral thoracentesis, which may include bilateral tube thoracotomy, pericardiocentesis, and umbilical venous catheter placement (generalized edema prohibits successful peripheral IV placement). Umbilical artery catheter placement can be obtained once initial stabilization is accomplished.

   b. Respiratory support as needed with acid–base determination and management. Paracentesis and additional thoracentesis or tube thoracotomy drainage may be required to enhance ventilation efforts. Frequent monitoring of breath sounds and chest movement and radiographs are essential.

   c. Anticipate and treat metabolic abnormalities.

   d. Exchange transfusion or partial exchange transfusion for severe anemia.

   e. Cardiovascular support: inotropes to improve cardiac output; pericardiocentesis; diuretic therapy.

   f. Fresh frozen plasma may be given for hypoalbuminemia.

   g. Assess for associated anomalies, syndromes, or malformations. Determine etiology of hydrops if unknown.

REFERENCES

Abrams, M. E., Meredith, K. S., Kinnard, P., and Clark, R.H.: Hydrops fetalis: A retrospective review of cases reported to a large national data base and identification of risk factors associated with death. *Pediatrics*, *120*(1):84-89, 2007.

Adamson, W. and Hebra, A.: Bowel obstruction in the newborn. 2004. Retrieved January 30, 2008, from http://www.emedicine.com/ped/topic2857.htm

American Academy of Pediatrics Task Force on Infant Sleep Position and Sudden Infant Death Syndrome. Changing concepts of sudden infant death syndrome: Implication for infant sleeping environment and sleep position. *Pediatrics*, *105*(3):650-656, 2000.

American Academy of Pediatrics Subcommittee on Hyperbilirubinemia: Management of hyperbilirubinemia in the newborn infant 35 or more weeks of gestation. *Pediatrics*, *114*(1):297-316, 2004.

American Academy of Pediatrics Task Force on Sudden Infant Death Syndrome: The changing concept of sudden infant death syndrome: Diagnostic coding shifts, controversies regarding the sleeping environment, and new variable to consider in reducing risk. *Pediatrics*, *116*(5):1245-1255, 2005.

American Academy of Pediatrics Section on Surgery and the Committee on Fetus and Newborn: Post-discharge follow-up of infants with congenital diaphragmatic hernia. *Pediatrics*, *121*(3):627-632, 2008.

Anderson, M.S., Wood, L.E., Keller, J., and Hay, W.W.: Enteral nutrition. In G.B. Merenstein and S.L. Gardner (Eds.): *Handbook of neonatal intensive care* (6th ed.). St. Louis, 2006, Mosby, pp. 391-428.

Askins, F.B. and Gilbert-Barness, E.: Respiratory system. In E. Gilbert-Barness (Ed.): *Potter's pathology of the fetus, infant and child* (2nd ed.). Philadelphia, 2007, Mosby, pp. 1073-1155.

Barclay, A.R.: Probiotics for necrotizing enterocolitis: A systematic review. *Journal of Pediatric Gastroenterology and Nutrition,* 45(5):569-576, 2007.

Bhat, R.Y., Rafferty, G.F., Hannam, S., and Greenough, A.: Acid gastroesophageal reflux in convalescent preterm infants: Effect of posture and relationship to apnea. *Pediatric Research,* 62(5):620-623, 2007.

Blackburn, S.T.: *Maternal, fetal, and neonatal physiology: A clinical perspective* (3rd ed.). St. Louis, 2007, Saunders.

Boucherat, O., Benachi, A., Chailley-Heu, B., et al.: Surfactant maturation is not delayed in human fetuses with diaphragmatic hernia. *PLoS Medicine,* 4(7):e237, 2007. doi:10.1371/journal.pmed.0040237

Caplan, M.: Neonatal necrotizing enterocolitis. In R.J. Martin, A.A. Fanaroff, and M.C. Walsh (Eds.): *Fanaroff and Martin's neonatal-perinatal medicine: Diseases of the fetus and infant* (8th ed.). Philadelphia, 2006, Mosby, pp. 1403-1417.

Colvin, J., Bower, C., Dickinson, J.E., and Sokol, J.: Outcomes of congenital diaphragmatic hernia: A population-based study in Western Australia. *Pediatrics,* 116(3):e356-e363, 2005.

Cortes, R.A., Keller, R.L., Townsend, T., et al.: Survival of severe congenital diaphragmatic hernia has morbid consequences. *Journal of Pediatric Surgery,* 40(1):36-45, 2005.

Dasgupta, R.: Evaluation and management of persistent problems after surgery for Hirschsprung disease in a child. *Journal of Pediatric Gastroenterology and Nutrition,* 46(1):13-19, 2008.

Deshpande, P.G. and Ramer, T.: Breast milk jaundice. 2006. Retrieved February 12, 2008, from http://www.emedecine.com/PED/topic282.htm

Diem, H.V., Evrard, V., Vinh, H.T., et al.: Pediatric liver transplantation for biliary atresia: Results of primary grafts in 328 recipients. *Transplantation,* 75(10):1692-1697, 2003.

Evers, D.B.: Alterations of digestive function in children. In K.L. McCance and S.E. Huether (Eds.): *Pathophysiology: The biologic basis for disease in adults and children* (5th ed.). St. Louis, 2006, Mosby, pp. 1447-1470.

Farrell, P.M. and Elias, S.: Prenatal diagnosis and neonatal screening. In E. Gilbert-Barness (Ed.): *Potter's pathology of the fetus, infant and child* (2nd ed.). Philadelphia, 2007, Mosby, pp. 611-644.

Frank, C.G. and Frank, P.H.: Jaundice. In G.B. Merenstein and S.L. Gardner (Eds.): *Handbook of neonatal intensive care* (6th ed.). St. Louis, 2006, Mosby, pp. 548-568.

Gabriela, A. and Gollinb, G.: Management of complicated gastroschisis with porcine small intestinal submucosa and negative pressure wound therapy. *Journal of Pediatric Surgery,* 41(11):1836-1840, 2006.

Goodwin, M.: Abdomen assessment. In. E.P. Tappero and M.E. Honeyfield (Eds.): *Physical assessment of the newborn: A comprehensive approach to the art of physical examination* (3rd ed.). Santa Rosa, CA, 2003, NICU Ink, pp. 97-105.

Goulet, O. and Sauvat, F.: Short bowel syndrome and intestinal transplantation in children. *Current Opinion*

in Clinical Nutrition and Metabolic Care, 9(3):304-313, 2006.

Gruslin, A.M. and Moore, T.R.: Erythroblastosis fetalis. In R.J. Martin, A.A. Fanaroff, and M.C. Walsh (Eds.): *Fanaroff and Martin's neonatal-perinatal medicine: Diseases of the fetus and infant* (8th ed.). Philadelphia, 2006, Mosby, pp. 389-407.

Hamdan, A.H.: Hydrops fetalis. 2007. Retrieved February 2, 2008, from http://www.emedicine.com/PED/topic1042.htm

Hansen, T.W.R.: Neonatal jaundice. 2007. Retrieved January 15, 2008, from http://www.emedicine.com/PED/topic1061.htm

Hartman, G.E., Boyajian, M.J., Choi, S.S., et al.: Surgical care of conditions presenting in the newborn. In M.G. MacDonald, M.K. Seshia, and M.D. Mullett (Eds.): *Avery's neonatology: Pathophysiology and management of the newborn* (6th ed.). Philadelphia, 2005, Lippincott Williams & Wilkins, pp. 1097-1134.

Hayakawa, M., Seo, T., Itakua, A., et al.: The MRI findings of the right-sided fetal lung can be used to predict postnatal mortality and the requirement for extracorporeal membrane oxygenation in isolated left-sided congenital diaphragmatic hernia. *Pediatric Research,* 62(1):93-97, 2007.

Holder, A.M., Klaassens, M., Tibboel, D., de Klein, A., Lee, B., and Scott, D.A.: Genetic factors in congenital diaphragmatic hernia. *American Journal of Human Genetics,* 80:825-845, 2007.

Jones, K.L.: *Smith's recognizable patterns of human malformation* (6th ed.). Philadelphia, 2006, Saunders.

Kalousek, D.K. and Oligny, L.L.: Pathology of abortion: The embryo and the previable fetus. In E. Gilbert-Barness (Ed.): *Potter's pathology of the fetus, infant and child* (2nd ed.). Philadelphia, 2007, Mosby, pp. 277-305.

Kee, J.L.: *Handbook of laboratory and diagnostic tests with nursing implications* (5th ed.). Upper Saddle River, NJ, 2005, Pearson Prentice Hall.

Kessman, J.: Hirschsprung's disease: Diagnosis and management. *American Family Physician,* 74(8):1319-1322, 2006.

Lally, K.P., Lally, P.A., Langham, M.R., et al.: Surfactant does not improve survival rate in preterm infants with congenital diaphragmatic hernia. *Journal of Pediatric Surgery,* 39(6):829-833, 2004.

Lees, C., Howie, S., Sartor, R.B., and Satsangi, J.: The hedgehog signaling pathway in the gastrointestinal tract: Implications for development, homeostasis, and disease. *Gastroenterology,* 129:1696-1710, 2005.

Levine, E., Taub, P.J., and Franco, I.: Laparoscopic-assisted abdominal wall reconstruction in prune-belly syndrome. *Annals of Plastic Surgery,* 58(2):162-165, 2007.

Louie, J.P.: Essential diagnosis of abdominal emergencies in the first year of life. *Emergency Medical Clinics of North America,* 25:1009-1040, 2007.

Magnuson, D.K., Parry, R.L., and Chwals, W.J.: Selected abdominal gastrointestinal anomalies. In R.J. Martin, A.A. Fanaroff, and M.C. Walsh (Eds.): *Fanaroff and Martin's neonatal-perinatal medicine: Diseases of the fetus and infant* (8th ed.). Philadelphia, 2006, Mosby, pp. 1373-1380, 1381-1403.

Meehan, J.J., Elliott, S., and Sandler, A.: The robotic approach to complex hepatobiliary anomalies in children: Preliminary report. *Journal of Pediatric Surgery,* 42(12):2110-2114, 2007.

Migliazza, L., Bellan, C., Alberti, D., Auriemma, A., Burgio, G., Locatelli, G., et al.: Retrospective study of 111 cases of congenital diaphragmatic hernia treated with early high-frequency oscillatory ventilation and presurgical stabilization. *Pediatric Surgery,* 42(9): 1526-1532, 2007.

Misiakos, E.P., Macheras, A., Kapetanakis, T., and Liakakos, R.: Short bowel syndrome: Current medical and surgical trends. *Journal of Clinical Gastroenterology,* 41(1):5-18, 2007.

Moukarzel, A.A., Abdelnour, H., and Akatcherian, C.: Effects of a prethickened formula on esophageal pH and gastric emptying of infants with GER. *Journal of Clinical Gastroenterology,* 41(9):823-829, 2007.

Neff, M.J.: Practice guidelines: CDC releases recommendations for state newborn screening programs for cystic fibrosis. *American Family Physician,* 71(8):1608-1610, 2005.

Nguyen, H. and Lund, C.: Exploratory laparotomy or peritoneal drain? Management of bowel perforation in the neonatal intensive care unit. *Journal of Perinatal & Neonatal Nursing,* 21(1):50-60, 2007.

Oligny, L.L.: Disorders of the anterior thoracic and abdominal walls. In E. Gilbert-Barness (Ed.): *Potter's pathology of the fetus, infant and child* (2nd ed.). Philadelphia, 2007, Mosby, pp. 919-942.

Roaten, J.B., Bensard, D.D., and Price, F.N.: Neonatal surgery. In G.B. Merenstein and S.L. Gardner (Eds.): *Handbook of neonatal intensive care* (6th ed.). St. Louis, 2006, Mosby, pp. 838-862.

Ross, A.J.: Organogenesis of the gastrointestinal tract. In R.A. Polin, W.W. Fox, and S.H. Abman (Eds.): *Fetal and neonatal physiology* (3rd ed.). Philadelphia, 2004, Saunders, pp. 1101-1110.

San Luis, V.A. and Btaiche, I.F.: Ursodiol in patients with parenteral nutrition-associated cholestasis. *Annals of Pharmacotherapy,* 41(11):1867-1872, 2007.

Seidel, H.M., Ball, J.W., Dains, J.E., and Benedict, G.W.: *Mosby's guide to physical examination* (6th ed.). St. Louis, 2006, Mosby.

Sharma, R., Hudak, M.L., Tepas III, J.J., Wludyka, P.S., Marvin, W.J., Bradshaw, J.A., and Pieper, P.: Impact of gestational age on the clinical presentation and surgical outcome of necrotizing enterocolitis. *Journal of Perinatology,* 26(6):342-347, 2006.

Siebert, J.R. and Kapur, R.P.: Back and perineum. In E. Gilbert-Barness (Ed.): *Potter's pathology of the fetus, infant and child* (2nd ed.). Philadelphia, 2007, Mosby, pp. 943-966.

Shih, H.-H., Lin, T.-M., Chuang, J.-H., et al.: Promoter polymorphism of the CD14 endotoxin receptor gene is associated with biliary atresia and idiopathic neonatal cholestasis. *Pediatrics,* 116(2):437-441, 2005.

Sondheimer, J.M.: Gastroesophageal reflux. In W.W. Hay, M.J. Levin, J.M. Sondheimer, and R.R. Deterding (Eds.): *Current diagnosis and treatment in pediat-* rics (18th ed.). New York, 2006, Lange, pp. 605-637.

Steinbach, M., Clark, R.H., Kelleher, A.S., et al.: Demographic and nutritional factors associated with prolonged cholestatic jaundice in the premature infant. *Journal of Perinatology,* 28(2):129-135, 2008.

Suchy, F.J.: Neonatal cholestasis. *Pediatrics in Review,* 25(11):388-396, 2004.

Thigpen, J.L. and Kenner, C.: Assessment and management of the gastrointestinal system. In C. Kenner and J.W. Lott (Eds.): *Comprehensive neonatal nursing: A physiologic perspective* (3rd ed.). St. Louis, 2003, Saunders, pp. 448-485.

Trainor, B. and Tubman, R.: The emerging pattern of hydrops fetalis: Incidence, aetiology and management. *Ulster Medical Journal,* 75(3):183-186, 2006.

Ukarapol, N., Wongsawasdi, L., Ong-Chai, S., Riddhiputra, P., and Kongtawelert, P.: Hyaluronic acid: Additional biochemical marker in the diagnosis of biliary atresia. *Pediatrics International,* 49(5):608-611, 2007.

U.S. Department of Health and Human Services: *Gastroesophageal reflux in infants.* NIH Publication No. 06-5419. Bethesda, MD, 2006, U.S. Department of Health and Human Services. Retrieved January 23, 2008, from http://digestive.niddk.nih.gov/ddiseases/pubs/gerdinfant/gerdinfant.pdf

Van Meurs, K. for the Congenital Diaphragmatic Hernia Study Group: Is surfactant therapy beneficial in the treatment of the term newborn infant with congenital diaphragmatic hernia? *Journal of Pediatrics,* 145(3):312-316, 2004.

Wang, J.X.: Detection and significance of serum protein marker of Hirschsprung disease. *Pediatrics,* 120(1):e56-e80, 2007.

Wert, S.E.: The lung. In R.A. Polin, W.W. Fox, and S.H. Abman (Eds.): *Fetal and neonatal physiology* (3rd ed.). Philadelphia, 2004, Saunders, pp. 783-794.

Winfield, R.D. and Beierle, E.A.: Pediatric surgical issues in meconium disease and cystic fibrosis. *Surgical Clinics of North America,* 86(2):317-327, 2006.

Wolf, R.B. and Moore, T.R.: Amniotic fluid and nonimmune hydrops fetalis. In R.J. Martin, A.A. Fanaroff, and M.C. Walsh (Eds.): *Fanaroff and Martin's neonatal-perinatal medicine: Diseases of the fetus and infant* (8th ed.). Philadelphia, 2006, Mosby, pp. 409-428.

Wong, R.J., DeSandre, G.H., Sibley, E., and Stevenson, D.K.: Neonatal jaundice and liver disease. In R.J. Martin, A.A. Fanaroff, and M.C. Walsh (Eds.): *Fanaroff and Martin's neonatal-perinatal medicine: Diseases of the fetus and infant* (8th ed.). Philadelphia, 2006, Mosby, pp. 1419-1465.

Woods, A.G. and Brandon, D.H.: Prune belly syndrome: A focused physical assessment. *Advances in Neonatal Care,* 7(3):132-143, 2007.

Wu, Y., Vogel, A.M., Sailhamer, E.A., et al.: Primary insertion of a silastic spring-loaded silo for gastroschisis. *The American Surgeon,* 69(12):1083-1086, 2003.

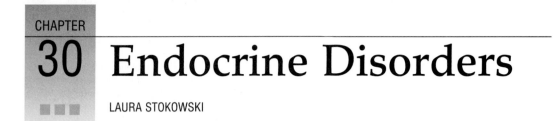

30 Endocrine Disorders

LAURA STOKOWSKI

OBJECTIVES
1. Define the endocrine system.
2. Describe endocrine system regulation.
3. Identify and discuss endocrine disorders that manifest in the neonatal period, including disorders of the thyroid, pituitary, adrenal gland, pancreas, and genital development.
4. List effective ways to help parents cope with the birth of an infant with ambiguous genitalia.

Neonatal Endocrine Disorders

Disorders of the endocrine system are relatively rare in neonates, but usually have lifelong consequences.

THE ENDOCRINE SYSTEM

The classic endocrine system is a group of nine ductless glands (Table 30-1), but in reality it includes every organ and cell in the body that produces and responds to hormones (Chrousos, 2002). A system of communication between different cells of the body, the endocrine system is intricately linked with the neurological and immune systems in a vast, interacting control network (Wilson, 2005). Regulation of growth and development, metabolic homeostasis, reproduction, control of energy metabolism, and response to environmental changes are a few of the tasks of this complex system.

A. **Hormones.**
  1. Hormones are the molecular messengers of the endocrine system, allowing communication between organs, tissues, and cells throughout the body. In composition, hormones are steroids, proteins, glycoproteins, peptides, or amines.
  2. Hormones bind to specific receptors on the surface of or within the cytoplasm or nucleus of target cells to produce physiologic actions. Sensitivity of a target cell to its hormones is critical to normal function.
  3. Many hormones are secreted directly into the circulation for transport to various target tissues. Hormones can also act on cells in the immediate vicinity of their release (paracrine action) or on the cell that produced the hormone (autocrine or intracrine action).
  4. Some hormones circulate partly in free form and partly bound to transport proteins. It is the free form that is available for receptor binding and that dictates regulatory influences on hormone release. Clinical states of hormone excess and deficiency correlate best with free hormone levels.
  5. Most hormones are secreted in their biologically active form, but some must be converted to their final active form in peripheral tissues.
B. **Endocrine system regulation** (Fig. 30-1).
  1. Many hormones are regulated by a negative-feedback loop involving the hypothalamic–pituitary axis and target endocrine glands. Beginning with hormonal or neural input, the hypothalamus produces one of two substances: releasing hormones or inhibiting hormones. These are transported via the pituitary portal system to the anterior pituitary, the gland that controls the secretory activity of most target organs. The anterior pituitary releases trophic hormones that in turn stimulate release of target gland hormones. As blood concentrations of target hormones reach certain thresholds, a negative message to the anterior pituitary inhibits further release of trophic hormones. Examples of hormones

■ TABLE 30-1
■ ■ **Major Glands and Hormones of the Endocrine System**

Endocrine Gland	Hormones Produced
Hypothalamus	Corticotropin-releasing hormone (CRH)
	Thyrotropin-releasing hormone (TRH)
	Gonadotropin-releasing hormone (GnRH)
	Somatostatin
	Growth hormone–releasing hormone (GHRH)
	Prolactin-releasing factor (PRF)
	Prolactin release–inhibiting hormone (PIH; dopamine)
Anterior pituitary	Adrenocorticotropic hormone (ACTH)
	Thyroid-stimulating hormone (TSH; thyrotropin)
	Follicle-stimulating hormone (FSH)
	Growth hormone (GH)
	Luteinizing hormone (LH)
	Prolactin (PRL)
Posterior pituitary	Antidiuretic hormone (ADH; arginine vasopressin)
	Oxytocin (OCT)
Thyroid gland	Thyroxine (T_4)
	Triiodothyronine (T_3)
	Calcitonin
Parathyroid gland	Parathyroid hormone (PTH)
Adrenal medulla	Epinephrine (adrenaline)
	Norepinephrine (noradrenaline)
Adrenal cortex	Cortisol (hydrocortisone)
	Aldosterone
Pancreas	Insulin
	Glucagon
	Somatostatin
Pineal gland	Melatonin

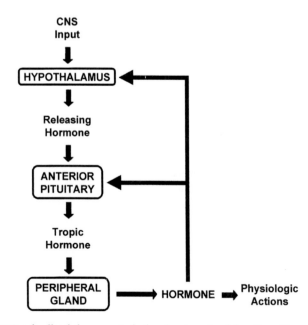

FIGURE 30-1 ■ Negative feedback-loop control of endocrine gland function. Hypothalamic-releasing hormones stimulate pituitary tropic hormones, which in turn act on peripheral glands to release hormones. Levels of circulating hormones then exert feedback control on the pituitary and hypothalamus, modulating further output by these glands.

regulated by negative feedback are thyroid hormone and cortisol. Negative feedback can be direct (at the level of the pituitary gland) or indirect (at the level of the hypothalamus).

2. Other endocrine glands, such as the parathyroids and the pancreatic islets, are not part of the hypothalamic–pituitary axis but have a "freestanding" control mechanism. These glands release hormones that stimulate a target tissue to produce an effect, which in turn directly modifies the output of the gland.

3. The neuroendocrine system plays a key role in body homeostasis. Hormones act as neurotransmitters, and neurotransmitters are involved in regulating endocrine function. Endocrine glands such as the hypothalamus, the pituitary, and the adrenal cortex respond to neural stimulation. The neuroendocrine system is important in the smooth adaptation of the neonate to the stresses of extrauterine life.

C. **Endocrine disruptors are synthetic or naturally occurring compounds that can mimic or block the body's endogenous hormones and disrupt endocrine function.** Estrogens, androgens, and thyroid hormones are particularly vulnerable to interference by endocrine disruptors. Exposure to an endocrine disruptor during embryonic gonadal sex differentiation can alter male germ-line epigenetics, a mechanism that can transmit adult-onset diseases, such as spermatogenic defects, prostate disease, kidney disease, and cancer to both current and future generations (Anway and Skinner, 2008). Sources of these chemicals include pharmaceuticals, dioxin and dioxin-like compounds, polychlorinated biphenyls, DDT and other pesticides, and plasticizers such as bisphenol A (National Institute of Environmental Health Science, 2008). Pesticides and plasticizers are among the chemicals suspected, based on animal studies, of being endocrine disruptors.

D. **Fetal origins of adult disease is a newly recognized phenomenon, describing effects of the maternal intrauterine environment on growth and development that can persist into adult life.** Chronic stress may induce the "thrifty phenotype fetus" and permanently alter the fetal hypothalamic–pituitary axis. In response to stressors, the fetus generates glucocorticoids and catecholamines that program the fetal endocrine system. Fetal endocrine programming has been associated with endocrine, metabolic, and cardiovascular disease in the adult.

E. **Endocrine disorders in the neonate.** Most endocrine disorders are caused by hormone overproduction, underproduction, altered receptor function, or altered tissue response to hormones. In addition to well-described neonatal endocrine disorders (hypothyroidism, congenital adrenal hyperplasia [CAH]), endocrine dysfunction can affect the preterm infant in a variety of ways as a function of maturation. Some of the more common endocrine alterations seen in term and preterm infants will be addressed here.

PITUITARY GLAND DISORDERS

The Pituitary Gland

A. **Anatomy and physiology.**
1. The pituitary gland has two distinct structures—the anterior and posterior glands. Although these two structures with different origins form a single gland, they are functionally separate.
2. Anterior pituitary arises from the oral ectoderm and its cells to differentiate into specific hormone-producing cells. The release of trophic hormones (GH, ACTH, FSH, TSH, LH, and PRL) is influenced by hypothalamic releasing/inhibiting hormones.
3. Posterior pituitary develops from neuroectoderm evaginating ventrally from the brain. The posterior pituitary produces oxytocin and antidiuretic hormone (ADH).

B. **Hypopituitarism.**
1. Although rare in the newborn, hypopituitarism can be caused by infection, hypovolemic shock, precipitous delivery, and low Apgar scores or it can be part of a syndrome such as septo-optic dysplasia. Congenital hypopituitarism can also be caused by mutations in transcription factors regulating pituitary gland development.
2. Types of hypopituitarism include absence of pituitary gland (pituitary agenesis), panhypopituitarism (deficiency of all pituitary hormones) or an isolated hormone defect, such as growth hormone deficiency. A primary hypothalamic disorder can also result in hypopituitarism.

3. Clinical signs and symptoms of hypopituitarism: hypoglycemia, dysmorphia/midline craniofacial defects, micropenis, prolonged jaundice), septo-optic nerve hypoplasia. Birth weight and length are often below the mean. Nonspecific signs such as poor feeding, failure to gain weight, hypothermia, hypotension, and lethargy may be evident (Dempsher, 2008). There is often a history of breech delivery (Brook and Brown, 2008).
4. Diagnosis is made by hormone testing (including insulin-like growth factor and insulin-like growth factor binding protein 3, ultrasound or MRI of anatomic structures, and genetic analyses. Tests of pituitary function include stimulation tests (ACTH, TRH, glucagon) to test the response of pituitary hormones.
5. Management involves correcting hypoglycemia and replacing deficient hormones.
C. **Diabetes insipidus.**
   1. Diabetes insipidus (DI) is a deficiency of antidiuretic hormone (vasopressin). DI can be associated with midline facial defects, central nervous system injury, hypoxia, or neoplasm.
   2. ADH secretion is normally triggered by changes in osmolality, increasing or decreasing to regulate urine output. In DI, ADH is deficient, resulting in free water loss.
   3. Clinical manifestations are vigorous sucking followed by vomiting, polyuria (high urine output with low specific gravity), irritability, fever, and evidence of dehydration.
   4. Diagnosis is made by reviewing serum electrolytes, osmolality, plasma ADH levels, urine output, and urinalysis. MRI may be done to visualize the posterior pituitary.
   5. DI is treated with cautious fluid management to correct dehydration without causing rapid shifts in serum sodium levels. Desmopressin (DDAVP) may be required to supplement ADH if the neonate is unable to concentrate his urine.
D. **Syndrome of inappropriate ADH.**
   1. Impairment of free water clearance caused by an uncontrolled release of ADH.
   2. Causes include central nervous system infection, birth asphyxia, intracranial hemorrhage, and meningitis.
   3. The release in ADH is inappropriate to the level of osmolality in the serum, causing fluid retention, oliguria, hyponatremia, weight gain, and edema.
   4. Diagnosis is made by finding an elevated circulating ADH level with low serum osmolality and hyponatremia.
   5. Treatment involves fluid restriction and monitoring of electrolytes, glucose, intake, and output.

THYROID GLAND DISORDERS

The Thyroid Gland

A. **Anatomy.**
   1. The thyroid gland comprises two lateral lobes connected by a band of tissue (isthmus) and contains densely packed colloid-rich follicular cells and parafollicular cells.
   2. Parafollicular cells (C-cells) produce the calcium-lowering hormone calcitonin.
B. **Normal physiology.**
   1. Functions of the thyroid gland.
      a. Concentrates and stores iodide, a trace element required for thyroid hormone synthesis.
      b. Synthesizes *thyroglobulin* (Tg), a thyroid hormone precursor.
      c. Synthesizes and releases the thyroid hormones *thyroxine* (T_4) and *triiodothyronine* (T_3), catalyzed by the enzyme thyroid peroxidase (TPO).
   2. Thyroid hormone metabolism.
      a. The thyroid gland produces T_4 and a small amount of T_3. Most of the plasma T_3 (the more potent hormone) is derived from peripheral metabolism (deiodination) of T_4.
      b. T_4 enters the cell and is converted to T_3 by enzymes.
      c. Deiodination of the outer ring of T_4 produces T_3. Deiodination of the inner ring of T_4 produces reverse T_3 (rT_3), a biologically inactive product.
   3. Thyroid hormone transport.
      a. Thyroid hormones circulate in the blood bound to *thyroid-binding globulin* (TBG) and other albumins. Only a tiny fraction is in equilibrium as free hormone, but it is this free fraction that is responsible for hormonal action.

    b. TBG, synthesized in the liver, has a high affinity for T_3 and T_4, carrying 70% of circulating hormone. When TBG is deficient, total thyroid hormone concentrations may be lower but free hormone levels are normal.

  4. Mechanisms of thyroid gland regulation.

    a. Hypothalamic–pituitary–thyroid (HPT) axis.

      (1) Hypothalamic thyrotropin-releasing hormone (TRH) is secreted in response to neural input, such as cooling of the skin. TRH stimulates synthesis and release of thyroid-stimulating hormone (TSH; thyrotropin) by the anterior pituitary. TSH secretion is inhibited by dopamine, somatostatin, and high doses of corticosteroids.

      (2) TSH binds to receptors on thyroid cell membranes and stimulates production of thyroid hormones.

      (3) As thyroid hormone levels rise, TSH and TRH secretion is inhibited.

    b. Deiodinase enzymes in the anterior pituitary, brain, heart, liver, and other tissues regulate intracellular T_3 availability.

    c. Autoregulation of hormone synthesis by the thyroid gland itself in relationship to its iodine supply.

    d. Stimulation or inhibition of thyroid function by TSH receptor antibodies.

  5. Physiologic effects of thyroid hormones.

    a. Metabolic processes such as oxygen consumption, thermogenesis, cardiac output, erythropoiesis, respiratory drive, gut motility, and metabolism of carbohydrates, proteins, and lipids.

    b. Growth and differentiation of organs and tissues, including the bones, lungs, and the central nervous system (CNS). Thyroid hormones induce differentiation and maturation of neural circuits during critical periods of brain development. Absence of thyroid hormone delays critical events by interrupting intercellular communication (Brook and Brown, 2008).

C. Fetal thyroid development.

  1. The thyroid is the first endocrine gland to develop in the fetus, originating at 3 to 4 weeks of gestation (Forghani and Aye, 2008).

  2. Fetal thyroid activity begins with synthesis of Tg (week 4), followed by trapping of iodide and limited synthesis of T_4 and T_3 (weeks 8 to 10).

  3. The HPT axis begins to function at midgestation (weeks 18 to 20), when iodide uptake increases and the fetal thyroid gland begins to release T_4. Total and free T_4, TSH, and TBG increase steadily until term. The T_3 level remains low until 30 weeks of gestation, rising only in the last 10 weeks as mechanisms for deiodination of T_4 in fetal tissues mature.

  4. The placenta is permeable to TRH, iodide, thyroid autoantibodies, and antithyroid drugs but impermeable to TSH. At about 4 weeks, small quantities of maternal thyroxine begin to cross the placenta and protect the fetal brain (Obregon et al., 2007).

  5. The fetus is also dependent on the maternal–placental system for adequate supply of iodide, a critical substrate for fetal thyroid hormone synthesis. Autoregulation of iodide uptake is not yet mature, so the fetal thyroid is susceptible to inhibitory effects of both iodide deficiency and iodide excess.

  6. Cord blood TSH and T_4 are directly proportional to birth weight and gestational age. At birth, 30% of thyroid hormone circulating in the infant is of maternal origin (Forghani and Aye, 2008).

D. Neonatal thyroid physiology.

  1. At birth in term and late preterm neonates, the cooling of the skin and a surge of circulating catecholamines stimulate a sharp rise in the serum TSH level. TSH peaks in the 70 to 100 mU/l range at 30 minutes of age and then falls to a normal (<20 mU/l) level during the first 3 days of life.

  2. The TSH surge stimulates an abrupt rise in thyroid hormone levels. T_4 and T_3 both increase in response to TSH, peaking at 24 to 36 hours after birth. This physiologic hyperthyroid state is temporary, and occurs in response to sudden exposure to a cold environment.

  3. Postnatal changes in TSH, T_4, and T_3 occur in some less mature infants as well but are quantitatively lower. In infants of less than 30 weeks of gestation, the postnatal surge of thyroid hormones does not occur (Biswas et al., 2002). The extremely preterm infant exhibits a dramatic fall in T_4 over the first 1 to 2 weeks of life, sometimes to undetectable levels (Brook and Brown, 2008).

Hypothyroidism

Hypothyroidism in the neonate can be considered either permanent (lifelong therapy required) or transient (spontaneously resolving in weeks or months; treatment is temporary or not required at all). Hypothyroidism can also be termed congenital (existing at birth) or acquired. Other labels indicate the origin of the hypothyroidism:

1. Primary hypothyroidism. A disorder involving the thyroid gland or some aspect of thyroid hormone synthesis, metabolism, or transport.
2. Central (also called secondary/tertiary). Deficient thyroid hormone secretion due to a disorder affecting pituitary control (TSH production) or hypothalamic control (TRH production).

A. **Etiology of permanent congenital hypothyroidism (CH).**
   1. Thyroid abnormalities.
      a. Thyroid dysgenesis: absent (agenesis), hypoplastic, and/or ectopic gland. Ectopic gland is the most common etiology of CH (LaFranchi and Austin, 2007).
      b. Familial dyshormonogenesis: inborn errors of thyroid hormone biosynthesis or metabolism, the most common of which is an organification defect related to a defective thyroid peroxidase (TPO) enzyme. The thyroid gland itself is usually normally positioned (Brook and Brown, 2008).
   2. Extrathyroid abnormalities.
      a. Defects of the pituitary gland (e.g., hypopituitarism) or the hypothalamus.
      b. TBG deficiency: X-linked disorder; more common in males.
      c. Thyroid hormone resistance. Resistance to the actions of endogenous and exogenous T_4 and T_3. All serum thyroid hormone levels are elevated and many patients have goiter.

B. **Etiologies of transient hypothyroid states.**
   1. Prenatally acquired:
      a. Maternal autoimmune thyroid disorders characterized by transplacental passage of TSH-receptor blocking antibodies, which inhibit the binding of TSH to the thyroid cell.
      b. Drugs given to the mother that cross the placenta and affect fetal thyroid production (propylthiouracil, methimazole, lithium, phenytoin, amiodarone, and radioiodine.)
      c. Ingestion of excess iodide or severe dietary iodide deficiency.
   2. Postnatally acquired: transiently impaired thyroid hormone production from exposure to iodine-containing topical disinfectants, ointments, drugs such as amiodarone, or intravenously administered contrast media. Preterm infants can absorb and excrete large amounts of iodine; thus, exposure to iodinated products should be minimized.

C. **The preterm infant.**
In addition to having the same incidence of permanent CH as full-term infants, several transient hypothyroid states have been described in preterm infants. Because two or more transient conditions can coexist, it is not always possible to determine the precise cause of low thyroid hormone levels in preterm infants.

   1. *Hypothyroxinemia of prematurity.* Serum levels of thyroid hormones in preterm neonates are significantly lower and more variable than those of term neonates and correlate with gestational age and birth weight (Fisher, 2007). T_4 levels of most preterms reach a nadir at 7 to 14 days of age and then climb to normal within 4 to 8 weeks (Oden and Freemark, 2002).

      Sicker preterm infants demonstrate more variability in their T_4 values than healthy preterms of the same gestational age. Preterm infants do have an initial TSH surge after birth, but it is blunted in comparison to more mature neonates (Clemente et al., 2007). The TSH of preterm infants with hypothyroxinemia is not consistently elevated, suggesting relative lack of hypothalamic response to the lower T_4 level. This condition is believed to be a developmental phenomenon caused by one or more of the following:
      a. Immaturity of thyroid hormone metabolism and the HPT axis.

    b. Loss of maternal contributions to the thyroid hormone pool at birth.

    c. Low TBG levels.

    d. Increased use of T_4 to meet the demands of extrauterine life.

    e. Insufficient enteral or parenteral iodine intake.

  2. *Atypical primary hypothyroidism.* Infants weighing less than 1500 g at birth have 14 to 20 times the incidence of a low T_4/high TSH profile (consistent with primary hypothyroidism) of infants weighing more than 2500 g (Larson et al., 2003; Mandel et al., 2000). The majority of these very low birth weight (VLBW) infants will have a delayed TSH rise: a normal TSH on initial screening, followed by an elevated TSH on repeat screen. In addition to immaturity of the HPT axis, possible etiologies include the following:

    a. Exposure to iodine (Larson et al., 2003). Unable to reduce iodide trapping in the presence of excess iodine, VLBW infants are more vulnerable to the effects of iodine.

    b. Exposure to dopamine (which suppresses TSH and the thyroid axis).

    c. Exposure to glucocorticoids.

    d. Effects of concurrent illness on thyroid function (see below).

  3. *Nonthyroidal illness (NTI) syndrome.* Nonthyroidal illnesses (e.g., respiratory distress syndrome or sepsis) can affect thyroid function in the neonate. NTI can lower serum TBG and total T_4 and T_3, and inhibit extrathyroidal conversion of T_4 to T_3 (Rapaport et al., 2001). Thus the small, sick infant who already has a low T_4 related to prematurity may suffer a further fall in T_4 levels as a result of concurrent illness. The TSH in such infants is inappropriately low because there is a poor pituitary response to TRH (Forghani and Aye, 2008). Cytokines produced in response to illness and inflammation may inhibit thyroid function, metabolism, and thyroid hormone action (Kok et al., 2001).

D. Trisomy 21 (Down syndrome). Higher frequency of thyroid dysfunction than the general population; include CH and compensated hypothyroidism with increased TSH levels. CH in children with trisomy 21 is mild yet persistent, and believed to be of thyroidal origin (Van Trotsenburg et al., 2006).

E. Clinical presentation and assessment.

  1. Few neonates are diagnosed with CH on clinical grounds, but 15% to 20% will have suggestive signs when carefully examined (Fisher, 2000). Early signs and symptoms reflect the wide-ranging actions of thyroid hormones on metabolism, intestinal motility, cardiac function, temperature regulation, neurologic function, and bone maturation (Box 30-1).

  2. Other features typical of hypothyroidism (e.g., macroglossia, dry skin, coarse hair, constipation) are not usually seen for several weeks after birth.

  3. Most preterm/VLBW infants will not have clinical signs and symptoms readily associated with hypothyroidism.

  4. Infants with hypopituitary hypothyroidism may present with midline facial defects (cleft lip and palate), microphallus, and hypoglycemia.

  5. Palpation of the neck will identify thyroid enlargement (goiter). A goiter indicates functional thyroid tissue with regard to iodine uptake and is associated with thyroid dyshormonogenesis. Small goiters can be difficult to detect in the short neck of the neonate; extending the neck is helpful.

F. Diagnostic studies in hypothyroidism (Table 30-2): Unless the infant is born to a mother with a history of thyroid dysfunction or has obvious clinical signs of hypothyroidism at birth, the diagnosis is usually made after the infant is identified by neonatal screening.

  1. Newborn screening for hypothyroidism.

    a. Screening for CH uses either a two-tiered T_4–TSH testing approach or primary TSH testing. In the two-tiered system, TSH is measured only if the T_4 level is low. Many screening programs are transitioning to primary TSH testing for CH.

    b. An elevated TSH level is presumed to be CH until further testing proves otherwise. Rapid confirmation is essential.

    c. The latest National Newborn Screening Report found the incidence of CH in the United States to be 1:2500, with a 2:1 female/male ratio (National Newborn Screening and Genetics Resource Center [NNSGRC], 2000).

■ BOX 30-1
■ **EARLY SIGNS AND SYMPTOMS OF CONGENITAL HYPOTHYROIDISM**

Large, open posterior fontanelle (>1 cm)
Birth weight greater than 4 kg; gestation longer than 42 weeks
Coarse features
Delayed bone age (identified on knee X-rays)
Umbilical hernia
Goiter
Thick skin
Poor perfusion (mottling, peripheral cyanosis)
Hypothermia
Abdominal distention
Poor feeding; sleepy and placid
Prolonged hyperbilirubinemia
Hoarse cry
Edema
Cardiomegaly, bradycardia

- d. False-positive results can occur when samples are drawn during the first 24 hours, when TSH levels are still physiologically elevated. Earlier discharge of newborns contributes to false-positive thyroid screens (Brook and Brown, 2008).
- e. Approximately 10% of infants with CH are missed on initial screening; they are detected only through routine second screening in states where this is required or on clinical grounds. Some of these infants have compensated hypothyroidism or delayed rise in the TSH level; most seem to have milder forms of hypothyroidism but still require treatment.
- f. Infants at risk of a missed or delayed diagnosis are those born at home, those who were extremely ill in the neonatal period, and those who were transferred to another hospital at an early age.
- g. The thyroid function of preterm infants with hypothyroxinemia should be individually evaluated during the first 2 months of life (Clemente et al., 2007).
2. Thyroid function tests.
   - a. When CH is suspected clinically or suggested by initial screening results, confirmatory serum T_4 and TSH measurements are obtained. Free T_4 and T_3 levels may also be measured, along with other tests, as needed, to determine the cause of abnormal screening results (see Table 30-2). Infants with an initial TSH of >50 mU/l are more likely to have permanent CH than those with TSH levels in the 20-49 mU/l range.
   - b. To rule out transient hypothyroidism, maternal serum may be analyzed for the presence of TSH receptor–blocking antibodies.
3. Further evaluation for the cause of a CH blood profile includes color Doppler ultrasonography of the neck, thyroid radionuclide imaging (to identify normal or ectopic thyroid tissue), and bone age radiography of the knee or foot (delayed bone ossification suggests long-standing thyroid deprivation).
G. **Patient care management.**
   1. Congenital hypothyroidism.
      - a. Thyroid replacement with synthetic T_4 (L-thyroxine), initially 10 to 15 mcg/kg/day (Ogilvy-Stuart and Midgley, 2006). The early goals of treatment are to raise the serum T_4 concentration into the upper half of the normal range as quickly as possible, and then normalize the TSH. Treatment must begin immediately; it should not be delayed to obtain radioisotope scans as every day without treatment can affect intelligence quotient (Ogilvy-Stuart and Midgley, 2006). Oral thyroxine tablets can be crushed and mixed with water or formula, but should not be administered at the same time as iron or soy, which can interfere with absorption of the hormone (Brook and

■ TABLE 30-2
■ ■ **Summary of Low Thyroid States in the Newborn Infant**

Screening Results	Possible Conditions	Further Diagnostic Tests	Treatment
T₄ low,* TSH elevated†	Congenital hypothyroidism (thyroid agenesis, ectopia dyshormonogenesis)	Serum TFTs‡, Tg§ level; thyroid scan; ultrasonography; bone age radiography	Thyroid replacement
	Transient hypothyroidism Maternal (autoimmune, drugs) iodine exposure	TSI, TBA Urinary iodine level	Monitoring
T₄ low, TSH normal or low-normal, TSH slightly elevated (borderline)	Congenital hypothyroidism	Repeat screen, other tests as for congenital hypothyroidism (above)	Thyroid replacement
	Early specimen collection (<24 hours) or false-positive	Repeat screen	
T₄ low, TSH normal	Hypothyroxinemia of prematurity	Serum TFTs or repeat screen to detect delayed TSH rise	Monitoring
	TBG deficiency	Serum TFTs; TBG level; T₃, resin uptake level‖	None
	Early specimen collection (<24 hours) or false-positive	Repeat screen	
T₄ low, delayed TSH rise	Atypical hypothyroidism	Serum TFTs	Close monitoring; possible treatment
	Some VLBW infants (nonthyroidal illness?)		
	Congenital hypothyroidism (some functional thyroid; ectopic or hypoplastic)	Serum TFTs and other tests as for congenital hypothyroidism (above)	Thyroid replacement
T₄ low, TSH low	Central hypothyroidism (hypothalamic–pituitary)	Serum TFTs; TRH stimulation test¶; other tests of pituitary function (cortisol, growth hormone)	Thyroid replacement; other hormonal therapy

TFTs, Thyroid function tests; *TSH*, thyroid-stimulating hormone; *TBG*, thyroid-binding globulin; *TSI*, thyroid-stimulating immuno-globulins; *TBA*, thyroid-blocking antibodies; *VLBW*, very low birth weight.
*T₄ low: <6 mcg/dl.
†TSH elevated: >40 mU/l; TSH normal: <10 mU/l; TSH borderline: 20 to 40 mU/l. Note that a slightly elevated TSH level may be normal in the first 2 days of life.
‡TFTs: May include assays of total and free T₄ and T₃ along with TSH.
§Tg: Thyroglobulin, a thyroid hormone precursor produced by the thyroid gland. A low level suggests thyroid agenesis.
‖T₃, resin uptake level: An indirect measure of protein binding. A high level suggests low binding capacity, as in TBG deficiency.
¶TRH stimulation is a test of hypothalamic or pituitary control of thyroid function. A dose of TRH is administered and TSH is measured serially. A subnormal TSH response suggests a deficient pituitary gland, and a delayed response suggests hypothalamic congenital hypothyroidism.

Brown, 2008). L-Thyroxine (T₄) should not be exposed to heat (LaFranchi and Austin, 2007).

    b. Although rapid normalization of T₄ is desirable, close monitoring of serum T₄ levels and clinical response is needed to prevent overtreatment or undertreatment.

        (1) Overtreatment can lead to advanced bone age, craniosynostosis, and thyrotoxicosis (tachycardia, irritability, hyperactivity, poor weight gain, and loose stools).

        (2) Undertreatment leads to clinical hypothyroidism, delayed bone maturation, and neurologic damage.

  2. Transient hypothyroidism.

    a. Hypothyroxinemia of prematurity is not routinely treated with T₄ supplementation (Root, 2007). Despite evidence of associations between low thyroxine levels and higher mortality, severity of lung disease (Biswas et al., 2002), intraventricular hemorrhage (Paul et al., 2001), cerebral white matter damage (Leviton et al., 1999), and worse cognitive and neuromotor outcome (van Wassenaer et al., 2002), causal relationships have not been established (Oden and Freemark, 2002). Furthermore, research to date has not demonstrated improvements in morbidity, mortality, or neurodevelopmental outcomes with T_4 supplementation in all infants (Osborn and Hunt, 2007). Neurodevelopmental benefits of thyroid supplementation have been demonstrated in the most immature (25 to 26 weeks) neonates (van Wassenaer et al., 2005), but more research is needed to confirm these findings (Ogilvy-Stuart and Midgley, 2006).

    b. Because hypothyroidism cannot always be confirmed as transient during the neonatal period, replacement therapy for a low T_4–high TSH profile is begun just as it is for established permanent hypothyroidism. Evaluation of the permanence of the disease is conducted after the child is 2 to 3 years of age.

    c. Infants who are not treated are reevaluated by repeated filter-paper specimen or thyroid function tests to ensure that thyroid function normalizes.

    d. Some preterm infants, especially those who have undergone surgery, sepsis workups, dopamine therapy, and gastrointestinal disorders, will exhibit a late rise in thyroid-stimulating hormone. Follow-up serum thyroid function tests in these infants will detect a late rise in TSH requiring treatment, or ensure normalization of the TSH (Hyman et al., 2007). Routine rescreening of thyroid function in VLBW infants, however, remains a subject of debate (Tylek-Lema ska et al., 2005; Vincent et al., 2002).

H. Outcome.

  1. Congenital hypothyroidism.

    a. CH is one of the most preventable causes of mental retardation. The majority of infants with early diagnosis and early and adequate treatment will have normal IQs. A delay in treatment after birth can lower IQ by several points per week (Fisher, 2000).

    b. Lifelong thyroid replacement therapy is necessary for normal growth and development.

  2. Transient hypothyroidism.

    a. Hypothyroxinemia of prematurity is transient, correcting spontaneously over 6 to 10 weeks as the infant matures.

    b. More research is needed to determine whether hypothyroxinemia of prematurity is a benign physiologic phenomenon or a cause of psychomotor and neurodevelopmental sequelae in the preterm population.

Hyperthyroidism

A. Etiologies.

  1. Maternal Graves disease (either active or inactive) causes neonatal Graves disease in 1 of 70 affected pregnancies. Most babies born to mothers with Graves disease have normal thyroid function (Brook and Brown, 2008).

  2. Rare causes of neonatal hyperthyroidism include McCune–Albright syndrome and activating mutations in the TSH receptor.

B. Pathophysiology of Graves disease.

  1. Graves disease is an autoimmune disorder that results in the production of TSH receptor antibodies. The mother produces thyroid-stimulating immunoglobulins (TSI) that mimic the action of TSH in stimulating fetal and neonatal thyroid growth and function. Some mothers also produce thyroid-blocking antibodies (TBAs), which inhibit the binding of TSH to the thyroid receptor. The effects on the fetus and neonate can therefore be highly variable, depending on the concentration and potency of the two opposing types of antibodies. The clinical picture also differs between untreated (active) and treated (inactive) maternal Graves disease.

  2. Effects of active, uncontrolled maternal Graves disease: Maternal TSI causes fetal hyperthyroidism with tachycardia, failure to thrive, and in some cases, development of a fetal goiter detectable by ultrasound. The neonate can exhibit early or delayed signs of hyperthyroidism, but these effects are usually self-limiting and disappear as the TSI are degraded in the first 3 to 12 weeks of life.

3. Effects of treated maternal Graves disease: Treatment of the mother is aimed at correcting her elevated thyroid hormone levels with antithyroid drugs, but this does not necessarily halt the production of thyroid antibodies. Antithyroid drugs cross to the fetus and block fetal thyroid production. Thus the neonate may actually be hypothyroid at birth, with a delayed onset (up to 10 days) of hyperthyroidism. As maternal antithyroid drugs leave the neonate's circulation, residual TSI stimulate the neonate's thyroid, and thyrotoxicosis can ensue. If there are coexisting TBA, even longer delays (up to 4 to 6 weeks) are possible before the onset of hyperthyroidism in the infant.

C. **Clinical presentation and assessment.**
   1. Many affected infants are born prematurely and/or exhibit intrauterine growth restriction.
   2. Signs and symptoms include irritability, tremor, hyperactivity, flushing of the skin, hyperthermia, sweating, gastrointestinal dysfunction (vomiting, diarrhea), and signs of cardiac stimulation (tachycardia, arrhythmias, congestive heart failure). Eye signs include exophthalmos, eye stare, and lid retraction. Early age of onset suggests a mutation in the TSH receptor, whereas later onset points to Graves disease (Ogilvy-Stuart and Midgley, 2006).
   3. Thyromegaly, if present, can worsen during the neonatal period.
   4. In severely affected infants, advanced skeletal maturation (craniosynostosis, frontal bossing) is seen.
   5. Rarely, affected neonates can present with thrombocytopenia, hepatosplenomegaly, jaundice, and hypoprothrombinemia (Brook and Brown, 2008).

D. **Diagnostic studies.**
   1. Total and free T_4 and T_3 are elevated (may initially be normal or low in neonates born to mothers with treated Graves disease).
   2. The TSH is low because of feedback-loop suppression.
   3. Levels of TSI, thyroid-binding inhibitory immunoglobulins (TBII), and TBA in the mother and infant are measured as indicated by clinical circumstances. It is advisable to take cord blood for TSH and free T_4 to measure values prior to the postnatal surge in thyroid hormones (Ogilvy-Stuart and Midgley, 2006).

E. **Patient care management.**
   Clinical and biochemical hyperthyroidism is a medical emergency; the use of some or all of the following can be anticipated:
   1. β-Adrenergic blockers, such as propranolol, to treat cardiovascular overstimulation.
   2. Digitalization may also be necessary.
   3. Agents to suppress hypersecretion of thyroid hormone:
      a. Propylthiouracil (PTU) inhibits TPO and the peripheral conversion of T_4 to T_3 (Peters and Hindmarsh, 2007). PTU is not effective until after 24 to 36 hours. Carbimazole (MMI) inhibits TPO and thyroid hormone synthesis.
      b. Lugol iodine (potassium iodide) solution has been used for acute inhibition of thyroid hormone release.
      c. Radiographic contrast agents (ipodate sodium and iopanoic acid) block peripheral conversion of T_4 to T_3 and inhibit thyroidal secretion of T_4 and T_3.
      d. Glucocorticoids are used to inhibit thyroid hormone secretion.
   4. A hypothyroid state could be induced by use of the agents mentioned above, making replacement with T_4 necessary.
   5. Sedatives are given for neurologic symptoms.
   6. If an enlarged thyroid gland is compressing the trachea and causing respiratory distress, elevation and extension of the infant's head will help maintain a patent airway. Rarely, surgery is necessary to relieve the obstruction.
   7. Infants with nonimmune hyperthyroidism related to an activating TSH receptor mutation are treated with thyroid ablation.
   8. In cases of maternal thyrotoxicosis, thyrotoxicosis should be anticipated in the neonate so diagnosis and treatment can be instituted without delay.

F. **Complications.**
   More severe manifestations of thyrotoxicosis, such as congestive heart failure, hepatosplenomegaly, thrombocytopenia, and hyperviscosity syndrome, may occur.

G. Outcome.

1. Neonatal hyperthyroidism is almost always transient. Rare, permanent neonatal hyperthyroidism is caused by a germline mutation in the TSH receptor (Brook and Brown, 2008).

2. The mortality rate of 12% to 16% is related to cardiovascular compromise, arrhythmia, tachycardia, and heart failure (Peters and Hindmarsh, 2007).

3. Survivors of severe, prolonged thyrotoxicosis often have permanent neurologic impairment from premature craniosynostosis and the direct effects of excess thyroid hormones on the brain.

ADRENAL GLAND DISORDERS

The Adrenal Gland

A. Anatomy and physiology.

1. The adrenal glands are located at the superior poles of the kidneys. Each highly vascular gland is composed of two endocrine organs: the inner adrenal medulla and the outer adrenal cortex.

2. The adrenal medulla produces and stores catecholamines (epinephrine, norepinephrine, dopamine) and is linked to the sympathetic nervous system.

3. All adrenocortical hormones (steroids) are synthesized from cholesterol. Three classes of steroids are produced by the adrenal cortex: glucocorticoids, mineralocorticoids, and androgens.

B. Adrenocortical hormones.

1. Cortisol, the primary glucocorticoid, has a major role in glucose homeostasis and key regulatory roles in development, growth, inflammatory responses, cardiovascular function, and response to stress.

2. Cortisol is closely regulated by adrenocorticotropic hormone (ACTH) and the hypothalamic–pituitary–adrenal (HPA) axis via an acute or chronic negative-feedback loop. Increased plasma cortisol inhibits secretion of corticotropin-releasing hormone and ACTH, whereas decreased plasma cortisol permits their release. Cortisol is also released in response to stress, hypoglycemia, surgery, extreme heat or cold, decreased oxygen concentration, infection, or injury.

3. Aldosterone, the most important mineralocorticoid, regulates renal sodium (Na^+) and water retention and potassium (K^+) excretion, thus affecting not only electrolyte balance but also blood pressure and intravascular volume. Aldosterone is regulated by the plasma renin–angiotensin system and by plasma K^+ concentrations. A drop in intravascular volume or the Na^+ concentration or a rise in the K^+ level stimulates the renin–angiotensin system, which in turn stimulates production of aldosterone.

4. Adrenal androgens include dehydroepiandrosterone (DHEA), DHEA sulfate, and androstenedione and are regulated by ACTH. These steroids have minimal androgenic activity but are converted in the peripheral tissues to two more potent androgens: testosterone and dihydrotestosterone.

C. Fetal adrenocortical development.

1. Early in gestation, the fetal adrenal cortex begins to differentiate into distinct zones: a large, unique fetal zone and an outer definitive ("adult") zone. The fetal zone is responsible for most of the steroids produced during fetal life. Fetal adrenal growth is rapid; at term the gland is twice the size of the adult's but shrinks in size after birth as the fetal zone involutes.

2. The fetal adrenal gland and the placenta are an integrated endocrine organ known as the fetoplacental unit. The fetal zone, deficient in a critical enzyme for cortisol synthesis, produces mostly DHEA and DHEA sulfate. These are the precursors for placental estrogen, which is vital to maintenance of the pregnancy and fetal well-being. In turn, the placenta provides substrates for fetal cortisol production.

3. Until about 30 weeks of gestation, fetal cortisol comes from both the fetal gland and transplacental transfer. In the placenta, 80% of maternal cortisol is rapidly metabolized to inactive cortisone to protect the fetus from very high cortisol levels. Near term, maturation of

fetal enzyme systems allows greater conversion of cortisone back to cortisol and synthesis of cortisol from cholesterol. Increases in circulating cortisol during the last 10 weeks of gestation (the prenatal cortisol surge) induce critical physiologic changes that prepare the fetus for extrauterine life, including maturation of pulmonary surfactant.

4. Aldosterone production increases throughout pregnancy, preparing the fetus to assume control of salt and water balance after birth.

D. Neonatal adrenocortical function.

1. Plasma cortisol levels are high at the time of birth but begin to fall in the first few days of life. In term infants a nadir is seen on day 4. Likewise, levels of a cortisol precursor, 17-hydroxyprogesterone (17-OHP), are high at birth but decrease to normal neonatal levels by 12 to 24 hours of age.

2. A diurnal pattern of cortisol secretion is evident at about 2 to 3 months of age in most infants, influenced more by environmental factors than genetic factors (Custodio et al., 2007).

3. In the neonate, aldosterone concentration and plasma renin activity are elevated compared with values for older infants, allowing for positive Na^+ balance until the kidneys fully mature. The hyponatremia and urinary Na^+ loss often seen in preterm infants during the early postnatal weeks are due to a relative mineralocorticoid deficiency as a consequence of immaturity of both the kidneys and the adrenal glands.

E. Adrenal disorders in the neonate: Adrenal insufficiency in the neonate is mainly attributed to hypopituitarism (secondary adrenal insufficiency) or to a single gene defect of adrenal development, steroid biosynthesis, or steroid responsiveness (Dempsher, 2008).

1. Congenital adrenal hyperplasia (see following section). Other enzymatic defects that result in adrenal insufficiency include P450 side-chain cleavage deficiency (congenital lipoid adrenal hyperplasia) and P450 oxidoreductase deficiency.

2. Adrenal hemorrhage (from hemorrhagic diathesis, shock, anoxia, birth trauma).

3. Hypopituitarism. The pituitary fails to produce ACTH, and the consequent lack of cortical stimulation results in hypoplasia of the adrenal cortex and adrenal insufficiency.

4. Adrenocortical insufficiency in ill extremely low birth weight (ELBW) infants.

   a. Low cortisol levels are most likely related to hypothalamic–pituitary–adrenal immaturity, a syndrome known as transient adrenocortical insufficiency of prematurity (TAP). In some infants, hypotension related to TAP is unresponsive to volume and inotropic support. Cortisol levels correlate with blood pressure, and adrenal function recovers by 14 days of life (Ng et al., 2004). ELBW infants continue to demonstrate low basal cortisol levels until about 8 months' corrected age, at which time their cortisol levels are higher than those of infants born at term. This suggests long-term resetting of endocrine stress syndromes, possibly caused by immaturity, cumulative stress, and other factors (Grunau et al., 2007).

   b. An inappropriately low cortisol level in the presence of significant stress (respiratory illness, mechanical ventilation, invasive procedures, etc.) indicates an inability to recognize stress owing to immaturity of brain regions involved in the stress response (Bolt et al., 2002).

5. Adrenal hypoplasia related to a loss-of-function mutation of the DAX1 gene; also associated with hypogonadotropic hypogonadism.

6. Adrenal suppression following steroid therapy (prenatal or postnatal).

7. Maternal Cushing syndrome (excess circulating glucocorticoids).

Congenital Adrenal Hyperplasia

A. Definition.

A group of autosomal recessive genetic disorders resulting from deficient activity of one of the enzymes required to synthesize cortisol from cholesterol in the adrenal cortex. Each enzyme is encoded by its own gene. Mutation of the 21-hydroxylase (21OHD) gene, CYP21, accounts for 95% of disorders, and is the most common cause of ambiguous genitalia in the neonate. The term *congenital adrenal hyperplasia* refers to the hypertrophy of the adrenal gland found at autopsy (Miller, 2002). CAH has a worldwide prevalence of 1:15,000 to 1:16,000,

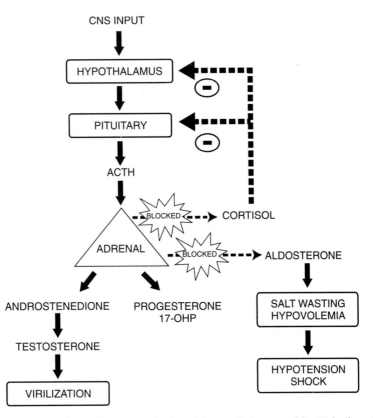

FIGURE 30-2 ■ Pathophysiology of congenital adrenal hyperplasia caused by 21-hydroxylase deficiency. In the absence of cortisol, adrenocorticotropic hormone (ACTH) stimulates the adrenal cortex to produce virilizing androgens. Diminished production of aldosterone leads to salt wasting and hypovolemia. (Adapted from Martin, R.J., Fanaroff, A.A., and Walsh, M.C.: *Fanaroff and Martin's neonatal-perinatal medicine: Diseases of the fetus and infant* [8th ed.]. Philadelphia, 2006, Mosby.)

      although higher frequencies have been documented in some geographical areas, including Alaska, Brazil, Reunion, and the Philippines (Therrell, 2001).

B. Pathophysiology (Fig. 30-2): Because the overwhelming majority of CAH cases are the result of 21-OHD deficiency, the remainder of the discussion will pertain to this form of CAH.

    1. Lack of fetal 21-hydroxylase prevents conversion of progesterone to its two end products: cortisol and aldosterone.

    2. By reduced negative-feedback regulation, the absence of cortisol causes oversecretion of ACTH, which chronically stimulates the adrenal cortex, resulting in hyperplasia.

    3. The cortisol precursor 17-OHP accumulates in the blood because its conversion to cortisol is blocked.

    4. The excess 17-OHP enters the unblocked androgen metabolic pathway, which results in an overproduction of androgens. At a critical stage in fetal development, androgens cause virilization of the external genitalia in female fetuses. Also important may be the effects of this androgen exposure on the developing CNS.

C. Clinical presentation. Three subtypes of CAH related to 21-OHD are traditionally recognized. Subtypes are based on the level of enzyme activity, and each can give rise to a different clinical picture. Two subtypes are known as "classic" CAH: a simple virilizing form and a salt-wasting form. A third, "nonclassic," milder subtype presents later in life. CAH is currently viewed as a disease continuum that reflects the severity of enzyme deficiency (Therrell, 2001).

    1. *Simple virilizing* (25% of patients). An incomplete enzyme block allows enough aldosterone production to maintain fluid and electrolyte homeostasis. Clinical signs are few or absent, depending on the degree of enzyme deficiency.

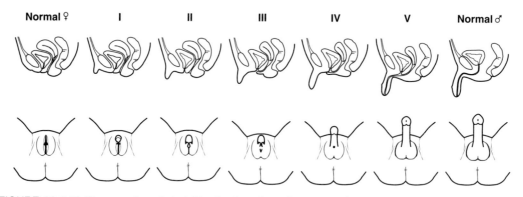

FIGURE 30-3 ■ Degrees of genital virilization based on the stages of Prader. The upper panel illustrates the sagittal view; the lower panel illustrates the perineal view. (From Scriver, C.R.: *The metabolic and molecular basis of inherited diseases* [7th ed.]. New York, 1995, McGraw-Hill Companies.)

    2. *Salt-wasting disease* (75% of patients).
        a. A complete deficiency of 21-hydroxylase activity halts both cortisol and aldosterone synthesis. High Na⁺ excretion occurring in the absence of aldosterone (called a "salt-losing" or "salt-wasting" state) results in profound hyponatremia. Dehydration and hyperkalemia are related to failure of both water conservation and K⁺ excretion. Glucocorticoid deficiency impairs carbohydrate metabolism resulting in hypoglycemia, hypotension, shock, and cardiovascular collapse.
        b. Onset of the salt-losing state is usually after day 7 of life. Although the newborn typically has a high aldosterone level in the first week secondary to slow hepatic clearance, in CAH when aldosterone is depleted, the deficient adrenal cortex cannot restore it.

D. Clinical assessment.
    1. The earliest signs and symptoms of CAH are lethargy, poor feeding, vomiting, diarrhea, dehydration, failure to thrive, apnea, and seizures.
    2. Appearance of the genitalia.
        a. In girls with 21-OHD (female karyotype, 46,XX), the external genitalia are virilized. The phenotype is mild to moderate clitoral hypertrophy, varying degrees of labioscrotal fusion, and a urogenital sinus. In the most severe cases, marked clitoral hypertrophy gives the appearance of a penile urethra, and labioscrotal folds are completely fused (Prader stage V virilization; Fig. 30-3). These infants can be mistaken for boys with bilateral cryptorchidism (undescended testes). There can also be hyperpigmentation of the genital skin resulting from excessive pituitary ACTH secretion.
        b. In boys with 21-OHD (male karyotype, 46,XY), external genitalia are male but sometimes overvirilized (enlarged penis and scrotum, hyperpigmentation).

E. Diagnosis of CAH related to 21-OHD. Genital ambiguity can be life-saving in females because it alerts the healthcare team to the possible diagnosis of CAH before a salt-losing crisis ensues with tragic consequences. With neonatal screening, the diagnosis of CAH before the advent of a salt-losing state has become more common.
    1. Diagnostic tests and findings in 21-OHD CAH are as follows:
        a. 17-OHP level is markedly elevated and is hyperresponsive to ACTH stimulation; levels of testosterone and its precursors are also increased. Blood for 17-OHP level must be drawn before any hormone replacement is administered.
        b. Serum aldosterone and plasma renin activity are measured to detect salt-losing states. The aldosterone level is low and plasma renin activity is high.
        c. Serum and urine electrolytes and steroid profiles are determined. Positive findings are hyponatremia, hyperkalemia, and high urine Na⁺ excretion. Other metabolic disturbances include hypoglycemia and metabolic acidosis.

    d. Fluorescence in situ hybridization (FISH) studies or karyotyping to establish genetic sex. It may be difficult for parents to accept that their severely virilized newborn is a genetic female without this testing. If genetic testing for CYP21B (gene for 21-OH) is to be done, blood samples should be taken from both the infant and the parents (Ogilvy-Stuart and Midgley, 2006).

    e. Ultrasonography and/or magnetic resonance imaging of the pelvis and abdomen are done to visualize the uterus and adrenal glands.

2. Neonatal screening for CAH is currently required in all 50 states and the District of Columbia (NNSGRC, 2008). In Canada, 5 of 15 provinces and territories currently require newborn screening for CAH (Canadian Organization for Rare Disorder, 2008).

    a. The goals of screening are the presymptomatic identification of infants at risk for life-threatening adrenal crisis and to prevent incorrect sex assignment of affected females.

    b. The basis of screening for CAH is measurement of 17-OHP, which is markedly elevated in neonates with the disorder. Random 17-OHP levels can reach 10,000 ng/dl (normal < 100 ng/dl). Diagnostic 17-OHP levels may not be reached until the second or third day of life, so a specimen drawn too early can be falsely negative. Blood samples drawn early in life (before 24 hours of age) can also give a false-positive screening result because 17-OHP is still physiologically elevated. False-positive results can occur in infants who have relatively higher 17-OHP levels related to illness or prematurity.

F. Management of CAH.

1. Restore physiologic level of cortisol, suppress ACTH and androgen overproduction, and maintain fluid and electrolyte homeostasis, especially any salt deficit that is present.

2. Administer hydrocortisone (glucocorticoid) and 9-α-fludrocortisone (mineralocorticoid). Medications such as androgen blockers and aromatase inhibitors remain under study.

3. Dietary sodium supplementation to prevent hyponatremia, if needed. Fludrocortisone is not effective without salt supplementation.

4. Additional measures. In a salt-losing state/adrenal crisis, these may include intravenous administration of fluids (glucose and sodium to correct dehydration and metabolic imbalances), treatment of shock, and correction of acidosis.

5. Genetic counseling.

    a. Prenatal diagnosis for subsequent pregnancies using direct molecular genetic analysis of the fetal DNA (Nimkarn and New, 2006).

    b. Intrauterine treatment can prevent some or all of the virilization of female fetuses. Dexamethasone given to the mother crosses the placenta and suppresses fetal ACTH. Treatment must begin before 8 weeks of gestation and continue to term in affected female fetuses.

6. Parent education. Parents need to understand that there is no cure for CAH, but it can be managed with medications and close monitoring. Their baby should receive care from a pediatric endocrinologist. Advise parents about immediate and long-term management of the disorder, the importance of compliance with therapy, and the need for follow-up of growth and development. Parents need to be aware of the requirement for double or even triple doses of steroids during illness and fever. Do not use the term *ambiguous genitalia* in discussions with parents as this term is disturbing to parents (Ogilvy-Stuart and Midgley, 2006).

G. Management of virilized genitalia in female neonates with CAH. Two issues that might be raised regarding the neonate with virilizing CAH are gender of rearing, the type of surgery that will be needed, if any, and the timing of that surgery.

1. Gender of rearing.

    a. The genetic female (46,XX) with 21-OHD, regardless of the degree of virilization of the external genitalia, has normal female reproductive structures: ovaries, uterus, fallopian tubes, and upper vagina, and is potentially fertile. The lower vagina is foreshortened, conjoining with the urethra to form a high urogenital sinus defect where the vagina enters the urethra (Schnitzer and Donahoe, 2001). Most 46,XX neonates with CAH are assigned to the female gender to preserve endogenous sex hormone production and fertility (Meyer-Bahlburg, 2001).

  b. Occasionally as a result of missed or delayed diagnosis, 46,XX neonates with severe virilization (complete fusion of the labia and a penile urethra) are raised as males, despite potential fertility as females. Choosing male sex of rearing at birth for similarly affected neonates has been suggested, based on the theory that significant prenatal brain virilization might have occurred, leading to the later adoption of a male gender identity. No studies have been done yet to evaluate this approach (Blizzard, 2002). It has not been established conclusively that gender identity is primarily formed through prenatal sex steroid exposure (Cohen-Kettenis, 2005).

 2. Surgical considerations.

  a. Typically, feminizing genitoplasty (clitoral recession and labioscrotal reduction) is performed early in life, often combined with vaginal exteriorization in a one-stage procedure to "normalize" the genitalia and spare the child the trauma of later genital surgeries. Data suggest, however, that this has not always had the desired outcome (Crouch et al., 2008).

   Some girls and women who have undergone surgical correction of their virilized genitalia in infancy have had poor results, including clitoral atrophy, vaginal stenosis, scarring, and persistent urogenital sinus. Virtually all required additional procedures after puberty (Alizai et al., 1999). Newer surgical techniques now in use might avoid these problems, but objective long-term outcome studies for these patients are not yet available (Schnitzer and Donahoe, 2001). Parents must be made aware of the irreversibility of surgery, the possible complications and the alternative of postponing surgery (Hughes et al., 2007).

  b. Lee and Witchel (2002) documented a shift away from early surgery, by parental choice, for female infants with CAH. They speculate that this might be the result of increased parental awareness of the variation of clitoral size and a desire to avoid unnecessary surgery.

   However, there is evidence that parents, even when well informed, would choose early genital surgery for their infants even at the risk of reduced genital sensitivity. (Dayner et al., 2004).

  c. Most surgeons now agree that infants with mild clitoromegaly should not undergo early surgery in anticipation that as the hormonal milieu normalizes with therapy, clitoral size will decrease and labial appearance will improve (Aaronson, 2001). Furthermore, Prader stages I and II require no surgical intervention (Hughes et al., 2007).

H. Complications of CAH.

 1. Adrenal crisis can occur with sudden signs of cortisol insufficiency (shock, hypotension, acidosis, hypoglycemia, seizures) plus sodium depletion. This can be triggered by episodes of illness or stress (such as systemic infection or surgery) in the neonatal period. Stress therapy to prevent this complication requires 2 or 3 times the usual dosage of hydrocortisone.

 2. Consequences of poorly controlled CAH:

  a. Failure to suppress ACTH and androgen production can result in signs of virilization and accelerated growth or bone maturation.

  b. Overtreatment, resulting in hypertension, pulmonary edema, congestive heart failure, growth failure, adrenal atrophy, and lowered resistance to infection.

I. Outcome.

 1. Lifelong hormonal replacement is usually necessary to improve chances for normal growth, pubertal development, and fertility.

 2. Missed or delayed diagnosis can result in sudden deterioration or death in infants with undiagnosed CAH.

 3. Differences in gender role behavior are seen in females with CAH, compared with those without CAH, such as toy preferences, rough-and-tumble play, aggressiveness, interest in sports, maternal behavior, and vocational preferences (Meyer-Bahlburg, 2001). In spite of this, females with CAH generally grow up with a female gender identity, provided that steroid treatment is started early and suppression of adrenal androgens is maintained (Warne and Kanumakala, 2002).

DISORDERS OF SEXUAL DEVELOPMENT

Sexual Differentiation

The earliest events in sexual differentiation are directed by genes. All embryos have bipotential gonads and structures for both male and female internal and external genitalia. Male-specific development requires the expression of the testis-determining gene (SRY) located on the short arm of the Y-chromosome. SRY directs the gonad to differentiate to a testis, the impetus for male sexual development. Further development along male lines requires the expression of specific genes and secretion of hormones at precise times. If the Y chromosome is absent, the gonad becomes an ovary. Appreciation of the bipotentiality of embryonic tissues is fundamental to understanding disorders of sexual development (DSDs).

A. **Internal genitalia.**
   1. By 7 weeks, the embryo has 2 sets of primitive ducts that will become the internal reproductive tracts: the müllerian (female) and wolffian (male) ducts.
   2. Embryonic testis has 2 types of hormone-producing cells: the Sertoli and the Leydig cells. Sertoli cells secrete müllerian-inhibiting hormone (MIH), causing the müllerian ducts to regress. At about 9 weeks, the Leydig cells secrete testosterone, which acts locally on the wolffian ducts to induce their development into epididymis, vas deferens, and seminal vesicles. If no testosterone is produced by the Leydig cells, the wolffian ducts regress and the müllerian ducts develop into Fallopian tubes, uterus, and upper vagina.

B. **External genitalia.**
   1. The primitive external genitalis are identical in both sexes (Fig. 30-4) and consist of a genital tubercle, and a urogenital sinus surrounded by inner urogenital folds and labioscrotal swellings. Between weeks 8 and 12 dihydrotestosterone (DHT), a potent metabolite of testosterone, binds to androgen receptors in the genital tissues and stimulates their differentiation to a penis, urethra, and scrotum.
   2. If there is no DHT, the primitive structures become a clitoris, labia majora, labia minora, lower vagina and urethra. Female external genital development is complete by 11 weeks; androgen exposure after this time can cause clitoral growth but not labial fusion (Houk and Lee, 2005).
   3. In the male, the testes descend to the scrotum at 25 to 35 weeks of gestation and penile growth continues to term under the influence of pituitary-produced luteinizing hormone.

Disorders of Sexual Differentiation

A DSD is defined as a congenital condition in which development of chromosomal, gonadal, or anatomical sex is atypical (Hughes et al., 2007). Most DSDs arise when there is either a failure in one of the steps along the male developmental pathway or when a genetically female fetus is exposed to an excess of androgens during a sensitive period of development. Current estimates place the collective incidence of DSDs at about 1 in 4500 births (Hughes et al., 2007). The more common disorders will be presented here; for a more comprehensive review, the reader is referred to a textbook of pediatric endocrinology.

A. **46,XY DSD.**
   1. Pure gonadal dysgenesis (46,XY). Complete or partial failure of testicular differentiation; affected neonates often have female internal genitalia.
   2. Mixed gonadal dysgenesis (45,XO/46,XY). These infants have ambiguous genitalia that are asymmetric, such as a scrotum on one side only.
   3. Klinefelter syndrome (usually 47,XXY), involving dysgenesis of the seminiferous tubules. This common disorder affects 1 in 1000 newborn male infants but is not generally diagnosed in the neonatal period.
   4. Turner syndrome (45,X or variation), a type of gonadal dysgenesis. Affected infants have the female phenotype, with classic somatic features and bilateral streak gonads. Affects 1 in 2500 live female births.

B. **Ovotesticular DSD.**
   1. Karyotype varies (46,XX, 46,XY mosaicism, or 46,XX/46,XY chimerism). Both ovarian and testicular tissues are present, either separately or combined in an ovotestis.

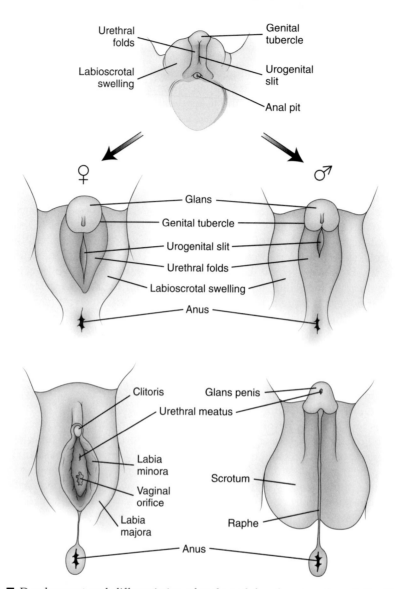

FIGURE 30-4 ■ Development and differentiation of male and female external genitalia. (Adapted from Spaulding, M.H.: The development of the external genitalia in the human embryo. *Contributions to Embryology of the Carnegie Institute, 13*:69-88, 1921; H.M. Kronenberg, S. Melmed, K.S. Polonsky, and P.R. Larsen [Eds.]: *Williams textbook of endocrinology* [11th ed.]. Philadelphia, 2008, Saunders.)

2. The internal ducts parallel the ipsilateral gonadal histology. The appearance of the external genitalia reflects the amount of testicular tissue in the gonads (Aaronson, 2001).

C. **Disorders of differentiation of the genital ducts/external genitalia.**

1. Genetic female (46,XX) with virilized external genitalia. Internal organs (gonads, genital ducts) are normal female structures. The degree of masculinization depends on the point during gestation when development was influenced by androgens. Etiologies include the following:

    a. CAH, caused by 21-hydroxylase deficiency, 11-β-hydroxylase deficiency, or 3-β-hydroxysteroid dehydrogenase deficiency. 21-OHD is the most common cause of genital ambiguity in the 46,XX neonate.

    b. Placental aromatase deficiency. The enzyme aromatase normally catalyzes the conversion of androgens to estrogens. In its absence, excess androgens can virilize both mother and fetus.

      c. Excessive androgen production by the mother (maternal CAH, androgen-producing tumors), ingestion of certain drugs, such as danazol.

  2. Genetic male (46,XY), with incomplete development of external genitalia as a result of defects in the synthesis, metabolism, or receptor sensitivity of androgens. Gonads are normal, but genital ducts may fail to fully develop and external genitalia are ambiguous. Etiologies include the following:

      a. Androgen insensitivity syndrome (AIS). This X-linked recessive disorder is caused by defects in androgen receptors, preventing binding of testosterone and DHT to genital tissues.

         DHT is present but is unable to effect its masculinizing action. AIS is a spectrum disorder, so there are complete and partial forms.

        (1) Partial AIS (PAIS) is the most common DSD in the 46,XY neonate. PAIS is extremely heterogeneous. Depending on the degree of androgen receptor function, a wide range of genital phenotypes, from a small phallus or hypospadias to extreme hypo-virilization, can be seen. Testes can be intraabdominal or in the inguinal canal.

        (2) Complete AIS may not be recognized at birth because the infant's genitalia are female. Many infants will present with an inguinal or labial hernia.

      b. Deficiency of 5-α-reductase. This enzyme is required for conversion of testosterone to DHT. Internal structures are normal male, but because of variable degrees of enzyme activity, the external phenotype ranges from ambiguous to female.

      c. Defect of testosterone biosynthesis. The most common disorder of testosterone biosynthesis causing ambiguous genitalia in the 46,XY neonate is 17-β-hydroxysteroid dehydrogenase deficiency (also termed 17-ketosteroid reductase deficiency).

      d. Persistent müllerian duct. The uterus and fallopian tubes fail to regress in an otherwise normal male fetus because of a defect in synthesis, secretion, or response to müllerian-inhibiting substance.

  3. Other conditions associated with DSDs:

      a. Cryptorchidism: unilateral or bilateral absence of testes in the scrotum, caused by failure of testicular descent. Occurring in 5% of term infants, it is one of the most common urogenital abnormalities of childhood.

      b. Hypospadias: incomplete fusion of the penile urethra. The urethral meatus is found proximal to the glans penis, somewhere along the ventral surface of the penis or, in severe cases, on the perineum. Hypospadias occurs in approximately 1 of 125 newborn male infants. Perineoscrotal hypospadias is frequently a feature of atypical sexual differentiation.

      c. Micropenis: an otherwise normally formed penis that measures less than 2.5 cm in stretched length from the pubic bone to the tip of the glans. Micropenis results from reduced androgen and/or growth hormone effects during the second or third trimester. Major causes of isolated micropenis include primary hypogonadism and hypopituitarism. With congenital hypopituitarism, neonates may have persistent hypoglycemia, hypothyroidism, hyperbilirubinemia, and midline craniofacial defects (cleft lip and palate) or septo-optic dysplasia.

D. Clinical presentation.

  1. Often, but not always, neonates with DSDs present with *ambiguous genitalia*, a term that refers to genitals that are anatomically in between what is typically considered male and typically considered female. In some DSDs, there may be only a single atypical genital feature; in still others, the genitalia appear "normal" at birth.

  2. Other presenting signs and symptoms may relate to a primary endocrine disorder (adrenal insufficiency, hypopituitarism, growth hormone deficiency).

  3. Dysmorphic features, such as those of Turner syndrome, can be associated with cases of gonadal dysgenesis. Many malformation syndromes and other nonendocrine conditions may be associated with genital ambiguity; among these are trisomy 13, cloacal exstrophy, Smith–Lemli–Opitz syndrome, and camptomelic dysplasia.

E. Assessment and physical examination.

  1. Examination of the genitalia: close scrutiny not only of infants with clearly atypical genitalia but also of apparent "girls" with inguinal masses, hernias, or clitoromegaly and of apparent "boys" with nonpalpable testes, hypospadias, or unusually small genitalia.

a. Phallus: size (length and width), presence of chordee (downward curvature of the penis, found in some forms of hypospadias), and location of the urethral meatus relative to normal position (may require observation of voiding).

b. Perineal openings (separate vaginal and urethral openings or a single urogenital sinus): presence of a vagina or a blind vaginal pouch.

c. Gonads: presence, location (scrotal sac, inguinal canal, groin), size, and symmetry.

d. Labioscrotal folds: location (posterior or anterior) and degree of fusion (partial or complete), rugosity.

e. Pigmentation of the genitalia.

2. Assessment findings. Possibilities include:

a. Virilization of a female neonate (Fig. 30-5) can be expressed by degrees of clitoral hypertrophy, partial or complete fusion of the posterior labia, a single urogenital orifice, and hyperpigmentation of the labia, which may also be rugose. Labial fusion can be determined by measuring the anogenital distance (the distance between the anus and the posterior fourchette divided by the distance between the anus and the base of the clitoris). Values greater than 0.5 support labial fusion (Calleghari et al., 1987). Because complete virilization can be mistaken for a male with bilateral cryptorchidism, any term infant with bilateral undescended testes should receive further evaluation.

b. Hypovirilization of a male neonate (Fig. 30-6) may be expressed by a micropenis (with or without chordee), absence of testes in the scrotum, or incomplete fusion of the genital folds (bifid scrotum, resembling labia majora). A urogenital orifice on the perineum may have a small vaginal pouch. A presumed female infant with unilateral or bilateral inguinal hernia(s) should be tested for complete AIS. One or both testes palpable in the scrotum or inguinal region usually indicates a male karyotype, suggesting an undervirilized male (Chi et al., 2008).

c. Infants with mixed gonadal dysgenesis (ovotesticular DSD) may present with marked ambiguity that is asymmetric.

d. When documenting findings of the physical exam, the term *ambiguous genitalia* should not be used, as this term is vague and nondescriptive. Instead, the structures that are present or absent should be noted in descriptive terms.

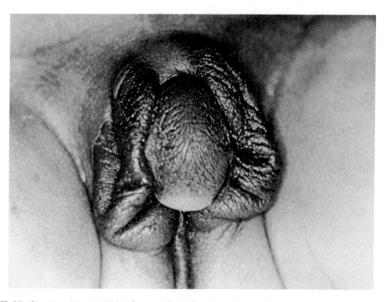

FIGURE 30-5 ■ Virilization in a 46,XX infant with 21-hydroxylase deficiency. Note clitoral hypertrophy and hyperpigmented and rugated labiosacral folds, resembling an empty scrotum. (Courtesy Michael S. Kappy, MD, PhD.)

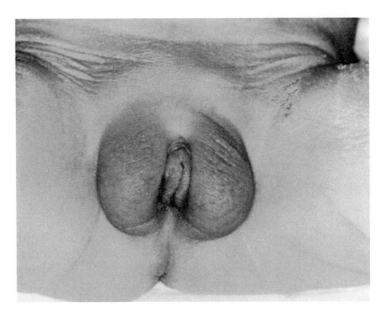

FIGURE 30-6 ■ Infant with karyotype 46,XY and ambiguous genitalia caused by 5-α-reductase deficiency. Note absence of a penis and lack of fusion of labiosacral folds, indicating incomplete virilization. (Courtesy Michael S. Kappy, MD, PhD.)

F. **Diagnosis: a combination of genetic evaluation, clinical and biochemical findings, and examination of internal structures.** It is important to note that in many cases, a precise diagnosis can never be established (Hughes et al., 2007). Numerous algorithms for evaluation of the neonate with a possible DSD have been published, but the evaluation is best tailored to the clinical findings (Hughes et al., 2007).

1. Family history: a similarly affected infant or family member, consanguinity, ingestion of androgens during pregnancy, maternal virilization, or uncontrolled CAH.

2. Karyotype and fluorescence in situ hybridization (FISH) analysis with X- and Y-specific DNA probes.

3. Hormonal studies for a possible underlying endocrine disorder and/or to evaluate response to exogenously administered human chorionic gonadotropin (hCG) or testosterone. This test is more valuable when delayed until the infant is about 4 weeks of age (Hughes et al., 2007). A steroid profile identifies an enzymatic block by revealing any steroid precursors that are elevated or diminished (Chi et al., 2008).

4. Evaluation of internal structures with ultrasonography, magnetic resonance imaging, and radiographic studies (genitography).

5. Laparoscopy/surgical exploration and gonadal biopsy.

6. More extensive tests (molecular genetic studies, enzyme assays of genital skin) for a definitive diagnosis.

G. **Care of the parents.** With advances in prenatal sonography and testing, some infants with genital anomalies are now being identified prior to birth and parents have already been counseled about their infant's condition (Pinhas-Hamiel et al., 2002). In another scenario, determination of fetal gender by routine prenatal ultrasound leads to delivery room confusion when the actual gender of the newborn is uncertain. And finally, parents who wish to be surprised by their infant's gender at birth might find it incomprehensible that doctors and nurses cannot immediately tell them the sex of their newborn infant. With very little time to consider their reply, caregivers are expected to respond to the "simple" question, "Is it a boy or a girl?"

1. Communication and education.

    a. There is little room for error in communications with parents regarding a possible DSD. What health care professionals say to parents in the early hours and days after a baby with a possible DSD is born has a long-lasting impact (Hughes et al., 2007). When faced with an infant of uncertain sex, staff in the delivery room should not announce a gender, no matter how much pressure they feel to do so, because reversing this gender assignment at a later time will be even more difficult for the parents. An alternative is to tell the parents that a difference in their infant's development prevents determination of the sex in the usual way (i.e., by examining the external genitalia).

b. Parents should be shown the infant while the differences from more typical features are explained. The health care professional should not say genitals are "unfinished" (Nabhan and Lee, 2007). Open communication regarding planned tests to determine the infant's sex, and when they may expect to hear results, is advocated.

c. Later, explanations of fetal sexual development, the bipotential nature of developing sexual organs, and critical influences during development are used to help parents understand what caused their infant's development to follow a different path. Important points to convey are as follows:

(1) Their child has the potential to become a well-adjusted person.

(2) A disorder of sexual development is not shameful, but privacy will be respected.

(3) Although the best course of action may not be obvious at first, the team will work with the parents to arrive at the best possible decision (Houk et al., 2006).

d. It is extremely important that the multidisciplinary team (pediatric endocrinologist, surgeon, urologist or gynecologist, psychiatrist, geneticist, neonatologist, social worker, nurse, and medical ethicist) communicate with one another in order to provide consistent, noncontradictory information to the family (Hughes et al., 2007). In addition, strict confidentiality must be maintained (Houk et al., 2006).

e. The Consortium on the Management of Disorders of Sexual Development has prepared a comprehensive, 131-page manual for families, "Handbook for Parents," available as a free download on their Web site, http://www.dsdguidelines.org/. The manual explains how DSDs develop, the treatment options (including surgery), how to talk with the child about his or her condition at different ages, obtaining information from medical professionals, how to talk to family and friends, and more.

2. Emotional support.

a. Anticipate parents' reactions, which may include shock, grief, anger, confusion, uncertainty, and disbelief (Frader et al., 2004). Frustration with long waits for test results may be expressed.

b. Provide guidance in dealing with friends and relatives, a significant source of distress for most parents.

c. Offer to put the parents in touch with people who have experienced similar situations (Frader et al., 2004).

d. It is suggested that parents delay naming the infant and registering the birth.

e. Every effort must be made to encourage parent–infant bonding from the moment of birth.

f. Counseling and professional support for the parents should begin immediately with a clinical psychologist knowledgeable about DSDs.

3. Decision making.

a. In the past, decisions regarding gender assignment and surgery for neonates with intersex disorders were often made primarily by teams of physicians. With parents excluded from full participation, such decisions could have reflected physicians' preferences, customs, or even biases and perpetuated a morally and legally unacceptable paternalism (Daaboul and Frader, 2001).

b. Complete disclosure of information to parents allows them to make fully informed decisions regarding gender assignment and surgery that are in the best interests of their child and family (Blizzard, 2002; Lee and Witchel, 2002).

c. Decisions about gender assignment and timing or type of medical intervention can only be made after full consideration of medical and psychosocial issues. A comprehensive assessment by professionals skilled in the management of DSDs must be made before a gender reassignment is imposed (Hughes et al., 2007).

H. Care of the infant.

1. Information gathering.

a. The birth of an infant with ambiguous genitalia is treated with urgency; diagnostic testing begins immediately. A multidisciplinary team (pediatric endocrinologist, geneticist, pediatric urologic surgeon, radiologist, psychiatrist) may be called to evaluate the infant or consult on the case.

b. It can take several days to get the information needed for some sex-of-rearing decisions. In the interim, sex assignment should not be guessed or made. Neither karyotype nor causative diagnosis can be reliably determined on the basis of the external features (Houk and Lee, 2005).

c. Sex assignment is not determined by any one factor in isolation, such as the chromosomes, gonads, or external anatomy. It is often mistakenly believed that the chromosomal sex of the individual has the greatest degree of influence on the development of gender identity, but in fact chromosomes have the lowest direct impact. Many other factors (e.g., underlying pathophysiology, prognosis for pubertal development, future sexual function and sensation, fertility, chances for a satisfactory surgical repair and need for additional procedures, and cultural beliefs and values of the family) are considered when sex-of-rearing decisions are made.

2. Gender assignment.

a. The majority of 46,XX neonates with CAH are raised as girls, regardless of the degree of virilization, because internal structures are female, fertility is possible, and most develop a female gender identity.

b. 46,XY neonates with defects of testosterone synthesis or gonadotropin deficiencies are usually raised as boys because they may respond to hormonal treatment with phallic growth and testicular descent. A stimulation test (hCG) may be given to evaluate this response. Neonates with 5-α-reductase deficiency are also assigned the male gender because they will virilize at puberty.

c. Gender assignment of 46,XY neonates with partial androgen insensitivity depends on the individual phenotype and in some cases, the results of additional testing conducted in the newborn period.

d. Occasionally, after considerable testing, consultation with experts, and discussions with parents, the decision is made to raise a severely undervirilized 46,XY neonate as a female. At the present time, data are insufficient to predict a child's eventual gender identity based on underlying condition or appearance of the genitalia, rendering these decisions difficult for parents and professionals alike.

3. Surgical considerations.

a. Decisions regarding surgery might not be finalized in the neonatal period, but the same issues faced during gender assignment decisions will have to be addressed when discussing surgical management. Although it is hoped that the child will adapt to the chosen sex of rearing, if surgery is carried out too early and a different gender identity becomes apparent, the outcome can be disastrous (Warne and Kanumakala, 2002).

b. Controversy exists regarding the performance of genital surgery on neonates with intersex conditions unless it is medically necessary. Former patients who were irreversibly harmed by gender reconstruction in infancy point out that such procedures are often done for cosmetic purposes only, and should be deferred until the child is old enough to give consent (Intersex Society of North America, 2006). The Intersex Society of North America recommends a patient-centered care approach that involves assigning a gender (boy or girl) and performing medically necessary procedures but postponing genital-altering surgery.

c. Parents must be advised about the consequences of surgical intervention: what can and cannot be accomplished with surgery, the irreversibility of surgery, and the possible complications. Parents must also be made aware of the alternatives to immediate surgery (Hughes et al., 2007).

d. The availability of a surgical technique that will normalize the appearance of the genitals does not alone provide justification for surgery (Frader et al., 2004), nor should surgery be performed on the infant to relieve parental anxiety (Crouch and Creighton, 2004).

e. Parents and child should receive ongoing counseling and psychological support.

I. **Complications.**

1. Inappropriate sex assignment when the ambiguity was not detected in the neonatal period.

2. Gonadal or genital duct malignancy.

J. Outcome.

1. Some children undergoing genital surgery will require staged reconstructive procedures and, at puberty, hormonal therapy to induce development of gender-appropriate secondary sexual characteristics. One-stage surgeries performed in infancy often have poor outcomes (Crouch and Creighton, 2004).

2. Reproductive capacity varies according to the condition. Fertility is possible in some circumstances (e.g., in a woman with CAH) but is rare or impossible in others (complete AIS, some forms of gonadal dysgenesis).

3. Outcome studies of intersex disorders are limited. Available data reveal that the affected child and the family face difficulties that extend well beyond the initial crisis in the neonatal period (Slijper et al., 1998). With patients sometimes "lost to follow-up," professionals may not always be fully aware of the lifelong implications of decisions that were made in the first days of life.

PANCREATIC DISORDERS

A. Anatomy and physiology.

1. The pancreas is both an endocrine and exocrine gland.
2. Endocrine pancreas controls blood glucose levels.
3. Specialized hormone-producing cells are called islets of Langerhans.
4. Hormones of the endocrine pancreas are glucagon, insulin, amylin, and somatostatin.

B. Fetal and neonatal pancreatic function.

1. Fetal insulin is produced at 8 to 10 weeks in response to glucose and amino acids. Insulin does not cross the placenta, so the fetus is dependent on its own insulin production. At birth, the supply of maternal glucose is ended, precipitating a fall in the neonate's blood glucose and plasma insulin levels.

   a. Counterregulatory hormones (epinephrine, glucagon) are released to stimulate glucose production by the neonate, protecting the neonatal brain until feeding is established.

C. Disorders of the pancreas: Rare congenital pancreatic disorders include pancreatic agenesis, pancreatic hypoplasia, and annular pancreas. Disorders of the endocrine pancreas include neonatal diabetes mellitus and hyperinsulinism. The most common disorder of the exocrine pancreas is cystic fibrosis.

1. Infant of a diabetic mother (IDM) (see Chapter 9, p. 177).
2. Neonatal diabetes mellitus (see Chapter 9, p. 179).
3. Congenital hyperinsulinism. Most frequent cause of severe persistent hypoglycemia in the newborn.

   a. Unregulated insulin release from the entire pancreas (diffuse β-cell hyperfunction) or from confined areas of the pancreas (focal adenomatous islet-cell hyperplasia).

   b. Excess insulin lowers circulating glucose and suppresses lipolysis and ketogenesis, reducing the availability of free fatty acids and ketone bodies for brain energy.

   c. Onset is within the first few days of life with severe hypoglycemia. Some are macrosomic at birth and those with Beckwith–Wiedemann present with macroglossia, abdominal wall defects, Wilms tumors, renal anomalies, and facial nevi.

   d. Diagnosis is made by finding an insulin level that is inappropriate to the blood glucose level. Blood samples must be taken during hypoglycemia.

   e. Management is to provide a high calorie intake; glucose infusions of 12 to 16 mg/kg/minute may be required via central line.

   f. Pharmacologic therapy includes diazoxide and octreotide. If there is no response to medical management, surgical removal of all or part of the pancreas may be necessary.

4. Cystic fibrosis (CF) is an autosomal recessive disorder caused by mutations in the gene encoding for the cystic fibrosis transmembrane conductance regulator. CF has an incidence of 1 in 2500 infants; most common among non-Hispanic whites.

   a. Deficient transport of chloride across epithelia, with compensatory excessive influx of sodium into the epithelial cells is the mechanism underlying the viscid mucus characteristic of CF. Nearly all organ systems are affected.

   b. CF is heterogenous; some patients have all the classical manifestations of multisystem organ involvement and a poor prognosis, whereas others have mild or atypical CF (De Boeck et al., 2006).

   c. Earliest indication of CF in the newborn is often a sticky plug of mucus (meconium ileus) caused by hyperviscous intestinal secretions and a deficiency of pancreatic enzymes.

   d. Typically not diagnosed in the neonatal period unless a meconium ileus is present. Affected babies may have signs of intestinal obstruction (abdominal distention, bilious vomiting, failure to pass meconium or passing gray-colored stools).

   e. Quantitative pilocarpine iontophoresis (sweat chloride test) can be done after the first two weeks of life. The sweat chloride test involves collecting sweat for 30 minutes onto a preweighed filter paper. The diagnosis is confirmed with mutation analysis. The American College of Medical Genetics has identified CF as one of 29 conditions that should be included in all state newborn screening panels (American College of Medical Genetics, 2006).

   f. Meconium ileus must be corrected as quickly as possible to prevent perforation, bowel necrosis, or volvulus. A Gastrografin enema used when the intestines are still intact evacuates inspissated meconium from the bowel.

REFERENCES

Alizai, N.K., Thomas, D.F., Lilford, R.J., Batchelor, A.G., and Johnson, N.: Feminizing genitoplasty for congenital adrenal hyperplasia: What happens at puberty? *Journal of Urology*, 161(5):1588-1591, 1999.

American College of Medical Genetics: Newborn screening: Toward a uniform screening panel and system. 2006. Retrieved March 10, 2008, from www.acmg.net/resources/policies/NBS/NBS_Exec_Sum.pdf

Anway, M.D. and Skinner, M.K.: Epigenetic programming of the germ line: Effects of endocrine disruptors on the development of transgenerational disease. *Reproductive Biomedicine Online*, 16(1):23-25, 2008.

Biswas, S., Buffery, J., Enoch, H., et al: Longitudinal assessment of thyroid hormone concentrations in preterm infants younger than 30 weeks gestation during the first 2 weeks of life and their relationship to outcome. *Pediatrics*, 109(2):222-227, 2002.

Blizzard, R.M.: Intersex issues: A series of continuing conundrums. *Pediatrics*, 110(3):616-621, 2002.

Bolt, R.J., van Weissenbruch, M.M., Lafeber, H.N., and Delemarre-van de Waal, H.A.: Development of the hypothalamic–pituitary–adrenal axis in the fetus and preterm infant. *Journal of Pediatric Endocrinology and Metabolism*, 15(6):759-769, 2002.

Brook, G.D. and Brown R.S.: *Handbook of clinical pediatric endocrinology*. Malden, MA, 2008, Blackwell.

Calleghari, C., Everett, S., Ross, M., and Brasel, J.A.: Anogenital ratio: Measure of fetal virilization in premature and full-term newborn infants. *Journal of Pediatrics*, 111(2):240-243, 1987.

Canadian Organization for Rare Disorders: *Newborn screening status report*. Retrieved March 5, 2008, from http://www.raredisorders.ca/index.php/site/resources/newborn_screening

Chi, C., Lee, H.C., and Kirk Neely, E.: Ambiguous genitalia in the newborn. *NeoReviews*, 9:e78-84, 2008.

Chrousos, G.P.: Organization and integration of the endocrine system. In M.A. Sperling (Ed.): *Pediatric endocrinology* (2nd ed.). Philadelphia, 2002, Saunders.

Clemente, M., Ruiz-Cuevas, P., Carrascosa, A., et al.: Thyroid function in preterm infants 27-29 weeks of gestational age during the first four months of life: Results from a prospective study comprising 80 preterm infants. *Journal of Pediatric Endocrinology & Metabolism*, 20(12):1269-1280, 2007.

Custodio, R.J., Junior, C.E., Milani, S.L., Simoes, A.L., de Castro, M., and Moreira, A.C.: The emergence of the cortisol circadian rhythm in monozygotic and dizygotic twin infants: The twin-pair synchrony. *Clinical Endocrinology (Oxford)*, 66(2):192-197, 2007.

Crouch, N.S. and Creighton, S.M.: Minimal surgical intervention in the management of intersex conditions. *Journal of Pediatric Endocrinology and Metabolism*, 17(12):1591-1596, 2004.

Crouch, N.S., Liao, M.L., Woodhouse, R.J., Conway, G.S., and Creighton, S.M.: Sexual function and genital sensitivity following feminizing genitoplasty for congenital adrenal hyperplasia. *Journal of Urology*, 179(2):634-638, 2008.

Daaboul, J. and Frader, J.: Ethics and management of the patient with intersex: A middle way. *Journal of Pediatric Endocrinology and Metabolism*, 14(9):1575-1583, 2001.

Dayner, J.E., Lee, P.A., and Houk, C.P.: Medical treatment of intersex: Parental perspectives. *Journal of Urology*, 172(4 Pt 2):1762-1765, 2004.

De Boeck, K., Wilschanski, M., Castellani, C., et al., for the Diagnostic Working Group: Cystic fibrosis: Terminology and diagnostic algorithms. *Thorax*, 61(7):627-635, 2006.

Dempsher, D.: Adrenal and pituitary insufficiency in the neonate. *NeoReviews*, 8(7):e72-e77, 2008.

Dewing, P., Bernard, P., and Vilain, E.: Disorders of gonadal development. *Seminars in Reproductive Medicine*, 20(3):189-197, 2002.

Fisher, D.A.: The importance of early management in optimizing IQ in infants with congenital hypothyroidism. *Journal of Pediatrics*, 136(3):273-274, 2000.

Fisher, D.A.: Thyroid function and dysfunction in premature infants. *Pediatric Endocrinology Reviews*, 4(4):317-328, 2007.

Forghani, N. and Aye, T.: Hypothyroxinemia and prematurity. *NeoReviews*, 9(2):e66-e71, 2008.

Frader, J., Alderson, P., Asch, A., et al.: Health care professionals and intersex conditions. *Archives of Pediatric and Adolescent Medicine*, 158(5):426-428, 2004.

Grunau, R.E., Haley, D.W., Whitfield, M.F., Weinberg, J., Yu, W., and Thiessen, P.: Altered basal cortisol levels at 3, 6, 8 and 18 months in infants born at extremely low gestational age. *Journal of Pediatrics*, 150(2):151-156, 2007.

Houk, C.P., Hughes, I.A., Ahmed, S.F., Lee, P.A., for the Writing Committee for the International Intersex Consensus Conference Participants: Summary of consensus statement on intersex disorders and their management. International Intersex Consensus Conference. *Pediatrics*, 118(2):753-757, 2006.

Houk, C.P. and Lee, P.A.: Intersexed states: Diagnosis and management. *Endocrinology and Metabolism Clinics of North America*, 34(3):791-810, 2005.

Hughes, I.A., Nihoul-Fekete, C., Thomas, B., and Cohen-Kettenis, P.T.: Consequences of the ESPE/LWPES guidelines for diagnosis and treatment of disorders of sex development. *Best Practice & Research Clinical Endocrinology & Metabolism*, 21(3):351-365, 2007.

Hyman, S.J., Greig, F., Holzman, I., Patel, A., Wallach, E., and Rapaport, R.: Late rise of thyroid stimulating hormone in ill newborns. *Journal of Pediatric Endocrinology and Metabolism*, 20(4):501-510, 2007.

Intersex Society of North America: *What does the ISNA recommend for children with intersex?* 2006. Retrieved February 28, 2008, from www.isna.org

Kok, J.H., Briet, J.M., and van Wassenaer, A.G.: Postnatal thyroid hormone replacement in very low birth weight infants. *Seminars in Perinatology*, 25(6):417-425, 2001.

LaFranchi, S.H. and Austin, J.: How should we be treating children with congenital hypothyroidism. *Journal of Pediatric Endocrinology and Metabolism*, 20(5):559-577, 2007.

Larson, C., Hermos, R., Delaney, A., Daley, D., and Mitchell, M.: Risk factors associated with delayed thyrotropin elevations in congenital hypothyroidism. *Journal of Pediatrics*, 143(5):587-591, 2003.

Lee, P.A. and Witchel, S.F.: Genital surgery among females with congenital adrenal hyperplasia: Changes over the past five decades. *Journal of Pediatric Endocrinology and Metabolism*, 15(9):1473-1477, 2002.

Leviton, A., Paneth, N., Reuss, M.L., et al.: Hypothyroxinemia of prematurity and the risk of cerebral white matter damage. *Journal of Pediatrics*, 134(6):706-711, 1999.

Mandel, S.J., Hermos, R.J., Larson, C.A., et al.: Atypical hypothyroidism and the very low birth weight infant. *Thyroid*, 10(8):693-695, 2000.

Meyer-Bahlburg, H.F.L.: Gender and sexuality in classic congenital adrenal hyperplasia. *Endocrinology and Metabolism Clinics of North America*, 30(1):155-171, 2001.

Miller, W.: The adrenal cortex. In M.A. Sperling (Ed.): *Pediatric endocrinology* (2nd ed.). Philadelphia, 2002, Saunders.

Nabhan, Z.M. and Lee, P.A.: Disorders of sex development. *Current Opinions in Obstetrics and Gynecology*, 19(5):440-445, 2007.

National Institute of Environmental Health Science: *Endocrine disruptors*. Retrieved January 16, 2008, from http://www.niehs.nih.gov/health/topics/agents/endocrine/docs/endocrine.pdf

National Newborn Screening and Genetics Resource Center: *National newborn screening report 2000*. Retrieved February 28, 2008, from http://genes-r-us.uthscsa.edu/resources/newborn/00chapters.html

National Newborn Screening and Genetics Resource Center: *National newborn screening status report, March 2008*. Retrieved from http://genes-r-us.uthscsa.edu/nbsdisorders.pdf

Ng, P.C., Lee, C.H., Lam, C.W., et al.: Transient adrenocortical insufficiency and systemic hypotension in very low birth weight infants. *Archives of Disease in Childhood, Fetal Neonatal Edition*, 89(2):F119-F126, 2004.

Nimkarn, S. and New, M.I.: Prenatal diagnosis and treatment of congenital adrenal hyperplasia. *Pediatric Endocrinology Reviews*, 4(2):99-105, 2006.

Obregon, M.J., Calvo, R.M., Del Ray, F.E., and de Escobar, G.M.: Ontogenesis of thyroid function and interactions with maternal function. *Endocrine Development*, 10:86-98, 2007.

Osborn, D.A. and Hunt, R.W.: Postnatal prophylactic thyroid hormones for prevention of morbidity and mortality in preterm infants. *Cochrane Database of Systematic Reviews*, 24(1):CD005948, 2007.

Oden, J. and Freemark, M.: Thyroxine supplementation in preterm infants. *Current Opinion in Pediatrics*, 14(4):447-452, 2002.

Ogilvy-Stuart, A.L. and Midgley, P.: *Practical neonatal endocrinology*. Cambridge, MA, 2006, Cambridge University Press.

Ogilvy-Stuart, A.L.: Neonatal thyroid disorders. *Archives of Disease in Childhood Fetal Neonatal Edition*, 87(3):F165-F171, 2002.

Paul, D.A., Leef, K.H., Voss B., et al.: Thyroxine and illness severity in very low-birth-weight infants. *Thyroid*, 11(9):871-875, 2001.

Peters, C.J. and Hindmarsh, P.C.: Management of neonatal endocrinopathies—Best practice guidelines. *Early Human Development*, 83:553-561, 2007.

Pinhas-Hamiel, O., Zalel, Y., Smith, E., et al.: Prenatal diagnosis of sex differentiation disorders: The role of fetal ultrasound. *Journal of Clinical Endocrinology and Metabolism*, 87(10):4547-4553, 2002.

Rapaport, R., Rose, S., and Freemark, M.: Hypothyroxinemia in the preterm infant: The benefits and risks of thyroxine treatment. *Journal of Pediatrics*, 139(2):182-188, 2001.

Root, A.: Thyroid function in extremely premature neonates: A reference database. *Journal of Pediatric Endocrinology and Metabolism*, 20(12):1267-1268, 2007.

Schnitzer, J.J. and Donahoe, P.K.: Surgical treatment of congenital adrenal hyperplasia. *Endocrinology and Metabolism Clinics of North America*, 30(1):137-154, 2001.

Selva, K.A., Mandel, S.H., Rien, L.R., et al.: Initial treatment dose of L-thyroxine in congenital hypothyroidism. *Journal of Pediatrics*, 141(6):786-792, 2002.

Slijper, F.M., Drop, S.L., Molenaar, J.C., and de Muinck Keizer-Schrama, S.M.: Long-term psychological evaluation of intersex children. *Archives of Sexual Behavior*, 27(2):125-145, 1998.

Therrell, B.L.: Newborn screening for congenital adrenal hyperplasia. *Endocrinology and Metabolism Clinics of North America*, 30(1):15-29, 2001.

Therrell, B.L., Berenbaum, S.A., Manter-Kapanke, V., et al.: Results of screening 1.9 million Texas newborns for 21-hydroxylase deficient congenital adrenal hyperplasia. *Pediatrics*, 101(4 Pt 1):583-590, 1998.

Tylek-Lema ska, D., Kumorowicz-Kopiec, M., and Starzyk, J.: Screening for congenital hypothyroidism: The value of retesting after four weeks in neonates with low and very low birth weight. *Journal of Medical Screening*, 12(4):166-169, 2005.

Van Trotsenburg, A.S., Kempers, M.J., Endert, E., Tijssen, J.G., de Vijlder, J.J., and Vulsma, T.: Trisomy 21 causes persistent congenital hypothyroidism presumably of thyroidal origin. *Thyroid*, 16(7):671-680, 2006.

van Wassenaer, A.G., Briet, J.M., van Baar, A., et al.: Free thyroxine levels during the first weeks of life and neurodevelopmental outcome until the age of 5 years in very preterm infants. *Pediatrics*, 109(3):534-539, 2002.

van Wassenaer, A.G., Westera, J., Houtzager, B.A., and Kok, J.H.: Ten-year follow-up of children born at <30 weeks' gestational age supplemented with thyroxine in the neonatal period in a randomized, controlled trial. *Pediatrics*, 116(5):e613-618, 2005.

Vincent, M.A., Rodd, C., Dussault, J.H., and Van Vliet, G.: Very low birth weight newborns do not need repeat screening for congenital hypothyroidism. *Journal of Pediatrics*, 140(3):311-314, 2002.

Warne, G.L. and Kanumakala, S.: Molecular endocrinology of sex differentiation. *Seminars in Reproductive Medicine*, 20(3):169-179, 2002.

Wilson, J.D.: The evolution of endocrinology. *Clinical Endocrinology*, 62(4):389-396, 2005.

31 Hematologic Disorders

WILLIAM DIEHL-JONES and DEBBIE FRASER ASKIN

OBJECTIVES

1. Understand the processes of hematopoiesis and erythropoiesis.
2. Recall erythrocyte and leukocyte development from pluripotent stem cells.
3. Relate the consequences of anemia to the management of the infant.
4. Evaluate the clinical presentation of disseminated intravascular coagulation in relation to the coagulation consumption and fibrinolysis.
5. Describe the etiologic factors of hemorrhagic disease of the newborn.
6. Describe key indicators for nursing assessment of the thrombocytopenic infant.
7. Evaluate the neonatal consequences of maternal immune thrombocytopenic purpura.
8. Discuss the role of partial exchange transfusion in the treatment of neonatal polycythemia.
9. Describe current recommendations for use of blood components.
10. Analyze the components of the complete blood cell count and describe the usefulness of each in the determination of neonatal sepsis.

To meet the objectives, the chapter presents an overview of blood cell development and coagulation factors, and includes normal birth values and common diagnostic tests. Blood products and transfusion therapies are discussed with current recommendations for use. Common hematologic problems and therapies affecting the newborn infant are outlined. An evaluation of the red blood cell indices, useful for diagnosis of hematologic disorders, is included.

DEVELOPMENT OF BLOOD CELLS

A. **Hematopoiesis:** formation, production, and maintenance of blood cells (Blackburn, 2007; Blanchette et al., 2005; Israels and Israels, 2002; Luchtman-Jones et al., 2006; Ohls, 2004).
1. Pluripotent stem cells, from which all blood cells derive, are present in the yolk sac at 16 days of gestation.
2. Circulation begins by day 22, with primitive cells arising intravascularly from vessel walls.
3. Extravascular liver hematopoiesis begins with migration of pluripotent stem cells from the yolk sac, well established by 9 weeks of gestation.
4. Liver hematopoiesis peaks at 4 to 5 months of gestation and then slowly regresses as medullary (bone marrow) hematopoiesis predominates from 22 weeks of gestation.
5. Sites of extramedullary hematopoiesis (spleen, lymph nodes, thymus, kidneys) aid production of cells during fetal life when long bones are small.
6. Pluripotent cells develop into either colony-forming unit–granulocyte, erythrocyte, monocyte, megakaryocyte (CFU-GEMM), or lymphoid stem cells, which evolve into specific cell lines (Fig. 31-1).
7. Hypoxia, bacterial infection, and other forms of physiologic stress can influence the rate of differentiation of pluripotent cells.
8. Hematopoietic factors include interleukins (e.g., IL-1, IL-3, and IL-5), growth and differentiation factors such as granulocyte colony-stimulating factor (G-CSF), monocyte colony-

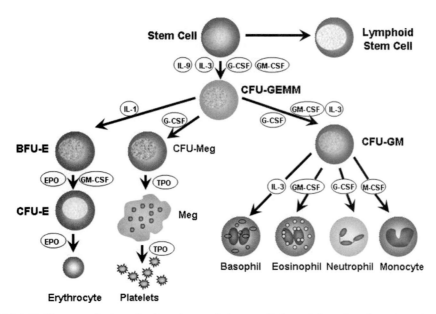

FIGURE 31-1 ■ Hematopoiesis and selected growth factors. (Adapted from Israels, L.G. and Israels, S.J.: *Mechanisms in hematology* [3rd ed.]. Toronto, 2002, Core Health Sciences, Inc., p. 402.)

stimulating factor (M-CSF), granulocyte–monocyte colony-stimulating factor (GM-CSF), thrombopoietin (TPO), and erythropoietin (EPO).

B. **Erythropoiesis:** production of erythrocytes (red blood cells [RBCs]).
   1. The erythrocyte precursor or burst-forming unit–erythroid (BFU-E) develops from a myeloid stem cell (CFU-GEMM), which also differentiates to produce a megakaryocyte precursor (CFU-Meg).
   2. Erythropoiesis and synthesis of hemoglobin are regulated by a hormone, erythropoietin, which is in turn regulated by hypoxia.
   3. Erythropoietin is produced postnatally in the kidneys, but during fetal life extrarenal sites (liver, submandibular glands) predominate.
   4. Erythropoietin levels are increased in response to anemia and low oxygen availability to tissues and are decreased in response to hypertransfusion.
   5. Erythropoietin levels are also elevated in infants with Down syndrome, intrauterine growth restriction, and those born to women with diabetes or pregnancy-induced hypertension (PIH).

C. **Hemoglobin:** major iron-containing component of the RBCs.
   1. Hemoglobin carries oxygen from the lungs to the tissue cells through the circulation.
   2. Hemoglobin synthesis begins around 14 days of embryonic life.
   3. Transition from predominant production of fetal hemoglobin (HbF) to production of adult hemoglobin (HbA) begins at the end of fetal life. RBCs contain 70% to 90% HbF at birth.
   4. Hemoglobin binds with 2,3-diphosphoglycerate (2,3-DPG), releasing an oxygen molecule.
      a. HbF has far less affinity for 2,3-DPG than does HbA, resulting in a greater affinity for oxygen.
      b. Levels of 2,3-DPG are directly proportional to gestational age.
   5. Normal birth values (Table 31-1).
      a. Values depend on gestational age, volume of placental transfusion (timing of cord clamping, infant position), and blood sampling site; Hb in capillary samples may be significantly higher than in venous samples.
      b. Peripheral vasoconstriction and stasis yield higher values from capillary samples.
      c. Hb levels are higher in newborns, and decrease by the end of the first week of life to values similar to cord blood.

■ TABLE 31-1
■ ■ **Normal Blood Values in Premature and Term Infants**

Value	Gestational Age (weeks)		Term Cord Blood	Day 1	Day 3	Day 7	Day 14
	28	34					
Hb (g/dl)	14.5	15	16.8	18.4	17.8	17	16.8
Hematocrit (%)	45	47	53	58	55	54	52
Red cells (mm^3)	4	4.4	5.25	5.8	5.6	5.2	5.1
MCV (μ^3)	120	118	107	108	99	98	96
MCH (pg)	40	38	34	35	33	32.5	31.5
MCHC (%)	31	32	31.7	32.5	33	33	33
Reticulocytes (%)	5 to 10	3 to 10	3 to 7	3 to 7	1 to 3	0 to 1	0 to 1
Platelets (1000 s/mm^3)			290	192	213	248	252

Hb, Hemoglobin; *MCH*, mean corpuscular hemoglobin; *MCHC*, mean corpuscular hemoglobin concentration; *MCV*, mean corpuscular volume.
From Klaus, M.H. and Fanaroff, A.A.: *Care of the high-risk neonate* (5th ed.). Philadelphia, 2001, Saunders.

    d. Increased Pao$_2$ following delivery and increase in HbA causes a decrease in erythro-poietin, leading to a gradual decline in hemoglobin (Kates and Kates, 2007).

D. Hematocrit: percentage of RBCs in a unit volume of blood.
    1. Values rise immediately after birth and then decline to cord levels in the first week.
    2. Normal birth values (see Table 31-1).
        a. Values depend on gestational age and volume of placental transfusion (timing of cord clamping, infant position).
        b. Peripheral vasoconstriction and stasis yield higher values from capillary samples.

E. RBCs.
    1. The erythrocyte BFU-E differentiates, under hormonal control, to form a CFU-E (colony-forming unit–erythrocyte), which loses its nucleus as it forms erythrocytes (see Fig. 31-1).
    2. The CFU-E (or reticulocyte), in the absence of physiologic stress, mature 1 to 2 days in the bone marrow and then another day in the circulation before maturing to erythrocytes.
        a. Reticulocyte count is inversely proportional to gestational age at birth (see Table 31-1) but falls rapidly to less than 2% by 7 days.
        b. Persistent reticulocytosis may indicate chronic blood loss or hemolysis.
    3. RBC function.
        a. Oxygen transport via oxyhemoglobin.
        b. Carbon dioxide transport via carboxyhemoglobin.
        c. Carbon dioxide reacts with water to form carbonic acid; reaction catalyzed by carbonic anhydrase in the cytoplasm of RBCs.
        d. Carbonic acid dissociation to form bicarbonate ions.
        e. Buffering protons via binding with hemoglobin to form acid hemoglobin and by reaction with bicarbonate ions.
    4. RBC count.
        a. Number of circulating mature RBCs per cubic millimeter (see Table 31-1).
        b. Count equals production versus destruction or loss.
        c. RBC life span proportional to gestational age.
            (1) Adult: 100 to 120 days.
            (2) Term infant: 60 to 70 days.
            (3) Premature infant: 35 to 50 days.
        d. Nucleated RBCs are circulating immature (prereticulocyte) red cells.
            (1) Number is inversely proportional to gestational age and declines rapidly in the first week.
            (2) Increase may indicate hemolysis, acute blood loss, hypoxemia, congenital heart disease, or infection.

5. RBC indices: measure of RBC size and hemoglobin content used for designation of anemias (see Table 31-1).
   a. Mean corpuscular volume (MCV): average size and volume of a single RBC.
      (1) MCV decreases as gestation progresses and continues to decrease after birth to adult size by 4 to 5 years.
      (2) Increased MCV: RBCs referred to as macrocytes.
      (3) Decreased MCV: RBCs referred to as microcytes.
   b. Mean corpuscular hemoglobin (MCH): average amount (by weight) of hemoglobin in each RBC.
      (1) A decrease in MCH parallels a decrease in MCV.
      (2) Increased MCH: RBCs appear hyperchromic.
      (3) Decreased MCH: RBCs appear hypochromic.
   c. Mean corpuscular hemoglobin concentration (MCHC): average concentration of hemoglobin per single RBC, calculated from the amount of hemoglobin per deciliter of cells.
      (1) Adult values for MCHC reached by 6 months.
      (2) Increased MCHC: RBCs appear hyperchromic.
      (3) Decreased MCHC: RBCs appear hypochromic.
   d. Erythrocyte mass: total mass of erythrocytes.
      (1) Best measure of anemia.
      (2) Direct correlation between erythrocyte mass and hemoglobin concentration.
      (3) Gold standard is use of chromium-labeled erythrocytes.
F. **White blood cells (WBCs).**
   1. Leukocyte precursors mature in the bone marrow and lymphatic tissues, in the absence of physiologic stress, through the CFU-GEMM and granulocyte macrophage (CFU-GM) stages (see Fig. 31-1).
   2. WBCs can leave the circulation to the extravascular tissues, where they function as an important part of the immunologic system in reaction to foreign protein.
   3. Granulocytes, lymphocytes, and monocytes are types of WBCs.
      a. Granulocytes: include basophils, eosinophils, and neutrophils.
         (1) Basophils.
            (a) Important in allergic and inflammatory responses.
            (b) Least numerous of the granulocytes: 0.5% to 1% of total WBC count.
         (2) Eosinophils.
            (a) Perform similar functions as neutrophils but are less effective in response.
            (b) Unlike neutrophils, can survive for prolonged periods in extravascular space.
            (c) Important in allergic and anaphylactic responses and most effective granulocyte for parasitic destruction.
            (d) Benign eosinophilia of prematurity, inversely proportional to gestational age, may reflect immaturity of barrier mechanisms in the gastrointestinal and/or respiratory tract (Blanchette et al., 2005).
            (e) Normally comprise 1% to 3% of total WBC count.
         (3) Neutrophils.
            (a) Neutrophils function as phagocytes that ingest and destroy small particles such as bacteria, protozoa, cells and cellular debris, and colloids.
            (b) Physiologic stress can increase production and bone marrow release of immature forms.
            (c) Neutrophils are increased at birth but decrease during the first week to reach percentages approximately equal to those of lymphocytes.
      b. Lymphocytes.
         (1) Thymus-derived (T) lymphocytes: important in graft-versus-host disease and delayed hypersensitivity reactions.
         (2) Bone marrow–derived (B) lymphocytes: important in the production and secretion of immunoglobulins and antibodies.
      c. Monocytes.
         (1) Circulating immature macrophages.

■ TABLE 31-2
■ ■ **Normal Leukocyte Values in Premature and Term Infants**

Age (hours)	Total White Cell Count	Neutrophils	Bands/Metas	Lymphocytes	Monocytes	Eosinophils
TERM INFANTS						
0	10.0 to 26.0	5.0 to 13.0	0.4 to 1.8	3.5 to 8.5	0.7 to 1.5	0.2 to 2.0
12	13.5 to 31.0	9.0 to 18.0	0.4 to 2.0	3.0 to 7.0	1.0 to 2.0	0.2 to 2.0
72	5.0 to 14.5	2.0 to 7.0	0.2 to 0.4	2.0 to 5.0	0.5 to 1.0	0.2 to 1.0
144	6.0 to 14.5	2.0 to 6.0	0.2 to 0.5	3.0 to 6.0	0.7 to 1.2	0.2 to 0.8
PREMATURE INFANTS						
0	5.0 to 19.0	2.0 to 9.0	0.2 to 2.4	2.5 to 6.0	0.3 to 1.0	0.1 to 0.7
12	5.0 to 21.0	3.0 to 11.0	0.2 to 2.4	1.5 to 5.0	0.3 to 1.3	0.1 to 1.1
72	5.0 to 14.0	3.0 to 7.0	0.2 to 0.6	1.5 to 4.0	0.3 to 1.2	0.2 to 1.1
144	5.5 to 17.5	2.0 to 7.0	0.2 to 0.5	2.5 to 7.5	0.5 to 1.5	0.3 to 1.2

Data modified from Xanthou (1970) by Glader (1977).
From Oski, F.A. and Naiman, J.L.: *Hematologic problems in the newborn* (3rd ed.). Philadelphia, 1982, Saunders.

    (2) Transformed into macrophages in tissues (i.e., lung, alveolar macrophage; liver, Kupffer cell macrophages).
    (3) Responsible for clearance of old blood cells, cellular debris, opsonized bacteria, antigen–antibody complexes, and activated clotting factors from the circulation.
  4. WBC count.
    a. WBC count is the number of circulating WBCs per cubic millimeter (Table 31-2).
    b. WBC count is proportional to gestational age, with the total counts of premature infants approximately 30% to 50% lower than those of term infants.
G. Platelets.
  1. Small, nonnucleated, disk-shaped cells aid in hemostasis, coagulation, and thrombus formation.
    a. Platelets are derived from megakaryocytes in the bone marrow.
    b. Disrupted endothelium stimulates platelet plug formation and initiates hemostasis.
  2. After release into the bloodstream, platelets will circulate 7 to 10 days before removal by the spleen. In the absence of injury, they circulate freely, without wall adhesion or aggregation with other platelets.
  3. Normal range is 150,000 to 400,000/mm^3 in the term and the premature infant. Counts are 20% to 25% lower in infants who are small for gestational age.
  4. Neonatal platelets are hypoactive in the first few days after birth; this property protects against thrombosis but may increase risk of bleeding and coagulopathy.
H. Blood volume.
  1. Volume of blood is measured in milliliters per kilogram of body weight.
  2. Factors affecting blood volume are as follows:
    a. Gestational age.
      (1) Term infant: approximately 80 to 100 ml/kg.
      (2) Preterm infant: approximately 90 to 105 ml/kg.
    b. Placental transfusion.
      (1) Timing of cord clamping.
      (2) Position of infant relative to placenta (above or below) before cord clamping.
      (3) Timing and strength of uterine contractions.
      (4) Onset of respiration and decrease in pulmonary vascular resistance.
      (5) Cord compression.
    c. Maternal–fetal or fetal–maternal transfusion.
    d. Twin–twin transfusion.

    e. Placenta previa or abruptio placentae.
    f. Nuchal cord.
    g. Iatrogenic loss.

COAGULATION

Hemostasis is accomplished by biochemical and physiologic events initiated to stop the flow of blood when vessel injury occurs (Israels and Israels, 2002).
A. Deficiencies in newborn clotting mechanisms.
    1. Transient diminished platelet function.
    2. Transient deficiency of clotting factors II, VII, IX, X, XI, and XII. Neonatal levels are approximately 50% of adult levels in the early weeks after birth (Blackburn, 2007).
        a. Immaturity of hepatic enzymes responsible for production.
        b. Transient deficiency of vitamin K, needed for synthesis of factors II, VII, IX, and X.
        c. Factor concentrations: proportional to gestational age.
B. Hemostatic mechanisms.
    1. Vascular: damaged vessel contracts, minimizing blood loss.
    2. Intravascular: platelet plug formation. Platelet function is stimulated by exposure to damaged endothelial lining. Platelets:
        a. Swell and develop thornlike projections.
        b. Adhere to subendothelial fibers.
        c. Secrete adenosine diphosphate to trigger swelling and adhesiveness in nearby platelets.
        d. Aggregate and form platelet plug.
    3. Extravascular.
        a. Compression by surrounding tissue.
        b. Release of tissue thromboplastin by injured tissue.
C. Coagulation process.
    1. Cascade of events, requiring both cellular and plasma components (Fig. 31-2).
    2. Culminates in the formation of fibrin-based clots, and requires serial activation of precursor zymogens.
    3. Calcium, iron, and phospholipids are key components of the coagulation cascade.
        a. Extrinsic system triggered by tissue injury and exposure of cell membrane tissue factor (TF).
        b. Intrinsic system triggered by vascular endothelial injury; amplifies factor X activation, which is a cofactor common to intrinsic and extrinsic pathways.
        c. Factor X activation begins the process of prothrombin-to-thrombin conversion. Conversion hydrolyzes fibrinogen (soluble protein in plasma) to fibrin (insoluble, threadlike polymer) and activates factor XIII, stabilizing fibrin threads into a meshwork to trap platelets and other cells to form the clot.
    4. Intravascular clotting is balanced by concurrent fibrinolysis.
        a. Inactive plasminogen synthesized by the liver is converted to plasmin, an active enzyme, when a fibrin clot is present.
        b. Plasmin begins fibrin clot dissolution, releasing fibrin degradation products (FDPs), also called fibrin split products (FSPs), into the circulation.
        c. FDPs exert an anticoagulant effect by interfering with clot formation and the function of platelets, thrombin, and fibrinogen.
D. Coagulation tests (Table 31-3).
    1. Platelet count is used to assess platelet number.
    2. Prothrombin time (PT) is used to assess extrinsic and common portions of the coagulation cascade.
    3. Partial thromboplastin time (PTT) is used to assess intrinsic and common portions of the coagulation cascade.
    4. Fibrinogen is used to assess the circulating level of this protein substrate, required for clot formation.

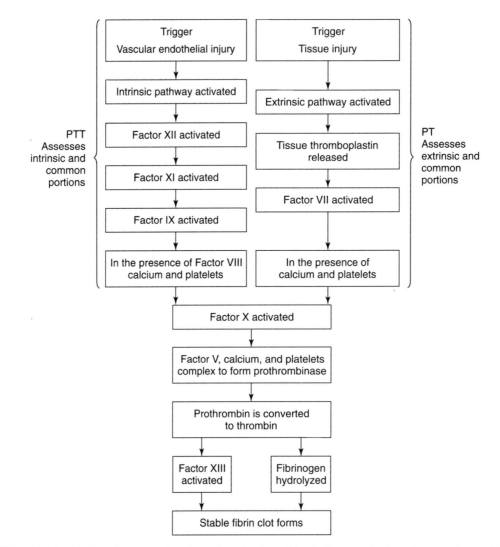

FIGURE 31-2 ■ Fibrin clot formation through activation of intrinsic or extrinsic pathways of coagulation process.

   5. FDP/FSP is used to assess fibrinolytic activity.
   6. Individual clotting factors may be assayed, depending on results of the tests cited above.
E. **Physiologic anemia of infancy** (Kates and Kates, 2007).
   1. Hemoglobin levels decline after birth, reaching a physiologic nadir at 8 to 12 weeks. Hemoglobin levels at this time are typically 9 to 11 g/dL.

ANEMIA

Low hemoglobin concentration and/or decreased number of RBCs diminishes the oxygen-carrying capacity of the blood and the level of oxygen available to the tissues (Oski et al., 2003). Anemia at birth can be classified into three major causes: (1) the result of blood loss (hemorrhage), (2) hemolysis, or (3) underproduction of erythrocytes (Bain and Blackburn, 2004; Blanchette et al., 2005).
A. **Etiologic factors.**
   1. Hemorrhage.
      a. Fetal–maternal. Occurs in 50% to 75% of all pregnancies. May be acute or chronic. In 1% of pregnancies, the exchange of blood exceeds 30 ml (Bagwell, 2007).
         (1) Spontaneous.

■ TABLE 31-3
■ **Normal Values for Tests of Hemostasis**

Parameter	Fetuses (Weeks of Gestation)			Newborns (n = 60)	Adults (n = 40)
	19 to 23 (n = 20)	24 to 29 (n = 22)	30 to 38 (n = 22)		
PT (s)	32.5 (19 to 45)	32.2 (19 to 44)†	22.6 (16 to 30)†	16.7 (12.0 to 23.5)*	13.5 (11.4 to 14)
PT (INR)	6.4 (1.7 to 11.1)	6.2 (2.1 to 10.6)†	3 (1.5 to 5)*	1.7 (0.9 to 2.7)*	1.1 (0.8 to 1.2)
APTT (s)	168.8 (83 to 250)	154 (87 to 210)†	104.8 (76 to 128)†	44.3 (35 to 52)*	33 (25 to 39)
TCT (s)	34.2 (24 to 44)*	26.2 (24 to 28)*	21.4 (17 to 23.3)	20.4 (15.2 to 25)†	14 (12 to 16)
Factor					
I (g/l, Von Clauss)	0.85 (0.57 to 1.50)	1.12 (0.65 to 1.65)	1.35 (1.25 to 1.65)	1.68 (0.95 to 2.45)†	3 (1.78 to 4.50)
I Ag (g/l)	1.08 (0.75 to 1.50)	1.93 (1.56 to 2.40)	1.94 (1.30 to 2.40)	2.65 (1.68 to 3.60)†	3.5 (2.50 to 5.20)
IIc (%)	16.9 (10 to 24)	19.9 (11 to 30)*	27.9 (15 to 50)†	43.5 (27 to 64)†	98.7 (70 to 125)
VIIc (%)	27.4 (17 to 37)	33.8 (18 to 48)*	45.9 (31 to 62)	52.5 (28 to 78)†	101.3 (68 to 130)
IXc (%)	10.1 (6 to 14)	9.9 (5 to 15)	12.3 (5 to 24)†	31.8 (15 to 50)†	104.8 (70 to 142)
Xc (%)	20.5 (14 to 29)	24.9 (16 to 35)	28 (16 to 36)†	39.6 (21 to 65)†	99.2 (75 to 125)
Vc (%)	32.1 (21 to 44)	36.8 (25 to 50)	48.9 (23 to 70)†	89.9 (50 to 140)	99.8 (65 to 140)
VIIIc (%)	34.5 (18 to 50)	35.5 (20 to 52)	50.1 (27 to 78)†	94.3 (38 to 150)	101.8 (55 to 170)
XIc (%)	13.2 (8 to 19)	12.1 (6 to 22)	14.8 (6 to 26)†	37.2 (13 to 62)†	100.2 (70 to 135)
XIIc (%)	14.9 (6 to 25)	22.7 (6 to 40)	25.8 (11 to 50)†	69.8 (25 to 105)†	101.4 (65 to 144)
PK (%)	12.8 (8 to 19)	15.4 (8 to 26)	18.1 (8 to 28)†	35.4 (21 to 53)†	99.8 (65 to 135)
HMWK (%)	15.4 (10 to 22)	19.3 (10 to 26)	23.6 (12 to 34)†	38.9 (28 to 53)†	98.8 (68 to 135)

INR, International normalized ratio; *TCT*, thrombin clotting time; *Ag*, antigenic value; *APTT*, activated partial thromboplastin time; *c*, coagulant activity; *HMWK*, high-molecular-weight kininogen; *PK*, protein kinase.

Values are the mean, followed in parentheses by the lower and upper boundaries including 95% of the population.

*$p = .05$.

†$p = .01$.

From Nathan, D.G. and Orkin, S.H., Ginsberg D., and Look, A.T. (Eds.): *Nathan and Oski's hematology of infancy and childhood* (6th ed.). Philadelphia, 2003, Saunders, p. 1855.

        (2) Traumatic amniocentesis.

        (3) External cephalic version.

    b. Twin-to-twin.

        (1) Monozygotic, monochorionic (single) placenta.

        (2) Hemoglobin difference between twins greater than 5 g/dl.

    c. Placental/cord.

        (1) Umbilical cord rupture.

        (2) Cord or placental hematoma.

        (3) Anomalous cord insertion.

        (4) Rupture of anomalous vessels of cord or placenta.

        (5) Accidental incision of cord or placenta.

        (6) Placenta previa or abruptio placentae.

    d. Internal.

        (1) Intracranial (subdural, subarachnoid, intraventricular), subgaleal.

        (2) Organ rupture (liver, spleen, adrenal, kidney).

        (3) Pulmonary.

    e. External.

        (1) Phlebotomy.

        (2) Iatrogenic (e.g., catheter losses).

  2. Hemolysis.

    a. Blood group incompatibilities.

        (1) Rh incompatibility: erythroblastosis fetalis (Glader and Allen, 2005; Liley, 2003).

            (a) Sequence of events. Fetal blood cells containing Rh antigen (Rh positive) enter the maternal circulation; maternal red cells have no antigen (Rh negative); maternal immune system produces antibodies against the foreign fetal antigens; in subsequent pregnancies maternal antibodies enter fetal circulation and destroy fetal red cells.

            (b) Predisposing factors.

                (i)   Previous pregnancy or abortion.

                (ii) Fetal–maternal hemorrhage during pregnancy.

                (iii) Delivery (vaginal, breech, cesarean).

                (iv) Amniocentesis, chorionic villus sampling.

                (v) External version.

                (vi) Manual removal of placenta.

            (c) Infant presentation.

                (i)   Anemia (caused by hemolysis, resulting in increased production of very immature red cells).

                (ii)   Tissue hypoxia, acidosis (decreased RBC count and decreased oxygen-carrying capacity of immature cells).

                (iii)   Congestive heart failure and hydrops fetalis (fetus attempts to expand blood volume and cardiac output, resulting in generalized edema).

                (iv)   Ascites, pleural effusion (fluid collecting in large cavities).

                (v)   Hepatosplenomegaly (increased extramedullary hematopoiesis).

                (vi)   Petechiae (thrombocytopenia accompanying severe anemia).

                (vii) Hypoglycemia (increased red cell destruction stimulates insulin secretion, resulting in hyperplasia of pancreatic islets and hyperinsulinemia).

                (viii) Positive direct Coombs test result.

            (d) Prophylactic therapy: anti-D immune globulin (RhoGAM).

                (i)   Anti-D antibodies injected into maternal circulation (one dose accommodates approximately 15 ml of fetal whole blood or approximately 30 ml of RBCs).

                (ii)   Destruction of fetal red cells in maternal circulation, blocking maternal antibody production.

                (iii)   90% effective in prevention of sensitization.

                (iv)   Recommended administration at 28 weeks of gestation, within 72 hours after delivery, and after amniocentesis, chorionic villus sampling, percuta-

■ TABLE 31-4
■ ■ **Potential Maternal–Fetal ABO Incompatibilities**

Maternal Blood Group	Incompatible Fetal Blood Group
O	A or B
B	A or AB
A	B or AB

neous umbilical blood sampling, or evidence or possibility of fetal–maternal hemorrhage.

    (2) ABO incompatibility (Blanchette et al., 2005).

        (a) More frequently occurring but less severe hemolytic disease than with Rh incompatibility.

        (b) Most often seen in mothers with O blood type (absence of antigen) carrying fetus with A or B blood type (see Table 31-4 for other potential incompatibilities).

        (c) Maternal exposure to naturally occurring A and B antigens in food, bacteria, and pollen initiates maternal production of anti-A, anti-B antibodies and accounts for severity of disease with first pregnancy.

        (d) ABO incompatibility protects against fetal Rh disease because of rapid destruction of fetal A/B cells, preventing Rh antigen exposure and maternal antibody production.

        (e) Infant presentation includes the following:

            (i)   Mild hemolysis, anemia, reticulocytosis.

            (ii) Hyperbilirubinemia (occasionally requiring exchange).

  b. Enzymatic defect: glucose-6-phosphate dehydrogenase (G6PD) deficiency (see also Chapter 29).

    (1) Most common inherited disorder of red cells (sex-linked disease affecting mainly male offspring, occasionally female carriers).

    (2) Interaction of intracellular abnormality (deficiency of red cell enzyme) and extracellular factor (exposure to oxidant stress: drugs, infection), causing hemolysis and shortened erythrocyte life.

    (3) Most common occurrence in American black infants (10% to 15%) and in infants of Mediterranean, African, and Asian descent.

  c. Hemoglobin disorders (Steiner and Gallagher, 2007).

    (1) α-Thalassemia.

        (a) Deletion of one or more of the four α-globin genes.

        (b) Severity of expression is related to the number of globin genes missing.

        (c) Ranges from asymptomatic to mild anemia to significant hemolytic anemia and hyperlipidemia.

        (d) Most common in infants of Southeast Asian, Middle Eastern, and Mediterranean descent.

    (2) β-Thalassemia.

        (a) Occurs as a result of deletion of β-globin.

        (b) Neonates occasionally present with hemolytic anemia.

        (c) Does not usually present before 2 months of age because of the presence of HbF.

  d. Infection. Intrauterine (viral, protozoan, spirochetal) and postnatal (bacterial) infection may cause neonatal hemolysis, anemia, thrombocytopenia, and disseminated intravascular coagulation.

3. Anemia of prematurity.

  a. Hemoglobin concentration at birth varies only slightly in relation to gestational age.

  b. During the first 2 to 3 months, hemoglobin concentration falls to the lowest value that occurs at any developmental period.

  c. Anemia of prematurity is considered physiologic because it is characteristic of healthy infants.

  d. Associated factors.

   (1) Rates of decline and nadir are inversely proportional to gestational age.

   (2) Iron concentration is low because of decreased blood volume and decreased concentration of circulating hemoglobin iron.

   (3) Improved extrauterine oxygen delivery causes a temporarily inactive stage of erythropoiesis.

   (4) Erythropoietin production in response to anemia is diminished.

   (5) Shortened red cell life span decreases red cell mass.

   (6) Growth causes dilutional anemia as a result of decreased hemoglobin concentration with expanding blood volume.

   (7) Despite rapid hemoglobin fall, tissue oxygenation is maintained by events responsible for right shift of the hemoglobin–oxygen dissociation curve.

  e. Some infants do manifest symptoms of hypoxemia (poor feeding and weight gain, dyspnea, tachypnea, tachycardia, diminished activity, pallor) in the absence of other problems and require transfusion.

  f. No direct correlation has been established between low hemoglobin levels and the occurrence of apnea (Westkamp et al., 2002).

 4. Iatrogenic postnatal phlebotomy. Critically ill infants who require frequent monitoring may have excessive amounts of blood removed for diagnostic studies, thereby inducing anemia. Removal of greater than 20% of the blood volume over 24 to 48 hours can produce anemia; in a 1500-g infant this represents approximately 25 ml (Blanchette et al., 2005).

B. Clinical presentation: varies with the volume of hemorrhage and the time period over which the blood is lost.

 1. Acute blood loss.

  a. Pallor initially, and then cyanosis and desaturation.

  b. Shallow, rapid, irregular respirations.

  c. Tachycardia.

  d. Weak or absent peripheral pulses.

  e. Low or absent blood pressure, low venous pressure.

  f. Hemoglobin concentration may be normal initially, with rapid decline over 4 to 12 hours with hemodilution.

 2. Chronic blood loss.

  a. Pallor without signs of acute distress.

  b. Possible signs of congestive heart failure with hepatomegaly.

  c. Normal blood pressure, normal or elevated venous pressure.

  d. Low hemoglobin concentration.

C. Clinical assessment.

 1. Family history.

  a. Bleeding, anemia, splenectomy.

  b. Consanguinity.

  c. Ethnic and geographic origins.

  d. Blood group incompatibilities.

 2. Maternal history.

  a. Blood type.

  b. Late third-trimester bleeding.

D. Physical examination.

 1. Signs of acute or chronic blood loss, as above.

 2. Jaundice.

 3. Cephalohematoma.

 4. Abdominal distention or mass: liver, spleen, adrenal, kidney rupture.

 5. Petechiae, purpura.

 6. Cardiovascular abnormalities: tachycardia, murmur, gallop rhythm.

 7. Hydropic changes.

■ TABLE 31-5
■ ■ Serial Hemoglobin Values in Low-Birth-Weight Infants

Birth Weight (g)	Hemoglobin Concentration (g/dl) by Age				
	2 weeks	4 weeks	6 weeks	8 weeks	10 weeks
800 to 1000	16 ± 0.6	10.2 ± 3.2	8.7 ± 1.5	8 ± 0.9	8 ± 1.1
1001 to 1200	16.4 ± 2.3	12.8 ± 2.5	10.5 ± 1.8	9.1 ± 1.3	8.5 ± 1.5
1201 to 1400	16.2 ± 1.3	13.4 ± 2.8	10.9 ± 1.2	9.9 ± 1.9	—
1401 to 1500	15.6 ± 2.2	11.7 ± 1	10.5 ± 0.7	9.8 ± 1.4	—

Hemoglobin values are presented as grams per deciliter.
From Oski, F.A.: Hematologic problems. In G.B. Avery (Ed.): *Neonatology: Pathophysiology and management of the newborn* (4th ed.). Philadelphia, 1994, Lippincott.

E. **Diagnostic studies.**
   1. Hemoglobin concentration. Normal hemoglobin values are dependent on gestation age, site of sampling and timing of sampling (Brugnara and Platt, 2003). Values vary according to birth weight and postnatal age (Table 31-5).
   2. Reticulocyte count. This reflects new erythroid activity and is persistently elevated with ongoing red cell destruction.
   3. Peripheral blood smear.
      a. Test evaluates alterations in size, shape, and structure of RBCs that might enhance destruction because of decreased deformability.
      b. Fragmentation of RBCs can be identified.
   4. Blood type to identify common blood group antigens: A, B, O, and Rh.
   5. Coombs test.
      a. Positive result on direct Coombs test indicates presence of maternal IgG antibodies on the surface of infant's red cells.
      b. Positive result on indirect Coombs test means that antibodies against the infant's RBCs are present in the maternal serum.
   6. Kleihauer–Betke test.
      a. Test identifies fetal hemoglobin in maternal blood.
      b. Calculations indicate volume of fetal–maternal hemorrhage and dose of immune globulin (RhoGAM) required to prevent sensitization.
F. **Differential diagnosis: diseases that diminish oxygen delivery to the tissues** (e.g., pulmonary, cardiac).
G. **Complications.**
   1. Inadequate tissue oxygenation, poor growth.
   2. Transfusion.
      a. Transfusion reaction.
      b. Overhydration with pulmonary congestion.
H. **Patient care management** (see Transfusion Therapies on pp. 686-690).
   1. Emergency treatment for acute blood loss resulting in hypovolemia.
      a. Whole blood or packed RBCs (PRBCs).
         (1) Type: group O, Rh negative.
         (2) Amount: 10 to 20 ml/kg.
      b. Albumin, or saline solution if blood is unavailable.
         (1) Amount: 10 to 20 ml/kg.
   2. Nonemergency replacement transfusion: clinical decision based on adequacy of tissue oxygenation in the individual infant.
      a. Advantages of transfusion must be weighed against risks, including infection, hypothermia, graft-versus-host disease, and other complications.
      b. Consider gestational and postnatal age, intravascular volume, and coexisting cardiac, pulmonary, or vascular conditions.

3. Exchange transfusion.
   a. Treatment of jaundice caused by blood group incompatibility.
   b. Partial exchange if necessary to treat severe anemia of hydrops without increasing intravascular volume.
I. **Outcome.**
   1. Improved tissue oxygenation and resolution of symptoms with replacement transfusion.
   2. Long-term outcome varies with degree of anemia and underlying cause.

HEMORRHAGIC DISEASE OF THE NEWBORN

Hemorrhagic disease of the newborn (HDN) is a hemorrhagic tendency caused by vitamin K deficiency and decreased activity of factors II, VII, IX, and X. A new term, vitamin K–dependent bleeding (VKDB), is thought to describe more accurately the link between vitamin K deficiency and spontaneous hemorrhage and to exclude newborn infants with bleeding from other causes (Blackburn, 2007; Monagle and Andrew, 2003; Tandoi et al., 2005).

A. **Etiologic factors:** primary vitamin K deficiency.
   1. Required for activation of clotting factors II, VII, IX, and X and of proteins C and S after liver synthesis.
      a. Vitamin K is important in the formation of calcium-binding sites, which are necessary for functional activation of clotting factors.
      b. In the absence of vitamin K, circulating proteins are decarboxylated; levels of protein induced by vitamin K absence (PIVKA) can be used as an indirect measure of bleeding risk.
   2. Suppression of bacterial synthesis.
      a. Intestinal flora is required for vitamin K synthesis.
      b. Newborn intestinal tract is virtually free of bacteria until feedings begin.
      c. Antibiotic therapy can alter normal intestinal bacterial colonization.
   3. Three forms of HDN are recognized.
      a. Early—within 24 hours in neonates born to women taking certain anticonvulsants.
      b. Classic or VKDB—seen at 2 to 6 days.
         (1) incidence is 0.4 to 1.7 per 100 live births if no vitamin K is given (Parker, 2005).
      c. Late onset—occurs at 2 to 12 weeks in infants not receiving vitamin K at birth or receiving an inadequate oral dose and breastfeeding or in infants with hepatobiliary disease.
B. **Clinical presentation:** bleeding.
   1. Begins at 24 to 72 hours of age.
   2. May be localized or diffuse.
   3. Rarely life threatening.
   4. Late-onset bleeding possible at approximately 2 to 3 weeks of age.
C. **Clinical assessment:** oozing.
   1. Localized: frequently gastrointestinal (hematemesis, melena).
   2. Diffuse: umbilical cord, circumcision, puncture sites.
D. **Physical examination.**
   1. Diffuse ecchymosis, petechiae.
   2. Oozing puncture sites.
   3. Abdominal distention.
   4. Jaundice.
E. **Diagnostic studies.**
   1. Response to vitamin K administration establishes the diagnosis.
   2. PT and PTT are prolonged.
   3. Levels of vitamin K–dependent clotting factors are low.
   4. PIVKA levels are elevated.
F. **Differential diagnosis.**
   1. Decreased absorption of vitamin K.
      a. Biliary atresia.

      b. Cystic fibrosis.

      c. Cholestasis.

  2. Pharmacologic antagonism of vitamin K (Abbott et al., 2006).

      a. Anticonvulsants (hydantoin, phenobarbital carbamazepine, diazepam), anticoagulants (coumarin, warfarin) and antibiotics (cephalosporins, isoniazid, quinolones, and rifampin).

        (1) Induce hepatic enzymes and increase vitamin K degradation.

        (2) Inhibit vitamin K transport across the placenta.

        (3) Depress vitamin K–dependent coagulation factors.

      b. Coumarol derivatives: replace with heparin during pregnancy.

      c. Maternal supplementation with oral vitamin K_1 from 36 weeks of gestation to delivery might prevent neonatal hemorrhage associated with anticonvulsant therapy; extra vitamin K given to the mother to increase vitamin K available to the fetus.

G. Complications.

  1. Anemia.

  2. Intraventricular/intracranial hemorrhage.

H. Patient care management.

  1. Prophylactic vitamin K at the time of delivery.

      a. Phytonadione (naturally occurring vitamin K), 0.5 to 1 mg, intramuscular (IM) administration: premature infants may require a lower initial dose with a supplemental dose given when breastfeeding is established (Clarke et al., 2006).

      b. The Canadian Paediatric Society (CPS, 2004) and the American Academy of Pediatrics (AAP, 2003) recommend the use of only IM vitamin K at birth, because of the history of prevention of life-threatening HDN with the parenteral preparation, the unproven risks of cancer, and the need for further research on the efficacy, safety, and bioavailability of oral preparations.

      c. Late HDN occurs primarily in breast-fed infants who have not received adequate vitamin K prophylaxis.

        (1) Parental concern with IM administration of vitamin K might stem from the following:

          (a) Need for injection.

          (b) Reports linking an earlier formulation of vitamin K to childhood cancer (Clarke and Shearer, 2007).

      d. Commercial formulas contain vitamin K supplement.

      e. Intestinal flora of breastfed infant may produce less vitamin K than that of formula-fed infant.

  2. Significant bleeding (hemoglobin concentration <12 g/dl). PRBC infusion may be indicated.

  3. Persistent bleeding in premature infant.

      a. FFP infusion may be indicated to replace clotting factors.

      b. Repeated doses of vitamin K are needed.

I. Outcome. Prophylactic treatment has virtually eliminated the disease.

DISSEMINATED INTRAVASCULAR COAGULATION

DIC is an acquired hemorrhagic disorder associated with an underlying disease manifested as uncontrolled activation of coagulation and fibrinolysis. Consumption of clotting factors is thought to be initiated by release of thromboplastic material from damaged or diseased tissue into the circulation. In DIC, fibrinogen converts to fibrin to form microthrombi. Neonates are at increased risk of DIC because of inherent imbalances between fibrinolytic, anticoagulant, and procoagulant factors, particularly decreased levels of antithrombin and protein C (Bick, 2003; Blackburn, 2007; Manco-Johnson, 2004; Monagle and Andrew, 2003; Parker, 2005).

A. Common precipitating factors.
　　1. Maternal.
　　　　a. Preeclampsia, eclampsia, placental abruption.
　　　　b. Placental abnormalities.
　　2. Intrapartal.
　　　　a. Fetal distress with hypoxia and acidosis.
　　　　b. Dead twin fetus.
　　　　c. Traumatic delivery.
　　3. Neonatal.
　　　　a. Infection (bacterial, viral, fungal).
　　　　b. Conditions causing hypoxia, acidosis, and shock.
　　　　c. Severe Rh incompatibility.
　　　　d. Thrombocytopenia.
　　　　e. Tissue injury (birth trauma, breech crush injury).
B. Clinical presentation (Fig. 31-3).
　　1. Hemorrhage: predominant symptom.
　　　　a. Clotting factors and platelets are depleted.
　　　　b. Fibrinolysis is stimulated.
　　　　c. Endogenous thrombin and plasmin are formed.
　　2. Organ and tissue ischemia. Microvascular thrombosis (occlusion) by fibrin thrombi causes potential ischemia and necrosis of any organ, particularly the kidneys.
　　3. Anemia.
　　　　a. Blood loss.
　　　　b. Red cell fragmentation by fibrin strands.
C. Clinical assessment.
　　1. Review the history for precipitating factors.
　　2. Concurrent evidence of coagulation and fibrinolysis.
D. Physical examination.
　　1. Variable signs, depending on underlying disease process.
　　2. Prolonged oozing from puncture sites or umbilicus.
　　3. Petechiae, purpura, ecchymosis.
　　4. Hemorrhage (pulmonary, gastrointestinal, cerebral).
　　5. Localized necrosis and gangrene resulting from microvascular thrombosis of peripheral vessels.

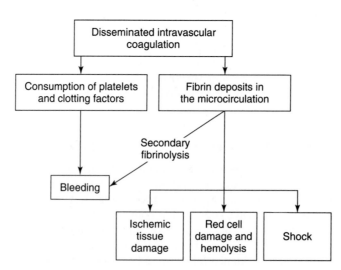

FIGURE 31-3 ■ Sequence of events in pathologic changes of disseminated intravascular coagulation (DIC).

E. **Diagnostic studies.**
   1. Variable diagnostic studies are performed for delineation of the underlying disease process.
   2. Platelet count is low.
   3. PT and PTT may be normal in early DIC then become significantly prolonged (Parker, 2005).
   4. Peripheral blood smear identifies microangiopathic hemolytic anemia, abnormalities of red cell shape, cell fragmentation, and decreased number of platelets.
   5. Fibrinogen level is low.
   6. Fibrinogen-degradation products are significantly increased but are not specific markers of DIC.
   7. D-Dimer is a sensitive marker for endogenous thrombin/plasmin production and can detect much milder forms of DIC.
   8. Additional factors and levels might be evaluated: factors VIII and II are decreased, as well as protein C, protein S, and antithrombin III.

F. **Differential diagnosis.**
   1. Parenchymal liver disease.
   2. Vitamin K deficiency.
   3. Microangiopathic disease.
   4. Primary fibrinogenolysis.

G. **Complications.**
   1. Microvascular thrombosis.
   2. Organ failure resulting from ischemia and necrosis, especially renal.
   3. Intraventricular and parenchymal hemorrhage.

H. **Patient care management.**
   1. Aggressive treatment of the underlying disease.
   2. Supportive care.
      a. Replacement transfusion with significant bleeding.
         (1) Whole blood for hypovolemia and shock.
         (2) PRBCs for isovolemic anemia.
         (3) Platelets for consumption.
      b. Maintenance of blood pressure.
   3. Measures to control DIC.
      a. Replacement of clotting factors.
         (1) FFP (replaces all factors, coagulation proteins, and coagulation inhibitors; small amount of fibrinogen).
         (2) Platelet concentrates.
         (3) Cryoprecipitate (replaces fibrinogen, factor VIII).
         (4) Antithrombin III (inhibits coagulation, controls fibrinolysis). High doses (120 to 250 units/kg/day) might attenuate organ failure and reverse coagulopathy in DIC without heparin therapy.
      b. Heparin therapy remains controversial; use if treatment of underlying disease and replacement of clotting factors fail to reverse the process or with evidence of significant large-vessel thrombosis.
         (1) Goals are to interrupt fibrin deposition and to achieve normal fibrinogen levels and platelet counts.
         (2) Continuous infusion is more physiologic and is safer because intermittent doses may aggravate existing hemorrhage.
         (3) Dosage is adjusted to maintain PTT within 60 to 70 seconds (once achieved, lower-dose heparin therapy may control ongoing consumption).

I. **Outcome: related to the prognosis of the underlying disease and the severity of the DIC.**

THROMBOCYTOPENIA

Thrombocytopenia is an acquired disease in which there is a significant decrease in the platelet count ($<150,000/mm^3$) of the term or premature infant (Blanchette et al., 2005; Blickstein and

Friedman, 2006; Wilson, 2003). It is the most common coagulation disorder in neonates (Manco-Johnson et al., 2006).

A. Etiologic factors.

1. Platelet destruction.
   a. Maternal autoantibodies (autoimmune): idiopathic thrombocytopenic purpura, systemic lupus erythematosus.
      (1) Maternal autoantibodies bind to platelet surface antigens, making them susceptible to premature destruction.
      (2) IgG antibodies cross the placenta and destroy fetal platelets.
         (a) Approximately 10% to 15% have cord platelet counts of less than 100,000/mm^3 (half of these have counts <50,000/mm^3).
         (b) Nadir usually occurs on the second day.
         (c) Counts can be depressed for 2 to 4 months (as long as maternal IgG antibodies remain in circulation).
      (3) Maternal platelet count is low.
   b. Neonatal conditions.
      (1) Neonatal alloimmune thrombocytopenia (Murphy and Bussel, 2007).
         (a) Analogous to Rh incompatibility.
            (i) Fetal platelets contain an antigen lacking in the mother.
            (ii) Fetal platelets enter the maternal circulation, resulting in maternal production of antibodies against foreign platelets.
            (iii) Maternal antibodies cross into the fetal circulation and coat fetal platelets, which are then destroyed.
         (b) Fetal thrombocytopenia can occur as early as by 20 weeks of gestation.
         (c) Nadir occurs in the first few days; counts normalize by the end of the first month.
         (d) About 15% to 25% have intracranial hemorrhage (approximately 10% occur in utero).
         (e) Maternal platelet count remains normal.
      (2) Infection: bacterial or congenitally acquired.
         (a) Megakaryocyte degeneration in bone marrow.
         (b) Can cause DIC (platelet consumption).
         (c) Activates reticuloendothelial system (increased platelet sequestration).
         (d) Platelets may form antigen–antibody complexes with infectious agent.
      (3) Thrombotic disorders.
         (a) Large-vessel disease (renal vein thrombosis).
         (b) Microvascular disease (necrotizing enterocolitis, respiratory distress syndrome, persistent pulmonary hypertension of the newborn).
         (c) DIC (platelet consumption).
      (4) Birth asphyxia. Fetal megakaryocytes may have increased sensitivity to hypoxic injury.
      (5) Giant hemangiomas.
         (a) Kasabach–Merritt syndrome. Vascular malformation results in platelet and fibrinogen consumption.
         (b) Mechanical destruction and sequestration.
      (6) Exchange transfusion: shortened survival of transfused platelets.
2. Impaired platelet production (rare, <5%) associated with congenital malformations.
   a. Trisomy syndromes (13, 18). Bone marrow hypoplasia affects megakaryocyte production.
   b. Thrombocytopenia with absent radii (TAR) syndrome.
      (1) Defective megakaryocyte progenitor cell.
      (2) Presentation at birth, improvement thereafter.
      (3) Anomalies of the radius but not the thumb.
   c. Fanconi anemia.
      (1) Thumb, skeletal, renal, and CNS anomalies; café-au-lait spots.
      (2) Thrombocytopenia: presentation rare in the neonatal period; worsens with time.
   d. Other, rare syndromes associated with unusually small or giant platelets.

3. Platelet interference: maternal drug ingestion.
    a. Interference with platelet aggregation.
    b. Meperidine (Demerol), promethazine (Phenergan), acetylsalicylic acid, sulfonamides, quinidine, quinine, thiazides.
B. **Clinical presentation** (platelet-type bleeding).
    1. Petechiae, purpura, epistaxis.
    2. Ecchymosis over presenting part.
    3. Cephalohematoma.
    4. Bleeding (mucous membranes, gastrointestinal tract, genitourinary system, umbilical cord, puncture sites, superficial cuts, or abrasions).
C. **Clinical assessment.**
    1. Family history: bleeding complications in previous children, other family members.
    2. Maternal history.
        a. History of bruising or bleeding, infections, collagen-vascular disease, splenectomy.
        b. Platelet count (low or normal).
        c. Peripheral blood smear (may show low platelet count, increased immature forms).
        d. Medication history.
    3. Birth history.
        a. Hypoxia.
        b. Infection risk.
D. **Physical examination.**
    1. Signs of clinical presentation.
    2. Jaundice.
    3. Intrauterine growth restriction, microcephaly, hepatosplenomegaly with infectious cause (absent with immune etiology).
    4. Congenital anomalies consistent with syndromes.
E. **Diagnostic studies.**
    1. Platelet count is low.
    2. Peripheral blood smear shows low platelet count and increased immature forms; may show abnormal size.
    3. PT and PTT are normal for age.
    4. Bleeding time is prolonged.
    5. Maternal blood can be tested for human platelet antigen (HPA) type and for the presence of platelet-specific antibody (up to 2 weeks postpartum).
    6. In severe cases, platelet typing of mother, father, and infant might be indicated.
F. **Differential diagnosis: DIC, vitamin K deficiency.**
G. **Complications.**
    1. Cranial hemorrhage with neurologic sequelae in alloimmune disease.
        a. Associated with approximately 12% mortality rate.
        b. Increased incidence in infants weighing less than 1500 g.
    2. Entrapped hemorrhage.
    3. Anemia.
    4. Hyperbilirubinemia.
H. **Infant management** (see Table 31-5).
    1. Supportive care and treatment of underlying disease. Majority of neonatal thrombocytopenias are secondary to other disease processes.
    2. Cesarean delivery.
        a. Autoimmune.
            (1) Rarely of benefit for infant.
            (2) Consider if:
                (a) Maternal disease is severe, with high antibody levels, or
                (b) Prior infant was severely affected.
        b. Alloimmune: maternal HPA typing not routinely done; infants identified postnatally.
    3. Platelet transfusion.
        a. Recommended goal: keep platelet count greater than 30,000 in the first 48 hours, and greater than 50,000 if surgery is necessary or infant is premature and at risk for intra-

ventricular hemorrhage. The need for multiple platelet transfusions has been shown to be a predictor of higher mortality rates (Baer et al., 2007).
   b. Autoimmune.
      (1) Rarely needed; platelet counts greater than 20,000/mm^3, usually benign course.
      (2) Consider cranial ultrasonography if platelet counts less than 50,000/mm^3.
      (3) Consider transfusion if platelet counts less than 20,000/mm^3.
   c. Alloimmune.
      (1) Serial transfusions may be necessary.
      (2) Obtain HPA type for infant before transfusion.
      (3) Transfusion of random donor platelets rarely results in sustained increase because of antibody destruction.
      (4) Transfuse maternal platelets (in absence of HPA) that have been washed and resuspended in AB-negative plasma.
   d. Production defects: repeated transfusions usually necessary.
   4. Intravenous immune globulin (IVIG).
      a. 80% effective in increasing platelet count.
      b. Effect delayed 12 to 24 hours.
      c. IgG pooled blood product from multiple donors.
   5. Steroids.
      a. May be used in infants with platelet counts less than 25,000/mm^3 and clinical bleeding.
      b. May be used for initial treatment of thrombocytopenia resulting from hemangioma.
I. Outcome.
   1. Varies with underlying disease, presence of congenital malformations.
   2. Autoimmune etiology: usually causes only mild, transient problems, with full recovery of platelet count in 8 to 12 weeks.
   3. Isoimmune etiology: causes mild to moderate problems with full recovery of platelet count in 6 to 8 weeks.

POLYCYTHEMIA

Polycythemia is a condition in which infants demonstrate an excess in circulating RBC mass. The venous hemoglobin concentration is 2 standard deviations above the mean for gestational and postdelivery age (Kates and Kates, 2007). Blood viscosity increases with hematocrits greater than 65% or when venous hemoglobin is >22 g/dl and leads to a reduction of blood flow to the organs. Occurs in 1% to 5% of healthy term newborns (Kates and Kates, 2007).
A. **Etiologic factors** (Schimmel et al., 2004).
   1. Intrauterine hypoxia, placental insufficiency. Hypoxia stimulates erythropoiesis, increasing the fetal red cell mass.
      a. Maternal preeclampsia/eclampsia.
      b. Postmaturity syndrome, intrauterine growth restriction.
      c. Maternal smoking.
   2. Maternal–fetal and twin-to-twin transfusion.
   3. Placental hypertransfusion.
   4. Maternal diabetes: possibly resulting from abnormal fetal erythrocyte deformability.
   5. Congenital syndrome resulting in increased red blood cell mass.
   6. Delayed cord clamping.
B. **Clinical presentation.**
   1. Many infants are asymptomatic.
   2. Plethora.
   3. Cyanosis.
   4. CNS abnormalities (lethargy, jitteriness, seizures).
   5. Respiratory distress (tachypnea, pulmonary edema, pulmonary hemorrhage).
   6. Tachycardia, congestive heart failure.
   7. Hypoglycemia.
   8. Poor feeding behaviors (poor nippling, regurgitation).

C. **Clinical assessment: history and physical examination usually identify cause.**
D. **Physical examination.**
   1. Findings may be normal except for plethora and occasionally cyanosis.
   2. Symptoms of clinical presentation cannot be attributed to other disease.
E. **Diagnostic studies.** Venous hemoglobin concentration and hematocrit are elevated. CT scan if stroke suspected.
F. **Complications.**
   1. Hyperbilirubinemia.
   2. Hypoglycemia—mechanism unknown.
   3. Hyperviscosity syndrome: elevated whole blood viscosity associated with reduced blood flow, vascular thrombosis (renal, cerebral, mesenteric), neurologic sequelae, fine motor abnormalities, speech delays up to 2 years of age (Drew et al., 1997).
G. **Patient care management.**
   1. Partial exchange transfusion.
      a. Controversial in asymptomatic infants. Has not been shown to decrease neurologic morbidity.
      b. Desired reduction of hematocrit to less than 60% (blood viscosity is thought to be relatively normal at this level).
      c. Crystalloid shown to be as effective as colloid for reduction exchange at less cost and with fewer risks related to blood product exposure (Dempsey and Barrington, 2005).
      d. Gastrointestinal symptoms: possibility of bleeding, poor feeding tolerance, and necrotizing enterocolitis after partial exchange transfusion (Capasso et al., 2003).
   2. Supportive treatment of persistent symptoms.
H. **Outcome** (Capasso et al., 2003; Murray and Roberts, 2004).
   1. Neonates with proven hyperviscosity (less than 50% of neonates exhibit hyperviscosity even when packed cell volumes >70%), are at risk of an adverse neurologic outcome.
   2. Adverse neurologic outcome may be independently related to underlying risk factors and race rather than polycythemia alone (Pappas and Delaney-Black, 2004).

INHERITED BLEEDING DISORDERS

Although inherited bleeding disorders were recognized as early as AD 600, the specific clotting abnormalities have been delineated only in this century, with the last (deficiency of factor XIII) documented in 1963. These gene disorders are rare, phenotypic expression is extremely variable, and only the most severely affected will be identified in the newborn period (Hagstrom, 2004; Manco-Johnson et al., 2006; Parker, 2005).
A. **Etiologic factors.**
   1. Hemophilia.
      a. Ninety percent of infants with hemophilia will have either classic hemophilia (hemophilia A, factor VIII deficiency) or Christmas disease (hemophilia B, factor IX deficiency).
         (1) Incidence of hemophilia A is 1 per 10,000 live births (Parker, 2005).
         (2) Incidence of hemophilia B is 1 per 100,000 live births (Parker, 2005).
      b. X-linked recessive inheritance.
         (1) Gene is located on the X chromosome.
         (2) Females are carriers; disease is present in male infants because they have only one X chromosome, which carries the abnormal gene (no normal X chromosome as counterbalance).
         (3) Each pregnancy carries a 25% chance of occurrence (50% of the male offspring will be affected).
         (4) 75% percent have a family history of a male with a bleeding disorder.
   2. von Willebrand disease.
      a. Autosomal dominant inheritance.
         (1) Males and females are equally affected.
         (2) Each pregnancy carries a 50% chance of occurrence.
         (3) Transmission is vertical (disease is seen in successive generations).

   b. Gene expression markedly variable (family history may be absent despite dominant inheritance).
   3. Factor XIII deficiency: autosomal recessive inheritance.
      a. Both parents are phenotypically normal carriers.
      b. Males and females are equally affected.
      c. In each pregnancy, 25% of the offspring will be affected, 50% will be carriers, and 25% will be normal.
      d. Expression is horizontal (deficiency is seen in siblings; skips a generation).
B. Clinical presentation.
   1. Rare newborn presentation except for factor XIII deficiency.
   2. Usually well infant with delayed bleeding.
   3. Clotting screening results usually normal.
C. Clinical assessment.
   1. Late bleeding.
      a. Delayed umbilical cord bleeding (>80% with factor XIII).
      b. Circumcision oozing (significant hemorrhage is rare).
      c. Rare intracranial hemorrhage.
   2. Family history.
D. Diagnostic studies.
   1. PT, PTT, platelet count, fibrinogen level (usually normal).
   2. Specific factor assays (identification by factor levels and DNA analysis).
      a. Factor VIII levels should be comparable to normal adult levels in the newborn period.
      b. Factor IX levels are normally low in the neonatal period; however, infants with bleeding presentation will be severely affected, with less than 2% activity (clearly abnormal level).
E. Patient care management.
   1. Initial correction is with FFP (contains adequate amounts of all clotting factors except factor VIII).
   2. Cryoprecipitate can be used if bleeding persists after use of FFP (enriched with approximately 20 units of factor VIII per milliliter).
   3. Diagnosis allows replacement of specific factor.
      a. Recombinant factor VIII is available for classic hemophilia.
      b. Purified (monoclonal antibody) factor IX is available for Christmas disease.
      c. Prothrombin concentrates are not recommended for neonatal use because of thrombogenicity.
   4. Use precautions to prevent bleeding.
      a. Immunizations should be given subcutaneously, with an ice pack applied to the site postinjection.
F. **Outcome: episodic bleeding requiring lifelong replacement.**

TRANSFUSION THERAPIES

A. Recommendations for use of blood components (Blanchette et al., 2005; CPS, 2002; Murray and Roberts, 2004; Quirolo, 2002; Wong and Luban, 2005).
   1. Develop and document criteria indicating need.
   2. Use only the blood components required for therapy.
   3. Use crystalloid or nonblood colloid whenever possible.
   4. Use universal precautions when handling blood products.
B. Written, informed consent has been recommended since 1986 to ensure that families understand risks and explore alternatives.
   1. Ethical or religious basis: autonomy—the right of choice.
   2. Legal basis: failure to inform adequately and to obtain consent constitutes negligence.
   3. Time consuming: start a few days in advance of need (i.e., include in discussion on the first day of life of sick preterm infants).

C. Informed consent includes discussion of the following:

1. Risks (American Cancer Society, 2006; American Red Cross, 2008; Galel and Fontaine, 2006).

   a. Infection.

      (1) Blood is screened for human immunodeficiency virus (HIV), hepatitis B virus (HBV), hepatitis C virus (HCV), human T-cell leukemia/lymphoma virus (HTLV), West Nile virus and *Treponema pallidum* (syphilis).

      (2) Cytomegalovirus transmission can be prevented by using CMV seronegative blood or leukocyte-depleted, irradiated products.

      (3) Major risks for transmission via transfusion.

         (a) HIV infection incidence is 1:2,135,000. Nucleic acid testing (NAT) based on polymerase chain reaction (PCR) is routine; a cheaper alternative (but not yet routine) is an enzyme-linked immunosorbent assay (ELISA)-based test for p24 antigen (Schupbach, 2002).

         (b) HBV (hepatitis B surface antigen [HBsAg]) infection incidence is 1:205,000; hepatitis B core antigen (HBcAg) is a marker for non-A, non-B hepatitis.

         (c) HCV infection incidence is 1:1,935,000.

      (4) Predonation questions foster self-elimination of prospective donors with high-risk behaviors.

      (5) Confidential unit exclusion allows donors to designate the elimination of their donation if they recognize risk but want to avoid the embarrassment of refusing to donate.

   b. Transfusion reactions (rare in neonates).

      (1) Febrile reactions (most common in adults but rare in neonates) (Galel and Fontaine, 2006).

         (a) Probably caused by transfused (passenger) WBCs and/or their cytokine products (RBC and platelet transfusions).

         (b) Leukocyte reduction might prevent reaction.

            (i) Expensive and time consuming.

            (ii) One unit of PRBCs can contain 1 billion WBCs.

            (iii) WBCs can be removed by centrifugation, or by filtering at donation (prestorage leukocyte depletion), or at transfusion (bedside filtration).

      (2) Allergic reactions.

         (a) Urticaria, angioedema, asthma.

         (b) Higher incidence with multiple transfusions.

      (3) Hemolytic reactions.

         (a) Usually ABO incompatibilities.

         (b) Possible acute or delayed hemolysis.

         (c) Most reactions can be eliminated by typing, screening, and crossmatching.

   c. Graft-versus-host disease (Wu and Stack, 2007).

      (1) Risk factors include neonates with congenital immunodeficiency syndromes, those receiving intrauterine or exchange transfusions, and low birth weight infants.

      (2) Immature immune system may not reject foreign lymphocytes (present in erythrocyte and platelet products); donor lymphocytes proliferate and damage the host (infection and neutropenia).

      (3) Clinical symptoms (within 100 days of transfusion) include rash, diarrhea, hepatic dysfunction, and bone marrow suppression with generalized reduction in all cell lines (pancytopenia).

      (4) Gamma irradiation of blood products will prevent lymphocyte proliferation.

         (a) Mature erythrocytes and platelets are resistant to radiation damage.

         (b) Enhances efflux of potassium ion from red cells (store <28 days, wash to remove excess potassium before transfusion).

   d. Fluid overload.

      (1) Volumes should not exceed 20 ml/kg.

2. Expected benefits.
   a. Whole blood (increases hematocrit approximately 35%).
      (1) Replacement of blood volume.
      (2) Treatment (massive hemorrhage, exchange transfusion).
   b. PRBC: 10 to 15 ml increases hemoglobin by 2 to 3 g/l (Wu and Stack, 2007).
      (1) Improved oxygen-carrying capacity and tissue oxygenation.
      (2) Relief of symptoms of anemia (tachypnea, apnea, periodic breathing, tachycardia, poor weight gain).
      (3) Treatment (active bleeding, hemolytic disease, extracorporeal membrane oxygenation).
      (4) Minimal fluid administration (approximate red cell mass of a whole unit of blood in one half fluid volume).
   c. Platelets.
      (1) Improved coagulation.
      (2) Treatment (hemorrhage caused by thrombocytopenia or platelet dysfunction).
   d. FFP: replacement of clotting factor deficiency.
   e. Albumin.
      (1) Volume expansion; improved oncotic pressure.
      (2) Treatment (for hypovolemia, third-space losses).
3. Alternatives.
   a. Directed donation.
      (1) Family and friends with compatible blood type can donate for infant.
      (2) Blood must be irradiated to prevent graft-versus-host disease.
      (3) There is no evidence of overall increased safety in comparison with anonymous volunteer donations.
         (a) Donors might be more truthful (i.e., regarding acceptability for donation) because they know the recipient.
         (b) Donors might be less truthful because they feel pressure to donate.
      (4) Parental donation.
         (a) Maternal plasma is unacceptable for transfusion to neonates because of the possible presence of antibodies directed against inherited paternal antigens on infant's cells.
         (b) Maternal platelets and RBCs can be used if washed before transfusion.
         (c) Paternal donation might be problematic if infant has circulating maternal antibodies produced by stimulation of inherited paternal antigens.
      (5) All blood products from directed donors should be irradiated. Potential antigen similarities between close family members may impede recognition and destruction of foreign lymphocytes.
   b. Erythropoietin (EPO) (Ohls, 2002; Ohls et al., 2001; Ohlsson and Aher, 2006; Strauss, 2006).
      (1) Recombinant human EPO (r-HuEPO) might be used to treat symptomatic anemia caused by physiologic decline in hematocrit or by blood loss from phlebotomy, or it might be used as a prophylactic therapy to minimize blood product exposure in preterm or sick neonates.
      (2) Plasma EPO levels are lower in anemic preterm infants, suggesting responsibility for hematocrit decline.
         (a) The liver, the initial site of EPO production at early gestation, is less responsive than the kidney to tissue hypoxia caused by anemia.
         (b) EPO pharmacokinetics differ in preterm infants: faster rate of clearance, larger volume of distribution, shorter elimination and mean residence times.
         (c) Clearance increases with duration of r-HuEPO therapy, suggesting the need for progressively higher doses.
      (3) Variable results and small sample sizes hamper clinical trials testing different doses and treatment schedules.
         (a) Therapy with r-HuEPO and iron stimulates erythropoiesis and increases reticulocyte counts.

(b) Increase in reticulocyte count is dose dependent.

(c) Oral iron supplement, adequate to support enhanced erythropoiesis, may not be tolerated. Intravenous iron therapy has not yet been adequately studied to ensure absence of oxidant injury and toxic metabolites; however, preterm infants appear to need a supplement of 4 to 4.5 mg/kg of dietary iron to prevent late anemia (CPS, 2002).

(d) The combination of r-HuEPO and iron stimulates erythropoiesis in infants of less than or equal to 1250 g birth weight; however, the lack of impact on transfusion requirements does not support routine use of r-HuEPO (Ohlsson and Aher, 2006; Strauss, 2006).

    c. Thrombopoietin. Recombinant human thrombopoietin is currently under development and testing for use as a megakaryocyte enhancer.

    d. G-CSF: currently under investigation; stimulates growth of neutrophil colonies and induces maturation of promyelocytes to mature neutrophils.

D. Transfusion volumes.

    1. Transfusions with PRBCs. For prevention of overhydration, replacement is usually given in increments of 15 to 20 ml/kg; 20 ml/kg results in a higher hemoglobin level and is associated with fewer transfusions than is 10 ml/kg (Murray and Roberts, 2004).

    2. Partial exchange transfusions.

        a. With normal saline solution: treatment of polycythemia (to reduce hematocrit without reducing blood volume).

        b. With PRBCs: treatment of hydrops fetalis (to correct anemia without increasing blood volume).

        c. Calculations for total exchange volume:

            (1) Volume of normal saline solution to exchange =

$$\frac{\text{Blood volume} \times (\text{Measured hematocrit} - \text{Desired hematocrit})}{\text{Measured hematocrit}}$$

            (2) PRBC volume to exchange =

$$\frac{\text{Blood volume} \times (\text{Desired hematocrit} - \text{Measured hematocrit})}{\text{PRBC hematocrit} - \text{Measured hematocrit}}$$

    3. Exchange transfusions.

        a. Single unit of blood (approximately 250 ml) will usually exchange twice the blood volume and remove 90% of the initial RBCs and 50% of the available intravascular bilirubin (Murray and Roberts, 2004).

        b. For treatment of hyperbilirubinemia.

        c. Because preservatives provide a significant glucose load, rebound hypoglycemia may occur.

        d. Preservatives contain citrate, which binds calcium and magnesium; hypocalcemia and hypomagnesemia may occur.

        e. Potassium level rises as blood ages; blood should be less than 5 days old. Washed RBCs may reduce the level of extracellular potassium and prevent hyperkalemia (Wu and Stack, 2007).

    4. Platelets.

        a. One unit (approximately 40 ml) provides approximately 5×10^{10} platelets; transfusion of 5 to 10 ml/kg of platelets should increase the platelet count by 50,000 to 100,000/mm^3 (Wu and Stack, 2007).

        b. Routine volume reduction (platelet concentration) before transfusion is not indicated in infants.

        c. Platelets are separated from single units of whole blood within 6 hours of collection and suspended in small amounts of plasma, or they are obtained by apheresis (single-donor platelets).

    5. FFP.

        a. FFP is usually transfused in increments of 10 ml/kg to minimize overhydration.

    b. Transfusion of 15 to 20 ml/kg replaces all coagulation proteins present in adult concentrations.

    c. Plasma is obtained from a unit of whole blood and frozen within 6 hours of collection.

6. Cryoprecipitate.

    a. Transfusion volume is usually 1 unit/kg (approximate volume, 15 ml).

    b. One unit contains approximately 100 to 250 mg of factor I (fibrinogen), approximately 80 to 100 units of factor VIII (von Willebrand), and 50 to 75 units of factor XIII.

7. Albumin.

    a. For volume expansion, 5% albumin is usually administered in increments of 10 ml/kg; for improvement of oncotic pressure, 25% albumin might be used in increments of 1 g/kg (4 ml/kg).

    b. Albumin is a major contributor to oncotic pressure because of molecular size and weight.

8. Granulocytes.

    a. Collected by leukapheresis and selectively harvested from whole blood.

    b. Granulocyte transfusions are now rarely used due to the difficulty in isolation and the efficacy of G-CSF in elevating neutrophil counts (Blanchette et al., 2005).

RECOMBINANT HEMATOPOIETIC GROWTH FACTORS

The identification, characterization, and molecular cloning of blood cell growth factors have facilitated production of therapeutic quantities of recombinant hematopoietic growth factors. These include G-CSF, M-CSF, EPO, and thrombopoietin (all of which act on committed cell lineages), as well as GM-CSF, IL-3, and IL-11, which act on earlier progenitor cells. The efficacy and safety of these growth factors are currently being evaluated (Clapp et al., 2001).

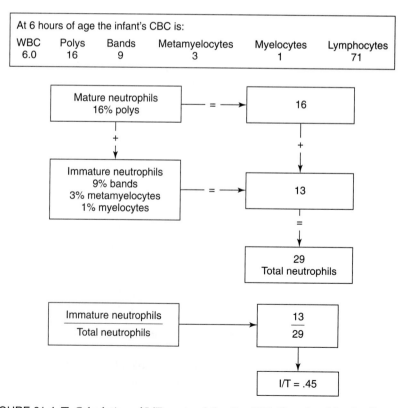

FIGURE 31-4 ■ Calculation of I/T neutrophil ratio. *CBC,* Complete blood cell count.

EVALUATION BY COMPLETE BLOOD CELL COUNT

The complete blood cell count is used in evaluating red blood cells, white blood cells, and platelets. The white blood cell indices are reviewed in Chapter 32.

A. Evaluation of RBC indices.

1. Identification of diseases affecting synthesis of hemoglobin.
2. RBC morphology.
   a. Anisocytosis: abnormal variation in size of erythrocytes (severe anemia).
   b. Macrocytosis: diameter greater than 9 mcm (increased cell volume: vitamin B_{12} and folic acid deficiencies).
   c. Microcytosis: diameter less than 9 mcm (decreased cell volume: iron deficiency, spherocytic and hemolytic anemias).
   d. Poikilocytosis: variation in shape (severe anemia).
   e. Spherocytosis: increased thickness and rounding (decreased deformability and greater susceptibility to destruction; seen in congenital spherocytosis, hemolytic anemias, after transfusion of stored blood).
   f. Target cells: thin, with large diameter, dark center and periphery, and a clear ring between the periphery and the center (hemoglobinopathies, sickle cell/thalassemia, liver disease).
   g. Burr cells: crenations; long spinous processes (hemolytic anemias, DIC, liver disease).
   h. Howell–Jolly bodies: spherical blue bodies in or on erythrocytes; nuclear debris (in asplenia, pernicious anemia).
   i. Nucleated red blood cells: immature red cells with nuclei still present (in chronic blood loss, significant hemolysis, chronic hypoxia, infection).

REFERENCES

Abbott, M.B., Levin, R.H., and Wu, S.: Medication potpourri. *Pediatrics in Review*, 27(8):283-288, 2006.

American Academy of Pediatrics Committee on Fetus and Newborn: Controversies concerning vitamin K and the newborn. *Pediatrics*, 112(1):191-192, 2003.

American Cancer Society: *Risks of blood product transfusion*. 2006. Retrieved March 5, 2008, from http://www.cancer.org/docroot/ETO/content/ETO_1_4x_Possible_Risks_of_Blood_Product_Transfusions.asp

American Red Cross: *Blood services national testing labs*. 2008. Retrieved March 5, 2008, from http://www.redcross.org/services/biomed/0,1082,0_494_,00.html

Baer, V.L., Lambert, D.K., Henry, E., Snow, G.L., Sola-Visner, M.C., and Christensen, R.D.: Do platelet transfusions in the NICU adversely affect survival? Analysis of 1600 thrombocytopenic neonates in a multihospital healthcare system. *Journal of Perinatology*, 27(12):790-796, 2007.

Bain, A. and Blackburn, S.: Issues in transfusing preterm infants in the NICU. *Journal of Perinatal and Neonatal Nursing*, 18(2):170-182, 2004.

Bick, R.L.: Disseminated intravascular coagulation current concepts of etiology, pathophysiology, diagnosis, and treatment. *Hematology/Oncology Clinics of North America*, 17(1):149-176, 2003.

Black, V.D., Lubchenco, L.O., Koops, B.L., et al.: Neonatal hyperviscosity: Randomized study of effect of partial plasma exchange transfusion on long-term outcome. *Pediatrics*, 75(6):1048-1053, 1985.

Blackburn, S.T.: *Maternal, fetal, and neonatal physiology: A clinical perspective* (3rd ed.). St. Louis, 2007, Saunders, pp. 242-266.

Blanchette, V., Dror, Y., and Chan, A.: Hematology. In M.G. MacDonald, M.D. Mullett, and M.M.K. Seshia (Eds.): *Avery's neonatology: Pathophysiology and management of the newborn*. Philadelphia, 2005, Lippincott Williams & Wilkins, pp. 1169-1234.

Blickstein, I. and Friedman, S.: Fetal effects of autoimmune disease. In R.J. Martin, A.A. Fanaroff, and M.C. Walsh (Eds.): *Fanaroff and Martin's neonatal-perinatal medicine: Diseases of the fetus and infant* (8th ed.). Philadelphia, 2006, Mosby, pp. 367-374.

Brugnara, C. and Platt, O.S.: The neonatal erythrocyte and its disorders. In D.G. Nathan, S.H. Orkin, D. Ginsberg, and A.T. Look (Eds.): *Nathan and Oski's hematology of infancy and childhood* (6th ed.). Philadelphia, 2003, Saunders, pp. 19-55.

Busfield, A., McNinch, A., and Tripp, J.: Neonatal vitamin K prophylaxis in Great Britain and Ireland: The impact of perceived risk and product licensing on effectiveness. *Archives of Disease in Childhood*, 92(9):754-758, 2007.

Canadian Paediatric Society (Fetus and Newborn Committee): Routine administration of vitamin K to newborns. *Pediatrics & Child Health*, 2(6):429-431, 1997. Reaffirmed 2004.

Canadian Paediatric Society (Fetus and Newborn Committee): Red blood cell transfusions in newborn infants: Revised guidelines. *Pediatrics & Child Health*, 7(8):553-558, 2002.

Capasso, L., Raimondi, F., Capasso, A., et al.: Early cord clamping protects at-risk neonates from polycythemia. *Biology of the Neonate, 83*(3):197-200, 2003.

Clapp, D.W., Shannon, K.M., and Phibbs, R.H.: Hematologic problems. In M.H. Klaus and A.A. Fanaroff (Eds.): *Care of the high-risk neonate* (5th ed.). Philadelphia, 2001, Saunders, pp. 447-480.

Clarke, P., Mitchell, S.J., Wynn, R., et al.: Vitamin K prophylaxis for preterm infants: A randomized, controlled trial of 3 regimens. *Pediatrics, 118*(6):e1657-1666, 2006.

Clarke, P. and Shearer, M.J.: Vitamin K deficiency bleeding: The readiness is all. *Archives of Disease in Childhood, 92*(9):741-743, 2007.

Delaney-Black, V., Camp, B.W., Lubchenco, L.O., et al.: Neonatal hyperviscosity in association with lower achievement and IQ scores at school age. *Pediatrics, 83*(5):662-667, 1989.

Dempsey, E.M. and Barrington, K.: Crystalloid or colloid for partial exchange transfusion in neonatal polycythemia: A systematic review and meta-analysis. *Acta Paediatrica, 94*(11):1650-1655, 2005.

Drew, J.H., Guaran, R.L., Cichello, M., and Hobbs, J.B.: Neonatal whole blood hyperviscosity: The important factor influencing later neurologic function is the viscosity and not the polycythemia. *Clinical Hemorheology and Microcirculation, 17*(1):67-72, 1997.

Edwards, T.J.: Hemophilia in the newborn: A case presentation. *Neonatal Network, 17*(2):67-71, 1998.

Galel, S.A. and Fontaine, M.J.: Hazards of neonatal blood transfusion. *NeoReviews, 7*(2):e69, 2006.

Hagstrom, J.N.: Pathophysiology of bleeding disorders in the newborn. In R.A. Polin and W.W. Fox (Eds.): *Fetal and neonatal physiology* (3rd ed.). Philadelphia, 2004, Saunders, pp. 1447-1460.

Israels, L.G. and Israels, S.J.: *Mechanisms in hematology* (3rd ed.). Toronto, 2002, Core Health Sciences, Inc., p. 402.

Kates, E.H. and Kates, J.S.: Anemia and polycythemia in the newborn. *Peds in Review, 28*:33-34, 2007.

Liley, H.G.: Immune hemolytic disease. In D.G. Nathan, S.H. Orkin, D. Ginsberg, and A.T. Look (Eds.): *Nathan and Oski's hematology of infancy and childhood* (6th ed.). Philadelphia, 2003, Saunders, pp. 56-85.

Luchtman-Jones, L., Schwartz, A.L., Wilson, D.B.: The blood and hematopoietic system. In R.J. Martin, A.A. Fanaroff, and M.C. Walsh (Eds.): *Fanaroff and Martin's neonatal-perinatal medicine: Diseases of the fetus and infant* (8th ed.). Philadelphia, 2006, Mosby, pp. 1287-1356.

Manco-Johnson, M., Rodden D.J., and Collins S.M.: Newborn hematology. In G.B. Merenstein and S.L. Gargner (Eds.): *Handbook of neonatal intensive care*. St. Louis, 2006, Mosby, pp. 521-547.

Manco-Johnson, M.: Pathophysiology of neonatal disseminated intravascular coagulation and thrombosis. In R.A. Polin, W.W. Fox, and S.H. Abman (Eds.): *Fetal and neonatal physiology* (3rd ed.). Philadelphia, 2004, Saunders, pp. 1460-1473.

Murphy, M.F. and Bussel, J.B.: Advances in the management of alloimmune thrombocytopenia. *British Journal of Haematology, 136*(3):366-378, 2007.

Monagle, P. and Andrew, M.: Acquired disorders of hemostasis. In D.G. Nathan, S.H. Orkin, D. Ginsberg,

and A.T. Look (Eds.): *Nathan and Oski's hematology of infancy and childhood* (6th ed.). Philadelphia, 2003, Saunders, pp. 1631-1667.

Murray, N.A. and Roberts, I.A.: Neonatal transfusion practice. *Archives of Disease in Childhood Fetal and Neonatal Edition, 89*(2):F101-F107, 2004.

Ohls, R.K.: Developmental erythropoiesis. In R.A. Polin, W.W. Fox, and S.H. Abman (Eds.): *Fetal and neonatal physiology* (3rd ed.). Philadelphia, 2004, Saunders, pp. 1397-1420.

Ohls, R.K.: Erythropoietin treatment in extremely low birth weight infants: Blood in versus blood out. *Journal of Pediatrics, 141*(1):3-6, 2002.

Ohls, R.K., Ehrenkranz, R.A., Wright, L.L., et al.: Effects of early erythropoietin therapy on the transfusion requirements of preterm infants below 1250 grams birth weight: A multicenter, randomized, controlled trial. *Pediatrics, 108*(4):1-18, 2001.

Ohlsson, A. and Aher, S.M.: Early erythropoietin for preventing red blood cell transfusion in preterm and/or low birth weight infants. *Cochrane Database of Systematic Reviews, 3*:CD004863, July 19, 2006.

Oski, F.A., Brugnara, C., and Nathan, D.G.: A diagnostic approach to the anemic patient. In D.G. Nathan, S.H. Orkin, D. Ginsberg, and A.T. Look (Eds.): *Nathan and Oski's hematology of infancy and childhood* (6th ed.). Philadelphia, 2003, Saunders, pp. 409-418.

Pappas, A. and Delaney-Black, V.: Differential diagnosis and management of polycythemia. *Pediatric Clinics of North America, 51*(4):1063-1086, 2004.

Parker, R.I.: Neonatal thrombosis, hemostasis, and platelet disorders. In A.R. Spitzer (Ed.): *Intensive care of the fetus and newborn* (2nd ed.). Philadelphia, 2005, Mosby, pp. 1295-1312.

Quirolo, K.C.: Transfusion medicine for the pediatrician. *Pediatric Clinics of North America, 49*(6):1-23, 2002.

Schimmel, M.S., Bromiker, R., and Soll, R.F.: Neonatal polycythemia: Is partial exchange transfusion justified? *Clinics in Perinatology, 31*:545-553, 2004.

Schupbach, J.: Measurement of HIV-1 p24 antigen by signal-amplification-boosted ELISA of heat-denatured plasma is a simple and inexpensive alternative to tests for viral RNA. *AIDS Reviews, 4*(2):83-92, 2002.

Steiner, L.A. and Gallagher, P.G.: Erythrocyte disorders in the perinatal period. *Seminars in Perinatology, 31*:254-261, 2007.

Strauss, R.G.: Controversies in the management of the anemia of prematurity using single-donor red blood cell transfusions and/or recombinant human erythropoietin. *Transfusion Medicine Reviews, 20*(1):34-44, 2006.

Strauss, R.G.: Neonatal red blood cell, platelet, plasma, and neutrophil transfusion. In T.L. Simon, W.H. Dzik, E.L. Snyder, et al. (Eds.): *Rossi's principles of transfusion medicine* (3rd ed.). Philadelphia, 2002, Lippincott Williams & Wilkins, pp. 486-498.

Tandoi, F., Mosca, F., and Agosti, M.: Vitamin K prophylaxis: Leaving the old route for the new one? *Acta Paediatrica, 94*(Suppl 449):125-128, 2005.

Westkamp, E., Soditt, V., Adrian, S., et al.: Blood transfusions in anemic infants with apnea of prematurity. *Biology of the Neonate, 82*(4):228-232, 2002.

Wilson, D.B.: Acquired platelet defects. In D.G. Nathan, S.H. Orkin, D. Ginsberg, and A.T. Look (Eds.): *Nathan and Oski's hematology of infancy and childhood* (6th ed.). Philadelphia, 2003, Saunders, pp. 1597-1630.

Wong, E.C. and Luban, N.L.: Intrauterine, neonatal, and pediatric transfusion. In P.D. Mintz (Ed.): *Transfusion therapy: Clinical principles and practice* (2nd ed.). Bethseda, MD, 2005, AABB Press, pp. 159-201.

Wu, Y., and Stack, G.: Blood product replacement in the perinatal period. *Seminars in Perinatology*, 31:262-271, 2007.

32 Immunology and Infectious Disease

▪▪▪

JUDY WRIGHT LOTT

OBJECTIVES

1. Describe the unique immunodeficiencies in the preterm and term infant.
2. Differentiate between humoral and cellular immunologic response in the neonate.
3. Differentiate the three categories of acquisition of infection.
4. Describe clinical signs and symptoms of early- and late-onset bacterial infection.
5. Calculate the absolute neutrophil count and immature/total cell ratio from a complete blood cell count and differential cell count.
6. Identify the common gram-positive and gram-negative organisms responsible for bacterial infections in the neonatal period.
7. Name common broad-spectrum antimicrobial agents used to treat neonatal sepsis and discuss indications for and risks of their use.
8. Differentiate between mucocutaneous, systemic, and cutaneous candidiasis.
9. List several clinical manifestations associated with congenital viral infection.
10. Describe the transmission of human immunodeficiency virus and its effect on the immune system.

▪
▪▪ Neonatal sepsis is a major cause of death during the first month of life. Neonatal sepsis is a general term used to define actual or potential infection. In the term infant early-onset bacterial infection occurs in 1 to 8 infants per 1000 live births. In several large multicenter studies from the National Institute of Child Health and Human Development Neonatal Research Network, 24% of very low birth weight (VLBW) infants were reported to have significant early-onset infections (Fanaroff et al., 1995, 1998; Hack et al., 1995; Stoll et al., 1996a). The diagnosis of early-onset sepsis, in the first 72 hours of life, remains one of the most difficult diagnostic tasks for neonatal nurses, advanced practice nurses, and physicians. Blood cultures may remain negative in the presence of pneumonia, meningitis, and even in clear indications of clinical signs suggesting fulminant blood-borne sepsis. In addition, secondary to the increasing use of intrapartum maternal antibiotics, one must not rely solely on the presence of a positive neonatal blood culture to confirm early-onset sepsis. In contrast to early-onset sepsis, late-onset sepsis or those neonatal infections acquired later by horizontal transmission (nosocomial) can occur in as many as 250 infants per 1000 live births. In late-onset sepsis there is an increased risk of developing meningitis (4 to 10 per 10,000 live births). Whereas this infection is rare in the neonate, the risk in the first month of life is the highest and 40% of the survivors of meningitis will have some neurologic sequelae. Early detection and implementation of therapy are critical.

Failure to identify early-onset sepsis contributes to morbidity, mortality, and increased health care costs. The mortality rate is high (4.2% to 26%), with the higher rates observed in premature infants and in those with early fulminant clinical signs (Stoll et al., 1996a). A review of the immune system and neonatal infection will aid in the understanding of the unique host-defense limitations of the term and premature infant. Accurate interpretation of hematologic and other studies and identification of risk factors and clinical signs of sepsis may facilitate early detection of neonatal infection.

Group B streptococci (GBS) and *Escherichia coli* are responsible for the majority of early-onset sepsis. Coagulase-negative staphylococci and *Candida albicans* are presently the most common nosocomial infections in hospitalized low birth weight infants. Antibiotic therapy for bacterial infections must be based on the susceptibility of the organism and the achievement of adequate bactericidal concentrations. Congenital viral infections may be asymptomatic at birth or may involve multiple systems depending on time of acquisition. Human immunodeficiency virus (HIV) has become a leading cause of immunodeficiency in the neonate, with maternal–infant transmission accounting for the majority of neonatal acquisitions.

This chapter provides the nurse with a comprehensive review of the neonatal immune system and common neonatal infections.

IMMUNE SYSTEM

A. Host defense mechanisms of the immune system.

1. Overall functions of the immune system.
   a. Defense—resistance to infection by microorganisms.
   b. Homeostasis—removal of worn-out cells.
   c. Surveillance—perception and destruction of mutant cells.
2. Components of the immune system.
   a. The nonspecific mechanisms, which include phagocytosis, the inflammatory response, and several amplification systems including complement, coagulation, and kinin systems.
   b. The specific immune responses, which consist of cell-mediated (T cell) and humoral (B cell) systems.
      (1) Both are interdependent and interrelated; for example, the activation of the complement system by immunoglobulins (IgM and IgG), or the production of chemotactic factors and other lymphokines, plays a significant role in the whole inflammatory response.
      (2) Nonspecific immune mechanisms—function without prior exposure, identified early in gestation, functional development at 32 to 33 weeks.
   c. Embryologic development (Table 32-1).
      (1) The maturation of specific immune responses begins in utero during the 7th to the 12th weeks of gestation.
      (2) Progenitor cells (stem cells) are initially located in the yolk sac, fetal liver, and bone marrow of the developing embryo.

■ TABLE 32-1
■ ■ **Development of Immune System in the Fetus**

Gestation (Weeks)	Findings
4	First blood centers appear in the yolk sac
5.5	Synthesis of complement is detected
7	Lymphocytes appear in peripheral blood, about 1000/mm^3
7 to 9	Lymphocytes appear in the thymus
11	T-cell receptors (E rosette) develop in thymus lymphocytes. B-cell maturation occurs in the liver and spleen, with IgG, IgA, IgM, and IgD surface markers. Serum IgG levels can be detected
12	Antigen recognition is demonstrable
13	Graft-versus-host reactivity is present
14	PHA response by thymus lymphocytes occurs
17	Serum IgM levels can be detected
20	Secondary lymphoid complex is present
20 to 25	Lymphocytes in blood number about 10,000/mm^3
22	Complement levels detectable in serum
30	IgA level detectable in serum

IgG, Immunoglobulin G; *PHA*, pituitary adrenal hypothalamus.
Adapted from Cauchi, M.N.: *Obstetrics and perinatal immunology.* London, 1981, Edward Arnold.

    d. Depending on the type of microchemical environment surrounding the tissue, the stem cells will differentiate along at least two pathways:

      (1) The hematopoietic.

      (2) The lymphopoietic.

        (a) The lymphopoietic system develops along two independent pathways leading to morphologically and functionally distinct populations of immune systems:

          (i) The thymus-derived or T system of cell-mediated immunity whose principal effector cells are the T lymphocytes.

          (ii) The bursal-dependent or B system of humoral or antibody-mediated immunity, which is displayed by the B lymphocytes.

      (3) The thymus gland is derived from epithelium of the third and fourth pharyngeal pouches at about 6 weeks.

      (4) Concomitantly, the parathyroids also begin their development at about this time from the same location.

      (5) Caudal migration occurs, and beginning at about 8 weeks bloodborne stem cells invade the gland and are induced into lymphoid differentiation.

      (6) With further development, the thymus is infiltrated by lymphocytes and differentiates into a dense cortex and a less dense loose central medulla with relatively more epithelial tissue.

      (7) Within the thymus gland, an intense rate of mitosis occurs, greater than in any other lymphatic organ.

B. Humoral immunity (Blackburn, 2007).

    1. Immunoglobulin (McCance and Huether, 2002; Polin et al., 2001).

      a. Humoral immunity is a specific antibody-mediated response that functions most effectively if there has been previous exposure.

      b. Antibodies are derived from B cells, which have been activated by T cells and antigens (Fig. 32-1).

        (1) B cells mature and are stored in lymph tissue and bone marrow.

        (2) B cells also produce memory cells that recognize antigens on subsequent exposures and initiate an antibody response.

        (3) Antibody functions include:

          (a) Recognition of bacterial antigens.

          (b) Neutralization or opsonization of foreign substances, rendering them susceptible to phagocytosis.

    2. Types of immunoglobulin.

      a. Immunoglobulin G (IgG).

        (1) Major immunoglobulin of serum and interstitial fluid.

        (2) Provides immunity against bacterial and viral pathogens.

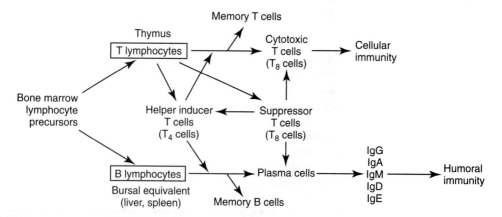

FIGURE 32-1 ■ Development of cellular and humoral immunity. (From Ganong, W.F.: *Review of physiology* [14th ed.]. East Norwalk, CT, 1989, Appleton & Lange.)

(3) Placental transfer to the fetus is either an active or a passive process.

(4) Increases gradually until 40 weeks of gestation (majority is passed in the third trimester).

(5) Decreased levels in preterm infants, proportional to their gestational age.

(6) Decreased levels in postmature and small for gestational-age infants, suggesting inhibition of transfer with placental damage.

b. Immunoglobulin M (IgM).

(1) Does not cross the placental barrier.

(2) Synthesis begins early in fetal life, with detectable levels at approximately 30 weeks of gestation.

(3) Levels may increase (>20 mg/ml) with intrauterine infection.

(4) Serum levels rapidly increase after birth.

c. Immunoglobulin A (IgA).

(1) Is the most common immunoglobulin in the gastrointestinal and respiratory tracts and is secreted in human colostrum and human milk.

(2) Does not cross the placental barrier.

(3) Intrauterine synthesis is minimal in an uninfected fetus.

(4) Does not become detectable in the infant until 2 to 3 weeks of postnatal life.

(5) Levels may increase with certain congenital viral infections.

d. Immunoglobulin E (IgE).

(1) Present in very small amounts in serum and secretions.

(2) Major role in allergic reactions.

C. Cellular immunity.

1. Specific cellular immunity is mediated by T lymphocytes, which enhance the efficiency of the phagocytic responses.

a. T lymphocytes migrate to the thymus, where they begin differentiation (see Fig. 32-1).

b. They are activated by antigens to which they have become sensitized and subsequently become memory or activated T cells. However, they must be "processed" and presented on the surface of antigen-presenting cells (i.e., macrophages and monocytes).

(1) Memory cells respond at a later time to the same antigen.

(2) There are three types of activated T cells.

(a) Cytotoxic: kill foreign or virus-infected cells.

(b) Helper: enable B or T cells to respond to antigens and activate macrophages.

(c) Suppressor: repress responses of specific T and B lymphocytes to antigens.

(3) T lymphocytes modify the behavior of phagocytic cells, produce a variety of cytokines, and increase their antimicrobial activity.

(4) Depressed T-cell function may occur as a consequence of neonatal viral infection, hyperbilirubinemia, corticosteroid therapy, or maternal medications taken late in pregnancy.

2. Nonspecific cellular immunity is an inflammatory response involving phagocytosis and includes neutrophils, monocytes, and complement. Neutrophilic cell invasion and platelet aggregation are aided by the activation of the three important plasma protein systems (the complement, clotting, and kinin systems) and immunoglobulins. Additionally, some host cells produce soluble factors that contribute to defenses by affecting other neighboring cells. These factors are known as cytokines and include interleukins, interferons, and other proteins. Cytokines are multifunctional proteins, often referred to as "hormones of the immune system."

a. Neutrophils are phagocytes and must detect them and move toward them (chemotaxis), adhere to them (adhesion), ingest them (phagocytosis), and kill them by intracellular generation of toxic oxygen metabolites such as superoxide ions (respiratory burst).

(1) Neutrophils mature from the bone marrow from the committed phagocyte stem cells.

(2) They are the first line of defense against bacterial infection.

(3) A neutrophil storage pool (reserve) is present and exceeds the circulating pool; however, in a septic neonate, the neutrophil reserve pool quickly becomes depleted because of the following:

    (a) Decrease in proliferation or reproduction.

    (b) Decrease in the immature neutrophil storage pool.

    (c) Decrease in the number of neutrophils that reach the site of infection.

  b. Monocytes are important in the defense against fungal and bacterial infections and are found primarily in the connective tissue.

  c. Complement is a series of proteins that interact or mediate a cascade of synthesis of other proteins responsible for chemotaxis, opsonization, and cell lysis.

    (1) Activation by an antibody-dependent mechanism (classic pathway) or antibody-independent mechanism (alternative pathway).

    (2) Purpose.

      (a) Increase neutrophil mobilization from the bone marrow.

      (b) Draw neutrophils to the site of infection.

      (c) Opsonize bacteria for improved phagocytosis.

      (d) Interleukins (ILs) are biochemical messengers produced by the macrophages or lymphocytes in response to stimulation by an antigen or by products of inflammation (Fig. 32-2). The analysis of immunologic mediators may greatly enhance timely diagnosis of sepsis. Concentrations of the cytokines interleukin-1 receptor antagonist (IL-1ra), interleukin-6 (IL-6), and the circulating adhesion molecule-1 (cICAM-1) are elevated in sepsis. IL-6 plays a critical role in the induction of C-reactive protein (CRP) in the liver. Interleukin-6 is an important mediator of the early inflammatory host response to infection; it reaches peak concentrations rapidly after the onset of bacteremia, several hours before the upregulation of CRP by IL-6 begins. IL-6 is a multifunctional polypeptide and is synthesized by an array of cells.

D. Summary of neonatal immunodeficiencies.

  1. Humoral immunity.

    a. Decreased antibody levels.

      (1) Poor response to antigenic stimuli.

      (2) No production of type-specific antibodies.

      (3) Fewer B cells recognize foreign antibodies.

      (4) Delay in the development of cytotoxic T lymphocytes, increasing the risk for viral infections.

    b. Decreased opsonic activity.

      (1) Impaired circulating antibody.

      (2) Maternal complement is not transferred.

      (3) Depressed complement (classical and alternate) pathways and decreased levels of components of the complement cascade (50% to 80%) of adult values and less in the premature infant.

  2. Neutrophil response.

    a. Diminished size of neutrophil storage and proliferative pools.

    b. Reduced numbers of immature neutrophils in the storage pool.

    c. Failure to increase stem cell proliferation during infection.

    d. Abnormal neutrophil function (adhesion, chemotaxis, phagocytosis, and bacterial killing).

TRANSMISSION OF INFECTIOUS ORGANISMS IN THE NEONATE

A. Vertical transmission: mother to infant.

  1. Transplacental acquisition.

    a. Transplacental hematogenous transmission (crosses from the placenta to the fetus).

      (1) *Treponema pallidum* and *Listeria monocytogenes*.

  2. Ascending acquisition: into the uterus near time of delivery, when the cervical mucous plug, chorion, and amnion are less than optimal barriers.

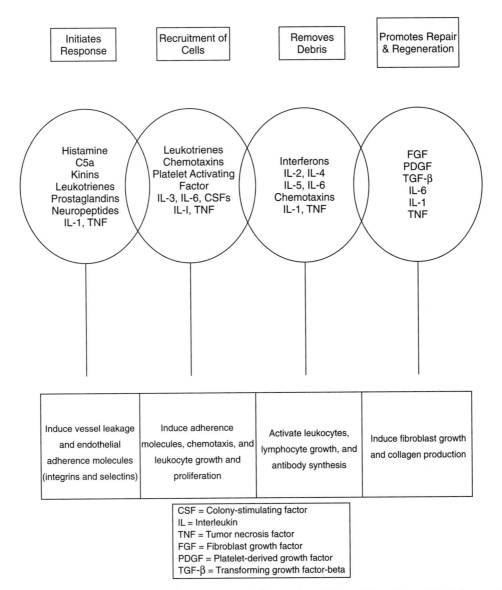

FIGURE 32-2 ■ Mediators associated with stages of inflammation. (Adapted from Rote, N.S.: Inflammation. In K.L. McCance and S.E. Huether [Eds.]: *Pathophysiology: The biologic basis for disease in adults and children* [4th ed.]. St. Louis, 2002, Mosby, p. 214.)

   3. Intrapartum acquisition: natal transmission at delivery, during passage of the fetus through a birth canal that is host to a variety of bacteria, as well as chlamydiae, fungi, yeast, and viruses. This mechanism implies colonization of the skin, mucous membranes, gastrointestinal tract, and respiratory tract during parturition.
B. **Horizontal transmission:** from nursery personnel and the hospital equipment to the infant; also known as a nosocomial infection.

DIAGNOSIS AND THERAPY

Clinical Assessment

Identification of Predisposing Risk Factors Found in the Maternal History
A. **Maternal.**
   1. Antepartum.
      a. Inadequate prenatal care.

      b. Inadequate nutrition.

      c. Low socioeconomic status.

      d. Recurrent abortion.

      e. Substance abuse.

      f. History of maternal sexually transmitted diseases.

  2. Intrapartum.

      a. Prolonged rupture of membranes (>12 to 18 hours).

      b. Vaginal group B streptococcal colonization.

      c. Low levels of maternal group B streptococcus (GBS) antibodies.

      d. Chorioamnionitis: sustained fetal tachycardia, uterine tenderness, purulent amniotic fluid, foul-smelling amniotic fluid, or unexplained maternal temperature higher than 38°C.

      e. Prolonged or difficult labor.

      f. Premature labor.

      g. Urinary tract infection.

      h. Invasive intrapartum procedures.

      i. Maternal fever.

      j. Elevated maternal heart rate (>100 beats per minute [bpm]).

      k. Elevated fetal heart rate (>160 bpm).

B. Neonatal.

  1. Prematurity (infants born <32 weeks of gestation have a 4 to 25 times increased risk).

  2. Low birth weight (<2500 g).

  3. Difficult delivery.

  4. Birth asphyxia.

  5. Meconium staining.

  6. Resuscitation.

  7. Congenital anomalies (i.e., abdominal wall and spinal defects).

  8. Black infants.

  9. Male infants.

 10. Multiple births.

C. Environmental.

  1. Hospital admission.

  2. Length of stay.

  3. Invasive procedures (i.e., peripheral IV punctures, endotracheal tubes, umbilical catheters, thoracostomy tubes, and other surgical interventions).

  4. Common use of broad-spectrum antibiotics.

  5. Use of humidification systems in ventilatory or incubator care.

Clinical Manifestations

A. Variable nonspecific presentation of sepsis: appearance of infant "just not right" to nurse or mother, accompanied by subtle changes in feeding and activity. Culture-proven sepsis is relatively rare in the newborn infant; many more infants have signs suggestive of infection at presentation.

B. Thermoregulatory instability.

  1. Temperature instability.

  2. Fever.

  3. Hypothermia.

C. Neurologic clinical signs.

  1. Lethargy.

  2. Jitteriness.

  3. Irritability.

  4. Seizures.

  5. Hypotonia or hypertonia.

  6. Bulging fontanelles.

  7. High-pitched cry.

D. Respiratory clinical signs: most common clinical sign occurring in 90% of infants with sepsis (Polin et al., 2001).

  1. Tachypnea.

    2. Grunting.
    3. Retractions.
    4. Cyanosis.
    5. Apnea.
E. Cardiovascular clinical signs.
    1. Tachycardia.
    2. Arrhythmias.
    3. Hypotension or hypertension.
    4. Cold, clammy skin.
    5. Decreased peripheral perfusion/vasoconstriction.
F. Gastrointestinal clinical signs.
    1. Poor feeding.
    2. Vomiting, diarrhea.
    3. Abdominal distention.
    4. Increasing feeding residuals.
G. Skin.
    1. Rash.
    2. Pustules.
    3. Jaundice.
    4. Pallor.
    5. Vasomotor instability.
    6. Petechiae.
H. Internal organ manifestations.
    1. Hepatomegaly.
    2. Splenomegaly.
I. Metabolic disturbances.
    1. Glucose instability.
    2. Metabolic acidosis.

Hematologic Evaluation

A. Complete blood cell count (CBC).
    1. White blood cell (WBC) count: interpretation is often difficult because of the wide range of normal values in the neonate (5000 to $30,000/mm^3$) (Oski and Naiman, 1966; Thureen et al., 2005).
        a. Leukocytosis: an elevated WBC count ($>25,000/mm^3$); may be a normal finding in the newborn infant.
        b. Leukopenia: a depressed WBC count ($<1750/mm^3$); generally is an abnormal finding in the newborn infant and may be due to sepsis or pregnancy-induced hypertension.
    2. Differential cell count (Fig. 32-3).
        a. Neutrophil count.
          (1) Absolute neutrophil count (ANC) is calculated as:
            (a) ANC = WBC × (% Immature neutrophils + % Mature neutrophils) × 0.01.
            (b) Manroe and colleagues (1979) developed a reference range for the absolute neutrophil count in term infants (Fig. 32-4).
          (2) Neutropenia: less than $1500/mm^3$.
            (a) Most accurate predictor of infection.
            (b) May be associated with maternal hypertension, confirmed periventricular hemorrhage, severe asphyxia, and reticulocytosis (after 14 postnatal days of life).
          (3) Neutrophilia.
            (a) Although less predictive, may also suggest presence of infection.
            (b) May be elevated at birth (as high as $26,000/mm^3$) because of birth stress, increased neutrophil production, and rates of release and demargination from the circulating neutrophil pool.
            (c) Other clinical conditions associated with neutrophilia include hemolytic disease, asymptomatic hypoglycemia, trisomy 21, use of oxytocin during labor, maternal

Neutrophil: Stages of Maturation

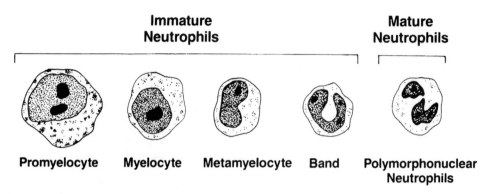

FIGURE 32-3 ■ Neutrophils represent a percentage of the total white blood cell count and are reported as the differential on a complete blood cell count.

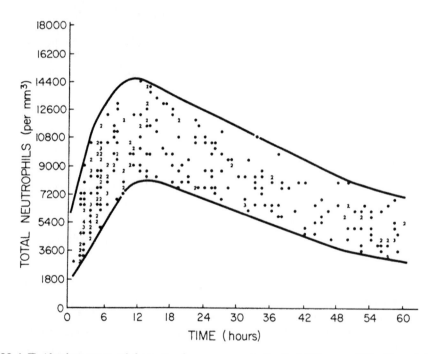

FIGURE 32-4 ■ Absolute neutrophil count reference range in the first 60 hours of life. (From Manroe, B.L., Weinberg, A.G., Rosenfeld, C.R., Browne, R., et al.: The neonatal blood count in health and disease. *Journal of Pediatrics, 95*[1]:89-98, 1979.)

       fever, stress during labor and birth, exogenous steroid administration, pneumothorax, and meconium aspiration.

b. Immature/total neutrophil (I/T) ratio.
  (1) Sensitivity is greater than 90%; however, less specific (having negative results when in fact there is no infection).
  (2) Increase in the I/T ratio also known as a left shift; reflects an increase in immature neutrophils.
  (3) I/T ratio greater than 0.20 is suggestive of infection (Fig. 32-5).
  (4) Calculation of I/T ratio:

$$\frac{\%\ \text{Bands} + \%\ \text{Immature forms}}{\%\ \text{Mature} + \%\ \text{Bands} + \%\ \text{Immature forms}}$$

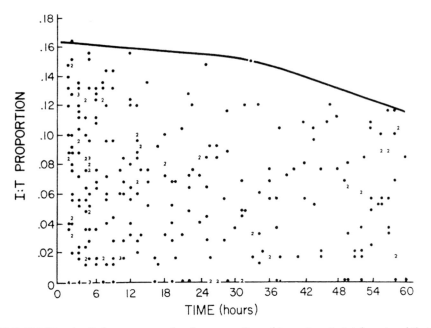

FIGURE 32-5 ■ I/T ratio. Reference range for the proportion of immature to total neutrophils in the first 60 hours of life. (From Manroe, B.L., Weinberg, A.G., Rosenfeld, C.R., Browne, R., et al.: The neonatal blood count in health and disease. *Journal of Pediatrics, 95*[1]:89-98, 1979.)

    c. Platelet count.
        (1) Normal count: 150,000 to 400,000/mm^3.
        (2) Thrombocytopenia (<100,000/mm^3): possible association with bacterial sepsis or viral infection.
        (3) Severe thrombocytopenia: possible association with disseminated intravascular coagulation (DIC).
B. Additional diagnostic screening tests.
  1. Detection of bacterial and viral deoxyribonucleic acid (DNA)–polymerase chain reaction (PCR).
    a. Provides a rapid and sensitive method of diagnosis of a specific bacterial or viral gene (DNA) segment.
    b. Identifies specific bacteria and viruses, such as *E. coli*, methicillin-resistant *Staphylococcus aureus* (MRSA), *Ureaplasma urealyticum*, herpes simplex virus, and hepatitis B virus.
        (1) May be performed on blood, catheter tips, cerebrospinal fluid, joint fluids, and other sterile body sites.
        (2) MRSA is an important cause of nosocomial infections. Nationally, 5% to 10% of all hospitalized patients will become colonized or infected with MRSA. In addition, coagulase-negative staphylococci are important causes of nosocomial bacteremia and catheter- or other iatrogenic device–associated infections. This PCR test amplifies a segment of the mecA gene. This PCR assay should be performed directly on all positive *S. aureus* blood cultures.
  2. Hematologic evidence of infection.
    a. Erythrocyte sedimentation rate. An indirect test of changes in serum proteins involved in the acute-phase reactant response. Although false-positive and false-negative results can occur and rates vary widely, levels may rise above the 95th percentile during an infectious process.
    b. CRP (Pourcyrous et al., 1993).
        (1) Nonspecific acute-phase reactant is synthesized by the liver in response to IL-6, which appears in the blood during an inflammatory process.

(2) Because of a latency period of 6 to 8 hours and a stabilization time of 1 to 2 days after the start of therapy, this test is best performed serially every 12 hours when infection is suspected. CRP is elevated in 50% to 90% of infected infants; however, it has a low positive predictive value (Malik et al., 2003).

(3) CRP is most useful in determining effectiveness of treatment, resolution of disease, and duration of antibiotic therapy.

c. IgM levels: may rise in the presence of bacterial and/or viral infections.

Diagnostic Evaluation

A. **Culture:** isolation of a pathogen in a blood culture obtained by using aseptic technique is the gold standard for diagnosing infection (Polin et al., 2001).

1. Blood.
    a. Culture specimen obtained from peripheral vein or umbilical vessel.
    b. Procedure.
        (1) Carefully clean infant's skin with an antiseptic such as povidone-iodine solution 10%.
        (2) For maximal bactericidal effect, allow skin to dry for 2 minutes before inserting needle and obtaining culture specimen.
        (3) A minimum of 1 ml of blood should be obtained to improve chances for detection of bacteremia. As many as 60% of culture results will be falsely negative if less than 1 ml is drawn (Schelonka et al., 1996).
    c. May be falsely negative if mother received antibiotics in labor.
    d. Blood culture results need to be followed at specified intervals, usually 24, 48, and 72 hours, and a final report at 5 to 14 days.
    e. 92% of positive blood culture will be positive by 24 hours (Byington et al., 2003).

2. Cerebrospinal fluid (CSF).
    a. Lumbar puncture. Routine use of lumbar puncture is controversial in early sepsis evaluation. It is frequently unsuccessful or bloody (Schwersenski et al., 1991) and may also compromise an unstable infant. Meningitis in the absence of bacteremia is uncommon, especially in the neonate with respiratory disease (Weiss et al., 1991). Lumbar puncture may be reserved for infants with central nervous system signs or proven bacteremia.
    b. Normal CSF findings.
        (1) A normal mean CSF leukocyte count of $9/mm^3$ (range $= 0$ to $22/mm^3$) in premature infants, and $8.2/mm^3$ (range $= 0$ to $25/mm^3$) in term infants.
        (2) A normal mean protein count of 57.2 mg/dl (range $= 65$ to 150 mg/dl) in premature infants, and a mean of 61.3 mg/dl (range $= 20$ to 170 mg/dl) in term infants.
        (3) CSF glucose concentration 55% to 105% in premature infants, 44% to 128% in term infants. Obtain serum level before spinal tap to allow for equilibrium to occur between CSF and blood.
        (4) Absence of microorganisms on Gram stain.
    c. Positive CSF culture.
        (1) Repeat the CSF tap every 24 to 36 hours until culture is sterile.
        (2) Duration of antibiotic therapy is based on when the first negative culture is documented.
        (3) There is a direct correlation between adverse neonatal outcome and persistence of bacteria in the CSF.

3. Urine.
    a. Incidence of contamination with urine obtained by an external collection bag is high. If urine is to be collected, the sample should be obtained by sterile catheterization or suprapubic needle aspiration to avoid contamination and false-positive results.
    b. If urine is obtained by urethral catheterization, a count greater than 50,000 to 100,000 organisms per milliliter suggests infection.
    c. When culture result is positive, a percutaneous suprapubic bladder tap should be performed because the urine is presumed to be sterile.

4. Superficial cultures: not recommended because
   a. Culture result may indicate colonization but does not show bacteremia or sepsis, and
   b. Infant may have sepsis in the absence of a positive surface culture result.
B. **Follow-up.**
   1. If a positive culture result has been obtained from blood, CSF, or urine specimen, a follow-up culture specimen should be obtained to document sterilization.
   2. Persistent bacteremia may be caused by
      a. Resistance to antibiotics,
      b. Incorrect administration of antibiotics,
      c. An occult site of infection that may require surgical intervention (e.g., abscess), or
      d. Central venous or peripherally inserted central catheters left in place during treatment for bacteremia.

Therapy

A. **Antibiotic therapy.**
   1. Appropriate antibiotic choice depends on the likely organisms, pharmacokinetics, efficacy, and potential toxicity of the antimicrobial agents used.
   2. Ampicillin is commonly used in combination with an aminoglycoside for initial broad-spectrum treatment of suspected or confirmed bacterial infection.
   3. If meningitis is suspected, ampicillin and cefotaxime are the antibiotics of choice until a specific organism has been identified.
   4. Third-generation cephalosporins, including cefotaxime and ceftazidime, have increased antimicrobial activity against gram-negative bacilli and enhanced penetration across the blood-brain barrier over gentamicin.
   5. Dosage and frequency of administration of antimicrobial agents vary with gestational age, birth weight, and postconceptual age.
   6. Duration of antibiotic therapy is 10 to 14 days for proven sepsis and 21 days for meningitis.
   7. If culture results are negative, antimicrobial agents may be discontinued after 48 to 72 hours.
   8. If the mother was treated before delivery, the antimicrobial course may be extended in the face of negative culture results (Polin et al., 2001).
B. **Immunotherapy:** The neonate is considered immunocompromised, and defense mechanisms to overcome infections are not yet mature. The administration of blood and tissue factors to enhance the neonatal immune system is under investigation.
   1. Intravenous immune globulin (IVIG).
      a. Administration of IVIG may be effective in reducing mortality from nosocomial infections, although there is insufficient evidence to support the routine administration of IVIG preparations investigated to date to prevent mortality in infants with suspected or subsequently proven neonatal infection (Ohlsson and Lacy, 2001).
      b. To be useful, IVIG transfusions must contain antibodies specific to the type of infection-causing organism.
      c. IVIG preparations contain protein and varying amounts of IgG, IgA, and IgM (Taketomo et al., 2002).
      d. IVIG acts to neutralize viruses, promote phagocytosis, increase opsonization, and enhance polymorphonucleocyte migration. It prevents neutrophil storage pool depletion by enhancing the neonate's IgG levels for protection against invading bacteria until the immune system is more mature.
      e. Studies continue to determine efficacy of treatment in neonatal infections.
   2. Granulocyte transfusion.
      a. Results in an increased number of polymorphonuclear neutrophils, which are responsible for phagocytic action in infection.
      b. May improve survival in infants with sepsis and a decreased neutrophil storage pool (Christensen et al., 1982).
      c. Process is both time consuming and expensive.

    d. Presumed risks include fluid overload, graft-versus-host disease, infections, and blood group sensitization.

    e. Studies continue to determine the potential for reducing morbidity and mortality rates for infection.

3. Exchange transfusion with fresh whole blood.

    a. Used in severe sepsis to remove bacterial endotoxins and decrease the bacterial burden, improve peripheral and pulmonary perfusion, and enhance the immune system.

    b. Used widely before 1980; however, limited prospective studies have been done to support effectiveness (Vain et al., 1980).

    c. Adverse reactions include hypoglycemia, acid–base imbalance, thrombocytopenia, and infection.

4. Granulocyte colony-stimulating factor (G-CSF).

    a. Acts to stimulate proliferation of neutrophils; primes neutrophils, thus enhancing their bactericidal and phagocytic activity.

    b. Early trials have demonstrated neutrophil enhancement in neonates without adverse hematologic, immunologic, or developmental defects.

    c. A Cochrane Review by Carr et al. (2003) concluded, "There is insufficient evidence to support the introduction of either G-CSF or granulocyte-macrophage colony-stimulating factor (GM-CSF) into current practice, either as a treatment of established systemic infection or as prophylaxis to prevent systemic infection."

HISTORY, SITES, AND TYPES OF NEONATAL INFECTION

A. Epidemiologic history.

    1. In 1930s and 1940s: high incidence of group A streptococcus.

    2. In 1940s and 1950s: *E. coli* responsible for majority of infections.

    3. In 1950s and 1960s: emergence of *S. aureus*.

    4. From 1970s to 1980s: GBS, *E. coli*, *L. monocytogenes*, and *Haemophilus influenzae* responsible for majority of sepsis during the first week of life.

    5. 1990s: *Staphylococcus epidermidis* and MRSA have emerged as nosocomial pathogens in the nursery.

B. Common sites of neonatal infection: blood, CSF, lungs, and urinary tract.

C. Types of neonatal infections.

    1. Sepsis.

        a. Incidence of neonatal sepsis varies between 1 to 8 in 1000 live term births and 1 in 250 live preterm births.

        b. Incidence of meningitis is 1 in 2500 live births.

        c. Most common organisms responsible for early-onset sepsis:

            (1) Early onset: *E. coli*, group B streptococcus (GBS), *L. monocytogenes*, and *H. influenzae*, *Enterobacter* spp., *Klebsiella pneumoniae*, *Pseudomonas aeruginosa*, and *S. aureus* (Polin et al., 2001; Stoll et al., 2002).

            (2) Nosocomial: Coagulase-negative staphylococci, *S. aureus*, *C. albicans*, *K. pneumoniae*, *P. aeruginosa*, and *Serratia marcescens* (Polin et al., 2001; Stoll et al., 1996b).

        d. Presentation is often nonspecific, with subtle signs of temperature instability, lethargy, poor feeding, and glucose instability.

    2. Meningitis.

        a. More frequent occurrence during the neonatal period than at any other time.

        b. GBS and *E. coli* are major pathogens identified in neonatal meningitis.

        c. Acquisition: direct invasion, contamination between CSF space and integumental surfaces, and bacterial dissemination from infected structures.

        d. Clinical manifestations.

            (1) General signs and symptoms of infection at presentation.

            (2) Specific CNS symptoms: increased irritability, alteration in consciousness, poor tone, tremors, seizures, and bulging fontanelle.

        e. CSF culture.

            (1) CSF culture result may be positive even though blood culture result is negative.

(2) If the CSF culture result is positive, culture must be repeated 24 to 36 hours after initiation of treatment to ensure adequate therapy.
   f. Antibiotic therapy.
      (1) Prompt initiation is crucial for optimal outcome, and antibiotic may be administered before CSF specimen is obtained.
      (2) Choose antimicrobial agents with good CSF penetration.
      (3) Duration of therapy is dependent on recovered pathogens and clinical response, generally 14 to 21 days.
   g. Significant sequelae in 20% to 50% of infants who survive: motor and mental disabilities, convulsions, hydrocephalus, and hearing loss.
3. Pneumonia.
   a. Transmission.
      (1) Vertical.
         (a) Onset usually from birth to 7 days.
         (b) Most common bacterial pathogen responsible for pneumonia: GBS; however, incidence of GBS is changing; any organism present in maternal genital tract can cause pneumonia in the neonate.
      (2) Horizontal.
         (a) Onset beyond 1 week of life.
         (b) Through human contact or contaminated equipment.
   b. Clinical manifestations: possibly general but usually specific symptoms of respiratory distress.
   c. Diagnosis.
      (1) May be difficult.
      (2) Chest x-ray examination.
         (a) Possible asymmetric densities and pleural effusion.
         (b) Pulmonary granularity present in GBS-related pneumonia; possibly indistinguishable from respiratory distress syndrome in premature infant.
4. Urinary tract infections.
   a. *E. coli*: most common organism responsible for urinary tract infections; *Klebsiella* and *P. aeruginosa*: less common; gram-positive bacteria: rare.
   b. Clinical manifestations.
      (1) General signs are often nonspecific and may include temperature instability, poor weight gain, poor feeding, cyanosis, abdominal distention, hyperglycemia, hematuria, and proteinuria.
      (2) Localized signs consist of a weak urinary stream and/or bladder distention.
   c. Antimicrobial agents: administer parenterally.
      (1) Oral absorption is erratic.
      (2) There is a 30% association between urinary tract infection and septicemia.
   d. Follow-up.
      (1) Repeat urine culture should be sterile within 36 to 48 hours after initiation of antimicrobial therapy.
      (2) If a urinary tract infection has been documented in an infant, voiding cystourethrogram should be performed to evaluate the possibility of any congenital abnormalities of the urinary tract.
5. Neonatal conjunctivitis.
   a. May be caused by a variety of organisms, including *S. aureus*, *P. aeruginosa*, *Neisseria gonorrhoeae*, and *Chlamydia trachomatis*.
   b. Manifestations usually include discharge from the eye and conjunctivitis.
   c. Diagnosis is made by a culture and Gram stain, which reveals leukocytes and the causative organism.
   d. Chemical conjunctivitis is usually due to instillation of prophylactic silver nitrate but may occur with topical antibiotics.
   e. Of the ophthalmic antibiotics, methicillin is the antibiotic of choice for *S. aureus*, and a combination of carbenicillin and gentamicin are used when *P. aeruginosa* has been identified (also refer to *N. gonorrhoeae* and *C. trachomatis*).

6. Gastrointestinal disease.
   a. Breastfeeding with the transmission of secretory IgA is important in the prevention of illness (Welsh and May, 1979).
   b. Specific gastrointestinal pathogens.
      (1) Rotavirus.
         (a) Virus is acquired by nosocomial transmission in the neonatal intensive care unit (NICU).
         (b) Infection may be asymptomatic; infant may exhibit signs and symptoms of severe gastrointestinal distress.
         (c) Symptoms include fever, vomiting, and watery yellow or green diarrhea.
         (d) Detection of the virus is by radioimmunoassay, immunofluorescence, and/or latex agglutination, enzyme-linked immunosorbent assay (ELISA).
         (e) Management includes:
            (i) Replacement of fluids and electrolytes.
            (ii) Elemental diet: may be needed for improved absorption if mucosal damage has occurred.
            (iii) Parenteral nutrition until feedings are well established.
            (iv) Handwashing after contact with infant is essential. Virus is shed in stool 2 to 3 days before illness is recognized.
            (v) Isolation: may decrease spread of virus.
         (f) Prevention: A rotavirus vaccine (Rv) is now available for the prevention of rotavirus. Rv is administered at 2, 4, and 6 months of age (American Academy of Pediatrics [AAP], 2003).
      (2) *Clostridium difficile.*
         (a) Gram-positive anaerobic bacillus.
         (b) Causative agent for necrotizing enterocolitis and pseudomembranous colitis.
         (c) Manifested by watery diarrhea, abdominal pain and tenderness, nausea and vomiting, fever, and blood in stool.
         (d) Complications: toxic megacolon, dehydration, and electrolyte disturbances.
         (e) Protective effect: possibly from human milk; neutralizing antibody against *C. difficile* in colostrum.
         (f) Associated with long-term administration of antibiotic therapy.
         (g) May be associated with necrotizing enterocolitis.
         (h) Intestinal colonization as high as 50% in neonates who generally remain well.
         (i) Treatment: fluid and electrolyte management, appropriate broad-spectrum antibiotics.

INFECTION WITH SPECIFIC PATHOGENS

Bacterial Infections

A. Gram-positive organisms.
   1. Group B streptococci (Centers for Disease Control and Prevention [CDC], 2002; Schrag et al., 2002).
      a. Gram-positive spherical bacteria that form pairs or chains during growth.
      b. Twenty identified strains. Groups A, B, and D and *Streptococcus pneumoniae* are responsible for most neonatal infections.
      c. Organism in maternal cervix, vagina, anus, and urethra.
      d. Colonization with GBS in 15% to 35% of women; there has been an overall 70% decline in GBS sepsis since the adoption of the 1996 CDC recommendations (Fig. 32-6) (AAP, 2003; Schrag et al., 2002).
      e. Recommendations for intrapartum penicillin therapy: although many of the recommendations in the 2002 guidelines are the same as those in 1996, they include some key changes (www.cdc.gov/mmwr/preview/mmwrhtml/rr5111a1.htm).
         (1) Recommendation of universal prenatal screening for vaginal and rectal GBS colonization of all pregnant women at 35 to 37 weeks of gestation, based on recent

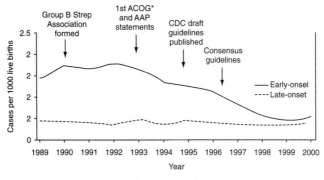

ACOG, American College of Obstetricians and Gynecologists;
AAP, American Academy of Pediatrics

FIGURE 32-6 ■ Incidence of early- and late-onset invasive group B streptococcal disease—selected active bacterial core surveillance areas, 1989 to 2000, and activities for prevention of group B streptococcal disease. (Adapted from Centers for Disease Control and Prevention: Early-onset group B streptococcal disease, United States, 1998-1999. *MMWR Morbidity and Mortality Weekly Report, 49*:793-396, 2000; Schrag, S.J., Zywicki, S., Farley, M.M., et al.: Group B streptococcal disease in the era of intrapartum antibiotic prophylaxis. *New England Journal of Medicine, 342*[1]:15-20, 2000.)

documentation in a large retrospective cohort study of a strong protective effect of this culture-based screening strategy relative to the risk-based strategy.
(2) Updated prophylaxis regimens for women with penicillin allergy.
(3) Detailed instruction on prenatal specimen collection and expanded methods of GBS culture processing, including instructions on antimicrobial susceptibility testing.
(4) Recommendation against routine intrapartum antibiotic prophylaxis for GBS-colonized women undergoing planned cesarean deliveries that have not begun labor or had rupture of membranes.
(5) A suggested algorithm for management of patients with threatened preterm delivery.
 f. Previous and current recommendations for intrapartum penicillin therapy:
(1) History of previous infant with invasive GBS disease.
(2) Maternal GBS bacteremia with current pregnancy.
(3) Intrapartum fever.
(4) Birth at less than 37 weeks of gestation.
(5) Rupture of membranes more than 18 hours before delivery.
 g. Colonization/disease ratio: approximately 100 to 200:1.
 h. Most common organism responsible for early-onset bacterial infection in the neonate.
 i. Manifestation of infection: asymptomatic bacteremia, septicemia, pneumonia, or meningitis.
 j. Early-onset infection with GBS.
(1) Fulminant presentation, typically within the first 24 hours of life.
(2) Most common presentation is with pneumonia and/or meningitis.
(3) Acquired by vertical transmission.
(4) Clinical manifestations: respiratory distress, hypotonia, lethargy, poor feeding, abdominal distention, pallor, tachycardia, temperature instability, shock, and seizures.
 k. Late-onset infection with GBS.
(1) Insidious presentation, usually after 7 to 10 days.
(2) Common complication: meningitis.
  (a) Mortality rate has declined significantly to 10% in 1997 (Harvey et al., 1999).
  (b) In 12% to 29% of survivors there may be serious neurologic damage such as mental retardation, spastic quadriplegia, cortical blindness, deafness, uncontrolled seizures, hydrocephalus, and diabetes insipidus, and in another 15% to 38% there may be mild neurologic impairment such as neuromotor loss without

functional loss, isolated hydrocephalus, epilepsy, and a cognitive IQ score of 70 to 80 (Stevens et al., 2003).

(3) Acquired by horizontal transmission.

(4) Symptoms: fever, lethargy, and bulging fontanelle.

l. Treatment.

(1) Antibiotic therapy.

(2) Fluid management.

(3) Volume expansion.

(4) Seizure control.

(5) Monitoring of electrolytes, fluid balance status, weight, and intake and output.

2. *Staphylococcus.* These bacteria are gram-positive spherical cells that appear as irregular clusters on a Gram stain. Some species are considered normal flora, and others are pathogenic. Staphylococcal infection can cause mild disease such as local infection from a scalp electrode, or may have widespread manifestations, including osteomyelitis, mastitis, and overwhelming sepsis.

a. *S. aureus.* A coagulase-positive organism. The major source of infection is through horizontal transmission from hospital personnel; it is also associated with umbilical catheters, endotracheal tubes, and central lines. Colonization occurs in 40% to 90% of neonates by the fifth day of life. May have widespread manifestations, including osteomyelitis, mastitis, and overwhelming sepsis. Treatment is with nafcillin or vancomycin. If methicillin resistant, vancomycin is the antibiotic of choice. In 2002, two cases of vancomycin-resistant *S. aureus* (VRSA) were documented in two different states. The guidelines for detecting these organisms and preventing the spread of VRSA are available at http://www.cdc.gov/ncidod/dhqp/ar_visavrsa_prevention.html (AAP, 2003).

b. *S. epidermidis.* A coagulase-negative staphylococcus (CoNS) organism that is part of the normal skin flora. Nearly all infants are colonized with CoNS by 2 to 4 days of life. In recent years CoNS has emerged as a serious pathogen in the premature low birth weight infant as a result of invasive procedures such as endotracheal tubes, umbilical catheters, chest tubes, and central lines. CoNS produces a slime-producing agent that can erode the surface of polyethylene catheters and cause colony growth. Many strains are methicillin resistant. Vancomycin is the antibiotic of choice (AAP, 2003).

3. *L. monocytogenes.*

a. Aerobic gram-positive bacillus.

b. Acquired transplacentally or from the vaginal canal, approximately 65% of women experience clinical symptoms of a prodromal illness prior to a diagnosis of listeriosis (AAP, 2003).

c. Should be suspected in the preterm infant who has passage of meconium or if the maternal history includes prior stillbirth, repeated spontaneous abortions, brown amniotic fluid or amnionitis (infection before 28 weeks of gestation frequently results in fetal death).

d. May result in fulminant, disseminated early-onset sepsis with multiorgan involvement.

e. Symptoms: hypothermia, lethargy, and poor feeding. The infant may have a characteristic salmon-colored rash.

f. Sensitive to ampicillin; an aminoglycoside is recommended for synergy (AAP, 2003).

B. **Gram-negative organisms.**

1. *E. coli.*

a. Most common gram-negative organism causing sepsis and meningitis in the neonatal period.

b. Found in the female genital tract, with high incidence of colonization in the neonate. Nosocomial acquisition from person to person; nursery environmental sites (i.e., sinks, multiple-use solutions, etc.) are also implicated.

c. Colonization of human gastrointestinal tract soon after birth; predominant fecal flora throughout life.

d. Many serotypes of *E. coli*. One form of *E. coli* antigen, K1, is associated with neonatal meningitis.

   e. Possible cause of severe, fulminant infection, leading to respiratory distress, cardiovascular collapse, meningitis, and multiorgan failure and death.
   f. In addition to septicemia, possible cause of localized infection, including cellulitis, pneumonia, septic arthritis, urinary tract infection, and otitis media.
   g. Sensitivity to aminoglycosides such as gentamicin and third-generation cephalosporins (such as cefotaxime). Initial treatment should include ampicillin and an aminoglycoside (AAP, 2003).

2. *P. aeruginosa.*
   a. Gram-negative, motile, aerobic rod.
   b. Known as "water bug"; inhabitant of respirators and moist oxygen circuits and humidified environments.
   c. Particular susceptibility to colonization and subsequent development of pneumonia in infant requiring ventilator and receiving antibiotics.
   d. Pathogenic organism in immunocompromised host or where normal defense mechanisms of the skin and mucous membranes are insufficient.
   e. Generally a cause of late-onset disease with respiratory distress.
   f. Treatment: combination of aminoglycoside and an anti-*Pseudomonas* penicillin such as carbenicillin, imipenem, piperacillin, or ticarcillin or by ceftazidime.
   g. Cause of conjunctivitis in newborn infant. Generally between 5 and 18 days after birth, mild conjunctivitis begins with edema and erythema of the lid, with purulent discharge. May progress quickly, causing corneal perforation, and may also result in virulent necrotizing endophthalmitis and blindness. Parenteral therapy is necessary—typically a parenteral aminoglycoside plus antipseudomonal penicillin or cephalosporin—plus topical aminoglycoside therapy for 7 to 10 days (Thureen et al., 2005).

3. *H. influenzae.*
   a. Gram-negative coccobacillus.
   b. Low rate of maternal genital colonization, although passage to fetus is via the ascending transcervical route.
   c. Chorioamnionitis occurs in all placentas but appears more severe among survivors. May also be spread nosocomially through respiratory droplet transmission.
   d. 50% chance of symptomatic infection in colonized infant.
   e. Early-onset fulminant presentation, with pneumonia, respiratory distress, hypotension, and leukopenia.
   f. Mortality rate may be as high as 50%, especially in the very low birth weight (VLBW) infant. Before introduction of the *H. influenzae* vaccine (HiB), *H. influenzae* was the most common cause of bacterial meningitis in children in the United States.
   g. Initial treatment includes a third-generation cephalosporin (cefotaxime or ceftriaxone). Some strains are resistant to ampicillin (AAP, 2003).
   h. The primary series of Hib vaccinations are recommended at 2, 4, and 6 months of age (AAP, 2003).

4. *N. gonorrhoeae.*
   a. Gram-negative diplococcal bacteria.
   b. Most frequently reported sexually transmitted disease in the United States: approximately 1 million cases annually. Concurrent infections with *C. trachomatis* or *T. pallidum* are common.
   c. Ophthalmia neonatorum presents in the first week of life with bilateral copious, mucopurulent eye drainage. Lid and conjunctival edema and erythema are common.
   d. Diagnosis made by Gram stain and confirmed with positive identification on chocolate agar culture. Evaluation for sepsis and meningitis is also necessary.
   e. Sequelae: rare, but permanent visual impairment and/or systemic infection possible.
   f. Treatment: third-generation cephalosporin, such as ceftriaxone, until susceptibility testing can be completed (AAP, 2003). Penicillin G is a secondary choice if the organism is not penicillin resistant. Many *N. gonorrhoeae* pathogens are penicillin and tetracycline resistant. Eye irrigation with saline solution until eye discharge clears is also recommended (Thureen et al., 2005).

    g. Recommended prophylaxis erythromycin (0.5%) ophthalmic ointment in the eyes of all vaginally delivered infants. (NOTE: eye prophylaxis only minimizes the risk of infection; it does not guarantee prevention.)

C. Bacterial parasite: *C. trachomatis.*

    1. Parasite is commonly found in the adult female genital tract. *C. trachomatis* has an incidence rate between 6% and 12% in most populations and may be as high as 37% in adolescents; it is the most common sexually transmitted disease in the United States (AAP, 2003).

    2. Delivery through an infected vaginal canal may result in neonatal infection.

    3. Conjunctivitis usually is manifested at 5 to 4 days of age but may be delayed with eye prophylaxis. Symptoms may be minimal. Findings include copious mucopurulent exudate with frequent pseudomembrane formation. Pneumonia, otitis media, and gastroenteritis may also develop.

        a. Diagnosis is by tissue culture isolation from conjunctival, oropharyngeal, genital, or rectal swabs of cells.

        b. Treatment for conjunctivitis includes ophthalmic and systemic erythromycin (50 mg/kg/day in four divided doses) for 14 days (AAP, 2003). Topical therapy is insufficient to eradicate nasopharyngeal colonization (Thureen et al., 2005).

    4. Chlamydial pneumonia is manifested between 4 and 11 weeks postnatally.

        a. Symptoms include a persistent cough, rales, and wheezing.

        b. Chest radiograph may reveal hyperinflation.

        c. Chronic disease may persist even after the acute phase of disease is over.

        d. Treatment is with erythromycin for 14 days.

Fungal Infection: Candidiasis

Candidiasis is caused by *Candida*, a significant neonatal pathogen. The most common species is *C. albicans.*

A. Mucocutaneous candidiasis.

    1. Most common form of candidiasis in the newborn infant.

    2. Acquired during passage through the birth canal or from mother during breastfeeding.

    3. Appears as pearly white material on the buccal mucosa, dorsum and lateral areas of the tongue, gingivae, and pharynx.

    4. Treatment is with oral nystatin suspension (100,000 units/ml) to each side of mouth every 6 hours for 3 days after symptoms have subsided (Taketomo et al., 2002).

    5. May need to treat mother if origin of infection is mother's breast.

B. Cutaneous candidiasis.

    1. Presence of oral Candida is strongly associated with development of cutaneous candidiasis in the perineal region.

    2. May appear initially as erythematous and vesiculopapular lesions, and then develop into fine white, scaly collarettes.

    3. Therapy.

        a. Use of topical agents such as nystatin four times a day and continued 2 to 3 days after the rash has cleared.

        b. Simultaneous treatment with oral nystatin to minimize the risk of recurrence.

        c. Maintenance of area free from moisture and stool.

C. Acute disseminated (systemic) candidiasis.

    1. A serious nosocomial infection occurring in VLBW infants less than 1500 g, with an incidence of 3% to 5% (Faix et al., 1989).

    2. Most frequent sites of infection include the lungs, kidneys, liver, spleen, and brain; several sites may be involved simultaneously.

    3. Risk factors include prematurity (immunocompromised state), use of total parenteral nutrition and intravenous fat emulsions, and prolonged use of broad-spectrum antibiotics.

    4. Presentation includes respiratory deterioration, abdominal distention, apnea, acidosis, carbohydrate intolerance, hypotension, skin abscesses, temperature instability, and/or erythematous rash.

    5. Formation of fungus in urine may lead to urinary tract infection.

6. Diagnosis is made by blood cultures, CSF cultures, microscopic examination of urine and the buffy coat of blood, determination of serum Candida antigen, ophthalmologic examination, and renal ultrasound.

7. Treatment.

   a. Amphotericin B: initial dose of 0.1 mg/kg IV over 20 to 60 minutes, followed by maintenance doses of 0.25 to 1 mg/kg/day every 24 hours as a daily infusion over 2 to 6 hours. Duration of therapy will vary with the clinical response. Requires close monitoring of hematologic and renal function (Taketomo et al., 2002).

   b. Flucytosine: 50 to 100 mg/kg/day in two divided doses for 3 to 4 weeks; may be used in combination with amphotericin B, especially if there is severe infection or CNS involvement.

Viral Infections

A. **Mode of transmission.**

   1. Congenital: acquired in utero during maternal viral infection with exposure to the fetus. Infant presents with disease at birth or shortly thereafter.

   2. Intrapartum: acquired at birth from organisms present in the maternal genital tract; onset of neonatal symptoms occurs within 5 to 7 days or later, depending on incubation period.

   3. Postnatal: acquired during neonatal period from breastfeeding (human immunodeficiency virus [HIV], hepatitis B virus, cytomegalovirus), through blood transmission (cytomegalovirus, hepatitis B virus), or from hospital personnel or family members (enterovirus, respiratory syncytial virus).

B. **Viral organisms.**

   1. Rubella virus.

      a. Generally causes a mild and often asymptomatic infection in children and adults. If acquired during pregnancy, can result in any of a wide range of fetal and neonatal outcomes: spontaneous abortion, congenital malformation, stillbirth, and neonatal disease (e.g., hepatitis, hepatosplenomegaly, jaundice, thrombocytopenia, "blueberry muffin" purpura), asymptomatic fetal infection, or no transmission of virus to the fetus (Cooper et al., 1995).

      b. Severity of neonatal disease is increased if infection occurs during the first trimester.

      c. There may be no initial symptoms, although most infected infants will have long-term sequelae such as endocrinopathies, deafness, eye damage, vascular disease, panencephalitis, and developmental delays (Overall, 1992; Sever et al., 1985).

      d. Early manifestations include intrauterine growth restriction, thrombocytopenia, hepatomegaly, jaundice, congenital heart disease (patent ductus arteriosus, peripheral pulmonary artery stenosis, atrial or ventricular septal defect), interstitial pneumonia, cataracts, bone lesions, microphthalmia, lethargy, irritability, bulging fontanelle, and late-onset seizures.

      e. Diagnosis is made by detection of specific rubella IgM; by demonstration of stable or rising rubella IgG titers in serial sera obtained for several months; and/or by cultivation of virus from nasal secretions, throat swab, urine, blood, or CSF. Special cell cultures are required for cultivation of rubella virus.

      f. Prevention measures are as follows:

         (1) Pregnant women should be screened for immunity whether or not they have received prior rubella immunization. Susceptible pregnant women should avoid exposure to infected persons. Pregnant women are not given the vaccine because of the small risk of transmission of virus to the fetus (1.2% to 1.8%) (CDC, 1987).

         (2) Seronegative women should be vaccinated postpartum, before discharge from the hospital. Vaccine virus is excreted in breast milk, but breastfeeding is not a contraindication to vaccination.

         (3) Routine rubella vaccination should be administered to all infants (AAP, 1998).

      g. Isolation procedures are carried out because respiratory and urinary secretion of virus may occur for several months or more after birth. Transmission-Based Precautions, in addition to Standard Precautions, should be used with all infants with suspected congenital rubella during hospitalization.

h. There is no specific antiviral therapy for congenital rubella or for amelioration of progressive disease after birth.

2. Cytomegalovirus (CMV).

a. CMV causes the most common congenital viral infection that is spread horizontally by salivary or urinary contamination or by sexual transmission. Infection is more common in crowded conditions, in lower socioeconomic groups, and in breastfed infants (Stagno, 1995). Up to 90% of the adult population and 70% of children in daycare are seropositive. Approximately 2% of women will have a primary CMV infection during pregnancy (Stagno and Whitley, 1985).

b. Infection may be acquired from cervical secretions at the time of delivery. After birth, the virus may be transmitted in infected maternal secretions or breast milk or through blood transfusions. Overall, with primary maternal infection, 40% of infants are infected, with symptoms manifested at birth in 10% and with late sequelae occurring in another 5% to 10% (Stagno and Whitley, 1985).

c. Clinical manifestations.

(1) Congenital infection.

(a) Symptomatic at birth: growth restriction, hepatosplenomegaly, microcephaly, jaundice, petechiae and purpura, pneumonia, chorioretinitis, and periventricular intracranial calcification. Prognosis is poor, with one third dying in infancy and up to 90% of survivors having severe neurologic sequelae.

(b) Asymptomatic at birth: 5% to 15% may have long-term sequelae, the majority having hearing loss and decreased IQ, microcephaly, visual difficulties, and school problems (Stagno, 1995).

(2) Perinatal or postpartum infection. The majority of infections remain asymptomatic and do not appear to result in any long-term sequelae (Stagno, 1995). Severe disease has occurred in premature infants infected with CMV by means of blood transfusion.

d. Diagnosis is made by viral isolation from the infant's urine or saliva or by a high anti-CMV IgM titer in the first 2 to 3 weeks of life or persistent or rising IgG titers in the first 6 months of life. Infants with both congenital and perinatal/postnatal CMV infection excrete virus in their urine for years (Stagno et al., 1983).

e. There is no proven treatment.

f. For prevention, pregnant women should be advised to use good handwashing technique. Blood products given to neonates should be treated to reduce the potential for CMV transmission or should be obtained from CMV-seronegative donors.

g. Neither infants with symptomatic CMV infection nor those with diagnosed but asymptomatic CMV infection require isolation, but Standard Precautions, particularly for pregnant caretakers, should be enforced.

3. Respiratory syncytial virus (RSV).

a. Most common respiratory pathogen in infants. It is the major cause of bronchiolitis and pneumonia in infants during the first 3 years of life. Almost all children have had RSV by age 2. About 30% to 40% of infants at first exposure develop signs of bronchiolitis or pneumonia, and about 0.5% to 2.0% require hospitalization (Moore, 2004).

b. Prevalence: Infection is most prevalent during winter and through early spring (November through April) and is highly contagious. It is transmitted through contact with infected secretions (droplet contamination) resulting from coughing and sneezing. Infection proceeds from the nasal mucosa and spreads from the upper to the lower respiratory tract.

c. Susceptibility: Initial infection and most serious illness generally occur during the first year of life, especially in infants who were premature or have either chronic lung disease or congenital heart disease.

d. Presentation.

(1) Nonspecific: poor feeding, lethargy, apnea, irritability.

(2) Respiratory symptoms: cough, wheezing, rales, rhonchi, dyspnea, pneumonia, cyanosis, pulmonary infiltrates.

(3) Increasing respiratory distress, which may result in respiratory failure.

e. Diagnosis.

(1) Clinical and epidemiologic findings.

(2) Rapid viral antigen detection isolated from nasopharyngeal aspirate.

f. Treatment. Supportive care includes oxygen, hydration, and isolation. High-risk infants may progress to assisted ventilation because of hypoxemia and hypercapnia.

g. Prophylaxis and treatment.

(1) Palivizumab (Synagis) has been established as the preferred method of RSV prophylaxis in infants with bronchopulmonary dysplasia (BPD), premature birth less than 35 weeks, and hemodynamically significant congenital heart defects (CHDs) (Johnson et al., 1997; Malley et al., 1998; The IMpact RSV Study Group, 1998). Synagis is a monoclonal antibody that is administered intramuscularly once monthly.

(2) RSV immune globulin (RSVIG): RSVIG has been approved by the U.S. Food and Drug Administration for use in infants for the prevention of RSV-induced lower respiratory tract disease. RSVIG is an IV preparation that is administered over 4 hours. Administration should be initiated before onset of the RSV season and administered monthly during the RSV season. It is ineffective in treating established RSV infection. The AAP (2003) recommended its use in infants and children younger than 24 months of age with a history of bronchopulmonary dysplasia and in infants born at less than 32 weeks of gestation without this disease.

h. Isolation procedures: Transmission-Based Precautions are used, in addition to Standard Precautions. May designate cohort of infected infants to prevent widespread infection.

4. Herpes simplex virus (HSV).

a. Cause of serious disease in fetus and neonate, with incidence estimated at 1 in 3000 to 1 in 20,000 births (AAP, 2003).

b. Types of HSV infection.

(1) HSV-1: nongenital type, although it can infect the genital area (accounts for 25% of neonatal disease).

(2) HSV-2: genital type; more often associated with neonatal disease (accounts for 75% of neonatal disease).

c. Transmission: 85% to 90% of infections are acquired at the time of delivery. More than 75% of infants who acquire neonatal HSV infection have been born to women who had no history or clinical findings suggestive of active HSV infection during pregnancy (AAP, 2003). Infections can also occur in utero or postnatally (Whitley and Arvin, 1995). Postnatal infections can be acquired from breast lesions during breastfeeding, from oral lesions through direct contact, and from other infants with HSV infection. The greatest risk to the neonate is in mothers with a primary infection at birth. Transmission occurs in 40% to 50% of these infants. With reactivation of the disease, transmission occurs in 4% to 5% of deliveries or fewer (Overall, 1992).

d. Presentation.

(1) Intrapartum or postnatal transmission: vesicular lesions, thermal instability, lethargy, respiratory distress, vomiting, poor feeding, cyanosis, and, if there is CNS involvement, irritability, bulging fontanelle, seizures, opisthotonos, and coma.

(2) Congenital transmission: early vesicular rash, small for gestational age, low birth weight, chorioretinitis, diffuse brain damage, microcephaly, and intracranial calcification.

e. Diagnosis: Positive culture result with specimen obtained from vesicular fluid, blood, or CSF results in a diagnosis. The diagnostic yield of CSF culture for neonates with CNS disease is less than 50%. The polymerase chain reaction (PCR) test has a much higher yield in CSF and should be performed if available. Other rapid identification tests include direct fluorescent antibody staining of vesicle scrapings and enzyme immunoassay antigen detection in vesicles or body fluids.

  f. Treatment.

   (1) Systemic infection: acyclovir, for premature infants, 10 mg/kg/dose every 12 hours for 14 to 21 days. In term infants 10 mg/kg/dose every 8 hours is recommended (Taketomo et al., 2002). Side effects are rare. Phlebitis may occur at the IV site because of alkaline pH of 10.

   (2) Ocular involvement: topical ophthalmic drug such as 3% vidarabine in addition to parenteral antiviral therapy. An ophthalmology consultation should be obtained.

  g. Prognosis: Approximately half of all infants with untreated infection die, with high morbidity rates in survivors. Morbidity and mortality rates are highest in infants with CNS or disseminated disease. Antiviral therapy improves prognosis, especially in infants with localized disease.

  h. Prevention.

   (1) Maternal history of HSV infection.

    (a) Weekly virologic and clinical screening beginning at 32 weeks.

    (b) Cesarean delivery if lesions are present or a culture result is positive at the time of delivery.

    (c) For known exposure to active recurrent infection at vaginal delivery or cesarean delivery, culture specimens should be obtained from the neonate 24 to 48 hours after birth. Treatment should be considered especially if the infant has symptoms, was born prematurely, acquired open wounds during delivery, or has other high-risk factors.

    (d) Delivery can be vaginal if no clinical or virologic evidence is present. Neonatal surface cultures can be considered but are not routinely recommended.

   (2) Primary infection: For infants born vaginally to women with suspected or documented active primary HSV infection at the time of delivery, give prophylactic acyclovir pending neonatal culture results. If delivery is cesarean, acyclovir administration should be considered, especially if rupture of membranes occurred more than 6 hours before delivery or if the neonate has symptoms.

   (3) Follow-up of at-risk infants: Infants who are at risk of HSV infection, even if culture result was negative after birth, should be followed up closely for a minimum of 6 weeks.

  i. Isolation procedures.

   (1) Mothers with HSV infections need to use strict handwashing techniques before touching their infant.

   (2) Infants born to mothers with active lesions should be physically separated from other infants and managed with Transmission Precautions in addition to Standard Precautions.

   (3) Infants born to mothers with a history of infection but without lesions at delivery do not require isolation. Good handwashing technique should be stressed.

   (4) Infants with HSV infection should be isolated and managed with Contact Precautions.

5. Hepatitis B.

  a. DNA double-shelled virus.

  b. Transmission: vertical. The virus is also found in any bodily secretion, including human milk. There is no added risk to the infant of acquiring HBV infection when the mother is hepatitis B surface antigen (HBsAg) positive; therefore, breastfeeding is not contraindicated if immunoprophylaxis recommendations are followed (Thureen et al., 2005).

  c. Presentation: Infants infected in utero are free of symptoms at birth. Infants infected at delivery or after birth do not have HBsAg present for at least 2 to 5 months. Infants who become chronically infected are at risk of having chronic hepatitis, cirrhosis, and/or other hepatocellular carcinoma.

  d. Prevention: Routine screening is used for all pregnant women and universal screening for all infants and children. Routine neonatal immunization is with hepatitis B vaccine: Engerix-B, 10 mcg, or Recombivax HB, 5 mcg (AAP, 2003).

   (1) Term infant is immunized at discharge and again at 2 and 6 months of age (AAP, 2003).

       (2) Preterm infant is immunized at discharge if weight is greater than 2 kg or at 2 months of age.

  e. Treatment: In the infant born to an HBsAg-positive mother, treatment is 85% to 95% effective in preventing the development of the hepatitis B carrier state and should include the following:

       (1) Careful bathing of the neonate to remove blood and secretions that may be contaminated.

       (2) Administration of hepatitis B immunoglobulin (HBIG), 0.5 ml intramuscularly, as soon as possible within 12 hours of birth, in addition to a hepatitis B vaccine: Engerix-B, 10 mcg, or Recombivax HB, 5 mcg (AAP, 2003).

  f. Isolation procedures: Infants born to mothers with HBsAg should be cared for with Standard Precautions. No isolation is required. Immediately after birth the infant should be handled with gloves until all maternal blood is removed.

6. HIV.

  a. Cytopathic human ribonucleic acid (RNA) retrovirus.

  b. Use of reverse transcriptase enzyme. HIV uses the enzyme to produce viral DNA and integrates this into the DNA of the T-helper cells.

  c. Suppression of T-helper lymphocytes. This results in B-cell and suppressor T-cell dysfunction, with subsequent defects in cell-mediated immunity and development of opportunistic infections.

  d. Infection of monocytes and macrophages—also possible.

  e. Symptom-free infection. An infant can have an HIV infection with an absence of symptoms, suggesting that other factors (e.g., genetic predisposition, nutritional status) may contribute to the development of infection.

  f. Transmission.

       (1) Transmission is through blood or blood products.

       (2) Vertical transmission is thought to be the most common method of transfer, although time of transmission is uncertain.

          (a) Transplacental transmission has been demonstrated.

          (b) Intrapartum transmission during drug exposure to infected maternal blood or genital tract secretions is presumed.

          (c) HIV may be transmitted through human milk.

          (d) Risk of infection to an infant born to an HIV-infected mother who did not receive antiretroviral therapy during pregnancy is estimated to be between 13% and 39% (Hutto et al., 1991).

  g. Presentation: Signs and symptoms are rare in the neonatal period but may be seen in infancy.

       (1) Failure to thrive.

       (2) Generalized lymphadenopathy, hepatomegaly, and splenomegaly.

       (3) Recurrent mucosal infections.

       (4) Systemic bacterial infections.

       (5) Recurrent candidiasis.

       (6) Lymphoid interstitial pneumonitis.

       (7) Parotitis, hepatitis, nephropathy, and cardiomyopathy.

       (8) Recurrent diarrhea.

       (9) Opportunistic infections.

      (10) Neurodevelopmental delay.

      (11) Malignancies.

  h. Diagnosis: Preferred diagnostic test for neonatal HIV is by PCR (AAP, 2003).

       (1) Antibody-based tests.

          (a) ELISA.

          (b) Western blot.

          (c) Indirect immunofluorescence assay.

       (2) Viral antigen detection: used to detect HIV antigen, usually the p24 antigen.

       (3) Viral nucleic acid detection: PCR and branched-chain DNA assays are used to diagnose and monitor disease progression and therapy efficacy.

(4) Viral culture.

(5) Combination of tests (usually PCR and/or viral isolation). A diagnosis can be made in more than 90% of infants by 2 months of age, and in nearly 100% by 4 months of age (AAP, 2003).

i. Management.

(1) Prompt intervention during bacterial and treatable opportunistic infections.

(2) Adequate nutrition.

(3) Combination antiretroviral therapy (current treatment recommendations for HIV-infected children can be found at www.aidsinfo.nih.gov). The Working Group on Pediatric HIV Infection for the Aids Education and Training Centers (AETC) has current updates of the medication recommendations for infants less than 12 months of age. Treatment recommendations for initial therapy have been revised, based on current clinical trial and pharmacokinetic data.

Several complete regimens are strongly recommended for initial therapy (Table 32-2).

Several protease inhibitor (PI)- and nonnucleoside reverse transcriptase inhibitor (NNRTI)-based regimens are listed as "alternative recommendations," as is one triple nucleoside reverse transcriptase inhibitor (NRTI) regimen. The guidelines also include discussion of regimens and individual drugs that are "not recommended" or that have "insufficient data to recommend." (Included in the latter category are the newer antiretrovirals tenofovir, emtricitabine, atazanavir, and enfuvirtide [www.aidsetc.org].)

(4) Perinatal prophylaxis (CDC, 2002).

(a) Zidovudine (ZDU), 200 mg by mouth three times per day, or 300 mg two times per day, initiated at 14 to 34 weeks of gestation and continued throughout the pregnancy.

(b) Intrapartum loading dose of ZDU is 2 mg/kg IV over 1 hour, followed by continuous infusion of 1 mg/kg/hour until delivery.

(c) Neonatal administration is 2 mg/kg/dose by mouth every 6 hours for 6 weeks, beginning at 8 to 12 hours of age (Taketomo et al., 2002).

(5) Prevention.

(a) Cesarean delivery has not been shown to prevent transmission of HIV to the infant.

(b) Breastfeeding concerns (AAP, 2003).

(i) Transmission of HIV infection to infants from breastfeeding occurs at rates of 27% to 40% in women with primary infection postpartum (Palasanthiran et al., 1993).

■ **TABLE 32-2**
■ ■ **Highly Active Antiretroviral Combination Regimens**

Mechanism of Action	Recommended Medication Combinations
Protease inhibitor-based	Lopinavir/ritonavir + 2 NRTIs* Nelfinavir + 2 NRTIs* Ritonavir + 2 NRTIs*
Nonnucleoside reverse transcriptase inhibitor (NRTI) based	Children >3 years: efavirenz + 2 NRTIs* Children ≤3 years or unable to take capsules: Nevirapine + 2 NRTIs*

*The nucleoside analog (NRTI) pairs of zidovudine + lamivudine, zidovudine + didanosine, and stavudine + lamivudine are strongly recommended for use in combination therapy regimens.

Data from Working Group on Antiretroviral Therapy and Medical Management of HIV-Infected Children convened by the National Pediatric and Family HIV Resource Center (NPHRC), The Health Resources and Services Administration (HRSA), and The National Institutes of Health. *Guidelines for the use of antiretroviral agents in pediatric HIV infection.* Washington, DC, 2003, Authors. Retrieved from www.aidsetc.org or http://aidsinfo.nih.gov

(ii) Women who are known to be HIV infected should be advised not to breast-feed (AAP, 2003).

(6) Isolation procedures. Standard Precautions should be strictly followed.

Other Infections

A. Toxoplasmosis.
1. Caused by intracellular protozoan parasite, *Toxoplasma gondii*, which is an important human pathogen.
2. Maternally acquired from consumption of poorly cooked meat or by exposure to infected cat feces. Only women who become acutely infected during pregnancy can give birth to a newborn infant with congenital toxoplasmosis. Estimated incidence of acute maternal infection in pregnancy is 1.1 in 1000 (Sever et al., 1988).
3. Congenitally acquired disease in the newborn infant by vertical transmission. Approximate neonatal incidence is 0.1 to 1 in 1000 live births.
4. Manifestations may include maculopapular rash, hepatomegaly, splenomegaly, jaundice, and thrombocytopenia.
5. CNS involvement includes microcephaly or hydrocephalus accompanied by convulsions; cerebral calcifications may be seen on radiographs.
6. Sequelae include mental retardation, learning disabilities, impaired vision, and blindness.
7. Toxoplasmosis may be asymptomatic at birth but may be manifested as intellectual impairment in late infancy or childhood.
8. Diagnosis may be made by a number of methods: isolation or histologic demonstration of the organism, detection of *Toxoplasma* antigens in tissues and body fluids, detection of *Toxoplasma* nucleic acid by PCR, and serologic tests.
9. Treatment consists of pyrimethamine, trisulfapyrimidines, and a folic acid supplement to prevent bone marrow suppression.
10. Isolation procedures consist of Standard Precautions.

B. Syphilis.
1. Cause: *T. pallidum*, a thin, motile spirochete.
2. Transmission: through sexual contact or by maternal-fetal transmission.
3. Presentation.
   a. Sometimes asymptomatic.
   b. Petechiae.
   c. Skin lesions: copper-colored maculopapular rash that is most severe on the hands and feet and appears at 1 to 3 weeks of age, with subsequent desquamation. Lesions present at birth may be bullous.
   d. Hepatosplenomegaly.
   e. Respiratory distress.
   f. CNS involvement.
   g. Rhinitis.
   h. Periostitis of long bones, with guarding of extremities.
4. Diagnosis.
   a. U.S. Public Health Service recommendation: all pregnant women screened with Venereal Disease Research Laboratory (VDRL) or rapid plasma reagin (RPR) test early in pregnancy and at the time of delivery.
   b. Diagnosis of active disease in the neonate.
      (1) High VDRL titer (4 times higher than maternal titer).
      (2) Reactive RPR.
      (3) Serum IgM level greater than 20 mg/dl.
      (4) Confirmation with a positive result on fluorescent treponemal antigen-antibody absorption (FTA-ABS) test.
   c. Prevention: Uninfected infants possess maternally acquired antibodies at concentrations similar to those of infected infants. It may be difficult to interpret neonatal laboratory data; therefore, it is important to determine adequacy of maternal treatment, possibility of reexposure, and family compliance with follow-up.

5. Treatment.
   a. Penicillin.
      (1) Benzathine penicillin G, 50,000 units/kg given intramuscularly once if infection is asymptomatic and CSF is normal (Bhatt et al., 1997).
      (2) Procaine penicillin G, 50,000 international units/kg/dose given intramuscularly once daily for 10 to 14 days if infection is symptomatic and CSF is abnormal (Young and Mangum, 2008); alternatively, aqueous crystalline penicillin G, 50,000 international units/kg/dose every 12 hours during the first 7 days of life, and every 8 hours thereafter, irrespective of gestational age (Young and Mangum, 2008).
      (3) Procaine and benzathine penicillins are administered intramuscularly only, providing tissue depots from which drug is absorbed for hours or days.
   b. Neonatal therapy: should be instituted if maternal treatment is uncertain or if treatment was given within the last 4 weeks of pregnancy.
6. Isolation procedures: Standard Precautions.

INFECTION CONTROL

A. **The CDC has published guidelines and recommendations for the prevention of healthcare-associated infections, including isolation precautions, guidelines for protecting healthcare workers, and guidelines for the prevention of postoperative and device-related infections.** These guidelines can be found on the CDC Web site http://www.cdc.gov/ncidod/dhqp/guidelines.html.
B. **Two major categories of infection control practices** (AAP, 2003; Garner, 1996):
   1. Standard Precautions: expanded set of previously designated Universal Precautions. Developed to protect patients and health care workers from bloodborne and other body fluid–borne infections; designed to prevent cutaneous and mucous membrane exposure to blood and body fluids. Guidelines include:
      a. Immediate handwashing or washing of other body surfaces if contaminated with blood and body fluids. This applies even if gloves are used, and hands should be washed immediately after glove removal. Hands should be thoroughly washed after all patient contact regardless of whether or not there was obvious contact with body fluids.
      b. Barrier precautions to prevent cutaneous and mucous membrane exposure to blood, body fluids, secretions, excretions, and contact with any items that might be contaminated with these fluids. Barriers include:
         (1) Gloves: should be worn when contacting blood and body fluids, mucous membranes, open skin, or items soiled by blood and body fluids. Hands should be washed immediately after glove removal. New gloves should be used with new patient contact and before touching noncontaminated items or surfaces.
         (2) Masks, face shields, and protective eyewear: should be used when patient contact or procedures can potentially generate splashes, sprays, or droplets of blood, body fluids, secretions, or excretions that might come in contact with the mucous membranes of the eyes, nose, or mouth.
         (3) Nonsterile gowns or aprons should be worn when patient contact or procedures are likely to generate splashes, sprays, or droplets of blood, body fluids, or secretions, which may contaminate the caregiver's skin or clothing.
      c. Cleaning of patient care equipment that might be contaminated, to prevent skin and mucous membrane exposure and clothing contamination.
      d. Correct handling, transport, and cleaning of soiled linen to prevent skin and mucous membrane exposure and clothing contamination.
      e. "Sharps program" in place to prevent exposure by needlestick and other sharp object injuries during cleaning, using, or disposing of these items.
      f. Avoidance of mouth-to-mouth resuscitation; replacement by readily available resuscitation and ventilation equipment.
   2. Transmission-Based Precautions: guidelines for the care of patients infected with specific pathogens or with syndromes in which the pathogenic organism may be spread by air-

borne, droplet, or contact routes. Measures additional to Standard Precautions are needed to prevent spread of infection. They are based on preventing transmission by one of three types of infection:

   a. Airborne transmission. Prevention requires special air handling and ventilation.

      (1) Private room with negative air pressure ventilation.

      (2) Required: masks.

      (3) Not required: gowns or gloves.

   b. Droplet transmission. Droplets do not remain suspended, so special air handling and ventilation measures are not required.

      (1) Private room preferred but not required; cohorting of infants with same infection is acceptable.

      (2) Required: masks.

      (3) Not required: gowns or gloves.

   c. Contact transmission. Contact is the most common type of transmission of hospital-acquired infections.

      (1) Direct contact: person-to-person transmission. This frequently involves transmission that occurs during patient care.

      (2) Indirect contact: contact with a contaminated object such as gloves, dirty dressings, dirty linen, or instruments, or transmission by personnel from one patient to another because of failure to wash hands thoroughly between patients.

      (3) Preferred but not required: private room. Cohorting of infants with same infection is acceptable.

      (4) Required: gowns and gloves.

      (5) Not required: masks.

   d. Nursery infection control measures (AAP and American College of Obstetricians and Gynecologists [ACOG], 2002). Standard universal precautions are generally considered effective in reducing nosocomial infections.

      (1) Routine, thorough handwashing: initially on entering the nursery, between patient contacts, and after touching contaminated objects.

      (2) Clothing worn by nursery personnel: short-sleeved hospital-provided attire or personal scrubs. The routine use of cover gowns has no proven value in infection control; however, current recommendations state that a long-sleeved gown should be worn over clothing when an infant is held by nursing staff, other personnel, or parents outside of the bassinet (Moore, 2004).

      (3) Cover gowns: to be worn when caring for infants with known or suspected infection. Gowns should be discarded before another patient is handled.

      (4) Sterile long-sleeved gowns, caps, and mask for surgical procedures.

      (5) Hand jewelry should not be worn in nursery while caring for patients.

      (6) Disposable, nonsterile gloves: use, if desired, for care of patients in isolation or to protect caregiver from contamination during procedures.

      (7) Artificial nails should not be worn by persons caring for newborns in the hospital setting. Studies have shown that hospital personnel with artificial nails harbor more potential pathogens both before and after handwashing than personnel with natural nails. Natural nail tips should be kept to $\frac{1}{4}$ inch in length (CDC, 2002).

      (8) Dirty diapers: handle with gloved hands. Gloving may not be necessary for changing diapers; however, in current practice, gloving is considered preferable.

   e. Screening of visitors for contagious infections before admission to the nursery.

 3. Linen and trash disposal (AAP and ACOG, 2002).

   a. Linen provided does not need to be sterile but should be clean.

   b. Cloth or disposable diapers are acceptable.

   c. Soiled linen should be placed in plastic bags in hampers.

   d. Linen and all diapers should be removed from the nursery at least once every 8 hours.

   e. Nursery linens and cloth diapers should be laundered separately from other hospital linen.

4. Intravascular flush solutions (AAP and ACOG, 2002).
   a. Sterile, unpreserved flush solution should be provided by the pharmacy.
   b. Flush solution containers should be timed and dated and kept no longer than 8 hours at room temperature before being discarded.

REFERENCES

American Academy of Pediatrics, Committee on Infectious Diseases: Age for routine administration of the second dose of measles-mumps-rubella vaccine. *Pediatrics, 101*(1 Pt 1):129-133, 1998.

American Academy of Pediatrics, Committee on Infectious Diseases: *2003 Red Book: Report of the Committee on Infectious Diseases* (24th ed.). Elk Grove Village, IL, 2003, AAP.

American Academy of Pediatrics and American College of Obstetricians and Gynecologists: *Guidelines for perinatal care* (5th ed.). Elk Grove Village, IL, and Washington, DC, 2002, Authors.

Bhatt, D.R., Reber, D.J., Wirtschafter, D.D., et al.: *Neonatal drug formulary* (4th ed.). Los Angeles, 1997, N. D.F. Los Angeles Publishers.

Blackburn, S.T.: *Maternal, fetal, and neonatal physiology: A clinical perspective* (3rd ed.). St. Louis, 2007, Saunders.

Byington, C.L., Rittichier, K.K., Bassett, K.E., et al.: Serious bacterial infections in febrile infants younger than 90 days of age: The importance of ampicillin-resistant pathogens. *Pediatrics, 111*(5 Pt 1):964-968, 2003.

Carr, R., Modi, N., and Doré, C.: G-CSF and GM-CSF for treating or preventing neonatal infections. *Cochrane Database of Systematic Reviews, 3*:CD003066, 2003.

Centers for Disease Control and Prevention: Guideline for hand hygiene in healthcare settings. *MMWR Morbidity and Mortality Weekly Report, 51*(RR-16):29, 2002.

Centers for Disease Control and Prevention: Rubella vaccination during pregnancy—United States, 1971-1986. *MMWR Morbidity and Mortality Weekly Report, 36*:457-461, 1987.

Centers for Disease Control and Prevention: Prevention of perinatal group B streptococcal disease in newborns. *MMWR Morbidity and Mortality Weekly Report, 51*(RR-11):1-12, 2002.

Christensen, R.D., Rothstein, G., Anstall, H.B., and Bybee, B.: Granulocyte transfusions in neonates with bacterial infection, neutropenia and depletion of mature marrow neutrophils. *Pediatrics, 70*(1):1-6, 1982.

Cooper, L.Z., Preblud, S.R., and Alford, C.A., Jr.: Rubella. In J.S. Remington and J.O. Klein (Eds.): *Infectious diseases of the fetus and newborn infant* (4th ed.). Philadelphia, 1995, Saunders, pp. 268-311.

Faix, R.G., Kovarik, S.M., Shaw, T.R., and Johnson, R.V.: Mucocutaneous and systemic candidiasis among very low birth weight (<1500 grams) infants in intensive care nurseries: A prospective study. *Pediatrics, 83*(1):101-107, 1989.

Fanaroff, A.A., Korones, S.B., Wright, L.L., et al.: Incidence, presenting features, risk factors and significance of late onset septicemia in very low birth weight infants. The National Institute of Child Health and Human Development Neonatal Research Network. *Pediatric Infectious Disease Journal, 17*(7):593-598, 1998.

Fanaroff, A.A., Wright, L.L., Stevenson, D.K., et al.: Very-low-birth-weight outcomes of the National Institute of Child Health and Human Development Neonatal Research Network, May 1991 through December 1992. *American Journal of Obstetrics and Gynecology, 173*(5):1423-1431, 1995.

Garner, J.S.: Hospital Infection Control Practices Advisory Committee: Guidelines for isolation precautions in hospitals. *Infection Control and Hospital Epidemiology, 17*(1):53-80, 1996.

Hack, M., Wright, L.L., Shankaran, S., et al.: Very-low-birth-weight outcomes of the National Institute of Child Health and Human Development Neonatal Network, November 1989 to October 1990. *American Journal of Obstetrics and Gynecology, 172*(2 Pt 1):457-464, 1995.

Harvey, D., Holt, D.E., and Bedford, H.: Bacterial meningitis in the newborn: A prospective study of mortality and morbidity. *Seminars in Perinatology, 23*(3):218-225, 1999.

Hutto, C., Parks, W.P., Laik, S., et al.: A hospital-based prospective study of perinatal infection with HI modifier virus type 1. *Journal of Pediatrics, 118*(3):347-353, 1991.

The IMpact RSV Study Group: Palivizumab, a humanized respiratory syncytial virus monoclonal antibody, reduces hospitalization from respiratory syncytial virus infection in high-risk infants. *Pediatrics, 102*:531-537, 1998.

Johnson, S., Oliver, C., Prince, G.A., et al: Development of a humanized monoclonal antibody (MEDI-493) with potent in vitro and in vivo activity against respiratory syncytial virus. *Journal of Infectious Diseases, 176*:1215-1224, 1997.

McCance, K.L. and Huether, S.E. (Eds.): *Pathophysiology: The biologic basis for disease in adults and children* (4th ed.). St. Louis, 2002, Mosby.

Malik, A., Hui, C.P., Pennie, R.A., and Kirpalmi, H.: Beyond the complete cell count and C-reactive protein. *Archives of Pediatrics and Adolescent Medicine, 157*(6):511-516, 2003.

Malley, R., DeVincenzo, J., Ramilo, O., et al: Reduction of respiratory syncytial virus (RSV) in tracheal aspirates in intubated infants by use of humanized monoclonal antibody to RSV F Protein. *Journal of Infectious Diseases, 178*:1555-1561, 1998.

Manroe, B.L., Weinberg, A.G., Rosenfeld, C.R., et al.: The neonatal blood count in health and disease. *Pediatrics, 95*:89-98, 1979.

Moore, D.: Nosocomial infections in newborn nurseries. In C. Glen Mayhall (Ed.): *Hospital epidemiology and infection control.* Baltimore, 2004, Lippincott Williams & Wilkins, pp. 851-884.

Ohlsson, A. and Lacy, J.B.: Intravenous immunoglobulin for suspected or subsequently proven infection in neonates. *Cochrane Database of Systematic Reviews, 2:* CD001239, 2001.

Oski, F. and Naiman, J.: *Hematologic problems in the newborn.* Philadelphia, 1966, Saunders.

Overall, J.C., Jr.: Viral infections of the fetus and neonate. In R.D. Feigin and J.E. Cherry (Eds.): *Textbook of pediatric infectious diseases* (3rd ed.). Philadelphia, 1992, Saunders, pp. 924-959.

Palasanthiran, P., Ziegler, J.B.V., Stewart, G.J., et al.: Breastfeeding during primary maternal human immunodeficiency virus infection and risk of transmission from mother to infant. *Journal of Infectious Disease, 167*(2):441-444, 1993.

Polin, R.A., Yoder, M.C., and Burg, F.D.: *Workbook in practical neonatology* (3rd ed.). Philadelphia, 2001, Saunders.

Pourcyrous, M., Bada, H.S., Korones, S.B., et al.: Significance of serial C-reactive protein responses in neonatal infections and other disorders. *Pediatrics, 92*(2):431-435, 1993.

Schelonka, R.L., Chai, M.K., Yoder, B.A., et al.: Volume of blood required to detect common pathogens. *Journal of Pediatrics, 129*(2):275-278, 1996.

Schrag, S.J., Zell, E.R., Lynfield, R., et al.: A population based comparison of strategies to prevent early-onset group B streptococcal disease in neonates. *New England Journal of Medicine, 347*(4):233-239, 2002.

Schwersenski, S., McIntyre, L., and Bauer, C.R.: Lumbar puncture frequency and cerebrospinal fluid analysis in the neonate. *American Journal of Diseases in Children, 145*(1):54-58, 1991.

Sever, J.L., Ellenberg, J.H., Ley A.C., et al.: Toxoplasmosis: Maternal and pediatric findings in 23,000 pregnancies. *Pediatrics, 82*(2):181-192, 1988.

Sever, J.L., South, M.A., and Shaver, K.A.: Delayed manifestations of congenital rubella. *Reviews of Infectious Diseases, 7*(Suppl 1):S164-S169, 1985.

Stagno, S.: Cytomegalovirus. In J.S. Remington and J.O. Klein (Eds.): *Infectious diseases of the fetus and newborn infant* (4th ed.). Philadelphia, 1995, Saunders, pp. 312-353.

Stagno, S., Pass, R.F., Dworsky, M.E., et al.: Congenital and perinatal cytomegaloviral infections. *Seminars in Perinatology, 7*(1):31-42, 1983.

Stagno, S. and Whitley, R.J.: Herpesvirus infections of pregnancy. Part I: Cytomegalovirus and Epstein-Barr virus infections. *New England Journal of Medicine, 313*(20):1270-1274, 1985.

Stevens, J.P., Eames, M., Kent, A., et al.: Long term outcome of neonatal meningitis. *Archives of Disease in Childhood, Fetal and Neonatal Edition, 88*(3):F179-F184, 2003.

Stoll, B.J., Gordon, T., Korones, S.B., et al.: Early-onset sepsis in very low birth weight infants: A report from the National Institute of Child Health and Human Development Neonatal Research Network. *Journal of Pediatrics, 129*(1):72-80, 1996a.

Stoll, B.J., Gordon, T., Korones, S.B., et al.: Late-onset sepsis in very low birth weight neonates: A report from the National Institute of Child Health and Human Development Neonatal Research Network. *Journal of Pediatrics, 129*(1):63-71, 1996b.

Stoll, B.J., Hansen, N., Fanaroff, A.A., and Wright, L.L.: Changes in pathogens causing early-onset sepsis in very-low-birth-weight-infants. *New England Journal of Medicine, 347*(4):240-247, 2002.

Taketomo, C.K., Hodding, J.H., and Kraus, D.M.: *Pediatric dosage handbook* (9th ed.). Hudson, OH, 2002, Lexi-Comp.

Thureen, P.J., Deacon, J.M., Hernandez, J., and Hall D.: *Assessment and care of the well newborn* (2nd ed.). St. Louis, 2005, Saunders.

Vain, N.E., Mazlumian, J.R., Swarner, O.W., and Cha, C.C.: Role of exchange transfusion in neonatal septicemia. *Pediatrics, 66*(5):693-697, 1980.

Weiss, M.G., Ionides, S.P., and Anderson, C.L.: Meningitis in premature infants with respiratory distress: Role of admission lumbar puncture. *Journal of Pediatrics, 119*(6):973-975, 1991.

Welsh, J.K. and May, J.T.: Anti-infective properties of breast milk. *Journal of Pediatrics, 94*(1):1-9, 1979.

Whitley, R.J. and Arvin, A.M.: Herpes simplex virus infections. In J.S. Remington and J.O. Klein (Eds.): *Infectious diseases of the fetus and newborn infant* (4th ed.). Philadelphia, 1995, Saunders, pp. 354-376.

Young, T.E. and Mangum, O.B.: *Neofax: A manual of drugs used in neonatal care* (21st ed.). Montvale, MJ, 2008, Thomson Healthcare.

33 Renal and Genitourinary Disorders

CAROL BOTWINSKI

OBJECTIVES

1. Relate congenital renal/genitourinary disorders to embryologic development.

2. Apply knowledge of normal renal anatomy and physiology to renal pathophysiology that presents in the neonatal period.

3. Explain the etiology of selected neonatal renal/genitourinary disorders.

4. Describe clinical manifestations and complications that may be associated with selected neonatal renal/genitourinary disorders.

5. Determine the appropriate management of each disorder discussed.

6. Formulate an appropriate plan of care for each disorder discussed.

■■■ Homeostasis of the newborn is dependent on a functioning renal system. In utero the placenta is the organ responsible for fluid and electrolyte homeostasis. Postnatally the kidney must assume its role as the regulator. However, the immature renal system of the newborn responds slowly and erratically to physiologic changes and demands that are placed on it. Knowledge of renal physiology and embryologic development is essential in caring for these newborns. This chapter presents information on the anatomy and physiology of the kidney as a base from which to discuss selected renal/genitourinary disorders.

EMBRYOLOGY

A. Introduction.

    1. Embryologic development of the urinary system begins within the first weeks after conception and progresses through three stages.

    2. Both the urinary and the genital systems develop from the same germ layer of the embryo.

B. Kidney.

    1. The kidneys develop in three sequential stages.

        a. Pronephros.

            (1) Plays a primary role in normal organogenesis.

            (2) Appears during 3 to 4 weeks of gestation.

            (3) Degenerates by the fifth week.

        b. Mesonephros.

            (1) Originates during 4 to 5 weeks of gestation, just before degeneration of the pronephros, and is fully developed by 37 days.

            (2) Consists of 30 to 40 glomerulotubular units.

            (3) Capsule and glomerulus form the mesonephros (renal) corpuscle.

            (4) Develops into genital glands.

            (5) Regresses at the end of the second month.

    c. Metanephros.

      (1) Develops early in the fifth week and functions within a few weeks.

      (2) Permanent kidney develops from the metanephric diverticulum (ureteric bud) and the metanephric mesoderm (metanephrogenic blastema).

      (3) Normal differentiation of the ureteric bud is essential for initiation of branching, which leads to formation of the urinary collecting system (ureter, pelvis, calyces, and collecting ducts) and to the start of nephron formation within the metanephric blastema.

      (4) Nephroblastic cells differentiate into the glomerulus, proximal convoluted tubule, loop of Henle, and distal convoluted tubule.

      (5) Nephrons form from the proximal end of the renal/metanephric tubules, beginning at about 8 weeks and continuing until approximately 34 to 36 weeks. Approximately 1 million nephrons result.

      (6) Minor calyces and their communicating papillary ducts are well delineated and resemble those of a mature kidney by 13 to 14 weeks of gestation.

      (7) By 4 months, the kidney contains 14 to 16 lobes, equivalent to the mature kidney.

      (8) The kidney begins urine production and glomerular filtration at 9 to 10 weeks of gestation.

C. Urinary tract.

  1. Differentiation of the urinary tract occurs synchronously with the early stages of metanephric development.

  2. Urinary bladder develops at approximately 6 weeks of gestation.

  3. Formation of the urethra is completed by the end of the first trimester.

  4. Fetal ureter does not open functionally into the bladder until the ninth week.

D. Development of vascular supply.

  1. The vascular pattern of the fetal kidney resembles that of the mature kidney by 14 to 15 weeks of gestation.

  2. Renal blood flow in the fetus is low because of high renal vascular resistance and low systemic blood pressure.

RENAL ANATOMY

A. Gross anatomy.

  1. Cortex: outermost portion of the kidney, which contains the glomeruli, proximal, and distal convoluted tubules, and collecting ducts of the nephron.

  2. Medulla: middle section of the kidney, which contains renal pyramids, straight portions of tubules, loops of Henle, vasa recta, and terminal collecting ducts.

  3. Renal sinus and pelvis: innermost portion of the kidney. The renal sinus contains the uppermost part of the renal pelvis and calyces, surrounded by some fat in which branches of the renal vessels and nerves are embedded.

  4. Ureter: excretory duct of the kidney, which transports urine from kidney to bladder.

B. Microscopic renal anatomy: the nephron.

  1. Structural and functional unit of the kidney.

  2. Composed of glomerulus, Bowman capsule, and the tubules.

  3. All nephrons are present by 32 to 34 weeks of gestation; functional maturation and hypertrophy continue into infancy (Huether, 2006; Vogt et al., 2006).

  4. Functional component of the nephron is the renal corpuscle, which consists of the glomerulus and the glomerular (Bowman) capsule.

    a. Glomerulus is formed by a capillary network.

    b. Glomerular/Bowman capsule is a membrane surrounding the glomerulus, which serves as a filter mechanism through which nonprotein components of blood plasma can enter the renal tubules.

  5. Tubular system consists of proximal convoluted tubule, loop of Henle, distal convoluted tubule, and collecting duct.

RENAL HEMODYNAMICS

A. Renal blood flow (Huether, 2006; Porth, 2007).
1. Renal blood flow comprises 4% to 6% of the cardiac output during the first 12 hours of life and 8% to 10% of the cardiac output during the first week of life.
2. The rate of renal blood flow is determined by the cardiac output and the ratio of renal to systemic vascular resistance. Developmental changes in these parameters contribute to the postnatal increase in renal blood flow.
3. The primary factor responsible for maturational increase in renal blood flow and redistribution of intrarenal blood flow from the inner cortex to the outer cortex is decreased renal vascular resistance.
4. Renal plasma flow.
   a. Flow is 150 ml/minute/1.73 m^2 at term and increases to 200 ml/minute/1.73 m^2 in the first weeks of life.
   b. The low renal plasma flow in the neonate is due mainly to high renal vascular resistance but also to low perfusion pressure.

B. Regulation of renal blood flow (Huether, 2006; Porth, 2007).
1. Autoregulation of renal blood flow.
   a. Autoregulation refers to the ability of the kidney to maintain a relatively constant glomerular filtration rate (GFR) over a range of systemic blood pressure.
   b. Mechanisms.
      (1) Myogenic mechanism is the dilation or constriction of the afferent arteriole in response to changes in vascular wall tension for the purpose of maintaining normal blood flow.
      (2) Tubuloglomerular feedback mechanism consists of afferent and efferent feedback mechanisms.
         (a) Afferent arteriolar vasodilator feedback mechanism is activated by decreased glomerular filtrate in the tubules, which results in dilation of the afferent arteriole and increased GFR. When renal blood flow increases, the afferent arterioles constrict and return GFR to normal.
         (b) Efferent arteriolar vasodilator feedback mechanism is activated by decreased volume. This stimulates renin release and causes constriction of the efferent arteriole to a greater degree than constriction of the afferent arteriole and thus maintains the GFR.
2. Hormonal regulation of renal blood flow.
   a. Renin–angiotensin–aldosterone system.
      (1) Major renal hormonal system.
      (2) Well developed in the newborn infant; renin is present from 3 months of gestation onward.
      (3) Responsible for regulation of systemic blood pressure, sodium, potassium, and regional blood flow.
   b. Prostaglandins.
      (1) Synthesized in both cortex and medulla, and by glomerulus and tubules.
      (2) Renal medulla seems to be the major site of prostaglandin synthesis in the kidney.
      (3) Most important prostaglandins in the kidney are prostaglandins E_2 and $F_{2-\alpha}$, prostacyclin (prostaglandin I_2, epoprostenol), and thromboxane A_2.
      (4) Role in regulation of renal function and control of systemic blood pressure.
         (a) Vasodilation.
         (b) Natriuresis.
         (c) Inhibition of the distal tubule's response to antidiuretic hormone.

RENAL PHYSIOLOGY

A. Postnatal changes (Swinford et al., 2006; Vogt et al., 2006).
1. GFR doubles in the first 2 weeks of life in term and preterm neonates to 30 to 40 ml/minute/1.73 m^2 and increases to adult values of 100 to 120 ml/minute/1.73 m^2 between 1 and 2 years of life. Factors responsible for this increase are as follows:

      a. Increasing mean arterial blood pressure.

      b. Increasing renal blood flow.

      c. Increasing glomerular permeability and filtration surface area.

  2. Fractional excretion of sodium decreases due to increasing tubular reabsorption.

  3. Infant has an increasing ability to concentrate urine.

  4. Renal vasoactive hormones are initially increased.

  5. Renal vascular resistance decreases.

  6. Renal blood flow increases.

B. Glomerular filtration (Swinford et al., 2006; Vogt et al., 2006).

  1. As blood passes through the capillaries, plasma is filtered through the glomerular capillary walls. Filtrate is collected in the Bowman space and enters the tubules, where composition is modified until it is excreted as urine.

  2. Glomerular filtration rate (GFR).

      a. Factors that may contribute to decreased GFR at birth are as follows:

        (1) Small glomerular capillary area available for filtration.

        (2) Structural immaturity of glomerular capillary, which is associated with decreased water permeability.

        (3) Decreased blood pressure.

        (4) Increased hematocrit.

        (5) Renal vasoconstriction, which results in decreased glomerular plasma flow.

      b. Neonates born at less than 34 weeks of gestation have low GFR (0.5 ml/min) until nephrogenesis is completed.

  3. Three primary factors determine GFR.

      a. Glomerular capillary hydrostatic pressure.

      b. Hydrostatic pressure in Bowman capsule.

      c. Capillary colloid osmotic pressure.

  4. Glomerular capillary hydrostatic pressure is the major controller of GFR.

  5. Additional factors that affect GFR are as follows:

      a. Capillary surface area.

      b. Permeability of capillary basement membrane.

      c. Rate of renal plasma flow.

      d. Changes in renal blood flow.

      e. Changes in blood pressure.

      f. Vasoactive changes in afferent or efferent arterioles.

      g. Ureteral obstruction.

      h. Edema of kidney.

      i. Changes in the concentration of plasma proteins.

        (1) Dehydration.

        (2) Hypoproteinemia.

      j. Increased permeability of the glomerular filter.

      k. Decrease in total area of glomerular capillary bed.

C. Tubular function (Swinford et al., 2006; Vogt et al., 2006).

  1. Components of tubular system include proximal tubule, loop of Henle, distal tubule, and collecting ducts.

  2. Tubules modify the glomerular ultrafiltrate, leading to production of urine, which is accomplished by the process of tubular reabsorption and secretion.

      a. Tubular reabsorption is the movement of substances into the peritubular capillary plasma from the tubular epithelium, which occurs by diffusion and active transport. The proximal tubule is the major site of reabsorption.

      b. Tubular secretion is the movement of substances into the tubular epithelium from the peritubular capillary plasma. Tubular secretion is necessary for regulation of fluid and electrolyte balance, along with other renal processes.

  3. Regulation of fluids and electrolytes is an important tubular function.

  4. Tubular function is altered in the neonate as a result of decreased renal blood flow and GFR.

5. Tubular portions of the neonatal nephron are smaller and less functionally mature, resulting in an altered ability to transport sodium, urea, chloride, and glucose, with decreased renal thresholds for many substances.
6. Rapid maturation of proximal tubular cells occurs between 32 and 35 weeks of gestation.

D. **Concentration and dilution mechanism** (Swinford et al., 2006; Vogt et al., 2006).
   1. Maintenance of osmolality. The term and preterm infant's ability to dilute urine is fully developed, but concentrating ability is limited. A major function of the kidney is to maintain osmolality of extracellular fluid within the narrow range compatible with optimal cellular function.
   2. Sites of urinary concentration and dilution.
      a. Loop of Henle.
      b. Collecting duct.
   3. Factors responsible for the limited ability of the neonatal kidney to concentrate urine:
      a. Anatomic immaturity of the renal medulla.
      b. Decreased medullary concentration of sodium chloride and urea.
      c. Diminished responsiveness of the collecting ducts to arginine vasopressin.
   4. Normal range of neonatal specific gravity: 1.002 to 1.010.
   5. Maximum concentrating ability.
      a. Term infants: 700 mOsm of water per kilogram of body weight.
      b. Preterm infants: 600 to 700 mOsm of water per kilogram of body weight.
   6. Capacity for urine dilution.
      a. 30 to 50 mOsm/kg of water.
      b. Ability of neonate to excrete a hypotonic load is limited, presumably because of the low GFR.

E. **Acid–base balance.**
   1. Regulation of acid–base balance by the kidneys occurs in conjunction with the lungs and blood buffers. The role of the kidneys in regulating acid–base balance involves regulating the plasma bicarbonate by reabsorbing filtered bicarbonate and affecting hydrogen ion secretion through the formation of titratable acids and ammonium (Porth, 2007).
   2. Renal response to acidosis.
      a. Reabsorption of bicarbonate in the proximal tubule.
      b. Increased secretion of hydrogen ions in the distal convoluted tubule.
      c. Production of ammonia.
   3. Renal response to alkalosis.
      a. Excretion of bicarbonate.
      b. Decreased production of ammonia.
      c. Decreased hydrogen ion secretion in the distal tubule.
   4. Neonatal limitations in maintaining acid–base homeostasis.
      a. Decreased ability to handle an acid load and compensate for acid–base abnormalities.
      b. Decreased renal threshold for bicarbonate, and decreased capacity to reabsorb bicarbonate results in slightly lower serum bicarbonate and pH.
      c. Decreased GFR.
      d. Decreased production of ammonia.
      e. Decreased ability to secrete organic acids.

ACUTE RENAL FAILURE

A. **Definition:** Acute renal failure (ARF) is the loss of the kidneys' ability to maintain water and electrolyte homeostasis. It is associated with an abrupt and severe decrease in GFR, a decrease in urine output, and a progressive increase in BUN and creatinine (Chua and Sarwal, 2005; Vogt et al., 2006).
B. **Incidence:** The incidence of acute renal failure in the neonatal intensive care unit (NICU) has been reported to range from 6% to 8%, with some estimates as high as 23% (Chua and Sarwal, 2005; Vogt et al., 2006).

C. **Etiology:** The causes of ARF in the newborn are multiple and can be divided into prerenal, intrinsic, and postrenal categories.

1. Prerenal: results from a state of relative hypoperfusion in an otherwise normal kidney. It is the most common cause of acute renal failure in the neonate (Chua and Sarwal, 2005; Vogt et al., 2006).
   a. Hemorrhage.
   b. Sepsis.
   c. Congestive heart failure.
   d. Dehydration.
   e. Necrotizing enterocolitis.
   f. Respiratory distress syndrome.
   g. Hypoxia.
   h. Drugs: angiotensin-converting enzyme (ACE) inhibitors, indomethacin, amphotericin B.

2. Intrinsic: renal cellular damage involving functional compromise to the glomerular, tubular, and collecting system owing to prolonged prerenal insult, use of nephrotoxic agents or congenital anomaly (Chua and Sarwal, 2005; Vogt et al., 2006). Perinatal asphyxia is the most common cause of acute tubular necrosis in the term neonate (65%); sepsis is the most common in the preterm neonate (35%). Conditions resulting in intrinsic failure can be categorized into four broad groups.
   a. Congenital anomalies.
      (1) Agenesis.
      (2) Renal dysplasia.
      (3) Polycystic kidney disease.
   b. Thromboembolic disease.
      (1) Renal vein thrombosis.
      (2) Renal artery thrombosis.
      (3) Disseminated intravascular coagulation.
   c. Infection/inflammatory disease.
      (1) Acute pyelonephritis.
      (2) Congenital syphilis and toxoplasmosis.
   d. Acute tubular necrosis.
      (1) Perinatal asphyxia.
      (2) Cardiac surgery.
      (3) Prolonged prerenal state.
      (4) Nephrotoxic drug administration.
      (5) Uric acid nephropathy.

3. Postrenal: obstruction to urinary flow distal to the kidney (Chua and Sarwal, 2005; Vogt et al., 2006).
   a. Posterior urethral valves.
   b. Bilateral ureteropelvic junction (UPJ) obstruction.
   c. Neurogenic bladder.
   d. Obstructive nephrolithiasis.

D. **Clinical presentation** (Chua and Sarwal, 2005; Swinford et al., 2006; Vogt et al., 2006).

1. Oliguric ARF is characterized by urinary excretion of less than 1 ml/kg/hour, whereas in nonoliguric ARF, the urinary flow rate is maintained above this level.
2. Azotemia with a blood urea nitrogen (BUN) greater than 20 mg/dl or rising more than 1 mg/dl/day.
3. Elevated serum creatinine greater than 1.5 mg/dl or rising more than 0.2 mg/dl/day.

E. **Clinical assessment.**

1. Careful review of perinatal history.
   a. History of renal disease in family.
   b. Perinatal asphyxia.
   c. Renal abnormalities on antenatal sonogram.
   d. History of oligohydramnios.

2. Careful physical examination of infant can be revealing.
   a. Abdominal palpation is important because renal masses are the most common abdominal masses in the newborn.
   b. Bilateral renal enlargement may reflect cystic disease, hydronephrosis, or renal vein thrombosis.
   c. Edema, ascites, or hydrops at birth, which may be associated with congenital renal disease.
   d. Isolated ear anomalies can be associated with obstructive uropathy.
3. Urine output less than 0.5 to 1 ml/kg/hour after the first 24 hours of life.
4. Increase in daily weight greater than that predicted on the basis of infant's condition and caloric intake.
5. Blood pressure.
   a. Hypotension: may contribute to acute renal failure.
   b. Hypertension: may be observed in cases of acute renal failure.
F. **Diagnostic studies can be useful to differentiate between prerenal, intrinsic, and postrenal failure** (Chua and Sarwal, 2005).
   1. Urine studies.
      a. Urinalysis.
         (1) Presence of casts, tubular cells, and proteinuria suggests intrinsic renal failure.
      b. Culture and Gram stain to rule out urinary tract infection/sepsis.
      c. Urine sodium and creatinine.
         (1) Used in determining the fractionated excretion of sodium (FeNa) (urine Na/plasma Na : plasma creatinine/urine creatinine × 100).
         (2) Values greater than 3% generally indicate intrinsic ARF, whereas those with a value of less than 2.5% indicate prerenal failure.
            (a) These values will have limited significance in neonates born at less than 32 weeks of gestation because of these infants' limited ability to conserve sodium.
            (b) Urinary indices lose their diagnostic usefulness after therapy for oliguria has begun, particularly with diuretics.
   2. Blood.
      a. BUN and creatinine.
         (1) BUN/creatinine ratio. A disproportionate rise in the BUN/creatinine ratio suggests a prerenal etiology, whereas a proportionate rise indicates an intrinsic etiology.
         (2) BUN greater than 20 mg/dl or rise greater than 1 mg/dl/day.
         (3) Creatinine concentration greater than 1.5 mg/dl or increase greater than 0.2 mg/dl/day. A rising serum creatinine level is never normal.
      b. Serum electrolytes to evaluate for metabolic abnormalities associated with ARF.
         (1) Hyperkalemia.
         (2) Hyponatremia.
         (3) Hypocalcemia.
         (4) Hyperphosphatemia.
   3. Renal ultrasound is helpful in identification of congenital renal disease and urinary tract obstruction.
   4. Voiding cystourethrography (VCUG) to rule out obstructive disease and reflux.
   5. Radionuclide renal scans may be used to evaluate renal perfusion and function.
      a. Fluid challenge should be administered to exclude prerenal ARF.
      b. 10 to 20 ml/kg of normal saline is administered over 1 hour.
      c. Rapid and sustained diuresis within 1 to 2 hours indicates a prerenal cause.
      d. Urine output of less than 2 ml/kg/hour after furosemide administration suggests an intrinsic or postrenal cause.
G. **Management.**
   1. Most important principle in treating ARF is to identify the cause and provide appropriate care for the primary condition (Chua and Sarwal, 2005; Vogt et al., 2006).
      a. Prerenal → treat specific causes of renal hypoperfusion.
      b. Intrinsic → supportive care until kidney function returns.
      c. Postrenal → surgery/nephrology.

  2. Strict management of intake and output.
   a. With intrinsic failure fluids are restricted to insensible water loss plus urine output.
   b. Full-term infants → 30 ml/kg/day urinary losses.
   c. Premature infants → up to 70 ml/kg/day urinary losses.
  3. Monitor body weight once or twice daily.
   a. Newborns with ARF should either maintain steady weight or lose 20 to 30 g per day.
  4. Monitor serum glucose and electrolytes.
   a. Sodium and potassium intake may need to be restricted.
   b. Newborns with anuria require no electrolyte intake.
   c. Treat acidosis.
  5. Provide adequate nutrition.
   a. Provide 100 cal/kg with fat and carbohydrates.
   b. Provide 1 to 2 g/kg/day of protein.
  6. Monitor blood pressure and treat hypertension.
   a. Hypertension occurs secondary to renal damage or fluid overload.
   b. Can be treated with restriction of sodium and fluid, or with antihypertensive agents.
  7. Observe for signs and symptoms of congestive heart failure.
  8. Assess for bleeding diathesis.
  9. Avoid nephrotoxic medications and those with a high sodium content.
  10. Dialysis treatment is indicated for a protracted course of ARF or if conservative treatment fails to prevent complications.
   a. Symptomatic hyponatremia.
   b. Hyperkalemia.
   c. Congestive heart failure.
   d. Hypertension.
   e. Hypervolemia.
H. **Outcome** (Vogt et al., 2006).
  1. Prognosis for neonates with ARF is variable, with mortality rates ranging from 14% to 73%.
  2. Reversal of underlying condition is the most important factor in determining prognosis.
   a. Best prognosis is for patients who receive prompt treatment for renal hypoperfusion.
   b. Long-term sequelae.
    (1) Chronic renal failure.
    (2) Decreased GFR.
    (3) Impaired tubular function.
    (4) Chronic hypertension.
    (5) Renal tubular acidosis.
    (6) Nephrocalcinosis.
    (7) Impaired renal growth.

HYPERTENSION

Blood pressures vary by gestational age, body weight, cuff size, and state of alertness. Hypertension is diagnosed when blood pressure is consistently greater than the 95th percentile (Ettinger and Flynn, 2002; Pejovic et al., 2007; Swinford et al., 2006).
A. **Etiology.**
  1. The most common causes of neonatal hypertension include renovascular anomalies and intrinsic renal disease (Ettinger and Flynn, 2002; Farnham et al., 2005).
  2. Additional causes include endocrine disorders, medications, and various other disease states.
B. **Incidence** (Ettinger and Flynn, 2002; Farnham et al., 2005).
  1. Incidence of neonatal hypertension is approximately 0.08%.
  2. Incidence of neonatal hypertension has been reported to be 2% of NICU admissions.
C. **Disease states** (Farnham et al., 2005; Swinford et al., 2006).
  1. Renal vascular.
   a. Thromboembolism.

   b. Renal artery stenosis.

   c. Renal vein thrombosis.

2. Cardiac.

   a. Coarctation of the aorta.

3. Pulmonary.

   a. Bronchopulmonary dysplasia.

4. Renal disease.

   a. Congenital.

   (1) Polycystic kidney disease.

   (2) Multicystic-dysplastic kidney disease.

   (3) Ureteropelvic junction obstruction.

   b. Acquired.

   (1) Acute tubular necrosis.

   (2) Hemolytic-uremic syndrome.

   (3) Obstruction by tumor.

5. Endocrine.

   a. Congenital adrenal hyperplasia.

   b. Pseudohypoaldosteronism type II.

   c. Thyrotoxicosis.

6. Medications/intoxications.

   a. Maternal.

   (1) Cocaine.

   (2) Heroin.

   b. Neonatal.

   (1) Dexamethasone.

   (2) Theophylline.

   (3) Caffeine.

   (4) Pancuronium.

   (5) Phenylephrine.

7. Neoplasms.

   a. Wilms tumor.

   b. Mesoblastic nephroma.

   c. Neuroblastoma.

8. Neurologic.

   a. Pain.

   b. Intracranial hypertension.

   c. Seizures.

9. Miscellaneous.

   a. Closure of abdominal wall defect.

   b. Fluid overload.

   c. Hypercalcemia.

   d. Adrenal hemorrhage.

   e. Birth asphyxia.

   f. Extracorporeal membrane oxygenation.

D. Clinical presentation (Swinford et al., 2006; Vogt et al., 2006).

1. Presenting symptoms may be nonspecific, including feeding difficulties, unexplained tachypnea, lethargy, mottling of skin; mild to moderate hypertension may be asymptomatic in 50% of infants.

2. Life-threatening presentations of hypertension include congestive heart failure and cardiogenic shock.

E. Clinical assessment.

1. Arterial blood pressure: persistent elevation of blood pressure (BP) to greater than 90/60 mm Hg in term infants and 80/50 mm Hg in preterm infants.

2. Careful review of perinatal history to identify history of umbilical artery catheter, renal disease, or congenital heart disease; maternal history of medications or illicit drug use during pregnancy; family history of renal or endocrine disease.

3. Physical examination should focus on cardiac and abdominal evaluations.
4. Obtain set of four extremity BPs and careful palpation of femoral pulses to rule out coarctation of aorta.
5. Dysmorphic features may indicate the diagnosis of congenital adrenal hyperplasia or Turner syndrome.
6. Presence of flank mass may indicate UPJ obstruction or renal cystic disease.

F. **Diagnostic studies** (Vogt et al., 2006).
1. Initial laboratory tests include urinalysis, complete blood count (CBC), electrolytes, BUN, creatinine, calcium, urine culture if infection is suspected, and plasma renin level.
2. Renal ultrasonography with Doppler flow study to rule out renovascular hypertension.
3. Renal scan to detect renal thrombosis and surgically amenable lesions (e.g., UPJ obstruction).
4. Magnetic resonance imaging or CT scan to detect tumors or masses.

G. **Management.**
1. Measure resting blood pressure, using a cuff of the appropriate size.
2. Correctable causes of hypertension should be addressed initially before considering medications (Ettinger and Flynn, 2002).
   a. Treat pain.
   b. Correct volume overload.
   c. Wean inotropic agents if present.
3. Antihypertensive medications (Young and Mangum, 2008).
   a. Hydralazine: 0.1 to 0.5 mg/kg/dose every 6 to 8 hours, IV bolus; or 0.25 to 1.5 mg/kg/dose every 6 to 8 hours. Administer with food to enhance absorption.
   b. Captopril: 0.01 to 0.5 mg/kg/dose every 8 to 12 hours, by mouth. Administer 1 hour before feeding.
   c. Enalapril: Begin at 0.04 mg/kg/dose every 24 hours, by mouth. Usual maximum dose 0.15 mg/kg/dose, as frequent as every 6 hours.
   d. Sodium nitroprusside: Initial dose 0.25 to 0.5 mcg/kg/minute by continuous infusion. Usual maintenance dose is <2 mcg/kg/minute.

H. **Complications.**
1. Congestive heart failure.
2. Left ventricular hypertrophy.
3. Hypertensive retinopathy.
4. Intracranial hemorrhage.
5. Cerebrovascular accident.
6. Encephalopathy.

I. **Outcome.**
1. Prognosis depends primarily on the etiology; however, time of diagnosis, presence of neurologic complications, and response to therapy are also factors (Vogt et al., 2006).
2. Poor renal growth may ensue on the side with renal artery pathologic changes, and renal scans may show abnormalities (Swinford et al., 2006).

POTTER SYNDROME (OLIGOHYDRAMNIOS SYNDROME)

A. **Bilateral renal agenesis with Potter facies** (Fig. 33-1).
B. **Etiology: failure of ureteric bud to divide and develop or abnormal development of the normal progression from pronephros to mesonephros to metanephros** (Huether, 2006).
C. **Incidence.**
1. Approximately 1:4,800 to 1:10,000 births (Vogt et al., 2006).
2. Male predominance.
3. Approximately 40% of affected infants are stillborn (Huether, 2006).
D. **Clinical presentation.**
1. Anuria.
2. Potter facies.
   a. Blunted nose.
   b. Receded chin.

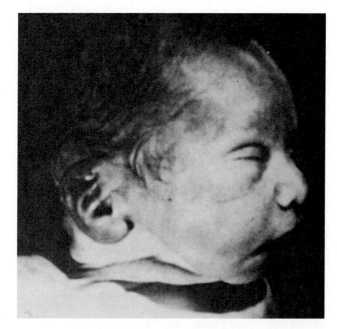

FIGURE 33-1 ■ Potter facies. Note epicanthal folds, hypertelorism, low-set ears, crease below lower lip, and receding chin. (From Martin, R.J., Fanaroff, A.A., and Walsh, M.C.: *Fanaroff and Martin's neonatal-perinatal medicine: Diseases of the fetus and infant* [8th ed.]. St. Louis, 2006, Mosby.)

    c. Prominent depression between lower lip and chin.
    d. Low-set ears.
    e. Widely spaced eyes.
    f. Depressed nasal bridge.
    g. Prominent skinfold arising from epicanthus, progressing interiorly, and extending laterally beneath the eyes.
  3. Small for gestational age.
  4. Pulmonary hypoplasia.
  5. Excessively dry skin.
  6. Relatively large and clawlike hands.
  7. Bell-shaped chest.
  8. History of oligohydramnios.
  9. Bowed legs and clubbed feet possible.
E. Clinical assessment.
  1. Urinary output: anuria after the first 24 hours without bladder distention.
  2. Potter facies.
  3. Signs and symptoms of respiratory distress.
  4. Perinatal history of oligohydramnios.
  5. Presence of other associated anomalies.
    a. Abnormal genitalia.
    b. Gastrointestinal malformations.
F. Physical examination: palpation of abdomen for presence of kidneys.
G. Diagnostic studies.
  1. Renal ultrasonography: to rule out renal agenesis.
  2. Renal scan: if ultrasonography is inconclusive.
H. Differential diagnosis.
  1. Bilateral polycystic kidney disease.
  2. Bilateral multicystic dysplastic kidney disease.
I. Complications.
  1. Respiratory distress.
  2. Pneumothorax.
  3. Complications associated with acute renal failure.

J. Patient care management.
  1. Palliative care measures for neonate.
  2. Support for the grieving family.
K. Outcome (Huether, 2006; Swinford et al., 2006).
  1. Death usually occurs within hours to several days.
  2. Most die of respiratory distress caused by associated pulmonary hypoplasia.

AUTOSOMAL RECESSIVE POLYCYSTIC KIDNEY DISEASE

A. Etiology: autosomal recessive.
B. Incidence: 1:10,000 to 1:40,000 (Vogt et al., 2006).
C. Clinical presentation (Swinford et al., 2006; Vogt et al., 2006).
  1. History of oligohydramnios.
  2. Bilateral flank masses.
  3. Oliguria.
  4. Abdominal distention from the massively enlarged kidneys.
  5. Respiratory distress and spontaneous pneumothorax.
  6. Hypertension.
  7. Renal insufficiency.
  8. Some degree of congenital hepatic fibrosis with biliary dysgenesis.
D. Diagnostic studies. Renal ultrasonography shows symmetrically enlarged hyperechoic kidneys with loss of corticomedullary junction.
E. Differential diagnosis.
  1. Multicystic dysplasia.
  2. Hydronephrosis.
  3. Renal vein thrombosis.
  4. Renal tumor.
  5. Autosomal dominant polycystic kidney disease.
  6. Tuberous sclerosis.
F. Complications.
  1. Renal failure.
  2. Hepatic failure.
  3. Hypertension.
  4. Portal hypertension with palpable liver and esophageal varices.
  5. Congestive heart failure.
G. Patient care management.
  1. Genetic counseling for parents.
  2. Supportive care.
     a. Treat hypertension.
     b. Treat congestive heart failure.
     c. Give adequate nutrition to support normal growth and development.
  3. Infants surviving neonatal period: close monitoring for inevitable decrease in renal function.
  4. Consideration of renal transplant once renal failure develops.
H. Outcome (Vogt et al., 2006).
  1. Those who survive the perinatal period have varying degrees of renal insufficiency and hypertension.
  2. Long-term consequences of hepatic fibrosis may include portal hypertension and liver failure.
  3. Death usually results from a combination of renal and respiratory failure.
  4. Survival time varies: 86% of affected children survive to 3 months; 79% to 1 year; 51% to 10 years; and 46% to 15 years.

MULTICYSTIC DYSPLASTIC KIDNEY DISEASE

A. Definition: a nonfunctional, dysplastic kidney with multiple large cysts and ureteral atresia. It is the most severe form of renal dysplasia (Vogt et al., 2006).

B. **Etiology.**
   1. Developmental anomaly.
   2. Nongenetic.
C. **Incidence.**
   1. Reported as 1:4300 (Vogt et al., 2006).
   2. Males and females equally affected.
   3. Most common form of renal cystic disease in neonates: unilateral multicystic dysplasia (Swinford et al., 2006).
D. **Clinical presentation.**
   1. Abdominal mass.
   2. History of oligohydramnios.
   3. Frequently associated with contralateral renal and extrarenal abnormalities, including cardiac, gastrointestinal, and central nervous system (CNS) abnormalities, and several malformation syndromes (Vogt et al., 2006).
E. **Physical examination:** abdominal palpation.
   1. Irregular mass.
   2. Usually unilateral.
      a. More often on the left side.
      b. Possible hypertrophy of the contralateral kidney; also risk of other abnormality, most commonly vesicoureteral reflux or ureteropelvic junction obstruction (Swinford et al., 2006).
F. **Diagnostic studies** (Vogt et al., 2006).
   1. Renal ultrasonography shows noncommunicating cysts of varying size; lack of normal renal parenchyma.
   2. Renal scan: absence of renal function.
   3. VCUG to rule out reflux.
G. **Differential diagnosis.**
   1. Polycystic kidney disease.
   2. Hydronephrosis.
   3. Renal vein thrombosis.
   4. Renal tumor.
H. **Complications.**
   1. Hypertension.
   2. Hematuria.
   3. Infection.
I. **Patient care management.**
   1. Nonoperative approach.
      a. Serial ultrasonography.
      b. Monitoring of blood pressure.
      c. Monitoring for infection.
      d. Monitoring for hematuria.
      e. Assessment for signs and symptoms of renal failure.
   2. Surgical removal of kidney may be indicated if its size causes severe abdominal distention preventing provision of adequate nutrition (Swinford et al., 2006).
J. **Outcome** (Vogt et al., 2006).
   1. Bilateral involvement is incompatible with life.
   2. Most unilateral disease undergoes spontaneous involution.
   3. Contralateral kidney (if unaffected) develops a compensatory hyperplasia.
   4. There is a small but increased risk of the development of Wilms tumor.

HYDRONEPHROSIS

A. **Definition:** dilation of the pelvis and calyces of one or both kidneys, resulting from obstruction of urine flow (Swinford et al., 2006).
B. **Etiology.** The etiology of most types of hydronephrosis is unclear. However, a urinary tract obstruction causes a retrograde increase in hydrostatic pressure and dilation above the lesion, resulting in impaired renal structure and function (Swinford et al., 2006).

C. **Incidence.**
  1. Most common congenital condition detected by prenatal ultrasound, occurring in 1 of 500 to 700 deliveries (Vogt et al., 2006).
  2. The abnormality occurs predominantly in males and most often on the left side.
D. **Clinical presentation.**
  1. Palpable abdominal mass.
  2. Decreased urinary output.
  3. Poor urinary stream.
  4. Urinary tract infection: common.
E. **Clinical assessment.**
  1. Urinalysis.
     a. Findings possibly within normal limits.
     b. Proteinuria.
     c. Hematuria.
     d. Leukocyturia.
  2. Serum creatinine: may be elevated.
  3. BUN: may be elevated.
  4. Antenatal ultrasonography: evidence of hydronephrosis.
F. **Physical examination.**
  1. Abdominal palpation reveals enlarged kidney.
  2. Observe for other genitourinary or associated anomalies that may occur outside the urinary tract.
     a. Imperforate anus.
     b. Congenital vertebral anomalies.
     c. Facial and skeletal anomalies.
     d. Malformed ears.
     e. Myelodysplasia.
     f. Absent or decreased abdominal musculature.
     g. Unexplained pneumonia.
     h. Absence or dysplasia of the radius.
     i. Hypoplasia of the pelvis.
     j. Unexplained septicemia.
G. **Diagnostic studies** (Lam et al., 2007; Vogt et al., 2006).
  1. Renal ultrasonography.
  2. Voiding cystourethrogram.
  3. Renal scan.
H. **Differential diagnosis.**
  1. Obstructive.
     a. Ureteropelvic junction obstruction: most common cause of hydronephrosis in neonates (Lam et al., 2007; Vogt et al., 2006).
     b. Ureterovesical junction obstruction.
     c. Multicystic dysplastic kidney disease.
     d. Ureterocele/ectopic ureter.
     e. Duplicated collecting system.
     f. Posterior urethral valves: most common cause of severe obstructive uropathy in neonates (Vogt et al., 2006).
     g. Urethral atresia.
  2. Nonobstructive.
     a. Physiologic dilation (Vogt et al., 2006).
        (1) Unassociated with anatomic abnormality of urinary tract.
        (2) May be caused by delay in maturation of the ureter leading to transient urinary flow obstruction.
     b. Vesicoureteral reflux.
     c. Prune-belly syndrome (also known as Eagle–Barrett syndrome).
I. **Complications.**
  1. Urinary tract infection.

2. Hypertension.
3. Damage to renal parenchyma.

J. Specific patient care management.

1. Ureteropelvic junction obstruction (Lam et al., 2007; Nelson, Park, et al., 2005).
   a. Management depends on age and affected kidney's function.
   b. Evidence of obstruction on diuretic renogram and preserved renal function may not require immediate pyeloplasty. Treat with antibiotics and follow up with a diuretic renogram in 3 months to determine any change in drainage pattern or deterioration in function of affected kidney.
   c. Pyeloplasty (excision of stenotic segment; normal ureter and renal pelvis are reattached) is indicated for obstruction with compromised renal function.
2. Posterior urethral valves.
   a. Catheterize initially to provide drainage of urinary tract.
   b. Correct fluid and electrolyte or other metabolic imbalances.
   c. Neonates whose diagnosis was made after 24 weeks of gestation or postnatally are treated in the neonatal period with endoscopic fulguration of the posterior urethral valves or decompression by various methods (i.e., percutaneous nephrostomy drainage, vesicostomy, or ureterostomies with later valve ablation).
3. Vesicoureteral reflux.
   a. Catheterize initially.
   b. Nonsurgical treatment.
      (1) Antibiotic prophylaxis: amoxicillin for first 2 months, followed by trimethoprim-sulfamethoxazole or nitrofurantoin daily.
      (2) Cystography should be repeated every 12 to 18 months to determine resolution of reflux.
      (3) Circumcision is recommended for male neonates to decrease the risk of urinary tract infection.
   c. Surgical repair is indicated for higher reflux grade and breakthrough infection, lack of compliance, and unlikely resolution.
4. For obstruction at the ureterovesical junction, management is similar to that for obstruction of the ureteropelvic junction.

K. Outcome (Lam et al., 2007).

1. Success rates for pyeloplasty: reported as 91% to 98%.
2. Posterior urethral valves.
   a. Neonates identified after 24 weeks of gestation or postnatally have a 5% mortality rate.
   b. Long-term outcome depends on degree of associated renal dysplasia.
   c. Thirty percent of boys with posterior urethral valves who present in infancy are at risk for progressive renal insufficiency in childhood (Vogt et al., 2006).
3. Vesicoureteral reflux.
   a. Most reflux resolves; 60% to 80% of grades 1 through 3 cases resolve spontaneously.
   b. The generally accepted rate for complication-free correction of reflux, including all grades, is more than 95% when carried out by an experienced urologist.

RENAL VEIN THROMBOSIS

A. Predisposing conditions (Marks et al., 2005; Vogt et al., 2006).

1. Hyperviscosity.
2. Polycythemia.
3. Hypovolemia.
4. Hypercoagulable states.
5. Dehydration.
6. Presence of indwelling umbilical arterial catheters.
7. Perinatal asphyxia.
8. Any condition resulting in decreased blood flow to the kidneys.

B. Clinical triad of symptoms (Vogt et al., 2006).
1. Hematuria.
2. Flank mass.
3. Thrombocytopenia.
4. Additional signs include
   a. Hypertension,
   b. Oliguria, and
   c. Gross hematuria.
C. Diagnostic studies (Marks et al., 2005).
1. Full thrombophilia screen to identify antithrombin, protein C and S deficiencies, and factor V Leiden and prothrombin 20210A gene defects.
2. Renal ultrasound shows enlarged kidney with diffuse homogeneous hyperechogenicity.
3. Doppler flow study may show renal venous or vena caval thrombosis and abnormal flow pattern in renal venous branches or evidence of venous collateral development.
4. Renal scan may show absent or decreased uptake, indicating nonfunctioning kidney.
D. Patient care management.
1. Treat underlying illness.
2. Supportive treatment.
   a. Correct electrolyte imbalances.
   b. Correct fluid imbalances.
   c. Treat for renal insufficiency.
   d. Treat coagulation disorders.
3. Thrombolytic therapy with streptokinase, urokinase, and recombinant tissue plasminogen activator remain controversial (Marks et al., 2005).
E. Outcome.
1. Kidney may recover or show signs of damage; depends in part on severity of underlying medical condition.
2. Long-term consequences can include renal insufficiency, renal tubular dysfunction, and systemic hypertension (Vogt et al., 2006).

URINARY TRACT INFECTIONS

A. Etiology.
1. Abnormality of the urinary tract.
2. Sepsis, although there is debate as to whether the urinary tract infection (UTI) is the cause or effect of bacteremia (Edwards, 2006).
3. *Escherichia coli* accounts for approximately 75% of the UTIs. Pathogens causing hospital-acquired infections also include other gram-negative bacilli (*Klebsiella, Enterobacter,* and *Proteus*), gram-positive cocci (enterococci, *Staphylococcus epidermidis, S. aureus*), and fungal organisms (Edwards, 2006; Kanellopoulos et al., 2006).
B. Incidence (Edwards, 2006).
1. Reported to range from 0.1% to 1% in all newborn infants and to be as high as 3% in low-birth-weight infants.
2. Occurs more frequently in males than females. Preponderance in males may reflect the increased risk of UTI in uncircumcised males because of increased preputial colonization with bacteria (Dulczak and Kirk, 2005; Singh-Grewal et al., 2005).
C. Clinical presentation (Dulczak and Kirk, 2005; Edwards, 2006).
1. May be asymptomatic.
2. Symptomatic manifestations are usually nonspecific.
   a. Abnormal weight loss during the first days of life.
   b. Poor feeding.
   c. Irritability.
   d. Lethargy.
   e. Jaundice.

D. **Diagnostic studies** (Dulczak and Kirk, 2005; Edwards, 2006; Kanellopoulos et al., 2006).
   1. Urine culture: urine specimen should be obtained for culture via suprapubic aspiration or bladder catheterization.
      a. Bacterial counts of 10^3 higher colony-forming units (CFUs) per milliliter of catheterized urine are considered significant.
      b. Isolation of any bacteria from a suprapubic tap is considered significant.
   2. Urinalysis may show pyuria (>10 to 15 white blood cells/high-power field [WBC/hpf] and hematuria).
   3. Blood culture.
   4. Complete blood cell count with differential cell count.
   5. Renal ultrasonography to rule out urologic abnormalities.
   6. VCUG to rule out reflux.
      a. Vesicoureteral reflux (VUR) occurs in 40% of neonates with UTIs.
      b. VUR is associated with renal scarring.
   7. If renal abnormalities are detected by VCUG, a renal scan to detect renal inflammation and scarring may be warranted.
E. **Management** (Dulczak and Kirk, 2005; Edwards, 2006).
   1. Administer antibiotic therapy for 10 days.
      a. Empiric treatment for neonatal UTI includes broad-spectrum antibiotics (e.g., ampicillin and aminoglycoside) in dosages used for sepsis.
      b. Consider vancomycin and an aminoglycoside for empiric treatment of nosocomial UTIs.
      c. Final choice of antibiotic is based on sensitivity of the cultured organism.
      d. Prophylaxis antibiotic coverage may be instituted in infants with an abnormal urinary tract after an initial urinary tract infection until VCUG is done.
   2. Sterilization of urine should be documented posttreatment.
   3. VCUG should be done as soon as infection has resolved to assess for VUR.
      a. Neonates who demonstrate reflux should be maintained on prophylaxis antibiotic therapy.
      b. VCUG should be repeated in 6 months if reflux was initially present.
F. **Outcome: excellent with prompt and adequate treatment.**

PATENT URACHUS

A. **Definition:** a communication between the bladder and the umbilicus, causing a leakage of urine from the umbilicus.
B. **Etiology:** failure of normal closure of epithelialized urachal tube, resulting in patent urachus.
C. **Incidence:** more common in males than in females (Lugo et al., 2006).
D. **Clinical presentation.**
   1. Discharge of urine from umbilicus at birth or later.
   2. Wet umbilicus.
   3. Enlarged/edematous umbilicus.
   4. Delayed sloughing of cord.
E. **Physical examination:** observation of umbilicus.
F. **Diagnostic studies.**
   1. Analysis of fluid for urea and creatinine.
   2. Bladder ultrasonography.
   3. VCUG.
   4. Transurethral injection of methylene blue.
G. **Differential diagnosis** (Lugo et al., 2006).
   1. Patency of vitelline/omphalomesenteric duct.
   2. Omphalitis.
   3. Simple granulation of a healing umbilical stump.
   4. Infected umbilical vessel.
   5. External urachal sinus.

H. Complications.
   1. Urinary tract infection.
   2. Excoriation.
   3. Infection.
I. Patient care management.
   1. Nonintervention: spontaneous closure may occur if defect is small and drainage is intermittent.
   2. Operative intervention.
      a. Treatment of distal obstructive uropathy, if present, before surgical closure of urachal duct.
      b. Extraperitoneal surgical excision of urachal tract with bladder cuff; laparoscopic approach is becoming the procedure of choice for management of uracheal pathology (Turial et al., 2006).
J. Outcome: good with surgical procedure.

HYPOSPADIAS

A. Definition: urethral meatus is located on the ventral surface or undersurface of penis (Fig. 33-2). The condition varies in severity from a slightly malpositioned meatus still within the glans and without chordee to extreme genital ambiguity with hypoplastic phallus, bifid scrotum, and scrotal or perineal meatus.
B. Etiology.
   1. Deficient anterior urethral development.
   2. Delay or arrest in normal sequence of development, causing the urethra to open proximally and the prepuce to be incomplete ventrally.
   3. Probably multifactorial mode of inheritance.
C. Incidence: reported as approximately 1:300 newborn boys, it is one of the most common anomalies of the penis (Huether, 2006).
D. Clinical presentation.
   1. Urinary meatus located on the undersurface of the penis.
   2. Deviation of urinary stream.
E. Clinical assessment.
   1. Direction of urinary stream.
   2. Voiding pattern.
F. Physical examination (Pulsifer, 2005).
   1. Observation of external genitalia.
      a. Meatal location.

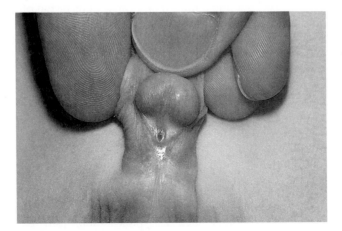

FIGURE 33-2 ■ Hypospadias. (Courtesy H. Gil Rushton, MD, Children's National Medical Center, Washington, DC. In M.J. Hockenberry and D. Wilson [Eds.]: *Wong's nursing care of infants and children* [8th ed.]. St. Louis, 2007, Mosby.)

      b. Quantity of ventral shaft skin and dorsal foreskin; usually incomplete formation of ventral prepuce.

      c. Chordee: downward curving of penis.

        (1) Association with chordee variable.

        (2) Severity of chordee generally proportional to degree of hypospadias.

      d. Assess for presence of associated anomalies (e.g., inguinal hernia, cryptorchidism, hydrocele, and meatal stenosis). Undescended testes and inguinal hernias are the most commonly associated anomalies.

   2. Palpation.

      a. Descent of testes.

      b. Presence of inguinal hernia.

G. Complications.

   1. Without repair.

      a. Difficulty in voiding while standing.

      b. The presence of chordee may cause painful erection.

   2. With postsurgical repair (Amukele et al., 2005).

      a. Urethrocutaneous fistula.

      b. Balanitis xerotica obliterans.

      c. Meatal stenosis.

      d. Urethral stricture.

      e. Urethral diverticulum.

H. Patient care management.

   1. Avoidance of circumcision.

   2. Genotypic evaluation if only one gonad is palpated; congenital adrenal disease must be ruled out when no gonads are palpable (Danish and Dahms, 2002).

   3. Surgical repair.

      a. Move meatus distally.

      b. Improve cosmetic appearance of genitalia.

      c. Straighten curved penis.

      d. Most cases can be corrected with single-stage repair (Huether, 2006).

      e. Repair between 6 and 12 months of age is generally recommended (Amukele et al., 2005; Huether, 2006).

I. Outcome: good for surgical correction of simple hypospadias (Pohl et al., 2007).

EXSTROPHY OF THE BLADDER

A. Definition: the bladder is exposed and protruding onto the abdominal wall because of failure of the anterior abdominal walls to close at the point of the bladder (Fig. 33-3). The umbilicus is displaced downward, and the pubic rami (bony projections of the pubic bone) are widely separated in the midline, and the rectus muscles are separated (Huether, 2006).

   1. Virtually all affected male infants have associated epispadias (opening of the urinary meatus onto the dorsal aspect of the penis).

   2. The remainder of the urinary tract is usually normal.

B. Etiology.

   1. Part of the spectrum of conditions resulting from abnormal development of the cloacal membrane.

   2. Failure of the mesoderm to invade cephalad extension of the cloacal membrane.

   3. Variant of exstrophy–epispadias complex determined by the position and timing of rupture of the cloacal membrane.

C. Incidence.

   1. Approximately 1:24,000 to 1:40,000 (Huether, 2006).

   2. More common in males by a ratio of 5:1 (Huether, 2006).

   3. Higher incidence of conditions such as spina bifida, cleft palate, preterm birth, and gastrointestinal anomalies are seen in infants with exstrophy (Nelson, Dunn, et al., 2005).

D. Clinical presentation: external presentation of bladder.

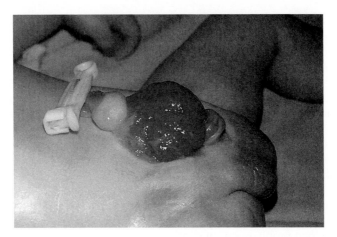

FIGURE 33-3 ■ Exstrophy of bladder. (Courtesy H. Gil Rushton, MD, Children's National Medical Center, Washington, DC. In M.J. Hockenberry and D. Wilson [Eds.]: *Wong's nursing care of infants and children* [8th ed.]. St. Louis, 2007, Mosby.)

E. **Physical assessment.**
   1. Observation of external presentation of bladder.
   2. Assessment of associated anomalies.
      a. Epispadias.
      b. Bifid clitoris.
      c. Anteriorly located vagina.
      d. Anteriorly located anus.
   3. Palpation.
      a. Testes: to assess descent.
      b. Groin: to assess for presence of inguinal hernias.
      c. Symphysis pubis: to assess widening.
F. **Differential diagnosis:** complete exstrophy–epispadias complex.
G. **Complications.**
   1. Infections.
   2. Postoperative hydronephrosis.
   3. Vesicoureteral reflux after bladder closure.
   4. Swelling and edema in the bladder wall after surgery, which obstructs ureteral drainage and can lead to anuria, hypertension, or hydroureteronephrosis.
   5. Urinary incontinence.
   6. Anal incontinence.
   7. Malignancy occurring 10 or more years later.
H. **Patient care management** (Ball and Bindler, 2008; Leung et al., 2005).
   1. Prevent cord clamp from damaging bladder by using cord tie.
   2. Cover exposed bladder with a clear plastic wrap.
   3. Irrigate bladder surface with sterile saline solution and replace the plastic wrap at each diaper change.
   4. Surgical closure is needed within 48 hours.
   5. Administer antibiotic therapy.
      a. Therapy continued for at least 7 days postoperatively.
      b. Forty-two percent of wound dehiscence is due to infections.
   6. Renal ultrasonography or radionuclide scan is performed to determine presence or absence of upper tract abnormalities.
   7. Assess for possible hydronephrosis and infections postoperatively.
   8. Modified Bryant traction for immobilization is used for 4 weeks in patients who have undergone closure without osteotomy or with only a posterior osteotomy; light Buck traction, with legs supported on a pillow, is used if the approach was anterior.

9. Bladder is drained with a 10F suprapubic Malecot catheter for 4 weeks and with 3.5F ureteral stents for 2 weeks to prevent ureteral obstruction hypertension.
10. Antispasmodics, analgesics, and sedatives are administered to prevent bladder spasm and excessive crying, which may disrupt closure.
11. Ultrasonography is performed to assess the upper tracts, and catheterization is performed to obtain residual urine and urine culture specimens before discharge.
12. The condition of the upper tracts is followed up with ultrasonography every 6 months.
13. Subsequent repair of epispadias is performed at about 2 to 3 years of age as are bladder neck reconstruction, ureteral implantation, and bladder augmentation (Huether, 2006; Leung et al., 2005).

I. **Outcome.**
1. Results of functional closure of bladder exstrophy can be expected to be as high as a 75% to 85% continence rate with preservation of renal function.
2. May have lifelong problem with incontinence.
3. Precise prognosis is directly related to the presence of other deformities (Nelson, Dunn, et al., 2005).

UNDESCENDED TESTICLES (CRYPTORCHIDISM)

A. **Etiology.**
1. Endocrine dysfunction of the hypothalamic–pituitary–gonadal axis.
2. Abnormal epididymal development, with failure to induce testicular descent.
3. Anatomic abnormality preventing descent.
B. **Incidence** (Palmert and Dahms, 2006).
1. Reported as 3.7% of term male infants.
2. Increased incidence of 21% in preterm infants, approaching 100% in the very preterm.
3. At 1 year of age: 0.8%.
C. **Disease states.**
1. Specific types of cryptorchidism.
   a. Abdominal: testes located inside the internal inguinal ring.
   b. Canalicular: testes located between the internal and external inguinal rings.
   c. Ectopic: testes located away from the normal pathway of descent, between the abdominal cavity and the base of the scrotum.
2. Genetic syndromes.
   a. Klinefelter syndrome.
   b. Noonan syndrome.
   c. Prader–Willi syndrome.
3. Vasal and/or epididymal abnormalities.
4. Prune-belly syndrome.
D. **Clinical presentation: absence of the testes in the scrotum.**
E. **Clinical assessment:** Associated abnormalities may be present. There is an increased incidence of CNS abnormalities and hypospadias.
F. **Physical examination** (Pulsifer, 2005).
1. Palpation of scrotum for presence of testes or associated hernia.
2. Palpation of inguinal area for presence of hernia.
G. **Diagnostic studies.**
1. Ultrasonography: identification of intraabdominal testes.
2. Magnetic resonance imaging: identification of intraabdominal testes.
3. Laparoscopy: identification of intraabdominal testes.
4. Complete endocrine and electrolyte evaluation and chromosome analysis to rule out hypothalamic-pituitary insufficiency, female adrenogenital syndrome, and anorchism in phenotypic male infants with bilateral impalpable gonads (Palmert and Dahms, 2006).

H. Differential diagnosis.
   1. Specific type of cryptorchidism.
      a. Abdominal.
      b. Canalicular.
      c. Ectopic or maldescended.
   2. Anorchia: absence of testes.
I. Complications (Palmert and Dahms, 2006).
   1. Testicular torsion.
   2. Hernia.
   3. Infertility.
   4. Postoperative complications.
      a. Obstruction of the testicular vascular supply by direct injury.
      b. Compression from twisting of the vascular supply resulting from direct injury.
      c. Tight closure of the abdominal musculature.
      d. Narrowing of vessels by placing them under significant tension as the testis is brought into the scrotum.
      e. Transient testicular swelling from partial obstruction of lymphatic and venous drainage.
   5. Increased risk of testicular cancer.
J. Patient care management.
   1. Orchiopexy.
      a. Surgical procedure that alters the course of the spermatic artery and creates a direct line from the renal pedicle to the scrotum.
      b. Surgical repair is to be performed at 1 to 2 years of age.
   2. Hormonal treatment (Palmert and Dahms, 2006).
      a. Consists of administration of human chorionic gonadotropin (hCG), and/or gonadotropin-releasing hormone (GnRH), also referred to as luteinizing hormone–releasing hormone (LH-RH).
      b. May be attempted in an effort to avoid orchiopexy.
      c. May make technical aspects of orchiopexy easier.
   3. Reevaluation of testicular location, size, and viability after 1 year.
K. Outcome (Palmert and Dahms, 2006; Pohl et al., 2007).
   1. Success rates for orchiopexy by anatomic testicular position have been reported as 74% for abdominal, 87% for canalicular, and 92% for those located beyond the external ring.
   2. Fertility may be impaired.

CIRCUMCISION

A. Indications. There are no absolute medical indications for routine circumcision in the newborn period. The advantages, disadvantages, and risks of the procedure have been reviewed in the literature (American Academy of Pediatrics [AAP] Committee Task Force on Circumcision, 1999; Singh-Grewal et al., 2005).
B. Incidence. Percentage of male infants circumcised varies by geographic location, by religious affiliation, and to some extent by socioeconomic classification (Nelson, Dunn, Wan, & Wei, 2005). The National Center for Health Statistics (2008) estimated that 65.3% of male infants were circumcised in the United States in 1999.
C. Physical examination.
   1. Observation. Assess for the presence of abnormalities of the glans, foreskin, or urethral meatus.
   2. Gestational age assessment. Circumcision should not be performed on premature infants until they meet discharge criteria.
D. Complications.
   1. Bleeding.
   2. Infection.
   3. Injury to the glans.

4. Meatal stenosis.
5. Urethrocutaneous fistula.
6. Formation of skin bridge.
7. Adhesions.
8. Phimosis.
9. Concealed penis.
10. Inflammation of the meatus or meatal ulcer.
11. Chordee.
12. Inclusion cysts.
13. Lymphedema.
14. Necrosis.

E. **Patient care management.**
1. Circumcision should not be performed on infants with bleeding disorders or on those with abnormalities of the glans, foreskin, or urethral meatus.
2. Vitamin K should be administered within 1 hour after birth.
3. Eutectic mixture of local anesthetic cream, dorsal penile nerve block, and a subcutaneous ring block have been shown to alleviate the discomfort associated with the procedure. The subcutaneous ring block may provide the most effective analgesia (Gardner et al., 2006; Razmus et al., 2004; Stork, 2006).
4. Risks and benefits should be discussed with parents and informed consent obtained.
5. Postoperative care.
   a. Check the site for bleeding, redness, or pus.
   b. Check for voiding.
   c. Avoid supine position.
   d. Change diapers frequently.
   e. Apply petroleum gauze to the site for 24 hours.
   f. Apply petroleum to site until healed.
6. Teach parent how to care for circumcision before discharge.

F. **Outcome.** The precise incidence of complications after circumcision is unknown; however, data indicate that the rate is low and that the most common complications are local infection and bleeding (AAP Committee Task Force on Circumcision, 1999; Singh-Grewal et al., 2005).

REFERENCES

American Academy of Pediatrics Committee Task Force on Circumcision: Circumcision policy statement. *Pediatrics*, 103(3):686-693, 1999.

Amukele, S., Stock, J., and Hanna, M.: Management and outcome of complex hypospadias repairs. *Journal of Urology*, 174(4):1540-1543, 2005.

Ball, J. and Bindler, R.: Alterations in genitourinary function. In J. Ball and R. Bindler (Eds.): *Pediatric nursing: Caring for children* (4th ed.). Upper Saddle River, NJ, 2008, pp. 972-1028.

Chua, A. and Sarwal, M.: Acute renal failure and management in the neonate. *NeoReviews*, 6:e369-376, 2005.

Danish, R.K. and Dahms, W.T.: Abnormalities of sexual differentiation. In A.A. Fanaroff and R.J. Martin (Eds.): *Neonatal-perinatal medicine: Diseases of the fetus and infant* (7th ed., vol. 2). St. Louis, 2002, Mosby, pp. 1416-1467.

Dulczak, S. and Kirk, J.: Overview of the evaluation, diagnosis, and management of urinary tract infections in infants and children. *Urologic Nursing*, 25(3):185-191, 2005.

Edwards, M.S.: Postnatal bacterial infections. In R.J. Martin, A.A. Fanaroff, and M.C. Walsh (Eds.): *Fanaroff and Martin's neonatal-perinatal medicine: Diseases of the fetus and infant* (8th ed., vol. 2). Philadelphia, 2006, Mosby, pp. 791-829.

Ettinger, L. and Flynn, J.: Hypertension in the neonate. *NeoReviews*, 3(8):e151-154, 2002.

Farnham, S., Adams, M., Brock, J., and Pope, J.: Pediatric urological causes of hypertension. *Journal of Urology*, 173:697-704, 2005.

Gardner, S., Enzman Hagedorn, M., and Dickey, L.: Pain and pain relief. In G.B. Merenstein and S.L. Gardner (Eds.): *Handbook of neonatal intensive care* (6th ed.). St. Louis, 2006, Mosby, pp. 223-272.

Huether, S.E.: Alterations of renal and urinary tract function in children. In K.L. McCance and S.E. Huether (Eds.): *Pathophysiology: The biologic basis for disease in adults and children* (5th ed.). St. Louis, 2006, Mosby, pp. 1337-1352.

Kanellopoulos, T., Salakos, C., Spilipoulou I., et al.: First urinary tract infection in neonates, infants and young children: A comparative study. *Pediatric Nephrology*, 21:1131-1137, 2006.

Lam, J., Breda, A., and Schulman, P.: Ureteropelvic junction obstruction. *Journal of Urology*, 177:1652-1658, 2007.

Leung, A., Robson, W., and Wong, A.: What's your diagnosis? Bladder exstrophy. *Consultant for Pediatricians*, 4:77-80, 2005.

Lugo, B., McNulty, J., and Emil, S.: Bladder prolapse through a patent urachus: Fetal and neonatal features. *Journal of Pediatric Surgery*, 41:E5-E7, 2006.

Marks, S., Masscotte, P., Steele, B., et al.: Neonatal renal venous thrombosis: Clinical outcomes and prevalence of prothrombotic disorders. *Journal of Pediatrics*, 146:811-816, 2005.

National Center for Health Statistics: *Trends in circumcisions among newborns*. Retrieved January 10, 2008, from http://www.cdc.gov/nchs/products/pubs/pubd/hestats/circumcisions/circumcisions.htm

Nelson, C., Dunn, R., Wan, J., and Wei, J.: The increasing incidence of newborn circumcision: Data from the nationwide inpatient sample. *Journal of Urology*, 173(3):978-981, 2005.

Nelson, C., Dunn, R., and Wei, J.: Contemporary epidemiology of bladder exstrophy in the United States. *Journal of Urology*, 173(5):1728-1731, 2005.

Nelson, C., Park, J., Dunn, R., and Wei, J.: Contemporary trends in surgical correction of pediatric ureteropelvic junction obstruction: Data from the nationwide inpatient sample. *Journal of Urology*, 173(1):232-236, 2005.

Palmert, M.R. and Dahms, W.T.: Abnormalities of sexual differentiation. In R.J. Martin, A.A. Fanaroff, and M.C. Walsh (Eds.): *Fanaroff and Martin's neonatal-perinatal medicine: Diseases of the fetus and infant* (8th ed., vol. 2). Philadelphia, 2006, Mosby, pp. 1550-1596.

Pejovic, B., Peco-Antic, A., and Marinkovic-Eric, J.: Blood pressure in non-critically ill preterm and full-term neonates. *Pediatric Nephrology*, 22:249-257, 2007.

Pohl, H., Joyce, G., Wise, M., and Cilento, B.: Cryptorchidism and hypospadias. *Journal of Urology*, 177(5):1646-1651, 2007.

Porth, C.: *Essentials of pathophysiology: Concepts of altered health states* (2nd ed.). Philadelphia, 2007, Lippincott Williams & Wilkins.

Pulsifer, A.: Pediatric genitourinary examination: A clinician's reference. *Urologic Nursing*, 25(3):163-168, 2005.

Razmus, T., Dalton, M., and Wilson, D.: Pain management for newborn circumcision. *Pediatric Nursing*, 30(5):414-417, 427, 2004.

Singh-Grewal, D., Macdessi, J., and Craig, J.: Circumcision for the prevention of urinary tract infections in boys: A systematic review of randomised trials and observational studies. *Archives of Disease in Childhood*, 90:853-858, 2005.

Stork, J.: Anesthesia in the neonate. In R.J. Martin, A.A. Fanaroff, and M.C. Walsh (Eds.): *Fanaroff and Martin's neonatal-perinatal medicine: Diseases of the fetus and infant* (8th ed., vol. 1). Philadelphia, 2006, Mosby, pp. 627-643.

Swinford, R.D., Bonilla-Felix, M., Cerda, R.D., and Portman, R.J.: Neonatal nephrology. In G.B. Merenstein and S.L. Gardner (Eds.): *Handbook of neonatal intensive care* (6th ed.). St. Louis, 2006, Mosby, pp. 736-772.

Turial, S., Hueckstaedt, T., Schier, F., and Fahlenkamp, D.: Laparoscopic treatment of urachal remnants in children. *Journal of Urology*, 177:1864-1866, 2006.

Vogt, B.A., MacRae Dell, K., and Davis, I.D.: The kidney and urinary tract. In R.J. Martin, A.A. Fanaroff, and M.C. Walsh (Eds.): Fanaroff and Martin's neonatal-perinatal medicine: Diseases of the fetus and infant (8th ed., vol. 2). Philadelphia, 2006, Mosby, pp. 1659-1685.

Young, T. and Mangum, B.: *Neofax 2007* (20th ed.). Montvale, NJ, 2007, Thomson Healthcare.

34 Neurologic Disorders

LYNN LYNAM and M. TERESE VERKLAN

OBJECTIVES

1. Identify the six primary stages of neurodevelopment and the congenital anomalies that result from defective development at each stage.
2. Define autoregulation.
3. Review a complete neurologic examination.
4. Examine birth injuries and patient care management.
5. Differentiate between the different types of intracranial hemorrhages and their origins, clinical presentation, and outcomes.
6. Recognize neonatal seizures, their distinguishing characteristics, and issues in patient care management.
7. Describe hypoxic–ischemic encephalopathy.
8. Describe the clinical implications of periventricular leukomalacia.
9. Distinguish pathophysiologic factors, clinical presentation, and patient care management of early- and late-onset meningitis.

■■ The human brain is an intricate, fragile organ requiring precise development from the moment of conception. Several crucial developmental landmarks pinpoint major events in the development of the human brain. If the process is interrupted, difficulties ranging from simple, easily treatable conditions to major neurologic malformations may occur. Neurologic problems account for a significant number of admissions into the neonatal intensive care unit each year. This chapter provides a comprehensive review of neurodevelopment, neurophysiology, and neuromalformations.

ANATOMY OF THE NEUROLOGIC SYSTEM*

A. **Embryologic development** (Table 34-1).
   1. Primary neurulation (dorsal induction).
      a. Occurs within the first month of life, ending between 24 and 28 days of gestation.
      b. Induction events of dorsal aspect of embryo.
      c. Neural tube is formed by the invagination and curling of the distal neural plate.
      d. Closure of the neural tube gives rise to the central nervous system, including the cranial nerves.
      e. This evolution results in the formation of the skull and vertebrae.
      f. Inaccuracies of primary neurulation result in craniorachischisis totalis, anencephaly, myeloschisis, encephalocele, myelomeningocele with Arnold–Chiari type II malformation.
   2. Prosencephalic development.
      a. Peak development is in the second and third months of gestation.
      b. Inductive interactive events that occur primarily at the rostral end on the ventral aspect of embryo.
      c. This influences the formation of the face, forebrain, corpus callosum and septum pellucidum, optic nerves/chiasm, the hypothalamic structures (thalamus and hypothalamus [diencephalon]), and the cerebral hemispheres (telencephalon).

*Moore and Persaud, 2007; Volpe, 2008.

■ TABLE 34-1
■ ■ **Major Events in Human Brain Development and Peak Times of Occurrence**

Major Developmental Event	Peak Time of Occurrence
Primary neurulation	3 to 4 weeks of gestation
Prosencephalic development	2 to 3 months of gestation
Neuronal proliferation	3 to 4 months of gestation
Neuronal migration	3 to 5 months of gestation
Organization	5 months of gestation to years postnatal
Myelination	Birth to years postnatal

From Volpe, J.J.: *Neurology of the newborn* (5th ed.). Philadelphia, 2008, Saunders.

    d. Absence of olfactory bulbs and tracts is not uncommon.
    e. Disturbance in prosencephalic development causes facial and forebrain alterations.
       (1) Holoprosencephaly (abnormal formation of telencephalon and diencephalon).
       (2) Midline and midfacial defects.
          (a) Hypotelorism (less common: hypertelorism).
          (b) Cyclopia.
          (c) Cleft lip with or without cleft palate.
       (3) Agenesis of corpus callosum, corpus pellucidum.
    f. Most common karyotype is normal (chromosomal disorder is possible).
  3. Neuronal proliferation.
    a. Occurs initially at 2 months, with peak between 3 and 4 months of gestation.
    b. Toxins and inherited diseases can significantly alter the number of neurons.
    c. Chemical and environmental substances can reduce the number of neurons, causing microcephaly vera.
    d. Insufficient neurons in absence of apoptotic events is primary micrencephaly; excess neurons can produce macrencephaly.
    e. Disorders of proliferation of small veins cause Sturge–Weber syndrome (6% unilateral, 24% bilateral facial lesions).
  4. Neuronal migration.
    a. Can occur as early as 2 months; peaks between 3 and 5 months.
    b. By 6 months of gestation, the neurons have migrated to their final, permanent place in the cortex.
    c. Neurons follow glial paths outward.
    d. Cells migrate and differentiate into six cortical layers.
    e. Migration is critical for development of the cerebral cortex and the deeper nuclear structures.
       (1) Basal ganglia.
       (2) Hypothalamus.
       (3) Thalamus.
       (4) Brainstem.
       (5) Cerebellum.
       (6) Spinal cord.
    f. Dysfunction at this stage results in cortical malformation with abnormalities of neurologic function.
    g. Seizures may be the first clinical manifestation in the early postnatal period.
    h. Defects associated with abnormal migration range in severity and may be associated with other neurologic development.
    i. Abnormal development of gyrus denotes a neuronal migration disorder.
    j. Disorders include lissencephaly ("smooth brain"), pachygyria, agenesis of the corpus callosum, and schizencephaly (clefts found in the cerebral wall).

5. Neuronal organization.
   a. Peaks at 5 months of gestation to several years after birth.
   b. Provides the basis for brain function and its complex circuitry.
   c. Includes cell differentiation, cell death, synaptic development, neurotransmitters, and myelination.
   d. Achieves stabilization of cell connections.
   e. Disorders due to organizational deficits and detrimental retardation (as with Down syndrome, fragile-X syndrome, and mild Duchenne muscular dystrophy).
6. Myelination.
   a. Begins in the second trimester and continues into adult life.
   b. Involves myelin deposition around axons.
   c. Myelin, a fatty covering, insulates the circuitry; prevents leakage of current and enables rapid, efficient transmission of nerve impulses.
   d. Enhances intercellular communication.
   e. Deficiencies occur in some acquired and inherited diseases.

B. **Brain anatomy** (Fig. 34-1) (Moore and Persaud, 2007; Volpe, 2008).
   1. Cerebellum.
      a. Promotes integrative muscle function.
      b. Maintains balance.
      c. Enables smooth, purposeful movements.
   2. Cerebrum: main components of cerebral hemisphere.
      a. Contains four lobes: frontal, parietal, occipital, and temporal.
         (1) Frontal lobes make up command center; concerned with decision making and other "executive" tasks.
         (2) Parietal lobes are responsible for hearing, understanding speech, and forming an integrated sense of self.
         (3) Occipital lobes process vision.
         (4) Temporal lobes are centers for smell with associative areas for memory and learning.

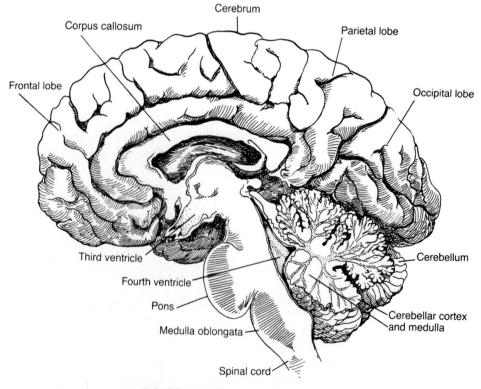

FIGURE 34-1 ■ Anatomy of the brain.

      b. Corpus callosum: fiber bundles connecting the cerebral hemispheres.

      c. Cerebral cortex.

         (1) Encompasses the mind, the intellect.

         (2) Gray matter.

      d. Lateral ventricles.

      e. Third ventricle: fluid-filled space.

      f. Thalamus: integrates sensory input.

      g. Hypothalamus: regulates body temperature.

  3. Brainstem.

      a. Relays input and output signals between higher brain centers and the spinal cord.

      b. Three main components.

         (1) Medulla oblongata.

            (a) Gives origin to cranial nerves VIII, IX, X, XI, and XII.

            (b) Controls areas of the abdomen, thorax, throat, and mouth.

         (2) Pons: carries information between the brainstem and the cerebellum.

         (3) Midbrain: involved in eye movements.

PHYSIOLOGY OF THE NEUROLOGIC SYSTEM*

A. Glucose metabolism.

  1. Cerebral metabolism is influenced by the availability of glucose and oxygen.

  2. Glucose is transported from blood to brain by a glucose transporter found in capillaries.

  3. Serum glucose provides the brain with a glucose pool.

  4. The neonatal brain is glucose dependent. The central nervous system (CNS) is quickly and significantly affected by hypoglycemia.

  5. Glycogen stores are minimal or nonexistent in the premature baby.

  6. The brain depends on adequate circulation to supply both oxygen and glucose to create enough energy for normal growth and metabolism.

  7. Anaerobic metabolism causes lactic acid buildup.

  8. Anaerobic metabolism produces significantly smaller amounts of energy.

  9. Newborn blood glucose levels less than 30 mg/dl are associated with significant increases in cerebral blood flow.

  10. Defining the lower limit of the neonatal blood glucose level is difficult because the infant's ability to present overt symptoms of hypoglycemia is not developed.

B. Cerebral blood flow.

  1. Cerebral blood flow is affected by pH (controlled by hydrogen ions and carbon dioxide levels), potassium, hypoxemia, osmolarity, and calcium ion concentrations.

      a. The brain increases cerebral blood flow to spare itself inadequacies.

      b. As pH decreases, cerebral blood flow increases.

      c. As potassium levels increase, cerebral blood flow increases.

      d. Hypoxemia causes an increase in cerebral blood flow to provide adequate oxygenated blood to the brain.

      e. Increased osmolarity causes increased cerebral blood flow.

      f. An increase in calcium ions causes a decrease in cerebral blood flow.

      g. Cerebral blood flow increases when blood glucose levels fall to less than 30 mg/dl; the hypoglycemic brain recruits previously unperfused capillaries to maintain glucose levels. Degree and duration of hypoglycemia are significant.

      h. Studies have shown that neonatal neurologic signs can be minimal or absent with subsequent abnormal cognitive development.

  2. Autoregulation.

      a. Maintains steady-state cerebral blood flow over a broad range of perfusion pressures.

---

*McLean et al., 2008; Volpe, 2008; Yager and Poskitt, 2008.

    b. Important vasoactive factors in the brain: hydrogen ions, potassium ions, adenosine, prostaglandins, osmolarity, calcium.

    c. Cerebral blood flow increases with advancing gestational age and concomitant cerebral metabolic demands.

    d. Normal arterial blood pressure in the preterm neonate is thought to be near or at the lower autoregulatory limit. This suggests an increased vulnerability to ischemic brain injury with modest hypotension, especially with decreasing gestational age.

    e. Cerebral vasculature vasodilates maximally in response to hypoxemia, hypercapnia, and acidosis.

        (1) Hypotension leads to ischemia.

            (a) Ischemia damages blood vessels and surrounding elements supporting the blood vessels.

            (b) Blood flow to cerebral white matter is restored only after reperfusion of other brain regions.

            (c) Once adequate blood supply resumes, hemorrhage can occur into ischemic areas.

        (2) Hypertension leads to hemorrhage.

NEUROLOGIC ASSESSMENT*

A. History.

B. Observation.

    1. Determine behavioral state.

    2. Note posture.

        a. Gestational age determines posture.

            (1) Premature infants: open, extended position reflecting diminished tone.

            (2) Term infants: flexed position reflecting adequate tone.

        b. Sequelae of intrauterine position may be evident.

        c. Abnormal findings are as follows:

            (1) Hyperextension.

            (2) Asymmetry.

            (3) Flaccidity.

    3. Note movements.

        a. Symmetric or asymmetric body movements.

        b. Note movement quality (jitteriness, seizures, tremors, and clonus).

        c. Quantity (absent or pronounced).

    4. Note respiratory activity.

        a. Signs of distress.

        b. Hypoventilation (apnea).

        c. Quality of cry.

            (1) High pitched (consider meningitis, drug withdrawal, neurologic abnormalities).

            (2) Stridor (consider vocal cord damage or paralysis).

    5. Observe skin.

        a. Lesions (note number, size, shape, color, and texture).

            (1) Café-au-lait spots (six or more lesions of ≥1.5 cm; may indicate neurofibromatosis).

            (2) Port-wine facial hemangioma (consider Sturge–Weber syndrome).

            (3) Areas of depigmentation.

        b. Abrasions, lacerations, bruises, and forceps marks (consider intracranial bleeding, injury).

C. Physical examination (Fenichel, 2007; Volpe, 2008).

    1. Check the skull size, shape, symmetry, hair whorls, fontanelles, and sutures.

    2. Measure frontal-occipital circumference (FOC).

        a. Document less than 10th percentile (symmetric vs. asymmetric compared with total body growth; may indicate microcephaly).

---

*Rennie, 2005a; Volpe, 2008.

      b. Document greater than 90th percentile (symmetric vs. asymmetric compared with total body growth; may indicate macrocephaly).

  3. Examine the face for abnormalities in structure.

      a. Placement of ears.

      b. Neck skinfolds.

  4. Spine (intact, openings, masses).

  5. Cranial nerve function.

      a. Refer to Table 34-2.

      b. May be difficult to assess in the preterm newborn.

      c. Blink reflex requires intact cranial nerves III and VII.

      d. Corneal reflex requires intact cranial nerves V and VII.

        (1) Generally elicited only if one suspects brain damage.

        (2) Consider testing integrity of reflex in the presence of eye damage.

      e. Cranial nerves IX, X, and XII regulate the tongue, swallow, gag, and cry.

      f. Rooting reflex starts at 28 weeks, with a complete response established by 32 weeks.

      g. Sucking reflex present at 28 to 30 weeks but slow, weak, and unsustainable; mature and robust by 34 to 36 weeks of gestation.

      h. Rooting and sucking reflexes test partial function of cranial nerves V, VII, and XII.

      i. Swallowing tests IX and X.

  6. Muscle tone.

      a. Evaluate head lag, ventral suspension, clonus, and recoil from extension.

      b. Check symmetry; briskness versus flaccidity.

  7. Reflexes.

      a. Check primitive reflexes (automatisms).

        (1) Blinking: An infant will close his or her eyes in response to bright lights.

        (2) Palmar and plantar grasp (bilaterally): An infant's fingers or toes will curl around a finger placed in the area.

        (3) Babinski: As the infant's foot is stroked, the toes will extend upward and fan outward.

        (4) Moro: A quick change in the infant's position will cause the infant to throw back his or her head, extend his or her arms outward, and open the hands.

        (5) Startle: A loud noise will cause the infant to extend and flex the arms, while the hands remain in a fist.

      b. Evaluate symmetry and strength of response of all primitive reflexes.

      c. Consider clavicular or humeral fractures or brachial plexus injury in the presence of an abnormal Moro reflex.

      d. Grasp varies with gestational age; if grasp is absent, consider nerve damage.

NEUROLOGIC DISORDERS

A. Anencephaly (Volpe, 2008).

  1. Risk factors: thought to be due to a combination of genetic and environmental influences.

      a. Risk appears to increase with low socioeconomic status, history of affected siblings.

      b. More common in whites.

      c. Females affected more often than males.

  2. Pathophysiology.

      a. Failure of anterior neural tube closure.

      b. Malfunction of the first stage of neurologic development, primary neurulation.

      c. Most commonly involves the forebrain and variable amounts of upper brainstem.

      d. Partial absence of skull bones, with absent cerebrum and with or without missing cerebellum, brainstem, and spinal cord.

  3. Incidence: Approximately 0.2 per 1000 live births.

  4. Clinical presentation.

      a. Exposed neural tissue with little definable structure.

■ TABLE 34-2
■ ■ **Cranial Nerves**

Number	Name	Type of Nerve	Function	Bedside Testing Mechanism	Expected Results and Comments
I	Olfactory	Sensory	Smell	Soak cotton pledget in strong odor and place under nares	Startle
II	Optic	Sensory	Conveys visual information from retina to brain	Check PERL; funduscopic examination	PERL intact; presence of red reflex
III	Oculomotor	Motor	Motor fibers to eyelid (lid elevation), some eye muscles, pupil (constriction and accommodation), and light reflex	Check EOM, PERL	PERL intact; EOM full and conjugate
IV	Trochlear	Motor	Movement of superior oblique muscles of eye, uvula movement	Check EOM	EOM full and conjugate
V	Trigeminal	Mixed	Sensation of face, scalp, and cornea; motor of jaw (mastication)	Touch cheek	Turns cheek toward stimulus
VI	Abducens	Motor	Lateral gaze; abducts eyeball	Rotate infant	Movement of eyes in direction of travel
VII	Facial	Mixed	Facial muscle movement, lid closure, taste	Elicit cry and observe facial movement	Symmetrical facial movements
VIII	Auditory	Sensory	Hearing	Talk softly to baby or clap loudly near baby's ear	Quiets to voice; blinks to clap
IX	Glossopharyngeal	Mixed	Taste, swallow, gag	Elicit gag response	Strong gag response
X	Vagus	Mixed	Most extensive innervation of any cranial nerve; motor, sensory, and autonomic innervation of neck, thorax, abdomen; swallow and gag	Elicit cry	Strong, lusty cry
XI	Accessory	Motor	Movement of head and neck	Turn supine infant's head to side	Attempts to bring head to midline; full range of shoulder and neck
XII	Hypoglossal	Motor	Tongue movement and symmetry	Insert gloved finger into baby's mouth while sucking	Suck should be strong and steady without fasciculations, tongue symmetry

EOM, Extraocular movements; *PERL,* pupils equal and reactive to light.
Adapted from Scanlon, J.W., Nelson, T., Grylack, L.J., and Smith, Y.F.: *A system of newborn physical examination.* Baltimore, 1979, University Park Press; in Whaley, L.F. and Wong, D.L.: *Nursing care of infants and children.* St. Louis, 1999, Mosby.
Adapted from Fletcher, M.A.: *Physical diagnosis in neonatology.* Philadelphia, 1997, Lippincott Williams & Wilkins.
Adapted from http://library.med.utah.edu/pedineurologicexam/html/newborn_n.html#02
Adapted from http://www.fpnotebook.com/Nicu/Exam/NwbrnNrlgcExm.htm

      b. The anomalous skull has a froglike appearance from an en face view.

      c. Amniotic fluid reveals high levels of alpha-fetoprotein late in the first trimester.

  5. Diagnostic evaluation.

      a. Identified by prenatal cranial ultrasonography in the second trimester.

      b. Apparent upon visual inspection after birth.

  6. Patient care management.

      a. Provide comfort measures for the infant.

      b. Obtain genetic consultation; encourage parents to seek genetic counseling.

      c. Support the grieving process.

      d. Encourage the family to see their baby because the family's imaginary impressions may be worse than reality.

  7. Outcome.

      a. Stillbirth occurs in 75%.

      b. Survival is unlikely beyond the neonatal period.

B. Microcephaly (Gleeson et al., 2006; Volpe, 2008).

  1. Definition.

      a. Frontal-occipital circumference ≥2 standard deviations below the mean for age and gender.

      b. Small brain implies neurologic impairment.

  2. Risk factors.

      a. Maternal:

          (1) Viral infections under the TORCH spectrum (*T*oxoplasmosis, *O*ther [syphilis], *R*ubella, *C*ytomegalovirus, or *H*erpes).

          (2) Exposure to radiation.

          (3) Metabolic conditions such as diabetes or phenylketonuria.

          (4) Use of prescription and/or street drugs, especially in the first trimester.

          (5) Genetic foundation may be autosomal recessive, autosomal dominant, or X-linked.

          (6) Malnutrition is the most common etiology worldwide.

      b. Fetal:

          (1) Prenatal/perinatal insult: inflammation; hypoxia; birth trauma.

      c. Neonatal:

          (1) Very low birth weight infant.

          (2) Hypoxic–ischemic encephalopathy.

          (3) Nutrition: most common worldwide cause.

  3. Pathophysiology.

      a. Neuronal proliferation defect.

      b. Occurs between 3 and 4 months of gestational age.

      c. Destructive microcephaly occurs when the normal brain suffers prenatal/perinatal insult.

  4. Clinical presentation.

      a. Small head, backward sloping of the forehead, small cranial volume.

      b. Neurologic deficits rarely evident at birth.

  5. Diagnostic evaluation.

      a. Perform a complete physical examination including neurologic assessment.

      b. Elicit a thorough maternal history.

      c. Use tests to confirm or rule out etiologic factors aligned with maternal history.

      d. Computed tomography (CT) or magnetic resonance imaging (MRI) is performed.

  6. Patient care management.

      a. Record accurate measurement of FOC, length, and weight weekly.

      b. Note percentiles and alert physician to abnormalities.

      c. Document clearly any deviations from normal.

      d. Obtain tests as ordered; note dates to follow up results.

      e. Ensure that the family is informed.

      f. Obtain consultations as needed: genetics, infectious diseases.

7. Outcome.
   a. Dependent on severity.
   b. May be associated with developmental delays.
C. **Hydrocephalus** (Bondurant and Jimenez, 1995; Volpe, 2008).
   1. Definition: excess cerebrospinal fluid (CSF) in the ventricles of the brain due to a decrease in reabsorption or overproduction.
      a. CSF is in balance between formation and absorption.
      b. CSF is produced at a rate of 0.35 ml/minute from brain parenchyma, cerebral ventricles, areas along the spinal cord, and the choroid plexus (70% is from the choroid plexus).
   2. Pathophysiology.
      a. Excessive CSF production (rare).
      b. Inadequate CSF absorption secondary to abnormal circulation.
      c. Excess ventricular CSF secondary to aqueductal outflow obstruction causes obstructive, noncommunicating hydrocephalus (refer to Fig. 34-2 for a simplified diagram of the brain).
         (1) The condition is most common in newborn infants.
         (2) Obstructive hydrocephalus may progress rapidly.
      d. Excess ventricular CSF with flow between the lateral ventricles and the subarachnoid space results in communicating, nonobstructive hydrocephalus.
   3. Congenital hydrocephalus.
      a. Risk factors.
         (1) Aqueductal stenosis.
         (2) Dandy–Walker cyst (cystic transformation of fourth ventricle).
         (3) Myelomeningocele with Arnold–Chiari malformation (herniation of the hindbrain, usually causing obstructive hydrocephalus).
         (4) Congenital masses and tumors.
         (5) Congenital infection (toxoplasmosis, cytomegalovirus [CMV] infection).
      b. Associated etiologies and/or congenital defects.
         (1) Spina bifida.
         (2) Encephalocele.
         (3) Holoprosencephaly.
      c. Clinical presentation.
         (1) Large head.
         (2) Widened sutures.
         (3) Full (bulging) and tense fontanelles.

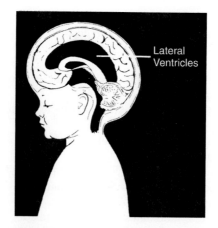

FIGURE 34-2 ■ Hydrocephalus. (From Ross Laboratories: *New perspectives on intraventricular hemorrhage.* Columbus, Ohio, 1988, Ross Laboratories.)

(4) Increasing FOC.

(5) Setting-sun eyes (may signify brain tissue damage).

(6) Vomiting, lethargy, irritability.

(7) Visible scalp veins.

d. Diagnostic evaluation.

(1) Serial intracranial ultrasonography.

(2) Neuroimaging techniques: CT, MRI, and cranial ultrasonography.

e. Patient care management.

(1) Intrauterine diagnosis affords the family more options and allows time for preparation and anticipation.

(2) Perform a thorough physical examination, assessing for further anomalies.

(3) Obtain neurosurgery and genetics consultation.

(4) Confirm diagnosis and cause.

(5) Consider the possible need for reservoir placement versus ventriculoperitoneal (VP) shunt placement.

(6) Support the infant by decreasing noxious stimuli (dim lights, minimal handling).

(7) Position the head carefully.

(8) Water-pillow beds diminish skin breakdown and may provide a source of comfort.

(9) Provide normal infant care as much as possible.

(10) Involve parents in infant's care as soon as family is ready.

(11) Position the infant prone for oral feedings.

(12) Allow parents to view an infant with a VP shunt or review pictured handouts.

(13) Review VP shunt with parents preoperatively and postoperatively.

(14) Prevent skin breakdown by not allowing the infant to put his or her head on the shunt side postoperatively.

(15) Relieve the infant's probable stiff neck by holding the child's neck on the shunt side during feedings.

(16) Review signs of infection or blocked shunt with the family.

(a) Irritability.

(b) Vomiting.

(c) Increasing head size.

(d) Lethargy.

(e) Changes in feeding patterns.

(f) Bulging fontanelle.

(17) If incision site reddens, position infant on opposite side to relieve pressure from this area.

4. Posthemorrhagic hydrocephalus (PHH) (Volpe, 2008).

a. Etiology.

(1) Progressive dilation of the ventricles after intraventricular hemorrhage (IVH) caused by injury to the periventricular white matter.

(2) Two types: acute and chronic.

(a) Acute.

(i) Rapidly appears—within days of the initial hemorrhage.

(ii) Probably occurs secondary to malabsorption of CSF secondary to a blood clot.

(b) Subacute, chronic.

(i) Inhibition of CSF flow.

(ii) Blood from IVH.

b. Incidence.

(1) Approximately 45% of infants with IVH have no evidence of hydrocephalus (Volpe, 2008).

(2) Acute ventricular dilation develops in approximately 50% of surviving infants with hemorrhage; in the majority, it resolves spontaneously or remains static (Papile, 2006).

    c. Clinical presentation.
      (1) Insidious following mild ventricular dilatation.
      (2) May be profound following severe ventricular dilatation.
        (a) Rapid increase in head size (begins days to weeks after ventricular dilatation present).
        (b) Episodic apnea and bradycardia.
        (c) Lethargy.
        (d) Increased intracranial pressure.
        (e) Tense, bulging anterior fontanelle.
        (f) Cranial sutures separating.
        (g) Ocular movement abnormalities.
    d. Diagnostic evaluation.
      (1) Graph of weekly FOC measurements.
      (2) CT scan.
      (3) Cranial ultrasonography.
      (4) MRI.
    e. Patient care management (Madsen and Frim, 2005).
      (1) Obtain daily FOC measurements.
      (2) Serial cranial ultrasonography.
      (3) Neurosurgical consultation.
      (4) Interventions to maintain lumbar or ventricular pressure at approximately 5 cm H_2O while evaluating for shunt placement.
        (a) Serial lumbar punctures or direct ventricular access may be helpful.
        (b) Administer medications that diminish CSF production rates:
          (i) Furosemide (Lasix): 1 mg/kg/day.
          (ii) Acetazolamide (Diamox): up to 100 mg/kg/day.
      (5) Consideration given to placing a reservoir or ventriculoperitoneal (VP) shunt.
      (6) Observe the infant for signs of increasing intracranial hemorrhage and hydrocephalus.
      (7) Support the family: neonate is very susceptible to shunt infections and shunt malfunction.
    f. Outcome (Volpe, 2008).
      (1) Poor outcomes are likely when cerebral decompression does not occur after VP shunt placement.
      (2) Initial IVH severity is the major determining factor in PHH development.
      (3) In slightly more than 50% of the cases, severe hemorrhage results in progressive ventricular dilatation.
      (4) Without therapy, a considerable number of infants exhibit halted progression, with or without resolution.
      (5) Deficits are motor and/or cognitive.
D. Myelomeningocele (Volpe, 2008).
  1. Definition.
    a. Neural tube defect.
      (1) Spina bifida occulta involves vertebral bone.
      (2) Defect is invisible (may be found if problems develop in later infancy or in childhood).
      (3) Meningocele is the protrusion of the meninges lying directly under the skin.
      (4) Myelocele is the exposure of the internal surface of the spinal cord or the nerve roots.
    b. In myelomeningocele, the spinal cord and meninges are exposed through the skin and onto the surface of the back.
    c. In myeloschisis, large areas of the spinal cord are without dermal or vertebral covering.
  2. Risk factors and/or associated disease states.
    a. Hydrocephalus.
      (1) With FOC at greater than the 90th percentile, 95% of infants will have hydrocephalus.

      (2) All newborn infants with myelomeningocele should be evaluated for hydrocephalus with CT scan and cranial ultrasonography shortly after birth.

  b. Arnold–Chiari malformation (Goddard-Finegold, 2004).

      (1) Hindbrain malformation with or without aqueductal atresia.

      (2) Almost always present with myelomeningocele.

      (3) Hydrocephalus present in 70% of babies with this malformation.

      (4) Common features.

        (a) Reflux and aspiration.

        (b) Laryngeal stridor.

        (c) Central hypoventilation, apnea.

3. Pathophysiology.

  a. Results from failure of posterior neural tube to close.

  b. 80% of cases occur in the lumbar region (the last region of the neural tube to close).

  c. Environmental factors, maternal nutrition, genetics, and teratogens, including maternal hyperthermia, are implicated.

4. Incidence: Approximately 0.2 to 0.4 per 1000 live births.

5. Clinical presentation.

  a. The majority of cases occur in the thoracolumbar, lumbar, and lumbosacral regions.

  b. A herniated sac, sealed or leaking, protrudes from the back.

  c. Defects include vascular networks surrounding abnormal neural tissue.

  d. Most lesions have incomplete skin coverage.

6. Diagnostic evaluation.

  a. Radiographic evaluation.

  b. Spinal ultrasound.

  c. MRI.

7. Patient care management.

  a. Prenatal diagnosis helpful.

  b. Examine lesion and measure size.

  c. Culture specimen from lesion if sac is open.

  d. Wrap lesion with sterile gauze moistened with warm sterile saline solution; place a sterile feeding tube within the gauze mesh for intermittent infusion of warm saline solution.

  e. Maintain the infant in a prone kneeling position, and protect the knees from skin breakdown.

  f. Place a drape over the buttocks below the lesion; utilize the drape's adhesive backing to secure the drape to the body.

  g. Obtain immediate consultation.

      (1) Neurosurgery.

      (2) Urology.

  h. Perform a thorough physical examination to assess the level of the injury, sensory involvement, and anal wink; include an FOC measurement.

  i. Encourage an open discussion among the family, the consultants, and the primary care team, providing the following:

      (1) Underlying physiology.

      (2) Physical examination findings.

      (3) Consultant reports.

      (4) Prognosis.

      (5) Complications.

      (6) Long-term care.

      (7) Options.

  j. Begin preparing the family for discharge.

      (1) Suggest that the parents contact a support group.

      (2) Involve the parents in their infant's care.

  k. Postoperatively, follow positioning instructions from the neurosurgeon.

  l. Spend time making eye contact with the infant.

  m. Observe for signs of hydrocephalus.

    n. Observe for development of Arnold–Chiari malformation that may present with feeding problems (reflux, aspiration), laryngeal stridor (due to vocal cord paralysis), or central hypoventilation or apnea.

    o. Maintain meticulous hygiene by clearing stool and urine quickly.

    p. Provide adequate nutrition.

    q. Orthopedic consultation is appropriate for maximal function of lower extremities.

    r. Physical therapy to encourage maximal range of motion.

8. Outcome (Volpe, 2008).

    a. Survival in 90%, with 80% or more having normal intelligence and 85% being ambulatory with or without special aids.

    b. Optimistic outlook with meningocele because of normal spinal cord.

    c. Varying degrees of paralysis: commonly in the lower extremities.

        (1) Lesions below the first sacral vertebra: infants can learn to walk unaided.

        (2) Lesions between the fourth and fifth lumbar vertebrae: infants may be able to walk with crutches or braces.

        (3) Lesions above the second lumbar vertebra: infants usually become wheelchair dependent.

    d. If surgery for defect closure is not performed, 80% die by 8 weeks and 100% are dead by 10 months.

E. Encephalocele (Volpe, 2008).

  1. Definition.

    a. Neural herniation.

    b. May or may not contain meninges or brain parenchyma.

  2. Risk factors.

    a. Environmental and genetic factors.

    b. May be multifactorial.

  3. Pathophysiology.

    a. Precise pathogenesis is unknown, but is thought of as a restricted disorder of neurulation that involves the closure of the anterior neural tube.

    b. About 70% to 80% of encephaloceles occur in the occipital region.

    c. About 10% to 20% of lesions in the occipital region contain no neural elements.

  4. Clinical presentation.

    a. Protruding midline skin-covered sac from the head or base of neck.

    b. Majority of sacs occur in the occipital region.

  5. Diagnostic evaluation.

    a. Second-trimester intrauterine ultrasonography.

    b. Cranial ultrasonography.

    c. CT scan.

    d. MRI.

  6. Patient care management.

    a. Examine the infant closely.

    b. Obtain neurosurgery consultation.

    c. Educate and support the family.

    d. Treat seizure activity.

  7. Outcome.

    a. Early surgery recommended.

    b. Prognosis more favorable if encephalocele is anterior.

    c. Possible motor deficits.

    d. Possible impaired intellectual function.

    e. 50% complicated by hydrocephalus.

F. Craniosynostosis (Sun and Persing, 2007).

  1. Definition.

    a. Premature closure of cranial sutures.

    b. Occurs along one or more suture lines (see Fig. 34-3 for names and placement of cranial sutures).

  2. Risk factors. Usually sporadic and without associated anomalies.

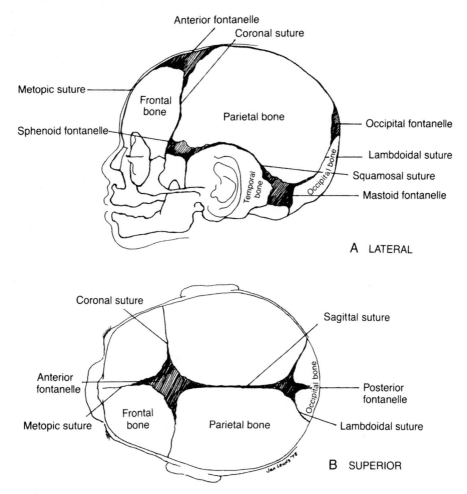

FIGURE 34-3 ■ **A** and **B**, Two views of neonatal skull, showing clinically important fontanelles and sutures. (From Scanlon, J.W., Nelson, T., Grylack, L., and Smith, Y.F.: *A system of newborn physical examinations.* Baltimore, 1979, University Park Press, p. 47.)

3. Pathophysiology.
   a. Cause unclear. May be a defect in the mesenchymal layer of the ossification center within the skull.
   b. Etiology includes developmental, mechanical, metabolic, and genetic factors that influence skull growth.
4. Incidence.
   a. Reported as 1 in 2000 to 2500 births.
   b. Sagittal craniosynostosis most common.
5. Clinical presentation.
   a. Asymptomatic.
   b. Cranial suture line reveals bony prominence; even and smooth bilaterally.
   c. Inability to move the suture.
   d. Abnormal cranial shape.
   e. Later signs:
      (1) Increased intracranial pressure.
      (2) Increased irritability.
      (3) Possible separation of other sutures.
6. Diagnostic evaluation.
   a. Skull x-ray examination.

    b. High resolution three-dimensional CT reconstruction scanning to determine the extent of premature bone fusion.

    c. Weekly graph of OFCs.

7. Patient care management.

    a. Thorough physical examination.

    b. Obtain neurosurgery consultation.

    c. Educate and support the family.

    d. Observe for signs of increased intracranial pressure.

        (1) Irritability.

        (2) Lethargy.

        (3) Vomiting.

        (4) Bulging fontanelle.

    e. Early surgical treatment is recommended.

8. Outcome.

    a. Surgically correctable.

    b. Good outcome; possible absence of sequelae.

    c. Cosmetically pleasing outcome.

    d. Multiple craniosynostosis associated with numerous syndromes.

G. Birth injuries.

1. Definition.

    a. Any injury that occurs during the entire phase of the birth process, comprising labor and delivery.

    b. Classification of the injury is anatomic or etiologic.

2. Risk factors.

    a. Abnormal labor time (long or short).

    b. Large size for gestational age.

    c. Cephalopelvic disproportion.

    d. Prematurity.

    e. Birth dystocia.

    f. Abnormal presentation (transverse, breech, face, and brow).

    g. Instrument-assisted extraction (vacuum or forceps).

3. Pathophysiology (see specific injury).

4. Incidence (Mangurten, 2006).

    a. Ranges from less than 2% of live births to about 6:1000 to 8:1000.

    b. Ranked eleventh in major causes of neonatal death (3.7 deaths per 100,000 live births).

    c. Varies with specific injury.

5. Specific injuries.

    a. Cephalohematoma.

        (1) Pathophysiology.

           (a) Subperiosteal hemorrhage.

           (b) Does not extend across the cranial suture lines.

           (c) Usually unilateral.

        (2) Incidence approximates 0.4% to 2.5% of deliveries (Mangurten, 2006).

        (3) Clinical presentation.

           (a) Enlarges during the first few days after birth.

           (b) Feels firm.

           (c) Does not transilluminate.

        (4) Diagnostic evaluation.

        (5) Patient care management.

           (a) Provide supportive care to the family and their baby.

           (b) Observe for hyperbilirubinemia.

           (c) If sudden enlargement occurs, question infection.

           (d) Educate the family.

           (e) Assess neurologic status.

(6) Outcome (Volpe, 2008).
    (a) Bony calcified ring may develop; usually disappears within 6 months.
    (b) Usually takes 2 weeks to 3 months for resolution.
    (c) Essentially all cases resolve.

b. Caput succedaneum.
  (1) Pathophysiology.
    (a) Hemorrhagic edema crossing cranial suture lines.
    (b) Commonly seen after vaginal delivery.
  (2) Clinical presentation.
    (a) Evident at birth.
    (b) Hemorrhagic scalp edema, causing discoloration at the site.
    (c) Does not grow in size after birth.
  (3) Diagnostic evaluation.
  (4) Patient care management.
    (a) No treatment is given.
    (b) Educate and counsel the family.
  (5) Outcome: resolution occurs during first few days of life.

c. Subgaleal hemorrhage (Levene, 2005).
  (1) Pathophysiology.
    (a) Hemorrhage beneath the scalp into the loose connective tissue below the aponeurotic membrane.
    (b) Possible entry of blood into the subcutaneous tissue of the neck.
    (c) Hematoma may cross suture lines in sufficient quantities to lead to exsanguination of the infant.
  (2) Incidence.
    (a) 1:1250 deliveries and 1:150 vacuum-assisted deliveries.
    (b) Occurs much less often than caput succedaneum.
    (c) Usually associated with a difficult delivery requiring midforceps or vacuum extraction (Mangurten, 2006).
  (3) Clinical presentation.
    (a) History of fetal distress noted in 50% of cases.
    (b) Often a fluctuant mass of the scalp.
    (c) May increase in size postnatally.
    (d) Hypotonia, pallor, lethargy, seizures.
    (e) Falling hematocrit levels.
  (4) Diagnostic evaluation.
    (a) Palpate: hemorrhage crosses suture lines, is firm but fluctuant to palpation.
    (b) Vital signs: monitor for symptoms of shock.
    (c) Serial hematocrit levels.
    (d) Monitor bilirubin levels during recovery.
  (5) Patient care management.
    (a) Rapid diagnosis and blood replacement is key to management.
      (i)   Observe for signs/symptoms of shock/hypovolemia.
      (ii) Monitor blood pressure, heart rate, and serial CBCs.
      (iii) Management for supporting organs, such as kidney, if shock occurs.
    (b) Infant may need blood transfusion on an emergent basis.
    (c) Ensure that infant receives vitamin K promptly.
    (d) Observe for hyperbilirubinemia.
  (6) Outcome: once the infant has survived the acute phase, recovery occurs in 2 to 3 weeks (Volpe, 2008).

d. Skull fractures.
  (1) Pathophysiology.
    (a) Linear fracture can occur.
    (b) Depressed fractures occur secondary to excessive force used with forceps and extreme molding.

(2) Incidence.
    (a) Unknown.
    (b) Linear fracture fairly common finding.
    (c) Depressed fracture much less common than linear.
(3) Clinical presentation.
    (a) Linear fracture: asymptomatic.
    (b) Depressed fracture.
        (i) Presents with depressed surface of skull; indented, without craniotabes.
        (ii) Does not cross the suture lines.
        (iii) Possible marked separation of adjacent sutures.
        (iv) Most often occurs in right parietal bone.
(4) Diagnostic evaluation.
    (a) X-ray examination.
    (b) CT scan.
(5) Patient care management.
    (a) Obtain neurosurgery consultation.
    (b) Assess closely for neurologic deficits.
    (c) If lesion is less than 2 cm and patient is without neurologic deficits, follow clinically; spontaneous resolution expected within a few weeks.
(6) Outcome.
    (a) Linear fractures usually heal completely within 3 months.
    (b) Depressed fracture outcome is dependent on degree of cerebral injury and success of therapy.

e. Brachial nerve plexus injuries (Smith and Ouvrier, 2006).
(1) Pathophysiology.
    (a) Excessive stretching of brachial plexus during delivery.
    (b) Erb palsy, involving cervical nerves V and VI. Denervation of the deltoid, supraspinatus, biceps, and brachioradialis leads to upper arm paralysis.
    (c) Klumpke paralysis, involving cervical nerve VI to thoracic nerve I. Denervation of the intrinsics of the hand, flexors of the wrist, fingers, and sympathetics (Horner syndrome) leads to lower arm paralysis.
    (d) Combination of Erb–Duchenne–Klumpke paralysis, involving the entire arm from cervical nerve V to thoracic nerve I (entire arm paralyzed). Paralysis of the diaphragm will occur if injury involves cervical nerve IV.
(2) Incidence: 0.38 per 1000 live births.
(3) Risk factors.
    (a) Multiparous mother.
    (b) Prolonged labor.
    (c) Large size for gestational age.
    (d) Shoulder dystocia.
(4) Clinical presentation.
    (a) Erb palsy.
        (i) Affected arm is abducted and internally rotated.
        (ii) The elbow is extended, with arm pronation and wrist flexion (waiter's tip position).
        (iii) Asymmetric Moro reflex (absent in the affected arm), with a normal grasp.
    (b) Klumpke paralysis.
        (i) Swelling in shoulder and supraclavicular fossa; clavicle may be fractured.
        (ii) Involves intrinsic muscles of the hand, with a claw-hand deformity.
        (iii) No grasp in the affected hand.
    (c) Erb–Duchenne–Klumpke paralysis.
        (i) A combination of the above.
        (ii) Occurs more often than isolated Klumpke paralysis.
        (iii) Entire affected arm is flaccid.
        (iv) Moro and grasp reflexes are absent.

(5) Diagnostic evaluation.
    (a) Obtain x-ray examination of affected arm and shoulder.
    (b) Obtain serial electromyographic studies.
    (c) Rule out fracture of the clavicle or humerus.
    (d) Rule out shoulder dislocation.
    (e) Rule out cerebral injury.
(6) Patient care management.
    (a) Obtain neurology consultation.
    (b) Obtain serial electromyographic examinations to note improvements.
    (c) Primary goal: avoid contractures of involved joints:
        (i)   Begin passive range of motion exercise, beginning after the swelling and inflammation subside.
        (ii) Exercise the arm with every diaper change.
        (iii) Request a physical therapy consultation (infant may be able to benefit from splints at some point).
        (iv) Educate the family about the importance of maintaining normal joint function.
            a. Reinnervated musculature needs supple joints.
            b. Will have wider choice of reconstructive procedures in the absence of contractures in the event there is no recovery.
(7) Outcome.
    (a) Generally spontaneous recovery occurs.
    (b) About 88% fully recover by 4 months, and 92% fully recover by 12 months (Volpe, 2008).
    (c) If no appreciable recovery is noted by 3 months, surgical exploration may be warranted (Volpe, 2008).

f. Phrenic nerve paralysis (Volpe, 2008).
(1) Pathophysiology.
    (a) Diaphragmatic paralysis involving overstretching of cervical nerves III, IV, and V.
    (b) Results from torn nerve sheaths with edema and hemorrhage.
    (c) 80% to 90% occur in association with brachial plexus injury, but it may also occur in isolation.
(2) Clinical presentation.
    (a) History of traumatic delivery, especially difficult breech delivery.
    (b) First hours after birth.
        (i)   Respiratory distress with cyanosis, tachypnea, hypoxemia, hypercapnia, and acidosis.
        (ii) Diagnosis may be missed as the elevated hemidiaphragm may not be present early in the course, especially with use of positive pressure ventilation.
    (c) Next several days.
        (i)   Improvement with oxygen and ventilatory support.
(3) Diagnostic evaluation.
    (a) Chest x-ray examination may not be useful, especially if positive pressure ventilation is in use.
    (b) Ultrasonographic or fluoroscopic examination will show elevated hemidiaphragm and the paradoxical movement of the affected side with breathing.
    (c) Serial ultrasonography to evaluate diaphragmatic function.
(4) Patient care management.
    (a) Administer oxygen and ventilatory support as needed.
    (b) Place the infant affected side down (splint the affected side).
    (c) Follow physical examination closely to note improvements.
    (d) Family education and support because prolonged ventilatory support may be required.
(5) Outcome.
    (a) Mortality rate 10% to 15%.

(b) Majority recover within the first 6 to 12 months.

(c) Prolonged ventilatory support associated with 50% mortality rate.

g. Traumatic facial nerve palsy (Volpe, 2008).

(1) Pathophysiology.

(a) Trauma causes hemorrhage and edema into the nerve sheath, rather than a true disruption of the nerve fiber.

(b) Site of the lesion typically at or near the exit of the nerve from the stylomastoid foramen.

(c) Weakness of the facial muscles results.

(2) Incidence: Approximately 0.75% of term infants.

(3) Clinical presentation.

(a) Varies with the degree of nerve involvement.

(b) Usually presents the first 2 days after birth.

(c) Persistently open eye on the affected side.

(d) Suck with drooling.

(e) Mouth drawn to normal side during crying.

(f) Corner of mouth does not pull down on affected side.

(g) Eyeball may roll up behind open eyelid.

(h) Usually does not increase in severity.

(4) Patient care management.

(a) Artificial tears for the open eye.

(b) Possible need to tape or patch affected eye to protect cornea.

(c) Support of parents.

(d) Necessary to watch for signs of improvement.

(5) Outcome.

(a) High rate of spontaneous recovery by 7 to 10 days, especially between 1 and 3 weeks of age.

(b) Detectable deficits rarely evident after several months.

(c) For persistence beyond a few weeks, pediatric neurology referral (Goddard-Finegold et al., 2004).

INTRACRANIAL HEMORRHAGES

A. Subdural hemorrhage.

1. Definition (Hill, 2005).

a. Due to laceration of the major veins and sinuses, usually associated with a tear of the dura overlying the cerebral hemispheres or cerebellum.

b. Occurs in both preterm and term neonates.

c. Occurrence with or without laceration of the dura.

2. Risk factors (Volpe, 2008).

a. Large fetal head in comparison with size of birth canal and with rigid pelvic structures.

b. Vaginal breech delivery.

c. Malpresentation (breech, face, brow, foot).

d. Skull is unusually compliant and/or pelvic structures unusually rigid.

e. Labor is either very short (not enough time for dilation) or too long (head subjected to prolonged compression/molding).

f. Forceps, vacuum extraction, or rotational maneuvers required to effect delivery.

3. Pathophysiology (Volpe, 2008).

a. Excessive vertical molding and frontal–occipital elongation, or oblique expansion of the head results in stretching of the falx and tentorium.

b. Venous sinuses are stretched, with possible rupture of the vein of Galen or cerebellar bridging veins.

c. Tear of the dura, including the falx or tentorium, may also occur.

4. Incidence.

a. Uncommon occurrence, accounts for <10% of intracranial hemorrhages.

5. Clinical presentation.
    a. Decreased level of consciousness.
    b. Seizure activity.
    c. Asymmetry of motor function.
    d. Determined by the extent of associated hypoxic–ischemic encephalopathy injury.
    e. Often minimal to no clinical symptoms for first 24 hours because of slowly enlarging hematoma.
    f. On day 2 or 3: signs of increasing intracranial pressure due to block in CSF flow in posterior fossa.
        (1) Full fontanel, irritability, lethargy.
    g. Signs of brainstem disturbance:
        (1) Dilated, poorly reactive pupil on same side as the hemorrhage.
        (2) Respiratory abnormalities, facial paralysis.
        (3) Doll's-eye reflex: normal to abnormal.
    h. Chronic subdural effusion: present within the first 6 months of life with enlarging FOC.
6. Diagnostic evaluation.
    a. CT scan.
    b. MRI scan more effective if hemorrhage is in the posterior fossa.
    c. Skull radiographs demonstrate skull fractures.
7. Outcome.
    a. Major laceration of tentorium and falx with massive hemorrhage have poor prognosis.
    b. Mortality rate approximately 45%.
    c. Survivors develop hydrocephalus and other sequelae.
    d. Concomitant hypoxic–ischemic injury critical factor in determining outcome.
B. **Primary subarachnoid hemorrhage** (Hill, 2005; Volpe, 2008).
    1. Definition: an intracranial hemorrhage into the CSF-filled space between the arachnoid and pial membranes on the surface of the brain.
    2. Pathophysiology.
        a. Bleeding of venous origin in the subarachnoid space as a result of rupture of small vessels in the leptomeningeal plexus or bridging veins in the subarachnoid space.
        b. Bleeding is not secondary to an extension of subdural hemorrhage, intraventricular hemorrhage, or cerebellar hemorrhage.
        c. Self-limited.
        d. May be precipitated by trauma (term infant) or hypoxia (preterm infant).
    3. Incidence: common type of neonatal intracranial hemorrhage.
    4. Clinical presentation.
        a. Most commonly no symptoms develop.
        b. Seizure activity may begin on day 2 of life, especially in the term infant.
        c. Infant looks healthy between seizures: "well baby with seizures" (Volpe, 2008).
        d. Recurrent apnea (more common in preterm infants).
    5. Diagnostic evaluation.
        a. Diagnosis of exclusion. Other forms of intracranial bleeding are eliminated by CT scan.
        b. Lumbar puncture demonstrates uniformly blood-stained CSF.
    6. Outcome.
        a. Sequelae very uncommon.
        b. 90% of term infants who exhibited seizures have normal follow-up.
C. **Intracerebellar hemorrhage.**
    1. Definition: hemorrhage(s) within the cerebellum resulting from primary bleeding or extension of intraventricular or subarachnoid hemorrhage into the cerebellum.
    2. Risk factors: association exists with respiratory distress, hypoxic events, prematurity, and traumatic delivery.
    3. Pathophysiology.
        a. Intravascular, vascular, and extravascular factors (Volpe, 2008).
            (1) Breech presentation and difficult forceps delivery secondary to a compliant skull, with external pressure causing occipital pressure.

      (2) Vitamin K deficiency, thrombocytopenia.

      (3) Vulnerable cerebral capillaries exposed to rapid colloid infusion, causing hypertensive spikes.

      (4) Richly vascularized subpial and subependymal locations.

      (5) Poor vascular support for subependymal and subpial germinal matrices.

      (6) Extension of blood into the cerebellum associated with:

          (i)   Large volume of blood present with IVH,

          (ii) Increased intracranial pressure, and

          (iii) Incomplete myelination of the cerebellum.

4. Incidence (Volpe, 2008).

   a. About 5% to 10% of neonatal deaths studied by autopsy.

   b. Higher in preterm infants than in term.

   c. Occurrence of 15% to 25% in premature infants born at less than 32 weeks of gestation or weighing less than 1.5 kg at birth.

5. Clinical presentation (Hill, 2005).

   a. May have a history of hypoxic–ischemic insult.

   b. Catastrophic deterioration with apnea, bradycardia, decreasing hematocrit values and bloody CSF may occur.

   c. Signs appear within the first 3 weeks, most commonly within the first 2 days of life.

   d. Term infants may have a history of difficult breech delivery.

6. Diagnostic evaluation.

   a. Cranial ultrasonography (lack of symmetric echogenicity may be important).

   b. CT scan necessary to define the hemorrhage.

   c. MRI provides definitive diagnostic information.

7. Outcome.

   a. More favorable in term infant than in premature infant.

   b. Poor outcome in premature infant.

   c. Probable neurologic deficits.

D. Periventricular–intraventricular hemorrhage (Volpe, 2008).

  1. Definition.

    a. Occurs once subependymal germinal matrix hemorrhage extends into lateral ventricles.

    b. Most extensive periventricular–intraventricular hemorrhage is a parenchymal intracerebral hemorrhage (Papile, 2006).

      (1) Involves bleeding into the periventricular (i.e., intracerebellar) white matter and may also precipitate cerebral infarction.

      (2) Only 10% to 15% of infants with hemorrhages.

      (3) With time, on follow-up scans, may see formation of porencephalic cyst at the original hemorrhage site.

    c. See Figure 34-4 for description and grading system (Papile, 2006).

      (1) Small hemorrhage: grade I or II.

      (2) Moderate hemorrhage: grade III.

      (3) Severe hemorrhage: grade IV.

  2. Risk factors.

    a. Prematurity: birth at less than 34 weeks of gestation; respiratory failure requiring mechanical ventilation.

    b. Associated with increasing arterial blood pressure and perinatal asphyxia.

    c. Associated clinical factors (Rennie, 2005b).

      (1) Maternal general anesthesia.

      (2) Low 5-minute Apgar score.

      (3) Asphyxia.

      (4) Low birth weight.

      (5) Acidosis.

      (6) Hypotension or hypertension.

      (7) Low hematocrit.

      (8) Respiratory distress requiring mechanical ventilation.

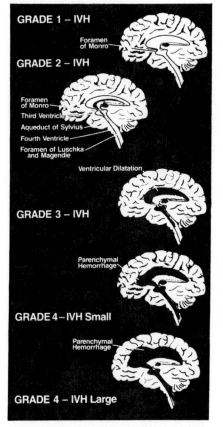

GRADE 1 – IVH

Foramen
of Monro

GRADE 2 – IVH

Foramen
of Monro
Third Ventricle
Aqueduct of Sylvius
Fourth Ventricle
Foramen of Luschka
and Magendie

Ventricular Dilatation

GRADE 3 – IVH

Parenchymal
Hemorrhage

GRADE 4 – IVH Small

Parenchymal
Hemorrhage

GRADE 4 – IVH Large

Grade I IVH: Subependymal hemorrhage in the periventricular germinal matrix. Often localized at the foramen of Monro.

Grade 2 IVH: Partial filling of lateral ventricles without ventricular dilatation.

Grade 3 IVH: Intraventricular hemorrhage with ventricular dilatation.

Grade 4 IVH (small and large): Parenchymal involvement or extension of blood into the cerebral tissue itself. Can be present to a lesser degree.

Correlation between the severity or extent of involvement and subsequent impairment is not absolute. Because outcomes are so varied, assessment of early symptoms and the practice of purposeful interventions are extremely important.

FIGURE 34-4 ■ Quantification of extent of intraventricular hemorrhage (IVH). Four grades of hemorrhagic involvement categorized IVH as differentiated by Papile and Burstein. (From Ross Laboratories: *New perspectives on intraventricular hemorrhage.* Columbus, Ohio, 1988, Ross Laboratories.)

    (9) Rapid administration of sodium bicarbonate.
    (10) Rapid volume expansion.
    (11) Infusion of hyperosmolar solution.
    (12) Coagulopathy.
    (13) Pneumothorax.
    (14) Ligation of patent ductus arteriosus.
    (15) Transport.
  3. Pathophysiology.
    a. Occurs once subependymal germinal matrix hemorrhage extends into lateral ventricles.
    b. Most extensive periventricular–intraventricular hemorrhage is a parenchymal intracerebral hemorrhage (Papile, 2006).
      (1) Involves bleeding into the periventricular (i.e., intracerebellar white matter) and may also precipitate cerebral infarction.
      (2) Only 10% to 15% of infants with hemorrhages.
      (3) With time, on follow-up scans, may see formation of porencephalic cysts at the original hemorrhage site.
  4. Incidence (Volpe, 2008).
    a. Occurs in 30% to 40% of infants weighing <1500 g or of approximately <30 weeks of gestation (Rutherford, 2002).
    b. Infants born at less than 28 weeks of gestation have a 3 times higher risk than infants born at 28 to 31 weeks of gestation.

    c. 2% to 3% of normal term infants have a periventricular–intraventricular hemorrhage.

        (1) More than half of these hemorrhages originated at the subependymal germinal matrix.

        (2) The remainder originated at the choroid plexus.

        (3) Timing of onset.

            (a) About 50% occur by 24 hours of age.

            (b) About 80% occur by 48 hours of age.

            (c) About 90% occur by 72 hours of age.

            (d) By 7 days of age, 99.5% have occurred.

            (e) 20% to 40% exhibit progression of the hemorrhage over 3 to 5 days.

5. Clinical presentation.

    a. Presentation ranges from unnoticeable to dramatic.

        (1) Sudden deterioration.

        (2) Oxygen desaturation.

        (3) Bradycardia.

        (4) Metabolic acidosis.

        (5) Significant decrease in hematocrit.

        (6) Hypotonia.

        (7) Shock.

        (8) Hyperglycemia.

        (9) Tense anterior fontanelle.

    b. Symptoms of worsening hemorrhage.

        (1) Full, tense fontanelles.

        (2) Increased ventilatory support.

        (3) Seizure activity.

        (4) Apnea.

        (5) Decrease in level of consciousness and/or activity.

6. Diagnostic evaluation.

    a. Optimal time to screen: 7 days of age because >90% of all hemorrhages have occurred.

        (1) If test result is normal, there is no need to recheck.

        (2) If test result is positive for periventricular–intraventricular hemorrhage, repeat test in 2 weeks.

    b. Serial cranial ultrasonography replaces CT as the principle diagnostic technique.

    c. Lumbar puncture (CSF studies show elevated red blood cells, increased protein concentration, xanthochromia, and decreased glucose concentration).

    d. Rule out septic shock or meningitis.

7. Patient care management.

    a. Prevent preterm birth, perinatal asphyxia, and birth trauma.

    b. Promote in utero transport.

    c. Promote nonstressful intrapartum course.

    d. Provide efficient, expedient intubation.

    e. Appropriate handling; minimal stimulation with clustering of care activities as tolerated.

    f. Minimize noxious stimuli (dim the lights, quiet the environment).

    g. Avoid noxious procedures when possible.

    h. Avoid events associated with wide swings in arterial and venous pressures.

        (1) Seizures.

        (2) Excess motor activity.

        (3) Apnea.

        (4) Crying.

        (5) Pneumothorax.

    i. Avoid administration of hyperosmolar solutions.

    j. Prevent blood pressure swings: give volume replacement slowly.

    k. Avoid overventilation leading to pneumothorax.

l. Use two people for endotracheal suctioning.

m. Use noninvasive monitoring of oxygen and carbon dioxide levels (maintain within normal limits).

n. Monitor and maintain normal pH.

o. Correct abnormal clotting.

p. Be alert to signs of a hemorrhage.

q. Educate and support the parents.

8. Outcome.

   a. Mortality rate is 50% with severe hemorrhage, 10% with moderate hemorrhage, and 5% with small hemorrhage.

   b. These hemorrhages are an important cause of morbidity and death in low birth weight infants.

   c. Hemorrhage alone does not account for all neurologic deficits.

   d. Approximately 50% of premature infants are free of neurologic symptoms.

   e. Approximately 25% to 30% of very low birth weight infants discharged from a level III neonatal intensive care unit (NICU) have a periventricular–intraventricular hemorrhage without major neurodevelopmental sequelae.

   f. Outcome depends on degree of severity of hemorrhage (Hill, 2005; Volpe, 2008).

      (1) Small hemorrhage.

         (a) Neurodevelopmental disability similar to that in premature infants without hemorrhage.

         (b) Major neurodevelopmental disability in 10%.

      (2) Moderate hemorrhage.

         (a) Major neurodevelopmental disability in 40% during infancy.

         (b) Mortality rate 10%, with progressive hydrocephalus in less than 20%.

      (3) Severe hemorrhage.

         (a) Major neurodevelopmental disability in 80%.

         (b) Mortality rate 50% with hydrocephalus common in survivors.

SEIZURES*

A. **Definition**: symptom of neurologic dysfunction (not a disease).

B. **Risk factors.**

1. Metabolic encephalopathies.

   a. Decreased production of adenosine triphosphate.

      (1) Ischemia.

      (2) Hypoxemia.

      (3) Hypoglycemia.

   b. Hyponatremia or hypernatremia.

   c. Hypocalcemia, hypomagnesemia.

   d. Inborn errors of metabolism.

   e. Pyridoxine dependency.

   f. Hyperammonemia.

2. Structural.

   a. IVH.

   b. Intrapartum trauma.

   c. Cerebral cortical dysgenesis: result of abnormal neuronal migration.

   d. Hypoxic–ischemic encephalopathy, the most common diagnosis of neonatal seizures.

3. Intracerebral meningitis.

   a. Bacterial infection.

      (1) Group B beta-streptococci and *Escherichia coli* may account for up to 65% of cases.

*Hill, 2005; Rennie, 2005b.

        (2) Many other bacterial organisms may be implicated and include but are not limited to other streptococci and staphylococci specie such as group D streptococci, *Staphylococcus epidermidis*, *S. aureus*, *Listeria monocytogenes*, *Haemophilus influenzae*, *Neisseria meningitidis*, and *Streptococcus pneumoniae*.

    b. Nonbacterial infection: TORCH.

  4. Withdrawal from maternal drugs.

    a. Uncommon cause of seizures (may cause jitteriness).

    b. Onset during first 3 days of life.

    c. Drugs.

        (1) Narcotic analgesics.

        (2) Sedative hypnotics.

        (3) Alcohol.

  5. Familial (genetic).

    a. Onset in second and third days of life.

    b. Infant appears well between seizures.

    c. Self-limiting: within 1 to 6 months, seizures stop.

    d. Autosomal dominant inheritance.

C. Pathophysiology: seizures result from excessive simultaneous electrical discharge or depolarization of neurons.

D. Incidence (Rennie, 2005a).

  1. 6% to 13% of very low birth weight infants.

  2. 1 to 2 per 1000 term infants.

E. Clinical presentation.

  1. Subtle.

    a. Most frequent of neonatal seizures.

    b. Present in most term and premature newborn infants having seizures.

    c. Often unrecognized.

    d. Presentation varies.

        (1) Horizontal deviation of the eyes.

        (2) Pedaling movements.

        (3) Rowing, stepping movements.

        (4) Eye blinking or fluttering.

        (5) Nonnutritive sucking.

        (6) Smacking of lips.

        (7) Drooling.

        (8) Apnea (convulsive apnea usually does not occur by itself).

  2. Tonic.

    a. Characteristic in premature infants weighing ≤500 g.

    b. Often seen with severe IVH.

    c. Generalized tonic extension of all extremities or flexion of upper limbs with extension of lower extremities.

    d. Often mimics decorticate posturing.

  3. Multifocal clonic.

    a. Characteristic in term infants with hypoxic–ischemic encephalopathy.

    b. Clonic movements migrating from one limb to another without a specific pattern.

  4. Focal clonic.

    a. Uncommon.

    b. Presents as localized clonic jerking.

  5. Myoclonic.

    a. Very rare in neonatal period.

    b. Multiple jerks of upper- or lower-limb flexion.

F. Diagnostic evaluation.

  1. Perform physical examination.

    a. Rule out jitteriness.

        (1) Characterized by trembling of hands and feet.

(2) No involvement of eye movements.

(3) Stopped by gentle, passive flexion of affected extremity.

b. Note infant's history, which may provide a predisposed underlying etiology.

2. Laboratory work.

   a. Serum glucose level.

   b. Electrolyte levels (sodium, potassium, chloride, calcium, magnesium).

   c. Arterial blood gas analysis.

   d. Urea, ammonia.

3. Diagnostic study for sepsis.

   a. Lumbar puncture.

   b. Culture of blood, urine, and CSF specimens; bacterial and viral.

   c. Complete blood cell count and platelet count.

4. Electroencephalography, CT scan, cranial ultrasonography, MRI.

5. Skull films if etiology is trauma.

6. Twelve-lead electrocardiography.

7. Consideration of following laboratory tests:

   a. Blood pyruvate.

   b. Lactate.

   c. TORCH.

   d. Urinary drug screen.

8. Neurology consultation.

G. Patient care management.

1. Determine underlying etiology.

2. Resuscitate as necessary.

3. Obtain diagnostic studies as ordered.

4. Provide pharmaceutical therapy (Young and Mangum, 2008).

   a. Phenobarbital.

      (1) Load: 20 mg/kg slow IV for 10 to 15 minutes.

      (2) Closely monitor respiratory status.

      (3) Maintenance dosage: 3 to 4 mg/kg/day, beginning 12 to 24 hours after the loading dose.

      (4) Therapeutic range: 15 to 40 mcg/ml.

      (5) Excretion.

         (a) Metabolized by liver: 50% to 70%.

         (b) Unchanged in urine: 20% to 30%.

      (6) Consider as the drug of choice.

   b. Phenytoin. Many facilities are replacing phenytoin with fosphenytoin. Check with your physician or pharmacist.

      (1) Load: 15 to 20 mg/kg IV (for 30 minutes or longer).

      (2) Maintenance dosage: 4 to 8 mg/kg/day.

      (3) Recommended administration routes, by slow IV push or by mouth.

      (4) Therapeutic range: 6 to 15 mcg/ml in the first weeks, then 10 to 20 mcg/ml because of changes in protein binding. First trough should be obtained 48 hours after the IV loading dose.

      (5) Excretion.

         (a) Protein bound (approximately 90%).

         (b) Displaced by bilirubin, increasing free drug levels.

   c. Fosphenytoin.

      (1) Load: 15 to 20 mg PE/kg IV over at least 10 minutes [PE = phenytoin equivalents; Fosphenytoin 1 mg PE = phenytoin 1 mg]. Consider continuous electrocardiographic, blood pressure, and respiratory monitoring with loading doses.

      (2) Maintenance.

         (a) Dosage: 4 to 8 mg PE/kg/day.

         (b) Rate of administration: up to 1.5 mg PE/kg/minute.

         (c) Flush the IV with saline before and after administration.

(d) Term infants > 1 week of age may need up to 8 mg PE/kg per dose every 8 to 12 hours.

(e) Therapeutic range and excretion. See section (b) Phenytoin, above.

    (i) Peak plasma concentrations: about the time that the IV infusion is complete; half-life is 4 to 10 minutes.

    (ii) Rapidly converted by the body to generate therapeutic levels of phenytoin.

  d. Lorazepam.

    (1) Administer: 0.05 to 0.1 mg/kg slow push IV (for status epilepticus).

    (2) Repeat dose based on clinical response.

    (3) Note routes of excretion.

      (a) By kidneys.

      (b) Lipid soluble.

    (4) Lorazepam produces anticonvulsant effect in minutes after administration.

    (5) Monitor oxygenation and vital signs.

    (6) Document precisely.

H. Outcome.

  1. Related to underlying etiology.

HYPOXIC–ISCHEMIC ENCEPHALOPATHY*

A. Definition of hypoxic–ischemic encephalopathy (HIE).

  1. Hypoxemia and anoxia (diminished oxygen in blood supply; partial or complete). Moderate to severe hypoxia leads to metabolic acidosis.

  2. Ischemia (diminished blood supply perfusing the brain).

    a. Systemic hypotension.

    b. Occlusive vascular disease.

  3. Hypoxia and ischemia, which lead to neurologic dysfunction.

  4. Asphyxia.

    a. Impairment of gas exchange of respiratory gases—oxygen and carbon dioxide.

    b. Mixed respiratory and metabolic acidosis.

    c. Failure of systemic multiorgan systems, including heart, lungs, liver, and kidneys.

B. Diagnosis.

  1. History and risk factors.

    a. Antepartum risk factors: socioeconomic status (SES), maternal thryroid disease, severe pregnancy-induced hypertension (PIH), fetal growth restriction, postdatism.

    b. Intrapartum risk factors: Maternal pyrexia, persistent occiput posterior (OP) fetal position, acute intrapartum events, such as cord accident, uterine rupture, abruption, evidence of intrapartum hypoxia defined by composite of abnormal fetal heart rate (FHR), fresh meconium, and low Apgar scores.

  2. Electroencephalography (EEG).

C. Incidence of HIE (Laptook, 2005; Lavery and Randall, 2008; Volpe, 2008).

  1. Prevalence of 1 to 6 per 1000 live births.

  2. About 2% to 4% of term infants.

  3. Approximately 60% of very low birth weight infants.

  4. Timing of insult occurrence.

    a. Antepartum occurrence: 20%.

    b. Intrapartum occurrence: 30%.

    c. Antepartum–intrapartum occurrence: 35%.

    d. Postpartum occurrence: 10%.

---

*Laptook, 2005, 2008; Volpe, 2008.

D. Clinical presentation and staging using Sarnat criteria (Hill, 2005; Volpe, 2008).
   1. Stage I (mild encephalopathy): characteristic features.
      a. Hyperalert state.
      b. Normal muscle tone, active suck, strong Moro reflex, normal/strong grasp, and normal doll's-eye reflex.
      c. Increased tendon reflexes.
      d. Myoclonus present.
      e. Hyperresponsiveness to stimulation.
      f. Tachycardia possible.
      g. Dilation of pupils, reactive.
      h. Sparse secretions.
      i. No convulsions (unless due to hypoglycemia or preexisting conditions that predisposed the infant to perinatal distress).
      j. Electroencephalographic findings: within normal limits.
   2. Stage II (moderate encephalopathy).
      a. Characteristic features.
         (1) Lethargy.
         (2) Hypotonia.
         (3) Increased tendon reflexes.
         (4) Myoclonus.
         (5) Seizure activity frequent.
         (6) Weak suck.
         (7) Incomplete Moro reflex.
         (8) Strong grasp.
         (9) Overactive doll's-eye reflex.
         (10) Pupils constrictive and reactive.
         (11) Respirations variable in rate and depth; respirations may be periodic.
      b. Critical period: infant's condition either improves or deteriorates.
      c. Indications of deterioration.
         (1) No signs of improvement.
         (2) Development of any of the following:
            (i)   Seizures.
            (ii) Cerebral edema.
            (iii) Lethargy.
            (iv) Abnormalities on electroencephalogram.
      d. Recovery.
         (1) No further seizure activity.
         (2) Electroencephalographic findings return to normal.
         (3) Transient jitteriness.
         (4) Improvement in level of consciousness.
   3. Stage III (severe encephalopathy).
      a. Clinical course.
         (1) Level of consciousness deteriorates from obtunded to stuporous to comatose.
         (2) Mechanical ventilation is required to sustain life.
      b. Clinical features.
         (1) Apnea/bradycardia.
         (2) Seizures appearing within the first 12 postnatal hours. 50% to 60% of patients who do ultimately seize do so within the first 6 to 12 hours. Premature infants present with generalized seizures. Term infants demonstrate multifocal clonic seizures. All these infants display subtle seizures (Volpe, 2008).
         (3) Severe hypotonia and flaccidity; suck, Moro, and grasp reflexes absent.
         (4) Stuporous to comatose.
         (5) Absent or depressed reflexes.
         (6) Doll's-eye reflex weak or absent.
         (7) Pupils often unequal; variable reactivity and poor light reflex.

    c. Deterioration (Volpe, 2008).

        (1) Deterioration occurs within 24 to 72 hours.

        (2) Severely affected infants often worsen, sinking into deep stupor or coma.

        (3) Death may ensue.

    d. Survivors.

        (1) Infants who survive to this point often improve in the next several days to months.

        (2) Feeding difficulties often develop secondary to abnormalities of suck and swallow. This is due to the poor muscle tone connected to involvement of cranial nerves for these functions.

        (3) Generalized hypotonia is common; hypertonia is uncommon.

        (4) Severe neurologic disabilities may ensue.

E. Diagnostic studies (Hill, 2005; Laptook 2005, 2008; Lavery and Randall, 2008; Volpe, 2008).

  1. Valuable in assessing the nature of the brain insult and the extent of the brain injury.

  2. Used to track the evolution of HIE.

    a. Precise history.

    b. Complete neurologic examination.

    c. Electroencephalography (EEG).

        (1) Confirm or deny clinical diagnosis of seizures.

        (2) Provide prognostic information regarding severity of permanent brain damage.

        (3) Two common types of EEG: conventional EEG (cEEG) or amplitude EEG (aEEG).

            (a) cEEG: Used to measure impact of neurologic insult and detect presence of seizure activity.

                (i) Twelve to 16 sensors applied by specialist technician. Sensors are usually invasive.

                (ii) Usually recorded for 40 to 60 minutes.

                (iii) Provides information about entire cerebral cortex.

                (iv) Logistically challenging to schedule technician to interpret and neurologist to interpret study.

            (b) aEEG: Measures, filters, and time-compresses raw EEG signal to create simplified pattern easy to interpret by nonneurologist.

                (i) May be single (2 sensors) channel to monitor single parietal channel or dual (4 sensors) channels in parietal and central positions.

                (ii) Usually recorded continuously.

                (iii) Provides hemispheric information of the cerebral cortex.

                (iv) No technician needed for sensor application, and nonneurologist can interpret study.

                (v) Abnormal aEEG is more specific (89% vs. 78%), has a greater positive predictive value (73% vs. 58%), and has a similar sensitivity (79% vs. 78%) as well as negative predictive value (90% vs. 91%) compared with abnormal neurologic examination by Sarnat criteria alone.

    d. Evoked potentials.

    e. Creatinine kinase and other biochemical/enzyme markers.

    f. Lumbar puncture, CSF analysis.

    g. CT scan.

    h. Cranial ultrasonography.

    i. Technetium scan.

    j. MRI.

    k. Intracranial pressure monitoring.

F. Patient care management.

  1. Prevent perinatal hypoxia, ischemia, and asphyxia (anticipation of risk factors, appropriate intervention).

  2. Perform prompt, efficient resuscitation by trained staff.

  3. Maintain physiologic oxygenation and acid–base balance.

  4. Correct fluid, electrolyte, and caloric abnormalities.

    5. Monitor blood volume; avoid blood pressure swings and hypotension.

    6. Maintain optimal perfusion.

    7. Treat seizures.

    8. Consider cerebral hypothermia (Laptook, 2008).

      a. Total body cooling.

      b. Selective head cooling.

      c. Goal of hypothermia: Maintenance of brain energy phosphorylated metabolites, improve coupling between blood flow and oxidative metabolism, decrease release of excitatory transmitters that lead to seizures, reduce nitric oxide production, and decrease apoptosis.

      d. See Table 34-3 for comparison between total body and selective cooling.

    9. Perform a thorough neurologic examination.

   10. Monitor and manage disturbances of other body organs.

      a. Pulmonary.

      b. Cardiac.

      c. Hepatic.

      d. Renal.

   11. Educate and support the family.

   12. Obtain neurology consultation.

G. Outcome (Volpe, 2008).

    1. Based on severity of brain insult; selective neuronal necrosis.

    2. Death within newborn period in 20% to 50% of asphyxiated infants who exhibit HIE.

    3. Overall neurologic sequelae with HIE at $3\frac{1}{2}$ years of age: approximately 17%.

    4. Factors associated with poor outcome.

      a. Apgar score.

        (1) If score is 0 to 3 for 20 minutes or more, approximately 60% die.

        (2) If score is less than 3 at 1 minute and less than 5 at 5 minutes, with abnormal neurologic signs (feeding difficulties, apnea, hypotonia, seizures):

          (a) About 20% die.

          (b) About 40% are normal.

          (c) About 40% have neurologic sequelae.

      b. Encephalopathy.

        (1) Mild: no subsequent deficits.

■ TABLE 34-3

■ ■ **Comparison of Brain Cooling Trials**

Parameter	CoolCap	Body Cooling
Mode of cooling	Head and systemic	Systemic only
Equipment	Cooling cap and radiant warmer	Cincinnati Sub-Zero Hyper-Hypothermia System
Target core: temperature	34° to 35°C	33.5°C
Target core: site	Rectum	Esophagus
Temperature control method at core site	Servo control of abdominal skin temperature 36.8° to 37.2°C; manual control of CoolCap to achieve target core temperature at rectum	Servo control of esophagus
Age at therapy initiation	<6 hours	<6 hours
Time to achieve target core temperature	2 hours	Approximately 1.5 hours
Duration of cooling therapy	72 hours	72 hours
Rate of rewarming after therapy cessation	0.5°C/hour	0.5°C/hour

From Laptook, A.R.: Brain cooling for neonatal encephalopathy: Potential indications for use. In J.M. Perlman (Ed.): *Neurology: Neonatal questions and controversies.* Philadelphia, 2008, Saunders, pp. 66-78.

  (2) Severe: 75% die, 25% have sequelae.

  (3) Term infants: 60% normal, 30% abnormal, and 10% die.

  (4) Premature infants: 50% normal, 20% abnormal, and 30% die.

  (5) Duration of abnormal neurologic signs: good indicator of severity of HIE injury.

  (6) Disappearance of abnormal neurologic signs by 1 to 2 weeks: good chance of being normal (possibility of learning disabilities not ruled out).

 5. Seizures early (first 12 hours of life) and/or difficult to control: associated with poorer prognosis.

 6. Hyperactivity and attention difficulties: in infants with less severe encephalopathy.

 7. Rapid initial improvement indicative of better outcomes.

 8. Long-term sequelae based on:

  a. Site,

  b. Extent of cerebral injury, and

  c. Duration of abnormal clinical presentation.

PERIVENTRICULAR LEUKOMALACIA*

A. Definition of periventricular leukomalacia (PVL).

 1. Ischemic, necrotic periventricular white matter.

 2. Principally ischemic lesion of arterial origin.

 3. Multicystic encephalomalacia with or without secondary hemorrhage into ischemic area.

B. Pathophysiology.

 1. Predisposition.

  a. Systemic hypotension severe enough to impair cerebral blood flow.

  b. Occurrence of focal cerebral infarction and cerebral ischemia.

  c. Major systemic hypotension.

  d. Episodes of apnea and bradycardia.

 2. Occurrence secondary to inadequate cerebral perfusion.

 3. Manifestation of hypoxic–ischemic encephalopathy in premature infants.

C. Incidence.

 1. Unknown.

 2. Approximately 3% to 10% of those with bilateral cystic leukomalacia.

 3. Increases to approximately 26% if noncystic PVL is included.

D. Clinical presentation.

 1. Acute phase: hypotension and lethargy.

 2. 6 to 10 weeks later characteristic picture:

  a. Irritable, hypertonic, increased flexion of arms and extension of legs.

  b. Frequent tremors and startles.

  c. Moro reflex may be abnormal.

E. Diagnostic evaluation.

 1. Cranial ultrasonography.

 2. CT scan.

 3. MRI.

F. Outcome.

 1. Spastic diplegia (major motor deficit common in premature infants with PVL).

 2. Motor deficits in premature infants; possible spontaneous resolution in first several years of life.

 3. Significant upper arm involvement associated with intellectual deficits.

 4. Visual impairment.

 5. Lower limb weakness.

 6. Outcome based on:

  a. Location and

  b. Extent of injury.

---

*Hill, 2005; Rennie, 2005a; Volpe, 2008.

MENINGITIS*

A. Definition.
1. Infection of central nervous system (CNS).
2. Early-onset infection from pathogens in vaginal flora (e.g., group B beta-streptococci and *E. coli*).
3. Late-onset infection from environmental microbes found in nursery environment (e.g., *Pseudomonas aeruginosa* and *S. aureus*).

B. Risk factors.
1. Maternal infection.
2. Prolonged ruptured membranes.
3. Prematurity.

C. Pathophysiology.
1. Organisms reach the fetus or newborn.
   a. Transplacental organisms lead to congenital infection.
   b. Ascending organisms from the vagina or cervix lead to early-onset infection.
   c. Late-onset infection develops in infants infected by passage through birth canal.
   d. Organism introduction after birth from surrounding environment leads to iatrogenic infection.
2. Organisms.
   a. Bacteria.
      (1) Aerobic.
         (a) Group B beta-streptococci (most common).
         (b) *E. coli* (second most common).
         (c) *L. monocytogenes* (third most common).
      (2) Anaerobic.
   b. Viruses.
      (1) TORCH infection.
      (2) Enterovirus.
   c. Fungi.

D. Clinical presentation.
1. Congenital viral infection.
   a. Preterm delivery.
   b. Possible low birth weight.
   c. Blueberry muffin rash.
   d. Inflammation of other affected organs.
   e. Microcephaly.
2. Early-onset bacterial meningitis.
   a. Presentation with shock in the first 24 hours.
   b. Possible rapid progression to shock.
   c. Respiratory distress.
   d. Hypotension.
   e. Apnea.
   f. Seizures.
   g. Temperature instability.
   h. Diarrhea.
   i. Hepatomegaly.
   j. Jaundice.
3. Late-onset meningitis.
   a. Nonspecific symptoms.
   b. Lethargy.
   c. Feeding intolerance.

---

*Fenichel, 2007; Volpe, 2008.

      d. Irritability.

      e. Posturing.

      f. Temperature instability.

      g. Apnea.

      h. Bradycardia.

      i. Bulging fontanelles.

      j. Nuchal rigidity.

E. Diagnostic evaluation.

   1. CSF.

      a. Organism found on Gram stain.

      b. Low glucose level.

      c. Elevated protein concentration and white blood cell count.

      d. Culture for specific identification of organism.

      e. Counterimmune electrophoresis.

   2. Complete diagnostic study for sepsis.

F. Patient care management.

   1. Detect early and treat.

   2. Perform thorough physical examination.

   3. Observe for seizure activity.

   4. Obtain infectious disease consultation.

   5. Provide pharmaceutical agents (Fenichel, 2007; Young and Mangum, 2008).

      a. Initial therapy.

         (1) Ampicillin or penicillin G.

         (2) *In addition*, aminoglycoside.

         (3) Ampicillin and cefotaxime recommended for aminoglycoside-resistant organism.

         (4) Treatment 7 to 10 days for sepsis without a focus; minimum of 21 days for gram-negative meningitis.

      b. Group B beta-streptococci.

         (1) Ampicillin or penicillin G.

         (2) *In addition*, gentamicin (discontinue if sensitivities warrant).

      c. Coliform bacteria (e.g., *E. coli*).

         (1) Cefotaxime.

         (2) Aminoglycosides are a suitable alternative.

      d. *L. monocytogenes* and enterococci.

         (1) Ampicillin.

         (2) *In addition*, aminoglycoside.

      e. *S. epidermidis*.

         (1) Vancomycin.

         (2) Methicillin resistance in many strains.

      f. *S. aureus*.

         (1) Methicillin.

         (2) Vancomycin if methicillin-resistant strain.

         (3) Rarely cause of meningitis in the newborn infant (vancomycin for meningitis).

      g. *P. aeruginosa*.

         (1) Mezlocillin or ticarcillin.

         (2) *In addition*, aminoglycoside.

      h. *Bacteroides fragilis* (anaerobic).

         (1) Metronidazole, clindamycin, mezlocillin, or ticarcillin.

         (2) For CNS infection, metronidazole recommended.

   6. Sample CSF at specific intervals until sterile.

   7. Treat at least 2 weeks after sterilization of CSF.

   8. Obtain and test CSF sample 48 hours after antibiotic therapy has been discontinued.

   9. Educate and support the family.

G. Outcome.

   1. Dependent on rapidity of detection and initiation of adequate drug therapy.

2. Survivors of bacterial meningitis: 50% have significant neurologic sequelae.
   a. Hydrocephalus.
   b. Seizures.
   c. Sensorineural hearing loss.
   d. Visual losses.
   e. Mental and motor disabilities.

REFERENCES

Bondurant, C.P. and Jimenez, D.F.: Epidemiology of cerebrospinal fluid shunting. *Pediatric Neurosurgery,* 23(5):254-258, 1995.

DeVries, L. and Rennie, J.M.: Preterm cerebral hemorrhage. In J.M. Rennie and N.R.C. Roberton (Eds.): *Roberton's textbook of neonatology* (4th ed.). Edinburgh, 2005, Churchill Livingstone, pp. 1148-1168.

Fenichel, G.M.: *Neonatal neurology* (4th ed.). Philadelphia, 2007, Churchill Livingstone, pp. 1-18.

Gleeson, J.G., Dobyns, W.B., Plawner, L., and Ashwal, S.: Congenital structural defects. In K.F. Swaiman, S. Ashwal, and D.M. Ferriero (Eds.): *Pediatric neurology: Principles and practice* (4th ed.). Philadelphia, 2006, Mosby, pp. 363-490.

Goddard-Finegold, J.: The intrauterine nervous system. In W.H. Taeusch, R.A. Ballard, and Christine Gleason (Eds.): *Avery's diseases of the newborn* (8th ed.). Philadelphia, 2004, Saunders, pp. 802-832.

Goddard-Finegold, J., Mizrahi, E.M., and Lee, R.T.: The newborn nervous system. In W.H. Taeusch, R.A. Ballard, and C. Gleason (Eds.): *Avery's diseases of the newborn* (8th ed.). Philadelphia, 2004, Saunders, pp. 839-891.

Hill, A.: Neurological and neuromuscular disorders. In M.G. MacDonald, M.D. Mullett, and M.M.K. Seshia (Eds.): *Neonatalogy: Pathophysiology and management of the newborn* (5th ed.). Philadelphia, 2005, Lippincott Williams & Wilkins, pp. 1384-1409.

Laptook, A.R.: Brain cooling for neonatal encephalopathy: Potential indications for use. In J.M. Perlman (Ed.): *Neurology: Neonatal questions and controversies.* Philadelphia, 2008, Saunders, pp. 66-78.

Laptook, A.R.: Hypoxic ischemic encephalopathy. In E.E. Lawson, C.U. Lehmann, L.M. Nogee, and L.A. Harbold (Eds.): *eNeonatal Review,* 2(5):1-9, 2005.

Lavery, S.V. and Randall, K.S.: Cerebral monitoring of the term infant. *Neonatal Network,* 27(5):329-337, 2008.

Levene, M.I.: Intracranial haemorrhage at term. In J.M. Rennie and N.R.C. Roberton (Eds.): *Roberton's textbook of neonatology* (4th ed.). Edinburgh, 2005, Churchill Livingstone, pp. 1120-1127.

McLean, C.W., Cayabyab, R.G., Noori, S., and Seri, I.: Cerebral circulation and hypotension in the premature infant: Diagnosis and treatment. In J.M. Perlman (Ed.): *Neurology: Neonatology questions and controversies.* Philadelphia, 2008, Saunders, pp. 3-36.

Madsen, J.R. and Frim, A.M.: Neurosurgery of the newborn. In M.G. MacDonald, M.D. Mullett, and M.M.K. Seshia (Eds.): *Neonatalogy: Pathophysiology and management of the newborn* (5th ed.). Philadelphia, 2005, Lippincott Williams & Wilkins, pp. 1410-1427.

Mangurten, H.H.: Birth injuries. In A.A. Fanaroff, R.J. Martin, and M.C. Walsh (Eds.): *Fanaroff and Martin's neonatal-perinatal medicine: Diseases of the fetus and infant* (8th ed.). Philadelphia, 2006, Mosby, pp. 425-454.

Moore, K.L. and Persaud, T.V.N.: The nervous system. In K.L. Moore and T.V.N. Persaud (Eds.): *Before we are born: Essentials of embryology and birth defects* (7th ed.). Philadelphia, 2007, Saunders, pp. 27-77; 343-370.

Papile, L.: Intracranial hemorrhage and vascular lesions. In A.A. Fanaroff, R.J. Martin, and M.C. Walsh (Eds.): *Fanaroff and Martin's neonatal-perinatal medicine: Diseases of the fetus and infant* (8th ed.). Philadelphia, 2006, Mosby, pp. 891-899.

Rennie, J.M.: Assessment of the neonatal nervous system. In J.M. Rennie and N.R.C. Roberton (Eds.): *Roberton's textbook of neonatology* (4th ed.). Edinburgh, 2005a, Churchill Livingstone, pp. 1093-1104.

Rennie, J.M.: Seizures in the newborn. In J.M. Rennie and N.R.C. Roberton (Eds.): *Roberton's textbook of neonatology* (4th ed.). Edinburgh, 2005b, Churchill Livingstone, pp. 1105-1119.

Rutherford, M.A.: Hemorrhagic lesions of the newborn brain. In M. Rutherford (Ed.): *MRI of the neonatal brain.* London, 2002, Saunders, pp. 171-200.

Smith, S.A. and Ouvrier, R.: Peripheral neuropathies. In K.F. Swaiman, S. Ashwal, and D.M. Ferriero (Eds.): *Pediatric neurology: Principles and practice* (4th ed.). Philadelphia, 2006, Mosby, pp. 1890-1892.

Sun, P.P. and Persing, J.A.: Craniosynostosis. In I.F. Pollack, P.D. Adelson, and A.L. Albright (Eds.): *Principles and practice of pediatric neurosurgery* (2nd ed.). New York, 2007, Theime Medical Publishers Inc., pp. 219-242.

Volpe, J.J.: *Neurology of the newborn* (5th ed.). Philadelphia, 2008, Saunders.

Yager, J.Y. and Poskitt, K.J.: Glucose and perinatal brain injury: Questions and controversies. In J.M. Perlman (Ed.): *Neurology: Neonatology questions and controversies.* Philadelphia, 2008, Saunders, pp. 153-171.

Young, T.E. and Mangum, B.: *Neofax* (21st ed.). Montvale, NJ, 2008, Thomson Reuters.

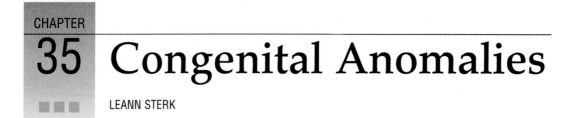

OBJECTIVES

1. Describe assessment strategies for diagnosis of infants experiencing a congenital defect.
2. Identify methods of initial management and care for individual congenital anomalies.
3. List possible causative factors that result in common congenital abnormalities.
4. Verbalize the importance of parental involvement on the development of infants affected with congenital anomalies.

In the United States, congenital malformations represent the most frequent cause of death within the first year of life (Jorde et al., 2003). The birth of an infant with a congenital anomaly represents a life-changing event for each family involved.

A congenital anomaly is defined as a physical, metabolic, anatomic, or behavioral deviation from the normal pattern of development (Moore and Persaud, 2007) (Box 35-1). This chapter presents information concerning the incidence, etiology, clinical presentation, and treatment modalities for some common abnormalities.

A. **Incidence.**
   1. The frequency of medically significant malformations diagnosed in the newborn period is documented as 2% to 3% of all live births (Jorde et al., 2003). These defects present as single or multiple defects, all with varying clinical significance.
      a. By 1 year of age, the incidence of congenital anomalies requiring surgery or interfering with normal functioning ranges from 4% to 7% (Lashley, 2005).
      b. Minor single anomaly rates are estimated to be as high as 10% to 12% (Lashley, 2005). Infants experiencing three or more minor abnormalities commonly have one or more major defects.
   2. Greater than 20% of infant deaths in North America are attributed to birth defects (Moore and Persaud, 2007).
   3. Birth defects are a significant cause of miscarriage and fetal death. Chromosomal abnormalities are present in 50% of first-trimester and 20% of second-trimester spontaneous abortions (Jorde et al., 2003).
      a. 6% to 7% of all zygotes have chromosomal abnormalities that will result in spontaneous abortion (McLean, 2005).

B. **Etiology.**
The etiology of 50% to 60% of congenital anomalies is unknown (McLean, 2005). Hudgins and Cassidy (2002) relate that congenital malformations may have more than one cause, are often associated with multiple associated anomalies, and have variable recurrence risks.
   1. Genetic factors.
      a. Genetic factors are numerically the most frequent cause of congenital anomalies and are responsible for approximately 0.5% to 0.7% of all anomalies (Matthews and Robin, 2006). Carey (2003) estimates the incidence of chromosomal abnormalities as 1 in 150 live births. Of anomalies with known causes, 85% are due to genetic factors (McLean, 2005).
      b. Abnormal chromosomes are produced in the germ line of either parent secondary to errors in fertilization, meiosis, or mitosis (Larsen, 2001).
      c. Embryos resulting from these events display missing or extra chromosomes (numerical abnormality) or rearranged segments (structural abnormalities). Chromosomal aberrations result in defective zygotes, blastocysts, and early embryos.

■ BOX 35-1
■ **TERMINOLOGY**

Consistent language, definitions, and accurate presentation of dysmorphology are vital to understanding congenital anomalies.
1. Malformation: A primary morphologic defect of an organ or body part that results from an intrinsic abnormal developmental process (Lashley, 2005), e.g., neural tube defect.
2. Deformation: Alteration of a previously normal body part by unusual forces on normal tissue (Dorland's, 2007). Timing of event usually occurs in the fetal period as a secondary alteration, often involving cartilage, joints, and bones (Lashley, 2005), e.g., club foot.
3. Disruption: Extrinsic breakdown or interruption of a normal developmental process resulting in a defect of an organ or larger body system, e.g., amniotic banding sequence.
4. Dysplasia: Abnormal organization of cells in tissue.
5. Syndrome: A recognized pattern of multiple anomalies derived from a single anomaly or mechanical factor (Dorland's, 2007), e.g., Down syndrome.

    d. Both sex chromosomes and/or autosomes may be affected.
    e. Categories of genetic factors:
        (1) Numerical abnormalities occur secondary to nondisjunction of genetic material, resulting in the loss or gain of one or more chromosomes (Matthews and Robin, 2006).
            (a) Trisomy: fertilization of an aneuploid gamete by a normal gamete resulting in a zygote with an extra chromosome.
            (b) Monosomy: zygote develops missing a specific chromosome.
            (c) Mosaicism: mixture of cells having cells with the normal number, whereas other cells have an abnormal number of chromosomes. Symptoms are generally less severe than if all the cells were abnormal.
    f. Numerical chromosomal abnormalities are frequently associated with intrauterine growth retardation, dysmorphic features, mental retardation, and physical malformations (Matthews and Robin, 2006).
    g. Structural abnormalities result as chromosomal material breaks, resulting in a loss or rearrangement of the broken segment to a different location on the chromosome or to a different chromosome.
        (1) Microdeletions are submicroscopic chromosomal abnormalities that involve specific minute portions of chromosomes. Their presence is detected by molecular cytogenic methods, e.g., FISH.
    h. Single gene or Mendelian disorders.
    i. Multifactorial disorders occurring secondary to interaction of genes and additive environmental influences. In order for an abnormality to be expressed, a threshold of traits must be exceeded.
    j. Disorders are familial but lack the inheritance traits of single-gene defects (Lashley, 2005).
    k. Most isolated single malformations, such as congenital heart defects, neural tube defects, and cleft lip and palate, develop secondary to multifactorial inheritance patterns (Matthews and Robin, 2006).
    l. Recurrence rates are higher for first-degree relatives, higher if a larger number of family members are affected, and are increased if the malformation is severe (Matthews and Robin, 2006).
  2. Disorders resulting from exposure to teratogens that affect the developing fetus.
    a. McLean (2005) describes environmental factors as causative for 7% to 10% of congenital anomalies.
    b. The majority of teratogenic agents exert their effect by interfering with cellular metabolic activity. The end result is death, failure of cellular replication, cell migration, or cellular fusion (Cole, 2001).

    c. The ability of a particular agent to exert a teratogenic effect are determined by the timing of the exposure (critical time once cellular differentiation has begun), dosage of the teratogen (higher the dose, greater the effect), the individual properties of the teratogen, and the genetic susceptibility of the mother and fetus (Matthews and Robin, 2006).

    d. McLean (2005) describes classifications of teratogens as infectious agents, chemical agents, radiation, and maternal factors.

C. Evaluation.

When a newborn is identified as having one or more malformations, a detailed history and physical examination is needed to aid in accurate diagnosis.

1. Family history should include the past three generations with health information about all relatives—parents, siblings, grandparents, uncles and aunts, as well as cousins.
    a. Reproductive losses and infertility.
    b. Relatives with mental retardation or known malformations.
    c. Infants within the family with malformations or birth defects.
    d. Neonatal deaths, childhood deaths, stillbirths.
    e. Familial disorders or physical features common to the family.
    f. Consanguinity in parents.
    g. Ethnic background.

2. Prenatal and perinatal history should detail information about maternal and fetal well-being.
    a. Maternal age, parity, and health—including maternal illness and medications.
    b. Pregnancy complications.
    c. Teratogenic exposures, including alcohol, drugs, medications, bacterial infections, viral infections, and parasitic infections.
    d. Duration of pregnancy, intrapartum course and duration.
    e. Fetal growth and behavior in utero—patterns of movement throughout pregnancy.
    f. Delivery mode, complications, condition of infant at delivery.
    g. Birth weight, length, and head circumference and whether measurements are appropriate for gestation.

3. Detailed physical examination is undertaken with attention to physical variations and malformations. Clinical photographs should be obtained.
    a. Growth parameters: weight, length, head circumference—assessment of proportionality and symmetry. Specific measurements of features that are abnormal in shape, size, or symmetry.
    b. Estimation of gestational age.
    c. General appearance: posture, tone, and position.
    d. Systematic examination of all body surfaces.
        (1) Skull: flattening or prominence.
        (2) Scalp: hair patterns, including placement of whorls, hairline, texture, pigmented areas, eye brow length, eyelash length.
        (3) Face: configuration, elfin, coarse, flat, triangular, round, birdlike, expressionless characteristics.
        (4) Eyes: iris color, palpebral fissures—length and degree of slanting, colobomas, hypotelorism, ptosis.
        (5) Nose: appearance—beaked, pinched, upturned, flattened bridge, position on face, number of nares.
        (6) Mouth: size of tongue, intact palate, teeth, shape of mouth, philtrum, and vermilion border.
        (7) Ears: location, rotation, unilateral/bilateral defect, protruding/prominent shape, patency.
        (8) Neck: length, webbed/redundant skin folds, posterior hairline, torticollis.
        (9) Chest: shape, size, symmetry, location and number of nipples.
        (10) Cardiovascular: murmurs, pulses, blood pressure.
        (11) Lungs: equality of breath sounds.

      (12) Abdomen: integrity of abdominal wall, location and appearance of umbilicus, presence of masses, abdominal tone.

      (13) Genitalia: presence of ambiguity, size, appearance.

      (14) Anus: location and patency.

      (15) Extremities: proportions, appearance, range of motion, number and placement of hands, feet, digits.

4. Diagnostic evaluation of a congenital abnormality.

    a. Radiographs, computed tomography, ultrasound, and magnetic resonance imaging are used to rule out structural abnormalities. These tests are also performed to investigate dysmorphic features that may be part of a syndrome or sequence.

    b. Chromosome analysis is useful in delineating a diagnosis when a genetic disorder is suspected. Several weeks may be required for results. For critically ill infants, analysis from bone marrow may be available within hours, results from blood lymphocyte culture can be obtained within 48 hours (Matthews and Robin, 2006). Postmortem, chromosome analysis can be obtained from any tissue—thymus, skin, gonad, and intracardiac blood in particular. Samples of tissue must be obtained under sterile conditions as soon as possible after the infant's death. Chromosome analysis should be obtained for all infants having two or more major malformations, for infants with growth restriction in association with anomalies, for infants having multiple minor abnormalities, and infants with ambiguous genitalia.

      (1) Routine karyotype on peripheral blood produces better resolution than karyotype from amniocentesis. This allows for detection of minute deletions and duplications (Hudgins et al., 2002).

    c. Molecular cytogenics allows for chromosomal abnormalities to be studied in greater detail. Diagnostic confirmation of microdeletion syndromes is possible, utilizing non-dividing cells including cells in fixed tissue.

      (1) FISH (fluorescent in situ hybridization) uses segments of fluorescently labeled DNA probes that attach to a specific segment of the chromosome and appear fluorescent under microscopic evaluation. Where material is missing from the segment, the probe cannot attach to the chromosome. Missing segments are termed microdeletions (Matthews and Robin, 2006).

    d. Biochemical studies are performed on ill neonates who have a condition that may be secondary to an inborn error of metabolism, or for whom a specific diagnosis cannot be made. Laboratory studies should be obtained before treatment is begun. Presenting symptoms guide the specific tests to be ordered. Newborn screening using tandem mass spectrometry allows for a single drop of blood to effectively screen for 40 inborn errors of metabolism.

D. Genetic counseling.

1. The diagnosis of a congenital anomaly places the family in a crisis. They must deal with the diagnosis, the immediate and long-term needs for care, financial concerns, and the dynamics of family life.

    a. Genetic counseling is offered to prospective parents to help them evaluate risks for hereditary or genetic conditions based on familial history, age, and other factors that may affect the birth of their offspring (Wynbrandt and Ludman, 2000).

    b. Goals of counseling center around provision of information concerning diagnosis, needed care, impact of the illness, and prognosis for the future. Counseling is aimed toward assisting parents to make informed decisions concerning their infants.

    c. Counseling can be offered by family physicians, neonatologists, or genetic specialists. Provide in a quiet location with all additional family members desired by the family present.

    d. Principles of genetic counseling.

      (1) Supportive, nonjudgmental attitude.

      (2) Respective of family privacy, confidentiality.

      (3) Sensitive to ethnic, cultural, and language differences.

      (4) Supportive of family's movement through the grieving process.

(5) Content of counseling should take into account medical issues, mechanisms causing the abnormality, a realistic prognosis, as well as a plan for treatment and support resources.

(6) Risk for recurrence and reproductive options.

(7) Assistance with family adjustment and social services as needed.

SPECIFIC DISORDERS

See Figure 35-1 for the division of congenital anomalies.

Abnormalities of Chromosomes

Trisomy 21

A. **Incidence and etiology.**

1. Most common autosomal chromosomal abnormality in live born infants; occurring in 1 in 700 to 800 infants (Lewanda et al., 2006).

2. Full trisomy 21 occurs in 94% of cases (all or large part of the chromosome). Affected individuals have 47 chromosomes (3 of chromosome 21) (Fig. 35-2).

3. Five percent are caused by translocation (women less than 30 years of age have a higher risk for translocation—6.9%).

4. One percent are mosaic (Matthews and Robin, 2006).

   a. Greater than 50% of trisomy 21 fetuses abort early in pregnancy.

   b. Recurrence risk approximately 1% overall. For those parents who are known translocation carriers, the risk is substantially higher. Risk for carrier parent is dependent on the type of translocation and the sex of the parent (Jones, 2006).

   c. Incidence of Down syndrome related to maternal age is as follows (Jones, 2006):

      (1) 15 to 29 years—1 in 1500.

      (2) 0 to 34 years—1 in 800.

      (3) 35 to 39 years—1 in 270.

      (4) 40 to 44 years—1 in 100.

      (5) Over 45 years—1 in 50.

B. **Clinical presentation.**

1. Craniofacial.

   a. Brachycephaly with flattened occiput.

   b. Upslanting palpebral fissures, iris speckled with Brushfield spots, colobomatous cataracts, and glaucoma.

   c. Prominent epicanthal folds.

   d. Flattened facial profile, micrognathia.

   e. Small rounded ears, low-set and malformed ears, hearing loss.

2. Musculoskeletal.

   a. Hypotonia: generalized—poor Moro reflex present in 80% of infants. Tendency to keep mouth open and protruding tongue (Jones, 2006).

   b. Hyperflexibility of joints, dysplasia of pelvis: narrow acetabular angle.

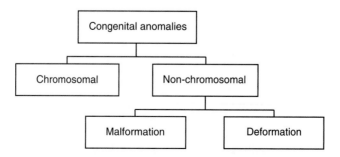

FIGURE 35-1 ■ Division of anomalies.

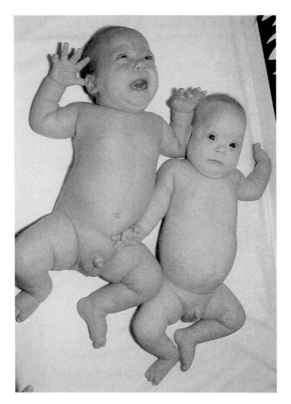

FIGURE 35-2 ■ Anterior view of dizygotic (fraternal) male twins discordant for Down syndrome (trisomy 21). The twin at right is smaller and hypotonic compared with the unaffected twin. The twin at right developed from a zygote that contained an extra 21 chromosome. (Courtesy Dr. A.E. Chudley, Department of Pediatrics and Child Health, University of Manitoba, Children's Hospital, Winnipeg, Manitoba, Canada.)

      c. Clinodactyly of fifth fingers, single or bilateral transverse simian crease.

      d. Prenatal growth restriction, short stature.

      e. Wide spacing between first and second toes (Matthews and Robin, 2006).

   3. Skin.

      a. Loose folds in posterior neck.

C. Associated findings.

   1. Prematurity.

   2. Mental retardation: all individuals are affected with mean IQ of 30 to 50 (McLean, 2005).

   3. Gastrointestinal: duodenal atresia/stenosis, imperforate anus.

   4. Hematologic: leukemoid reaction, polycythemia, congenital leukemia.

   5. Cardiac anomalies in approximately 40% to 50% of infants: endocardial, cushion defect, ventral septal defect, patent ductus arteriosus, atrial septal defect (Lewanda et al., 2006).

D. Diagnosis.

   1. Chorionic villus sampling at 9 to 12 weeks of gestation.

   2. Amniocentesis at 16 weeks.

   3. Maternal serum screening for low values of alpha-fetoprotein.

   4. Ultrasound targeting growth, polyhydramnios, heart defects.

   5. Standard chromosome banding techniques provide confirmation of trisomy 21 and to differentiate those infants having nondisjunctional trisomy from a translocation. In those infants with confirmed translocation, each parent should have karyotype analysis done to rule out carrier status as recurrence risk is significantly increased (Lewanda et al., 2006).

   6. FISH: Region on chromosome affected is q22.2.

E. Treatment.
  1. Initial treatment geared to expressed symptoms.
  2. Aimed at optimizing potential for intellectual and social growth.
  3. Parent education and support are essential for treatment of continuing health issues.
     a. Frequent upper respiratory and ear infections.
     b. Cardiac sequelae, including congestive heart failure.
     c. Developmental delays—muscle tone increases with age, rate of developmental progress slows with age (Jones, 2006). Early developmental enrichment programs seem to be of the most value.
     d. Social performance is usually above the expected level. Emotional problems are apparent in many affected individuals.
  4. Parents should be provided with resources for emotional and medical support.

Trisomy 18

A. Incidence and etiology.
  1. Affected infants have 47 chromosomes (3 of chromosome 18) (Fig. 35-3).
  2. Occurs in 1 in 600 births; females more often than males (3:1) (Jones, 2006). Trisomy 18 is the third most common autosomal disorder.
  3. Eighty percent of cases are caused by chromosomal nondisjunction (Lewanda et al., 2006); 95% of infants have three copies of entire chromosome 18, and 5% have either partial trisomy or mosaicism of most of the long arm of 18 (Carey, 2003).
  4. Occurs more frequently as maternal age advances: mean maternal age is 32 (Jones, 2006).
  5. Gilbert (2000) describes three patterns of presentation:
     a. Severe: most body cells display abnormality. Handicaps are severe, with a short life expectancy.
     b. Mosaic form: some cells have the normal complement of genetic material, the remaining cells having the typical pattern for trisomy 18. Infants are less severely affected and have a longer life expectancy.
     c. Partial: dependent on the portion of the chromosome affected. Trisomy of the short arm of the chromosome have minimal handicaps and few abnormalities are expressed. Trisomy involving the entire long arm of the chromosome display the full spectrum of the syndrome. Trisomy of the distal one third of the chromosome demonstrate a partial syndrome with less profound mental deficit and longer survival (Jones, 2006).

B. Clinical presentation.
  1. General: growth deficiency, hypoplasia of skeletal muscle, subcutaneous and adipose tissue (Jones, 2006).
  2. Craniofacial: prominent occiput, low-set malformed auricles, atresia of auditory canals, narrow palpebral fissures, microphthalmia, corneal opacities, colobomas, micrognathia, microstomia and high, arched palate (Lewanda et al., 2006).
  3. Musculoskeletal: clenched hand, with index finger overlapping the third finger and the fifth finger overlapping the fourth, abnormal creases, low arch dermal ridge pattern on six or more fingertips, hypoplasia of nails, short sternum, narrow pelvis with hip dislocation, rocker bottom appearance to feet, hammer toes, and syndactyly between toes 2 and 3 (Jones, 2006).
  4. Skin: redundant skin, mild hirsutism of back and forehead.

C. Associated findings.
  1. Cardiac anomalies: varied. Occurs in 95% of cases (Gilbert, 2000). Ventricular septal defects and patent ductus arteriosus most common.
  2. Renal anomalies: horseshoe kidneys, ectopic kidneys, double ureters, and cystic kidneys. Incidence in approximately 50% of affected individuals (Gilbert, 2000).
  3. Genital abnormalities: cryptorchidism in males. Hypoplasia of labia and prominent clitoris in females.
  4. Umbilical hernias.
  5. Severe psychomotor retardation.

D. Diagnosis.
  1. Chorionic villus sampling.

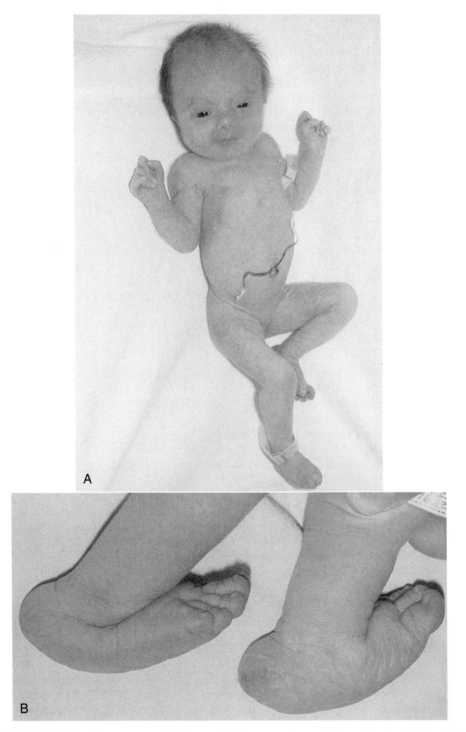

FIGURE 35-3 ■ **A,** Female neonate with trisomy 18. Note growth retardation, clenched fists with characteristic positioning of fingers (second and fifth digits overlap third and fourth digits). **B,** Feet of another trisomy 18 infant showing characteristic rocker-bottom appearance as a result of vertical position of tali (ankle bones). Also observe prominent calcanei (heel bones). (Courtesy Dr. A.E. Chudley, Department of Pediatrics and Child Health, University of Manitoba, Children's Hospital, Winnipeg, Manitoba, Canada.)

2. Amniocentesis at 16 weeks.
3. Maternal serum triple screening revealing low levels of alpha-fetoprotein, estradiol, and human chorionic gonadotropin.
4. Ultrasound targeting growth retardation, oligohydramnios, and polyhydramnios.
5. Following delivery, standard chromosomal banding assay or FISH.

E. **Treatment.**
   1. Infants with full Trisomy 18 are usually fragile, with a history of feeble fetal activity (Jones, 2006). Capacity for survival is limited—50% of infants with trisomy 18 die within the first week of life (Carey, 2003); 90% die within the first year of life.
   2. Children who survive the first year of life deal with feeding issues secondary to hypotonia, growth issues, and significant developmental disability. These children generally do not walk unsupported or develop expressive language, but can be capable of limited verbal communication and some social interaction. Carey (2003) describes some children as attaining some psychomotor maturity, recognizing family members, and demonstrating skills comparable to that of a 2-year-old child.
   3. Once a diagnosis has been confirmed, decisions about extraordinary medical means for prolongation of life present nearly overwhelming challenges for families. Individual circumstances for each family must be considered (Jones, 2006).
   4. For those infants surviving the immediate newborn period, care is supportive and individualized to the infant's needs.
   5. Parents should be offered genetic counseling and provided with resources for support.

Trisomy 13

A. **Incidence and etiology.**
   1. Affected infants are born with 47 chromosomes instead of the usual 46, with the extra genetic material located on chromosome 13.
   2. Defect occurs in 1 in 5000 live births (Jones, 2006), making it the fourth most common autosomal dominant disorder.
      a. Older mothers are more likely to have an infant with this aneuploidy defect.
      b. Slightly more boys than girls are affected (Jones, 2006).
   3. Seventy-five percent of cases result from chromosomal nondisjunction (Lewanda et al., 2006).
   4. The etiology for this disorder is trisomy of all or part of chromosome 13.
      a. Eighty percent of affected infants have three complete copies of chromosome 13.
      b. Mosaicism accounts for 5% of cases, these infants demonstrating a wide range of expression from near normal to severe full pattern malformation.
         (1) Survival for infants with mosaicism is usually longer.
         (2) Degree of mental deficit is variable (Jones, 2006).
      c. Partial trisomy of the proximal segment is characterized by infants with severe mental deficiency and an overall pattern of full trisomy 13.
      d. Partial trisomy of the distal segment results in severe mental deficiency and characteristic phenotype (Jones, 2006).

B. **Clinical presentation.**
   1. General: growth deficiency.
   2. Craniofacial: microcephaly, microphthalmia, colobomata, glaucoma, midline scalp defects, retinal dysplasia, cleft lip and/or palate (60% to 80%) (Jones, 2006), malformed ears, atresia of external auditory canals, deafness, prominent nasal bridge, short neck with excessive skin.
   3. Musculoskeletal: polydactyly, single simian crease, overlapping of fingers, flexion deformities of hands and wrists, prominent heel resulting in rocker bottom feet, thin posterior ribs with or without missing rib, and hypoplasia of pelvis with shallow acetabular angle.
   4. Genital abnormalities: males—cryptorchidism, abnormal scrotum: females—bicornate uterus.
   5. Central nervous system: holoprosencephaly type of defect with incomplete development of the forebrain, olfactory and auditory nerves, seizure activity, apnea in early infancy, and severe mental deficiency (Jones, 2006).
   6. Capillary hemangiomas, localized scalp defects.

C. **Associated findings.**
   1. Cardiac anomalies occur in approximately 80% of infants: ventral septal defects, dextro-position, patent ductus arteriosus.
   2. Renal abnormalities: polycystic kidneys.
   3. Inguinal or umbilical hernias, single umbilical artery.
D. **Diagnosis.**
   1. Chorionic villus sampling between 9 and 12 weeks of pregnancy.
   2. Amniocentesis at 16 weeks.
   3. Ultrasound targeting growth parameters, abnormalities of heart and kidneys, brain.
   4. Following delivery, standard chromosome banding assay, FISH.
E. **Treatment.**
   1. The presence of holoprosencephaly is the single most important finding predicting survival. The range of expression for this defect is wide—from cyclopedia, to cebocephaly, to premaxillary agenesis (Carey, 2003).
   2. The median survival for these infants is 7 days (Jones, 2006), with greater than 90% dying within the first year of life. Survivors frequently have seizures, severe mental retardation, and failure to thrive.
      a. Feeding issues are related to the smallness of the lower jaw and poor muscle tone.
      b. For those infants with cleft lip/or palate, feeding issues present additional challenges (Gilbert, 2000).
   3. The high rate of early mortality for this syndrome requires the parents to prepare for the infant's death as well as plan for supportive care. The desires of the parents must be taken into account as care is designed for each patient.

   22q11.2 Deletion Syndrome   This syndrome has been referred to as DiGeorge syndrome, Sprintzen syndrome, or velocardiofacial syndrome.
A. **Incidence and etiology.**
   1. Occurs in 1 in 4000 to 5000 infants (Carey, 2003). This syndrome is extremely variable in expression and varies from patient to patient.
      a. Inherited as an autosomal dominant pattern.
      b. Individuals have an interstitial deletion of 22q11.2; 80% to 90% of patients have the same large deletion (Saitta and Zackai, 2005).
      c. This disorder is the most common deletion syndrome (Saitta and Zackai, 2005).
      d. Most 22q11 deletions occur as de novo lesions—less than 10% are inherited from an affected parent. Both parents must be tested to determine carrier status (Jones, 2006).
B. **Clinical presentation.**
   1. Growth: postnatal onset of short stature (Jones, 2006).
   2. Craniofacial: microcephaly, velopharyngeal insufficiency, cleft palate, small or absent adenoids, prominent nose with bulbus tip, narrow palpebral fissures, long face, retruded mandible with chin deficiency, small mouth, hooded eyelids, hypertelorism, hearing deficits, and minor auricular abnormalities.
   3. Musculoskeletal: limbs are slender, hypotonic, hands and fingers are hyperextensible (Jones, 2006).
C. **Associated findings.**
   1. Cardiac defects are present and usually significant in 85% of patients. Most common defects include ventral septal defects, right interrupted aortic arch, tetralogy of Fallot, and truncus arteriosus (Jones, 2006).
   2. Atresia or hypoplasia of the thymus and parathyroid glands (Saitta and Zackai, 2005).
   3. Functional T-cell abnormalities.
   4. Hypocalcemia: occurs as a transient finding in neonates (60%). Seizures can occur—usually as a result of the hypocalcemia.
   5. Learning disabilities: 62% of patients will have normal or mild learning issues, with severe or moderate learning difficulties in 18% (Jones, 2006).
      a. IQ range 70 to 90.
      b. Psychiatric disorders—schizophrenia.
      c. Speech and language is often delayed. Speech pattern is frequently nasal secondary to poor pharyngeal musculature.

D. Diagnosis.
  1. Defect is detected by FISH.
E. Treatment.
  1. Death primarily secondary to cardiac defects—occurs in approximately 8% of infants (Jones, 2006). Majority of affected patients die before 6 months of age.
  2. Hypotonia is common, resulting in developmental delays. Early intervention, physical and speech therapy, is helpful.
  3. Infants may require surgical intervention to improve speech.
  4. Infants frequently demonstrate greater socialization skills than intellectual skills.
  5. Onset of psychiatric symptoms is usually between 10 and 21 years of age—ongoing assessment and support are essential (Jones, 2006).

Sex Chromosome Abnormalities

Turner Syndrome
A. Incidence and etiology.
  1. Affected individuals have monosomy—loss of all or part of one copy of the X chromosome in a female. Most 45,X conceptuses die early—0.1% survive to term, the majority are spontaneously aborted (Saitta and Zackai, 2005).
     a. Loss of the entire chromosome occurs in approximately 50% of cases (Lewanda et al., 2006).
  2. Occurs in approximately 1 in 2500 live-born phenotypic females.
  3. Most often, the paternal X chromosome is missing.
  4. Mosaicism is associated with complex karyotypes, ring chromosomes, and deletions.
  5. Disorder generally occurs as a sporadic event in a family (Jones, 2006).
B. Clinical presentation.
  1. Growth: small stature.
  2. Craniofacial: narrow palate, low-set ears with anomalous auricles, hearing loss, ptosis of eyelids, epicanthal folds, broad nasal bridge, low posterior hairline with appearance of a short neck.
  3. Musculoskeletal: broad chest with wide-spaced nipples, pectus excavatum, short fourth metacarpal/metatarsal, marked lymphedema of extremities, bone dysplasia, dislocation of the hip, knee abnormalities (Lewanda et al., 2006).
  4. Skin: excessively pigmented nevi, loose skin—especially posterior folds of neck.
C. Associated anomalies.
  1. Cardiac defects: Bicuspid aortic valve, coarctation of aorta, valvular aortic stenosis, and mitral valve prolapse (Jones, 2006).
  2. Renal: horseshoe kidney, unilateral renal agenesis.
  3. Gonads: Ovarian dysgenesis with hypoplasia owing to lack of germinal elements (Jones, 2006).
  4. Performance issues: delayed motor skills, poor coordination, clumsiness, problems with nonverbal problem solving, depression and poor self-esteem in young adults (Jones, 2006).
D. Diagnosis.
  1. Ultrasound for short stature, monitoring of growth throughout gestation.
  2. Standard chromosome banding assay or FISH.
E. Treatment.
  1. Growth issues persist throughout childhood and adolescence. Growth is commonly normal within the first 3 years of life, then decreases during school-age years, more dramatically during teenage years when these girls do not get their usual growth spurt at puberty. Growth hormone therapy is generally begun at around 4 to 5 years of age. Significant improvement in final height has been achieved (Saitta and Zackai, 2005).
  2. Congenital lymphedema requires symptomatic treatment initially, presenting with edema of hands and feet secondary to faulty lymph drainage. Recedes in early infancy (Gilbert, 2000).

3. Ovarian function is affected, with primary ovarian failure occurring secondary to gonadal dysplasia. The result can be delay in development of secondary sex characteristics and primary amenorrhea (Saitta and Zackai, 2005). Treatment options include estrogen replacement therapy for hypogonadotropic girls beginning at ages 13 to 14 (Jones, 2006).
4. Ongoing evaluation of congenital heart defects is necessary secondary to the increased risk for dissection of the aorta. Coarctation of aorta must be surgically repaired.
5. With increasing age, a greater incidence of osteoporosis, autoimmune thyroid disease, and chronic liver disease have been reported (Jones, 2006). Close monitoring for these conditions is needed.
6. For those infants for whom their physical appearance would be aided by plastic surgery, concerns for the formation of keloid scars must be considered.
7. School performance may be affected primarily in word comprehension and presentation (Gilbert, 2000). Intelligence is usually normal.

Klinefelter Syndrome
A. **Incidence and etiology.**
 1. Affects approximately 1 in 500 males, making it the most common single cause of hypogonadism and infertility in males (Jones, 2006).
 2. Chromosomal analysis reveals a 47,XXY karyotype.
    a. Parental nondisjunction errors account for one half of the affected infants; maternal meiosis errors accounting for the majority of remaining cases (Lewanda et al., 2006).
    b. Advanced maternal age is related to an increased incidence for those whose defect is secondary to maternal factors.
    c. According to Jones (2006), older fathers are at higher risk for producing a higher number of XY sperm, resulting in a higher risk of having an infant with Klinefelter syndrome.
 3. Infants with XXY/XY mosaicism may have a greater potential for testicular function.
 4. Infants carrying XXYY karyotype are more often developmentally delayed.
B. **Clinical presentation.**
 1. General: affected males frequently have long limbs, reduced upper to lower segment ratio (Jones, 2006). Tall and slim stature.
 2. Musculoskeletal: elbow dysplasia, fifth finger clinodactyly.
 3. Genital: hypogonadism, cryptorchidism, hypospadias, gynecomastia.
C. **Associated findings.**
 1. Cancers: teratoma, leukemia, breast (Grottkau and Goldberg, 2005).
 2. Scoliosis during adolescent years (Jones, 2006).
 3. School performance and behavioral issues: delayed speech and language development, difficulties with auditory processing and auditory memory.
D. **Diagnosis.**
 1. Prepubertal males have no significant dysmorphism. Minor abnormalities are helpful in providing clues for diagnosis: penile size, skeletal defects (Lewanda et al., 2006).
 2. Chromosomal testing, FISH to determine XXY or XXYY or XXXY status.
E. **Treatment.**
 1. As adolescence progresses, screening for scoliosis is needed.
 2. Deficient testosterone and elevated gonadotropin levels signal the need for hormone replacement. Boys must be monitored for prospective testosterone replacement as they near ages 10 to 12. As some males have incomplete or inadequate puberty, replacement will assist in development of a more masculine physique, increase pubic and facial hair, and improve bone density and muscle mass (Jones, 2006). Delays in treatment can increase risk for osteoporosis.
 3. The incidence of breast cancer for affected infants is 20 times higher than the general population, but only 1 in 5000 affected men. Routine mammography is not required (Jones, 2006). Incidence of mediastinal teratomas is 34 to 40 times that of nonaffected populations. Ongoing assessment of these individuals is needed.
 4. IQ range for affected individuals is variable, from well below to well above average. Assistance in school is commonly required, especially in the areas of reading and spelling.

5. Emotional and behavioral problems persist and may increase throughout childhood. Formation of peer relationships may be difficult secondary to insecurity, shyness, and poor judgment activity. Support with psychological adjustment is needed.

NONCHROMOSOMAL ABNORMALITIES

Malformation Disorders

Malformation sequences occur with a single, localized, poor formation of tissue that initiates a chain of subsequent defects (Jones, 2006). Expressed manifestations range from nearly normal to severe and carry a variable recurrence risk.

Osteogenesis Imperfecta   Clinically and genetically heterogenous hereditary disease involving connective tissue and bone (Zaleske, 2001).
A. **Incidence and etiology.**
  1. Disorder is caused by mutations of COL1A1 and COL1A2 genes on chromosomes 17q21 and 17q22.1. The result of the mutation is an abnormality of type I collagen (Kaplan, 2005). Overall incidence is 3 to 4 per 100,000.
  2. Six clinical types are identified:
     a. Type I: autosomal dominant, resulting from mutations of COL1A1 gene on chromosome 17q21 (Jones, 2006). Most common form found in most populations. Characterized by bone fragility with onset of fractures following birth.
     b. Type II: autosomal dominant, inheritance pattern occurring secondary to a sporadic, dominant mutation in one of the two collagen genes (Jones, 2006).
        (1) Frequency 1 in 20,000 to 60,000 (Kaplan, 2005). Lethal in the perinatal period—either as stillborn or secondary to respiratory failure; 80% die within the first month of life.
        (2) Recurrence risk is described as 6%.
     c. Type III: primarily an autosomal dominant inheritance pattern, although rare autosomal recessive pattern has been identified (Jones, 2006). Progressive and deforming, perinatal death is common.
     d. Type IV: autosomal dominant pattern resulting from mutations of the two collagen genes. Significant bone deformities are common.
     e. Type V: autosomal dominant inheritance pattern that is not associated with collagen type I mutations (Jones, 2006). Moderate tendencies to fracture long bones.
     f. Type VI: pattern of inheritance is unknown. Results from a mineralization defect; fractures occurring later between 4 and 18 months.
B. **Clinical presentation.**
  1. Type I.
     a. Growth: near normal or normal growth pattern.
     b. Craniofacial: macrocephaly, triangular appearing facies, hearing impairment, altered dentition with hypoplasia of dentin and pulp (Jones, 2006).
     c. Musculoskeletal: postnatal onset of mild limb problems; bowing of femur, tibia, scoliosis, hyperextensibility of joints, and osteopenia.
     d. Skin: translucent, easy bruising, blue sclerae secondary to partial visualization of the choroid.
  2. Type II.
     a. Growth: short limbed growth deficiency with prenatal onset, low birth weight.
     b. Craniofacial: head is soft and boggy, with minimal calvarial bone palpable, large fontanels, deep blue sclerae, shallow orbits, and variable hydrocephalus (Kaplan, 2005).
     c. Musculoskeletal: shortened and bowed limbs with extra skin, flexed and abducted hips, flattened vertebrae (Jones, 2006).
  3. Type III.
     a. Growth: prenatal onset of growth deficiency, extremely short stature.
     b. Craniofacial: macrocephaly, triangular facies, deep blue sclera, hearing loss, dentinogenesis imperfect.
     c. Musculoskeletal: kyphoscoliosis, which may lead to respiratory distress (Jones, 2006), multiple fractures, and deformations of limbs at birth.

4. Types IV to VI.
   a. Presentation less severe for these forms. Stature and growth may be mildly affected; fractures, if they occur, present later. Sclerae may be mildly affected or absent. Dentition is less commonly affected.

C. **Associated findings.**
   1. Conductive hearing loss secondary to deformity of the small bones of the ear (Gilbert, 2000).
   2. Platelet function is decreased due to defects in adhesion and clot retraction.
   3. Corneal clouding and keratoconus, megalocornea (Jones, 2006).
   4. Cardiac: floppy mitral valve.
   5. Scoliosis developing later, progressing during puberty, sometimes resulting in severe deformity in adulthood. Loss of height may occur secondary to progressive spinal osteoporosis in adults.

D. **Diagnosis.**
   1. Prenatal diagnosis is possible with ultrasonography and mutation analysis.
   2. Radiographs: Type I = femurs are short, broad, or crumpled. Fibulas may be thin.
      Type II = femurs are short and deformed, but not crumpled. The long bones appear thin with bowing and deformations. Cranial bones are undermineralized, with wormian bones.
   3. Chromosomal study confirming genetic mutation on 17q 21 and 17q22.1.
   4. Diagnosis can be confirmed with collagen studies performed on cultured fibroblasts from skin biopsy (Kaplan, 2005).

E. **Treatment.**
   1. Depending on the type of osteogenesis, treatment will vary extensively. Type I patients may require little or no treatment, whereas type II patients may die before any treatment is begun. Types III and IV are the most complex, requiring intensive support.
      a. Initial treatment of fractures are aimed toward alignment of bones to avoid deformity, comfort measures, prevention of further deformity, optimizing function following healing, and prevention of further fractures.
      b. Laxity of ligaments and previous fracture abnormalities complicate the healing process.
      c. Lightweight splints or braces provide the first-line treatment; depending on previous bone damage, surgical procedures may be necessary to provide strengthening and support.
      d. Stabilization of limbs that have received multiple fractures may be necessary. Placement of rods may provide needed support (Gilbert, 2000).
   2. Early intervention for hearing loss is essential for development of language and later learning.
   3. Dentition may be difficult or delayed; these children are more prone to cavities. Ongoing examination and treatment is vital.
   4. Scoliosis may progress quickly for those nearing puberty—bracing is often ineffective. Early surgical fusion may provide the best option for treatment.
   5. If a diagnosis has been made prenatally, operative delivery to avoid fractures and intracranial bleeding is recommended.
   6. Careful handling of the neonate is necessary to minimize pain and prevent further fractures.

Achondroplasia

A. **Incidence and etiology.**
   1. Achondroplasia occurs with a frequency of 1 in 15,000 live births (Jones, 2006).
      a. Most common skeletal dysplasia in humans (Lewanda, 2006).
   2. Defect has an autosomal dominant inheritance pattern with 90% secondary to a de novo mutation of FGFR3 (Fibroblast Growth Factor receptor 3) on chromosome 4p16.3 (Carey, 2003).
      a. New mutations occur in the father's sperm and are associated with advanced paternal age (Lewanda et al., 2006).

   b. Transmitted as a fully penetrant autosomal dominant trait; each person who inherits the mutant gene will show the condition (Kaplan, 2005).
B. Clinical presentation.
   1. General: Small stature. Small at birth, with increasingly apparent growth deficiency secondary to failure of endochondral ossification.
   2. Craniofacial: Megalocephaly, small foramen magnum, low nasal bridge, flat midface, short flat nose with broad tip, anteverted nares, long philtrum, hypotelorism (Jones, 2006).
   3. Musculoskeletal: Short limbs, lumbar lordosis, mild thoracolumbar kyphosis, short tubular bones, vertebral anomalies, short, trident hand, hyperextensible joints, shortened upper limbs, and flexion contractures at elbows.
C. Associated findings.
   1. Mild hypotonia, especially in the trunk and extremities with delayed milestones.
   2. Predisposition to serous otitis media.
   3. Bowing of the legs after ambulation has started (Carey, 2003).
   4. Orthodontic problems related to maxillary hypoplasia.
   5. Stenosis of the magnum and spine leading to compression of the upper cord and resultant symptoms of apnea, growth delays, hydrocephalus, quadriparesis, and sudden death (Carey, 2003).
D. Diagnosis.
   1. Chromosomal studies to confirm mutation on 4p16.3 chromosome.
   2. Diagnosis is confirmed for achondroplasia through radiographic survey: iliac bones are short and round, lumbar vertebrae have short pedicles and scalloping, long bones have mildly flared metaphyses and are shortened.
E. Treatment.
   1. Infants with known achondroplasia must be closely monitored for developmental delay, hypotonia, and growth patterns.
   2. Unsupported sitting is associated with development of kyphosis. Infants should not be allowed to be carried in flexed positions before trunk muscle strength is adequate (Kaplan, 2005).
      a. Bracing or surgical correction may be needed to manage kyphosis.
   3. Hydrocephalus may develop within the first 2 years of life. Radiologic imaging of the skull as a baseline is recommended for monitoring; monthly head circumference should be obtained and plotted to determine abnormal growth.
   4. Sleep apnea may be a sign of foramen magnum stenosis and must be evaluated.
   5. Treatment for severe bowing of the legs is often deferred until full growth has occurred. Osteotomies provide needed corrections (Jones, 2006).
   6. Close monitoring of auditory performance is needed as shortened eustachian tubes may lead to middle ear infections and resultant hearing loss. Many infants require placement of tympanic membrane tubes.
   7. Dental crowding is frequently encountered, requiring removal of one or more teeth.
   8. Obesity develops toward late childhood and should be monitored closely.

Neural Tube Defects

As the neural tube develops, developmental processes can be altered by intrinsic or extrinsic factors, resulting in defective closure or a reopening of the neural tube.
A. Incidence and etiology.
   1. Neural tube defects are among the most commonly occurring congenital malformation of the central nervous system (Paige and Carney, 2002).
      a. Incidence of neural tube defects in the United States is estimated as 1:1000 live births (Paige and Carney, 2002).
   2. The risk for a neural tube defect is influenced by race, geographic area, ethnicity, and socioeconomic status.
      a. Risks for recurrence are significantly higher if a previous pregnancy has resulted in a child with a neural tube defect. The risk may actually be nearly triple for subsequent pregnancies (Buck, 2005).

3. The etiology of neural tube defects is multifactorial. Genetic and environmental factors operate independently to determine individual and population risk.
   a. Genetic syndromes may be associated with neural tube defects, but such syndromes account for a small percentage of cases.
   b. Environmental risk factors most commonly identified with development of a neural tube defect include: maternal febrile illness, maternal heat exposure in the first trimester, lower socioeconomic status, dietary factors, and prenatal exposure to drugs (Buck, 2005).
4. The defects result from a failure in closure of the neural groove to form an intact neural tube. The type and severity of the defect is dependent on the location and extent of failure of neurulation.
   a. The spinal column and brain develop from a process called neurulation.
      (1) Primary neurulation occurs between 18 and 28 days of gestation, beginning with folding of the neural plate to form the neural tube. Neural folds meet and fuse with the anterior and posterior ends of the neuropore.
      (2) Secondary neurulation begins at approximately 26 days and continues till 8 weeks postovulatory. Differentiation and cavitation of lower sacral and coccygeal segments occur during this period (Volpe, 2001).
   b. Complete failure of the neural groove to close often results in spontaneous abortion during embryogenesis or early in fetal development.

Specific Neural Tube Defects

Anencephaly

Anencephaly is a primary defect in neural tube closure.
A. **Incidence and etiology.**
   1. Anencephaly is the most common and severe of disorders of anterior neural tube closure, comprising over half of the neural tube defects (Buck, 2005).
      a. Girls are more frequently affected than boys.
      b. The majority of infants are stillborn; of the infants who do survive into the neonatal period, it is uniformly lethal within the first months of life.
   2. Incidence in the United States is estimated at 1:1000 live births.
   3. Recurrence risk for parents who have had one affected child is 1.9% (Jones, 2006).
B. **Clinical presentation.**
   1. General: no documented growth deficiency.
   2. Craniofacial: commonly involves the forebrain and upper brainstem, resulting in absence of the calvaria; cerebral hemispheres are frequently missing, lower brainstem is present, varied facial features, cleft palate and/or lip, altered auricular development, and cervical abnormalities (Jones, 2006).
   3. Musculoskeletal: malformation of the ribs, thoracic cage, abdominal wall, anterior spina bifida, and short neck.
C. **Associated findings.**
   1. Polyhydramnios.
   2. Diaphragmatic defects with/without herniation, hypoplastic lung.
D. **Diagnosis.**
   1. Fetal ultrasound or radiographs in the second trimester to detect absence of vital structures.
   2. Alpha-fetoprotein: major serum protein in the early embryo and is fetus specific. Leakage of fetal serum through an open neural tube defect directly into the amniotic fluid results in elevation of AFP levels. These increases are detected by maternal serum and amniocentesis evaluation.
E. **Treatment/prevention.**
   1. U.S. Public Health Service recommends that women of childbearing age consume 0.4 mg of folic acid daily to decrease their risk for conceiving a child with a neural tube defect. Periconceptional use of vitamins and folate have resulted in a 70% reduction in the recur-

rence of these malformations when given to women who had previously given birth to an infant with a neural tube disorder (Jorde et al., 2003).
   2. As most anencephalic infants are stillborn or die within a few days of delivery, the parents must prepare for the death of their infant at a time when they would be anticipating the birth. Support for the family must take into account their individual preferences and needs. Counseling must be made available short-term as well as long-term, with attention to future pregnancy risks.
   3. The opportunity for these infants to serve as organ donors is complex. Ethical and legal concerns over the diagnosis of brain death and persistent clinical signs of brainstem function have limited the donation of organs from anencephalic infants.
   4. Following delivery, care is supportive, reflecting the desires of the family.

Encephalocele

Defects are secondary to restricted failure of the anterior neuropore to close at approximately day 26 of gestation, resulting in extension of the brain tissue through a defect in the skull.
A. **Incidence and etiology.**
   1. 1:2000 to 1:5000 live births (Wynbrandt and Ludman, 2000).
   2. Precise mechanism for development is unclear; geographic or ethnic genetic factors appear to influence location of the lesion (Buck, 2005).
   3. Genetic factors may be indicated; autosomal recessive patterns of inheritance have been reported, that is, Meckel syndrome, Walker–Warburg syndrome (Buck, 2005).
   4. Environmental factors, including maternal teratogens have been linked to development of encephalocele.
      a. Maternal febrile illness resulting in temperatures of 38.9° C (102.2° F) or greater within the first one third to one half of gestation to be teratogenic (Jones, 2006).
B. **Clinical presentation.**
   1. Craniofacial: cranial defect through which brain protrudes. Defects are commonly occipital (80%), with frontal, temporal, and parietal composing the remainder. Lesions generally are covered by skin or membrane.
C. **Associated findings.**
   1. Microcephaly, arrhinencephaly, cleft lip/palate, craniosynostosis occur in approximately one half of the affected children (Buck, 2005). Small midface, micrognathia, cleft lip/or palate, ear anomalies (Jones, 2006).
   2. Hydrocephalus is present in 50% of infants.
   3. Partial or complete agenesis of the corpus callosum (Buck, 2005).
   4. Mental deficiencies.
   5. Hypotonia.
D. **Diagnosis.**
   1. Evaluation of these defects is supported through the use of radiographs of the skull, transillumination of the defect, cranial ultrasound, and CT or MRI imaging.
   2. Chromosomal studies should be undertaken if suspicion of a genetic syndrome is present.
   3. Careful history of maternal exposure to teratogens or adverse environmental events may provide clues to etiology.
E. **Treatment.**
   1. Based on the individual position and extent of the lesion.
      a. Neurosurgical relief is indicated for most lesions, especially if cerebrospinal fluid is leaking from the lesion. Mortality and morbidity are dependent on the individual lesion. Of those children surviving initial repair, a significant number will have neurologic defects, paralysis, seizures, and deficits in muscular coordination.
   2. For those families who experience a child with an encephalocele, genetic counseling is essential as recurrence risk is estimated at 3% to 5%, depending on the etiology of the defect.
   3. Decisions for supportive care must include the parents.

4. Education concerning the individual patient's primary defect, associated defects, and needs for long-term care must be provided.

Spina Bifida

Defects of the spinal cord resulting from restricted failure of the posterior neuropore to close at approximately day 26 of gestation, resulting in failure of the neural plate to join together to form an intact neural tube.

A. **Incidence and etiology.**
   1. The overall incidence in the United States is estimated to be 0.2 to 0.4 per 1000 live births (Buck, 2005).
   2. Precise etiology is unknown, believed to multifactorial in origin.
      a. A greater number of females than males are affected (Volpe, 2001).
      b. Ethnic and racial group differences exist, with Egyptians, Irish, and English demonstrating higher occurrence rates.
      c. Rates for recurrence are higher for mothers who have had a child with a neural tube defect; from between 1% and 5% to 4% to 9%.

B. **Clinical presentation.**
   1. Defects are divided into two categories:
      a. Spina bifida occulta: Mildest form of the defect presenting with skin covering the opening in the spinal column.
         (1) Defect is often limited to the dermal sinus between adjacent vertebrae.
         (2) Hairy patch or birthmark may be present above the defect.
         (3) Defect may present as a bulge under the skin as the spinal cord ends terminate in fatty tissue.
   2. Spina bifida manifesta: Defects occur most often in the lumbar or lumbosacral area (69%) (Buck, 2005). The defect is clearly evident as a protrusion on the infant's back.
      a. Defects are divided into two categories:
         (1) Meningocele: restricted herniation of meninges at the site of defect. Defect is usually covered by skin; neurologic function is usually normal.
         (2) Myelomeningocele: characterized by herniation of meninges and spinal cord at the site of the defect. Lesions may or may not have vertebral or dermal covering. These defects are 4 times more common than meningoceles (Buck, 2005).

C. **Associated findings.**
   1. Hydrocephalus is a common associated development either at birth or shortly after.
      a. Development correlates with the site of the lesion: 60% in patients with occipital, cervical, or thoracic lesions; 90% in infants with thoracolumbar, lumbar, or lumbosacral lesions.
   2. Chronic bladder infections and subsequent kidney deterioration.
   3. Kyphosis at birth; scoliosis later in childhood.
   4. Club feet secondary to neurologic and orthopedic abnormalities.
   5. Dislocation of hips.
   6. Arnold–Chiari malformation occurs in 95% of patients with a lumbar lesion (Buck, 2005).
   7. Mental retardation in 30% of infants with myelomeningocele (Volpe, 2001).

D. **Diagnosis.**
   1. Serum alpha-fetoprotein elevation in maternal serum at 16 to 18 weeks.
   2. Amniotic fluid acetylcholinesterase and amniotic AFP at 14 to 16 weeks.
   3. Fetal ultrasound.
   4. Radiographs and CT and MRI imaging following delivery.

E. **Treatment.**
   1. Clinical management is individualized to the type and position of the lesion.
      a. Early surgical repair is advocated for most infants to preserve cognitive function, improve prognosis for ambulation, and decrease mortality.

    b. Assessment of function at the level of the lesion allows for estimates of potential capabilities; motor, sensory, and sphincter function.

2. Periconceptual administration of folic acid has demonstrated improvement in the rate and development of neural tube defects.
3. Secondary to the extensive associated finding for these defects, parents must be made aware of the need for continuing care and support. Often a team approach is needed to ensure that complications are minimized.

       a. Kyphosis may worsen over time, especially as the child enters puberty. Scheduled developmental exams are needed to track growth and maintain ambulation.

Cleft Lip and Cleft Palate

Cleft lip and palate result as a failure of mesenchymal masses in the medial nasal and maxillary prominences and palatal shelves to meet and fuse (Moore, 2003).

A. Etiology and incidence.
1. Defects represent one of the most common structural defects; overall frequency is approximately 1:1000 (Lewanda et al., 2006).
2. Racial predilection exists, with Native American and Asian populations experiencing rates as high as 1:250 to 1:350 births (Carey, 2003).
3. Male infants are affected more often than female infants.
4. Multifactorial inheritance with a hereditary component is believed to be causative for these lesions. Most cases represent sporadic events, but recurrence within families has been documented. Mothers who have a first child with orofacial clefts carry a 4% risk for the next child (McLean, 2005). Severity of defect raises the risk for recurrence (Jones, 2006).

B. Clinical presentation.
1. Presentation of the defect is variable, with cleft lip and palate frequently occurring together (Jones, 2006).
2. Defect may occur as a part of a syndrome of anomalies.
3. Unilateral cleft lip most commonly occurs on the left side.
4. Bilateral cleft lip is usually accompanied by a cleft palate.

C. Associated findings.
1. Defects of tooth development in the area of the cleft.
2. Incomplete growth of nasal structures.
3. Mild ocular hypertelorism.
4. Speech deficits and language delay.
5. Frequent episodes of otitis media secondary to palatal incompetence and conductive hearing loss (Jones, 2006).
6. Airway obstruction issues; especially if Robin sequence is associated.

D. Diagnosis.
1. Ultrasound evaluation with close attention to the oral and facial areas may provide a clue to the presence of the defect prenatally.
2. Careful physical examination following delivery; as many as 42% of infants with cleft palate may have an associated syndrome (Jones, 2006).

E. Treatment.
1. The degree of defect may markedly alter the ability for the infant to bottle-feed effectively. A variety of feeding systems and nipples are available, and trial of many types may be needed to find the appropriate system.

       a. Dental appliances can be helpful to provide a palatal surface.

       b. Dentition patterns should be monitored closely, timing interventions with surgical intervention.
2. Development of speech must be closely monitored and therapy provided as an ongoing portion of care.
3. Surgical correction of the lip occurs first—usually when the infant is gaining weight and weighs 8 to 10 pounds. Palatal repair occurs later at 1 to 2 years of age.

4. Airway management is a primary concern. Safety of the infant must be ensured before the infant is discharged. Those infants with associated micrognathia and glossoptosis may require protective positioning and possible tracheostomy.

Developmental Dysplasia of the Hip

Wide Spectrum of Abnormalities That Affect the Femoral Head and Acetabulum

A. **Incidence and etiology.**
1. Defect occurs in 1 of 800 live births (Sniderman and Taeusch, 2005).
2. Female infants are affected more commonly than males: 19:1000 (Grottkau and Goldberg, 2005).
3. Genetic and ethnic factors play a role, with white females having the highest number of affected infants (Sniderman and Taeusch, 2005).
4. Etiology is multifactorial, though genetic factors may be involved as recurrence rates for siblings of an affected neonate are increased.
   a. Prenatal breech positioning, especially frank breech with hips flexed and knees bent, increases the risk.
   b. Ligamentous laxity secondary to circulating maternal hormone (relaxin) exerts an effect, resulting in hip dislocation. Familial ligamentous laxity has also been described.
5. In utero conditions that limit movement as well as specific syndromes and chromosomal disorders may be associated with hip dysplasia.
6. Left hip alone is affected 60% of the time, the right hip 20%, and both hips 20% (Grottkau and Goldberg, 2005).

B. **Clinical presentation.**
1. The defect is variable in expression from the dislocatable hip to fixed dislocations.
2. Anatomic changes are minimal in the neonate. As the hip becomes permanently dislocated, pathologic changes of the acetabulum, femoral head, hip capsule joints, and ligaments can occur. End result is degenerative changes in femoral head and acetabulum.
3. Physical examination will demonstrate differences in adduction, apparent shortening of the affected femur, and extra skin folds.

C. **Associated findings.**
1. Associated with other postural adductus deformities such as torticollis, talipes equinovarus, and metatarsus deformities.
2. A strong correlation with Larsen syndrome (multiple joint dislocations) exists (Jones, 2006).
3. Unilateral defects often have secondary problems with limb-length inequality, ipsilateral knee deformity, scoliosis, and disturbances in gait.

D. **Diagnosis.**
1. Physical tests are aimed at determining if the femoral head is fixed in the acetabulum. Tests should be repeated at intervals within the first year of life as a dislocation may not be demonstrated for several months following delivery.
   a. Barlow's test: determines if the femoral head can be dislocated posteriorly.
   b. Ortolani test: determines if femoral head is dislocated laterally.
   c. If the dislocation is a fixed type of lesion, Barlows and Ortolani tests are not helpful as the femoral head is locked outside of the acetabulum. Diagnosis is made by palpation of the femoral head posteriorly (Sniderman and Taeusch, 2005).
   d. Galeazzi's sign: presence of asymmetrical thigh and/or buttock folds.
2. Radiographs are helpful but are difficult to obtain secondary to the high percentage of cartilage in newborn infants. Beginning at 4 to 6 months, the gold standard is the AP pelvic radiograph.
   a. In early infancy, real-time ultrasound may provide the best diagnostic evidence of the deformity.

E. **Treatment.**
1. Following delivery, unstable hips must be monitored closely. A percentage of unstable hips will stabilize, whereas others progress to subluxation or dislocation. The outcome

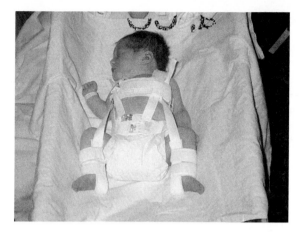

FIGURE 35-4 ■ Infant with dislocated hips in a Pavlik harness. (Courtesy Jane Deacon, RNC, MS, NNP, The Children's Hospital, Denver, Colorado.)

of hip stability cannot be predicted: all newborns with clinical hip instability should be treated.

2. Initial goal of treatment is reduction of the displaced femoral head and support of acetabular and femoral head growth. Reduction and stability of the femoral head are needed for normal growth and development of the hip joint.

3. The Pavlik harness is the most commonly used device to prevent adduction while allowing flexion and abduction. Treatment is provided on a full-time basis for a period of 6 weeks. The harness encourages deepening and stability of the acetabulum. Treatment is successful in 90% of patients (Grottkau and Goldberg, 2005) (Fig. 35-4).

4. For those infants for whom harnessing is not effective or the lesion is fixed, surgical intervention may be required.

5. Ongoing developmental assessment of these infants is needed to monitor the infant for secondary deformities.

6. Parents play a pivotal part in the success in management of harnessing therapy. It is vital for parents to have a clear understanding of the deformity and plan for care.

Talipes Equinovarus

Developmental deformity of the hindfoot.

A. **Incidence and etiology.**
   1. Defect occurs in 1:1000 to 2:1000 live births (Grottkau and Goldberg, 2005).
   2. Club foot is bilateral in 50% of cases, with males affected twice as often as females.
   3. Inheritance is believed to be multifactorial in nature.
      a. Mendelian: usually as part of a syndrome. Autosomal dominant and X-linked recessive.
      b. Extrinsic causes: related to changes within the uterine environment, uterine abnormalities, oligohydramnios, and effects of uterine pressure during critical periods of development.
      c. Neural origin: neuromuscular pathologic conditions, resulting in muscle fibrosis, shortening of muscles, and development of contractures.
   4. Recurrence rates are increased for subsequent children.

B. **Clinical presentation.**
   1. Clinically, the foot has a medial crease, with toes pointing toward midline; the sole of the foot is angulated medially; and the hindfoot is plantar flexed (Grottkau and Goldberg, 2005) (Fig. 35-5).
      a. The calf and foot are smaller than the contralateral side.

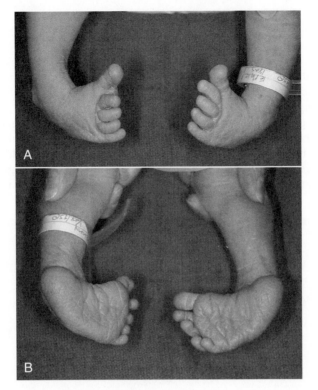

FIGURE 35-5 ▪ Bilateral talipes equinovarus. Note structural deformity of hind part of foot. (Courtesy Jane Deacon, RNC, MS, NNP, The Children's Hospital, Denver, Colorado.)

   b. Associated dysplasia of osseous, muscular, tendons, cartilage, skin, and neurovascular tissues distal to the knee of the affected extremity (Grottkau and Goldberg, 2005).
   c. Weight bearing is not possible secondary to position of the foot.
C. Associated anomalies.
   1. Deformity is associated with Smith–Lemli–Opitz, Larsen, Freeman–Sheldon, and Poland syndromes.
   2. Congenital hip dysplasia, neural tube defects, particularly myelomeningocele.
   3. Myotonic dystrophy.
D. Diagnosis.
   1. Physical examination and manipulation of the foot through range of motion.
   2. Radiographs are helpful, assist with diagnosis of other bony abnormalities.
E. Treatment.
   1. Initial treatment for all congenital clubfoot is nonoperative; early treatment is more successful secondary to pliability of tissues and resilience to immobilization.
      a. Manipulation, serial casting, and taping are first-line treatment, lasting for 3 to 4 months.
      b. Surgical intervention, if needed, is done at 9 to 12 months of age—before the infant begins to walk (Grottkau and Goldberg, 2005).
      c. 15% of cases will demonstrate recurrence; further surgical intervention is needed.
   2. Parents must be educated to the importance of their role in ongoing treatment.

Polydactyly

A. Incidence and etiology.
   1. Inherited as an autosomal dominant trait.
   2. Incidence is common: anomaly results from a duplication error in which a stimulus induces excessive limb bud formation.

B. Clinical findings.
  1. Commonly involves the ulnar aspect of the hand; affected digits are often incomplete and lack muscular development. Defects are often bilateral (Fig. 35-6).
  2. Abnormalities are divided into three classifications: soft tissue mass connected by a tissue pedicle; partial duplication involving the phalanges; and complete duplication of the digit with bony formation (Mosca, 2001).
C. Associated findings.
  1. The anatomic placement of the digit varies and is associated with genetic syndromes.
    a. Preaxial or duplicate thumbs occur most commonly as an isolated lesion. Defect has been associated with Holt–Oram, Fanconi, and Ellis–van Crevald syndromes.
    b. Triphalangeal thumb; also referred to as a thumbless, five-fingered hand. Defect is associated with trisomies 13 and 15, and Blackfan–Diamond and Fanconi syndromes.

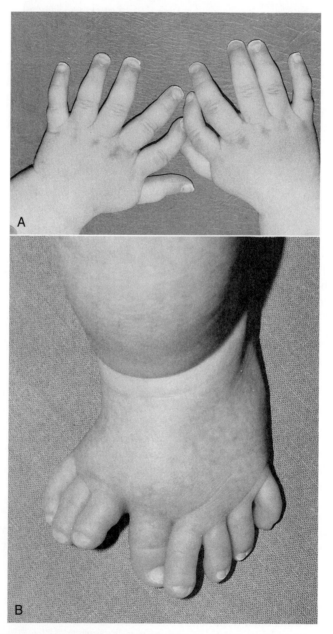

FIGURE 35-6 ■ Polydactyly of hands (**A**) and feet (**B**). This condition results from formation of one or more extra digital rays during the embryonic period. (Courtesy Dr. A.E. Chudley, Department of Pediatrics and Child Health, University of Manitoba, Children's Hospital, Winnipeg, Manitoba, Canada.)

D. Diagnosis.
1. Physical examination.
2. Radiologic exam to identify bony defects.

E. Treatment.
1. Treatment is dependent on defect.
2. Therapy is aimed toward preservation of function and motion, as well as provision of cosmetic remedy.
3. Education of parents as to the risks for recurrence and associated syndromes is essential.

DEFORMATION ABNORMALITIES

Amniotic Band Syndrome

A. Incidence and etiology.
1. Amniotic band sequence occurs in 1 in 1200 to 1 in 1500 newborns (Lewanda et al., 2006).
2. Etiology is sporadic, with little risk of recurrence. Secondary to amnion rupture, strands of amnion encircle developing structures (Jones, 2006).
   a. Defects are dependent on the degree of entanglement, timing of insult, and the body part involved (Lewanda et al., 2006).
   b. Maternal trauma has been related to development.

B. Clinical findings.
1. Constriction bands commonly involve the distal portion of limbs, resulting in Annular constrictions, pseudosyndactyly, intrauterine amputations, and umbilical cord constriction (Jones, 2006) (Fig. 35-7).
   a. Deformational defects occur secondary to the primary insult.
   (1) Loss of fetal movement can occur following tethering of a limb, resulting in foot or hand abnormalities.
   (2) Constraint deformities result from a lack of amniotic fluid.
   (3) Neurologic defects distal to the defect may occur.
   (4) Defect may involve veins, arteries, and nerves, compromising circulation and growth of affected extremities.

C. Associated findings.
1. Club feet occurring in 12% to 56% of affected infants. Treatment may be difficult owing to the rigid position and paralysis secondary to nerve damage.
2. Angular deformity, bone dysplasia, pseudoarthrosis, and anterolateral bowing of the tibia may occur secondary to deep constriction bands in extremities.
3. Leg length discrepancy exceeding 2.5 cm occurs in 25% of children (Mosca, 2001).
4. Syndactyly, brachydactyly.
5. Cranial vault defects.

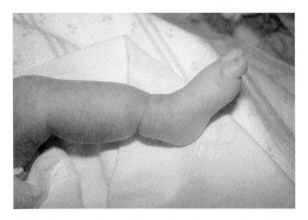

FIGURE 35-7 ■ Amniotic band constriction of lower leg. (Courtesy Jane Deacon, RNC, MS, NNP, The Children's Hospital, Denver, Colorado.)

6. If amniotic fluid has been leaking, features of oligohydramnios deformation may occur (Jones, 2006).

D. **Diagnosis.**
 1. No one feature consistently occurs as this is a disruption sequence abnormality. No two infants will present with exactly the same defect.
    a. Physical examination, including vascular supply, joint function.
    b. Examination of the placenta for aberrant bands or strands of amnion, or rolled-up remnants of amnion at the placental base of the umbilical cord (Jones, 2006).
 2. Radiographs assist with definition and classification of defect.

E. **Treatment.**
 1. Dependent on anatomic position, associated abnormalities.
    a. If constriction is severe, early surgical relief is needed to preserve vascular, lymph and nerve integrity.
    b. Deformities that pose no emergent threat are best repaired at ages 1 to 2 years. Repair may require a staged approach; repair is seldom completed in one surgery.
 2. Genetic counseling is necessary to educate parents as to the rare likelihood of recurrence. The appearance of some defects is significantly severe as to discourage further pregnancies, and accurate diagnosis of these defects is essential.
 3. Life expectancy is normal unless brain malformation or deep facial clefts are present.

Talipes Calcaneovalgus

A. **Incidence and etiology.**
 1. Thought to be a postural defect secondary to intrauterine positioning, characterized by marked dorsiflexion of the entire foot at the ankle joint (Mosca, 2001).
 2. Incidence of defect is estimated at 0.4 to 1 per 1000 births (Grottkau and Goldberg, 2005).
    a. More common following breech deliveries.
    b. Girls are affected more often than boys.

B. **Clinical findings.**
 1. Dorsum of the foot is, or is easily, positioned directly apposed to the anterior aspect of the leg.
    a. Soft tissues of the dorsal and lateral aspects of the foot are often contracted, limiting plantar flexion and inversion (Mosca, 2001).

C. **Associated findings.**
 1. Increased association with hip dysplasia; no hip dysplasia present initially.
 2. May occur with external rotation of the tibia, and posteromedial bowing of the tibia.

D. **Diagnosis.**
 1. Physical examination provides the diagnosis for this condition.
    a. Reveals free mobility of the foot to passive manipulation.
    b. Hindfoot is in the dorsiflexed position so that the plantar aspect of the forefront is in line. Plantar flexion of the foot is limited.
 2. Must be differentiated from congenital vertical talus.

E. **Treatment.**
 1. Evaluation for hip dysplasia is essential; repeated exams are needed.
 2. Gentle stretching exercises, done with diaper changes, will usually resolve this positional deformity within 3 to 6 months (Grottkau and Goldberg, 2005).
 3. Infrequently, serial casting may be required; rarely ankle–foot orthoses are needed.
 4. Parents provide an active part in resolution of this condition and must be aware of the need for ongoing treatment and follow-up examinations.

CONGENITAL METABOLIC PROBLEMS

The process by which the body converts food into energy is complex. Disturbances in these processes result in a wide array of medical problems. The following section will review some of the more common inborn errors that affect the newborn.

Inborn Errors of Metabolism

A. **Incidence and etiology.**
   1. Inborn errors of metabolism are genetic biochemical disorders that left untreated can cause brain damage and death.
   2. In newborns, metabolic diseases are secondary to malfunctioning of both maternally and paternally inherited alleles at one specific gene locus (Berry, 2005).
      a. Errors of metabolism are usually inherited as autosomal recessive or X-linked recessive traits.
      b. Gene mutations produce deficiencies in enzymes, cofactors, transport proteins, and cellular functions.
   3. Newborn metabolic diseases can be classified into two groups:
      a. Defects involving complex molecules—storage diseases.
      b. Defects concerning the intermediary metabolism of small molecules—glucose, lactate, amino acids, organic acids, and ammonia (Berry, 2005).
B. **Clinical presentation.**
   1. The fetus is afforded protection as the placenta effectively removes circulating toxins. The newborn appears normal at birth but may quickly present with life-threatening symptoms as the underlying metabolic defect is manifested.
   2. Symptoms of inborn errors commonly include the following:
      a. Metabolic encephalopathy: lethargy, changes in muscle tone, seizures, irritability, weak suck, and apnea.
      b. Respiratory: tachypnea and apnea secondary to underlying metabolic acidosis and metabolic encephalopathy.
      c. Gastrointestinal symptoms: vomiting secondary to protein intolerance, failure to gain weight despite adequate intake and formula changes.
      d. Cardiac symptoms: cardiomyopathy, arrhythmias.
      e. Hepatic symptoms: appear within the first 2 weeks of life. Jaundice: usually direct reacting associated with vomiting, diarrhea, poor weight gain, hepatomegaly, cataract formation, and hypoglycemia.
      f. Unusual body or urinary odor. In phenylketonuria, infant's urine has a musty odor, whereas the urine of infants with maple syrup urine disease has a sweet odor secondary to isovaleric acidemia.
      g. Ocular findings: cataracts, glaucoma, corneal clouding, and dislocated lenses.
C. **Diagnosis.**
   1. Goals of treatment include identification, treatment, and prevention of major sequelae (Matthews and Robin, 2006).
      a. Mandatory screening of newborns: tandem mass spectrometry enables a single spot of blood to test for more than 40 inborn errors of metabolism.
         (1) All states require screening for PKU, hypothyroidism, and galactosemia.
         (2) Expanded newborn screening is mandated by individual states.
         (3) This technology allows for low-cost, high efficiency testing.
         (4) Collection of samples must be undertaken early (before 7 days of age) and repeated at prescribed intervals (Matthews and Robin, 2006).

DISORDERS OF METABOLISM

Errors of Protein Metabolism

Phenylketonuria

A. **Incidence and etiology.**
   1. PKU is the most common inborn error of amino acid metabolism that may result in mental retardation (Matthews and Robin, 2006).
      a. Occurs in 1:12,000 live births.
      b. Gene location: chromosome 12q22-q24.1. Inherited as an autosomal recessive trait.
      c. Results from a deficiency of the liver enzyme phenylalanine hydrolase to convert phenylalanine to tyrosine. Lack of this enzyme is responsible for brain disease.

B. Clinical findings.
   1. Symptoms occur following birth to 6 months of age; early symptoms include vomiting, poor feedings, overactivity, and irritability.
   2. After 6 months of age, developmental delays are evident; seizures, infantile spasms, and musty-smelling urine (Berry, 2005).

C. Diagnosis.
   1. Standard newborn screening.
   2. DNA sequencing and mutational analysis are used to identify carriers in families, and assist with family genetic counseling (Berry, 2005).

D. Treatment.
   1. Therapy consists of a low protein diet and use of special amino acid–containing formula that does not have phenylalanine.
   2. Parents must be counseled to understand the importance of continued dietary restrictions.

Errors of Carbohydrate Metabolism

Galactosemia

A. Incidence and etiology.
   1. Three enzymes of the galactose metabolic pathway convert galactose to glucose. GALT (one of the enzymes) deficiency is the most common of these disorders (Berry, 2005).
     a. Lactose is a disaccharide composed of galactose and glucose—deficiency of GALT enzyme blocks conversion, so infants are unable to metabolize lactose.
   2. Incidence 1 in 35,000 to 60,000 (Berry, 2005).
   3. Inherited as an autosomal recessive condition (Gilbert, 2000).

B. Clinical findings.
   1. Initial signs of deficiency include poor growth, vomiting, poor feeding, irritability, or lethargy.
   2. Jaundice; presenting in the first weeks of life, persisting.
   3. Later signs: multiorgan toxicity, with liver disease that progresses to cirrhosis, anemia, lethargy, and cataracts.
     a. *Escherichia coli* sepsis occurs as a complication in 50% of the affected infants (Berry, 2005).

C. Associated findings.
   1. Speech defects—especially expressive speech.
   2. Convulsions.
   3. Infertility.

D. Diagnosis.
   1. Chorionic villus sampling at 9 to 12 weeks, amniocentesis at 16 weeks: either one demonstrating deficiency of enzyme.
   2. Newborn screening demonstrating absence of the enzyme necessary for breakdown and metabolism of galactose.
   3. Laboratory: serum blood galactose levels, RBC galactose-1 phosphate levels, and elevated urine galactitol. Albuminuria, hyperbilirubinemia, elevated ALT and AST levels.
     a. Positive reducing substances in urine are present in severe hypergalactosemia.

E. Treatment.
   1. Initiation of a lactose-free diet is essential. This reflects a life-long change; parents must receive appropriate counseling to ensure long-term success.
   2. With treatment, intellectual development may be normal or near normal. But even for infants who receive treatment, rates of mental retardation remain higher.
   3. Communication problems continue throughout life despite speech therapy.

Inborn Errors of Amino Acid Metabolism

Maple Sugar Urine Disease

A. Incidence and etiology.
   1. MSUD is a rare inborn error occurring in 1 of 200,000 live births.
     a. Exception: Pennsylvania Mennonites, in whom the frequency is 1 in 358 (Berry, 2005).

2. Inherited as an autosomal recessive trait. Males and females equally affected.
3. Results from a deficiency of the liver enzyme branched-chain 2-keto-dehydrogenase complex (BCAA).

B. **Clinical findings.**
   1. Infants are usually well at time of delivery, but after 2 to 3 days of feedings, infants demonstrate poor feeding and lethargy. The infant worsens with high pitched cry, hypotonia and hypertonia, eventually becoming obtunded and lapsing into a coma.
   2. Odor of maple syrup is evident on breath, in urine and feces, and in saliva.

C. **Diagnosis.**
   1. Laboratory findings include metabolic acidosis, ketonuria. Elevation of plasma BCAAs, leucine, isoleucine, and valine (Berry, 2005).
   2. Standard metabolic screening.
   3. Molecular diagnosis may be useful in target populations.

D. **Treatment.**
   1. Initial therapy in the acute crisis includes parenteral nutrition modified to be BCAA-free and insulin therapy to manage catabolic stress. Peritoneal dialysis has also been utilized to decrease circulating plasma BCAAs.
      a. For those infants treated within 7 days of life, incidence of mental retardation is diminished. Delays beyond this time result in significant IQ deficiencies, with spastic diplegia or quadriplegia (Berry, 2005).
   2. Long-term management requires a special formula devoid of BCAAs. The intake of formula must be carefully monitored. Supplemental isoleucine and valine may be needed.
   3. The long-term management of these infants requires that parents are vigilant in the provision of the diet and the need for follow-up.

Errors of Fatty Acid Oxidation

Medium-chain Acetyl-CoA Dehydrogenase Deficiency

A. **Incidence and etiology.**
   1. Defect involves an abnormality in the enzyme that facilitate mitochondrial beta oxidation of fatty acids.
      a. Fatty acid oxidation provides energy during periods of caloric deprivation. When normal metabolism is disrupted, the quickly depleted glycogen stores lead to hypoglycemia.
   2. Medium-chain acetyl-CoA dehydrogenase deficiency (MCAD) is the most commonly occurring fatty acid oxidation disorder, occurring in 1 in 20,000 infants.
      a. MCAD gene has been cloned and sequenced, several mutations have been identified (Berry, 2005).
      b. Inherited as an autosomal recessive trait (Gilbert, 2000).

B. **Clinical findings.**
   1. Presentation of symptoms is frequently in later infancy: following an infection, the infant experiences anorexia, vomiting, dehydration, lethargy, and hypoglycemia associated with seizures (Berry, 2005).
      a. High mortality rates are common with initial episodes.
   2. Symptoms may mimic Reye syndrome, death occurring from brain edema.

C. **Associated findings.**
   1. Carnitine deficiency develops as a result of excess excretion of acylcarnitine.
   2. In infants who die suddenly and have fat accumulation in the liver suggests a disorder of fatty acid oxidation.

D. **Diagnosis.**
   1. Chorionic villus sampling, amniocentesis, DNA analysis.
   2. Newborn screening.
   3. Laboratory studies: hypoglycemia, absence of moderate to large ketones in urine.
   4. MCAD enzyme may be assayed in cultured skin fibroblasts (Berry, 2005).

E. **Treatment.**
   1. Symptomatic hypoglycemia is treated aggressively. IV glucose and caloric support must be provided quickly.

2. Prevention of hypoglycemia is the cornerstone of therapy; avoid free fatty acid mobilization during times of catabolic stress and relative insulin deficiency.
3. Diagnosis and treatment of associated carnitine deficiency.
4. Infants having MCAD often have a sibling who has died of sudden infant death syndrome. Accurate diagnosis and genetic counseling are essential.

Fetal Endocrine Disorders

Normal adrenal function is vital for maintenance of intrauterine well-being, organ maturation, and adaptation to extrauterine life (Bethin and Muglia, 2005).

Congenital Adrenal Hyperplasia

A. **Incidence and etiology.**
1. Disorder results secondary to enzyme defect involved with the synthesis of cortisol from cholesterol, resulting in the impaired production of cortisol.
   a. Ninety percent of CAH cases are caused by a 21-hydroxylase deficiency (Bethin and Muglia, 2005).
   b. Inherited as an autosomal recessive genetic trait, believed to be located on the short arm of chromosome 6.
2. Incidence is approximately 1 in 15,000 worldwide, but is as high as 1 in 300 in ethnic populations, e.g., the Yupic Eskimos in Alaska (Bethin and Muglia, 2005).
3. Cortisol production is blocked, resulting in high adrenocorticotropic hormone levels.
      These elevated levels of ACTH stimulate the adrenal glands inappropriately. The end result of this process is adrenal hypertrophy, buildup of cortisol precursors, and excesses of adrenal androgens (Gilbert, 2000).

B. **Clinical findings.**
1. Genital ambiguity—nearly all female infants will display degrees of virilization.
   Infants with severe CAH may have a single perineal orifice that originates from a fused vagina and urethra. Males have no apparent genital defects.
2. Two forms of classic 21-hydroxylase deficiencies exist:
   a. Salt losing: both cortisol and aldosterone production are blocked, resulting in excess sodium loss through the kidneys—accounts for 75% of cases (Gilbert, 2000).
   b. Electrolyte imbalances are common: elevated serum potassium and decreased sodium levels may not be evident for 1 week. As aldosterone is depleted, effects become evident.
   c. Symptoms of acute adrenal insufficiency and salt-losing crisis include weakness, vomiting, dehydration, hyponatremia, hypokalemia, and hypoglycemia.
   d. Non–salt losing: only cortisol production is blocked. Aldosterone production is usually adequate.
      (1) Mild deficit of aldosterone production presents as an elevated plasma rennin activity or mild hyponatremia in times of stress (Gilbert, 2000).
      (2) Affected infants are frequently undiagnosed for years: they are frequently unable to handle stress—illnesses may become protracted for minor illness or may develop acute adrenal insufficiency when stressors are severe.

C. **Associated findings.**
1. Growth abnormalities.
2. Seizure activity.
3. Infertility.

D. **Diagnosis.**
1. Pelvic ultrasound examination to determine if a uterus is present.
2. Abdominal ultrasound to evaluate the adrenals—usually longer and wider in affected infants, greater echogenicity than normal infants, and have unusual surface characteristics (Bethin and Muglia, 2005).
3. Chorionic villus sampling at 9 to 10 weeks, amniocentesis at 14 to 16 weeks. DNA analysis to determine sex of the infant or presence of deficiency status in female.
4. Newborn screening, repeat if presumptive.
5. Serum cortisol levels.

E. Treatment.

1. All infants with ambiguous genitalia must be screened for CAH.

2. Intrauterine therapy is provided for fetuses when a diagnosis is made, or if the pregnancy is complicated by a previous infant with CAH, as soon as possible.

    a. Fetal therapy should prevent occurrence of associated structural defects; therapy should begin as soon as possible, preferably before 6 weeks of gestation. The degree of structural deformity in the female is related to the timing of therapy. Maternal dexamethasone is the drug of choice.

3. For infants with classic deficiency syndrome, sodium and mineralocorticoid replacement is required.

4. For female infants suffering with genital abnormalities, the possibility of incorrect gender assignment is a possibility. Correct diagnosis is vital for long-term support and acceptance of these individuals.

5. Genetic counseling must be provided, especially if the family desires additional children. Parents must be screened for carrier state as recurrence risk is elevated for these families.

REFERENCES

Berry, G.: Congenital metabolic problems. In H. Taeusch, R. Ballard, and C. Gleason (Eds.): *Avery's diseases of the newborn* (8th ed.). Philadelphia, 2005, Saunders, pp. 217-226.

Bethin, K. and Muglia, L.: Disorders of the adrenal gland. In H. Taeusch, R. Ballard, and C. Gleason (Eds.): *Avery's diseases of the newborn* (8th ed.). Philadelphia, 2005, Saunders, pp. 1366-1373.

Buck, S.: Congenital malformations of the central nervous system. In H. Taeusch, R. Ballard, and C. Gleason (Eds.): *Avery's diseases of the newborn* (8th ed.). Philadelphia, 2005, Saunders, pp. 938-963.

Carey, J.: Chromosome disorders. In C. Rudolphs, A. Rudolph, M. Hostetter, G. Lister, and N. Sigel (Eds.): *Rudolph's pediatrics* (21st ed.). New York, 2003, McGraw-Hill, pp 731-741.

Cole, W.: Genetic aspects of orthopaedic conditions. In R. Morrissy and S. Weinstein (Eds.): *Lovell and Winter's pediatric orthopaedics*. Philadelphia, 2001, Lippincott Williams & Wilkins, pp. 158-176.

Dorland's illustrated medical dictionary (31st ed.). Philadelphia, 2007, Saunders.

Gilbert, P.: *A-Z syndromes and inherited disorders* (3rd ed). United Kingdom, 2000, Stanley Thornes, pp. 83-86, 92-94.

Grottkau, B. and Goldberg, M.: Common neonatal orthopedic ailments. In H. Taeusch, R. Ballard, and C. Gleason (Eds.): *Avery's diseases of the newborn* (8th ed.). Philadelphia, 2005, Saunders, pp. 1423-1435.

Hudgins, L. and Cassidy, S.: Congenital anomalies. In R. Morrisy and S. Weinstein (Eds.): *Neonatal perinatal medicine: Diseases of the fetus and in infant*. St. Louis, 2002, Lippincott Williams & Wilkins, pp. 158-176.

Jones, L.: *Smith's recognizable patterns of human malformation* (6th ed.). Philadelphia, 2006, Saunders.

Jorde, L., Carey, J., Bamshed, M., and White, R.: *Medical genetics* (3rd ed.). St. Louis, 2003, Mosby.

Kaplan, P.: Skeletal dysplasias and connective tissue disorders. In H. Taeusch, R. Ballard, and C. Gleason (Eds.): *Avery's diseases of the newborn* (8th ed.). Philadelphia, 2005, Saunders, pp. 279-299.

Larsen, W.: Gametogenesis, fertilization, and the first week of life. In *Human embryology* (3rd ed.). Philadelphia, 2001, Churchill Livingstone, pp. 1-35.

Lashley, F.: Birth defects and congenital anomalies. In *Clinical genetics in nursing practice*. (3rd ed.). New York, 2005, Springer, pp. 147-160.

Lewanda, A., Boyadjiev, S., and Jabs, E.: Dysmorphology: Genetic syndromes and associations. In J. McMillan, R. Feigin, C. DeAngelis, and M. Jones (Eds.): *Oski's pediatrics* (4th ed.). Philadelphia, 2006, Lippincott Williams & Wilkins, pp. 2629-2669.

Matthews, A. and Robin, N.: Genetic disorders and malformations and inborn errors of Metabolism. In G. Merenstein and S. Gardner (Eds.): *Handbook of neonatal intensive care*. St. Louis, 2006, Mosby, pp. 812-837.

McLean, S.D.: Congenital anomalies. In M.G. MacDonald, M.D. Mullett, and M.M. Seshia (Eds.) *Avery's neonatology: Pathophysiology and management of the newborn* (6th ed.). Philadelphia, 2005, Lippincott Williams & Wilkins, pp. 892-913.

Moore, K. and Persaud, T.: Human birth defects. In *The developing human: Clinically oriented embryology* (8th ed.). Philadelphia, 2007, Saunders, pp. 158-186.

Mosca, V.: The foot. In R. Morrissy and S. Weinstein (Eds.): *Lovell and Winter's pediatric orthopaedics*. Philadelphia, 2001, Lippincott Williams & Wilkins, pp. 1151-1215.

Paige, P. and Carney, P.: Neurologic disorders. In G.B. Merenstein and S.L. Gardner (Eds.): *Handbook of neonatal intensive care* (5th ed.). St. Louis, 2002, Mosby, pp. 644-655.

Saitta, S. and Zackai, E.: Specific chromosome disorders in newborns. In H. Taeusch, R. Ballard, and C. Gleason (Eds.): *Avery's diseases of the newborn* (8th ed.). Philadelphia, 2005, Saunders, pp. 204-215.

Sniderman, S. and Taeusch, H.: Initial evaluation: History and physical examination of the newborn. In H. Taeusch, R. Ballard, and C. Gleason (Eds.): *Avery's diseases of the newborn* (8th ed.). Philadelphia, 2005, Saunders, pp. 301-322.

Volpe, J.: Neural tube formation on prosencephalic development. In J. Volpe (Ed.): *Neurology of the newborn* (5th ed.). Philadelphia, 2008, Saunders, pp. 3-44.

Wynbrandt, J. and Ludman, M.: *The encyclopedia of genetic disorders and birth defects* (2nd ed.). New York, 2000, Facts on File, Inc, pp. 237-239, 293, 295.

Zaleske, D.: Metabolic and endocrine abnormalities. In R. Morrissy and S. Weinstein (Eds.): *Lovell and Winter's pediatric orthopaedics*. Philadelphia, 2001, Lippincott Williams & Wilkins, pp. 177-241.

36 Neonatal Dermatology

CATHERINE L. WITT

OBJECTIVES

1. Name three functions of the skin.

2. Describe two ways in which the skin of a newborn or preterm infant differs from that of an adult.

3. Identify three factors that affect the appearance of the neonate's skin.

4. Identify two nursing interventions that provide protection for the preterm infant's skin.

5. Recognize three common skin lesions that are normal variations in the newborn infant. Describe their appearance and treatment, if any.

6. Describe three common vascular lesions in the neonate, their appearance, and appropriate treatment.

7. Identify two syndromes associated with vascular lesions.

8. Evaluate two pigmented lesions occurring in the newborn infant and list implications associated with each.

9. Name two types of infectious skin lesions and select the appropriate treatment.

Careful assessment of the skin is an important element of the neonatal physical examination. The appearance of the skin gives the nurse important clues regarding gestational age, nutritional status, function of organs such as the heart and liver, and the presence of cutaneous or systemic disease. It is important for the clinician to be familiar with normal variances in the skin of the newborn infant as well as those variances that signify disease.

Proper care of the neonate's skin can directly affect mortality and morbidity, especially in the preterm infant. The skin is the first line of defense against infection. Proper skin care can protect the integrity of the skin and prevent breakdown.

ANATOMY AND PHYSIOLOGY OF THE SKIN

A. **Anatomy of the skin—three main layers** (Fig. 36-1).

1. Epidermis: outermost layer, which functions as a barrier from outside penetration. The epidermis is subdivided into the following:

   a. Stratum corneum: outermost layer, consisting of closely packed dead cells that are consistently brushed off and replaced by lower levels of the epidermis. These cells are flatter and have thicker walls than other cells. The cells are held together by intracellular lipids, which aid in forming the protective barrier of the skin.

   b. Lower layers of epidermis: contain keratin-forming cells that create the outer layer of skin as well as melanocytes, which produce melanin, or pigment. Despite racial differences in pigmentation, the number of melanocytes in a given surface area of skin is the same (Weston et al., 2007).

2. Dermis: directly under epidermis; 2 to 4 mm thick at birth. The dermis is composed of

   a. Collagen and elastic fibers that connect the epidermis and dermis and provide the skin with the ability to stretch and then to return to normal shape;

   b. Blood vessels and nerves that carry sensations of heat, touch, pain, and pressure from the skin to the brain and provides protection against injury, infections, or other invasions; and

   c. Sweat glands, sebaceous glands, and hair shafts.

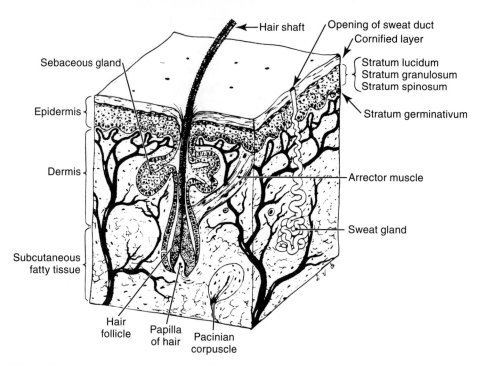

FIGURE 36-1 ■ Several layers and structures of human skin. (From Francis, C.C. and Martin, A.H.: *Introduction to human anatomy* [7th ed.]. St Louis, 1975, Mosby.)

3. Subcutaneous layer: fatty tissue functions as insulation, protection of internal organs, and calorie storage.

B. **Functions of the skin.**
   1. Physical protection.
      a. Mechanical.
         (1) Tightly packed, thick-walled cells, held together by intercellular lipids, provide a protective barrier against transepidermal water loss and external invasions.
         (2) Process of constant sloughing and replacement of stratum corneum prevents colonization of the skin surface by bacteria and other organisms.
      b. Chemical/bacterial.
         (1) Acidic surface of skin (pH 5 to 6) provides defense against bacteria and other microorganisms (Larson and Dinulos, 2005).
         (2) Production of melanin protects against damage from ultraviolet-light radiation.
   2. Heat regulation.
      a. Production and evaporation of sweat.
      b. Dilation and constriction of blood vessels.
      c. Insulation of body by subcutaneous fat.
   3. Sense perception: heat, touch, pain, and pressure.

C. **Differences in newborn/preterm skin.**
   1. Basic structure is same as that of the adult; the less mature the infant, the less mature is the functioning of the skin.
   2. Skin matures rapidly during the first few weeks after birth. The full-term infant will achieve a stratum corneum that is structurally and functionally equivalent to the adult by approximately 3 weeks of age. The preterm infant will also experience accelerated skin maturity, although it may take longer (Loomis et al., 2008).
   3. The earlier the gestational age, the more thin and gelatinous is the skin, with fewer layers in the stratum corneum and a thinner dermis with fewer elastic fibers. The skin gradually matures after birth; however, even at 4 weeks of age, a 25-week infant has twice the transepidermal water loss as a term infant (Agren et al., 2006; Hammarlund and Sedin, 1979;

Hoeger and Enzmann, 2002). Maturation of skin is accelerated after preterm delivery but may take as long as 8 weeks in an infant of 24 to 25 weeks (Agren et al., 2006; Gilliam and Williams, 2008).
4. Subcutaneous fat is accumulated predominantly during the third trimester.
   a. Preterm babies have little fat, resulting in an inability to maintain body temperature and blood glucose level.
   b. Brown fat, which is important for temperature regulation in the newborn infant, begins to differentiate during the seventh month of gestation (Loomis et al., 2008).
5. Immature skin is thinner and therefore more permeable.
   a. An infant, especially a preterm infant, quickly absorbs topically applied medications and chemicals (Blumer and Reed, 2005; Loomis et al., 2008).
   b. Greater permeability allows for greater insensible water loss in the preterm infant.
   c. Higher surface area–body weight ratio allows for greater absorption of chemicals and greater transepidermal water loss.
6. Fewer fibrils connect the dermis and epidermis, and they are more fragile in term and preterm skin than in the skin of an adult. The stratum corneum is thinner in the term and preterm infant. Risk of injury from tape, monitors, and handling is increased, especially in the preterm infant; this type of injury includes removal of the outermost layer of the dermis with removal of tape or electrodes (Lund et al., 1997).
7. Sweat glands are present at birth, but full adult functioning is not present until the second or third year of life. Although present in the preterm infant, sweat glands are immature and function poorly before 36 weeks of gestation (Gilliam and Williams, 2008).
   a. The newborn infant has limited ability to tolerate excessive heat.
   b. Vasodilatation to increase heat loss can result in hypotension and dehydration caused by increased insensible water loss.

CARE OF THE NEWBORN INFANT'S SKIN

A. **Term newborn infant.**
   1. Initial bath with water and a mild soap.
      a. Avoid strong alkaline soaps to minimize alteration of surface pH.
      b. Soaps containing hexachlorophene should not be used. The hexachlorophene has been shown to be absorbed through the skin (Kopelman, 1973).
      c. Safety of other bacteriostatic soaps has not been determined. These products may be too harsh for the neonate's skin and may negatively affect normal skin colonization (Association of Women's Health, Obstetric and Neonatal Nurses [AWHONN], 2007).
      d. As soon as the body temperature is stable (>36.5° C [97.7° F]), it is advisable to bathe the healthy term infant to decrease the caregiver's risk of exposure to blood-borne pathogens. Standard precautions, including the use of gloves, should be adhered to when handling the infant who has not been bathed after delivery and during any invasive procedure in which the caregiver may be exposed to body fluids (Centers for Disease Control and Prevention, 2006; Watson, 2006).
   2. Parents may prefer to give the first bath themselves.
   3. Vernix caseosa contains large amounts of fats, which protect the skin from the amniotic fluid and bacteria in utero. Vernix insulates the stratum corneum and should not be scrubbed off during the initial bath (Akinbi et al., 2004; Moraille et al., 2005; Tollin et al., 2005).
   4. When possible, avoid puncturing the skin of babies with suspected maternal infections.
   5. Routine use of emollients is not recommended in the term infant. Creams and emollients that contain perfumes are drying and may irritate the infant's skin. Products that change the pH of the skin decrease the bacteriostatic properties (Larson and Dinulos, 2005). If cracking or fissures develop in the skin, a nonperfumed emollient may be used (AWHONN, 2007).
B. **Preterm infant.**
   1. Keep skin clean with water. Mild, nonalkaline soap may be used, but is not necessary and may damage healing skin (Da Cunha and Procianoy, 2005; Wilson et al., 2005). Preterm

infants should be bathed infrequently during the first 2 months of life to avoid excessive drying of the skin and to avoid overstimulation, stress, and fatigue (AWHONN, 2007; Quinn et al., 2005).

2. Handle infant gently and minimally to avoid trauma.
3. Minimize use of tape and other adhesives as much as possible. Use care when removing tape to avoid stripping the epidermis (AWHONN, 2007).
   a. Safety of adhesive solvents is uncertain. Cotton balls soaked with warm water can be used effectively for removing tape and other adhesives.
   b. Gelled adhesives and pectin-based barriers have been found to be helpful in avoiding trauma to the skin during their removal (Lund et al., 1997).
   c. Pectin or hydrocolloid layers applied before adhesives may protect the skin from damage when endotracheal tubes or catheters are secured (Lund et al., 1997).
   d. Benzoin and other adhesive bonding agents form a strong bond between the adhesive and the epidermis, increasing the risk of stripping the epidermis when the adhesive is removed. Use of these agents with preterm infants should be avoided.
4. Increased permeability of the skin allows absorption of some medications and products such as alcohol and povidone–iodine (Linder et al., 1997). When these substances are used for an invasive procedure, it is recommended that they be removed completely with water as soon as possible to prevent absorption or chemical burns.
5. The skin should be disinfected before any invasive procedure. Although chlorhexidine gluconate (CGH) has been shown to be more effective than other agents in reducing skin colonization, it has not been approved for use in infants less than 2 months of age. Chlorhexidine gluconate is available in single-use applicators that contain 70% alcohol but may be drying to the neonate's skin or cause burning or other injury (AWHONN, 2007; Reynolds et al., 2005). Aqueous CHG products are not yet available in the United States as single-use applicators (AWHONN, 2007).
6. Emollient creams that are free of preservatives and perfumes may be of benefit to the preterm infant as they decrease transepidermal water loss and skin breakdown when cracking, excessive dryness, or fissures are present (AWHONN, 2007; Lund and Kuller, 2007). Humidity at levels of 70% to 90% during the first week after birth reduces insensible water loss and evaporative heat loss in extremely low birth weight infants. Humidity should be gradually decreased to 50% after the first week. Transepidermal water loss in extremely low-birth-weight infants decreases after the first week after birth. Decreasing humidity to around 50% may improve skin barrier maturation (Agren et al., 2006).
7. Transparent adhesive dressings can be used over wounds and abrasions and to secure intravenous (IV) catheters and central lines (Lund and Kuller, 2007).

C. **Umbilical cord care.**
   1. Sterile cutting of cord at delivery, rapid drying of umbilical cord, and keeping cord clean is the most effective way to prevent umbilical infections. The use of antimicrobial creams or ointments has not been shown to be more effective in preventing infection than keeping the cord clean and dry (Zupan et al., 2004).
   2. Isopropyl alcohol and triple dye (a solution containing crystal violet, brilliant cresyl green, and proflavine hemisulfate) are the agents most commonly used for cord care. These agents have not demonstrated any beneficial effect on the frequency of cord infections or in cord separation time.
   3. Bathing does not increase the rate of omphalitis or cause a delay in cord separation (Bryanton et al., 2004).
   4. It is normal for the cord to appear slightly mucky, with small amounts of cloudy, mucus-like material at the junction of the cord and abdominal skin.
   5. Omphalitis is characterized by serosanguineous drainage, inflammation of the surrounding tissues, and a foul odor. Poor feeding, lethargy, and fever may also be associated.

ASSESSMENT OF THE NEWBORN INFANT'S SKIN

A. **Factors affecting the appearance of the skin.**
   1. Gestational age.

2. Postnatal age.
3. Nutritional status and hydration.
4. Racial origin.
5. Type and amount of available light.
6. Hemoglobin and bilirubin levels.
7. Environmental temperatures.
8. Oxygenation status.

B. **Definitions used to describe skin lesions** (Weston et al., 2007).
1. Macule: a pigmented, flat spot that is visible but not palpable. Macules greater than 1 cm in diameter may be referred to as a patch.
2. Papule: a solid, elevated, palpable lesion, with distinct borders less than 1 cm in diameter.
3. Plaque: a solid, elevated, palpable lesion, with distinct borders, greater than 1 cm in size.
4. Nodule: a solid lesion, elevated with depth, up to 2 cm in size.
5. Tumor: a solid lesion, elevated with depth, greater than 2 cm in size.
6. Vesicle: an elevated lesion or blister filled with serous fluid and less than 1 cm in diameter.
7. Bulla: a fluid-filled lesion larger than 1 cm.
8. Pustule: a vesicle filled with cloudy or purulent fluid.
9. Petechiae: subepidermal hemorrhages, pinpoint in size. They do not blanch with pressure.
10. Ecchymosis: a large area of subepidermal hemorrhage.
11. Wheal: area of edema in the upper dermis, creating a palpable, slightly raised lesion.
12. Ulcer: erosion of skin with damage of the epidermis into the dermis. Will leave a scar after healing.

COMMON SKIN LESIONS

A. **Normal variations in newborn skin.**
1. Cutis marmorata.
   a. Bluish mottling or marbling effect of the skin.
   b. Physiologic response to chilling caused by dilation of capillaries and venules.
   c. Disappears when infant is rewarmed.
   d. May be a sign of stress or overstimulation in newborn infant.
   e. Common in infants with trisomies 18 and 21.
   f. If condition persists in infants 6 months of age or older, it may be a symptom of hypothyroidism or a vascular abnormality such as cutis marmorata telangiectasia (Mazereeuw-Hautier et al., 2002).
2. Harlequin color change (Fig. 36-2).
   a. A difference in the amount of blood flow in the right and left sides of the body results in a sharply demarcated difference in color between one side and the other. This is most often seen in the dependent half of the body when the infant is lying on its side. When the infant's position is reversed, the color changes to the other side. This condition may also be seen when the infant is lying flat. It is most often visible in the trunk. It may last from a few seconds to a few minutes and changes with activity or changes in position.
   b. Caused by immaturity or temporary disturbance of the autonomic regulation of the cutaneous vessels. It is more common in preterm neonates.
3. Erythema toxicum (newborn rash) (Fig. 36-3).
   a. Small white or yellow pustules surrounded by an erythematous base (erythematous base is caused by histamine release) (Lucky, 2008).
   b. Benign, found in up to 70% of newborn infants (Lucky, 2008).
   c. Seen in neonates and infants up to 3 months of age.
   d. Lesions come and go on various sites of face, trunk, and limbs, although they are never seen on the palms of the hands or soles of the feet.

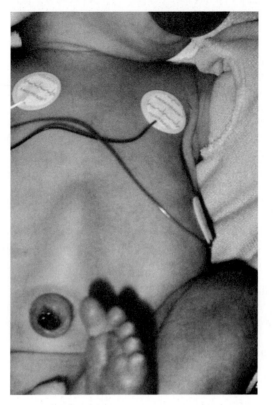

FIGURE 36-2 ■ Harlequin color change. (Courtesy Jane Deacon, RNC, MS, NNP, The Children's Hospital, Denver, Colorado.)

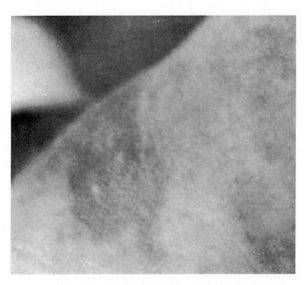

FIGURE 36-3 ■ Erythema toxicum. (Courtesy Jacinto Hernandez, MD, The Children's Hospital, Denver, Colorado.)

    e. Cause unknown, but condition may be exacerbated by handling or by chafing from linen.

    f. Differential diagnosis: may resemble a staphylococcal infection. Diagnosis can be confirmed by smear of aspirated pustule showing numerous eosinophils.

    g. No treatment is necessary. Lotions or creams may exacerbate condition.

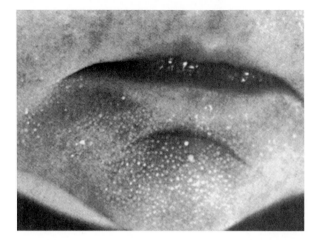

FIGURE 36-4 ■ Milia. (Courtesy Jacinto Hernandez, MD, The Children's Hospital, Denver, Colorado.)

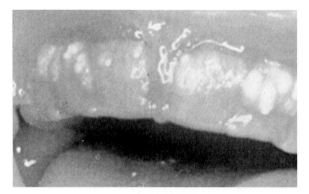

FIGURE 36-5 ■ Epstein pearls. (Courtesy Jacinto Hernandez, MD, The Children's Hospital, Denver, Colorado.)

4. Milia (Fig. 36-4).
   a. Multiple yellow or pearly white papules about 1 mm in size; epidermal inclusion cysts composed of laminated, keratinous material. They occur on the brow, cheeks, and nose.
   b. Milia are observed in about 40% of term infants (Weston et al., 2007).
   c. No treatment is necessary. They resolve spontaneously during the first few weeks after birth.
5. Epstein pearls (Fig. 36-5).
   a. Oral counterpart of facial milia. They can be seen on the midline of the palate or on the alveolar ridges.
   b. Epstein pearls occur in approximately 60% of neonates (Weston et al., 2007).
6. Sebaceous gland hyperplasia.
   a. Tiny (<0.5 mm) white or yellow papules found on the nose, cheeks, and upper lips of newborn infants.
   b. Common in term infants but rarely seen in preterm infants.
   c. Represent overactivity of the sebaceous follicles and are a manifestation of maternal androgen stimulation.
   d. They resolve without treatment within a few weeks.
7. Miliaria. Caused by occlusion of sweat ducts by keratin, resulting in retention of sweat. There are four types of miliaria.
   a. Miliaria crystallina: clear, thin vesicles 1 to 2 mm in diameter that develop in the epidermal portion of the sweat glands. They are seen over the head, neck, and upper aspect of the trunk in newborn infants. Can be present at birth (Haas et al., 2002).

    b. Miliaria rubra: commonly referred to as prickly heat; results from prolonged occlusion of pores, leading to release of sweat into the lower epidermis. Condition appears as pink or white papules and vesicles 2 to 4 mm in diameter, with an erythematous base. The lesions are generally found in the flexure areas, such as the neck, groin, and axillae, as well as on the face and the upper aspect of the chest.

    c. Miliaria pustulosa: resulting from continued exposure to heat, which leads to infiltration of the vesicles with leukocytes. This is rare in most climates and resolves with change to a dry, cool environment.

    d. Miliaria profunda: rare in infants; infection of lower portion of sweat glands in the dermis. Treatment consists of avoidance of further sweating and keeping the skin cool and dry.

8. Diaper dermatitis.

    a. May be caused by chafing from diapers, by prolonged contact with urine or feces, or by sensitivity to chemicals in disposable diapers or in detergent used in laundering cloth diapers.

    b. The best treatment is prevention by frequent diaper changes and by protection of the skin with a barrier product containing zinc oxide. The skin should be cleansed with warm water after voiding or stooling. Avoid diaper wipes that contain alcohol (Atherton, 2004; Scheinfeld, 2005).

    c. Cornstarch and baby powder should not be used. They provide a medium for growth of bacteria and yeast, and inhaled particles are irritating to the respiratory tract (AWHONN, 2007).

    d. Candida diaper dermatitis: see item 2 under section E, Infectious Lesions, page 826.

B. Lesions resulting from trauma.

1. Forceps marks.

    a. Forceps marks are red or bruised areas seen over the cheek, scalp, or face of infants after forceps delivery.

    b. The infant should be examined for underlying tissue damage or other signs of birth trauma such as scalp abrasions, fractured clavicles, or facial palsy.

2. Subcutaneous fat necrosis.

    a. A hard, circumscribed, red or purple nodule under the dermis in the subcutaneous tissue. Nodules appear on the trunk, extremities, or face, usually during the first 2 weeks of life. They may grow larger initially and then resolve spontaneously within several weeks.

    b. Subcutaneous fat necrosis has been attributed to trauma, cold stress, shock, and asphyxia and is caused by crystallization of the subcutaneous fat cells (Mahe et al., 2007).

    c. Hypercalcemia may be associated with subcutaneous fat necrosis in infants with multiple nodules. Hypocalcemia has also been reported, possibly because of the underlying cause of the nodules. Serum calcium levels should be monitored (Karochristou et al., 2006; Mahe et al., 2007).

3. Scalp lacerations.

    a. Scalp lacerations may be caused by trauma during delivery, placement of scalp electrodes, or fetal blood pH sampling.

    b. Treatment consists of keeping the area clean and dry and assessing for infection.

4. Intravenous extravasations.

    a. Vascular access sites in the infant should be assessed hourly to evaluate line patency and detect extravasation. The IV catheter should be removed immediately if patency is not certain or if signs of extravasation are apparent. If an infiltration of a vesicant medication has occurred, treatment should be determined before removing the catheter (AWHONN, 2007; Sawatzky-Dicksson and Bodnaryk, 2006).

    b. If extravasation occurs, the extremity should be elevated (Ramasethy, 2004). Using a multiple-puncture technique has been reported to help avoid swelling at the site and further tissue damage (AWHONN, 2007). Using aseptic technique, make several puncture holes with a 25-gauge needle over the area of swelling and gently squeeze fluid out of the tissue, or allow the fluid to leak out on its own. Hyaluronidase injected into the tissue surrounding the site may decrease tissue damage (AWHONN, 2007; Sawatzky-Dicksson and Bodnaryk, 2006), and phentolamine can be used as an antidote for infiltration of vasoconstrictive agents such as dopamine or norepinephrine (AWHONN, 2007).

   c. Application of an occlusive hydrocolloid dressing may aid in healing (AWHONN, 2007; Cisler-Cahill, 2006).

C. Pigmented skin lesions.

   1. Hyperpigmented macules (mongolian spots) (Fig. 36-6).

   a. Large macules or patches, gray or blue-green, seen most commonly over the buttocks, flanks, or shoulders.

   b. Most common pigmented lesion seen at birth, occurring in 80% of black, Asian, and Hispanic infants and only occasionally in lighter-skinned infants (Gibbs and Makkar, 2008).

   c. Hyperpigmented macules are caused by the increased presence of melanocytes dispersed in the dermis.

   d. The spots fade somewhat during the first few years after birth, particularly as surrounding skin darkens, but may persist into adulthood.

   e. It is important to document size and location to avoid question of nonaccidental trauma.

   2. Congenital melanocytic nevi (pigmented nevi) (Fig. 36-7).

   a. Dark brown or black macules that may or may not be hairy. Nevi may occur anywhere on the body, with the "bathing trunk" area being the most common site.

   b. Caused by collection of melanocytes under the skin.

   c. Most are small, less than 2 cm, with smooth surfaces. Large nevi (>10 cm) are rare (Weston et al., 2007).

   d. Pigmented nevi are generally benign. Malignant changes may occur but are rare before puberty in small nevi (Gibbs and Makkar, 2008; Weston et al., 2007).

   e. Close observation for changes in size or shape is indicated, with possible surgical excision. Large, unusually shaped nevi may be difficult to assess for changes and should be followed closely (Weston et al., 2007).

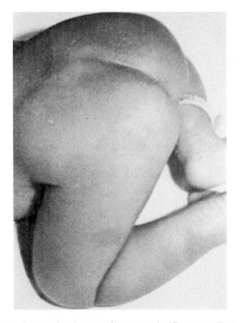

FIGURE 36-6 ■ Hyperpigmented macules (mongolian spots). (Courtesy Jacinto Hernandez, MD, The Children's Hospital, Denver, Colorado.)

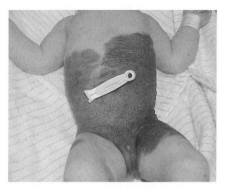

FIGURE 36-7 ■ Giant pigmented nevus. (Courtesy Catherine L. Witt, Aurora, Colorado.)

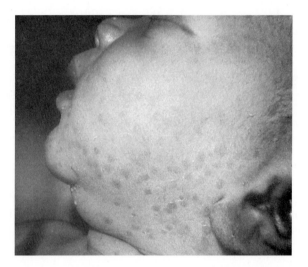

FIGURE 36-8 ■ Neonatal pustular melanosis. (Courtesy Jane Deacon, RNC, MS, NNP, The Children's Hospital, Denver, Colorado.)

    f. Pigment specific lasers such as the Q-switched or ruby laser have been used with some success, although complete clearance is rare. Dermabrasion, cryosurgery, and electro-cautery have been used with some success (Gibbs and Makkar, 2008).

    g. A hairy nevus present over the spine may be associated with spina bifida or meningo-cele (Gibbs and Makkar, 2008).

    h. Pigmented nevi may also be associated with neurofibromatosis or tuberous sclerosis.

  3. Transient neonatal pustular melanosis (Fig. 36-8).

    a. Superficial vesiculopustular lesions that rupture during the first 12 to 48 hours after birth, leaving small, brown, hyperpigmented macules. The macules may be surrounded by very fine white scales. They often rupture before delivery, presenting as macules.

    b. Benign; found in up to 5% of black infants and in about 0.2% of white neonates (Ramamurthy et al., 1976).

    c. No treatment is necessary. The macules generally fade during the first few weeks or months after birth.

    d. Aspirating the contents of the vesicles will reveal a variable number of neutrophils and few or no eosinophils.

  4. Café-au-lait spots (Fig. 36-9).

    a. Tan or light-brown patches with well-defined borders.

    b. When less than 3 cm in length and fewer than six in number, they are of no pathologic significance.

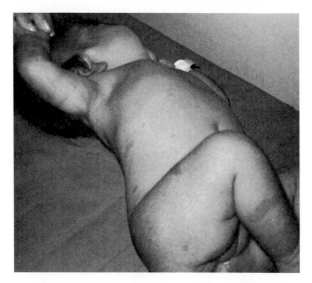

FIGURE 36-9 ■ Café-au-lait spots. (Courtesy Jacinto Hernandez, MD, The Children's Hospital, Denver, Colorado.)

    c. Six or more spots may be an indication of neurofibromatosis (Gibbs and Makkar, 2008).
        (1) Neurofibromatosis is a condition in which tumors form on cutaneous nerves and along the thoracic, brachial, and lumbar nerve trunks. Cranial nerves may also be affected.
        (2) It is an autosomal dominant disorder.
        (3) Café-au-lait spots may be the only finding of this disease in the neonatal period.
  5. Ash leaf macules.
    a. White macules in the shape of an ash leaf or thumbprint; seen primarily over the trunk or buttocks.
    b. Found in 90% of infants with tuberous sclerosis, although up to 5% of Caucasians will have hypopigmented macules (Weston et al., 2007).
    c. May be difficult to see in fair-skinned infants. Use of a Wood (ultraviolet) lamp will aid in examination.
    d. Infants with unexplained seizures should be examined for these macules.
    e. May also be a normal finding or may be associated with neurofibromatosis.
D. Vascular lesions.
  1. Nevus simplex.
    a. Nevus simplex (stork bite) refers to macular pink areas of distended capillaries found on the nape of the neck, the upper eyelids, the nose, or the upper lip. They have diffuse borders, blanch with pressure, and become pinker with crying.
    b. These are the most common of vascular birthmarks, seen in 30% to 50% of newborn infants (Weston et al., 2007).
    c. The lesions tend to fade by the first or second year, with the exception of those on the nape of the neck, which may persist.
  2. Port-wine stain.
    a. A flat vascular nevus is present at birth. It is usually pink in infancy, but may be red or purple. The nevus may be small or may cover almost half of the body. It is flat, sharply delineated, and blanches minimally. Facial lesions are the most common.
    b. Port-wine stains consist of mature capillaries that are dilated and congested directly below the epidermis. The cause is unknown.
    c. The nevus does not grow in area or size. It will not resolve and should be considered permanent. The lesion may become darker and thicker with age.

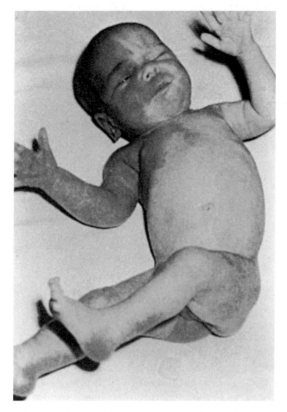

FIGURE 36-10 ■ Sturge–Weber syndrome. (Courtesy Jacinto Hernandez, MD, The Children's Hospital, Denver, Colorado.)

    d. The pulsed-dye laser has been successful in lightening most port-wine stains by up to 50%. The laser works by causing intravascular coagulation (Alster and Railan, 2006). Light-colored facial lesions have the best results; red or purple lesions that are thick and nodular respond less well. Most infants require several treatments. Recurrence or darkening of the lesion several years after treatment has been reported (Huikeshoven et al., 2007; Soulid and Waters, 2006). Other methods of surgical excision have been largely unsatisfactory.

    e. Sturge–Weber syndrome (Fig. 36-10).

        (1) Port-wine stains are confined to a pattern similar to that of the branches of the trigeminal nerve.

        (2) Their central feature is disordered proliferation of endothelial cells, particularly in the small veins. It is associated with atrophic changes in the cerebral cortex and calcium deposits in the walls of small vessels and areas of affected cortex (Weston et al., 2007).

        (3) Manifested by glaucoma, focal seizures, hemiparesis, and mental retardation (Weston et al., 2007).

  3. Strawberry hemangioma (Fig. 36-11).

    a. Raised, lobulated, soft, bright red tumor located on the head, neck, trunk, or extremities. These lesions may also occur in the throat, where they can cause airway obstruction, requiring a tracheostomy in extreme cases.

    b. Caused by dilated capillaries occupying the dermal and subdermal layers, in association with endothelial proliferation.

    c. About 50% to 60% are present at birth, and 90% are evident by 2 months of age (Enjolras and Garzon, 2008). The lesions occur in approximately 1% to 2% of newborn infants and are more common in preterm infants (10% to 15% will have lesions), with females predominating (Blei et al., 1998; Haggstrom et al., 2007). They are also more

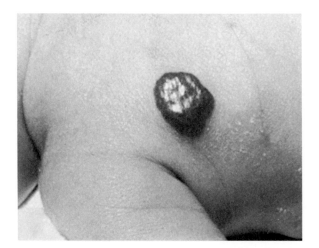

FIGURE 36-11 ■ Strawberry hemangioma. (Courtesy Jacinto Hernandez, MD, The Children's Hospital, Denver, Colorado.)

common in Caucasian infants and in twins or higher-order multiples. The lesions may also be familial (Blei et al., 1998).
   d. Strawberry hemangiomas will generally increase in size during the first 6 months, and then become stable in size before undergoing gradual spontaneous regression, with most leaving no trace. This may take several years. Infants will often have more than one lesion.
   e. Treatment of choice is to allow the lesion to regress spontaneously. If the lesion is interfering with vision, is bleeding or ulcerating, or is impinging on other vital functions, treatment should be considered.
      (1) Systemic corticosteroid therapy is the treatment of choice for most hemangiomas (Enjolras and Garzon, 2008).
      (2) Flashlamp-pumped pulsed-dye laser may be effective on some lesions (Enjolras and Garzon, 2008).
      (3) Cryosurgery may be used with small lesions, but concerns about scarring have prevented this option from becoming widespread (Enjolras and Garzon, 2008).
      (4) Interferon-α-2b may be effective in treating steroid-resistant lesions (Enjolras and Garzon, 2008).
   f. The infant should be monitored for signs of impingement on vital organs or functioning, such as stridor, poor feeding, and difficulty in swallowing, which would make treatment necessary.
   g. The cosmetic concerns of parents require a caring, supportive approach. Pictures illustrating spontaneous regression may be helpful.
4. Cavernous hemangioma.
   a. This lesion is composed of large venous channels and vascular elements lined by endothelial cells.
   b. It involves the dermis and subcutaneous tissue and appears as a bluish red discoloration under the overlying skin.
   c. The cavernous hemangioma has poorly defined borders and may feel cystic, like a "bag of worms," when palpated. Like the strawberry hemangioma, the cavernous hemangioma will increase in size during the first 6 to 12 months and then involute spontaneously (Enjolras and Garzon, 2008).
   d. Treatment is not indicated unless the lesion is interfering with vital functions, including airway obstruction, in which case systemic corticosteroid treatment or interferon-α may be helpful (Enjolras and Garzon, 2008).
   e. Kasabach–Merritt phenomenon.
      (1) Vascular anomalies resembling a hemangioma may be associated with sequestration of platelets and thrombocytopenia (Enjolras et al., 1997).

(2) Treatment consists of systemic corticosteroid therapy. Transfusions of platelets and blood are frequently necessary (Enjolras and Garzon, 2008; Weston et al., 2007). The lesions may resolve spontaneously.

(3) Surgical excision has been successful in isolated cases.

f. Klippel–Trenaunay–Weber syndrome.

(1) Syndrome consists of hypertrophy of a limb with associated vascular anomalies and hypertrophy of underlying bone and soft tissue.

(2) No specific treatment for the disease. Severe limb hypertrophy may require orthopedic consultation, with possible amputation of the affected limb.

E. Infectious lesions.

1. Thrush.

a. A fungal infection of the mouth or throat, caused by *Candida albicans*.

b. Very common in infants.

c. Manifested as patches of adherent white material scattered over the tongue and mucous membranes.

d. Treated with an oral antifungal preparation such as nystatin (Mycostatin).

2. *Candida* diaper dermatitis.

a. Fungal infection of skin in the diaper area; may include buttocks, groin, thighs, and abdomen.

b. Caused by *C. albicans*.

c. Manifested as a moist, erythematous eruption, often with white or yellow satellite pustules.

d. Treatment consists of an antifungal cream or ointment preparation such as nystatin, applied to the rash several times per day. Oral antifungal treatment may be recommended in cases of persistent *Candida* dermatitis.

3. Systemic *Candida* infection.

a. Very low birth weight infants are at risk of having systemic, invasive fungal infections, with invasion of the fungus beyond the stratum corneum.

b. Improving the barrier function of the skin by minimizing trauma and maintaining a sterile environment may help prevent onset of this infection.

4. Herpes.

a. Neonatal herpes simplex infection is one of the most serious viral infections in the neonate.

b. Rash appears as vesicular or pustular rash (Fig. 36-12).

c. Seventy percent of infants with herpes will have subsequent rash but not necessarily before other signs and symptoms of illness develop. Therefore, the absence of vesicles does not eliminate the possibility of disease (Friedlander and Bradley, 2008).

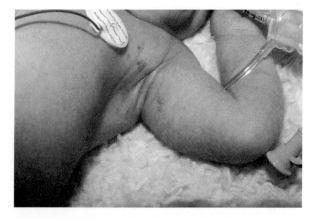

FIGURE 36-12 ■ Herpes simplex vesicles in axilla. (Courtesy Jane Deacon, RNC, MS, NNP, The Children's Hospital, Denver, Colorado.)

    d. Treatment with an antiviral agent such as acyclovir should begin immediately. The earlier treatment is begun, the better the outcome (Weston et al., 2007).

5. "Scalded skin" syndrome (also known as bullous impetigo, toxic epidermal necrolysis, Ritter disease, and nonstreptococcal scarlatina).

    a. An inflammatory skin disorder generally caused by the phage strain of group II staphylococcus. May follow an upper respiratory tract infection or otitis media.

    b. Manifested as a widespread, tender erythema, followed by blisters ranging from small vesicles to large bullae. Caused by the release of an endotoxin that acts on the stratum granulosa of the epidermis. The blisters, which frequently begin in the diaper area and spread to the rest of the body, rupture, leaving large, raw, scaldlike areas.

    c. Treatment includes isolation and aseptic handling to prevent further infection in the infected infant and the spread of bacteria to others. The infant is treated systemically with methicillin because of the number of penicillin-resistant strains in the phage strain of group II staphylococcus. A topical antibiotic ointment such as bacitracin may be applied locally.

6. Congenital viral infection.

    a. Petechiae and purpuric macules erupt on the head, trunk, and extremities of affected infants. The lesions are often described as "blueberry muffin" spots and are caused by dermal erythropoiesis (Fig. 36-13).

    b. The lesions generally disappear in 2 to 3 weeks. Treatment is based on the underlying disorder.

    c. Although the lesions are most often associated with rubella, they are also seen in association with other congenital infections such as cytomegalovirus, toxoplasmosis, syphilis, and herpes.

    d. Affected infants may also have growth restriction, jaundice, hepatosplenomegaly, and thrombocytopenia.

F. Hereditary and miscellaneous lesions.

1. Epidermolysis bullosa.

    a. Disease characterized by the formation of vesicles and bullae over various parts of the body. Skin is extremely fragile. The underlying genetic defect may be autosomal dominant or recessive (Fine et al., 2008).

    b. Vesicles may appear spontaneously or in response to minor trauma such as routine handling.

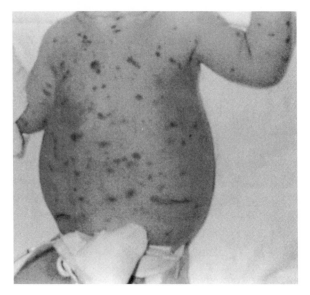

FIGURE 36-13 ■ Blueberry muffin rash. (From Clark, D.: *Atlas of neonatology*. Philadelphia, 2000, Saunders, p. 56.)

    c. Lesions may appear at birth or a few weeks later.

    d. Three types of vesicles may appear at birth.

       (1) Simple, nonscarring: bullae form in small numbers throughout childhood and heal without scarring. Often disappear at puberty. Prevention of trauma and infection is important.

       (2) Dystrophic, scarring: more severe form of the disease, with lesions forming scars, loss of nails, and contractures. Death may result from secondary infections.

       (3) Epidermolysis bullosa lethalis: most severe form, with large, numerous lesions, usually present at birth. Large areas of epidermis are lost, leaving red, weeping erosions. Esophageal lesions may also occur. The life span of these patients is generally short. Treatment is supportive care, minimizing trauma and infection (Weston et al., 2007).

  2. Collodion baby.

    a. Term describes an appearance rather than a disease. These babies are born covered with a tight, shiny, transparent membrane that cracks and peels off after a few days. A few infants will have no underlying disorder, but many will have some form of ichthyosis (Weston et al., 2007) (Fig. 36-14).

    b. Treatment consists of liberal application of sterile olive or mineral oil several times a day to hydrate and lubricate the skin, careful handling, and prevention of infection.

  3. Ichthyosis.

    a. Ichthyosis is a disease involving excessive scaling of the skin, caused by excessive production of stratum corneum cells or faulty shedding of the stratum corneum (Weston et al., 2007). There are four types of ichthyosis.

       (1) Ichthyosis vulgaris: an autosomal dominant disease, usually appearing after 3 months of age. This is the most common and most benign of the ichthyosis

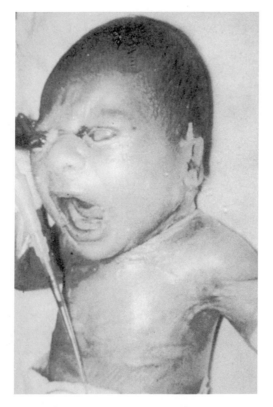

FIGURE 36-14 ■ Collodion infant. (From Solomon, L.M. and Esterly, N.B.: *Neonatal dermatology.* Philadelphia, 2001, Saunders, p. 115.)

disorders, occurring in approximately 1 in 250 infants (Weston et al., 2007). It consists of fine white scales and excessively dry skin.

(2) X-linked ichthyosis: appears at birth or during the first year of life. It occasionally occurs in a collodion baby. The disorder consists of large, thick, dark-brown scales over the entire body, with the exception of the palms and soles. It occurs in males only.

(3) Lamellar ichthyosis: an autosomal recessive trait that is manifested at birth as bright red erythema and universal desquamation. Some infants resemble collodion babies. Scales are large, flat, and coarse and may be less prominent in infancy than later in childhood. Eversion of the lips and eyelids may occur, and the palms and soles may be thickened. Hyperkeratosis may be seen on skin biopsy, although this is not diagnostic of the disorder (Weston et al., 2007).

(4) Bullous ichthyosis: autosomal dominant disorder characterized by recurrent formation of bullous lesions, erythroderma, and excessive dryness and peeling. As the child grows, the involvement generally becomes limited to small, thick, hard scales, most often found in the flexure regions. Hyperkeratosis may be seen on the palms and soles. Infection in the neonatal period with *Staphylococcus aureus* is of primary concern because of the widespread skin breakdown.

  b. Treatment of ichthyosis is limited to use of topical preparations to hydrate and lubricate the skin. Daily baths with a water-dispersible bath oil, with use of alpha-hydroxy acid ointments, may be helpful (Weston et al., 2007).

  c. Drying soaps and detergents should be avoided.

  d. Care must be taken to prevent infection of dry or cracked skin.

4. Harlequin fetus.

  a. The harlequin fetus previously was considered to have a severe form of ichthyosis but may in fact have a separate rare autosomal recessive disease (Weston et al., 2007). The harlequin fetus has hard, thick, gray or yellow scales that cause severe deformities of skeletal and soft tissues.

  b. The condition is untreatable, and most infants die within a few hours or days of life.

5. Cutis aplasia.

  a. Term refers to congenital absence of skin, either as a midline defect, a posterior scalp defect, or several small or large defects involving the upper and lower extremities (Fig. 36-15).

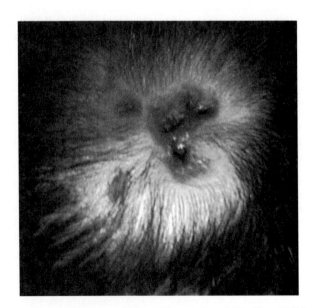

FIGURE 36-15 ■ Cutis aplasia. (Courtesy Jacinto Hernandez, MD, The Children's Hospital, Denver, Colorado.)

   b. Lesions heal slowly over several months, leaving a hypertrophic or atrophic scar.
   c. May be associated with other defects such as cleft lip and palate, heart disease, tracheoesophageal fistula, and other midline defects. It is seen in approximately 50% infants with trisomy 13 (Jones, 2006).

REFERENCES

Agren J., Sjors, G., and Sedin, G.: Ambient humidity influences the rate of skin barrier maturation in extremely premature infants. *Journal of Pediatrics*, 148(5):613-617, 2006.

Akinbi, H., Narendran, V., Pass, A., Markart, P., and Hoath, S.: Host defense proteins in vernix caseosa and amniotic fluid. *American Journal of Obstetrics and Gynecology*, 191(6):2090-2096, 2004.

Alster, T. S. and Railan, D.: Laser treatment of vascular birthmarks. *Journal of Craniofacial Surgery*, 17(4):720-723, 2006.

Association of Women's Health, Obstetric, and Neonatal Nurses: *Neonatal skin care* (2nd ed.). Washington, DC, 2007, AWHONN.

Atherton, D.J.: A review of the pathophysiology, prevention and treatment of irritant diaper dermatitis. *Current Medical Research and Opinion*, 20(5):645-649, 2004.

Blei, F., Walter, J., Orlow S.J., and Marchuk, D.A.: Familial segregation of hemangiomas and vascular malformations as an autosomal dominant trait. *Archives of Dermatology*, 134(6):718-742, 1998.

Blumer, J.L. and Reed, M.D.: Principles of neonatal pharmacology. In S.J. Yaffe and J.V. Aranda (Eds.): *Neonatal and pediatric pharmacology: Therapeutic principles in practice* (3rd ed.). Philadelphia, 2005, Lippincott Williams & Wilkins, pp. 146-158.

Bryanton, J., Walsh, D., Barrett, M., and Gaudet, D.: Tub bathing versus traditional sponge bathing for the newborn. *Journal of Obstetric, Gynecologic, and Neonatal Nursing*, 33(6):704-712, 2004.

Centers for Disease Control and Prevention: Leads from the *MMWR*. Update: Universal precautions for prevention of transmission of human immunodeficiency virus, hepatitis B virus, and other bloodborne pathogens in health care settings. *Journal of the American Medical Association*, 260:462-465, 2006.

Cisler-Cahill, L.: A protocol for the use of amorphous hydrogel to support wound healing in neonatal patients: An adjunct to nursing skin care. *Neonatal Network*, 25(4):267-273, 2006.

Da Cunha, M.L. and Procianoy, R.S.: Effect of bathing on skin flora of preterm newborns. *Journal of Perinatology*, 25(6):375-379, 2005.

Enjolras, O. and Garzon, M.C.: Vascular stains, malformations, and tumors. In L.F. Eichenfield, I.J. Frieden, and N.B. Esterly (Eds.): *Neonatal dermatology* (2nd ed.). Philadelphia, 2008, Saunders, pp. 343-374.

Enjolras, O., Wassef, M., Mazoyer, E., et al.: Infants with Kasabach-Merritt syndrome do not have "true" hemangiomas. *Journal of Pediatrics*, 130(4):631-640, 1997.

Fine, J.D., Johnson, L.B., Weiner, M., and Suchindran, C.: Cause-specific risks of childhood death in inherited epidermolysis bullosa. *Journal of Pediatrics*, 152(2):276-280, 2008.

Friedlander, S.F. and Bradley, J.S.: Viral infections. In L.F. Eichenfield, I.J. Frieden, and N.B. Esterly (Eds.): *Neonatal dermatology* (2nd ed.). Philadelphia, 2008, Saunders, pp. 193-227.

Gibbs, N.F. and Makkar, H.S.: Disorders of hyperpigmentation and melanocytes. In L.F. Eichenfield, I.J. Frieden, and N.B. Esterly (Eds.): *Neonatal dermatology* (2nd ed.). Philadelphia, 2008, Saunders, pp. 397-421.

Gilliam, A.E. and Williams, M.L.: Skin of the premature infant. In L.F. Eichenfield, I.J. Frieden, and N.B. Esterly (Eds.): *Neonatal dermatology* (2nd ed.). Philadelphia, 2008, Saunders, pp. 45-57.

Haas, N., Henz, B.M., and Weigel, H.: Congenital miliaria crystallina. *Journal of the American Academy of Dermatology*, 47(5 Suppl):S270-S272, 2002.

Haggstrom, A., Drolet, B., Baselga, E., et al.: Prospective study of infantile hemangiomas: demographic, prenatal and perinatal characteristics. *Journal of Pediatrics*, 150(3):291-294, 2007.

Hammarlund, K. and Sedin, G.: Transepidermal water loss in newborn infants. Relation to gestational age. *Acta Paediatrica Scandinavica*, 68(6):795-801, 1979.

Hoeger, P.H. and Enzmann, C.C.: Skin physiology of the neonate and young infant: A prospective study of functional skin parameters during early infancy. *Pediatric Dermatology*, 19(3):256-262, 2002.

Huikeshoven, M., Koster, P.H., deBorgie, C.A., Beck, J.F., van Gemert, M.J., van der Horst, C.M.: Redarkening of port-wine stains 10 years after pulsed dye laser treatment. *New England Journal of Medicine*, 356(12):1235-1240, 2007.

Jones, K.L.: *Smith's recognizable patterns of human malformation* (6th ed.). Philadelphia, 2006, Saunders, pp. 18-19.

Karochristou, K., Siahanidou, T., Kakourou-Tsivitanidou, T., Stefanaki, K., and Mandyla, H.: Subcutaneous fat necrosis associated with severe hypocalcaemia in a neonate. *Journal of Perinatology*, 26(1):64-66, 2006.

Kopelman, A.E.: Cutaneous absorption of hexachlorophene in low birth weight infants. *Journal of Pediatrics*, 82(6):972-975, 1973.

Larson, A. and Dinulos, J.: Cutaneous bacterial infections in the newborn. *Current Opinion in Pediatrics*, 17(4):481-485, 2005.

Linder, N., Davidovitch, N., Reichman, B., et al.: Topical iodine-containing antiseptics and subclinical hypothyroidism in preterm infants. *Journal of Pediatrics*, 131(3):434-439, 1997.

Loomis, C.A., Koss, T., and Chu, D.: Fetal skin development. In L.F. Eichenfield, I.J. Frieden, and N.B. Esterly (Eds.): *Neonatal dermatology* (2nd ed.). Philadelphia, 2008, Saunders, pp. 1-17.

Lucky, A.W.: Transient benign cutaneous lesions in the newborn. In L.F. Eichenfield, I.J. Frieden, and N.B.

Esterly (Eds.): *Neonatal dermatology* (2nd ed.). Philadelphia, 2008, Saunders, pp. 85-97.

Lund, C.H. and Kuller, J.M.: Integumentary system. In C. Kenner and J.W. Lott (Eds.): *Comprehensive neonatal care: An interdisciplinary approach* (4th ed.). St. Louis, 2007, Saunders, pp. 65-91.

Lund, C.H., Nonato, L.B., Kuller, J.M., et al.: Disruption of barrier function in neonatal skin associated with adhesive removal. *Journal of Pediatrics, 131*(3):367-372, 1997.

Mahe, E., Girszyn, N., Hadj-Rabia, S., Bodemer, C., Hamel-Teillac, D., and De Prost, Y.: Subcutaneous fat necrosis of the newborn: A systematic evaluation of risk factors, clinical manifestations, complications, and outcome of 16 children. *British Journal of Dermatology, 156*(4):709-715, 2007.

Mazereeuw-Hautier, J., Carel-Caneppele, S., and Bonafe, J.L.: Cutis marmorata telangiectatica congenital: Report of two persistent cases. *Pediatric Dermatology, 19*(6):506-509, 2002.

Moraille, R., Pickens, W., Visscher, M., and Hoath, S.: A novel role for vernix caseosa as a skin cleanser. *Biology of the Neonate, 87*(1):8-14, 2005.

Quinn, D., Newton, N., and Piecuch, R.: Effect of less frequent bathing on premature infant skin. *Journal of Obstetric, Gynecologic, and Neonatal Nursing, 34*(6):741-746, 2005.

Ramamurthy, R.S., Reveri, M., Esterly, N.B., Fretzin, D. F., and Pildes, R.S.: Transient neonatal pustular melanosis. *Journal of Pediatrics, 88*(5):831-835, 1976.

Ramasethy, J.: Prevention and management of extravasation injuries in neonates. *NeoReviews, 5*:491-497, 2004.

Reynolds, P.R., Banerjee, S., and Meek, J.H.: Alcohol burns in extremely low birthweight infants: Still occurring. *Archives of Disease in Childhood, Fetal and Neonatal Edition, 60*:F10, 2005.

Sawatzky-Dicksson, D. and Bodnaryk, K.: Neonatal intravenous extravasation injuries. Evaluation of a wound care protocol. *Neonatal Network, 25*(1):13-19, 2006.

Scheinfeld, N.: Diaper dermatitis: A review and brief survey of eruptions of the diaper area. *American Journal of Clinical Dermatology, 6*(5):273-281, 2005.

Soulid, A. and Waters, R.: Re-emergence of port wine stains following treatment with flashlamp-pumped dye laser 585 nm. *Annals of Plastic Surgery, 57*(3):260-263, 2006.

Tollin, M., Bersson, G., Kai-Larsen, Y., et al. Vernix caseosa as a multi-component defense system based on polypeptides, lipids, and their interactions. *Cellular and Molecular Life Science, 62*(19-20):2390-2399, 2005.

Watson, J.: Community-associated methicillin-resistant *Staphylococcus aureus* infection among healthy newborns—Chicago and Los Angeles County, 2004. *MMWR Morbidity and Mortality Weekly Report, 3*:329, 2006.

Weston, W.L., Lane, A.T., and Morelli, J.T.: *Color textbook of pediatric dermatology* (4th ed.). St Louis, 2007, Mosby.

Wilson, J.R., Mills, J.G., Prather, I.D., and Dimitrijevich, S.D.: A toxicity index of skin and wound cleansers used on in-vitro fibroblasts and keratinocytes. *Advances in Skin and Wound Care, 18*:373-378, 2005.

Zupan, J., Garner, P., and Omari, A.A.A.: Topical umbilical cord care at birth. *Cochrane Database of Systematic Reviews, 3*:CD001057, 2004. DOI: 10.1002/ 14651858.CD001057.

37 Ophthalmologic and Auditory Disorders

DEBBIE FRASER ASKIN and WILLIAM DIEHL-JONES

OBJECTIVES

1. Describe the normal anatomy of the eye.
2. Identify the normal anatomy of the ear.
3. Identify the major function(s) of each structure.
4. Describe the components of a nursing assessment of the eyes and ears in the neonate.
5. Describe the nurse's role in assisting the physician with neonatal eye examinations.
6. Discuss the factors to consider in universal hearing screening of newborns.
7. For each of six types of eye disorders in the neonatal period—traumatic injuries to the eye, conjunctivitis, nasolacrimal duct obstruction, cataracts, infections (TORCH diseases), and retinopathy of prematurity—(1) provide an overview of the pathogenesis and (2) describe commonly used treatment modalities, outlining the specific nursing care measures designed to meet the needs of neonates with these disorders.
8. Outline the most common causes of hearing loss in the newborn.
9. Outline teaching points for the family of a newborn at risk for hearing or vision problems.

An examination of the neonate's eyes and ears is an important, though often neglected, portion of a physical assessment. There is a great deal of clinically significant information that the astute nurse can glean from a thorough evaluation of these systems. Evidence of intrauterine infection, birth trauma, congenital malformations, disease, and a variety of genetic abnormalities can be detected during the course of the nurse's assessment of the neonate's eyes and ears.

This chapter provides the neonatal nurse with a review of normal anatomy of the eye and ear, together with the major function(s) of each structure; the essential components of an assessment of the newborn's eyes and ears; an overview of the most common eye disorders in the neonate; and common treatment modalities and nursing measures used in the treatment of various ocular disorders in the newborn infant. The essential elements of a universal hearing screening program for newborns is addressed as are the most common causes of hearing loss in neonates.

ANATOMY OF THE EYE (Fig. 37-1)

Protective Structures

A. **Eyelids:** shade the eyes during sleep; protect from excessive light or foreign objects; spread lubricating secretions over the eyeball.
B. **Conjunctiva:** mucous membrane lining the inner aspect of the eyelids (palpebral) and onto the eyeball to the periphery of the cornea (bulbar).
C. **Lacrimal system:** manufactures and drains away tears; cleans, lubricates, and moistens the eyeball.
D. **Bony orbit or socket:** surrounds and protects the eyeball. Most important opening within the orbit is the optic foramen, through which the optic nerve, ophthalmic artery, and ophthalmic vein from each eye pass en route to the brain.

The Eyeball

A. **Outer layer (fibrous tunic).**
1. Cornea: transparent; reflects light rays.

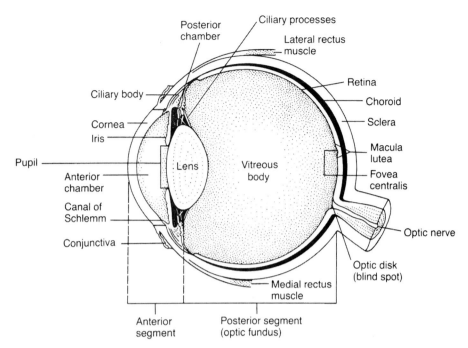

FIGURE 37-1 ■ Cross section of eyeball. (From Boyd-Monk, H.: The structure and function of the eye and its adnexa. *Journal of Ophthalmic Nursing and Technology*, 6[5]:176-183, 1987.)

2. Sclera: the "white" of the eye; normal bluish appearance in newborn infants; gives shape to the eyeball and protects the inner parts.

B. Middle layer (vascular tunic): the uveal tract.
1. Iris and pupil: a circular pigmented diaphragm with a central hole; controls the amount of light entering the eye.
2. Ciliary body: the anterior portion of the choroid.
3. Choroid: a vascular, pigmented membrane that lines most of the internal surface of the sclera, absorbs light rays, and nourishes the retina.

C. Inner layer: the retina.
1. Extends from the ora serrata to the optic nerve.
2. Functions in image formation.
   a. Photoreceptors: rods and cones.
   b. Bipolar cells.
   c. Ganglion cells.
3. Optic disc: retinal blood vessels enter the eye, and optic nerve exits the eye. Blind spot in field of vision because optic disc has no photoreceptors.
4. Optic nerve: second cranial nerve.
5. Macula: exact center of the retina and location of sharpest vision.

D. Anterior cavity (filled with aqueous humor).
1. Anterior chamber: behind the cornea, in front of the iris.
2. Posterior chamber: behind the iris, in front of the suspensory ligament and lens.

E. The lens: a biconvex, transparent capsule that refracts light; the most important focusing mechanism of the eye.
1. Lens remains cloudy until 30 to 34 weeks of gestation.

F. Posterior cavity (filled with vitreous humor): lies between the lens and the retina. Contributes to intraocular pressure, gives shape to the eyeball, and holds the retina in place.

Extraocular Muscles

A. Musculature. Six muscles move each globe. The muscles of each eye work in conjunction with each other.

B. **Innervation.** The extraocular muscles are innervated by the oculomotor (third cranial) nerve, the abducens (sixth cranial) nerve, and the trochlear (fourth cranial) nerve.
  1. Pupillary reflex is functional by 36 weeks.
C. **Function** (Blackburn, 2007; Gardner and Goldson, 2006).
  1. At birth newborns are able to see an object best at a distance of 8 to 10 inches.
  2. A healthy term newborn is able to fix on an object and follow it up to 90° in a horizontal arc.
  3. Newborns prefer black and white patterns and the human face.
  4. Color discrimination develops at 2 to 3 months of age (Graven, 2004).

PATIENT ASSESSMENT

History

A. **Pregnancy:** first-trimester infections (e.g., rubella), unknown rashes, fever, venereal disease, vaginal discharge, medications.
B. **Birth history:** gestational age, duration of labor, use of forceps.
C. **Family history:** incidence of ocular disorders, especially retinoblastoma; systemic diseases.
  Examination (Johnson, 2003; Strodtbeck, 2007)   The examination is performed with the baby in a quiet, alert state. To facilitate the spontaneous eye-opening, use an auditory stimulus, change the infant's position from supine to upright, or dim the lights (Johnson, 2003). Eye prophylaxis may make the examination more difficult.
A. **External assessment.**
  1. General facial configuration: should be symmetric. Note distance between the eyes; increased width between the eyes is referred to as hypertelorism and decreased width hypotelorism.
  2. Spontaneous eye movements: note range of motion and conjugation (the ability of the eyes to move together). Infants can track and follow objects with both eyes. Erratic or purposeless movements may be observed during the first few weeks of life. Median focal distance for the term neonate is about 8 inches (20 cm).
B. **Reaction to light or visual stimuli:** strong blink reflex to bright light or stimulation of the lids, lashes, or cornea. A somewhat unsteady gaze can be observed shortly after birth, with ability to fixate on a stimulus for 4 to 10 seconds and refixate every 1 to 1.5 seconds. Ability to maintain fixation and to follow does not occur until 5 to 6 weeks of age.
C. **Pupils:** shape should be round and reaction to light should be equal; constriction to both direct and contralateral stimulation should occur. The red reflex should be elicited bilaterally; normally appears as a homogeneous bright red-orange. Opacities or interruptions may indicate cataracts or retinoblastoma.
D. **Eyelids:** note symmetry, epicanthal folds, bruising or edema, lacerations, ptosis, and presence of lacrimal puncta.
E. **Conjunctiva:** should be pink and moist; redness or exudate is abnormal.
F. **Cornea:** may be somewhat less than transparent or slightly hazy in the first few days of life in both premature and term infants. Sclerae may be bluish in premature or small babies as a result of thinness.
G. **Irises:** should be similar in appearance; note pigmentation. A coloboma, or keyhole pupil, may be associated with congenital anomalies. Brushfield spots are silvery gray spots scattered around the circumference of the iris—strongly associated with Down syndrome.
H. **Lens:** should be clear and black with direct illumination. Examination of the anterior vascular capsule of the lens is a useful adjunct to determination of gestational age in preterm infants between 27 and 34 weeks.
I. **Doll's-eye reflex:** as head is turned toward each shoulder, eyes move in the opposite direction.

PATHOLOGIC CONDITIONS AND MANAGEMENT

Birth Trauma

Pathophysiology
A. **Direct result of duration and difficulty of delivery.**

B. **Improperly applied forceps.**

C. **Compression of cranial nerves.**
   Clinical Presentation

A. **Petechiae, ecchymoses, edema, and/or lacerations of pinna, lids, conjunctiva, or globe.**

B. **Bright-red patches on conjunctiva (subconjunctival hemorrhage):** occurs in up to 13% of births (Isenberg, 2005).

C. **Droopy eyelids.**
   Complications   These injuries are generally mild and transient, often resolving spontaneously.

Conjunctivitis

Conjunctivitis is an inflammatory reaction resulting from invasion of conjunctiva by pathologic organisms.

   Etiology   A wide variety of infectious agents are capable of producing conjunctivitis in the newborn infant. The most common causes in North America include the following:

A. *Neisseria gonorrhoeae*: peripartum transmission.

B. *Chlamydia trachomatis*: peripartum transmission.

C. *Staphylococcus aureus*: acquired during the neonatal period.

D. **Enteric pathogens.**

NEISSERIA GONORRHOEAE

A. **Incidence:** 30% to 35% of neonates born vaginally to infected women develop ophthalmic gonococcal infection (Embree, 2006). May be higher in areas with poor perinatal care or irregular antibiotic eye prophylaxis after birth.

B. **Onset of infection:** onset of symptoms usually between days 2 and 5 of life.

C. **Clinical presentation.**
   1. Edema of the eyelids.
   2. Purulent discharge.
   3. Redness/hyperemia of the conjunctiva.

D. **Diagnostic findings.**
   1. History.
      a. Maternal history of sexually transmitted disease.
      b. Age at onset of infection.
   2. Physical examination.
      a. Clinical signs of inflammation.
      b. Purulent discharge.
   3. Laboratory.
      a. Gram stain shows gram-negative diplococci.
      b. Culture positive for gonococci from conjunctival surface or exudate.

E. **Nursing care.**
   1. Isolate infant in accordance with infection control guidelines.
   2. Irrigate eyes with sterile normal saline solution hourly until discharge is eliminated.
   3. Promptly administer appropriate systemic therapy. Topical antimicrobial therapy is not required.
      a. Penicillin-sensitive *N. gonorrhoeae*: aqueous crystalline penicillin G, intravenous (IV) or intramuscular (IM), 50,000 to 100,000 units/kg/day in two or three divided doses for 7 days based on postconceptional and postnatal age (consult a drug manual for specific information).
      b. Penicillin-resistant *N. gonorrhoeae*: ceftriaxone, 50 mg/kg (maximum 125 mg) IV or IM in a single daily dose (Zenk, 2003).
   4. Parents of infected infant should be referred for evaluation and treatment.

F. **Complications.**
   1. Infants with gonococcal conjunctivitis are at risk of having corneal ulceration, perforation, and subsequent visual impairment.
   2. Systemic complications involving the blood, joints, or central nervous system (CNS) may occur in a small number of infants.

CHLAMYDIA TRACHOMATIS

A. **Incidence.**
1. The most common cause of conjunctivitis in the neonatal period, especially in areas with poor perinatal care or irregular administration of erythromycin eye prophylaxis after delivery. Chlamydial eye infections occur in up to 1% of births in developed countries (Isenberg, 2005).
2. About 20% to 50% of babies born to mothers who are colonized with *C. trachomatis* will develop the disease (Darville, 2006).
3. Prevention of infection in the newborn infant is dependent on prenatal detection and treatment of the mother or on the use of an effective form of eye prophylaxis at birth (e.g., erythromycin ointment).

B. **Onset:** symptoms are usually observed between 5 and 14 days of age.

C. **Clinical presentation:** symptoms vary from mild conjunctivitis to intense edema of the lids with purulent discharge.

D. **Diagnostic findings.**
1. Identification of Chlamydia antigen.
2. Stains of conjunctival scrapings.
3. Culture of conjunctival scrapings.

E. **Patient management.**
1. Therapy of choice is ophthalmic and oral erythromycin (estolate preparation), 20 mg/kg/day (Zenk, 2003).
2. Topical therapy alone is inadequate to eradicate the organism from the upper respiratory tract.
3. Parents of infected infants should be referred for evaluation and therapy.

F. **Complications:** infection is spread via the nasolacrimal system to the nasopharynx, leading to Chlamydia-related pneumonia.

Nasolacrimal Duct Obstruction

Pathophysiology

A. **Lacrimal apparatus** consists of structures that produce tears (lacrimal glands) and structures responsible for drainage of tears (upper and lower puncta, canaliculi, lacrimal sac, and nasolacrimal duct). System functions to clean, lubricate, and moisten the eyeball.

B. **Term and preterm newborn infants have the capacity to secrete tears** (reflex tearing to irritants) but usually do not secrete emotional tears until 2 to 3 months of age.

C. **Congenital obstruction** is usually caused by an imperforate membrane at the distal end of the nasolacrimal duct.

D. **Congenital nasolacrimal obstruction is the most common abnormality of the neonate's lacrimal apparatus.** Incidence of this condition ranges between 2% and 6% of all newborn infants.

Clinical Presentation

A. **Usually within the first few weeks of life.**

B. **Persistent tearing (epiphora):** need to rule out congenital glaucoma.

C. **Crusting or matting of the eyelashes:** "sticky eye."

D. **Spilling of tears over the lower lid and cheek:** a "wet look" in the involved eye(s).

E. **Absence of conjunctival infection.**

F. **Mucopurulent material refluxing from either punctum when gentle pressure is applied over the involved nasolacrimal sac.**

Complications

A. **Acute dacryocystitis:** inflamed, swollen lacrimal sac.

B. **Fistula formation.**

C. **Orbital or facial cellulitis.**

Nursing Care

A. **Conservative management,** with daily massage of the nasolacrimal sac in an attempt to rupture the membrane at the lower end of the duct.

B. **Technique** consists of placing the index finger over the common canaliculus to block the exit of material through the puncta, and stroking downward firmly.

C. **Digital pressure increases hydrostatic pressure in the nasolacrimal sac,** which may cause a rupture of the membranous obstruction.

D. **If a mucopurulent discharge is present,** antibiotic eyedrops (sodium sulfacetamide) or ointment (erythromycin) may be required.

E. **Cleansing of eyes:** eyes should be cleaned with moist compresses, with secretions mechanically removed.

F. **Duration of conservative management:** conservative management is advocated for the first year of life.

G. **Resolution:** the majority of nasolacrimal obstructions resolve spontaneously or with massage by 1 year of age.

H. **Surgical treatment:** unresolved obstructions can be successfully treated surgically; tear duct probing is done, with the infant under general anesthesia, after the first year of life.

Cataracts

Congenital cataracts are the main treatable cause of visual impairment in infancy. The sooner in life the cataracts are removed surgically and proper optics are restored, the better the child's visual prognosis.

Pathophysiology

A. **Lens:** The lens is a biconvex, transparent capsule that refracts light. It is the most important focusing mechanism of the eye.

B. **Cataract:** A cataract is an opacity of any size or degree in the lens of the eye.

C. **Path of light:** Normally the light from an object passes directly through the lens to a focal point on the retina, producing a sharp image. Cataracts result in a degraded image or no image at all.

D. **Visual impairment:** Cataracts lead to varying degrees of visual impairment, from blurred vision to blindness, depending on the location and extent of the opacity. In neonates, cataracts are often transient, disappearing spontaneously within a few weeks.

Etiology or Precipitating Factors

A. **Idiopathic:** developmental variation, not associated with other abnormalities.

B. **Genetically determined:** most common mode of inheritance—autosomal dominant.

C. **Congenital rubella:** cataracts in 50% of newborn infants with congenital rubella syndrome.

D. **Other congenital infections.**
1. Toxoplasmosis.
2. Cytomegalovirus infection.
3. Herpes simplex.
4. Varicella.

E. **Metabolic disorders** (e.g., galactosemia).

F. **Chromosomal abnormalities** (e.g., Down syndrome).

G. **Clinical syndromes** (e.g., Crouzon disease, Pierre Robin syndrome).

H. **Prematurity.**

Clinical Presentation

A. **White pupil** (leukocoria).

B. **Searching nystagmus** (at 1 to 2 months of age).

Diagnostic Findings

A. **History.**
1. Family history of ocular disease or systemic disorders.
2. Pregnancy, especially first-trimester intrauterine infections.

B. **Physical examination.**
1. Normally the pupils look black to the bare eye of the examiner when light is directed at them.
2. Examine to detect a white pupil by shining a light into each eye, with the light source held to one side.

3. If the opacity is small, it may be identified only when the pupils are dilated and with the use of an ophthalmoscope.
4. Consider other diseases of the eye that may produce a white pupil (e.g., retinoblastoma).

Complications

A. **Varying degrees of visual impairment, leading to developmental delay.**
B. **Presence and/or severity of associated ocular defects, such as microphthalmos and glaucoma.**

Nursing Care

A. **Eye examination:** Assist the physician in carrying out a thorough eye examination of the newborn infant. This includes administering drops to dilate the pupils before the examination and supporting the infant's head to facilitate examination.
B. **Parental education:** In collaboration with the physician, assist parents in understanding the nature, possible cause, and treatment of cataracts in the newborn infant, together with the prognosis for future vision. Surgery is indicated whenever the cataract is likely to interfere with vision.
C. **Explore any feelings of guilt the parents may have** in relation to the cause of the cataracts; provide appropriate support.
D. **Encourage parent–infant attachment:** Neonate may not be able to see the parents but can learn to know their voices, smell, and touch.
E. **Care for the patient postoperatively.**
   1. Prevent increased intraocular pressure. Keep the neonate comfortable, well fed, and free of pain to decrease crying.
   2. Administer eyedrops or ointments as ordered postoperatively.
   3. Apply clean eye patches or protective shields to protect the eye from rubbing or bumping and to prevent irritation from light.
   4. Monitor for complications of cataract surgery. These are relatively infrequent but include infection within the eye, glaucoma, and retinal detachment. Note any increased redness or haziness of the eye, increased tearing, photophobia, or cloudiness of the cornea. Increased crying, irritability, disruption in sleeping patterns, or rubbing of the eye may indicate pain.
   5. Assist the parents in understanding the essential role of optical correction devices, such as glasses or contact lenses, on their infant's vision and development.
   6. Promote appropriate visual stimulation and foster normal infant development by teaching parents about newborn visual preferences (e.g., black-and-white contrast or medium-intensity colors, the human face, geometric shapes, checkerboard designs).

   Outcome   Visual prognosis depends not only on the extent of cataracts, age at removal, surgical outcome, and rapid optical correction but also on the nature of other associated anomalies of the eye or syndromes.

   Congenital Infections   The developing eyes are highly vulnerable to the damaging effects of prenatal infection (Allen et al., 2006), and ocular abnormalities may in fact be the predominant manifestation of the disease. A number of the congenitally acquired infections are associated with abnormal ocular conditions, including cataracts, chorioretinitis, corneal opacities, and glaucoma.

   The most common of these infections are toxoplasmosis, rubella, cytomegalovirus, and herpes (see also Chapter 33).

Congenital Rubella Syndrome

Pathophysiology

A. **Timing of infection:** Consequences of the transplacental infection are determined primarily by the timing of the viral insult.
B. **Infection in the first trimester of pregnancy presents the greatest hazard to organogenesis, including that of the eyes.**

Incidence   Ocular abnormalities are the cardinal manifestations of congenital rubella, occurring in 50% to 75% of patients, with cataracts being the most common ocular abnormality (Cooper and Alford, 2006).

Clinical Presentation

A. **Gestational age:** Findings in the infant exposed to rubella in utero depend on the gestational age at which the infection occurred.

B. **Ocular manifestations.**
   1. Cataracts: in approximately 50% to 75% of patients.
   2. Pigmentary retinopathy.
   3. Microphthalmos.
   4. Glaucoma: in 20% to 50% of patients.
C. **Other common manifestations** include intrauterine growth restriction, hepatomegaly, thrombocytopenia, and cardiac anomalies (see also Chapter 33).

   Nursing Care
A. **Virus shedding may continue for months after birth.** Infants with suspected congenital rubella should be isolated from other newborn infants and from pregnant women (both in the hospital and at home after discharge).
B. **Parents need to understand the immediate and long-term effects of this disease.**
C. **See Nursing Care section,** under Cataracts, on p. 838.

   Outcome
A. **Prognosis:** depends on severity of symptoms and number of organ systems involved.
B. **Mortality rate:** in first year of life may approach 80% when multisystem involvement occurs.
C. **Multiple disabilities:** common in surviving infants.
D. **Consequences of congenital rubella:** may not be evident at birth but may become apparent in subsequent months.
E. **Follow-up:** ongoing follow-up and evaluation after discharge of infant from hospital. Major problems after the neonatal period include communication disorders, hearing defects, and mental or motor retardation.

Cytomegalovirus

Pathophysiology
A. **Cytomegalovirus (CMV)** can cause a perinatal viral infection.
B. **Congenital illness is most severe if infection occurs early in pregnancy,** the period of greatest susceptibility of the developing fetus.

   Etiology
A. **Ubiquitous virus:** CMV can cause infection in all age groups.
B. **Route of transmission:** Infection may be acquired transplacentally, during birth (via the cervix), or through breast milk.
C. **Transfusion:** An important possible cause of morbidity in premature infants is transfusion-acquired CMV. All premature infants should receive seronegative blood products.

   Incidence
A. **The most common congenital viral infection.**
B. **In the presence of primary acute maternal infection, 40% of fetuses are affected, with a range of 24% to 75%** (Freij and Sever, 2005; Stagno and Britt, 2006).

   Clinical Presentation
A. **A diagnosis of congenital CMV infection can rarely be made on the basis of clinical findings alone.** Only 5% to 10% of neonates infected with CMV will have symptoms at birth.
B. **Laboratory diagnostic methods** (e.g., isolation of the virus from the urine) must be used if this condition is suspected.
C. **Chorioretinitis is present in 10% to 20% of infants with symptoms and is the single most common finding in congenitally infected infants.**
D. **Other eye abnormalities include conjunctivitis, corneal clouding, cataracts, and optic atrophy.**
E. **Other manifestations include intrauterine growth restriction, hepatosplenomegaly, and bleeding disorders** (see also Chapter 33).

Complications

A. **Cytomegalic inclusion disease.**
B. **Sensorineural hearing loss, the most important late sequela, and the most common cause of congenital hearing loss** (Freij and Sever, 2005; Stagno and Britt, 2006).

Nursing Care

A. **No effective treatment exists.** Supportive nursing care measures, aimed at specific symptoms, are employed.

B. **Use of gowns and good handwashing technique are essential** to prevent the spread of infection.

C. **Seronegative pregnant women should not care for infants with known or suspected infection.**

D. **These infants require long-term follow-up.**

Outcomes

A. **Mortality rate:** Overall mortality rate for symptomatic congenital infection is up to 30% (Freij and Sever, 2005; Stagno and Britt, 2006).

B. **Few survivors are normal.** In 10% to 20% of infants who are free of symptoms at birth, neurologic sequelae, such as mental retardation or sensorineural deafness, may develop in the first years of life.

Toxoplasmosis (Remington et al., 2006)

Pathophysiology   Fetal damage occurs as a direct result of inflammation caused by the presence of cysts in the tissues, including the eyes.

Etiology

A. **Maternal infection by the protozoan** *Toxoplasma gondii* in the first and second trimesters of pregnancy is often associated with transplacental infection of the fetus.

B. **Infection is acquired through contact with the excrement of infected cats and ingestion of improperly cooked meat.**

Incidence

A. **The incidence of maternal infection ranges from 2 to 12 per 1000** (Freij and Sever, 2005).

B. **Congenital infection rates are approximately 1 to 7 per 1000 live births** (Freij and Sever, 2005).

Clinical Presentation

A. **Chorioretinitis** is the most common manifestation.

B. **Other manifestations** include hepatosplenomegaly, jaundice, and bleeding disorders (see also Chapter 33).

Specific Nursing Care

A. **Nursing care includes pharmaceutical treatment of** Toxoplasma infection by administering sulfadiazine and pyrimethamine. These agents will eradicate the cysts but will not reverse the damage already done.

B. **Give supportive care to the family,** with sensitivity to feelings of guilt they might have.

C. **Teach parents to recognize the signs of visual impairment in infancy** (e.g., failure to fix and focus on objects or faces).

Outcome

A. **Prognosis for infants with congenital infection:** poor.

B. **Mortality rate:** roughly 10% to 15% of infected infants.

C. **Psychomotor retardation:** severe in 85% of survivors.

D. **Visual disturbances:** develop in 50% of surviving infants.

Retinopathy of Prematurity   Formally referred to as retrolental fibroplasia, retinopathy of prematurity (ROP) is a vasoproliferative retinopathy that occurs primarily in premature infants less than 28 weeks of gestational age (American Academy of Pediatrics [AAP], 2006).

Pathophysiology

A. **Human retina is avascular until 16 weeks of gestation.** After this time a capillary network begins to grow, starting at the optic nerve and branching outward toward the ora serrata (edge of the retina).

B. **Nasal periphery is vascularized by about 32 weeks of gestation,** but the process is not complete in the more distant temporal periphery until 40 to 44 weeks.

C. **After premature birth,** this process of normal vasculogenesis may be arrested as a result of injury from some noxious agent(s) or stressor(s).

D. **Vasoproliferation:** This arrest of normal vasculogenesis is later followed by a phase of rapid, excessive, irregular vascular growth and shunt formation (vasoproliferation), stimulated by vascular endothelial growth factor (VEGF) and interleukin growth factor (ILGF).

E. **Area of new growth generally forms an abrupt ridge between the vascular and avascular retina,** particularly in the temporal periphery.

F. **ROP may resolve if the vasculature in the area recovers and resumes advancing normally,** allowing the retina to become completely vascularized.

G. **If the new vasculature proceeds to develop abnormally,** these capillaries may extend into the vitreous body and/or over the surface of the retina (where they do not belong). Leakage of fluid or hemorrhage from these weak, aberrant blood vessels may occur.

H. **Blood and fluid leakage** into various parts of the eye can result in scar formation and traction on the retina.

I. **Traction may pull the macula out of its normal position, thus affecting visual acuity.** If the macula is slightly out of position, vision will be mildly affected.

J. **Tractional exudative retinal detachment results in blindness.**

Etiology

A. **Complex multifactorial disorder.**

B. **Possible risk factors** (Hagedorn et al., 2006).
   1. Prematurity/low birth weight: most important clinical factor associated with ROP.
   2. Hyperoxia.
   3. Hypoxia.
   4. Multiple births.
   5. Blood transfusions.
   6. Intraventricular hemorrhage.
   7. Apnea/bradycardia episodes.
   8. Sepsis.
   9. Hypercapnia/hypocapnia.
   10. Patent ductus arteriosus.
   11. Vitamin E deficiency.
   12. Lactic acidosis.
   13. Prenatal complications: maternal hypertension, diabetes, bleeding, smoking.
   14. Duration of mechanical ventilation and oxygen therapy.
   15. Exposure to bright light.

Incidence

A. **Incidence of ROP appears to increase significantly as birth weight and gestational age decrease.** Up to 82% of neonates weighing less than 1 kg will develop ROP; 9.3% of these infants will progress to vision-threatening disease (Isenberg, 2005).

Stages of Retinopathy

A. **Standardized approach for describing ROP,** developed by the International Committee for the Classification of Retinopathy of Prematurity (2005) according to five stages.
   1. Stage 1: demarcation line within the plane of the retina separating the avascular and vascular retinal regions.
   2. Stage 2: ridge or elevation extending out of the plane of the retina.
   3. Stage 3: ridge with extraretinal fibrovascular proliferation, either
      a. Continuous with the posterior edge of the ridge,
      b. Posterior but disconnected from the ridge, or
      c. Into the vitreous.
   4. Stage 4: subtotal retinal detachment.
      a. Extrafoveate.
      b. Involving the foveae.
   5. Stage 5: total retinal detachment.

B. **"Plus" disease:** an indicator of activity. Signs (in increasing severity) include the following:
   1. Engorgement and tortuosity of the posterior pole retinal vessels.
   2. Iris vessel engorgement.
   3. Pupil rigidity.
   4. Vitreous haze.

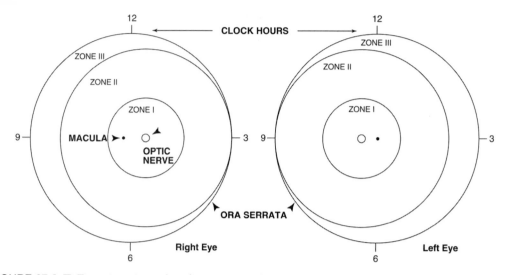

FIGURE 37-2 ■ Zones in retinopathy of prematurity. (From George, D.S.: The latest on retinopathy of prematurity. *MCN American Journal of Maternal/Child Nursing, 13*[4]:254-258, 1988.)

C. **Rush disease,** an aggressive type of ROP. Rush disease develops between 3 and 5 weeks after delivery and may progress rapidly to severe ROP.
D. **Zones for classification of ROP** (Fig. 37-2).
   1. Zone 1: extends from the optic disc to twice the disc-foveal distance—a radius of 30 degrees.
   2. Zone 2: extends from the periphery of the nasal retina (ora serrata) in a circle around the anatomic equator.
   3. Zone 3: anterior to zone 2; present temporally, inferiorly, and superiorly but not in the nasal retina.

   Physical Examination
A. **Examination of the high-risk neonate:** All newborn infants born at less than 32 weeks of gestation or with a birth weight of less than 1500 g, and selected infants between 1500 and 2000 g or gestational age greater than 32 weeks with an unstable clinical course should have their eyes examined by a trained pediatric ophthalmologist when in stable clinical condition, 4 to 6 weeks after birth (approximately 31 to 33 weeks of postconceptional age) (AAP, 2006).
B. **Dilation of pupils:** Infant's pupils should be dilated with a mydriatic agent before examination, to facilitate optimal evaluation. Cycloplegic mydriatic agents (e.g., cyclopentolate, tropicamide) have rapid onset of action, with peak ophthalmic effects between 20 and 60 minutes. The excess eyedrops should be wiped away promptly to avoid systemic absorption. Absorption can also be minimized by applying gentle pressure over the nasolacrimal duct for 1 minute following instillation of the eyedrops. It is necessary to protect eyes from bright light after mydriasis. Assess for symptoms of systemic absorption (e.g., tachycardia, restlessness) and notify physician immediately if symptoms are present.
C. **Documentation:** Location and extent of any retinopathy should be precisely documented and classified according to the guidelines developed by the International Committee for the Classification of Retinopathy of Prematurity (2005).
D. **Follow-up.**
   1. Infants who are found to have areas of retinal immaturity on initial examination should have repeated examinations every other week and, subsequently, every 2 to 3 weeks until vascularization has reached the ora serrata.
   2. If ROP is present during the initial examination, the infant should be examined weekly or every other week, depending on the severity of clinical findings.

Prevention

A. **Precautions while using oxygen:** Although the role of oxygen in the pathogenesis of ROP is unclear, cautious and judicious administration and monitoring of oxygen remains one possible preventive measure.

1. Continuous assessment and monitoring of the infant receiving oxygen to control arterial oxygenation. Cautious administration of oxygen while carrying out nursing procedures such as suctioning.

2. Ongoing assessment of the oxygen delivery system, including calibration of oxygen analyzers, monitoring fractional inspired oxygen, checking/recording ventilator settings, circuit, and oxygen saturation monitors.

3. Use of oxygen blenders to deliver precise oxygen concentrations.

4. Lowering oxygen saturation alarm limits to 85% to 93% for neonates who weigh ≤1250 g at birth for the first week of life may decrease the incidence of threshold ROP (Vanderveen et al., 2006).

B. **Sensory stimulation:** Provide a variety of forms of sensory stimulation to the infant, appropriate to level of development and behavioral cues.

C. **Assessment:** Assess newborn infant's ability to fix and focus.

D. **Assistance:** Assist the physician in carrying out a safe, minimally stressful eye examination of the newborn infant.

E. **Protection against bright light:** Protect the infant's eyes from bright light by shielding the incubator with a blanket and reducing the light in the nursery. The use of eye pads should be evaluated according to the principles of developmental care.

F. **Parent education:** Provide accurate parent education about the possibility of ROP (when parents are ready to receive information about potential non–life-threatening complications). Ensure that parents understand that ROP is essentially a problem of immaturity whose cause is yet unknown (AAP, 2006).

Treatment

A. **Timing of treatment:** Threshold ROP may no longer be the preferred time for intervention (Early Treatment for Retinopathy of Prematurity Cooperative Group, 2003). Ablative treatment may be initiated for the following (AAP, 2006):

1. Zone I ROP: Any stage with plus disease.

2. Zone I ROP: Stage 3 with no plus disease.

3. Zone II: Stage 2 or 3 with plus disease.

4. The number of clock hours may not always be the determining factor for the strong consideration of ablative treatment.

5. Treatment should be started within 72 hours of the finding of treatable disease to decrease the risk of retinal detachment.

B. **Laser photocoagulation.**

1. Uses either an argon or diode laser to coagulate the avascular periphery of the retina.

2. With results similar to those from cryotherapy, laser surgery can be performed in the nursery with sedation and analgesia rather than general anesthesia.

3. Is more difficult when the retina is not readily visualized (pupils cannot be dilated, presence of hemorrhage)

4. Has fewer systemic and ocular side effects than cryotherapy and carries less risk of damage to adjacent structures (Isenberg, 2005). Is less painful than cryotherapy.

5. Complications: cataracts (Isenberg, 2005); burns to the cornea, iris, or lens; retinal, periretinal, or vitreous hemorrhage; photocoagulation of the fovea; and late-onset retinal detachment.

C. **Nursing care for the infant undergoing laser photocoagulation.**

1. Preoperatively, the infant should be given nothing by mouth for 4 to 6 hours; phenylephrine with cyclopentolate (Cyclomydril) and sedation and analgesia should be given as ordered.

2. Intraoperatively, monitor the baby and give medications as indicated.

3. After laser photocoagulation, the infant's respiratory status, oxygen saturation, and vital signs should be monitored.

4. Assess the eyes for drainage and edema.

5. Medications such as cyclopentolate and the combination dexamethasone, neomycin, and polymyxin B sulfate (Maxitrol) may be ordered to reduce postoperative complications.

D. **Cryotherapy.**
1. Although the use of cryotherapy is decreasing, it continues to be used in some centers. Cryotherapy can be used in special circumstances (Isenberg, 2005).
2. Supercooled probe is used to freeze the avascular retina, preventing vessel proliferation.
3. Invasive procedure requires anesthesia.
4. Complications include scarring of the retina; periorbital edema; conjunctival hematoma or laceration; elevation of intraocular pressure; retinal, periretinal, or vitreous hemorrhage; central renal artery occlusion; freezing of the optic nerve; and late-onset retinal detachment (Isenberg, 2005).

E. **Nursing care of the infant undergoing cryotherapy.**
1. Monitor the infant closely for possible risks of the procedure.
   a. Risks of undergoing general anesthesia.
   b. Arrhythmias induced from the use of lidocaine (Xylocaine).
   c. Bradycardia caused by vagal stimulation created by pressure on the eyeball.
   d. Edema of the eyelids.
   e. Infection.
   f. Intraocular bleeding.
2. Ensure patient safety and comfort during the treatment.
   a. Place baby in supine position.
   b. Maintain adequate heat source throughout the procedure.
   c. Monitor vital signs and oxygenation status throughout the procedure.
   d. Provide comfort measures and analgesia as needed.
3. Provide postoperative care after the treatment.
   a. Administer eyedrops or ointments as ordered.
   b. Shield infant from unnecessary direct light.
   c. If mydriatic agents were used, observe infant for signs of feeding intolerance, gastric distention, and/or aspirates when feedings are resumed.

F. **Vitreoretinal surgery** results in reattachment of the retina in 30% of cases; however, following macular detachment visual prognosis is poor even if the retina is successfully reattached (Isenberg, 2005).

G. **Provide emotional support and appropriate community referrals** for parents whose infant will have significant visual impairment.

Complications

A. **Mydriatic eyedrops and eye examinations can produce hypertension, reflex bradycardia, and apnea as a result of drug effects and vagal stimulation.**

B. **Varying degrees of visual impairment** (e.g., myopia) may require corrective lenses to improve visual acuity.

C. **Additional complications include the following:**
1. Strabismus.
2. Glaucoma.
3. Cataracts.
4. Amblyopia.
5. Retinal detachment and blindness.

Outcome

A. **Ninety percent (or more) cases of acute ROP resolve spontaneously, with little or no visual loss.**

B. **Laser and cryotherapy have been shown to decrease the risk of blinding complications of ROP by 50%.** A significant number of visual impairments may result, especially in the presence of disease in zone 1.

ANATOMY OF THE EAR (Fig. 37-3)

External Ear

A. **Auricle.**
1. Thin plate of elastic cartilage covered by skin.
2. Collects air vibrations.

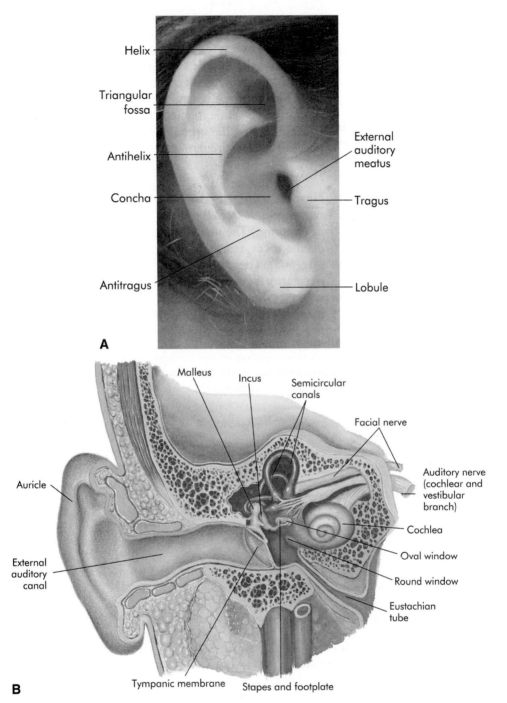

FIGURE 37-3 ■ **A**, Different parts of the auricle of the external ear. **B**, Anatomy of the ear. (From Seidel, H.M., Ball, J.W., Dains, J.E., and Benedict, G.W.: *Mosby's guide to physical examination* [6th ed.]. St Louis, 2006, Mosby.)

3. Possesses extrinsic and intrinsic muscle.
4. Supplied by branches of facial nerve.
5. Consists of tragus, helix, concha, and lobule.

B. **External auditory meatus.**
   1. Curved tube leading to tympanic membrane.
   2. Framework composed of elastic cartilage (outer one third) and bone (inner two thirds).

3. Lined by skin; outer one third has hair, sebaceous, and ceruminous glands.
4. Auriculotemporal nerve and auricular branch of vagus nerve provide sensory output.
5. Lymph drainage is to parotid, mastoid, and cervical lymph nodes.
6. At birth, meatus is shorter and less curved than in the adult.

Middle Ear

A. **Slitlike air-containing cavity within petrous (bony) portion of the temporal bone.**
B. **Has roof, floor, anterior, posterior, medial, and lateral walls.**
C. **Lateral wall is the tympanic membrane.**
   1. Tympanic membrane is thin, fibrous membrane.
   2. Sound waves move tympanic membrane medially.
   3. Obliquely placed, concave laterally.
      a. Depression in concavity is called the umbo.
      b. Umbo is produced by the tip of the handle of the malleus ("hammer").
D. **Contains the auditory ossicles.**
   1. Ossicles include malleus, incus (anvil), and stapes (stirrup).
   2. Malleus and incus can be recognized on otoscopic examination.
      a. Tensor tympani muscle inserts on malleus; dampens vibrations.
   3. Stapes inserts on the oval window of the semicircular canal.
      a. Stapedius muscle inserts on stapes; dampens vibrations.
   4. Movement of tympanic membrane moves ossicles.
   5. Movement of ossicles induces compression waves in fluid (perilymph) in cochlea.
E. **Communicates to the nasopharynx via the eustachian (auditory) canal.**
   1. Eustachian tube equalizes air pressure between the middle ear and the nasopharynx.

Inner Ear

A. **Cavity in petrous portion of temporal bone, medial to middle ear.**
B. **Consists of bony labyrinth and membranous labyrinth; the latter is lodged within the former.**
   1. Membranous labyrinth filled with endolymph.
   2. Bony labyrinth consists of vestibule, semicircular canals, and cochlea.
      a. Vestibule forms base of semicircular canals.
      b. Semicircular canals (superior, posterior, and lateral) arise from vestibule; filled with perilymph.
      c. Movement of perilymph in semicircular canals induced by axial movement.
      d. Transduced by vestibular branch of cochlear nerve.
      e. Cochlea composed of two continuous chambers (scala tympani and scala vestibule) filled with perilymph and a medial chamber (cochlear duct) filled with endolymph.
      f. Sensory ("hair") cells stimulated by compression waves that cause relative movement of membranes within cochlea.

INNERVATION

A. **Sensory afferents from cochlea and vestibule transmitted by branches of vestibulocochlear (eighth cranial) nerve.**
   1. Vestibular branch forms vestibular ganglion, which receives nerves from different regions of the vestibule.
   2. Cochlear nerve has motor and sensory branches.
B. **Motor efferents to tensor tympani and stapedius muscles.**
   1. Tensor tympani supplied by mandibular branch of trigeminal nerve.
   2. Stapedius supplied by the facial nerve.
C. **Vestibulocochlear and facial nerves enter the inner ear via the internal acoustic meatus.**

PATIENT ASSESSMENT

History

A. **Pregnancy:** first-trimester infections (e.g., cytomegalovirus), unknown rashes, fevers, flu-like illnesses.

B. **Family history:** incidence of hearing loss, ocular disorders.

C. **History of risk factors:** identified below.

Examination

During all interactions care providers should observe the neonate's response to sound. A more focused assessment is performed with the baby in a quiet, alert state.

A. **General assessment.**
1. General facial configuration: the ears should be symmetrically positioned with the helix of the ear on or above an imaginary line drawn from the inner to the outer canthus of the eye toward the ear. Ears that fall below that line are termed *low-set* and often associated with genetic syndromes and other congenital malformations.
2. The development of the pinna correlates with the infant's gestational age. The pinna of a term infant is firm, with prompt recoil.
3. Presence of preauricular pits or skin tags may be familial or associated with other anomalies, especially of the renal system. Pits may also communicate with the brain or inner ear and lead to infection.
4. Poorly developed or malformed ears are associated with hearing loss and other anomalies (Johnson, 2003).
5. Otoscopic examination of the newborn ear is not part of a routine examination. Visually inspect the auditory canal to ensure patency.
6. As part of a complete assessment, physical features of syndromes associated with sensorineural hearing loss should be identified.

    Hearing Loss　Hearing loss in the newborn population is estimated to occur at a rate of between 1 and 2 in 1000 live births (Matthews and Robin, 2006). Low birth weight neonates demonstrate failure rates of 20% to 25% when tested at term (Volpe, 2008). Hearing loss occurs across a continuum and can be classified as mild, moderate, or severe. Some types of hearing loss such as those caused by congenital infections are progressive or manifest well beyond the newborn period. Ongoing monitoring is needed for those infants with risk factors but who have normal hearing at birth (Kaye and the Committee on Genetics, 2006; Volpe, 2008).

Pathophysiology

A. **Conductive:** dysfunction of the outer or middle ear prevents sound transmission.

B. **Sensorineural:** results from damage to the sensory nerve endings in the cochlea or impairment of the auditory nerve.

C. **Mixed:** a combination of conductive and sensorineural hearing loss.

Etiology

RISK FACTORS (Kaye and the Committee on Genetics, 2006; Volpe, 2008)

A. **Familial.**

B. **Craniofacial anomalies: especially those involving the pinna and ear canal.**

C. **Hyperbilirubinemia:** at levels requiring exchange transfusion.

D. **Bacterial meningitis.**

E. **Low Apgar scores** (less than 5 at 1 minute, less than 6 at 5 minutes).

F. **Ototoxic drugs.**
1. Gentamicin.
2. Vancomycin.

G. **Intrauterine infections.**
1. Cytomegalovirus.
2. Rubella.
3. Syphilis.
4. Herpes.
5. Toxoplasmosis.

H. Syndromes associated with hearing loss.

I. Idiopathic (up to 50% of cases).

Hearing Screening

Examination of all newborns. The AAP and the Joint Committee on Infant Hearing recommend universal hearing screening for all newborns (AAP, 1999; Joint Committee on Infant Hearing, 2007). Prompt detection of hearing loss facilitates interventions aimed at preventing speech, language, and cognitive development impairments.

Methodology

A. **Evoked otoacoustic emissions (EOAE).**

   1. Measures sound waves generated in the inner ear in response to clicks or tone bursts generated by small microphones placed in the infant's auditory canals.

   2. Advantages: results are specific to each ear; not dependent of the infant's state; short test time.

   3. Disadvantages: inaccurate in the presence of debris in the ear canal; infant must be relatively inactive during the test; does not test neural transmission of sound.

B. **Auditory brainstem response (ABR).**

   1. Using three scalp electrodes, measures brain waves generated in response to mechanically generated ticks.

   2. Advantages: ear-specific results; unaffected by ear canal debris.

   3. Disadvantages: infant must be in a quiet state.

C. **Follow-up:** hearing screening identifies infants at risk for hearing loss but is not diagnostic. Infants who fail screening tests must be referred for further testing and intervention.

REFERENCES

Allen, M.C., Donohue, P.K., and Porter, M.: Follow-up of the NICU Infant. In G.B. Merenstein and S.L. Gardner (Eds.): *Handbook of neonatal intensive care* (6th ed.). St Louis, 2006, Mosby, pp. 953-969.

American Academy of Pediatrics: Newborn and infant hearing loss: Detection and intervention. *Pediatrics*, 103(2):527-530, 1999.

American Academy of Pediatrics: *Report of Committee on Infectious Diseases*. Elk Grove Village, IL, 2006, American Academy of Pediatrics.

Blackburn, S.T.: *Maternal, fetal, and neonatal physiology: A clinical perspective* (3rd ed.). Philadelphia, 2007, Saunders.

Cooper, L.Z. and Alford, C.A.: Rubella. In J.S. Remington and J.O. Klein (Eds.): *Infectious diseases of the fetus and newborn infant*. Philadelphia, 2006, Saunders, pp. 893-926.

Darville, T.: Chlamydia Infections. In J.S. Remington and J.O. Klein (Eds.): *Infectious diseases of the fetus and newborn infant*. Philadelphia, 2006, Saunders, pp. 385-392.

Early Treatment for Retinopathy of Prematurity Cooperative Group: Revised indications for the treatment of retinopathy of prematurity: Results of the early treatment for retinopathy of prematurity randomized trial. *Archives in Ophthalmology*, 121:1684-1694, 2003.

Embree, J.E.: Gonococcal infections. In J.S. Remington and J.O. Klein (Eds.): *Infectious diseases of the fetus and newborn infant*. Philadelphia, 2006, Saunders, pp. 393-401.

Freij, B.J. and Sever, J.L.: Viral and protozoal infections. In M.G. MacDonald, M.D. Mullet, and M.M.K. Seshia

(Eds.): *Avery's neonatology. Pathophysiology and management of the newborn* (6th ed.). Philadelphia, 2005, Philadelphia, pp. 1274-1356.

Gardner, S.L. and Goldson, E.: The neonate and the environment: Impact on development. In G.B. Merenstein and S.L. Garner (Eds.): *Handbook of neonatal intensive care* (6th ed.). St. Louis, 2006, Mosby, pp. 273-349.

Graven, S.: Early neurosensory visual development of the fetus and newborn. *Clinics in Perinatology*, 31:199, 2004.

Hagedorn, M.I., Gardner, S.L., and Abman, S.: Respiratory diseases. In G.B. Merenstein and S.L. Gardner (Eds.): *Handbook of neonatal intensive care* (6th ed.). St. Louis, 2006, Mosby, pp. 595-698.

International Committee for the Classification of Retinopathy of Prematurity: The International Classification of Retinopathy of Prematurity revisited. *Archives in Ophthalmology*, 123:991-999, 2005.

Isenberg, S.J.: Eye disorders. In G.B. Avery, M.A. Fletcher, and M.G. MacDonald (Eds.): *Neonatology: Pathophysiology and management of the newborn* (6th ed.). Philadelphia, 2005, Lippincott Williams & Wilkins, pp. 1469-1484.

Johnson, C.B.: Head, eyes, ears, nose, mouth and neck assessment. In E. Tappero and M.E. Honeyfield (Eds.): *Physical assessment of the newborn* (3rd ed.). Santa Rosa, CA, 2003, NICU Ink.

Joint Committee on Infant Hearing: Year 2007 Position Statement: Principles and guidelines for early hearing detection and intervention program. *Pediatrics*, 120(4):898-921, 2007.

Kaye, C.I. and the Committee on Genetics: Newborn screening fact sheets. *Pediatrics, 188*(3):e934-e963, 2006.

Matthews, A.L. and Robin, N.H.: Genetic disorders, malformations, and inborn errors of metabolism. In G.B. Merenstein and S.L. Gardner (Eds.): *Handbook of neonatal intensive care* (6th ed.). St. Louis, 2006, Mosby, pp. 812-837.

Remington, J., McLeod, R., Thulliez, P., and Desmonts, G.: Toxoplasmosis. In J.S. Remington, J.O. Klein, C.B. Wilson, and C.T. Baker (Eds.): *Infectious diseases of the fetus and newborn* (6th ed.). Philadelphia: Saunders, 2006, pp. 947-1091.

Stagno, S. and Britt, W.: Cytomegalovirus infections. In J.S. Remington and J.O. Klein (Eds.): *Infectious diseases of the fetus and newborn infant*. Philadelphia, 2006, Saunders, pp. 739-782.

Strodtbeck, F.: Ophthalmic system. In C. Kenner and J.W. Lott (Eds.): *Comprehensive neonatal care: A multidisciplinary approach*. Philadelphia, 2007, Saunders, pp. 313-332.

VanderVeen, D.K., Mansfield, T.A., and Eichenwald, E.C.: Lower oxygen saturation alarm limits decrease the severity of retinopathy of prematurity. *Journal of AAPOS, 10*:445-448, 2006.

Volpe, J.J.: *Neurology of the newborn* (5th ed.). Philadelphia, 2008, Saunders.

Zenk, K.: *Neonatal medications and nutrition* (3rd ed.). Santa Rosa, CA, 2003, NICU Ink.

38 Foundations of Neonatal Research

KAREN A. THOMAS

OBJECTIVES

1. Identify roles of nurses engaged in research according to educational preparation.
2. Describe the research process and key components of research studies.
3. Identify nurses as research consumers who implement research utilization strategies in clinical practice.
4. List questions to ask when critiquing research literature.
5. Be informed about the rights of research subjects and the ethical conduct of research.

RESEARCH AND GENERATION OF NURSING KNOWLEDGE*

Research refers to systematic inquiry or investigation governed by scientific principles and conducted to expand knowledge and increase understanding. The research process describes a logical and orderly progression from development of a question through the conduct of a study and resultant findings and dissemination of conclusions. The questions asked and the methodology that guide inquiry reflect underlying values and beliefs, worldview, or philosophy. Scientific method describes prescribed rules of logic and imposed controls, ensuring that the knowledge generated is truthful. Research generates empirical (i.e., experienced) knowledge. Although nursing, as a science-based profession, strongly subscribes to empirical research, the body of nursing knowledge is enriched by diversity in ways of knowing. Nonresearch bases for nursing knowledge—tradition, authority, trial and error, personal experience, intuition, and common-sense reasoning—have a powerful influence and are part of nursing tradition; however, nonresearch knowledge does not permit scientific predictability, nor does it provide for scientific rationale and justification for nursing actions. Within the nursing profession, research promotes health and well-being of client populations through a variety of applications. Research improves practice by providing answers to clinical questions, evaluating the effectiveness of nursing interventions, and expanding the body of nursing knowledge. Increasing emphasis on evidence-based practice, research-based practice, best practices, practice guidelines, and outcomes focus mandate that research occupy a central role in nursing. "There is a research role for every practicing nurse" (LoBiondo-Wood and Haber, 2006, p. 9).

Every nurse is a consumer of research, an extremely important function. Research roles vary from using research findings in practice to independently planning and conducting research. Assuming that any nurse can do research is like assuming any nurse can insert a peripherally inserted central catheter (PICC) line. Both require specific education and skill development. The conduct of research requires expertise in research design and methods as well as statistical analysis. Research is differentially emphasized in the curriculum of nursing academic programs. Table 38-1 illustrates general research roles based on educational preparation. The American Association of Colleges of Nursing specifies emphasis on critical thinking, application of research-based knowledge, and data-driven evaluation of nursing care outcomes as essentials in baccalaureate education (American Association of Colleges of Nursing, 1998). The American Association of Colleges of Nursing (1996) also specifies a central core of research for the utilization of new knowledge to provide high-quality health care, initiate change, and improve nursing practice in master's education. More recently, the Association has outlined the research focus of the doctor-

---

*Houser and Bokovoy, 2006; DiCenso et al., 2005; Guiliano et al., 2005; LoBiondo-Wood and Haber, 2006.

■ TABLE 38-1
■ ■ **Research Roles of Nurses and Educational Preparation**

Associate degree in nursing	Appreciates the importance of research in nursing and assists in problem identification and data collection
Baccalaureate in nursing	Critically applies research findings to practice, participates in development and conduct of research projects, and uses research approaches to improve nursing practices
Master's degree in nursing	Facilitates the conduct of research in clinical settings, collaborates with other investigators, develops research problems based on practice expertise, evaluates quality of care and best practices, promotes research utilization in nursing practice
Doctoral degree	Capable of independently planning and conducting theory-based research, provides leadership in research activities, and expands scientific basis for nursing

Adapted from American Nurses Association, Commission on Nursing Research: *Guidelines for the investigative function of nurses.* Kansas City, Missouri, 1989, American Nurses Association.

■ BOX 38-1
■ **STANDARDS FOR RESEARCH IN NURSING**

- Understand and appreciate the research process
- Identify researchable questions in nursing practice
- Use professional literature to examine nursing problems
- Work collegially in solving identified problems
- Participate in research activities, based on educational preparation
- Support nursing research activities
- Share research outcomes through presentation and publication
- Comply with ethical standards in the conduct of research
- Advocate for protection from harm for research participants
- Use research findings to implement change in nursing practice

Adapted from Canadian Orthopaedic Nurses Association: *Orthopaedic Nursing Standards,* 2002.

ate of nursing practice (DNP) to include integrative practice experience and practice application-oriented final project, evaluation of care delivery and clinical outcomes, translational research, quality improvement, and analysis of practice data (American Association of Critical-Care Nurses [AACN], 2006).

Various nursing organizations have published standards emphasizing the importance of research in nursing practice. Box 38-1 illustrates the research standards of the Canadian Orthopaedic Nurses Association. Nurse practitioner professional role competencies, written by the National Organization of Nurse Practitioner Faculties (2002) and AACN, speak of using research to implement the nurse practitioner role.

RESEARCH PROCESS AND COMPONENTS OF A RESEARCH STUDY

The nursing process and research process both represent an organized approach to critical thinking and share several similarities (Table 38-2). Regardless of the topic investigated, a research study contains several key elements (DiCenso et al., 2005; Houser and Bokovoy, 2006; LoBiondo-Wood and Haber, 2006):

A. **Question:** All research begins with a problem or general question, which is refined to form specific research questions or hypotheses.

    1. The research questions or hypotheses are the focal point of a research study, driving all other aspects of the investigation, including choice of design and analysis.

    2. Each element of a research project fits the stated questions or hypotheses.

■ TABLE 38-2
■ ■ **Similarities of the Research Process and the Nursing Process**

Nursing Process	Research Process
Client assessment	Identification of problem
Nursing diagnosis	Questions or hypotheses
Plan of care	Method
Evaluation	Findings
Revision of plan	Implications and dissemination

Adapted from Gillis, A. and Jackson, W.: *Research for nurses: Methods and interpretation.* Philadelphia, 2002, F.A. Davis.

B. **Background:** Framework is derived from a review of the literature that establishes what is currently known regarding the study topic and identifies the gaps in knowledge that the study will address.
   1. When a study is derived from an existing theory the theoretical framework portrays the variables and their relationships as prescribed by the theory.
   2. A conceptual framework is a description of concepts, defined for the purposes of the research and their relationships.
C. **Method:** In some readings the term *method* is used to define what was done to collect the data (e.g., observation, questionnaire, interview, physiologic measure); however, here *method* is defined as the entire description of how the study is conducted.
   1. Design: the plan for data collection, much like a recipe or pattern. There are two general types of research design:
      a. Descriptive (sometimes divided into descriptive and exploratory).
         (1) Designs involve depicting the study sample "as is."
      b. Experimental.
         (1) The investigator manipulates independent variables and measures the response in dependent variables.
      c. The design determines the number of subject groups, the timing of data collection, and control of extraneous variables.
      d. These design choices reduce bias in the study and are related to how subjects are selected, the degree of the investigator's control over the independent variables, and whether the outcome of interest was present at the time of enrollment (Jacob and Carr, 2000).
      e. Designs are described according to internal and external validity. Designs offer differing strengths and weaknesses relative to internal and external validity (Table 38-3).
         (1) Internal validity refers to lack of bias and random variation that support obtaining accurate results obtained in the population studied.
         (2) External validity refers to the generalizability of results to a wider population.
   2. Sample: represents who or what is studied.
      a. Made up of units of analysis, such as individuals, nursing units, or hospitals.
      b. Typically selected from a larger population.
      c. Specific strategies for sampling determine if results from a sample can reasonably be generalized to the larger population.
         (1) Probability sampling: each individual in the population has an equal chance of being included in the sample. Probability sampling is not always feasible, particularly in nursing research dealing with small client populations. In this situation, nonprobability sampling is employed.
      d. Sample size is a factor in the selection of analysis strategies.

■ TABLE 38-3
■ ■ **Levels of Bias Control in Research Design**

Level	Designs	Independent Variable Control*	Control Group	Outcomes Present at Enrollment
A	Randomized concurrent controlled trial Quasi-randomized concurrent trial Randomized pre–post design	Yes	Yes (concurrent)	No
B	Cohort concurrent study Pre-post study	No	Yes (may or may not be concurrent)	No
C	Ex post facto study Case control study	No	Yes (may or may not be concurrent)	Yes
D	Descriptive	No	No	Yes or no

*Independent variable or intervention controlled by investigator.
Adapted from Jacob, R.F. and Carr, A.B.: Hierarchy of research design used to categorize the "strength of evidence" in answering clinical dental questions. *Journal of Prosthetic Dentistry, 83*(2):137-152, 2000.

3. Variables: the attribute or property measured in a research study.
   a. Variables are defined both conceptually and operationally.
      (1) Conceptual definition: variable is described in the abstract, e.g., hypertension.
      (2) Operational definition defines the variable in measurable terms. For example, hypertension will be defined as a systolic blood pressure greater than 100 mm Hg in the term neonate.
   b. Instruments and tools are terms used interchangeably to indicate operational measures.
   c. The quality of measurement is critical to research. Validity and reliability describe instrument measurement characteristics.
      (1) Validity is the degree to which an instrument measures what it is purported to measure.
      (2) Reliability refers to ability of the instrument to obtain consistent results (i.e., reproducibility).
4. Setting: portrays where the study is conducted and the conditions surrounding the study.
5. Procedure: describes in stepwise fashion how the study was carried out.
6. Analysis: uses statistical or analytic techniques on the data collected to answer the research questions or compare findings with stated hypotheses.
7. Results: include a description of the study sample as well as findings from the analysis.
8. Conclusion: includes discussion of study findings, implications, limitations, and recommendations for future research.

QUANTITATIVE RESEARCH

A. **Numerical data are analyzed using a statistical approach specified as part of the planning for the research project.**
B. **Descriptive statistics include measures of central tendency (mean, median, mode) and dispersion (standard deviation, variance, range).**
C. **Inferential statistics are based on probability and allow judgments to be made about the population and to test hypotheses.** In general, inferential statistics test either how things differ or how things are related.
D. **Statistical significance means that the particular finding is not likely due to chance alone.**
   1. The investigator sets an alpha or probability level that will be acceptable in interpreting results (often alpha is set at $p < 0.05$).

2. The *p* value is the probability associated with the test statistic calculated from the study data. If the *p* value is less than alpha, the test is statistically significant.
3. Statistical significance is not always consistent with clinical significance, meaning that the magnitude of the effect is not relevant or important in clinical practice.

QUALITATIVE RESEARCH

A. **Maintains the same rigor as quantitative research.**
B. **Focus is in-depth understanding of a phenomenon with particular emphasis on the subject's reports of personal experience.**
C. **Participant observation, focus groups, and interviews are methods frequently employed in qualitative research.**
D. **The specific research approach stems from an underlying philosophical perspective.** Three perspectives commonly used in nursing qualitative research include phenomenology, grounded theory, and ethnography (Gillis and Jackson, 2002).
   1. Phenomenology: seeks to understand the lived experience of individuals.
   2. Grounded theory: symbolic interaction forms the basis for understanding social processes and behavior.
   3. Ethnographic: describes a cultural group.
E. **The analysis is inductive and interpretive.**
F. **The process of conducting qualitative research and components of the research project are parallel with those of quantitative research.**

AREAS OF EXPLORATION IN NEONATAL NURSING

A. **Research supports generation of knowledge guiding evidence-based practice.**
B. **Contemporary topics in neonatal nursing research include the following:**
   1. Pain management.
   2. Initiation of oral feeding in preterm infants.
   3. Promotion of breastfeeding in preterm infants.
   4. Empowerment of families and support of parent–infant interaction.
   5. Safe care delivery.
   6. Cost containment.
   7. Promotion of optimal developmental outcomes.
   8. NICU nursing staff recruitment, training, and retention.
   9. NICU environment effects on infants and nursing staff.
   10. Ethical challenges in NICU care.
   11. Prevention of antibiotic-resistant infection.
   12. Care of drug-exposed neonates.
   13. Reduction of medication errors.
   14. Patient safety.

NURSES AS CONSUMERS OF RESEARCH

A. **Every nurse is a consumer of research whether or not direct participation in research activities occurs** (Box 38-2).
B. **Consumption of research may occur informally or formally and varies in scope** (Kirchhoff, 1999).
   1. Reading current research articles and attending conference research presentations expand nurses' knowledge base, supporting practice.
   2. Conducting a focused literature review provides information addressing a clinically defined problem area. In an integrated literature review, the findings from several research publications are summarized and synthesized, establishing the current knowledge base for a specific topic.
   3. Skill in searching the literature and critical appraisal are essential to nurses (Jennings and Loan, 2001). Research critique is a systematic approach to reading and assessing research

■ BOX 38-2
■ **RESEARCH APPLICATIONS IN PRACTICE**

- Clinical practice committee
- Quality improvement committee
- Process improvement protocol
- Policies
- Procedures
- Standards

- Critical pathways
- Protocols
- Guidelines
- Journal club
- Product review committee

■ BOX 38-3
■ **RESEARCH CRITIQUE**

- Is there a clear statement of the problem and purpose?
- Are the research questions or hypotheses unambiguous and stated in measurable terms?
- Does the background establish a theoretical or conceptual framework and show gaps in knowledge?
- Does the background define key concepts and their measures and describe relationships among study concepts?
- Is the literature review comprehensive and current?
- Do the purpose, questions/hypotheses, design, method, and analysis fit together logically?
- Is the design clearly described?
- Are possible extraneous variables identified and controlled?
- Are the sample characteristics described and sampling exclusion and inclusion criteria reported?
- To whom can study results be generalized?
- Is the sample size adequate to address the research questions or hypotheses?
- Is loss of subjects explained?
- Is the measurement of study variables described?
- Are study measures valid and reliable?
- Are study procedures described?
- How were extraneous variables controlled?
- Is the analysis described and are the statistics appropriate for addressing the questions/hypotheses?
- Do the reported results address the research questions/hypotheses?
- Are the findings interpreted and compared with current knowledge?
- Are conclusions justifiable on the basis of the stated findings?
- Are statistically significant findings also clinically significant?
- Are limitations of the study presented?
- Is application of findings discussed?
- Are future research directions outlined?

articles to assess applicability of knowledge in practice and use in further research. Key questions to ask when reviewing a research article are provided in Box 38-3.

C. **There are several formal, structured ways of using research findings in nursing.**

1. The concept of evidence-based practice (EBP) is that research studies produce knowledge on which to base our clinical decisions. The principles guiding evidence-based medicine entail assessment of intervention effectiveness through systematic review of data-based literature, grading studies according to level of evidence, with highest priority given to randomized controlled trials (Box 38-4), and aggregation of findings, typically using meta-analysis.

2. Evidence-based medicine is exemplified by the Cochrane Collaboration, an organization that has established robust criteria for the systematic evaluation of research studies resulting in production of practice.

3. Evidence-based practice in general refers to established criteria for sources of knowledge and acceptable research methods (LoBiondo-Wood and Haber, 2006). Unfortunately there

■ BOX 38-4
■ **LEVELS OF RESEARCH EVIDENCE**

- Meta-analysis of randomized controlled trials
- Single randomized controlled trial
- Single well-designed controlled study without randomization
- Single well-designed quasi-experimental study
- Well-designed nonexperimental study
- Expert opinions, committee reports, consensus panels

Adapted from Agency for Health Care Policy and Research: *Clinical practice guideline*, Number 9, Management of cancer pain (AHCPR Publication No. 94-0592). Rockville, MD, 1994, Department of Health and Human Services; Jennings, B.M. and Loan, L.A.: Misconceptions among nurses about evidence-based practice. *Journal of Nursing Scholarship, 33*(2):121-127, 2001.

is confusion and misconception within the nursing community regarding evidence-based medicine, evidence-based practice, research utilization, best practices, and research-based practice (DiCenso et al., 2006). Jennings and Loan (2001) suggest that research use and research-based practice are subsets of the wider term *evidence-based practice*. Evidence-based practice has been criticized for negating the full range of knowledge used in practice and the multiple sources of knowledge that constitute nursing.

D. **Research utilization refers to specific application of research findings, irrespective of research method, in practice and includes critique of studies, synthesis of findings, assessing applicability to practice, development and implementation of research-based guidelines, and evaluation of practice change** (Titler et al., 2001).

1. Several models of research utilization have been implemented in nursing:
   a. The Iowa Model (Fig. 38-1) is an example of research-based practice that includes generation of practice-related questions and systematic assessment of research findings used to change caregiving.
      (1) The Iowa Model emphasizes a variety of research sources of data and is not limited to randomized controlled trials.
      (2) AWHONN has been instrumental in establishing research-based practice programs, addressing such issues as transition of the preterm to an open crib and neonatal skin care (AWHONN, 2002).

ETHICS IN RESEARCH AND NURSES AS ADVOCATES

A. **Whether nurses are investigators conducting research or caring for clients who are research participants, careful consideration of ethics in research is essential.**

B. **It is important that nurses maintain a clear distinction between research and practice and of role of researcher and care provider** (AACN, 2001). Practice is aimed at caregiving to aid the well-being of an individual, whereas research involves gathering of data to generate knowledge (AACN, 2001).

C. **The ethical principles guiding human research include autonomy, beneficence, and justice** (AACN, 2001).

1. Autonomy: the ability to make an informed choice, free of coercion, regarding participation in research. The components of informed consent are provided in Box 38-5. Consent for research participation must be obtained by a member of the research team who is qualified to explain the study and answer questions. In neonatal research, parents provide consent for infant participation.

2. Beneficence: the research benefits must outweigh the risks. Children are considered to be a vulnerable group and federal mandates require that risks to a child must be minimal when there is no direct benefit to the child. When a research project involves more than minimal risk, the direct benefit to the child must outweigh the risk.

3. Justice: relates to who is represented in the research sample. Groups that bear the burden for research participation should also be groups that will ultimately benefit from the results.

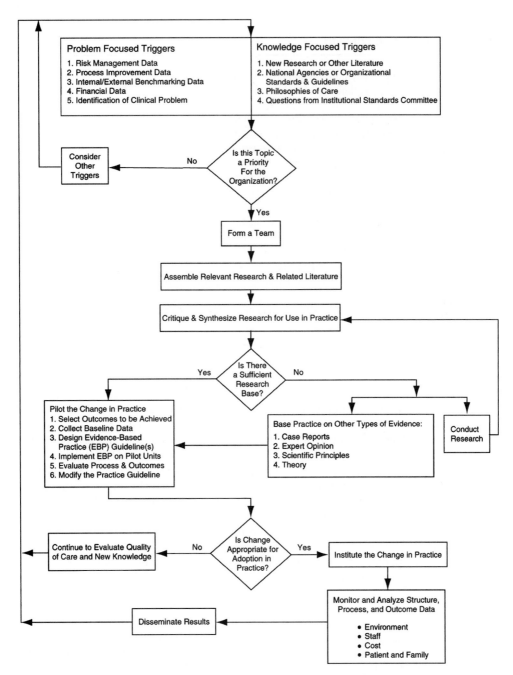

FIGURE 38-1 ■ Iowa Model of research-based practice to promote quality care. (From Titler, M.G., Steelman, V.J., Budreau, G., et al.: The Iowa Model of evidence-based practice to promote quality of care. *Critical Care Nursing Clinics of North America, 13*[4]:497-509, 2001.)

D. Subject selection should be free of discrimination and represent a broad population.
E. Several documents provide guidelines for the protection of human subjects in the United States.
   1. The Belmont Report (National Commission for the Protection of Human Subjects of Biomedical and Behavioral Research, 1979) was developed within the Department of Health and Human Services (DHHS).
   2. All research sponsored by any of 17 federal agencies, including the National Institute for Nursing Research (an institute under the National Institutes of Health and part of the

■ BOX 38-5
■ **ELEMENTS OF INFORMED CONSENT**

- Complete explanation of study purpose and procedures
- Duration of involvement and time commitment clearly stated
- Full disclosure of study risks
- Potential adverse effects described and how they will be treated
- Identification of any costs that are subject's responsibility
- Accurate description of potential benefit to self and/or society
- Description of deviations from standard care
- Indication of alternatives if an intervention is to be tested
- Permission for use of medical records
- Protection of confidentiality
- Specify possible limits to confidentiality (e.g., mandatory reporting)
- Duration of identifiable data retention
- Permission to withdraw at any time
- Permission to refuse to answer any questions
- No coercion including assurance that refusal will not change care or other entitlements
- Opportunity to ask questions
- Consent language and literacy at the level of signatory's understanding
- Receive copy of consent

DHHS), must comply with standards for human participation in research listed under Title 45, Code of Federal Regulations, Part 46, "Protection of Human Subjects" (Code of Federal Regulations, 1991).

3. The Office for Human Research Protections (OHRP) is specifically charged with ensuring the safety and welfare of people participating in DHHS research (OHRP, 2003).

4. To ensure the protection of human subjects all research should be approved by a peer review group. All research supported by federal funds requires review by an internal review board (IRB), a specific type of peer review group established according to federal regulations.

5. Nurses conducting research should become familiar with regulations protecting human subjects. For nurses in practice, understanding of rights in research, particularly informed consent, provides a basis for advocacy and ensuring the protection of clients who are also research participants (AACN, 2001). Concerns about research ethics should be raised with the local peer review group or IRB.

REFERENCES

American Association of Colleges of Nursing: *The essentials of master's education for advanced practice nursing.* Washington, DC, 1996, AACN.

American Association of Colleges of Nursing: *The essentials of baccalaureate education for professional nursing practice.* Washington, DC, 1998, AACN.

American Association of Critical-Care Nurses: *Research: Ethics in critical care nursing research.* 2001. Retrieved March 16, 2003, from wysiwyg://64/ https://www.aacn.org

American Association of Critical-Care Nurses: *The essentials of doctoral education for advanced nursing practice.* Washington, DC, 2006, AACN.

AWHONN: *Research-based practice programs.* 2002. Retrieved March 16, 2003, from www.awhonn.org/awhonn/?pg=0-874-2190

Code of Federal Regulations: Title 45 Public Welfare, Part 46 Protection of Human Subjects, Washington,

DC, 1991, DHHS. Retrieved March 16, 2003, from http://ohrp.osophs.dhhs.gov/humansubjects/guidance/45cfr46.htm

DiCenso, A., Guyatt, G., and Ciliska, D.: *Evidence-based nursing. A guide to clinical practice.* St. Louis, 2005, Mosby.

Gillis, A. and Jackson, W.: *Research for nurses: Methods and interpretation.* Philadelphia, 2002, F.A. Davis.

Guiliano, K.K., Tyer-Viola, L., and Lopez, .P.: Unity of knowledge in the advancement of nursing knowledge. *Nursing Science Quarterly,* 18(3): 243-248, 2005.

Houser, J. and Bokovoy, J.: *Clinical research in practice. A guide for the bedside scientist.* Boston, 2006, Jones and Bartlett.

Jacob, R.F. and Carr, A.B.: Hierarchy of research design used to categorize the "strength of evidence" in answering clinical dental questions. *Journal of Pros-*

thetic Dentistry, 83(2):137-152, 2000. Retrieved March 16, 2003, from www.us.elsevierhealth.com

Jennings, B.M. and Loan, L.A.: Misconceptions among nurses about evidence-based practice. *Journal of Nursing Scholarship*, 33(2):121-127, 2001.

Kirchhoff, K.T.: Strategies in research utilization, one form of evidence-based practice. In M.A. Mateo and K.T. Kirchhoff (Eds.): *Using and conducting nursing research in the clinical setting* (2nd ed.). Philadelphia, 1999, Saunders, pp. 56-63.

LoBiondo-Wood, G. and Haber, J.: *Nursing research: methods, critical appraisal, and utilization* (6th ed.). St. Louis, 2006, Mosby.

National Commission for the Protection of Human Subjects of Biomedical and Behavioral Research: *The Belmont Report: Ethical principles and guidelines for the protection of human subjects of research*. Washington, DC, 1979, DHHS. Retrieved March 16, 2003, from http://ohrp.osophs.dhhs.gov/humansubjects/guidance/belmont.htm

National Organization of Nurse Practitioner Faculties: *Nurse practitioner primary care competencies in specialty areas: adult, family, gerontological, pediatric, and women's health*. Washington, DC, 2002, The U.S. Department of Health and Human Services, Health Resource and Services Administration, Bureau of Health Professions, Division of Nursing, pp. 1-84.

Office for Human Research Protections. 2003. Retrieved February 11, 2004, from http://ohrp.osophs.dhhs.gov/

Titler, M.G., Steelman, V.J., Budreau, G., et al.: The Iowa Model of evidence-based practice to promote quality of care. *Critical Care Nursing Clinics of North America*, 13(4):497-509, 2001.

39 Ethical Issues

■ ■ ■ TANYA SUDIA-ROBINSON

OBJECTIVES

1. Explore how the principles of biomedical ethics can be applied in the neonatal intensive care unit (NICU).
2. Identify alternate theoretical and case analysis approaches to examining ethical issues in the NICU.
3. Examine the nurse's role when ethical issues arise in the NICU.
4. Recognize the role of hospital ethics committees in exploring and resolving ethical issues in the NICU.

■
■ ■ Ethical issues are ever present in the NICU. Each technologic advance brings ethical questions to the forefront of care. How far can and should the limits of viability be extended? How can we minimize the social, emotional, and financial costs associated with NICU care? Are we providing adequate palliative care in the NICU? These are just a few of the poignant questions that warrant ongoing ethical analysis.

Nurses, nurse practitioners, physicians, and other members of the NICU health care team have professional obligations to patients. For nurses and physicians, these obligations are based on the professional codes of practice and means of ethical conduct. For example, the practice of medicine evolved from the founding obligation of *Primum non nocere*, a Latin phrase meaning "First, do no harm." This has become a guiding ethical obligation for health care professionals, regardless of their practice setting.

EXAMINING ETHICAL ISSUES IN THE NICU

In the NICU, ethical dilemmas arise when ethical principles and well-intended actions compete. For example, when a neonate with overwhelming sepsis and IVH begins to exhibit multisystem failure, an ethical dilemma can arise between avoiding causing harm while ensuring that actions taken are in the best interest of this neonate at this point in time. What are those actions, who decides, and what happens if members of the healthcare team and/or the parents disagree about the best interests of the neonate? Ethical issues can be very complex situations that are best addressed by a team approach.

Nurses, physicians, and other members of the NICU health care team need to have a framework for understanding and resolving the ethical issues that arise in the NICU. Although there are many different philosophical perspectives one can use to examine ethical issues, health care professionals need to be able to directly translate those theories to bedside care. Thus this chapter's discussion of ethical approaches focuses on models from the field of applied ethics. The following sections are designed to assist the bedside caregiver to recognize and examine ethical issues as they arise in the NICU.

PRINCIPLES OF BIOMEDICAL ETHICS

The most well-known framework for examining biomedical ethical issues was developed by Beauchamp and Childress in 1979. Commonly referred to as the Principle Approach or the Principles of Biomedical Ethics, this model provides the health care team with four key principles to examine: beneficence, nonmaleficence, autonomy, and justice. All four principles must be taken into account when examining an ethics case.

Beneficence

The principle of beneficence focuses on the act of doing good or performing actions with the intent of benefiting another person (Beauchamp and Childress, 2001). Under this principle, the health care team must examine their actions and overall plan of care to determine the intended direct benefit for the neonate. An important point to remember is that as the neonate's condition changes, an ongoing consideration of beneficence should occur.

To illustrate the principle of beneficence in the NICU, consider the case of a neonate who is born extremely premature and with an extremely low birth weight. The parents are in agreement with a plan of aggressive treatment. However, at approximately 4 days of age, the neonate has a grade IV intraventricular hemorrhage, severely distended abdomen, poor perfusion, and signs of failing organs. The plan of care that was benefiting this neonate several days ago no longer has the same effect. The care measures are not having a direct beneficial effect and must be reexamined with the parents.

Nonmaleficence

The principle of nonmaleficence obligates health care providers to avoid directly causing harm to a patient. Specifically, the plan of care must avoid causing intentional harm. Using the above example, the NICU team would need to evaluate the continuing use of aggressive therapies when the neonate is in the dying process. The plan of care should not involve measures directly intended to cause the neonate's death, nor should the care plan cause harm without any direct benefit.

The key aspect of this principle resides in the intent of the action. The health care provider cannot perform an action that is intrinsically wrong to yield a positive outcome. This is known as the principle of double effect or the rule of double effect (RDE) (Beauchamp and Childress, 2001). According to Beauchamp and Childress (2001), for an act to be considered morally justifiable under the RDE, the following four conditions must be met: (1) the actual act must be good or morally neutral; (2) the intent must be limited to the good effect; (3) the bad effect cannot serve as the means to the good effect; and (4) the good effect must outweigh the bad effect.

The RDE is best illustrated by the administration of increasing amounts of morphine in a dying patient. A nurse administers morphine with the intent of relieving the patient's pain and in the process the patient's respirations slow considerably to the point of cessation. The nurse's intent was not to cause the patient to stop breathing and die. Rather, the nurse's intent was to ease the patient's pain. Thus, this nurse did not act in a maleficent manner toward the patient.

Autonomy

The principle of autonomy emphasizes the right of an individual to make decisions for himself/herself. In health care, this principle is reflected in both the right to make decisions about a treatment plan as well as the right to refuse treatment. When an adult is the patient, the healthcare team seeks permission for treatment by means of informed consent. True informed consent is an actual process that involves more than obtaining a signature on a form or legal document. During the informed consent process, the patient should be provided with accurate, sufficient, and understandable information. The patient can then weigh the pros and cons of the proposed treatment options and express an informed decision regarding his or her preferences.

In the NICU, parents serve as the legal surrogate decision makers for their neonate. NICU staff can assist parents in their decision-making role by keeping them well informed of the neonate's condition and by objectively presenting treatment options. Parents' preferences for care must be reassessed as the neonate's condition warrants, because their preferences may change in either direction. For example, parents who expressed a desire for very aggressive treatment may later decide that deceleration of care may not be in the infant's best interest. Other parents may decide to continue care as planned, even though a grim prognosis is present. Regardless, in order for parents to act in their infant's best interest, they need to be kept informed of all options as well as the likely outcomes of the options.

Justice

The principle of justice focuses on the fair distribution of the benefits, risks, and costs among members of society in relation to health care needs. In the NICU, questions of justice frequently arise. For example, two mothers are about to give birth to neonates who will require care in the NICU. The births will occur within an hour of each other. One neonate is extremely premature and will have a less than 20% chance of survival. The other neonate will have a 75% chance of survival. If the neonate with only a 20% chance of survival is born first, should he or she occupy the last available NICU bed or should that bed be reserved for the more viable neonate?

Questions of justice are difficult to resolve at the bedside. Yet pursuing these questions is an important step in achieving balance in health care. Furthermore, moving toward examining justice from a societal perspective provides an opportunity to develop and refine health policy that will shape hospital policy and translate back to the bedside.

Utilization of Principle Approach in the NICU

When ethical issues arise in the NICU, the principle approach can assist the health care team to organize its assessment and analysis of the situation. Examining the proposed plan of care with full consideration of benefits and burdens to the neonate can provide insight into competing goals. Fully engaging the parents in the decision-making process as early as possible will assist them in exercising their rights as surrogate decision makers for their neonate. Raising justice-related questions will help clarify how this neonate's case affects the institution and how related cases affect public policy.

OTHER APPROACHES TO ETHICAL ISSUES

In addition to the principle approach to ethical issues, there are many ethical theories and case analysis models. It is beyond the scope of this chapter to adequately address all of these perspectives. However, NICU nurses should be encouraged to further explore these in any clinical ethics textbook.

Ethical Theories

Three of the theories commonly referenced in bioethics are Kantianism, utilitarianism, and liberal individualism. Whereas these theories can assist nurses in examining ethical issues broadly, they do not provide direct guidance for resolving issues at the bedside.

Kantianism

Kantianism, or deontology, is an obligation-based theory from the 1700s. This theory requires that individuals act with a sense of obligation, yet does not address how to act when there are conflicting obligations (Beauchamp and Childress, 2001). For example, a father may have a child who needs a kidney donation as well as his own parent who needs a kidney. The father may wish to donate, and may have an obligation to donate. Yet to whom does he owe the greatest obligation? This theory does not directly help resolve such dilemmas.

Utilitarianism

The focus of utilitarianism is on utility, or the maximization of the goodness of an act (Beauchamp and Childress, 2001). According to this theory, the decision maker has to identify greatest good while balancing the interests of all affected individuals. For example, the health care team may desire to provide aggressive treatment to a neonate who will require a succession of expensive surgical repairs. The family may be unable to pay for any of the treatment. Under utilitarianism, it may be determined that providing care for this infant would not maximize utility of resource allocation for the community and thus this infant would not receive the extensive care recommended. Although this theory provides a means of examining issues, it was developed in the late 1700s and is not easily adapted to daily NICU decision making.

Liberal Individualism

Liberal individualism addresses the rights, both positive and negative, that individuals in our society possess. A positive right requires someone to do something for another individual, such as a health care provider's duty to treat those in need of immediate care. A negative right keeps individuals from being directly harmed by others. For example, an individual requests that no experimental treatments be performed on him. Without his or her explicit consent, his right cannot be overridden.

CASE ANALYSIS MODEL

Apart from ethical theories and principles, a model for analyzing ethical cases was developed and refined for bedside use by Jonsen et al. (2002). Their model provides four components that health care providers should examine for each case: the medical indications, patient preferences, quality of life, and contextual features.

Medical Indications

Health care providers can begin by summarizing the neonate's diagnosis and prognosis. The treatment plan, along with the benefits and burdens, would also be discussed.

Patient Preferences

In the NICU, the health care providers would obtain the parents' preferences for their neonate's treatment plan. It would be important to ask the parents what their goals are for the infant. In light of the current and/or proposed treatment plan, the NICU team should also ask parents how they view the benefits and burdens for their infant.

Quality of Life

This component of the model provides an opportunity to examine the quality of life from the perspective of the health care team and to relate those to the stated parental preferences. This may require additional conversation with the parents to ensure correct interpretation of their values by the NICU team.

Contextual Features

The contextual features incorporate a variety of factors, including religious beliefs and practices, financial concerns, family issues, potential conflicts of interest among the care providers or the institution, and the legal implications of treatment options (Jonsen et al., 2002).

The case analysis model can be useful as an initial step in examining or identifying ethical issues in the NICU. It does not provide a directive for decision making, but it illuminates the issues so that further steps can be taken toward resolution.

THE NURSE'S ROLE IN ETHICAL ISSUES

The NICU nurse plays a critical role in both direct care of the neonate and support for the parents. The nurse can help prevent some ethical issues from arising by engaging the parents from the time of admission throughout the neonate's hospitalization. Parents will need help understanding and coping with their infant's NICU admission.

Adequate Communication with Parents

In the NICU, nurses along with other members of the health care team have an obligation to keep the parents thoroughly informed of the options for care and the associated risks and benefits (Sudia-Robinson and Freeman, 2000). To adequately involve parents in the decision-making process, health care providers need to move beyond merely imparting information. Parents must have the information but also know how to interpret the information they receive. This has been described in various health care situations as the transparency model (King, 1992).

Nurses can assist in this process by incorporating the transparency model into their daily interactions with parents. Telling parents what the neonate's ventilator settings or latest blood gas results were represent simply giving information, which parents may or may not know how to interpret. However, when a nurse explains what the ventilator settings mean for this particular neonate in relation to the course of the neonate's disease process, then parents can begin to better understand and think about the information. Nurses need to remember that knowledge is different than comprehension or understanding. Therefore when parents are helped to understand their neonate's condition, they will be better prepared to make decisions for their neonate.

Not all parents will want to be fully engaged in the decision-making process for their neonate. Sometimes parental preferences for involvement will change during the course of the neonate's hospitalization. For example, some parents may be so intimidated by the NICU initially that they may not ask many questions and agree with whatever is presented to them. As time passes they may begin to ask more questions and become more involved in daily care. It is important to recognize differences in parental preferences while reassessing parental desire for involvement as the neonate's condition changes.

Supporting the NICU Team

At times the NICU nurse may feel torn between support for the parents and support for the health care team. This can occur when the health care team advocates one plan of care and the parents disagree with the team's recommendation. For example, the NICU team may recognize that the neonate is in multiorgan system failure and that death is imminent, yet the parents continue to request that aggressive medical intervention continue. The nurse has an obligation to support the team and the parents while ensuring that the infant's best interests are being met. This is where ethical dilemmas arise, and the nurse may find it helpful to seek ethical consultation.

CONSULTING THE HOSPITAL ETHICS COMMITTEE

When significant differences in the desired plan of care arise between the parents and NICU team, it can be beneficial to initiate an ethics consultation. In most institutions, a nurse, physician, social worker, other staff, or a parent can request an ethics consultation. The focus of the consultation should be the actual process rather than the outcome. Ethics committee members can sometimes aid in clarifying the issues and various perspectives presented. The process must be respectful of all perspectives and give full consideration of all possible options. The product of an ethics consultation will be a set of recommendations, not a mandate for a particular trajectory of care.

The ethics committee can be of assistance to the NICU in situations other than actual case consultation. Hospital ethics committees can serve as important resources about both ethically and legally permissible courses of action that can guide policy development in the NICU. Some ethics committees also prepare educational materials for families to make them aware of the process and how to access committee members (Mitchell and Truog, 2000).

REFERENCES

Beauchamp, R.L. and Childress, J.F.: *Principles of biomedical ethics* (6th ed.). New York, 2001, Oxford University Press.

Jonsen, A.R., Siegler, M., and Winslade, W.J.: *Clinical ethics* (5th ed.). New York, 2002, McGraw-Hill.

King, N.M.: Transparency in neonatal intensive care. *Hastings Center Report*, 22(3):18-25, 1992.

Mitchell, C. and Truog, R.D.: From the files of a pediatric ethics committee. *Journal of Clinical Ethics*, 11(2):112-120, 2000.

Sudia-Robinson, T. and Freeman, S.B.: Communication patterns and decision-making among parents and health care providers in the neonatal intensive care unit: A case study. *Heart & Lung*, 29(2):143-148, 2000.

Legal Issues

M. TERESE VERKLAN

OBJECTIVES

1. Identify how an attorney may use the nursing process for litigation.
2. Define standards of care and guidelines for establishing the standard of care.
3. Define malpractice and the conditions that constitute malpractice.
4. Define concepts of liability and negligence.
5. Discuss the importance of documentation in the patient's record and guidelines for charting.
6. Discuss the nurse's role in informed consent.
7. Identify scope of practice issues in providing patient care functions.
8. Identify the risks and benefits of possessing professional liability insurance.

■■ In the past, the specialty of obstetrics was considered the "high risk" area for malpractice suits and loss of licensure. Today litigation is not uncommon in our own area of specialization. Neonates are seen as a "special" population that are afforded extra protection (Verklan, 2007). Thus neonatal nurses must be cognizant of the minimum standards of professional conduct that they, as health care providers, must adhere to. The purpose of this chapter is to familiarize the nurse with the concepts and ramifications of legal concerns as they pertain to the realm of neonatal intensive care nursing. Topics that will be discussed include standards of care, liability, documentation, informed consent, scope of practice, and professional liability insurance.

NURSING PROCESS

A. **The nursing process forms the foundation for nursing education, practice, and documentation, regardless of whether the nurse graduated from a diploma, associate degree, or baccalaureate program.** Although the phrase "nursing process" is often omitted from practice standards and teaching strategies, nursing documentation should continue to be reflective of the nursing process. Failure to follow the following five steps of the nursing process is the number one cause of all patient injuries:
   1. Assessment: gathers data related to the neonate's physiologic and psychosocial status.
      a. Vital sign records, flow sheets, and nursing progress records.
      b. Body and organ-system findings (e.g., cardiopulmonary findings).
      c. Laboratory and diagnostic reports.
      d. Medical progress notes.
      e. Intake and output.
      f. Progress notes from other disciplines (e.g., respiratory, social work, pharmacy).
      g. Information from the family.
   2. Diagnosis: correctly identifies the neonate's condition using the data obtained from the assessment step, documents on the nursing care plan, and in the progress notes.
   3. Planning: develops a plan of care that incorporates all aspects of the neonate's condition.
      a. Uses a multidisciplinary approach.
      b. Documents interventions and anticipated outcomes for the targeted diagnosis on the nursing care plan.
      c. Incorporates research-based findings into practice.

4. Implementation: carries out the plan of care.
   a. Follows neonatologist and/or advanced practice nurse orders, provides direct care, supervises the care given by another, teaches and/or counsels the family, provides referrals for care by other disciplines.
   b. Documents all pertinent information on the neonate's medical record.
5. Evaluation: evaluates the neonate's response to the plan of care as outlined by the multidisciplinary team, noting any revisions or changes to the plan.
   a. Implementation process is not complete without evaluating the effectiveness of the intervention.
   b. Communicates patient response to treatment to members of the multidisciplinary team.
   c. Documents pertinent findings in the patient's medical record.
   d. Revises plan of care based on the patient's response and anticipated outcomes.
B. **The attorney, as well as all interested parties involved in the legal process, will use the steps of the nursing process to**
   1. Interpret the medical record,
   2. Identify possible deviations from the standard of care,
   3. Speak the same language as the nurse,
   4. Generate questions that will be used to depose a nurse defendant, and
   5. Use the reports of expert witnesses who will outline how the nurse did or did not follow the nursing process.

STANDARD OF CARE

The standard of care outlines the minimum criteria by which proficiency is defined in the clinical area. When the standard is not specifically referred to in the state nurse practice act, it becomes a guideline for practice rather than law. In the legal system, the standard of care is established by defining what a reasonable and prudent nurse would have done in the same or similar circumstances (Ferrell, 2007). The issue of excellence in practice or quality of care given does not pertain to the argument—what is being sought is reasonableness and prudence. A reasonable and prudent nurse is a nurse with like education, background, and experience who would behave in a corresponding manner, given a parallel set of events. The plaintiff attorney has the burden to prove that the standard(s) does exist and that the defendant nurse failed to meet the standard(s).

In addition, it is expected that the standard of care given to neonates everywhere is the same. "A neonatal nurse is a professional nurse who provides skilled nursing care for low-risk, high-risk and critically ill neonates, high-risk neonates, and their families. The neonatal nurse has specialized knowledge and develops and maintains clinical competence through standardized practice and continuing education" (Association of Women's Health, Obstetric and Neonatal Nurses [AWHONN] and National Association of Neonatal Nurses [NANN], 1997, p. 8). "Although neonatal nurses may provide basic neonatal care, they may also focus on an area of expertise, as for example, intensive or critical neonatal care, transport, lactation, grief, extracorporeal membrane oxygenation or developmental care" (AWHONN and NANN, 1997; AWHONN, 2003; American Nurses Association [ANA], 2004a).

Ewing v. Aubert (1988) set out that a maternal–child nurse is held to the standard of care of a nurse practicing in the maternal–child specialty. Neonatal nurses, a subspecialty within maternal–child nursing, must be cognizant of what the professional practice standards are for that subspecialty:

> A nurse who practices her profession in a particular specialty owes to her patients the duty of possessing the degree of knowledge or skill ordinarily possessed by members of her profession actively practicing in such a specialty under similar circumstances. It is the nurse's duty to exercise the degree of skill ordinarily employed, under similar circumstances, by members of the nursing profession in good standing who practice their profession in the same specialty and to use reasonable care and diligence, along with his/her best judgment, in the application of his/her skill to the case. (*King v. Department of Health & Hospitals*, 1999)

The quality of the nursing care provided is judged according to national standards, making obsolete the "locality rule." The locality rule permitted nurses to be judged according to the standard of care evidenced by nurses working in the same geographic area, reflecting the community's accepted practices. Recognition of national standards by professional neonatal nursing organizations and accreditation agencies is reflected in clinical policy and procedure manuals. In addition, accredited schools of nursing across the nation have similar curricula and textbooks, and nurses attend similar continuing education conferences. Thus it is expected that the professional nurse will be and remain competent and continually updated on the standards of care and practice (ANA, 2004a, 2004b).

Five basic types of evidence are used to establish the legal standard of care: (1) state and federal regulations, (2) institutional policies, procedures, and protocols, (3) testimony from expert witnesses, (4) standards of professional organizations, and (5) current professional literature.

State and Federal Regulations

These agencies establish the standards of care and scope of practice. The national standards tend to be written in broad language to permit flexibility without compromising standards to accommodate differences within each state. The standard of practice is also defined by the state nurse practice act as mandated by each state's legislature. Here the scope of practice is delineated for each level of nursing (e.g., licensed vocational nurse, registered nurse, advanced practice nurse). For example, a registered nurse may not delegate the act of assessment and the formulation of a nursing diagnosis to any assistive personnel who are unqualified to perform this task (ANA, 2005). In addition, standards of nursing practice are also regulated by the state board of nursing, the department of health, The Joint Commission (TJC), and the Health Care Financing Administration, in addition to other regulatory agencies (Iyer, 2007a).

Institutional Policies, Procedures, and Protocols

The hospital's policies, procedures, and protocols also outline the standard of care. The policy establishes the purposes for performing a procedure, whereas the procedure is the guideline for how that procedure should be carried out. These guidelines must reflect the national and state standards of care, should be reviewed at least annually, and should be revised to reflect current acceptable nursing practice (TJC, 2006). In addition, these guidelines must also be (1) prepared by a qualified committee of professionals who practice in the specialty, (2) consistent with current research and practice literature, (3) archived for the length of liability, and (4) accessible to staff (Rottkamp, 2007). The policy and procedure manual should be approved by both the unit and the hospital's nursing and medical administrations.

Being unaware of the policy and procedures for the standard clinical practice at your institution is not an acceptable excuse for not being held accountable for your practice. The policy and procedures manual is often one of the first documents requested by both the plaintiff and defense attorneys because it is the best source for specific standards by which to evaluate a specific nurse's care. Because the statutes of limitations endure for 18 to 21 years and standard care practices change dramatically across the years, keeping the policy and procedures manual will also help to determine what the standard of care was at the time the neonate was hospitalized.

Testimony from Expert Witnesses

A nurse expert is typically required to articulate what the standard of care is or was in the situation in which the nurse has deviated from the usual and customary standard of care. A nursing expert opinion requires that the person expressing that opinion possess special skill, knowledge, and experience in the neonatal area and knowledge of the standards applicable at the time of the occurrence (Zerres et al., 2007). The judge and jury have little knowledge related to neonatal physiology, pathophysiology, and the relevant neonatal nursing care. They therefore need assistance in understanding just what a reasonable and prudent nurse would have done in the given circumstances. (e.g., Did the nurse meet the accepted standard of care?)

Both liability and damages have to be proved in nursing malpractice cases. Thus two types of experts are usually necessary: a nurse to address the nursing standard of care and a physician to determine causation, that is, to link the breach of standard to the injuries suffered by the neonate. Professional nursing philosophies dictate that nurses be the only witnesses permitted to testify as experts outlining what the nursing standard of care is in a nursing malpractice suit. However, it is the quality of the expert's experience and education that determines the competency and credibility of the testimony (Zerres et al., 2007).

Standards of Professional Organizations

Professional associations represent the interests of nurses. The ANA has developed standards with measurable criteria that define professional nursing practice (2004b) as well as neonatal nursing (2004a). Specialty organizations such as the NANN, AWHONN, American Association of Critical Care Nurses (AACN), and National Association of Pediatric Nurse Associates and Practitioners (NAPNAP) have adapted these standards to define the standards of care and professional practice guidelines applicable to the care of neonates. For example, AWHONN publishes *Standards for Professional Nursing Practice in the Care of Women and Newborns* (2003).

Current Professional Literature

Current texts and journal articles, although technically hearsay, aid in establishing the legal standard of care. A number of journals specific to the care of neonates focus on clinical, management, and research articles. Clinical articles are useful in helping to determine the applicable standard of care at the time of the malpractice suit, whereas nursing textbooks provide information related to the standard of care associated with nursing techniques and care (Iyer, 2007a). Research articles are beginning to assume more importance in the legal arena because of the desire to document evidence-based practice. Evidence-based practice is defined as the incorporation of the current best evidence in clinical decision making. Increased use of Web sites for research/clinical information such as MEDLINE and CINAHL have led to an increase in the critique of published literature by nurses. Hospitals holding Magnet status must demonstrate that nurses participate in research utilization or they will lose their designation. Despite this, the integration of research findings into clinical practice is slow, taking as long as 10 to 15 years. However, keeping theory and clinical practice on par with the literature and remaining current with regard to continuing education will assist the nurse in ensuring that his or her professional standards are synonymous with those of his or her peers.

Further Issues: Practice Guidelines and Ethical Standards

Standards of care are often confused with practice guidelines. Standards of care are the basis for proving that the nurse had a duty to the patient and that there was a breach of that duty. Clinical practice guidelines, with reference to the standards of care, are meant to assist the health care provider in the delivery of care in specific clinical circumstances. For example, *Guidelines for Perinatal Care* outlines recommendations regarding nurse providers, nursing ratios, staffing guidelines, and outreach education for inpatient perinatal care facilities providing basic, specialty, and subspecialty care (American Academy of Pediatrics and American College of Obstetricians and Gynecologists, 2006). Critical pathways are another example of a practice guideline that is modified to reflect the neonate's clinical progress. Therefore the difference between a standard of care and a practice guideline is that the standard always must be adhered to, whereas the guideline suggests a voluntary approach to achieve a desirable patient outcome (Iyer, 2007a).

The ethical standards of nursing practice may also be the issue in a malpractice suit:

> The Mississippi Board of Nursing charged Terry Lynn Hanson, a registered nurse, with abuse of neonatal patients. It was noted that her clinical practices included holding a baby around its neck with only one hand, carrying babies by holding them under their axillae, carrying naked babies around the NICU and washing them in the unit's sinks, and that she endangered the babies by rapidly flipping the levers on the incubators when attempting to stimulate them. The Board, finding her guilty on all charges, revoked her license. Nurse Hanson appealed to the Supreme Court of Mississippi, who held that her behavior constituted a reckless disregard of the health and safety of the neonates. The Court also ruled that she was negligent by holding babies under the axillae, permitting their bodies to dangle, removing

them naked from incubators to bathe and weigh them in different areas of the NICU compromised thermoregulation and exposed them to risks of infection, and that overstimulation increased the risk of intraventricular hemorrhage. (Tammelleo, 1998, p. 1)

MALPRACTICE

The term *malpractice* means negligence on the part of the nurse, in that she or he has violated the standards of ordinary nursing practiced by nurses of similar background in the same specialty of nursing. Malpractice is professional misconduct that may be intentional or unintentional (Seidman, 2007). If the individual is acting in a personal capacity, then the individual would be subject to negligence, as malpractice is limited to the omission, lack, or misuse of a professional skill.

> By undertaking professional services to the patient, a nurse represents that she/he possesses, as a duty, the degree of learning and skill ordinarily possessed by nurses of good standing practicing in the same community under similar circumstances. It is the nurse's further duty to use the care ordinarily exercised in like cases by reputable members of the profession practicing in the same or a similar locality and under similar circumstances. The nurse is to use reasonable diligence and best judgment in the exercise of her or his skills and learning in an effort to accomplish the purpose of employment. A defendant nurse must violate one of these duties before being found to have committed malpractice. (Fulginiti et al., 2007, p. 1375)

It must be emphasized that the nurse need possess only the knowledge and skill possessed by the average reasonable, prudent nurse and to exercise reasonable care, skill, and judgment in carrying out her or his professional work. The nurse need not be perfect or able to predict every single difficulty or uncertainty regarding the patient. However, the nurse must act in a reasonable fashion in the delivery of professional care while exercising reasonable care, skill, and judgment (Fulginiti et al., 2007). Occasionally an unexpected situation arises so quickly that one's actions on hindsight may not be considered to have been the perfect course of action.

A mistake in judgment is not considered malpractice:

> A mistake in judgment on the part of the nurse is not evidence of negligence. If a nurse possesses reasonable and ordinary skill and uses care ordinarily used in like or similar situations by nurses of reasonable and average skill, practicing in the community at the time in question, she/he is not guilty of negligence even though her/his judgment may be subsequently proven incorrect. (Fulginiti et al., 2007, p. 1375)

LIABILITY

Today nurses are recognized as professionals who are responsible and accountable for the care they give to their patients. If the nurse is liable to the patient because of negligent conduct, that nurse can be held legally responsible for the harm caused to that patient (Verklan, 2007). Harm must result from the act, because without damage, no legal wrong has been committed.

> Baby R was born after a difficult labor including the presence of meconium and episodes of hypoxia. Routine orders for the admission were given despite the presence of risk factors for hypoglycemia. Over the next three hours of life, the baby's glucose values decreased from 104 mg/dL to 28 mg/dL. The nurse fed the baby, but did not notify the physician. The neonate continued to experience hypoglycemia throughout the night. The glucose level increased to normal parameters after a feeding in the morning. The physician examined the baby shortly after the feeding, noting that she was at risk for hypoglycemia. No further orders were given such as the need to begin intravenous glucose. A neonatologist was not consulted. Later that day profound hypoglycemia was evidenced by seizure activity. Nursing did not notify the physician of the seizure activity until later in the evening when the seizures became worse. The physician returned to the nursery and examined Baby R. Once the seizures were observed, the baby was transferred to another hospital. The hospital settled for $1.75 million prior to trial. (Laska, 2005)

The plaintiff, the party bringing the suit, must prove the following four elements in a malpractice case:

1. The nurse had a duty to her or his patient.
2. There was a breach of that duty.
3. Harm or damages did occur to the patient.
4. Breach of that duty resulted in harm (proximal cause).

An infant, born in a depressed state, had Apgar scores of 3 and 8 at 1 and 5 minutes, respectively. Although his condition was improving, he continued to have raspy breathing that required suctioning. It was alleged that the defendants failed to provide adequate special care and observation, causing the baby to suffocate on its own secretions. The neonate was discovered in a cyanotic state two hours after birth. Resuscitative techniques restored the heartbeat in eighteen minutes. He was transferred to another hospital, declared to be brain-dead, and was removed from life support four days later. The plaintiff claimed that resuscitation was both delayed and improperly performed. The defendants argued that the baby appeared normal, that the cause of the respiratory arrest was unknown, and that inborn errors of metabolism caused the death. They also countered that failure to respond to resuscitation does not imply negligence (Du Page County [IL] Circuit Court, Case No. 94L-318 [Laska, 1997]).

In this case the plaintiff proved that the defendant owed a duty to the neonate, in that the baby and his parents should expect the care received to be at least equal to the standard of care. However, the plaintiff was not able to prove that the defendant breached the duty (failure to respond to resuscitation does not imply negligence) or that there was proximal cause (inborn errors of metabolism may have contributed to or caused the injury). Thus, despite the neonate's death (damages), a malpractice suit cannot be won if all four elements are not present.

A. **The costs of liability when a neonate is involved are high for three reasons:**
  1. The costs of health care for a damaged infant with a normal life expectancy are high.
  2. The longer statute of limitations for minors may permit charges to be made years later, applicable to other medical malpractice actions.
  3. There is sympathy toward the family, who may not be able to afford the needed care for the child, as opposed to the deep pockets of a corporation, who may be seen as uncaring and will not miss the money anyway.

B. **Although an individual nurse is accountable only for his or her own practice, there are three additional theories of liability that may be pursued against a facility or its management** (Lewis and Krulewicz, 2007; Rottkamp, 2007):
  1. *Respondeat superior*, which, in essence, says that the employer is given the responsibility and accountability for the actions or intentions of the employee. This doctrine:
     a. Holds an employer liable for the negligent acts of employees that arise in the course of the employment (i.e., employers are held responsible for the acts of those whom they have a right to supervise or control).
     b. Holds the institution responsible for ensuring that the policies and procedures meet the standard of care, and that employees follow these policies.
     c. Will not impose liability in most circumstances on a nursing supervisor for negligent acts of the nursing personnel he or she is supervising. This responsibility rests with the person who makes changes in the policies and procedures.
     d. Obligates the nursing supervisor to ensure that the licensed and unlicensed nursing personnel under his or her supervision is able to provide patient care safely. If the supervisor does not document the personnel's deficiencies and use the chain of command, she or he can be held liable for any damages that befall a patient.
     e. Holds that negligent employees are always liable for their own conduct.
  2. *Corporate negligence* holds the institution's management and board of trustees liable for any breach of its duties:
     a. The institution must provide a safe physical setting and monitor the quality of care provided, along with the equipment necessary for patient care.
     b. An equipment standard must be implemented.
        (1) The institution must have a management plan documenting competency validation for the proper use of medical equipment by the institution's employees (JCAHO, 2006).
        (2) The institution may also name the equipment manufacturer as a third-party defendant in an attempt to shift the blame (Verklan, 2007).

Shortly after birth, Baby Wright's blood pressure decreased, necessitating a transfer to the Special Care Unit. Dr. Bloom ordered a bolus of normal saline (unconcentrated) to be given over 30 minutes. Nurse Diltz offered to prepare the bolus. The hospital stocked both the unconcentrated and the concentrated normal saline solutions in the same place. Nurse Diltz obtained a vial of the concentrated sodium chloride, that had "CONCENTRATE" and "CAUTION: MUST BE DILUTED FOR I.V. USE" in large red letters. There was also a written warning in red letters that the fluid was a 14.6% solution. Nurse Diltz did not read the physician's order nor did she note the label on the sodium chloride vial. The fluid bolus was subsequently administered to Baby Wright. After the second bolus, Baby Wright suffered severe brain damage. The Wrights sued Abbott Laboratories, the suppliers of the concentrated sodium chloride solution. Abbot never sent a warning letter to the hospital despite the Food and Drug Administration's warning to change the labeling and package inserts for the concentrated and unconcentrated normal saline products. The plaintiffs argued that Abbott had a duty to warn the hospital about the dangers of inadvertent administration of the wrong solution and that the failure to warn the hospital was the proximate cause of Baby Wright's brain injury. The court granted summary judgment for Abbott (not guilty). It also found the hospital and its staff should have been aware of the dangers of stocking the look alike products together, and therefore, Abbott Laboratories did not have a duty to warn the hospital of the risk. The Court also found that had Nurse Diltz simply read the physician's orders and the label on the vial, the concentrated solution would not have been given (*Wright v. Abbott Lab.*, No. 99-333 I, 2001).

    c. The facility may be found liable for advertising a service for which it lacks the proper equipment or personnel or for failure to keep these services at the acceptable standard of care.

    d. The institution must verify the credentials of those who apply for clinical privileges (e.g., advanced practice nurses) and must also query the National Practitioner Data Bank at the time clinical privileges are requested, and subsequently every 2 years, regarding those who hold practice privileges. The data bank maintains records of disciplinary action taken on licenses, hospital privileges, and payment in conjunction with malpractice suits. In addition to health care organizations, professional societies and attorneys have access to the data bank. Each advanced practice nurse should be familiar with the data bank and should periodically verify that the information it contains regarding herself/himself is accurate.

    e. Clinical competencies must also be evaluated and documented every 2 years (TJC, 2006).

  3. *Apparent/ostensible authority* holds an institution liable for the acts and omissions of an independent contractor (Lewis and Krulewicz, 2007; Rottkamp, 2007).

    a. The hospital should maintain a file for each agency nurse that contains her or his nursing license, required certifications, and a current competency skills checklist.

    b. Advanced practice nurses working within the hospital must be aware that patients view them as hospital employees even if they are in private practice, and as such the hospital may be held liable for their acts.

C. **An area of considerable controversy in the liability arena relates to risk management and quality assurance activities** (Liang, 2007).

  1. Quality assurance, more commonly called quality management today, focuses on evaluation of the quality of patient care, continuous quality improvement, and total quality management. The department and its activities may or may not be integrated with risk management.

  2. Risk management is an internal systematic process aimed at preventing injuries and accidents, and reducing financial liability for the institution. Occurrence, variance, or incident reports are reviewed to evaluate and anticipate risk associated with the provision of services.

    a. By documenting occurrences and maintaining related records, such as the organization's claims history, quality assurance and utilization review activities, and risk management and analysis, this area may have information valuable for a plaintiff's malpractice case.

    b. Many jurisdictions have provided a protective shield for quality assurance and risk management activities, which renders the materials generated and the thought processes engaged in during those activities "privileged" or otherwise nondiscoverable (defendant cannot be asked to produce the materials).

  3. Risk management works closely with quality assurance as information from risk management activities may be helpful in improving the quality of patient care. TJC links these areas in that such information must be accessible to all components of the quality assessment departments (TJC, 2006).

D. Scope of practice. Each state has its own nurse practice act, composed of statutes passed by its legislature and defining the boundaries of nursing practice. These laws vary from state to state in their demarcation of nursing practice. In contrast to state medical practice acts, the nurse practice statutes delineate nursing responsibilities in broad, universal nomenclature that generally must be examined with reference to the pertinent local law. The crucial issue regarding the scope of practice is whether the procedure performed by the nurse is legally within or beyond the scope of a nursing license to practice (Verklan, 2007).

There are numerous areas of medical and nursing practice that overlap one another, especially in the NICU. Depending on the unit and its written protocols, the same procedure may be considered within the realm of medicine when performed by a physician and within the realm of nursing when performed by a nurse. These gray areas have evolved partly in response to the nurse's increased level of educational preparation and advanced practice role and partly in response to the high-tech environment found in the NICU. Neonatal nursing is considered a specialty area of practice, and the high-risk neonatal nursing in the NICU is considered a subspecialty area of practice. Certification for both the low-risk and the high-risk neonatal nurse is available through several specialty organizations (ANA, AACN, National Certification Corporation [NCC], NAPNAP).

Increasing the scope of practice, autonomy, and authority is likely to result in greater exposure to liability situations. Critical legal-liability and scope-of-practice problems arise whenever the nurse assumes patient care functions of an independent nature that:

1. Have long been held to be solely within the province of physicians.
2. Are not the subject of standing orders.
3. Lack definition in the nurse practice act.
4. Are not generally recognized as legitimate nursing functions by accredited professional organizations.

The standard of care and liability for negligence may be determined by (Brent, 2001):

1. Nurse's level of training and experience.
2. Manuals and textbooks written for the specialty.
3. Actions and inactions of the nurse.
4. Protocols and instructions referred to by the nurse.
5. The accepted professional nursing practice.

The following case highlights many of these principles.

> Dr. Seal remained with Baby T, born at 0130 after a difficult labor and traumatic forceps delivery, for approximately 1 hour before the baby was taken to the nursery. He left the hospital at approximately 0300, with instructions to the nurse that the medical student was in charge, but that he was to be called if needed. Nurse Bowles was concerned about Baby T from the outset, taking vital signs every 15 minutes. She called the medical student at 0345 and 0400, both times at which she was reassured that the baby looked "fine." Nurse Bowles did not call Dr. Seal. The nurse's aide assigned to Baby T did not take vital signs as ordered, and fell asleep twice during the shift. Baby T's condition required transport to another hospital, where he was diagnosed with hypovolemic shock related to a subgaleal hematoma, likely the result of the forceps delivery. The plaintiffs brought a negligence suit against the hospital after the baby's death alleging that the hospital personnel failed to take proper action when Baby T displayed signs of distress. The jury returned a verdict against the hospital of $800,000, which was reduced to $650,000 because Dr. Seal agreed to a pretrial settlement of $150,000. (Tammelleo, 1995)

The reasonable, prudent nurse, besides being responsible to the patient, is also accountable to herself or himself and to the profession (Verklan, 2007). Both the nurse and the employer have the responsibility to determine the level of competence of the nurse who is asked to provide care outside her or his specialty area. The right of a nurse's refusal to "float" has been upheld by the Wisconsin Supreme Court (*Winkelman v. Beloit Memorial Hospital*) (Tammelleo, 1992):

> A nursery nurse, Nurse Winkelman, was asked to float to a unit that provided postoperative and geriatric care. She discussed the situation with the supervisor, indicating that she had never floated, that she was exclusively a nursery nurse, and that she was not qualified to provide the type of care being requested. It was her opinion that the floating would put the patients and her license at risk, and thus, the hospital in jeopardy. The supervisor gave her three options, (a) float; (b) find another nurse to float; or (c) take an unexcused absence day. Nurse Winkelman left the hospital, and later received a letter informing her that the hospital took her actions to be a voluntary resignation. Although she denied that

she had ever resigned, the hospital refused to reinstate her. Nurse Winkelman filed a complaint of wrongful discharge against the hospital. The case was decided in her favor, and the hospital appealed. The Supreme Court affirmed that she had identified the fundamental policy that provides for only qualified nurses to render care, and that nurses who provide care for which they are not qualified are subject to sanctions under the law (Tammelleo, 1992).

ADVANCED PRACTICE

Coincident with evolving health care delivery systems, neonatal advanced practice nurses can be found in hospitals, ambulatory care centers, and private practice. The advanced practice nurse (APN) is often the only health care provider in many rural areas. According to the American Nurses Association (ANA), APNs are those who have further knowledge and practice experiences that have prepared them for specialization, expansion, and advancement in the practice role (ANA, 2004a).
1. Specialization: focusing on one aspect of the field of nursing.
2. Expansion: acquisition of new practice skills.
3. Advancement: encompassing both specialization and expansion and involving:
   a. New integration of theories and skills.
   b. Graduate education.

The licensing statute in each state controls advanced practice and thereby protects the use of the title of APN. All states have defined the scope of the APN by the board of nursing, with several states having the state board of nursing and the state medical board jointly oversee licensing and scope of practice for APNs. An APN is a nurse with a graduate degree in nursing who is practicing in an advanced clinical role. They are able to conduct comprehensive health assessments and demonstrate expert skill in the diagnosis and treatment of complex clinical issues evidenced by individuals, their families, and communities. The APN functions with a high degree of autonomy in the formulation of clinical decision to manage acute and chronic illness and promote wellness. Education, research, management, leadership, and consultation are integrated into their clinical role. They collaborate with nursing, physicians, pharmacists, and others who influence the health-care arena (ANA, 2004a).

In the neonatal area, the two recognized APNs are the neonatal nurse practitioner (NNP) and the clinical nurse specialist (CNS). As APN roles continue to expand, there will be further debate on what constitutes nursing functions.

A. **Neonatal nurse practitioner** (ANA, 2004a; AWHONN, 2003).
1. One of the most common APNs found in the tertiary care setting.
2. Is responsible for managing a caseload of neonatal patients with general supervision, collaboration, and consultation from a physician.
3. Exercises independent judgment in the assessment, diagnosis, and initiation of delegated medical processes and procedures by using extensive knowledge of pathophysiology, pharmacology, and physiology.
4. Is involved in education, consultation, and research.
5. Has successfully graduated from a master's program (after year 2000) with certification through the NCC.

B. **Clinical nurse specialist.**
1. Focuses on patient care, staff education, research, and consultation.
2. Responsibilities are (ANA, 2004a; AWHONN, 2003):
   a. Acting as a resource for neonatal nurses, NNPs, and other care providers.
   b. Establishing and evaluating patient care standards.
   c. Assessing and identifying educational needs of the family, nursery, and community.
   d. Designing and implementing appropriate educational programs based on identified needs.
   e. Providing consultation to health care providers.
   f. Initiating research projects, participating in data collection, and instituting changes based on research findings (evidence-based practice).

By virtue of the necessary education and training required to become an APN, they are held to a higher standard than a registered nurse. Thus the standard of care expected of the APN is the degree of care expected of any reasonable and prudent APN who practices in the same specialty.

A major legal issue relates to the permissible scope of practice and how independent of physician oversight the APN may be. The nurse practice act, in reference to the APN, has been broadened to include diagnosis and treatment, areas that were exclusive to those holding medical credentials. All states have passed legislation that defines the scope of practice.

Most common areas in which APNs have incurred liability (Guido, 2001; Iyer, 2007b):

1. Conduct exceeding their scope of expertise resulting in damages.
2. Conduct exceeding physician-delegated authority resulting in damages.
3. Practicing independently in a state that stipulates that APNs must have a sponsoring physician.
4. Failure to refer the patient to a physician when the APN's skills are exceeded.
   a. Is the most common cause of action.
   b. APNs must also refer the patient in a timely manner when they recognize the patient's condition requires increased medical attention.
5. Negligence in their delivery of health care.
6. Failure to adequately diagnose the patient's condition.

DOCUMENTATION

A. **It is a professional responsibility of the nurse to document on the medical record. This will:**
   1. Facilitate care.
   2. Enhance continuity and coordination of care.
   3. Assist in the evaluation of the patient's response to treatment.
   4. Provide a legal and official record of the care provided.
B. **Thus the medical record is used by the attorney as a tool to provide evidence in legal proceedings because it also verifies that the nurse** (Iyer, 2007b; Iyer and Koob, 2007):
   1. Provided the standard of care.
   2. Did so within the scope of his or her nursing practice act.
   3. Provided "routine care." Negligence could be proved if this information is absent or inappropriate. Flow sheets that list these routines, along with times, dates, patient and caregiver identification, and nursing care outcomes are valuable in providing a means of documenting repetitious nursing activities.
C. **Although nursing notes need to be as complete as possible, the comment "If it's not documented, then it wasn't done" doesn't always hold true.** Patient care is always the number one priority. Once the emergency is past, the nurse should strive to document the events, using as much detail as possible. However, if the needs of other patients were placed on hold during a crisis, those needs must be met immediately once the crisis is past. When the medical record is incomplete, the nurse may testify as to what constitutes her or his usual practice.
D. **The most common charting systems in the NICU are** (Iyer and Koob, 2007):
   1. Flow sheets.
      a. Decrease the need to document repetitive, routine nursing functions in the narrative notes.
      b. Have column-and-row format organized according to time and/or shift.
      c. Use abbreviations, symbols, and checkmarks to enter information.
   2. Narrative charting.
      a. Patient care is documented by using chronologic format.
      b. Entries describe the neonate's status, interventions, evaluation of care, medical treatments, and equipment (e.g., ventilator, bed, phototherapy lights) used, and the neonate's response to care.
   3. Problem-oriented charting.
      a. Problem list outlines the patient's priority problems.
      b. Updates should be entered on a regular basis as problems resolve and new ones emerge.
      c. Documentation may be directly on the care plan or in the narrative notes.
      d. Specific format is followed:
         (1) S = subjective information that the patient tells the nurse.

      (2) O = objective information the nurse observes (including laboratory results).

      (3) A = assessment of the above-mentioned data, leading to a nursing diagnosis.

      (4) P = plan that the nurse will implement to address the care issue.

  4. Problem, intervention, and evaluation of problems (PIE) charting: uses flow sheets, progress notes, and nursing diagnoses.

  5. Charting by exception.

    a. Narrative notes are completed only when the neonate's progress and/or condition deviates from the expected or when an untoward occurrence arises.

    b. Charting system contains nursing care plans, nursing database, flow sheets, and progress notes.

    c. Standards of practice, determined by the institution, are incorporated into the charting system to record routine, repetitive nursing interventions (e.g., observation of intravenous site, checking ventilator settings).

E. **Table 40-1 outlines the advantages and disadvantages of each charting strategy.**

F. **Guidelines for documentation** (Iyer and Koob, 2007).

  1. Sign at the end of every entry by using full name and credentials or only initials (full name and credentials noted in the appropriate space). Ensure that no vacant lines are left. An empty space may later prompt someone to fill in a "missing" piece of information.

■ TABLE 40-1
■ ■ **Advantages and Disadvantages of Charting Systems**

Charting Systems	Advantages	Disadvantages
Flow sheets	Easy to use Decrease time spent	No note on narrative sheet Duplication of documentation on narrative sheet
Narrative charting	Easy to document events as they occur in time	Information may be disorganized and may not contain all elements of nursing process Key patient issues may vary from shift to shift and from nurse to nurse; thus it may be difficult, years later, for hospital, nurse, and/or attorney to tease out relevant information related to specific patient complaint
Problem-oriented charting	Documentation is organized All disciplines use same progress notes, permitting increased collaboration and continuity of care	Continuing same format on all patient problems becomes redundant, with same information appearing over and over Time consuming because of repetitious nature of note
PIE charting	Documentation is organized Evaluation of each problem requires only the information that is specific to that particular problem, intervention, and evaluation	Novice nurses may have difficulty where there is no traditional care plan but instead an ongoing plan of care that is documented daily
Charting by exception	Complete, detailed patient information is easily accessible to the health care provider Standard of practice for documentation outlines expected normal findings	Exceptions to the standards of practice may not be documented because nurses become accustomed to "checking off" the flow sheets

PIE, Problem, intervention, and evaluation.
Data from Iyer, P.W. and Koob, S.L.: Nursing documentation. In P.W. Iyer (Ed.): *Nursing malpractice.* Tucson, AZ, 2007, Lawyers & Judges Publishing, pp. 181-227.

2. Cosigning means that you have observed and/or approved the care given and that you are accepting joint responsibility (and liability) for that care. Nurses who are required by hospital policy routinely to countersign documents or information in the patient's chart should protect themselves in one of two ways:
    a. By personally verifying the information being recorded.
    b. By noting in the record that the signature is included in accordance with hospital policy and is not based on personal knowledge of the information in question.
3. Illegible, sloppy handwriting with spelling and grammatical errors will convey a negative impression of the nurse.
4. Late charting is always suspect because it is typically key information that is added. Chart the information as soon as possible, beginning with the words "late entry for [date and time]."
5. To correct a mistaken entry:
    a. Draw one line through the entry.
    b. Write "mistaken entry" above the line. (The term *error* is no longer advised because juries tend to associate it with a clinical error.)
    c. Initial or sign document and add date next to "mistaken entry."
    d. What if a nurse is instructed not to chart an error by the attending physician? Nurses who accede to the demands of a physician to cover up the true facts of an unusual clinical episode by deliberately not mentioning it in the patient's chart not only may be subject to possible loss of licensure but also, in flagrant circumstances, even subject themselves to criminal action, leading to a fine or jail sentence.
6. Avoid inappropriate comments concerning:
    a. The patient's or family's personality traits or idiosyncrasies (unless such remarks are relevant to the infant's treatment).
    b. Subjective views to the effect that the patient or family is a potential litigant.
    c. Admissions of legal liability with respect to untoward medical or nursing events. Examples are:
        (1) "The IV infiltrated because the night staff forgot to check it" (Solberg, 1986, p. 13).
        (2) "Patient going into shock. Could not get Dr. Jones to come. We never can!!!" (Fox and Imbiorski, 1979).
7. Document occurrences accurately and concisely. For example, the neonate's parents (plaintiffs) may have a different view of what actually took place. In a malpractice action the burden of proof rests with the plaintiff. In the case of *Coleman v. Touro Infirmary of New Orleans* (1993), the plaintiff alleged that the defendants had been negligent by failing to treat an abruptio placentae before the premature delivery of the infant and that the defendants' actions or inaction had caused the child's death. There were several discrepancies between the patient's recollection of events and the medical record. The court consulted the chart and the physician, determined that the nurses' notes stated another set of events, and concluded that the plaintiff failed to prove any act or omission by the obstetrician or hospital that resulted in the wrongful death of the Coleman infant.
8. Document objectively.
    a. Avoid using "appears to be" and "seems to be." These phrases are not consistent with the judgments/diagnosis made by the critical thinking nurse of today.
    b. Quantify in measurable aliquots when possible. For example, "approximately 30 cc emesis" gives more information than "large emesis."
    c. The patient record is not an appropriate place to refer to an incident report's having been made. What should be documented is a factual account of what transpired and what was done. Incident reports enable the hospital or agency to make necessary investigations of the situation while the patient is still hospitalized, to identify situations of increased risk, and to trend these events to determine whether they are preventable (Iyer and Koob, 2007).
9. Document promptly:
    a. Any significant changes in the patient's status.
    b. Nursing actions undertaken to intercede in the situation, including notifying the physician of the concern. Note the time of the phone call notifying the physician, the information relayed, any orders received, and what you did next.

The case of *Mark and Debbie Easter, etc. v. Baylor University Medical Center* (Laska, 1993) illustrates the way in which nurses can place themselves in a liability situation by ignoring the above-noted standard of conduct.

> The defendant was a 29-week gestational age neonate delivered by cesarean section at the defendant hospital. His serum potassium was not measured during the first 6 days of his life, and the blood glucose level was measured once on the day of his birth. As a result, hyperkalemia and hypoglycemia were undetected until he had a severe episode of bradycardia and/or cardiac arrest, stopped breathing, and required cardiopulmonary resuscitation. He suffered permanent brain damage. A subsequent laboratory report revealed severe hyperkalemia and hypoglycemia; however, the report was not forwarded to the neonatologists for approximately 7 hours. The plaintiff brought a complaint of gross negligence for failure to properly diagnose and timely treat the hyperkalemia and hypoglycemia. The jury returned a $4,500,000 verdict.

Medical records are crucial in a court case because they provide the sequence of events, the time frame in which they occurred, and the participants in the care of the patient.

> Dylan Keene was born at 0107 May 15, 1986. He was discharged from the NICU to the regular nursery at 0630 with a one-page discharge note that noted "watch for sepsis, hold antibiotics pending complete blood count [CBC] results and cultures." The medical records for the next 24 hours went missing. Dylan was diagnosed with septic shock and seizures at 0230 May 16, 1986. Testing determined he had sepsis and meningitis that resulted in profound brain damage. He was discharged from the hospital June 18, 1986. His parents brought a malpractice suit against the hospital on May 12, 1995, alleging that there was a failure to properly diagnose and treat for sepsis and meningitis. The plaintiffs requested names of health care providers involved in the treatment and care of Dylan on May 14, 15 and 16, 1986, including those involved in the decision to not give antibiotics on those dates. The hospital records for these dates could not be located. The judge applied a default sanction against the hospital as the loss of the records for which the hospital was responsible had deprived the plaintiffs of their day in court. The plaintiffs were awarded $4,108,311.66 (*Keene v. Brigham and Women's Hospital*, 755 N.E.2d 725-MA 2002) (Tammelleo, 2002).

If a nurse is named in a suit or is called to testify with regard to what took place, sometimes many years later, the chart serves as a memory aid. Statements contained in the medical record are not, in themselves, admitted into evidence; rather, the testimony of the witness concerning the particular event, as reinforced by the medical record, becomes the direct evidence given under oath. Most cases in which the hospital records cannot be located appear to be those in which the amount of damages in question is significant and the hospital appears to be liable; seldom do "missing" records ever favor the defendant hospital (Tammelleo, 2002).

INFORMED CONSENT

Legally, for a person to be able to give informed consent, that person must have the capability of "capacity." This usually entails that the person (1) has reached the age of majority and (2) can understand the information that is being given by the health care provider. Neonates therefore do not meet the criteria to give informed consent legally. Thus the parents typically are the surrogate decision makers for the neonate, as long as they appear to be acting in the best interests of their infant. If the parents are married (to each other), either may consent on behalf of the neonate. However, in situations involving divorce, custody battles, and teenaged and foster parenting, issues related to informed consent and patient privacy can become convoluted (Guido, 2001). A guardian ad litum may be appointed by the court to act in the neonate's best interests, instead of or in addition to the parent(s). To meet the legal standard of informed consent, the surrogate decision maker must receive sufficient information regarding the proposed plan of treatment, including the risks and benefits of treatment, alternative treatment strategies, and the repercussions of not consenting (Brent, 2001). The only exception to treating before obtaining informed consent is when delay of treatment could place the neonate at risk of further harm, such as in an emergency situation.

It is outside the boundaries of nursing practice to provide the patient and/or family with information regarding medical-surgical risks and benefits of treatment or to suggest alternative medical-surgical therapies. It is appropriate for the nurse to inform the physician that the family members need further clarification to enable them to come to a decision comfortably. Obtaining the informed consent is the responsibility of the physician providing the treatment. Ideally, the treating physician should also be responsible for obtaining the signatures on the appropriate form once the parent(s) has consented, because she or he is truly the only one who can ensure that the parent(s) has no further questions and fully comprehends all treatment issues.

A. **If nurses are required to obtain patient and/or family signatures on consent forms, they should limit their clarification of patient and/or family understanding to two questions:**
   1. Has your physician discussed your baby's surgery (i.e., treatment approach) with you?
   2. Are you ready to sign this consent form? This means that you consent to the procedure.

B. **It is recommended that the name of the person able to give informed consent on behalf of the neonate be recorded in the medical record or nursing care plan once identified** (Scott, 2000).

C. **What if the parents or guardian will not give consent?**
   1. If physicians heed the parents' wishes and do not treat the infant, they may be guilty of child abuse or neglect, because laws stipulate that parents must provide needed medical care. Denial of this care can constitute a form of child neglect or abuse.
   2. If physicians proceed to treat the infant, ignoring parental objections, they could be liable for battery because their touching of the infant was intentional and there was a lack of consent.
   3. Physicians may petition the court for an authorization to provide the infant with the necessary treatment (i.e., obtain a court order). The most common example of physicians' seeking court orders to intervene in treatment is that of refused consent for blood transfusions based on religious beliefs. This request is almost always granted—certainly in emergency situations.

D. **When parents refuse treatment for other reasons, the court will base its decision on several factors** (Brent, 2001; Guido, 2001; Scott, 2000).
   1. The infant's overall health and development.
   2. The immediacy of danger to the infant if treatment is withheld.
   3. The risks and benefits of the proposed treatment.

PROFESSIONAL LIABILITY INSURANCE

There is a growing trend to hold nurses personally liable for their acts of negligence, especially when they have assumed additional responsibility as APNs. Some believe that nurses should not carry insurance because this only provides them with "deep pockets," making them more attractive to the plaintiff. Others insist that being well insured will serve as good protection. How much insurance is enough? Is the insurance coverage provided by the employer enough, or should nurses also invest in a personal policy for additional protection? These questions need to be answered by the individual nurse after examination of her or his practice.

A. **Principal benefits afforded by an individual malpractice policy** (Guido, 2001).
   1. Insurer's agreement to defend all malpractice claims filed against the nurse. Also generally included are claims alleging assault, battery, invasion of privacy, and defamation of character and claims that the nurse/APN practiced outside the scope of his or her license.
   2. Insurer's agreement to pay the amount that the nurse is legally liable to pay the plaintiff, up to the limits of the policy.
   3. Coverage of all costs associated with an appeal of an adverse verdict.
   4. Coverage for instructional and supervisory activities, as well as off-duty and non–hospital-related nursing activities, such as volunteer work.

B. **Reasons to obtain malpractice insurance** (Guido, 2001).
   1. The hospital may have liability insurance policies that limit coverage and cover employees only when they work as hospital employees. No institutional policy covers a nurse for any acts or omissions that occur outside the normal work environment.
   2. Hospital's policy is designed to meet its needs, and may not be able to protect the nurse's best interests.
   3. If the hospital decides that what you did was not covered under its policy, it will not defend you. In fact, the hospital may actually assume an adversarial position to demonstrate that you are the legally responsible party. The institution may bring an indemnity

claim against the nurse for monetary contributions if the nurse's actions or failure to act resulted in the patient's original injury. You will now have to defend yourself on your own.

4. Hospital policies do not have supplementary payments for the nurse's additional expenses related to investigating the claim or loss of work while defending the claim. The nurse will have to pay for his or her own out-of-pocket expenses.

5. You will be protected if the hospital is not insured.

The case of *Wake County Hospital System v. National Casualty Co.* (1992) involved alleged nursing malpractice of a neonatal nurse. The hospital had a self-insured retention, or a deductible, of up to $750,000 per person/event before its commercial insurance coverage became effective. The defendant nurse's policy was deemed to be excess coverage over other valid and collectible insurance. The U.S. District Court ruled that self-insurance by a hospital is not really insurance in the legal sense. It also ruled that the nurse's insurer had to pay the full amount awarded in the case. This case is a good illustration of a nurse's needing her or his own malpractice coverage.

6. When an insurance carrier makes payment to a plaintiff on the basis of malpractice, the insurer is legally entitled to sue the nurse to obtain reimbursement for the amount paid.

7. Cost of a policy for staff nurses is low; however, the insurance for the APN may cost several hundred dollars a year.

C. **Most health care providers do carry their own professional liability insurance. There are two types of insurance policies** (Guido, 2001).

1. Claims-made policy: covers damages only when the damages occurred during the policy period (when the policy was in effect) and only if the claim is reported to the insurance company during the policy period or the extending reporting endorsement (tail). This is typical of policies held by institutions.

2. Occurrence-basis policy: covers damages occurring during the period covered by the policy, even if the claim is made after the policy period has ended. This is typical of policies held by individuals.

   a. Preferable for neonatal nurses because the lawsuit may not be filed until an extended period after the infant is discharged from the hospital.

D. **There are differences in coverage between an institutional and an individual liability policy** (Guido, 2001).

1. Institutional liability policy.

   a. Employer purchased and provided as typical "claims-made" coverage.

   b. Institution is the primary insured party, holding fullest rights and responsibilities.

   c. Policy covers specific professional activities in the work environment.

   d. Institution may be able to sue the nurse for all or part of the money paid in settlement, judgment, and legal fees.

   e. Insurance company employs the attorney; the individual nurse may not have a right to select counsel.

   f. Individual nurse has no right to refuse or authorize settlement.

2. Individual liability policy.

   a. Commercially purchased insurance that typically has an "occurrence" coverage.

   b. Individual nurse is the primary insured party.

   c. Policy covers specific professional activities of the insured at any time and place.

E. **All nurses can practice preventive legal maintenance by avoiding eighteen legal pitfalls** (Guido, 2001; Monarch, 2002; Scott, 2000):

1. Neglecting to make safety a high priority.

2. Failing to spot and report possible violence. For example, the number of kidnapping occurrences has increased in recent years. Nurses play a role in the security plan by wearing photographic identification badges, enforcing visiting policies, and, along with risk management, developing a preventive program to anticipate neonatal kidnapping.

3. Not following institutional policies and standards of care.

4. Responding unwisely in a short-staffing or floating situation. Courts have generally upheld the validity of the hospital's floating policy; thus a nurse's refusal to accept the assignment may place the nurse in jeopardy. It is suggested that the prudent course is to accept the assignment after clearly informing the nurse manager or charge nurse concerning your limitations and concerns.

5. Neglecting to use due care in physical procedures, such as the dispensing of medications.
6. Not checking equipment.
7. Assuming that others are responsible for your duties.
8. Assuming responsibility for informed consent.
9. Wrongfully disclosing confidential information.
10. Making reckless accusations.
11. Failing to act like a professional.
12. Confusing licensure issues with malpractice.
13. Failing to communicate.
14. Failing to monitor and assess.
15. Failing to listen to information provided by family and friends, and to patient's or parent's requests for assistance.
16. Neglecting to follow principles of risk management.
17. Not following documentation principles.
18. Confusing legal and ethical questions.

REFERENCES

American Academy of Pediatrics and the American College of Obstetricians and Gynecologists: *Guidelines for perinatal care* (6th ed.). Elk Grove Village, IL, 2006, American Academy of Pediatrics.

American Nurses Association: *Principles for delegation.* Washington, DC, 2005, Author.

American Nurses Association: *Neonatal nursing: Scope and standards of practice.* Washington, DC, 2004a, Author.

American Nurses Association: *Standards of clinical nursing practice.* Washington, DC, 2004b, Author.

Association of Women's Health, Obstetric and Neonatal Nurses and National Association of Neonatal Nurse: *Neonatal nursing: Orientation and development for retired and advanced practice nurses in basic and intermediate care settings.* Washington, DC, 1997.

Association of Women's Health, Obstetric and Neonatal Nurses: *Standards for professional nursing practice in the care of women and newborns* (6th ed.). Washington, DC, 2003, Author.

Brent, J.N.: *Nurses and the law: A guide to principles and applications* (2nd ed.). Philadelphia, 2001, Saunders.

Coleman v. Touro Infirmary of New Orleans, 506 So.2d 571-LA, 1993.

Ewing v. Aubert, 532 S.2d 876 (Lo. App. 1988).

Ferrell, K.G.: Documentation, part 2: The best evidence of care. *American Journal of Nursing,* 107(7):61-64, 2007.

Fox, L. and Imbiorski, W.: *The record that defends its friends.* Chicago, 1979, Care Communications.

Fulginiti, K.F., Davis, S.L., Chalierl, H.G., and Neggers, W.: Trial techniques. In P.W. Iyer (Ed.): *Nursing malpractice* (3rd ed.). Tucson, AZ, 2007, Lawyers & Judges Publishing, pp. 1343-1384.

Guido, G.W.: *Legal and ethical issues in nursing* (3rd ed.). Upper Saddle River, NJ, 2001, Prentice Hall, pp. 44-46.

Iyer, P.W.: Foundations of nursing practice. In P.W. Iyer (Ed.): *Nursing malpractice* (3rd ed.). Tucson, AZ, 2007a, Lawyers & Judges Publishing, pp. 127-147.

Iyer, P.W.: The roots of patient injury. In P.W. Iyer (Ed.): *Nursing malpractice.* Tucson, AZ, 2007b, Lawyers & Judges Publishing, pp. 13-30.

Iyer, P.W. and Koob, S.L.: Nursing documentation. In P.W. Iyer (Ed.): *Nursing malpractice.* Tucson, AZ, 2007, Lawyers & Judges Publishing, pp. 181-227.

The Joint Commission: *2006 Hospital accreditation standards.* Oakbrook Terrace, IL, 2006, Author.

Keene v. Brigham and Women's Hospital, 755 N.E.2d 725-MA, 2002.

King v. Department of Health & Hospitals (1999). 728 So. 2d 1027, 1030 (La. Ct. App.), writ denied, 741 So. 2d 656 (La. 1999).

Laska, L. (Ed.): Failure to treat newborn's hypoglycemia. *Medical Malpractice Verdicts, Settlements & Experts,* 4:26, 2005.

Laska, L. (Ed.): Failure to timely diagnose and treat hyperkalemia and hypoglycemia in premature infant: Brain damage—$4.5 million Texas verdict. *Medical Malpractice Verdicts, Settlements & Experts,* 9:1, 1993.

Laska, L. (Ed.): Newborn suffers cyanosis soon after birth due to lack of suctioning: Brain damage leads to death—defense verdict. *Medical Malpractice Verdicts, Settlements & Experts,* 1:25-26, 1997.

Lewis, T. and Krulewicz, E.D.: The intersection of nursing and employment law. In P.W. Iyer (Ed.): *Nursing malpractice* (3rd ed.). Tucson, AZ, 2007, Lawyers & Judges Publishing, pp. 175-180.

Liang, B.A.: Moving from traditional law and medicine to promote safety and effective risk management. In P.W. Iyer (Ed.): *Nursing malpractice* (3rd ed.). Tucson, AZ, 2007, Lawyers & Judges Publishing, pp. 59-72.

Monarch, K.: The nurse as a civil litigation defendant. In K. Monarch (Ed.): *Nursing and the law: Trends and issues.* Washington, DC, 2002, pp. 53-94.

Rottkamp, J.: Inside the healthcare environment. In P.W. Iyer (Ed.): *Nursing malpractice.* Tucson, AZ, 2007, Lawyers & Judges Publishing, pp. 149-174.

Scott, R.W.: *Legal aspects of documenting patient care* (2nd ed.). Gaithersburg, MD, 2000, Aspen Publishers.

Seidman, S.F.: Professional misconduct and ethics. *Clinics in Perinatology,* 34(3):461-471, 2007.

Solberg, D.: Legal implications of patient charting. Fayetteville, North Carolina, 1986, *Nursing Business News*, p. 13.

Tammelleo, A.D.: Court upholds nurse's refusal to float. *Regan Report on Nursing Law*, 33(2):2, 1992.

Tammelleo, A.D.: Nurses fail to "go over doctor's head": Death results. *Regan Report on Nursing Law*, 36(4):4, 1995.

Tammelleo, A.D.: Neonatal nurse's reprehensible conduct results in revocation. *Regan Report on Nursing Law*, 38(9):4, 1998.

Tammelleo, A.D.: "Lost" hospital records lead to default and 4 million-dollar award. *Nursing Law's Regan Report*, 43(5):2, 2002.

Verklan, M.T.: Neonatal and pediatric malpractice issues. In P.W. Iyer (Ed.): *Nursing malpractice* (3rd ed.). Tucson, AZ, 2007, Lawyers & Judges Publishing, pp. 1279-1318.

Wake County Hospital System v. National Casualty Co., 804 F. Supp. 768 (N.C. 1992).

Wright v Abbott Lab. Inc., No.99-333 I (10th Circ. Aug. 6, 2001)

Zerres, M., Iyer, P., and Banes, C.: Working with nursing expert witnesses. In P.W. Iyer (Ed.): *Nursing malpractice* (3rd ed.). Tucson, AZ, 2007, Lawyers & Judges Publishing, pp. 1217-1247.

A Newborn Metric Conversion Tables

■ TABLE A-1
■ ■ **Temperature Conversion: Fahrenheit (F) to Centigrade (C)**

°F	°C	°F	°C	°F	°C	°F	°C
95.0	35.0	98.0	36.7	101.0	38.3	104.0	40.0
95.2	35.1	98.2	36.8	101.2	38.4	104.2	40.1
95.4	35.2	98.4	36.9	101.4	38.6	104.4	40.2
95.6	35.3	98.6	37.0	101.6	38.7	104.6	40.3
95.8	35.4	98.8	37.1	101.8	38.8	104.8	40.4
96.0	35.6	99.0	37.2	102.0	38.9	105.0	40.6
96.2	35.7	99.2	37.3	102.2	39.0	105.2	40.7
96.4	35.8	99.4	37.4	102.4	39.1	105.4	40.8
96.6	35.9	99.6	37.6	102.6	39.2	105.6	40.9
96.8	36.0	99.8	37.7	102.8	39.3	105.8	41.0
97.0	36.1	100.0	37.8	103.0	39.4	106.0	41.1
97.2	36.2	100.2	37.9	103.2	39.6	106.2	41.2
97.4	36.3	100.4	38.0	103.4	39.7	106.4	41.3
97.6	36.4	100.6	38.1	103.6	39.8	106.6	41.4
97.8	36.6	100.8	38.2	103.8	39.9	106.8	41.6

Note: $°C = (°F - 32) \infty \frac{5}{9}$. Centigrade temperature equivalents are rounded to one decimal place by adding 0.1 when second decimal place is 5 or greater. The metric system replaces the term "centigrade" with "Celsius" (the inventor of the scale).

■ TABLE A-2
■ ■ **Length Conversion: Inches to Centimeters**

1-inch increments. Example: to obtain centimeters equivalent to 22 inches, read "20" on top scale, "2" on side scale; equivalent is 55.9 cm.

Inches	0	10	20	30	40
0	0	25.4	50.8	76.2	101.6
1	2.5	27.9	53.3	78.7	104.1
2	5.1	30.5	55.9	81.3	106.7
3	7.6	33.0	58.4	83.8	109.2
4	10.2	35.6	61.0	86.4	111.8
5	12.7	38.1	63.5	88.9	114.3
6	15.2	40.6	66.0	91.4	116.8
7	17.8	43.2	68.6	94.0	119.4
8	20.3	45.7	71.1	96.5	121.9
9	22.9	48.3	73.7	99.1	124.5

One-quarter (¼) inch increments. Example: to obtain centimeters equivalent to 14¾ inches, read "14" on top scale and "¾" on side scale; equivalent is 37.5 cm.

10 to 15 Inches

	10	11	12	13	14	15
0	25.4	27.9	30.5	33.0	35.6	38.1
¼	26.0	28.6	31.1	33.7	36.2	38.7
½	26.7	29.2	31.8	34.3	36.8	39.4
¾	27.3	29.8	32.4	34.9	37.5	40.0

16 to 21 Inches

	16	17	18	19	20	21
0	40.6	43.2	45.7	48.3	50.8	53.3
¼	41.3	43.8	46.4	48.9	51.4	54.0
½	41.9	44.5	47.0	49.5	52.1	54.6
¾	42.5	45.1	47.6	50.2	52.7	55.2

Note: 1 inch = 2.540 cm. Centimeter equivalents are rounded one decimal place by adding 0.1 when the second decimal place is 5 or greater; for example, 33.48 becomes 33.5.

■ TABLE A-3
■ ■ **Weight (Mass) Conversion: Pounds and Ounces to Grams**

Example: to obtain grams equivalent to 6 pounds, 8 ounces, read "6" on top scale, "8" on side scale; equivalent is 2948 g.

	Pounds														
Ounces	**0**	**1**	**2**	**3**	**4**	**5**	**6**	**7**	**8**	**9**	**10**	**11**	**12**	**13**	**14**
0	0	454	907	1361	1814	2268	2722	3175	3629	4082	4536	4990	5443	5897	6350
1	28	482	936	1389	1843	2296	2750	3203	3657	4111	4564	5018	5471	5925	6379
2	57	510	964	1417	1871	2325	2778	3232	3685	4139	4593	5046	5500	5953	6407
3	85	539	992	1446	1899	2353	2807	3260	3714	4167	4621	5075	5528	5982	6435
4	113	567	1021	1474	1928	2381	2835	3289	3742	4196	4649	5103	5557	6010	6464
5	142	595	1049	1503	1956	2410	2863	3317	3770	4224	4678	5131	5585	6038	6492
6	170	624	1077	1531	1984	2438	2892	3345	3799	4252	4706	5160	5613	6067	6520
7	198	652	1106	1559	2013	2466	2920	3374	3827	4281	4734	5188	5642	6095	6549
8	227	680	1134	1588	2041	2495	2948	3402	3856	4309	4763	5216	5670	6123	6577
9	255	709	1162	1616	2070	2523	2977	3430	3884	4337	4791	5245	5698	6152	6605
10	283	737	1191	1644	2098	2551	3005	3459	3912	4366	4819	5273	5727	6180	6634
11	312	765	1219	1673	2126	2580	3033	3487	3941	4394	4848	5301	5755	6209	6662
12	340	794	1247	1701	2155	2608	3062	3515	3969	4423	4876	5330	5783	6237	6690
13	369	822	1276	1729	2183	2637	3090	3544	3997	4451	4904	5358	5812	6265	6719
14	397	850	1304	1758	2211	2665	3118	3572	4026	4479	4933	5386	5840	6294	6747
15	425	879	1332	1786	2240	2693	3147	3600	4054	4508	4961	5415	5868	6322	6776

Note: 1 pound = 453.59237 g; 1 ounce = 28.349523 g; 1000 g = 1 kg. Gram equivalents have been rounded to whole numbers by adding 1 when the first decimal place is 5 or greater.

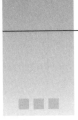

Index

A

Abdomen
  assessment, 591–592
  auscultation, 592
  characteristics, 287
  distention, 292
  muscular development, 591
  palpation, 592
  percussion, 592
  size/shape/color, 591
Abdominal ascites
  bilateral pleural effusions,
    inclusion, 293f
  radiographic evaluation, 293
Abdominal cavity exposure, 159
Abdominal circumference, usage, 8
Abdominal contents, herniation,
  104, 281
Abdominal CVS, 405
Abdominal distention, 290
Abdominal girth, increase, 30
Abdominal viscera, distention/
  enlargement, 327
Abdominal wall defect, 595–599
  care, 597–599
  definition, 595
  observation, 146
  postoperative care, 598–599
  primary repair, 598
  staged repair, 598
Abdominal wall defects, 105
  clinical risks, 105
  definition/characteristics, 105
  management, 105
ABG. *See* Arterial blood gas
Abnormal fetal growth, 121–122
ABO incompatibility, 675. *See also*
    Maternal-fetal ABO
    incompatibilities
ABR. *See* Auditory brainstem
  response
Abruptio placentae, 29–31, 43
  assessment, 25
  blood volume impact, 671
  cause, 30
  clinical presentation, 30
  complications, 30
  etiology/predisposing factors, 30

Abruptio placentae *(Continued)*
  fetal distress, 30
  incidence, 30
  management decisions, 30
  maternal signs/symptoms, 30
Absolute neutrophil count
  reference range, 702f
Absorption
  biochemical/physiologic
    capacities, 183
  photometry, usage, 175
Absorptive barriers, bypass, 238
Acetabulum. *See* Femoral head/
  acetabulum
Acetyl-coenzyme A, oxidization,
  156–157
Achondroplasia, 795–796
  associated findings, 796
  clinical presentation, 796
  diagnosis, 796
  treatment, 796
Acid-base balance, 107–108, 728
  disorders, 169–170, 517
Acid-base balance/disorders, 168–
  170
  compensation, 169
Acid-base physiology, 168–169
Acid-neutralizing agents, 622
Acidosis, 25, 517
  avoidance, 581
  causes, 518t
  correction, 164
  impact, 457
Acoustics, structural modifications,
  219–220
Acoustic stimulation, physiologic
  responses, 219
Acquired positioning
  malformations, 215
Acrocyanosis, 77
  questions, answering, 89
ACTH. *See* Adrenocorticotropic
  hormone
Action, goodness (maximization),
  862
Activated clotting time (ACT)
  monitoring, 526
Active bacteremia, 311
Active immunization, 249
Acute adrenal insufficiency,
  symptoms, 810

Acute bilirubin encephalopathy,
  626
Acute blood loss, 159
  emergency treatment, 677
Acute dacryocystitis, 836
Acute disseminated candidiasis,
  712–713
Acute enteropathy, 327
Acute gestational hypertension, 24
Acute hypovolemic shock, 85
Acute renal failure (ARF), 30, 728–
  731
  clinical assessment, 729–730
  clinical presentation, 729
  definition, 728
  diagnostic studies, 730
  etiology, 729
  incidence, 728
  management, 730–731
  outcome, 731
Acute/reversible respiratory/
  cardiac pathology, 522
Acute systemic candidiasis, 712–
  713
Acyanotic lesions, 85
Addiction, definition, 247
A-delta fibers, 335
Adenosine triphosphate (ATP),
  generation, 172
ADEs. *See* Adverse drug events
Adhesive solvents, safety
  (uncertainty), 816
ADM. *See* Automated dispensing
  machines
Adolescence, turning point/change
  period, 349
Adolescent pregnancy
  family ties, disruption, 351
  infant risk, 351–352
  maternal health problems, 351
  paternal problems, 351
  peer group, loss, 351
  problems, 351–352
Adolescents
  developmental tasks, 349
  needs, 349
Adrenal androgens, 649
Adrenal gland, 649–650
  anatomy/physiology, 649
  disorders, 649–654
  location, 649

Page numbers followed by *f*
indicate figures; *t*, tables; *b*, boxes.

Adrenal hemorrhage, 650
Adrenal hypoplasia, 650
Adrenal suppression, 650
Adrenocortical hormones
    (steroids), 649
    synthesis, 649
Adrenocortical insufficiency, 650
Adrenocorticotropic hormone
    (ACTH), cortisol regulation,
    649
ADUs. See Automated drug-
    dispensing units
Advanced practice, 873–874
    licensing statute, 873
Advanced practice nurses (APN),
    362–363
    availability, 873
    education/training, requirement,
    873
Advancing enteral feedings,
    evidence, 200
Advancing feeds, initiation
    (contraindications), 200–201
Adventitious breath sounds, 143
Adverse drug events (ADEs),
    prevention, 368–369
Adverse events (AE)
    elimination, 361
    family support strategies, 373
    triggers/clues, 372
Afferent fiber neurotransmitters,
    stimulation, 335
Afferent traffic, decrease, 485
AFI. See Amniotic fluid index
AFP. See Alpha-fetoprotein
Afterload, 541, 579
    changes, low cardiac output, 579
    reduction. See Right ventricular
    afterload
Agency for Healthcare Research
    and Quality (AHRQ), 370–
    371
Air, inspiration, 77
Airborne transmission, 721
Air bronchogram, 270
    illustration, 275f
    usage, 275
Aircraft. See Fixed-wing aircraft
Air leak, 84. See also Pulmonary air
    leaks
Air transport
    altitude, impact, 430
    considerations, 430
    dysbarism, impact, 430
    extubation, evaluation, 430
    motion, effects, 430
    noise/vibration, impact, 430
    pulmonary air leaks, evaluation,
    430
Airway
    assist devices. See Very low birth
    weight
    management, 517
        head positions, 98f
    obstruction. See Upper-airway
    obstruction
    opening, 98

Airway (Continued)
    patency, assessment, 438
    suctioning, 503
    support, continuation, 98
Airway procedures, 299–307
    complications, 301–302
    contraindications, 300
    equipment/supplies, 300
    indications, 299–300
    precautions, 300
    procedure, 300–301
AIS. See Androgen insensitivity
    syndrome
Alanine aminotransferase (ALT),
    594
Albumin, usage, 690
Albumin-binding sites, 113
Albumin test, 593
Alcohol, 44–46
    anxiolytic analgesic, 44
    behavioral/cognitive
        abnormalities, evidence, 45
    breastfeeding impact, 64
    dosage, 44
    exposure, effects (diagnostic
        categories), 45
    neonatal withdrawal, 45
    nursing considerations, 45–46
    pharmacology, 44
    teratogen, 44
    usage, 543
    use, incidence, 44
Alcohol-like intoxication
    symptoms, 53
Alcohol-related birth defects
    (ARBD), 45
    maternal risk factors, 45
Alcohol-related
    neurodevelopmental
    disorder (ARND), 45
    maternal risk factors, 45
Aldosterone, regulation ability,
    649
Alimentary tract, maternal
    physiologic changes, 1–2
Alkaline phosphatase (ALP), 593
Alkalosis, 517
    causes, 518t
Allele, definition, 399
Allen's test, performing. See
    Modified Allen's test
Allow a natural death (AND), 354–
    355
Alpha$_1$-adrenergic receptor
    response, 245
Alpha$_2$-adrenergic receptor
    response, 245
Alpha-fetoprotein (AFP), 403
Alpha-thalassemia, ethnic
    predisposition, 7
Alternate-site testing (AST), 256
Aluminum-containing PN
    solutions, 194
Alveolar dead space, definition, 494
Alveolar overdistention, 275
Alveolar stability, maintenance,
    454

Alveoli
    overdistention, 475–476
    surface-tension force (reduction),
        surfactant (impact), 454
Ambulances
    equipment/articles, securing, 428
    transport, 418–419
American Academy of Pediatrics
    (AAP), online practice
    management web site, 371
Amino acids
    intestinal transport, 183
    metabolism, inborn errors, 808–
    809
Aminophylline, dosage, 490
Aminotransferase activity, 594
Ammonia, examination, 594
Amniocentesis, 122, 404–405
    analysis, 405
    care. See Postamniocentesis care
    fluid analysis, 404
    indications, 404
    invasive screening, 9
    performing, 27
    preparation, 404
    procedure, timing, 404
    risks, 404–405
    ultrasonography safety, 404
    usage, 597
Amniotic band construction, 805f
Amniotic band syndrome, 150,
    805–806
    associated findings, 805–806
    clinical findings, 805
    diagnosis, 806
    incidence/etiology, 805
    treatment, 806
Amniotic fluid
    appearance, 123
    clarity, 97
    decrease, 25
    evaporation, 114
    measurement, 10
    phospholipids, pattern (change),
    454
    removal, 404
    surfactant/albumin ratio,
        measurement, 10–11
    volume, 122
Amniotic fluid index (AFI), 10
Amphetamines, 48–49
    breastfeeding impact, 64
    fetus, effects, 49
    incidence, 48
    neonate
        effects, 49
        withdrawal, 49
    nursing considerations, 49
    pharmacology, 49
    pregnancy effects, 49
    usage, 543
Amplitude, determination, 510
Amyl nitrites (poppers/snappers),
    53
Analgesia, induction, 343
Analgesic medication, 246
Anal manometry, 610

Anatomic dead space, definition, 494
Anatomic landmarks,
        identification, 305
AND. *See* Allow a natural death
Androgen insensitivity syndrome
        (AIS), 657. *See also* Complete
        AIS; Partial AIS
Anemia, 26, 30, 85, 672–678. *See also*
        Infancy
    clinical assessment, 676
    clinical presentation, 676
    complications, 677
    diagnostic studies, 677
    differential diagnosis, 677
    etiologic findings, 672–676
    exchange transfusion, 678
    impact, 262
    outcome, 678
    patient care management, 677–
        678
    physical examination, 676
Anemia of prematurity, 675–676
Anencephaly, 105, 753–755, 797–798
    associated findings, 797
    clinical presentation, 753–755
    diagnosis, 797
    diagnostic evaluation, 755
    etiology, 797
    incidence, 753, 797
    outcome, 755
    pathophysiology, 753
    patient care management, 755
    prevention, 797–798
    risk factors, 753
    treatment, 797–799
Anesthetic medication, 246
Animals, pain (long-term effects),
        336
Anisocytosis, 691
Annular pancreas, 290
Anocutaneous reflex (anal wink),
        153
Anomalies. *See* Congenital
        anomalies
    division, 786f
Anorectal agenesis, 611–612
Antagonistic substances, amounts
        (variation), 235
Antenatal steroids, role, 455
Antepartum care, 6–11
Antepartum fetal surveillance, 9–10
Antepartum-intrapartum
        complications
    anatomy/physiology, 20–24
Antepartum period conditions, 24–
        27
Antepartum visits, 11–17
    assessments, 9
    frequency, 9
    lab/diagnostic assessments, 9
Anterior fontanelles, 137
Antiarrhythmics, 246
Anticipatory grief, definition, 355
Anticonvulsants, usage, 543
Antidepressants, 53–58
    fetus/neonate effects, 54
    pharmacology, 53–54

Anti-D immune globulin, 674–675
Antihypertensives
        (antihypertensive
        medications), 245, 733
    usage, indication, 25
Antimicrobial activity (measure),
        vernix caseosa (usage), 436
Antimicrobial agents, 243–244
    definitions, 243
    selection, consideration, 244
Antimicrobial medications,
        definition, 243
Antimicrobials, removal, 437
Antimicrobial use, principles, 243–
        244
Antineoplastic medications, usage,
        543
Antiretroviral combination
        regimens, 718t
Aorta
    development, 538
    list, 539t
    division, 538f
Aorta, coarctation, 287, 560–561
    anatomy, 560
    clinical manifestations, 560–561
    hemodynamics, 560
    illustration, 560f
    incidence, 560
    management, 561
    prognosis, 561
Aortic arches
    abnormalities, 549
    development, 535
Aortic atresia, 286–287
Aortic branches, development, 538
    list, 539t
Aortic insufficiency, 549
Aortic stenosis, 287, 561–562
    anatomy, 561
    clinical manifestations, 562
    hemodynamics, 562
    illustration, 562f
    incidence, 561
    management, 562
Aortopulmonary septum defects,
        risk (increase), 43
Apert syndrome, 590
Apgar scores, 17, 133
    checklist, 97t
    impact, 847
    questions, answering, 89
    scoring, 95–97
Apnea, 142. *See also* Central apnea;
        Idiopathic apnea; Mixed
        apnea; Obstructive apnea;
        Primary apnea; Secondary
        apnea
    aminophylline, dosage, 490
    barium swallow, usage, 489
    caffeine
        dosage, 490
        theophylline, contrast, 491
    cardiovascular disorders, impact,
        487
    causes, 487–488
    chemoreceptors, 486

Apnea *(Continued)*
    CNS disorders, impact, 487
    control, 489–490
    CPAP, providing, 490
    cranial ultrasound, usage, 489
    CXR, usage, 489
    definition, 484
    doxapram
        side effects, 491
        usage, 491
    drugs, impact, 487
    echocardiogram, usage, 489
    electroencephalogram, usage, 489
    environmental factors, impact,
        488
    episodes, documentation, 488–489
    evaluation, 488–489
    hematopoietic disorders, impact,
        488
    history, 488
    home monitoring, 491–492
        effectiveness, 491–492
        follow-up care, 492
        indications, 492
        technology, 492
    hypoxia, impact, 487
    infection, impact, 487
    laboratory evaluation, 489
    management techniques, 489–491
    mechanoreceptors, 486
    metabolic disorders, impact, 488
    methylxanthine, usage, 490–491
    monitor teaching, 393
    pathogenesis, 485–487
    periodic breathing, 484
    pharmacokinetics, usage, 490
    pharmacologic therapy, 490–491
    pH study, usage, 489
    physical examination, 488
    pneumogram, usage, 489
    prematurity, impact, 487
    presence, 200
    protective reflexes, 486
    reflex stimulation, impact, 488
    respiratory disorders, impact,
        487
    respiratory problems, 484
    sleep state, 486–487
    theophylline
        caffeine, contrast, 491
        dosage, 490
    thermal afferents, 486
    types, 484–485
Apnea of prematurity, 485
Apparent/ostensible authority, 871
Appropriate-for-gestational-age
        (AGA) infants, 161
Apt test, 592
Aqueous humor, 833
ARBD. *See* Alcohol-related birth
        defects
Areolas, enlargement/darkening, 4
ARF. *See* Acute renal failure
Arm recoil, 124
ARND. *See* Alcohol-related
        neurodevelopmental
        disorder

Arnold-Chiari malformation, development, 760
Arterial blood gas (ABG)
  determinations, 83
  measurements, 457
    obtaining, 526
    syringe, usage, 323
    values, 550–551
Arterial blood sampling, 314
Arterial cannulation methods, 319f
Arterial catheterization, 314
Arterial changes, schematic drawings, 540f
Arterial pressure, invasive monitoring, 577
Arterial puncture, 256, 261
  technique, 324f
Arterial switch operation, 568
Arteries, dilation, 316
Artifact, definition, 270
Ascending infection, *Escherichia coli* (impact), 11
ASD. *See* Atrial septal defect
Ash leaf macules, 823
Aspartate transaminase (AST), 594
  increase, 193
Asphyxia
  history, 465
  impact, 464
Aspiration
  risk, decrease, 104
  syndromes, 84–85
Assessment, nursing process step, 865
Assist/control mode of ventilation (A/C), 502
Assisted ventilation
  auscultation, 511
  breathing, control, 497
  concepts, 495
  CPAP, usage, 499–501
  definitions, 494–495
  equipment functions, 512
  indications, 516
  noninvasive monitoring, 512–513
  nursing care, 511–513
  oxygen transport, 503
  patient care assessment/care, 508–509
  physical assessment, 511–512
  physiology, 494–499
  requirement, 494
  techniques, 516
  therapy, medications (usage), 513–516
  treatment modalities, 499–502
  types, 501
  weaning, 516–517
    process, nursing care, 517
Association, definition, 409
Association of Paediatric Anaesthetists of Great Britain and Ireland, neonatal procedural pain prevention/treatment guidelines, 334

Association of Women's Health, Obstetric and Neonatal Nursing (AWHONN), CPG provision, 370
AST. *See* Alternate-site testing
Asymptomatic bacteriuria, increase, 4
Atelectasis, 468
ATP. *See* Adenosine triphosphate
Atrial septal defect (ASD), 286, 557–558
  anatomy, 557
  clinical manifestations, 558
  hemodynamics, 557–558
  illustration, 558f
  incidence, 557
  management, 558
  prognosis, 558
Atrial septation, 537f
Atrial septum
  formation, 535
  radiofrequency perforation, 552
Atrioventricular canal (AVC)
  defect, 286
  illustration, 559f
At-risk infants, incidence, 158
Attachment
  behaviors, development (identification), 357
  definition, 357
Attorneys
  medical record usage, 874
  nursing process usage, 866
Atypical primary hypothyroidism, 644
Auditory brainstem response (ABR), 848
Auditory canal, usage, 846
Auditory environment, exposure, 219–220
Auditory memory, 219
Auditory ossicles, 846
Auricle, 844–845
  parts, 845f
Auscultation, 511
Authority, increase, 872
Automated dispensing machines (ADM), 368–369
Automated drug-dispensing units (ADUs), 369, 377
Autonomic functioning, infant abilities/sensitivities/thresholds, 209
Autonomy, 856
  ethics principle, 861
    emphasis, 861
  impact, 68
  increase, 872
Autosomal disorders, 400–401
Autosomal dominant disorders, 400
  characteristics, 400
Autosomal recessive disorders, 400–401
  characteristics, 400–401
Autosomal recessive polycystic kidney disease, 735
  clinical presentation, 735

Autosomal recessive polycystic kidney disease (*Continued*)
  complications, 735
  diagnostic studies, 735
  differential diagnosis, 735
  etiology, 735
  incidence, 735
  outcome, 735
  patient care management, 735
Autosome, definition, 399
AVC. *See* Atrioventricular canal
Avoidance behaviors, observation, 213
Axilla, herpes simplex vesicles, 826f
Axillary temperature, 110
  checking, 78
  measurement, safety/ease, 110–111

B

Babinski reflex, 153
Babson and Benda fetal-infant growth, graph, 129–130
Back/return transport, 418
Bacterial colonization, 613
Bacterial flora, 237
Bacterial infections, 708–712
Bacterial meningitis, 847
Bacterial parasites, 712
Bacterial sepsis, impact, 464
Bag-and-mask ventilation, 99–100, 501
  ineffectiveness/undesirability, 302
Ballard, tool, 123
Balloon valvuloplasty, 552
Ball-valve air trapping, 468
Banding. *See* High-resolution banding; Prometaphase banding
Barbiturates, 52
Bar-code medication administration (BCMA) technology, 369, 377
Barcode scanning medication administration (BSMA), 369
Bar coding, usage, 369–370
Barium enema
  diagnostic imaging, 297
  usage, 291
Barotrauma exposure, 438
Barrier precautions, 720
Basal metabolic rate, increase, 6
Basophils, 669
BAT. *See* Brown adipose tissue
Bathing trunk area, nevi occurrence, 821
Bayley Scales of Infant Development, Infant Behavior Record, 48
BCAA. *See* Branched-chain 2-keto-dehydrogenase complex
BCMA. *See* Bar-code medication administration
Beckwith-Wiedermann syndrome, 132, 140, 175
  defect percentage, 542
  history, 590

Bed rest, left lateral position, 30
Bed sharing, avoidance, 218
Behavioral state assessment, 224
Belmont Report, 857
Beneficence, 68, 856
    ethics principle, 860–861
    focus, 860–861
Benzodiazepines, short-acting
        barbiturate replacement, 52
Benzoin, bonding, 816
Beractant (Survanta), usage, 458
Best Practice Sheets, 370–371
Beta$_1$-adrenergic receptor response,
    245
Beta$_2$-adrenergic receptor response,
    245
Beta-thalassemia, ethnic
        predisposition, 7
BFU-E. See Burst-forming unit-
        erythroid
Bicarbonate (HCO$_3$-), 168
    adverse effects, 170
    gain, 170
    laboratory assessment, 203
    loss, 169
    renal conservation, 169
Bilateral diffuse alveolar infiltrates,
    275
Bilateral hearing loss, rate, 531–532
Bilateral pleural effusions, 293f
Bilateral renal agenesis, 733
Bilateral talipes equinovarus, 803f
Bile acid
    secretion, 183
    synthesis, 183
Bile-stained aspirate, insufficiency,
    200
Bile-stained vomiting, clinical
        presentation, 290
Biliary atresia, 617–618
    considerations, 617–618
    definition, 617
    diagnosis, 617–618
    etiology, 617
    incidence, 617
    laboratory studies, 618
    physical examination, 617
    postoperative care, 618
    preoperative care, 618
    prognosis, 618
    radiologic examination, 617
    surgical procedures, 618
Bilirubin
    examination, 594
    metabolism, 627
Bioavailability, definition, 233
Biochemical hyperthyroidism,
        medical emergency, 648
Biochemical markers,
        interpretation, 8
Biochemical mediators, release, 335
Biomedical ethics, principles, 860–
    862
Biophysical profile, 10
    usage, 27
Biparietal diameter, usage, 8
Bipolar cells, 814

Birth
    asphyxia, 83–84
    blood glucose concentration, 80
    cardiopulmonary adaptation, 75–
        77
    circulation, representation, 76f
    defect, definition, 399
    expediting, 34
    fluid adjustments, 156
    weight, 127
        specific mortality, 384t
Birth injuries, 27, 762–766
    definition, 762
    incidence, 762
    outcome, 763
    pathophysiology, 762
    risk factors, 762
Birth trauma, 83, 834–835
    clinical presentation, 835
    complications, 835
    pathophysiology, 834–835
Bladder
    exstrophy, 105
    palpation, 146
    puncturing, 327
    reservoir, 525
Bladder, exstrophy, 742–744
    clinical presentation, 742
    complications, 743
    definition, 742
    differential diagnosis, 743
    etiology, 742
    incidence, 742
    outcome, 744
    patient care management, 743–
        744
    photograph, 743f
    physical assessment, 743
Bladder aspiration
    advanced practice procedure,
        326–328
    complications, 328
    contraindications, 326–327
    equipment/supplies, 327
    indications, 326
    precautions, 327
    procedure, 327
Bladder catheterization
    complications, 326
    contraindications, 324
    equipment/supplies, 324–325
    fundamental procedure, 324–326
    indications, 324
    precautions, 324
    procedure, 325
Bleeding, 581
    sedation, providing, 581
Blind proximal pouch, 600
Blood
    accumulation, 30
    bank tests, 254–255
    cells, development, 666–671
    components
        body compartments, 239–240
        use, recommendations, 686
    culture, 83, 704–705
    diagnostic evaluation, 704

Blood (Continued)
    drug screening, 64
    extravasation, 628
    group, incompatibility, 121, 674–
        675
    oxygenation, 72
    oxygen saturation, 73f, 76f
    pH, body compartment, 240
    pH, increase, 102
    products, administration
        problems, 374
    sampling. See Percutaneous
        umbilical blood sampling
        necessity, decrease, 159–160
        procedures, 320–324
    transfusions, 439
    typing/crossmatch, 255
Blood-brain barrier, body
        compartment, 240
Blood flow, 23, 72–74
    concepts, 541
    impact, 526
    medication movement, 240
    results, complications, 27
Blood gases
    changes, 300
    measurement, 513
    monitoring, 526
    tension, ventilation-perfusion
        ratio (effects), 496f
    values
        interpretation, 517–518
Blood glucose
    concentration, 80
        postnatal drop, 174
    levels, monitoring, 176
    screening, 177
Blood pressure, 549–550
    birth weight, 145f
    cuff, usage, 576
    monitoring, 513, 581
    values, 549
Blood-surface interface, 527
Blood urea nitrogen (BUN), 158
    laboratory assessment, 203–204
    level, validity, 204
Blood volume, 541, 670–671
    factors, 670–671
    inadequacy, 581
    indicators, 582–583
    replacement, 526, 580
    requirement, 264
Blow-by oxygen, 499
Blueberry muffin
    rash, photograph, 827f
    spots, 827
Blue tube (laboratory specimen
        tube), 257
Body
    compartments, 239–240
    measurements, 77
    surface area/weight, ratio,
        238
    surfaces, examination, 784–785
Body water, compartments, 440
Bonding, definition, 356
Bony dysplasias, 294

Bony labyrinth, 846
  composition, 846
Bony orbit/socket, 832
Bottle oral feeding, 202
Bowel atresia, 26–27
Bowel (distal portion), air
  (absence), 291f
Bowel gas pattern, 288f
Bowel loops, 591
Bowel sounds, auscultation, 146
BPD. *See* Bronchopulmonary
  disease; Bronchopulmonary
  dysplasia
Brachial nerve plexus injuries, 764–
  765
  clinical presentation, 764
  diagnostic evaluation, 765
  incidence, 764
  outcome, 765
  pathophysiology, 764
  patient care management, 765
  risk factors, 764
Brachial palsy, 27
Brachial plexus injury, 150
Bradycardia, 143
  complication, 306
  hemodynamic management, 578
  presence, 200
Bradypnea, 142
Brain
  anatomy, 750–751
    illustration, 750f
  cooling trials, comparison, 777t
  development, events/peak times,
    749t
  growth, indication, 127
Brainstem, 751
Branched-chain 2-keto-
  dehydrogenase complex
  (BCAA), 809
Breastfeeding, 17–18, 64–65
  alcohol, impact, 64
  amphetamines, impact, 64
  cocaine, impact, 64
  commercial term infant formulas,
    contraindication, 195
  contraindications, 81
  counsel/education, 58
  establishment, 18
  HBV/HCV, impact, 65
  heroin, impact, 65
  HIV impact, 65
  hypnotics, impact, 65
  jaundice, 629–630
    management, 633
  management. *See* Late preterm
    neonate
  marijuana, impact, 65
  methadone, impact, 65
  nicotine, impact, 64
  sedatives, impact, 65
  smoking, impact, 64
  usage, 342
Breast milk
  dilution, 200
  fortification, 197
    requirement, 442

Breast milk (*Continued*)
  jaundice, 629
    management, 633
  mother, providing (opportunity),
    358
  odor, NNS increase, 223
Breasts
  cancer, 194
  development, 126
  early changes, 4
  engorgement, occurrence, 18
  herpetic lesions, 194
  lactogenesis, capability, 5
  maternal physiologic changes, 4–
    5
  oral feeding, 202
  tissue, hyperplasia, 4–5
Breathing, control, 497
Breath sounds, 78
Breech position, continuation, 35
Breech presentation, 34–35
  assessment/management, 34–35
  clinical presentation, 34
  complications, 35
  etiology/predisposing factors, 34
  fetal/neonatal complications, 35
  incidence, 34
  maternal complication, 34
  placental/fetal complication, 34
Bronchodilators, usage, 474, 514
Bronchogenic cyst, 479
Bronchopulmonary disease (BPD),
  197
Bronchopulmonary dysplasia
  (BPD), 160, 470–475
  AAP recommendations, 474–475
  alveoli, involvement, 472
  appearance, 277f
  bronchodilators, usage, 474
  clinical evolution, injury
    pathways, 471
  clinical presentation, 472
  clinical significance, 280
  complications, 473
    cardiac evaluation, 474
  definition, 470
  development, contribution, 471
  diagnosis, 472–473
  diagnostic criteria, 470t
  etiology, 470–472
  incidence, 470
    decrease, 473
  large airways, involvement, 472
  long-term follow-up, 475
  management, 473–475
  neurologic/developmental
    sequelae, 475
  nutrition, 474
  outcome, 475
  oxygen toxicity, impact, 471
  pathophysiology, 472
  prevention, 473
  pulmonary vascular bed,
    involvement, 472
  radiographic evaluation, 276–277
  respiratory support,
    continuation, 473

Bronchopulmonary dysplasia
  (BPD) (*Continued*)
  risk, increase, 162
  shunting, increase, 471
  small airways, involvement,
    472
  steroids, usage, 473
Brown adipose tissue (BAT)
  metabolism, 113
    nonesterified fatty acids
      release, 113
    thermal receptor stimulation,
      113
  properties, 113
  termistors, placement
    (avoidance), 111
Brushfield's spots, 412
BSMA. *See* Barcode scanning
  medication administration
Buffering system, 168
Bulla, 817
Bullous ichthyosis, 829
Bullous impetigo, 827
BUN. *See* Blood urea nitrogen
Burr cells, 684
Burst-forming unit-erythroid (BFU-
  E), development, 667
Butyl nitrite, 53

C

Café au lait spots, 135, 822–823
  photograph, 823f
Caffeine
  dosage, 490
  theophylline, contrast, 491
  usage, 514
CAH. *See* Congenital adrenal
  hyperplasia
Calcifications, 292
Calcium, 165–167. *See also* Free
  ionized calcium; Inactivated
  calcium
  functions, 165
  homeostasis, 165
  levels, 204
  medications, negative effect, 204
  metabolism. *See* Fetal calcium
    metabolism; Neonatal
    calcium metabolism
  regulation, 165
  transportation. *See* Serum
    calcium
Calfactant (Infrasurf), usage, 458–
  459
CAM. *See* Cystic adenomatoid
  malformation
Camptomelic dysplasia, 657
Canavan, ethnic predisposition, 7
Candida diaper dermatitis, 826
Candidiasis, fungal infection, 712–
  713
Cannabinoids, 49–50
Cannulas, circuit component, 524
Cannulation
  requirement, 527
  success, 308
Caphalohematoma, 138

Capillaries
  blood sampling, 255–256
  heel sticks, usage, 261
  hydrostatic pressure, increase, 160
  permeability, increase, 160
  refill/perfusion, assessment, 145
Capillary blood sampling
  complications, 321
  contraindications, 320
  equipment/supplies, 320
  fundamental procedure, 320–321
  indications, 320
  precautions, 320
  procedure, 320–321
Caput succedaneum, 138, 763
  clinical presentation, 763
  diagnostic evaluation, 763
  outcome, 763
  pathophysiology, 763
  patient care management, 763
Carbamazepine (Tegretol), usage, 543
Carbohydrate metabolism
  alteration, 26
  errors, 808
  maternal physiologic changes, 6
Carbon dioxide (CO_2)
  diffusion, 526
  retention, elevation, 179
Cardiac anomalies, 26–27
Cardiac catheterization, 314
  laboratory data, 553
  pressure valves, 576t
  treatment modalities, 553
  usage, 552–553
Cardiac contractility, decrease, 579
Cardiac cycle, 541
  timing, 548
Cardiac defects, 160
Cardiac depolarization, 539–540
Cardiac development, 535–537
Cardiac disease
  clinical presentation, 545–550
  diagnosis, approach, 544–553
  familial history, 545
  gestational age, 545
  history, 545
  maternal history, 545
  perinatal history, 545
  risk assessment, 544–553
Cardiac dysfunction, 160
Cardiac function, indicators, 583
Cardiac lesions, sex preferences, 544
Cardiac malposition, 285
Cardiac output, 540–541
  calculation, 541
  maximization, 583–584
Cardiac septation, 535–537
Cardiac sounds, alteration, 4
Cardiac stun, 530
Cardiac tamponade, indication, 279
Cardiac teratogenesis, 543
Cardiac transplantation, 573
Cardiac tube, 535
Cardiogenic shock, 582

Cardiomegaly, appearance, 284f
Cardiomyopathy, 177
  congestive heart failure, inclusion, 26
Cardiopulmonary arrest, risk, 91
Cardiopulmonary bypass third spacing, 580
Cardiopulmonary failure, 24
Cardiopulmonary status, changes, 582
Cardiorespiratory monitor, 303
Cardiothoracic ratio, definition, 270
Cardiovascular adaptation, 75
Cardiovascular agents, 244–246
Cardiovascular clinical signs, 701
Cardiovascular disorders, 480
  alcohol, 543
  amphetamine, 543
  anticoagulants, 543
  anticonvulsants, 543
  antineoplastic medications, 543
  apnea cause, 487
  developmental care, 584–585
  diagnostic adjuncts, 550–553
  heart sounds, 546–549
  long-term outcomes, 585
  maternal disease, 543–544
  mixed defects, 567–573
  neurodevelopmental outcomes, 585
  operative factors, 585
  outcomes, factors, 585
  pain assessment, 584
  parental support/education, 585
  postoperative pain management, 584
  preoperative factors, 585
  respiratory pattern, 546
  thalidomide, 543
  viral infections, 543–544
Cardiovascular embryology/anatomy, 535–541
Cardiovascular medications
  lithium, 543
  retinoic acid, 543
  types, 245–246
  use, principles, 245
Cardiovascular physiology, 539–541
Cardiovascular system
  maternal physiologic changes, 4
  radiographic evaluation, 284–287
Care maps, 385
Care standard. See Standard of care
Carina, definition, 270
Car seat
  guidelines/testing, 391b
  usage, 392
Case analysis model, 863
  components, 863
Cataracts, 837–838
  clinical presentation, 837
  complications, 838
  congenital infections, 838
  diagnostic findings, 837–838
  etiology, 837
  nursing care, 838

Cataracts (Continued)
  outcome, 838
  parental education, 838
  pathophysiology, 837
  postoperative patient care, 838
  precipitating factors, 837
Catecholamines
  production/storage, 649
  release, 178
Catheter disruption, avoidance, 314
Catheter knotting, 326
Cation exchange resin, 164
Caudal regression, 160
  syndrome, 26–27
Cavernous hemangioma, 825–826
  borders, 825
  treatment, 825
CDH. See Congenital diaphragmatic hernia
CDSS. See Clinical Decision Support System
Cell membrane permeability, change, 234
Cellular immunity, 697–698. See also Nonspecific cellular immunity
  development, 696f
Cellular metabolism, glucose (importance), 172
Center of gravity, alteration, 5
Central apnea, 485
  definition, 485
Central cyanosis, 545
  capillaries/hemoglobin saturation, 133
  peripheral cyanosis, differentiation, 545
  presence, 99
Central hypothyroidism, 643
Central line-associated bloodstream infections (CLABSIs), 378
Central nervous system (CNS)
  abnormalities, 45, 111
  depressants, 53
  deterioration, 530
  disorders, 480
    apnea cause, 487
  injury, 160
  irritability, signs, 47
  malformations, 43
  medications, 246–250
    definitions, 246–247
    neonatal population considerations, 247–248
    use, principles, 247
Central venous line, radiographic evaluation, 296
Cerebellum, 750
Cerebral blood flow, 751–752
  autoregulation, 751–752
  impact, 751
Cerebral cortex, 751
Cerebral fuel deficiency, seizures, 178
Cerebral palsy (CP), 459
Cerebral vasculature, vasodilation, 752

Cerebrospinal fluid (CSF)
  diagnostic evaluation, 704
  drop, allowance, 330
  excess, 756
  obtaining, 328
Cerebrovascular accident, 24
Cerebrum, 750–751
Cervix, ultrasonographic
    evaluation, 29
Cesarean birth, preparation, 31
Cesarean delivery, 38–39
  assessment/management, 39
  complications, 39
  fetal indications, 38–39
  fetal/neonatal complications, 39
  incidence, 38
  indications, 38–39, 82
  maternal complications, 39
  maternal indications, 38
  placental indications, 38
Cesarean section, 43
CF. *See* Cystic fibrosis
C fibers, 335
CFU-GEMM. *See* Colony-forming
    unit-granulocyte,
    erythrocyte, monocyte,
    megakaryocyte
CGH. *See* Chlorhexidine gluconate;
    Comparative Genomic
    Hybridization
CH. *See* Congenital
    hypothyroidism
CHARGE. *See* Coloboma, Heart
    defects, choanal Atresia,
    Restriction of growth and
    development, Genital
    anomalies, Ear anomalies
Charting
  problems. *See* Late charting
  systems, 874–875
    advantages/disadvantages,
    875t
    components, 875
Charting by exception, 875
CHD. *See* Congenital heart defect
Chemical concentrations, changes
    (measurement), 252–254
Chemical resuscitation, 102–103
Chemical substances, presence, 254
Chemistry analysis, 252–254
Chemoreceptors, 486
Chest
  normal appearance, 274
  physiotherapy, helpfulness, 474
  rise/fall, observation, 100
  shapes, differences, 142f
  wall
    profile, change, 2
    vibration, 508
Chest compressions
  compression/ventilation ratio,
    101–102
  techniques, 101f
  thumb technique, 101
  two-finger technique, 101–102
Chest tube, radiographic
    evaluation, 295

Chest x-ray (CXR), 457
  examination, 83, 457
    usage, 551
  film, normal appearance, 274f
  findings, variability, 461
  helpfulness, 465
CHF. *See* Congestive heart failure
Children, ADEs, 374
Chlamydia trachomatis, 712, 835–836
  clinical presentation, 836
  complications, 836
  diagnostic findings, 836
  incidence, 836
  onset, 836
  patient management, 836
Chlamydia trachomatis, impact, 79
Chloasma, impact, 3
Chlorhexidine gluconate (CGH),
    effectiveness, 816
Chloride, laboratory assessment,
    203
Chlorothiazide (Diuril), usage, 575
Choanal atresia, 103
  impact, 478
Cholecystokinin, presence, 183
Cholestasis, 618–620
  considerations, 618–619
  definition, 618
  diagnosis, 619
  enteral feeding management,
    620
  etiology, 619
  incidence, 619
  laboratory studies, 619
  management, 620
  medications, 620
  prognosis, 619
  radiologic examination, 619
  result, 193
  TPN management, 620
Cholestatic jaundice, result, 193
Chondrodystrophies, 480
Chorioamnionitis, 11
  symptoms, 122
Chorion, infection, 11
Chorionic villus sampling (CVS),
    405. *See also* Abdominal
    CVS; Vaginal CVS
  care. *See* Post-CVS care
  contraindications, 405
  fetal cell analysis, 405
  indications, 405
  invasive screening, 9
  preparation, 405
  procedure, timing, 405
  risks, 405
  techniques, 405
  transvaginal/transabdominal
    sampling, 405
Chorioretinitis, 840
Choroid, 833
Chromosomal abnormalities, 837
  noninvasive screening, 8–9
Chromosomal defects, 402
Chromosomal DNA (cDNA)
    clones/sequences, 406–407
Chromosome 21, translocation, 412

Chromosomes
  abnormalities, 786–792
  abnormal number, 402
  abnormal structure, 402
  analysis, 406
  combinations, 400
  definition, 399
Chronic disorders/disabilities,
    120
Chronic grief, definition, 355
Chronic hypertension, 24, 122
Chronic illness, history, 120
Chronicity, 79
Chronic lung disease (CLD), 223
  risk, decrease, 459
Ciliary body, 833
Circuit components, 524–526
Circulatory access procedures, 307–
    320
Circulatory compromise,
    precipitation, 95
Circulatory development, 539
Circumcision, 334, 745–746
  complications, 745–746
  incidence, 745
  indications, 745
  outcome, 746
  patient care management, 746
  physical examination, 745
CISM. *See* Critical incident stress
    management
CLABSIs. *See* Central line-
    associated bloodstream
    infections
Claims-made policy, 879
Classic HDN, 79
Clavicle, radiographic evaluation,
    293
CLD. *See* Chronic lung disease
Cleft lip/cleft palate, 800–801
  associated findings, 800
  clinical presentation, 800
  diagnosis, 800
  etiology/incidence, 800
  treatment, 800–801
Cleft upper lip, 140
Clinical Decision Support System
    (CDSS), 368
Clinical hyperthyroidism, medical
    emergency, 648
Clinical intervention,
    implementation, 266
Clinical nurse specialist (CNS), 873
  recognition, 873
Clinical pathways, 385
Clinical practice guidelines (CPGs),
    370
Cloacal exstrophy, 657
Closed-system suction catheter kits,
    availability, 301
Clot observation, 25
Clustered care, recommendation,
    213
CMV. *See* Conventional mechanical
    ventilation; Cytomegalovirus
CNS. *See* Central nervous system;
    Clinical nurse specialist

Coagulase-negative staphylococcus (CoNS) organisms, 710
Coagulation, 671–672
defects, evidence, 582
hemostatic mechanisms, 671
process, 671
tests, 671–672
Coagulopathy, assessment/treatment, 581
Coaxial diffusion, 506f
Cocaine, 46–48. *See also* Crack cocaine
admissions, increase, 46
adverse effects, 46
behavioral changes, display, 47
breastfeeding impact, 64
derivation, *Erythroxylon coca*, 46
fat solubility, 46
follow-up studies, 48
incidence, 46
inhibition, 46
metabolism, 46
neonatal withdrawal, 47
neuromotor deficits, 47
nursing considerations, 48
obstetric effects, 47b
pharmacology, 46
pregnancy effects, 46–47
STDs/STIs, presence, 47
Cochlea, 846
sensory afferents, 846
Cochrane Neonatal Database, resource, 212
Cochrane Review, 514
Coleman v. Touro Infirmary of New Orleans, 876
Collaboration, impact, 227
Collaborative caregiving, 227
Collaborative care postdischarge, 395
Collagen, 813
Collateral circulation, assessment, 323
Collodion baby, 828
Collodion infant, photograph, 828f
Coloboma, Heart defects, choanal Atresia, Restriction of growth and development, Genital anomalies, Ear anomalies (CHARGE), 542
Colon
abnormalities, 291–292
aganglionosis, 291
functional immaturity, 291
Colonic obstruction, plain films (usage), 291
Colony-forming unit-granulocyte, erythrocyte, monocyte, megakaryocyte (CFU-GEMM), 666
Colorado Intrauterine Growth Chart
development, 128
illustration, 128f
Color-flow Doppler echocardiography, 552

Colostrum
expression, 5
importance, 198
Comments, inappropriateness (avoidance), 876
Commercial infant formulas, human milk (comparison), 194–195
Commercially prepared human milk fortifiers/formulas, 199t
Commercial milk formulas, 194–199
Commercial term infant formulas, contraindication, 195
Common trisomies, 411–412
Communicable diseases, 16t
maternal infection, 11
Communication
adequacy, 863–864
devices, types, 429
equipment, 429
methods, effectiveness, 366
Comparative Genomic Hybridization (CGH), 406
Complement, protein series, 698
Complete AIS, 657
Complete blood count (CBC), 25, 701–703
evaluation, 691
usage, 83
Complicated meconium ileus, 607
Complicated meconium ileus, surgical repair, 608
Compression/ventilation ratio, 101–102
Computed tomography (CT), diagnostic imaging, 297
Computerized provider order entry (CPOE), 368–369
adoption, barriers, 369
Concentration gradient, 20–23
increase, 23
maintenance, 23
Concomitant angiography, 553
Conductive hearing loss, 847
Conductive heat loss, reduction, 114–115
Confinement. *See* Estimated date of confinement
estimated date, 121
Congenital abnormality, diagnostic evaluation, 785
Congenital adrenal hyperplasia (CAH), 650–654, 810–811
associated findings, 810
clinical assessment, 652
clinical findings, 810
clinical presentation, 651–652
complications, 654
definition, 650
diagnosis, 652–653, 810
diagnostic tests/findings, 652–653
genetic counseling, 653
genitalia, appearance, 652
incidence/etiology, 810

Congenital adrenal hyperplasia (CAH) *(Continued)*
management, 653
neonatal screening, 653
outcome, 654
parent education, 653
pathophysiology, 651
flowchart, 651f
subtypes, 651–652
surgical considerations, 654
treatment, 811
21-OHD, relationship, 652–653
virilized genitalia, management, 653–654
Congenital anomalies
biochemical studies, 785
body surfaces, examination, 784–785
definition, 782
disorders, 783–784, 786–794
etiology, 782
evaluation, 784
family history, 784
genetic counseling, 785–786
genetic factors, 782–783
incidence, 782
molecular cytogenics, 785
multifactorial disorders, 783
numerical chromosomal abnormalities, 783
physical examination, 784–785
prenatal/perinatal history, 784
structural abnormalities, 783
terminology, 783b
Congenital cataracts, 788
Congenital diaphragmatic hernia (CDH), 104, 624–625
clinical presentation, 624
definition, 624
diagnosis, 624
etiology, 624
incidence, 624
laboratory tests, 624
management, 625
physical examination, 624
postnatal surgery, 625
postoperative care, 625
prenatal surgery, 625
prenatal treatment, 625
preoperative care, 625
prognosis, 625
radiographic evaluation, 281–283
structural heart defects, impact, 574
surgical procedures, 625
survival diagnosis, 522
Congenital heart defect (CHD), 542–544
genetic factors, 542–543
incidence, 542
occurrence, 542–544
treatment, 534
Congenital heart disease, 85, 160
conduction disorders, 106
impact, 464
structural defects, 106
Congenital hydrocephalus, 756–757

Congenital hyperinsulinism, 662
Congenital hypothyroidism (CH)
early signs/symptoms, 645b
etiology, 643
clinical presentation/
assessment, 644
outcome, 647
patient care management, 645–646
Congenital infection, 121, 838
Congenital lobar emphysema
appearance, 283f
impact, 479
radiographic evaluation, 283
Congenital malformation, 26–27
impact, 177
risk, increase, 43
Congenital melanocytic nevi, 821–
822
occurrence, bathing trunk area,
821
Congenital metabolic problems,
806–807
Congenital nasolacrimal
obstruction, 786
Congenital pneumonia, 461
Congenital rubella, 837
Congenital rubella syndrome, 838–
839
clinical presentation, 838–839
gestational age, 838
incidence, 838
mortality rate, 839
nursing care, 839
ocular manifestations, 839
outcome, 839
pathophysiology, 838
Congenital spine defects, 149
Congenital viral infection, 827
Congestive heart failure (CHF), 26,
160, 573–576
cardiology consultation, 576
causes, 574t
clinical manifestations, 574–575
clinical presentation, 550
clinical signs/symptoms, set,
573–574
definition, 550
digoxin therapy, 575
diuretic therapy, 575–576
etiology, 573–574
fluid/nutritional support, 575
management, 575–576
measures, 575–576
pharmacologic therapy, 575–576
signs, 574–575
symptoms, presentation, 550
in utero, 574
Conjugated hyperbilirubinemia,
629–630
management, 632–633
Conjunctiva, 832, 835
characteristic, 784
patches, 835
redness/hyperemia, 835
Conjunctival infection, absence, 836
Conjunctivitis, 835–836
etiology, 835–836

Consanguinity, 408
Consortium on the Management of
Disorders of Sexual
Development (family
manual), 660
Containment, usage, 214–215
Contextual features, case analysis
model component, 863
Continuous arterial blood gas,
monitoring, 314
Continuous arterial blood pressure,
monitoring, 314
Continuous arteriovenous
hemofiltration, 164
Continuous murmur, presence, 554
Continuous positive airway
pressure (CPAP), 106. See
also Endotracheal CPAP;
Mask CPAP; Nasal CPAP;
Nasopharyngeal CPAP
avoidance, 107
providing, 459, 490
usage, 437, 499–501
Continuous skin temperature
monitoring, 111
Continuous-wave Doppler
echocardiography, 552
Contractility, 541
changes, low cardiac output, 579
Contraction stress test (CST), 10, 25
Contract transmission, 721
Contrast echocardiography, 552
Contrast-enema study, 290
Convection, 114
Convective heat loss, reduction,
116
Conventional mechanical
ventilation (CMV), usage,
466
Cord prolapse, 122
Cord stump, stabilization, 316
Cornea, 832
characteristic, 834
Corporate negligence, 870–871
Corpus callosum, 751
Corrective medical/nursing action,
usage, 268
Corticosteroids
impact, 176
therapy, 178
usage, 25, 515, 584
Cortisol, homeostasis role, 649
Cosigning, term (meaning), 876
Couvelaire uterus, 30
CPAP. See Continuous positive
airway pressure
C-peptide levels, 180
CPGs. See Clinical practice
guidelines
Crack cocaine, 46
Cranial/cardiac ultrasonography
findings, 522
Cranial nerves, 153–154, 754t
compression, 835
function, 753
Cranial size, decrease, 45
Craniofacial anomalies, 847

Craniosynostosis, 760–762
clinical presentation, 761
definition, 760
diagnostic evaluation, 761–762
incidence, 761
outcome, 762
pathophysiology, 761
patient care management, 762
risk factors, 760
Craniotabes, 137
Creatinine, laboratory assessment,
203–204
Credentials, verification, 871
Crew resource management
(CRM), 366
Crib safety, 379
CRIES. See Crying Requires oxygen
Increased vital signs
Expression Sleeplessness
Criminal model, harm-reduction
model (contrast), 68
Crisis
definition, 348
origins, understanding, 350–351
Critical incident stress management
(CISM), 428
Crossing the Quality Chasm (IOM),
368
Crouzon disease, 788
Crown-rump measurement,
gestational age reflection, 8
Crown-to-heal measurement, 127
Crying Requires oxygen Increased
vital signs Expression
Sleeplessness (CRIES)
neonatal postoperative pain
measurement score, 338t
postoperative pain tool, 338–339
Cryoprecipitate, usage, 255, 690
Cryosurgery, usage, 825
Cryotherapy, 844
Cryptorchidism, 657, 744–745
CSF. See Cerebrospinal fluid
CST. See Contraction stress test
CT. See Computed tomography
Cue-based feeding practices, 227
Cultural differences, consideration,
386
Cultural values/beliefs, role, 349–
350
Culture. See Blood
Culture of safety
board of trustees, role, 363
development/sustaining,
organizational/individual
approaches, 361–373
establishment, 363
just culture, 363
nurses, role, 363
patients/families, role, 363–364
person-centered approach, 363
physicians, role, 363
safe practices, NQF
identification, 368–369
senior leader promotion/
establishment, 362–363
simulation/debriefing, 365–366

Culture of safety *(Continued)*
  staffing, 367–368
  stakeholders
    engagement, 363–364
    role, 363
  systems approach, 363
  teamwork/communication,
    relationship, 364
  workforce, aging, 367
Current pregnancy, history, 7
Cutaneous candidiasis, 712
Cutis aplasia, 829–830
  photograph, 829f
Cutis marmorata, 134, 817
  telangiectasia, 817
CXR. *See* Chest x-ray
Cyanosis
  impact, 545
  observation, 545
Cyanotic congenital heart disease,
  497
Cyclopentolate, usage, 843
Cysteine, instability, 192
Cystic adenomatoid malformation
  (CAM), 479
  appearance, 283f
  radiographic evaluation, 283–284
  types, 479
Cystic fibrosis (CF), 120, 662–663
  screening, 8
Cystic hygroma, 478–479
Cytogenetic tests, 255
Cytomegalic inclusion disease, 839
Cytomegalovirus (CMV), 714, 839
  clinical manifestations, 714
  clinical presentation, 839
  diagnosis, 714
  etiology, 839
  incidence, 839
  infection, 837
  pathophysiology, 839
  transmission, route, 839

D

Daily fetal movement counting,
  usage, 27
DAT. *See* Direct antiglobulin test
DDAVP. *See* Desmopressin acetate
Decannulation, 530–531
Defect, causation, 410
Define, measure, analyze, improve
  (DMAI), 374
Deformation
  abnormalities, 805–806
  definition, 409, 783b
Degenerative CNS disease, 408
Degenerative placental changes,
  24
Dehydration, signs, 163
Dehydroepiandrosterone (DHEA),
  649
Deiodinase enzymes, regulation
  activity, 642
Deletion, definition, 402
Delivery
  admission, assessments, 33
  complications, 82

Delivery *(Continued)*
  drug withdrawal symptoms,
    onset, 55t
  history, 122–123
  information, 6
  mode, 122
  parental support, 88
  parent teaching, 88–89
  room
    preparation. *See* Extremely low
      birth weight infants;
      Neonatal delivery room
      resuscitation
    resuscitation, preheat surfaces,
      115
  stress, 80
  unknown maternal HBsAg
    status, 80
Dendritic sprouting, causes, 335
Dental eruptions, 140
Dentition, defectiveness, 306
Deontology, 862
Deoxygenated blood, drainage, 522
Deoxyribonucleic acid (DNA)
  detection, 703
  hybridization, 406
Dependence, definition, 247
Dermis, 813
Descending aorta, 74
Descriptive research (design), 852
Descriptive statistics, 853
Desmopressin acetate (DDAVP),
  requirement, 641
Detector contamination, 303
Development, synactive theory,
  210t–211t
Developmental care, 584–585
  standards, 209–227
Developmental dysplasia, 150
Developmental feeding,
  framework, 221
Developmental follow-up clinic,
  referrals, 397
Developmentally supportive
  environment, provision, 218
Developmental morbidities,
  increase, 397
Dexamethasone (Decadron), usage,
  515, 843
Dextrocardia, 285. *See also* Mirror
  image dextrocardia
  situs solitus, inclusion, 285
Dextrose 5%, usage, 81
DHEA. *See*
  Dehydroepiandrosterone
DHT. *See* Dihydrotestosterone
Diabetes insipidus (DI), 159, 641
  vasopressin deficiency, 641
Diabetes mellitus, 26–27
  assessment/management, 27
  complications, 26–27
  incidence, 26
Diabetic retinopathy, evidence, 27
Diagnosis, nursing process step, 865
Diagnostic adjuncts, 550–553
Diagnostic imaging, 296–298
Diagnostic screening tests, 703–704

Diaper dermatitis, 820. *See also*
  Candida diaper dermatitis
Diaphragm
  anatomic/pathologic x-ray
    changes, 273
  eventration
    appearance, 281f
    radiographic evaluation, 280
  placement, 294
  right side, paralysis, 281f
  upward displacement, 2
Diaphragmatic disorders, 480
Diaphragmatic excursion, 142
Diaphragmatic hernia, presence, 302
Diaphragmatic paralysis,
  radiographic evaluation, 280
Diastolic filling, 579
Diastolic murmur, 548
Diazoxide, usage, 176
DIC. *See* Disseminated
  intravascular coagulation
Differential cell count, 701–703
Diffusing distance, 23
DiGeorge syndrome, 543, 791–792
Digestion, biochemical/physiologic
  capacities, 183
Digitalis consideration, 584
Digitalis glycosides, 245
Digoxin therapy, 575
Dihydrotestosterone (DHT),
  binding, 655
Dipalmitoylphosphatidylcholine
  (DPPC), 454
Diploid, definition, 399
Direct antiglobulin test (DAT), 255
Direct bilirubin (DB) level, 193
Direct care adjustments, 212
Disaster preparation, 429
Discharge
  alternative setting, 392
  anticipatory guidance, 393
  community agencies/resources,
    links, 397
  criteria, establishment, 385–386
  durable medical equipment,
    selection, 390–392
  feeding/formula, 390
  home nursing agency, selection,
    390–392
  home oxygen teaching, 392
  home/parental capabilities,
    assessment, 385–386
  infection prevention, 395b
  parents, advice, 394b
  plan, success, 395
  prematurity-related problems,
    396b
  primary health care practitioner,
    selection, 390–392
  readiness criteria, 386b
  safety instruction, 379–380
  stability, requirement, 385
  summary, 387–389
  teaching, 387
  time, parents/care providers
    (information), 390b
  web sites, 394b

Discharge-focused care conference, completion, 387
Discharge planning, 387–392
  importance, 385
  inclusion, 385
  initiation, 383
  principles, 383–384
  technology, usage, 388t
Disorders, examples, 411
Disorders of sexual development (DSDs), 655–662
  assessment, 657–658
    findings, 658
  clinical presentation, 657
  complications, 661
  conditions, 657
  decision making, 660
  definition, 655
  diagnosis, 659
  emotional support, 660
  family manual (Consortium on the Management of Disorders of Sexual Development), 660
  gender assignment, 661
  infant, care, 660–661
  outcome, 662
  parents, care, 659–660
  physical examination, 657–658
  surgical considerations, 661
  understanding, 655
Disruption, definition, 409, 783b
Disseminated intravascular coagulation (DIC), 25, 30, 679–681
  acquired hemorrhagic disorder, 679
  association, 703
  clinical assessment, 680
  clinical presentation, 680
  complication, 462, 681
  control, measures, 681
  diagnostic studies, 681
  differential diagnosis, 681
  pathologic changes, events (sequence), 680f
  patient care management, 681
  physical examination, 680
  precipitating factors, 680
  supportive care, 681
Distal ischemia, complication, 317
Distribution, 239
Distributive shock, 582
Diuretics, 248–249
  impact, 164
  neonatal population considerations, 248–249
  usage, 514–515
    principles, 248
  usefulness, 161
Dizygotic (fraternal) male twins, anterior view, 787f
DMAI. See Define, measure, analyze, improve
Dobutamine (Dobutrex), usage, 467–468, 584

Doctorate of nursing practice (DNP), 850–851
Documentation, 874–877. See also Interfacility neonatal transport; Intrafacility neonatal transport; Logistical documentation; Patient care
  accuracy/concision, 876
  entry problem, correction, 876
  guidelines, 875–876
  necessity, 427
  objectivity, 876
  promptness, 876
Doll's-eye reflex, 834
Dominance, 400
Dominant gene, definition, 400
Do not resuscitate (DNR) order, 354–355
Do Not Use abbreviations, 375t
Dopamine, usage, 467, 583–584
Dopamine and norepinephrine reuptake inhibitor (DNRI), 54
Dopamine receptors, location, 245
Dopamine reuptake, cocaine inhibition, 46
Double bubble pattern, 289
Double effect. See Principle of double effect; Rule of double effect
Double ureters, 26–27
Double-walled incubators, usage, 116, 440
Down Syndrome, 411–412, 788
  genetic screening, 9
  photograph, 787f
Doxapram
  side effects, 491
  usage, 491
DPPC. See Dipalmitoylphosphatidylcholine
Droopy eyelids, 835
Droplet transmission, 721
Drugs
  abuse, 42–46
  apnea cause, 487
  categories, 42b
  screening, 63–64
    maternal characteristics, 63b
    method, 63
    policy, 63
  substances, presence, 254
DSDs. See Disorders of sexual development
Dubowitz, tool, 123
Ductless glands, 638
Ductus arteriosus, 74–75
  blood oxygenation, 75
  hemodynamic significance, 555
  patency, persistence, 554
Ductus venosus, 72, 75
Duodenal abnormalities, 289–290
Duodenal atresia, 289, 603–604
  definition, 603

Duodenal atresia (Continued)
  diagnosis, 603
  double bubble pattern, 289f
  etiology, 603
  postoperative care, 604
  preoperative care, 604
  prognosis, 603
  surgical repair, 604
Duodenal stenosis, 603–604
  definition, 603
  diagnosis, 603
  etiology, 603
  incidence, 603
  postoperative care, 604
  preoperative care, 604
  prognosis, 603
  surgical repair, 604
Duodenal villi, hypertrophy, 2
Duplication, definition, 402
Durable medical equipment
  agency, criteria, 392
  selection, 390–392
Dying infants, families (assistance), 354
Dysbarism, impact, 430
Dysplasia, definition, 783b

E
E. coli, 710–711
Eagle-Barrett syndrome, 623
  definition, 623
  diagnosis, 623
  etiology, 623
  incidence, 623
  prognosis, 623
  radiologic examination, 623
Early discharge. See Postpartum period
Early HDN, 79
Early-onset infection, GBS (impact), 709
Early-onset invasive group B streptococcal disease, incidence, 709f
Early-onset sepsis, identification failure, 694
Early radiation effects, 272
Ears. See External ear; Inner ear; Middle ear
  anatomy, 844–846
  assessment, 847
  examination, 847–848
  family history, 847
  history, 847
  malformation, risk (increase), 43
  patient assessment, 847–848
  physical examination, 126
  risk factors, history, 847
EBM. See Expressed breast milk
Ecchymosis, 135, 817, 835
ECF. See Extracellular fluid
Echocardiograms, types, 552
Echocardiograph (ECHO), diagnostic imaging, 297
Echocardiography, color flow mapping, 571

Eclampsia, 24–26
  assessment/management, 25–26
  clinical presentation, 24
  complications, 24–25
  etiology/predisposing factors, 24
  grand mal seizure, 24
ECMO. *See* Extracorporeal membrane oxygenation
Economic pressures, 385
Ectopia cordis, 285
EDC. *See* Estimated date of confinement
Edema, 784
  presence, 158
  salt retention, impact, 24
EHRs. *See* Electronic health records
Ejection clicks, 547
Elastic recoil, 495
Elbow flexion, 152
ELBW. *See* Extremely low birth weight
Elective abortions, number, 6
Elective endotracheal intubation, 106
Electrical conduction system, functionality, 539
Electrical monitoring, vibration (interference), 510
Electrocardiography, 551, 576
  values, 551
Electrochemical glucose meters, usage, 175
Electroencephalogram (EEG) characteristics, 211
Electrolytes
  abnormalities, 179
  balance, 161–168, 439–441
    elements, 440
    maintenance, 581
  disorders, 161–168
  disturbance, 540
  glucose/fluid imbalance, 530
  imbalance, 810
  laboratory assessment, 203
  losses, replacement, 180
  support, 108
Electronic fetal monitoring, 17
Electronic health records (EHRs), 370
Embolism, complication, 317
Embryologic development, 748–750
Embryology, 724–725
Embryonic vessels, 124
Emergency contact form, staff completion, 429
Emergency medical technicians (EMTs), transport involvement, 421
Emesis, result, 200
EMLA. *See* Eutectic mixture of local anesthetics
Emollients (usage), recommendation (absence), 815
Emptying time, delay, 2

Encephalocele, 105, 760, 798–799
  associated findings, 798
  clinical presentation, 760, 797–798
  definition, 760
  diagnosis, 798
  diagnostic evaluation, 760
  incidence/etiology, 798
  outcome, 760
  pathophysiology, 760
  patient care management, 760
  risk factors, 760
Endocardial cushion defect (atrioventricular canal), 26–27, 286
  anatomy, 559
  clinical manifestations, 559
  hemodynamics, 559
  incidence, 559
  management, 559–560
  prognosis, 560
Endocardial tube dislocation, observation, 101
Endocrine changes, maternal physiologic changes, 6
Endocrine disorders. *See* Neonates
  adult disease, fetal origins, 640
Endocrine disruptors, 640
Endocrine glands
  freestanding control mechanism, 640
  function, negative feedback-loop control, 639f
Endocrine system, 638–640
  glands/hormones, 639t
  regulation, 638–640
End of life, pain management, 344–345
Endotracheal CPAP, 500
Endotracheal intubation, 100–101
  performing, 100
Endotracheal tube (ETT), 294
  extubation, 379
  insertion depth, determination, 304
  observation, 512
  placement, 295f
    landmarks, identification, 305f
  securing, 303
  selection, 304
  size, 302
  usage, 502–503
  visible secretions, 300
Endotracheal tube (ETT) suctioning, 299–302
  complications, 301–302
  contraindications, 300
  equipment/supplies, 300
  indications, 299–300
  precautions, 300
  procedure, 300–301
End-tidal CO$_2$
  detector, 303
  monitoring, 513
Endurance, 224

Enteral feedings, 194–199, 613
  achievement, 199
  contraindications, 81
  ELBW maintenance, 442
  initiation, 184
  methods, 199–202
  minimum, 199–200
  tolerance, facilitation (nursing interventions), 202–203
Enteral nutrition, minimum, 200
Enteric pathogens, 835
Enterohepatic circulation, increase, 628
Entrainment, 507
Environmental checklist, 379
Environmental factors, impact, 543
Environmental influences, definition, 402
Environmental modifications, usage, 218
Environmental risk factors, 700
Environmental temperature, 79
Environmental tobacco smoke (ETS), 43
Enzymatic defect, 675
Enzymatic reagent strips, usage, 175
Enzyme maturity, induction, 241
EOAE. *See* Evoked otoacoustic emissions
Eosinophils, 669
Epicardial pacing wires, invasive monitoring, 578
Epidermis, 813
  lower layers, 813
Epidermolysis bullosa, 136, 827–828
Epidermolysis bullosa lethalis, 828
Epidural anesthesia, 37
Epidural fever, 37
Epidural shakes, 37
Epinephrine, usage, 468
Epiphora, 836
Episiotomy, performing/extension, 34
EPO. *See* Erythropoietin
Epstein pearls, 819
  photograph, 819f
Erb-Duchenne-Klumpke paralysis, 764
Erb palsy, 764
Errors. *See* Medication errors
Erythema toxicum (newborn rash), 135, 817–818
  photograph, 818f
Erythrocyte
  hemolysis, 27
  mass, 669
  Rosette test, 255
  sedimentation rate, 703
Erythropoiesis, 667
Erythropoietin (EPO), 666–667
  usage, 688–689
Escherichia coli, UTI percentage, 739
Esophageal abnormalities, radiographic evaluation, 287–289

Esophageal atresia, 104, 600–602
  absence, 289
  appearance, 288f
  definition, 600
  diagnosis, 601
  postoperative care, 602
  postoperative complications, 602
  preoperative care, 601
  prognosis, 601
  radiographic evaluation, 287–288
  surgical repair, 601
  tracheoesophageal fistula,
    inclusion, 288–289
Esophageal lesions, occurrence, 828
Esophageal malformations, 600f
Esophageal pouch, oral/nasogastric
    decompression, 104
Esophageal sphincter, presence, 182
Esophageal temperature
    monitoring, 110
Esophagus
  contrast medium, usage, 288f
  perforation, 306
  radiographic evaluation, 287
Estimated date of confinement
    (EDC), 8
Estrogen, levels (elevation), 3
EtCO$_2$ detector, attachment, 306
Ethical issues
  approaches, 862–863
  nurses, roles, 863–864
  presence, 860
Ethical standards, 868–869
Ethical theories, 862
ETS. See Environmental tobacco
    smoke
ETT. See Endotracheal tube
Eustachian canal, usage, 846
Eutectic mixture of local anesthetics
    (EMLA) cream, usage, 344
Evaluation, nursing process step,
    866
Evaporation, 114
Evaporative heat loss
  increase, 114
  reduction, 116
Evaporimeter, usage, 440
Evidence-based care, provision, 385
Evidence-based clinical practice
    interventions, usage, 361
Evidence-based medicine, 855
Evidence-based practice (EBP),
    370–371
  concept, 855
  definition, 868
  guidance, 854
  reference, 855–856
Evoked otoacoustic emissions
    (EOAE), 848
Ewing v. Aubert, 866
Exchange transfusion, 314
  fresh whole blood, usage, 706
Executive walk rounds, definition,
    362b
Exogenous surfactant,
    administration, 302
Experimental research (design), 852

Expert witnesses, testimony, 867–
    868
Expiratory film, definition, 270
Exposure, definition, 270
Expressed breast milk (EBM),
    administration problems,
    374
Exstrophy of the bladder, 742–744
External auditory meatus, 845–846
External ear, 844–846
  auricle, parts, 845f
External genitalia
  differentiation, 655
  disorders of differentiation, 656–
    657
  edema, 35
Extracellular fluid (ECF)
  contraction, 159
  distribution, 156
  physiologic contraction, 156
Extracorporeal circulation,
    physiology, 526–527
Extracorporeal Life Support
    Organization (ELSO),
    International Registry
    Report, 522
Extracorporeal membrane
    oxygenation (ECMO), 104
  ACT monitoring, 526
  blood gas monitoring, 526
  bubble detector, 526
  cannulation, 527
  circuit, 524–525
    components, 524f
  emergencies, 527–530
  flow, servomechanism
    regulation, 525
  follow-up/outcome, 531–532
  gas exchange devices, 525
  heat exchanger, 525
  historical perspective, 521–522
  infant care, 527–531
  medical morbidity, 531
  nursing responsibilities/
    interventions, 528t–529t
  parental support, 531
  parent-to-parent support, 531
  patient
    complications, 530
    criteria. See Neonatal ECMO
      patient criteria
  perfusion, 526
  prolongation, 521
  pumps, 525
  run, 527–530
  specialist responsibilities, 527
  survivors, scrutiny, 531
  usage, 467
    criteria, 522
  weaning/decannulation, 530–531
Extrahepatic bile duct, 619
Extrahepatic biliary atresia, 617
Extraocular muscles, 833–834
  function, 815
  innervation, 815
  musculature, 815
Extrapulmonary shunt, 497–499

Extraretinal fibrovascular
    proliferation, 793
Extrathoracic anomaly, 285
Extrathyroid abnormalities, 643
Extrauterine life
  adaptation, 72, 94
  anatomy/physiology, 72–77
  fetus transition, 93
Extravasation. See Intravenous
    extravasations
  treatment, 309–310
Extremely low birth weight
    (ELBW) infants
  barotrauma/oxygen exposure,
    438
  bed type, usage, 436
  birth, preparation, 435
  blood transfusions, 439
  body water, compartments, 440
  breathing
    changes, assessment, 438
    patterns, assessment, 438
  cardiovascular support, 439
  challenges, 434
  clinical assessment, parameters,
    437–445
  clinical stability, 178
  cues, learning, 443
  decision making, parent
    participation, 434–435
  delivery, 434–435
  delivery room management, 435
  developmentally appropriate
    care, 442–443
  electrolyte balance, 439–441
  electrolyte imbalances, 440
  enteral nutrition, 442
  environmental risk factors, 441
  evaporative heat loss, 114
  family-centered environment,
    support, 444
  feeding, goal, 441–442
  fluid balance, 439–441
  fluid imbalances, 440
  fluid intake, increase, 160
  hearing screens, 444
  hyperbilirubinemia, 441
  hypernatremia, 440
    prevention, 163
  hyponatremia, 440
  immunizations, usage, 444
  maintenance, 444
  management considerations,
    116–118
  MAP, persistence, 439
  mechanical ventilation, usage,
    437–438
  metabolic demands (decrease),
    supportive measures
    (usage), 438
  monitoring, 444
  NICU monitoring, 436
  NICU transfer, 435
  nonoliguric hyperkalemia, 440
  nosocomial bloodstream
    infections, risk reduction,
    441

Extremely low birth weight
(ELBW) infants *(Continued)*
nursing assessment, principles,
439
nursing management, 438–439
parameters, 437–445
principles, 439
NUS, usage, 444
nutrition, 441–442
opioid infusions, treatment, 443–
444
oxygen consumption,
minimization, 438
pain management, 443–444
palliative care, 444–445
PDA, congenital heart lesion, 439
prenatal considerations, 434–435
probe, usage, 436
respiratory support, 437–438
ROP screening, 444
screening, 444
sedatives, safety, 444
sepsis, 441
susceptibility, increase, 441
skin adhesives/solvents,
avoidance, 437
skin care, 436–437
stratum corneum, barrier
effectiveness, 436
stress
impact/signs, 442–443
minimization, 443
supplemental oxygen,
maintenance, 438
TEWL, estimation, 440–441
thermoregulation, 436
ventilatory support,
maintenance, 438
warming table placement, 435
Extubation
evaluation, 430
preparation, 517
signs, 512
Eyeball, 832–833
anterior cavity, 833
cross section, 833f
extraocular muscles, 833–834
function, 834
inner layer, 833
innervation, 834
lens, 833
middle layer (vascular tunic), 833
musculature, 833
outer layer (fibrous tunic), 832–
833
pathologic conditions/
management, 834–844
posterior cavity, 833
Eyelashes, crusting/matting, 836
Eyelids, 832
characteristics, 834
edema, 835
Eyes
anatomy, 832–834
care, 79
cleansing, 837
examination, 838, 844

Eyes *(Continued)*
malformation, risk (increase), 43
physical examination, 126
protective structures, 832

F

Face
petechiae, 77
sun-sensitive hyperpigmentation, 3
Facial bruising, 77
Facial cellulitis, 836
Facial configuration, 834
Facial milia, oral counterpart, 819
Facial nerves, 846
paralysis, 27
Facilitated tucking, usage, 443
Factor XIII deficiency, 686
FAE. *See* Fetal alcohol effects
False diagnosis, impact, 262
Familial dysautonomia, ethnic
predisposition, 7
Familial dyshormonogenesis, 643
Familial recurrence risks, 546t
Families
acceptance/openness/
availability, 355
assistance. *See* Dying infants
care, management, 410–411
crisis, 349–359
assessment, 349–351
intervention, 352–354
developmentally supportive
environment, promotion,
353
discharge criteria, 385–386
dynamics, alteration, 383
history, 409
notification system,
establishment, 429
postdischarge, 395–397
signatures, obtaining, 878
support systems, determination,
350
ties, disruption, 351
Family-centered care (FCC), 363–
364
core concepts, 363–364
Family-centered developmental
care, promotion, 358
Family-centered environment,
establishment, 364
Family history, 120
Family-infant bonding, 356–357
assessment, 357
definitions, 356–357
discussion, 357
encouragement, interventions,
357–359
Fanconi anemia, 682
Fasting basal gastric residuals, 200
Fasting hypoglycemia, 6
Fat, body compartment, 239
Fat emulsification, 183
Fatigue, shift work (relationship),
366–367
Fat-soluble vitamins, newborn
deficiencies, 187

Fatty acid oxidation, errors, 809–810
FDPs. *See* Fibrin degradation
products
Fecal fat, 593
Feeding
accomplishment, 201
contraindications, 81
demand, 223
guidelines, 81
initiation, contraindications
(potential), 200–201
modalities, 226–227
parents, relationship, 224
readiness behaviors, recognition,
221
success
evaluation, 224
relationship, 222
tolerance/intolerance,
contraindications, 200–201
Feet, polydactyly, 804f
Female bladder catheterization,
landmarks (usage), 326f
Female catheterization, 325–326
Female external genitalia,
development/differentiation,
656f
Female neonates
CAH presence, virilized genitalia
(management), 653–654
trisomy 18, 789f
Femoral head/acetabulum,
abnormalities, 801–802
associated findings, 801
clinical presentation, 801
diagnosis, 801
incidence/etiology, 801
treatment, 801–802
Fentanyl (Sublimaze), usage, 303,
343
Fetal adrenocortical development,
649–650
Fetal alcohol effects (FAE)
incidence, 45
maternal risk factors, 45
Fetal alcohol syndrome (FAS)
maternal risk factors, 45
occurrence, 44
socioeconomic group occurrence,
45
Fetal Alcohol Syndrome
Surveillance Network
(FASSNet), 44
Fetal anomaly, 122
Fetal assessment, 27
Fetal blood glucose concentrations,
74
Fetal bradycardia, 24
Fetal breathing, 74
Fetal calcium metabolism, 165
Fetal capillaries, distance (increase),
23
Fetal cardiac development,
occurrence, 535
Fetal cardiovascular system,
maternal diseases
(classification), 544b

Fetal cell analysis, 405
Fetal circulation
  adult circulation, difference, 539
  characteristics, 72–74
  establishment, 539
  scheme, 73f
Fetal complications, 25
Fetal death, 26
Fetal descent/pushing, 17
Fetal distress, 25, 30, 83
Fetal ductal closure, 464
Fetal echocardiography (ECHO), 122
  advances, 534
  usage, 552
Fetal endocrine disorders, 810–811
Fetal energy needs, lipids
    (contribution), 184
Fetal factors, 24
Fetal femur length, usage, 8
Fetal fibronectin test, performing, 29
Fetal GA, overestimation, 132
Fetal glucose homeostasis, 173
Fetal growth, abnormality, 121–122
Fetal heart
  continuous monitoring, 31
  development, timeline, 535t
  monitoring, 25
  motion (detection), real-time
    ultrasonography (usage), 8
  movement, loss, 30
  tones, 8
    loss, 30
Fetal heart rate (FHR)
  baseline, evaluation, 17
  decelerations, 10
  detection. See Nonreassuring
    FHR
  patterns, 17
  variability, decrease, 30
Fetal hematology, 72
Fetal hemoglobin, oxygen affinity,
    74
Fetal hyperinsulinemia, 160
Fetal hypoxia, 488
  sign, 35
Fetal insulin, detection, 173
Fetal kick counts, 9
Fetal lung fluid, chloride
    concentration, 462
Fetal lung maturity (FLM), 122, 455
  assay, 10–11
  documentation, laboratory
    assessments, 10–11
  increase, corticosteroids (usage),
    25
Fetal lungs
  blood flow, decrease, 74
  characteristics, 74
Fetal magnesium homeostasis, 167
Fetal-maternal infusion, 670
Fetal metabolism, 74
Fetal movement
  counting, 27
  counts, 9
  decrease, 9
  first feeling, quickening, 8
Fetal pancreatic function, 662

Fetal pH, labor value, 24
Fetal phosphorous levels, increase,
    185
Fetal shunts, 72–74
  persistence, 85
  types, 75
Fetal sound experience, 219
Fetal tachycardia, 24
Fetal thyroid development, 642
Fetal weight, estimation, 35
Fetal zinc levels, midpregnancy
    increase, 185
Fetamaternal hemorrhage, 30
Fetomaternal hemorrhage,
    Kleihauer-Betke test, 255
Fetus
  alcohol
    effects, 44–45
    risk, 44
  amphetamines/MDMA, effects,
    49
  anatomy/physiology, 20
  cocaine, effects, 47
  enzyme maturity, induction, 241
  fluid homeostasis, 156
  glucose, active transport, 6
  immune system, development,
    695t
  inhalants, effects, 53
  marijuana, effects, 50
  narcotics/opioids, effects, 51–52
  neurobehavioral effects, 43
  sedatives/hypnotics, effects, 53
  smoking, impact, 43
  transition, predisposition, 93
FFP. See Fresh frozen plasma
FGFR3. See Fibroblast Growth
    Factor receptor 3
FHR. See Fetal heart rate
Fibrils, dermis/epidermis
    connection, 815
Fibrin clot dissolution, 671
Fibrin clot formation, flowchart, 672f
Fibrin degradation products
    (FDPs), release, 671
Fibrinogen, usage, 671
Fibrin split products (FSPs), 671
Fibroblast Growth Factor receptor
    3 (FGFR3), 795–796
Fibrous tunic. See Eyeball
Fight-or-flight mechanism,
    compensation, 337–338
Finnegan Score. See Neonatal
    Abstinence Scoring System
Finnegan's NAS, 54
First-born children, FAS, 45
First feeding, 80–81
First heart sound, 546–547
First pain, association, 335
First-pass effect, 241
First-trimester integrated screening,
    8
FISH. See Fluorescence in situ
    hybridization
Fistula formation, 836
5-α-reductase, deficiency, 657
Five rights, definition, 362b

Fixed-wing aircraft
  equipment/articles, securing, 428
  transport, 419
Fixed-wing transports, 422
Flashlamp-pumped pulsed-dye
    laser, effectiveness, 825
FLM. See Fetal lung maturity
Flotation vests, usage, 428
Flow sheets, usage, 874
Fluid adjustments, 156
Fluid balance, 156–158
  assessment, 158
    considerations, 156–158
    parameters, 158
  body weight, 158
  disorders, 159–161
  elements, 440
  maintenance, 581
  physiologic considerations, 156–
    158
  regulation, 156–157
  urine
    specific gravity, 158
    volume, 158
Fluid constituents, 158
Fluid depletion, 159–160
  causes, 159
  complications, 160
  diagnostic studies, 159
  pathophysiology, 159
  patient care management, 159
  precipitating factors, 159
Fluid excess, 160–161
  clinical presentation/assessment,
    161
  complications, 161
  diagnostic studies, 161
  etiologies, 160–161
  hemodynamic changes, 161
  pathophysiology, 160
  patient care management, 161
  precipitating factors, 160–161
Fluid homeostasis, 156
Fluid intake, recalculation, 163
Fluid overload, avoidance, 581
Fluid requirements, quantification,
    158
Fluid therapy, 158
  goal, 158
Fluid volume decisions, principles,
    158
Fluorescence in situ hybridization
    (FISH), 406
  requirement, 542
Focal clonic seizure, 772
Focal intestinal perforation, 613
Focus, in-depth understanding, 854
Focus groups, 854
Folic acid, supplementation, 2
Follow-up care, components, 397
Fontanelles, 136–138
  illustration, 761f
Foramen ovale, 75
  formation, 535
  pulmonary vascular resistance,
    decrease, 75
  sealing, 75

Forceps, application, 816
Forceps marks, 820
Forcing functions, 377
  definition, 362b
Foreign fetus, accommodation, 5–6
Formula milk, fortification, 197
46,XY DSD, 655
46,XY infant, virilization (21-
  hydroxylase deficiency), 658f
Fosphenytoin, usage, 773–774
Fourth heart sound, 547
Fourth trimester. *See* Puerperium
Fractured left clavicle, 293f
Fractured ribs, appearance, 294f
Fractures, radiographic evaluation,
  293–294
FRC. *See* Functional residual
  capacity
Free air, radiolucent halo, 279
Free fatty acids, body
  compartment, 240
Free-flow oxygen, usage, 302
Free ionized calcium (iCa), 165
Freeze milk, usage (absence), 198
Frenulum, 140
Fresh frozen plasma (FFP), 689–690
Frog-leg position, 152
FSPs. *See* Fibrin split products
Full disclosure, 372–373
Functional morbidities, increase,
  397
Functional placental area, decrease
  (outcome), 20
Functional residual capacity (FRC),
  definition, 494
Fundal height, 8
  measurements, 8
Fungal infection, 712–713
Furniture safety, 379
Furosemide (Lasix), usage, 473–474,
  514–515, 575

G

GA. *See* Gestational age
Gag reflex, maturation, 202
Galactosemia, 194, 197, 808
  associated findings, 808
  clinical findings, 808
  diagnosis, 808
  incidence/etiology, 808
  treatment, 808
Gallbladder, muscle tone/motility
  (decrease), 2
Gamete, definition, 399
Gamma-aminobutyric acid (GABA),
  balance (alteration), 52
Ganglion cells, 814
Gases, humidification, 508
Gas exchange, 526
  devices, 525
  effectiveness, 507
  mechanisms, 505
Gas trapping, 495
Gastric aspirates, 200
  significance, determination, 200
Gastric contents, aspiration, 304
Gastric decompression, 598

Gastric emptying, delay, 184
Gastric gland secretion activity,
  presence, 183
Gastric intubation, procedure, 201
Gastric lipases, presence, 183
Gastric perforation, 289
Gastric tests, 592
Gastric tube feeding, transition, 202
Gastrin, presence, 183
Gastroesophageal reflux (GER),
  183, 620–622
  conservative measures, 621–622
  considerations, 620–621
  definition, 620
  diagnosis, 621
  etiology, 620
  incidence, 621
  management, 621–622
  pharmacologic measures, 622
  prognosis, 621
  spectrum, 620
  surgical measures, 622
Gastrointestinal (GI) clinical signs,
  701
Gastrointestinal (GI) defects, 26–27
Gastrointestinal (GI) disease, 708
Gastrointestinal (GI) embryonic
  development, 589–590
Gastrointestinal (GI) enzyme
  activity, 237
Gastrointestinal (GI) function,
  postnatal development
  (influences), 184
Gastrointestinal (GI) involvement,
  multisystem disorders, 623–
  635
Gastrointestinal (GI) losses,
  increase, 163
Gastrointestinal (GI) medication
  administration, 236–237
Gastrointestinal (GI) motility
  limitation, reference, 183–184
  reference, 183
Gastrointestinal (GI) system
  abdominal assessment, 591–592
  assessment, 590–595
  auscultation, 592
  diagnostic tests, 592–593
  endoscopy, 593
  evaluation, laboratory tests, 594t
  fecal fat, 593
  history, 590–591
  illness, history, 590–591
  laboratory tests, 593–595
    list, 594t
  palpation, 592
  percussion, 592
  pH probe test, 593
  radiographic evaluation, 287–293
  radiologic studies, 593
  scintigraphy, 593
  stool examination, 593
  ultrasonography, 593
Gastrointestinal (GI) tract
  acidity, 237
  anatomic/functional
    development, 182–183

Gastrointestinal (GI) tract
  (Continued)
  anatomic/pathologic x-ray
    changes, 273–274
  embryologic features, 589
  functions, 590
  medication excretion, 242
  obstructions, 599–612
    considerations, 599–600
  perfusion, 237
  postnatal development, 183–184
Gastroschisis, 105, 146, 596–597
  amniocentesis, usage, 597
  definition, 596
  diagnosis, 596–597
  etiology, 596
  incidence, 596
  omphalocele, comparison, 597t
  photograph, 596f
  prognosis, 597
  risk, increase, 43
Gastrotomy tube feeding, 202
Gavage feedings, provision, 202–203
GBS. *See* Group B streptococci;
  Group B streptococcus
G-CSF. *See* Granulocyte colony-
  stimulating factor
GDM. *See* Gestational diabetes
  mellitus
Gelled adhesives, helpfulness, 816
Gender/race differences, 129
Gene, definition, 400
Gene expression, regulation, 234
General anesthesia
  assessment/management, 36–37
  complications, 36
Generalized edema, complication,
  530
Generalized subcutaneous edema,
  104
Genetic brain disorder, 120
Genetic counseling, 407–408
  definition, 407
  encouragement, 410
  goal, 407
  indications, 407–408
  information, obtaining
    (methods), 408
  medical facts, provision, 408
  parents, discussion, 408
  principles, 407
  usage, 542–543
Genetic heterogeneity, 409
Genetic history, information, 6–7
Genetics, 399–401
  terminology, 399–400
Genetic screening, 8–9
Genetic syndromes/disorders,
  family care management,
  410–411
Genital ducts, disorders of
  differentiation, 656–657
Genitalia, physical examination,
  126
Genital virilization, degrees, 652f
Genitourinary anomaly, 327
Genotype, definition, 400

Gentle human touch (GHT), 213
Genu recurvatum, 150
GER. *See* Gastroesophageal reflux
Gestation, calculation, 1
Gestational age (GA)
  assessment, 7–8, 27, 77
    abdominal circumference,
      usage, 8
    grading system, 124f
  blood volume impact, 670
  clinical estimate, 126–127
  clinical presentation, 838
  defining, 97
  establishment, biparietal
    diameter (usage), 8
  estimation, 128f
  examination, 124–126
  growth parameters, comparison,
    130
  history, 545
  impact, 816
  instruments, 123–127
  invasive procedure frequency,
    inverse relationship, 333
  weight, comparison, 130
Gestational diabetes, treatment
  (goal), 178
Gestational diabetes mellitus
  (GDM), 26
  clinical presentation/screening,
    26
  female risk, 26
    ACOG indication, 26
  glucose challenge test, 9
  predisposing factors, 26
GFR. *See* Glomerular filtration rate
GHT. *See* Gentle human touch
Giant pigmented nevus,
  photograph, 822f
Gibbon, John, 521
GIR. *See* Glucose infusion rate
Glaucoma, 839
Global system for mobile
  communication (GSM), 429
Glomerular capillary hydrostatic
  pressure, 727
Glomerular filtration, 727
Glomerular filtration rate (GFR),
  156
  determination, factors, 727
  doubling, 726–727
  medication excretion, 242
Glottis, anterior position, 92
Glucagon
  secretion, 173
  usage, 176
Gluconeogenesis, 172
  stimulation, 178
Gluconeogenic pathways,
  adequacy, 173
Glucose
  carbohydrate source, 184
  concentration, 74
    monitoring, 108
  consumption, delivery excess,
    174
  delivery, 174

Glucose *(Continued)*
  electrolyte/fluid imbalance, 530
  excretion, renal threshold, 4
  homeostasis, 172–173. *See also*
    Fetal glucose homeostasis;
    Neonatal glucose
    homeostasis
    hormonal regulation, 173
  infusion, 175
  IV administration, 88
  levels, monitoring, 180
  metabolism, 172, 751
  molecules, transport, 172
  needs, 80–81
  oral administration, 87–88
  production, 172
  status, assessment, 175
  supply, 87–88
Glucose challenge test, 9
Glucose infusion rate (GIR)
  decrease, 179
  receiving, 178
Glucose polymers (Polycose),
  usage, 575
Glutamine, inclusion (absence), 192
Gluteal fold, asymmetry, 149
Glycogenolysis, stimulation, 178
Glycogen storage disease, 174
  type I, 197
Glycogen stores, energy reserves, 74
Glycosuria, 180
Glycosylated hemoglobin tests, 27
GM-CSF. *See* Granulocyte-
    monocyte colony-stimulating
    factor
Gonococcal conjunctivitis, 835
Graft-*versus*-host disease, 687
Gram-negative diplococci, 835
Gram-negative organisms, 710–712
Gram-positive organisms, 708–710
Grand mal seizure, 24
Granulocyte colony-stimulating
    factor (G-CSF), 666–667, 706
Granulocyte-monocyte colony-
    stimulating factor (GM-CSF),
    666–667
Granulocytes, 669
  transfusion, 705–706
  usage, 255, 690
Graves disease, 647
  pathophysiology, 647–648
Gravidity, pregnancy indication, 6
Gravity, center (alteration), 5
Great vessels, development, 537–
    539
Great vessels, transposition, 26–27
  anatomy, 567
  clinical manifestations, 568
  corrective surgery, 568
  hemodynamics, 567
  illustration, 568f
  incidence, 567
  management, 568
  prognosis, 569
  radiographic evaluation, 285
Green tube (laboratory specimen
    tube), 257–258

Grief, 354–356. *See also* Anticipatory
    grief; Chronic grief
  assessment, 355
  counseling, information
    (providing), 355
  definitions, 355
  facilitation, interventions, 355
  response. *See* Parents
Gross anatomy, 725
Group B streptococcal pneumonia,
    278f
  x-ray diagnosis, difficulty, 278
Group B streptococci (GBS)
  gram-positive organisms, 708–
    710
  impact, 694–695
Group B streptococcus (GBS)
  colonization, intrapartum
    chemoprophylaxis, 122
  infection, 11
  screening. *See* Rectal-genital
    GBS
Group II staphylococcus, phage
    strain, 827
Growth. *See* Infants
  classification, 127–132
  curve charts, 205
  factors, illustration, 667f
  measurement, 127
    obtaining, 127
  parameters, GA comparison, 130
Guardian consent, absence, 878
Guidelines for Cardiopulmonary
    Resuscitation and
    Emergency Cardiovascular
    Care of Pediatric and
    Neonatal Patients (AAP/
    AHA), 94
Gut-regulating polypeptides,
    presence, 183
Gut trophic factors, 184

H
H. influenzae, 711
Hair cells, 846
Hair shafts, 813
Hairy nevus, presence, 822
HAIs. *See* Health care-associated
    infections
Half-life, definition, 234
Handling
  considerations, 214
  usage, 213–214
Hands, polydactyly, 804f
Handwriting, problems (impact),
    876
Haploid, definition, 400
Harlequin color change, 817
  photograph, 818f
Harlequin fetus, 829
Harlequin sign, 134
Harm-reduction model, criminal
    model (contrast), 68
Hashish, potency, 50
HBIG. *See* Hepatitis B
    immunoglobulin
HBV. *See* Hepatitis B virus

hCG. *See* Human chorionic gonadotropin
HCV. *See* Hepatitis C virus
HD. *See* Hirschsprung disease
HDN. *See* Hemorrhagic disease of the newborn
Head, physiologic changes, 78
Head circumference (HC), 127
    decrease, 43
    measurements, obtaining, 136
    occipital-frontal circumference, 204
Head-sparing IUGR, 130
Head-to-toe physical examination, 77–78
Healthcare-associated infections, prevention, 720
Health care-associated infections (HAIs), 377
    risk reduction, improvement strategies, 378–379
Health care errors, 373–379
Health care providers
    professional liability insurance, carrying, 879
    training, 364–366
Health care trends, 384–385
Health information technology (HIT), 368
    addition, 370
Health Insurance Portability and Accountability Act (HIPAA), 58, 425
Healthy People 2010, objectives, 44
Hearing loss, 847
    etiology, 847–848
    intrauterine infections, 847
    ototoxic drugs, impact, 847
    pathophysiology, 847
    risk factors, 847–848
Hearing screening, 848
    methodology, 848
Heart
    contractions, 539
    development, 538f
        identification, 535
        ventral views, sketches, 536f
    physiologic changes, 78
    positional anomalies, 285
    size, 284
    sounds, 78, 546–549, 561
        auscultation, 144
    tube, elongation, 535
Heart failure
    afterload, 579
    cardiac contractility, decrease, 579
    causes, 578–579
    contractility, 579
    etiology, 578–579
    low cardiac output, recognition, 579–580
    postoperative disturbance, 578–581
    postoperative event, commonness, 578
    preload/diastolic filling, 579

Heart failure *(Continued)*
    pulmonary vascular resistance, increase, 579
    risk, increase, 160
    systemic venous return, inadequacy, 579
Heart rate, 102
    disturbances, 550
    fluctuation, 541
    increase, 102
Heat conservation, physical methods, 112
Heat exchange, 525
Heat gain, balance, 111–113
Heat loss
    balance, 111–113
    conversion, impact, 114
    decrease, strategies, 114–116
    increase, 113
    mechanisms, 114
    reduction, 116
Heat production
    balance, 111–113
    physical methods, 112
Heat transfer, 113
    air currents, impact, 114
    increase, 114
    mechanisms, 113–114
    occurrence, 113–114
Heel stick, usage, 334
Helicopters, transport, 419
Hematocrit, 668
    determination, 83
    levels, increase/decrease, 159
Hematologic changes, maternal physiologic changes, 5–6
Hematologic disorders, 480
    diagnosis, 666
Hematologic evaluation, 701–704
Hematologic tests, 254
Hematopoiesis, 666–667
    illustration, 667f
Hematopoietic disorders, apnea cause, 488
Hemithorax, loops (filling), 281
Hemodynamic changes, occurrence, 4
Hemodynamic instability, 193
Hemodynamic management, 578
Hemodynamics, 85
Hemoglobin, 667–668
    binding, 667
    birth values, 667–668
    disorders, 675
    oxygen affinity, 74
    oxygen binding, 496–497
Hemoglobin-oxygen dissociation curve, 497f
Hemolysis, 674–675
    prophylactic therapy, 674–675
Hemolysis elevated liver function test results and low platelet count (HELLP syndrome), 25
Hemophilia, 685
Hemorrhage, 672–674
    complication, 530

Hemorrhagic disease of the newborn (HDN), 79, 678–679
    clinical assessment, 678
    clinical presentation, 678
    complications, 679
    deficiency results, 79
    diagnostic studies, 678
    differential diagnosis, 678–679
    etiologic factors, 678
    factors, 678
    outcome, 679
    patient care management, 679
    physical examination, 678
    prophylactic vitamin K, usage, 679
Hemostasis, test values, 673t
Hemostatic mechanisms, 671
Heparin, usage, 543
Heparin solution, titration, 526
Hepatic biotransformation, 241
Hepatic enzyme systems, hypoxic/ischemic insult (vulnerability), 241
Hepatic function, decrease, 628
Hepatic glucose production, 178
Hepatic glycogen
    depletion, 157
    mobilization, 80
Hepatic rupture, 24
Hepatitis B, 716–717
    presentation, 716
    prevention, 716–717
    transmission, 716
    treatment, 717
Hepatitis B immunoglobulin (HBIG), 79–80
Hepatitis B virus (HBV)
    breastfeeding, impact, 65
    rate, 79
Hepatitis C virus (HCV), breastfeeding impact, 65
Hepatitis vaccine, 79–80
Hepatocyte, 619
Hereditary anemia, 120
Hereditary lesions, 827–830
Heroin
    breastfeeding impact, 65
    methadone, comparison, 52
    semisynthetic opiate, 51
    use, increase, 50
Herpes, 826–827
Herpes simplex vesicles, 826f
Herpes simplex virus (HSV), 715–716
    diagnosis, 715–716
    infection, maternal infection, 716
    isolation procedures, 716
    presentation, 715
    prevention, 716
    prognosis, 716
    transmission, 715
    treatment, 716
Herpetic lesions, 194
Heterogeneous chromosomes, definition, 400
HFJV. *See* High-frequency jet ventilation

HFOV. *See* High-frequency oscillatory ventilation
HFV. *See* High-frequency ventilation
Hiatal hernia (repair), Nissen fundoplication (usage), 622f
HIE. *See* Hypoxic-ischemic encephalopathy
High-alert medications, 376b
ISMP creation, 376
High-flow nasal cannula, 499
High-frequency jet ventilation (HFJV), 467, 507–509
entrainment, 507f
weaning, 508
High-frequency oscillatory ventilation (HFOV), 467, 507
usage, 509–511
High-frequency ventilation (HFV), 467, 473, 505–511
gas exchange mechanisms, 505
gas exchange theories, 505–507
tidal volumes, usage, 505
trial, 522
types, 507–511
High-resolution banding, 406
High-risk infants
physiological instability, 213–214
postpartum depression, 386
High-risk neonate, examination, 842
High spinal complication/management, 38
Hips, 150
developmental dysplasia, 150, 801–802
Hirschsprung disease (HD), 291, 297, 609–611
anal manometry, 610
clinical presentation, 610
complications, 611
definition, 609
diagnosis, 610
etiology, 609–610
illustration, 291f
incidence, 610
postoperative care, 610–611
preoperative care, 610
prognosis, 610
radiologic examination, 610
surgical repair, 610
History. *See* Families; Newborn infants; Prenatal history
HIT. *See* Health information technology
Holt-Oram syndrome, 542
Home, infant positioning, 215–218
Home blood glucose monitoring, 27
Home care nursing, inclusion, 395–396
Home care transition, principles, 383–384
Home contraction monitoring systems, effectiveness, 29

Home monitoring, 491–492
effectiveness, 491–492
follow-up care, 492
indications, 492
technology, 492
Home nursing agency, selection, 390–392
Home oxygen teaching, 392
Home process, discharge/transition (parental needs/role), 386–387
Home safety topics, 379
Home team, interdisciplinary discharge planning/transition, 384b
Home transition, 387–392
multidisciplinary approach, 387
plan, family members (active participants), 387
Homologous chromosomes, definition, 400
Hormonal mechanisms, 157
Hormonal regulatory mechanisms, 184
Hormonal therapy, 176
Hormones, 638
Hospital ethics committee, consultation, 864
Hospitalization, cost (increase), 43
Hospitalized children, ADEs, 374
Hospitalized infants, phototherapy guidelines, 449f
Howell-Jolly bodies, 691
HPA. *See* Human platelet antigen; Hypothalamic-pituitary-thyroid
HSV. *See* Herpes simplex virus
H-type TEF, 600
Human brain. *See* Brain
Human chorionic gonadotropin (hCG), 403
Human factor engineering, 366–368
Human Genome Project, 406–407
definition, 406–407
ethical/legal/social issues program, 407
goals, 406–407
Human immunodeficiency virus (HIV), 717–719
breastfeeding, impact, 65
breastfeeding risks, 194
diagnosis, 717–718
management, 718–719
perinatal prophylaxis, 718
presentation, 717
prevention, 718–719
testing, consideration, 58
transmission, 717
Human milk
benefits, 198
collection/storage/handling, 198
commercial infant formulas, comparison, 194–195
consumption, contraindications, 194–195
formulas, 194–199
fortifiers, 198

Human milk (*Continued*)
host resistance factors/antimicrobial properties, 194–195
term infant usage, 195
Human platelet antigen (HPA), test, 683
Human retina, avascular characteristic, 792
Human skin. *See* Skin
Human T-cell lymphotropic virus, 194
Humidification, requirement, 116–117
Humidified oxygen, delivery, 499
Humoral immunity, 696–698
development, 696f
Hyaline membrane disease, 522
radiographic evaluation, 275
reticulogranular lung pattern/air bronchograms, 275f
surfactant
postadministration appearance, 276f
preadministration appearance, 276f
white-out appearance, 275f
Hyaluronidase (Vitrase)
indication/usage, 310
subcutaneous injection, 176
Hybrid incubator, usage (consideration), 116
Hydralazine (Apresoline), usage, 25
Hydramnios, 26
Hydration status, laboratory evaluation, 158
Hydrocephalus, 756–758. *See also* Congenital hydrocephalus
definition, 756
diagnostic evaluation, 757
illustration, 756f
pathophysiology, 756
patient care management, 757
Hydrochlorothiazide, spironolactone (combination), 515
Hydrogen (H_2) antagonists, 622
Hydronephrosis, 736–738
clinical assessment, 737
clinical presentation, 737
complications, 737–738
definition, 736
diagnostic studies, 737
differential diagnosis, 737
etiology, 736
incidence, 737
outcome, 738
patient care management, 738
physical examination, 737
Hydrophilic surfactant proteins A/D (SP-A) (SP-D), 454
Hydrophobic surfactant proteins B/C (SP-B) (SP-C), 454
Hydrops, 633–635. *See also* Immune hydrops; Nonimmune hydrops
care, 635

Hydrops (*Continued*)
conditions, 634
definition, 633
diagnosis, 634–635
etiology, 633–634
incidence, 634
postnatal care, 635
postnatal diagnosis, 634–635
prenatal care, 635
prenatal diagnosis, 634
Hydrops fetalis, 104, 161
Hydrostatic pressure, increase, 160, 837
Hyperbilirubinemia, 26, 625–630, 847. *See also* Conjugated hyperbilirubinemia; Late preterm neonate; Pathologic unconjugated hyperbilirubinemia
clinical feature, 193
conditions, 629
definitions, 625–627
diagnosis, 630
ELBW treatment, 441
etiology, 627–629
exchange transfusion, 631–632
incidence, 629
management, 630–632
ranking, 631t
nonpathologic characteristic, 627–629
Hypercalcemia, 167
causes/precipitating factors, 167
clinical presentation/assessment, 167
complications, 167
pathophysiology, 167
patient care management, 167
subcutaneous fat necrosis, association, 820
Hypercalciuria, 193
Hypercapnia. *See* Permissive hypercapnia
sense, 486
Hypercarbia. *See* Permissive hypercarbia
Hypercoagulable state, 5
Hyperexpanded lungs, definition, 270
Hyperglycemia, 178–179
aggravation, 176
clinical presentation/assessment, 179
complications, 179
correction, 180
definition, 178
diagnostic studies, 179
etiologies/precipitating factors, 178
incidence, 178
outcome, 179
pathophysiology, 178
patient care management, 179
Hyperinflation, avoidance, 300
Hyperinnervation, causes, 335
Hyperinsulinemia, 6

Hyperinsulinism, suspicion, 159
Hyperkalemia, 164–165
causes/precipitating factors, 164
clinical presentation/assessment, 164
complications, 164–165
pathophysiology, 164
patient care management, 164
Hyperlucent lung fields, appearance, 285f
Hypermagnesemia, 168
causes/precipitating factors, 168
clinical presentation/assessment, 168
complications, 168
pathophysiology, 168
patient care management, 168
signs, 25–26
Hypernatremia, 163
causes/precipitating factors, 163
clinical presentation/assessment, 163
complications, 163
impact, 440
incidence, decrease, 157
pathophysiology, 163
patient care management, 163
Hypernatremic hyperosmolar dehydration, fluid management, 160
Hyperosmolar hypernatremic dehydration, occurrence, 159
Hyperoxia test, 465
Hyperoxygen test, 551
Hyperpigmented macules (mongolian spots), 821
photograph, 821f
Hypertension, 731–733
clinical assessment, 732–733
clinical presentation, 732
cocaine, impact, 46
complications, 530, 733
diagnostic studies, 733
disease states, 731–732
etiology, 731
incidence, 731
management, 733
outcome, 733
Hypertensive disorders, 121
impact, 122
Hyperthermia
cocaine, impact, 46
dislodged temperature probe, impact, 111
impact, 464
infant risk, 111
prevention, 97–98
Hyperthyroidism, 647–649
clinical presentation/assessment, 648
complications, 648
diagnostic studies, 648
etiologies, 647
outcome, 649
patient care management, 648
Hypertonic uterine contractions, 24

Hyperviscosity, 26–27
impact, 464
Hypnotics, 52–53, 246–247
breastfeeding impact, 65
pharmacology, 52
pregnancy effects, 53
use, incidence, 52
Hypocalcemia, 26–27, 165–166. *See also* Late hypocalcemia
causes/precipitating factors, 165–166
clinical presentation/assessment, 166
complications, 166
impact, 177
pathophysiology, 165
patient care management, 166
problem, 581
Hypoexpanded lungs, definition, 270
Hypoglycemia, 27, 86, 173–176
clinical presentation/assessment, 175
clinical signs, 175
complications, 176
definition, 173
diagnostic studies, 175
etiologies/precipitating factors, 174–175
glucose, IV administration, 88
impact, 464
incidence, 173
infant risk, identification, 130–132
metabolic rate, impact, 131
occurrence, 177
outcome, 176
pathophysiology, 174
patient care management, 175–176
persistence, 176
prevention, 175
problem, 581
prolongation, 174
Hypoglycemic reactions, 26
Hypokalemia, 163–164
clinical presentation/assessment, 164
complications, 164
pathophysiology, 163
patient care management, 164
problem, 581
Hypomagnesemia, 26–27, 168
causes/precipitating factors, 168
clinical presentation/assessment, 168
complications, 168
impact, 177
pathophysiology, 168
patient care management, 168
Hyponatremia, 162
causes/precipitating factors, 162
clinical presentation/assessment, 162
complications, 162
impact, 440
pathophysiology, 162
patient care management, 162

Hypopituitarism, 640–641, 650
  clinical signs/symptoms, 641
  diagnosis, 641
  management, 641
  types, 640
Hypoplastic left heart syndrome,
      286–287, 571–573
  anatomy, 571
  cardiac transplantation, 573
  clinical manifestations, 572
  hemodynamics, 571
  illustration, 572f
  incidence, 571
  management, 572–573
  prenatal diagnosis, 572
  prognosis, 573
  staged surgical report, 572–573
Hypospadias, 657, 741–742
  clinical assessment, 741
  clinical presentation, 741
  complications, 742
  definition, 741
  etiology, 741
  incidence, 741
  outcome, 742
  patient care management, 742
  photograph, 741f
  physical examination, 741–742
  risk, increase, 43
Hypotension, regional anesthetics,
      37–38
Hypothalamic-pituitary-thyroid
      (HPA) axis, 642, 649
Hypothermia. See Very low birth
      weight
  impact, 464
  importance, 114–118
  infant risk, 111
  prevention, 97–98, 597
  rewarming, impact, 118
Hypothyroidism, 140, 643–647
  confirmation, 647
  consideration, 643
  diagnostic studies, 644–645
  newborn screening, 644–645
  outcome, 647
  patient care management, 645–647
Hypovolemia, 159
  acute blood loss, emergency
      treatment, 677
  prevention, 597
Hypovolemic shock, 30, 582
Hypoxemia
  avoidance, 581
  sense, 486
Hypoxia, 25
  apnea cause, 487
  complication, 306
  history, 465
  impact, 464
  premature infant, biphasic
      response, 486
Hypoxic-ischemic damage, 84
Hypoxic-ischemic encephalopathy
      (HIE), 774–778
  clinical presentation, 775–776
  definition, 774

Hypoxic-ischemic encephalopathy
      (HIE) (Continued)
  diagnosis, 774
  diagnostic studies, 776
  evolution, tracking, 776
  incidence, 774
  outcome, 777–778
  patient care management, 776–777
  staging, 775–776

I

IASP. See International Association
      for the Study of Pain
IAT. See Indirect antiglobulin test
Iatrogenic anemia, 262
Iatrogenic hyperthermia,
      avoidance, 107
Iatrogenic loss, 671
Iatrogenic NAS, 58
iCa. See Free ionized calcium
ICF. See Intracellular fluid
Ichthyosis, 828–829
  treatment, 829
ICP. See Intracranial pressure
Icterus, 626
Idiopathic apnea, 485
IDM. See Infant of diabetic mother
IgA. See Immunoglobulin A
IgG. See Immunoglobulin G
IgM. See Immunoglobulin M
IH. See Immune hydrops
Ileal atresia, 604–605
  definition, 604
  diagnosis, 605
  etiology, 605
  incidence, 605
  postoperative care, 605
  preoperative care, 605
  prognosis, 605
  surgical repair, 605
ILGF, stimulation, 841
Illicit drug abuse, 195
Illicit drug use
  ranking, 41
  urine drug screen, 63t
  women, percentage, 41–42
Illness severity, invasive procedure
      frequency (inverse
      relationship), 333
Immature central respiratory
      center, 485
Immature skin, permeability, 815
Immature/total (I/T) neutrophil
      ratio, 702
  calculation, 690f
  representation, 703f
Immune hydrops (IH), 633
Immune system, 695–698
  antibiotic therapy, 705
  clinical assessment, 699–701
  development. See Fetus
  diagnosis/therapy, 699–706
  diagnostic evaluation, 704–705
  host defense mechanisms, 695–696
  microchemical environment,
      dependence, 696
  therapy, 705–706

Immunizations, 18, 249–250
  CDC Advisory Committee on
      Immunization Practices
      guidelines, 249
  neonatal population,
      considerations, 250
  types, 249
  usage. See Extremely low birth
      weight infants
  use, principles, 249
Immunoassays, 255
Immunoglobulin, 696
  types, 696–697
Immunoglobulin A (IgA), 697
Immunoglobulin G (IgG), 696–697
Immunoglobulin M (IgM), 697
Immunology tests, 255
Immunotherapy, 705–706
Imperforate anus (anorectal
      agenesis), 26–27, 611–612
  definition, 611
  diagnosis, 611
  etiology, 611
  illustration, 612f
  incidence, 611
  postoperative care, 612
  preoperative care, 612
  prognosis, 611
  surgical repair, 612
Implementation, nursing process
      step, 866
Inactivated calcium, 165
Inadvertent PEEP, 495
Inborn errors of amino acid
      metabolism, 808–809
Inborn errors of metabolism (IEM),
      196–197, 807
  clinical presentation, 807
  diagnosis, 807
  incidence/etiology, 807
  treatment, goals, 807
Incubator covers
  illustration, 117f
  usage, 116
Incubators, usage, 160
Incus, recognition, 846
Indirect antiglobulin test (IAT), 255
Individualized developmental care,
      212
Individual liability policy, 879
  institutional liability policy,
      coverage differences, 879
Individual malpractice policy,
      benefits, 878
Individual rights, liberal
      individualism (impact), 862–
      863
Indomethacin (Indocin)
  management, 555–556
  rectal/oral administration, 29
Indwelling catheter, requirement
      (absence), 577
Indwelling lines/tubes, 294–296
Infancy, physiologic anemia, 672
Infant Behavior Record, 48
Infant Development, Bayley Scales
      (Infant Behavior Record), 48

Infant-driven feedings, 227
  readiness scales, 227
Infant of diabetic mother (IDM),
    131, 177–178, 662
  clinical presentation/assessment,
    177
  incidence, 177
  pathophysiology, 177
  problems, anticipation, 178
Infants
  abilities/sensitivities/thresholds,
    responsiveness, 209
  admission procedures,
    completion, 89
  altered fluid requirements, 197
  anthropometric measurements,
    204
  anticipatory guidance, 393
  assessment, 223–224
  autopsy, parental discussion, 356
  baptism, option, 356
  biliary atresia, 618
    postoperative care, 618
    preoperative care, 618
    surgical procedures, 618
  birth, crisis. See Premature infant;
    Sick infant
  body, parental disposition, 356
  BPD, caloric requirements, 197
  calorie intake requirements, 197
  cardiac problems, 197
  care
    experience, impact, 386–387
    postdischarge, 395–397
    practices, education, 392
    specifics, 389–390
  CDH, 625
    prenatal treatment, 625
    preoperative care, 625
    surgical procedures, 625
  cholestasis
    enteral feeding management,
      620
    management, 620
    medications, 620
    TPN management, 620
  clinical examination, change,
    263–264
  condition, parent perception, 352
  cryotherapy, 844
  death
    parental understanding, 356
    sibling information, 356
  definition, 91
  development
    barriers, 208–209
    synactive theory, 210t–211t
  discharge
    criteria, establishment, 385–386
    timing, 385
  dislocated hips, Pavlik harness,
    802f
  endurance, 224
  environmental temperature, 79
  extremities, anatomical
    irregularities, 311
  facial appearance, 131

Infants (Continued)
  families
    assistance. See Dying infants
    impact, 386
    visit, nurse (assignation), 357
  feedings
    contraindications, 81
    demand, 80–81
    evaluation, 81
    position, 203
  first bath, 78
  first feeding, 80–81
  formula/feeding teaching, 392
  GER
    conservative measures, 621–622
    management, 621–622
    pharmacologic measures, 622
    surgical measures, 622
  glucose needs, 80–81
  gonococcal conjunctivitis, 835
  growth
    charts, 204–205
    nutritional assessment/
      standards, 203–205
  heel stick, performing, 321f
  home arrival, preparation, 348
  homeothermic characteristic, 111
  hydrops, 635
    postnatal care, 635
    prenatal care, 635
  hyperbilirubinemia, 630–633
    exchange transfusion, 631–632
    management, 630–632
  hyperthermia risk, 111
  hypothermia risk, 111
  inborn errors of metabolism
    (IEM), usage, 196–197
  in-home care, 395–396
  interaction, resumption, 348
  intermittent home visits, 395–396
  karyotype 46,XY/ambiguous
    genitalia, 659f
  laser photocoagulation, 843
  Level II/III setting, transfer, 89
  loss, preparation, 348
  memorial/funeral service, 356
  mother, attendance, 89
  NEC, 614–615
    medical management, 614
    postoperative care, 615
    surgical management, 614–615
    surgical repair, 615
  nutritional requirements, 196–198
  nutritional support, goals, 196
  opioid doses, 345
  oral feeding
    fatigue, intervention, 222
    transition, nurse preparation,
      221
  organized sleep, development,
    211–212
  pain, nursing care, 340–344
  parental holding/cuddling,
    assistance, 358
  parent bond, 220
  parent understanding,
    assessment, 352

Infants (Continued)
  perinatal substance abuse
    interventions, 59
  physiologic assessment, 223
  PN, receiving (monitoring
    schedule), 193t
  positioning, 215–218
  positive attitude, conveyance,
    358
  prenatal drug exposure, caring
    strategies, 59t–62t
  privacy/comfort, 226
  prune belly syndrome
    management, 623–624
    medical management, 623–624
    surgical procedures, 624
  readiness, assessment, 203
  recognition. See Sick newborn
    infant
  recovery, 264
  retained fetal lung fluid risk,
    462–463
  risk, 351–352
    identification, 130–132
  sensory capabilities, discussion,
    89
  short bowel syndrome, 616–617
    medical management, 616
    surgical management, 616–617
  siblings, parents (maintenance),
    353
  stable condition, family member
    visits, 89
  stroking, 213
  suck-swallow-breathe
    coordination, demonstration,
    202
  temperature, 78
    physiologic response, 111
  thermal instability, risk
    (identification), 110–111
  thrombocytopenia, management,
    683–684
  transfer, 89
  transition, parent teaching, 89
  transport, family notification
    system (establishment), 429
  vascular access sites, assessment,
    820
  Vitamin K_1 (phytonadione),
    administration, 79
Infection
  airborne transmission, 721
  apnea cause, 487
  contact transmission, 721
  control, 107, 720–722
    practices, 720–722
  droplet transmission, 721
  hematologic evidence, 703–704
  pathogens, impact, 708–720
  risks, 122
  screening, 108
Infectious lesions, 826–827
Infectious organisms
  horizontal transmission, 699
  transmission, 698–699
  vertical transmission, 698–699

Inferential statistics, 853
Inferior vena cava (IVC), blood flow, 72
Infertility, history, 120
Infiltration, treatment, 309–310
Inflammation stages, mediators (association), 699f
Informed consent, 877–878. *See also* Transfusion therapies
  capacity, 877
  defining, 877
  elements, 858b
Infusion pumps, usage. *See* Smart infusion pumps
Inguinal hernia, risk (increase), 43
Inhalants, 53
  fetus/neonate effects, 53
  pharmacology, 53
  pregnancy effects, 53
Inhalation, medication administration, 237–238
Inhaled nitric oxide (iNO). *See* Very low birth weight
  usage, 467, 516
Inherited bleeding disorders, 685–686
  clinical assessment, 686
  clinical presentation, 686
  diagnostic studies, 686
  etiologic factors, 685–686
  outcome, 686
  patient care management, 686
Inhibin A, 403
In-home care, 395–396
Initial antepartum visit, 6–7
Initial communication, caregiver (presence), 373
In-line suction devices, 503
Inner ear, 846
Innervation, 834, 846
Inotropic agents, 245
  usage, 583
Insensible water loss (IWL), 92
  decrease, 157
  environmental influences, 157b
  factors, 157–158
  reductions, 160
Inspiration, work, 77
Inspiratory/expiratory (I/E) ratio, 504–505
Inspiratory film, definition, 271
Institutional liability policy, 879
  individual liability policy, coverage differences, 879
Insulin
  administration, 162
  peripheral resistance, 6
  pump therapy, 27
  secretion, 173
Insurance. *See* Professional liability insurance
  policies, types, 879
Intake measurements, usage, 251
Intensive care environment, infant adaptation, 348
Interdisciplinary discharge planning/transition, 384b

Interfacility neonatal transport, 417–418
  back/return transport, 418
  documentation, 427–428
  ethical considerations/issues, 430–431
  historical aspects, 415–416
  legal considerations/issues, 430–431
  preaccident planning, 429
  quality indicators, 431
  safety, 428–429
  three-way transport, 418
  total quality management, 431–432
  two-way transport, 417–418
  types, 417–418
  uniforms, usage, 428
Interferon-α-2b, effectiveness, 825
Interlobar fissure, definition, 271
Intermittent care conferences, 387
Intermittent home visits, 395–396
Intermittent mandatory ventilation, 501
  rate, 504
Internal acoustic meatus, 846
Internal anatomic structures, evaluation, 296
Internal diameter (ID), measurement, 302
Internal genitalia, differentiation, 655
Internal organ manifestations, 701
Internal review board (IRB), 858
International Association for the Study of Pain (IASP), pain definition, 333
International Evidence-Based Group for Neonatal Pain, neonatal procedural pain prevention/treatment guidelines, 334
International Liaison Committee on Resuscitation (ILCOR), 94
International transport, 430
Interstitial fluids, lymphatic drainage, 160
Intervention strategies, 212
Interviews, 854
Intervillous spaces, maternal blood flow (decrease), 24
Intestinal ischemia, 612
Intestinal obstruction, causes, 599t
Intestines, physiologic sounds, 78
Intracellular fluid (ICF), distribution, 156
Intracerebellar hemorrhage, 767–768
  clinical presentation, 768
  definition, 767
  diagnostic evaluation, 768
  incidence, 768
  outcome, 768
  pathophysiology, 767–768
  risk factors, 767
Intracerebral meningitis, 771–772
Intracranial bleeding, 27

Intracranial hemorrhages, 107, 766–771
Intracranial pressure (ICP), increase, 300
Intrafacility neonatal transport, 416–417
  communication, 417
  documentation, 427–428
  equipment, 417
  ethical considerations/issues, 430–431
  historical aspects, 415–416
  legal considerations/issues, 430–431
  preaccident planning, 429
  preparation, 416
  quality indicators, 431
  safety, 417, 428–429
  staffing, 416–417
  total quality management, 431–432
  uniforms, usage, 428
Intrahepatic bile duct, 619
Intrahepatic biliary atresia, 617
Intramuscular medication administration, 238
Intrapartum care, terminology, 1
Intrapartum labor management, 11–17
  admission, 11–17
  physical examination, 11–17
  prenatal records, review, 11
Intrapartum period, conditions, 28–35
Intrapulmonary shunt, 497
Intrauterine asphyxia, 464
Intrauterine GI perforation, results, 292
Intrauterine growth, estimate (growth curves), 129f
Intrauterine growth restriction (IUGR), 25
  appearance, 180
  factors, 121–122
Intrauterine hypoxia, 684
Intrauterine infection, 460
  impact, 847
Intrauterine life, adaptation, 94
Intravascular clotting, balance, 671
Intravascular flush solutions, 722
Intravascular volume, restoration, 180
Intravenous extravasations, 820–821
  occurrence, 820–821
Intravenous immune globulin (IVIG), 705
Intravenous (IV) fluids, vascular access, 314
Intravenous (IV) infusion, medication errors, 369
Intravenous (IV) medication administration, 238–239
Intraventricular hemorrhage (IVH), extent (quantification), 769f
Invasive monitoring, 577–578
Invasive screening, 9

Inversion, definition, 402
Iowa Model, 857f
Irises, 833
    characteristics, 834
    vessel engorgement, 841
Iron requirements, increase, 5
Isolated esophageal atresia, 600
Isopropyl nitrite (rush/locker
        room), 53
Isoproterenol (Isuprel), usage, 583
I/T. *See* Immature/total
IUGR. *See* Intrauterine growth
        restriction
IV glucose infusion, indications,
        81
IVH. *See* Intraventricular
        hemorrhage
IVIG. *See* Intravenous immune
        globulin
IWL. *See* Insensible water loss

J

Jatene procedure, 568
Jaundice, 134, 626. *See also*
        Breastfeeding; Breast milk
    clinical features, 193
Jejunal atresia, 604–605
    definition, 604
    diagnosis, 605
    etiology, 605
    incidence, 605
    postoperative care, 605
    preoperative care, 605
    prognosis, 605
    surgical repair, 605
    types, 604f
Jet injector, usage, 507
Jet ventilation, efficiency, 509
Joanna Briggs Institute (JBI), 371
    resources, 212
Joint articulation, 215
Joint Commission, The, 365t, 867
Joint compression, NICU
        production, 215
Judgment mistake, malpractice
        consideration, 869
Just culture, 363
Justice, 856
    ethics principle, 861–862
        focus, 861–862
        questions, 861–862
Juvenile insulin-dependent
        diabetes, development, 178

K

Kangaroo care (KC), 213–214, 220
    benefits, 213–214
    encouragement, 115
Kantianism (deontology), 862
Kartagener syndrome, 542
Karyotype
    analysis, 406
    definition, 400
Karyotype 46,XY/ambiguous
        genitalia, 659f
Kasabach-Merritt phenomenon,
        825–826

*Keeping Patients Safe—Transforming
        the Work Environment of
        Nurses* (IOM), 366–367
Keratinization, problem, 157
Kernicterus, 626–627
Ketoacidosis, 27
Ketosis, 179
Kidneys
    development, sequential stages,
        724–725
    medication excretion, 242–243
    palpation, 146
    regulation, 169
Kleihauer-Betke test, 255
Klinefelter syndrome, 793–794
    associated findings, 793
    clinical presentation, 793
    diagnosis, 793
    incidence/etiology, 793
    treatment, 793–794
Klippel-Trenaunay-Weber
        syndrome, 826
Klumpke paralysis, 764
Knowledge. *See* Nursing
    generation, research support,
        854

L

Labetalol hydrochloride, usage, 25
Labor, 75
    admission, assessments, 33
    history, 122–123
    induction, 27
Laboratory assessment, 203–204
Laboratory collection
    process, 255–258
    types, 255–257
Laboratory contact, specimen
        verification, 267
Laboratory data interpretation,
        importance, 264–268
Laboratory interpretation
    decision tree, 264–268
    normalcy, 267b
    reliability/believability, 265b
    test follow-up, 268b
Laboratory result, reference range
        (appropriateness), 267
Laboratory sample
    handling, correctness, 265
    problem, 264
    source, inappropriateness, 266
Laboratory sampling, needle
        puncture, 261
Laboratory specimens
    collection, 255–258
    drawing, timing, 266
    sampling, patient care practice
        (review), 267
    site condition, importance, 266
    tubes, 257–258
    verification, 267
Laboratory testing
    anemia, impact, 262
    cost factor, 262
    false diagnosis, impact, 262
    goal, 260–262

Laboratory testing (*Continued*)
    iatrogenic sequelae, preventive
        strategies, 260–262
    infection, impact, 261
    organ/nerve injury, impact, 261–
        262
    pain, impact, 260–261
    physiologic stress, impact, 260
    purpose, 255
    skin injury, impact, 261
    U.S. national health budget,
        portion, 252
Laboratory tests
    abnormalities, significance, 259
    accuracy, 258
    artifacts, impact, 259
    benefit/risk, 264
    blood volume requirement, 264
    clerical errors, 259
    drugs, impact, 259
    follow-up, 268
    interpretation, concepts, 258
    medical history, usefulness, 263
    obtaining, questions, 262–264
        list, 263b
    ordering, quality, 264
    patient requirement, 263
    precision, 258
    reference ranges, 258
        variation, 259
    repetition
        consideration, 266–267
        waste, 259
    result
        abnormality, 268
        impact, 263
        normalcy, 267–268
        reliability, 265–267
    sensitivity, 258
    so what question, answering, 263
    specificity, 258
    timing
        appropriateness, 264
        issue, 265
    usage, judiciousness, 262–264
    utilization, principles, 259
Laboratory work (labwork),
        obtaining (timing), 264
Lacrimal apparatus, 836
Lacrimal system, 832
Lactase activity, appearance, 183
Lactic acid, elevation, 174
Lactiferous ducts, development, 4–
        5
Lamellar body (LB) counts,
        surfactant (storage form), 11
Lamellar ichthyosis, 829
Lanugo, 126, 135
Large-for-gestational-age (LGA)
        infant, 122, 177
    hypoglycemia, incidence, 173
    identification, 131–132
Laryngeal mask airway, 100
Laryngeal tissues, trauma/edema,
        306
Laryngoscope blade, usage, 302
Laryngoscope bulb, ingestion, 307

Laryngoscope hand position, 305f
Larynx, obstruction, 479
Laser photocoagulation, 843
  nursing care, 843
Last menstrual period (LMP), 7–8
Late charting, problems, 876
Late HDN, 79
Late hypocalcemia, 166
Late metabolic acidosis, 169
Late-onset infection, GBS (impact),
  709–710
Late-onset invasive group B
  streptococcal disease,
  incidence, 709f
Late preterm neonate
  breastfeeding management, 450
  definition, 447
  development, 451
    anatomy/physiology, 451
    clinical management, 451
  discharge criteria, 451
  drug toxicity, 451
    anatomy/physiology, 451
    clinical management, 451
  hospitalized infants,
    phototherapy guidelines,
    449f
  hyperbilirubinemia, 448
    anatomy/physiology, 448
    clinical management, 448
    risk factors, 448
  hypoglycemia/feeding
    anatomy/physiology, 449–451
    challenges, 449–451
    clinical problems, 450
    considerations, 450
  immature neurobehavioral
    development, 450
  infection, 448
    anatomy/physiology, 448
    clinical management, 448
  long-term outcome, 452
  nonsupportive feeding
    interventions, 451
  parent education, 451–452
  respiratory issues, 448
    anatomy/physiology, 448
    clinical management, 448
    conditions, 448
    risk factors, 448
  risk designation, nomogram, 449f
  thermoregulation, 447
    anatomy/physiology, 447
    clinical management, 447
    risk factors, 447
Lateral ventricles, 751
Lavender tube (laboratory
  specimen tube), 258
Lecithin concentration, 454
Lecithin/sphingomyelin (L/S)
  ratio, 10
  determination, 27
Left atrium blood, 74
Left clavicle, fracture, 293f
Left diaphragmatic hernia, 282f
Left-sided cardiac pressures, left
  atrial line monitoring, 578

Left-sided obstruction, 286–287
Left tension pneumothorax, 279f
Left ventricular blood, 74
Legal issues, professional literature,
  868
Length conversion, 883
Lens, characteristics, 834
LES. See Lower esophageal
  sphincter
Lesions, 827–830. See also Acyanotic
  lesions; Obstructive lesions
  admixture, 85
  pulmonary vascularity
    decrease, 287
    increase, 285–287
  trauma, impact, 820–821
Leukocoria, 837
LGA. See Large-for-gestational-age
Liability, 869–873. See also
  Negligence
  costs, 870
  insurance. See Professional
    liability insurance
  policy differences, 879
  quality assurance activities,
    controversy, 871
  risk management, controversy,
    871
  theories, pursuit, 870–871
Liberal individualism, 862–863
Licensure, loss (risk), 865
Lidocaine, usage, 344
Life Port endotracheal tube
  adapter, 509f
Limb/digit amputation, 150
Linen disposal, 721
Lingual lipases, presence, 183
Lipids
  emulsification, 183
  infusion, 178
  postnatal caloric intake, 185
  stores, 184–185
Liposomoal lidocaine cream (LMX),
  usage, 344
Lithium, usage, 543
Live births, premature percentages,
  415
Liver
  medication
    excretion, 242
    metabolism, 241
  upward displacement, 2
Liver function tests, 25
Live vaccines, usage, 249
Lobular alveolar tissue,
  development, 4–5
Locality rule, obsolescence, 866–
  867
Locus, definition, 400
Logistical documentation, 427
Long-term glucose monitoring,
  enabling, 159
Long-term morbidity, 131
Lorazepam, usage, 774
Loss. See Parents
  assessment, 355
  definitions, 355

Low birth weight infant
  caloric requirements, estimation,
    189t
  hyperbilirubinemia,
    management, 631t
  serial hemoglobin values, 677t
Low cardiac output
  bleeding, 581
  blood pressure, monitoring,
    581
  color, 579
  extremities, 579–580
  management, 580–581
  metabolic derangement, 580
  observation, 579
  oliguria, 580
  pharmaceutical agents,
    consideration, 580–581
  rate/rhythm disturbance,
    treatment, 580
  recognition, 579–580
  right ventricular afterload,
    reduction, 580
  sedation, providing, 581
  severity, factors, 579
  tachycardia, 580
  volume challenge, 580
  volume replacement, blood
    (usage), 580
  weight gain, 580
  x-ray findings, 580
Low-dose dopamine therapy, 164
Lower esophageal sphincter (LES),
  relaxation, 183
Lower-extremity pulses, 549
Lower GI series, 593
Lower leg, amniotic band
  constriction, 805f
Low-risk patient, management, 17
L/S. See Lecithin/sphingomyelin
Lubchenco data, limitations, 128–
  129
Lumbar puncture, 83, 256
  advanced practice procedure,
    328–331
  anxiety/pain management,
    providing, 329
  complications, 330–331
  contraindications, 328
  equipment/supplies, 328
  indications, 328
  positioning/landmarks, 329f
  precautions, 328
  pressure measurement reading,
    obtaining, 330
  procedure, 328–330
Lung development, 453–455
  alveolar period, 454
  anatomic events, 453–454
  antenatal steroids, role, 455
  biochemical events, 454–455
  canalicular period, 453
  embryonic development, 453
  pseudoglandular period, 453
  terminal sac period, 453–454
Lung fluid, delayed clearance,
  463

Lungs
  aeration, 75
  air entry, 75–77
  compliance, 495
  compression, 104
  disease. *See* Wet lung disease
  expansion, 77
  fields
    homogeneous pattern, 275
    x-ray anatomic/pathologic
      changes, 273
  fluid retention, 84
  fluid secretion, 74
  gas exchange, 75
  medication excretion, 241–242
  recovery, 531
  regulation, 169
  resistance, 495
  tissue (damage), sodium
    bicarbonate (impact), 102
Lymphocytes, 669

M
Macrocytosis, 691
Macroglossia, 132
Macrosomia, 131, 177
Macrostomia, 140
Macula, 833
  traction, impact, 841
Macule, 817. *See also* Ash leaf
    macules
  eruption. *See* Purpuric macules
Magnesium (Mg), 167–168
  concurrent use, 168
  functions, 167
  homeostasis, 167–168. *See also*
    Fetal magnesium
    homeostasis; Neonatal
    magnesium homeostasis
Magnesium sulfate, IV
    administration, 29
Magnetic resonance imaging (MRI)
  diagnostic imaging, 297
  nurses, role, 297
  usage, 552
Maintenance laboratory
    surveillance, implementation
    plan (consideration), 268
Male bladder catheterization, 325f
Male catheterization, 325
Male external genitalia,
    development/differentiation,
    656f
Male neonates, hypovirilization,
    658
Malformation
  definition, 409, 783b
  disorders, 794–795
Malleus, recognition, 846
Malposition, types, 285
Malpractice, 869
  elements, proof elements
    (necessity), 869
  insurance, obtaining (reasons),
    878–879
  policy, benefits. *See* Individual
    malpractice policy

Malpractice *(Continued)*
  professional misconduct, 869
  suits, risk, 865
  term, meaning, 869
Malrotation, 605–606
  definition, 605
  diagnosis, 606
  etiology, 605
  incidence, 606
  postoperative care, 606
  preoperative care, 606
  prognosis, 606
  surgical repair, 606
Mammary glands, medication
    excretion, 241
MAOIs. *See* Monoamine oxidase
    inhibitors
MAP. *See* Mean airway pressure;
    Mean arterial pressure
Maple sugar urine disease (MSUD),
    808–809
  clinical findings, 809
  diagnosis, 809
  incidence/etiology, 808–809
  treatment, 809
Maple syrup urine disease, 197
Marginal placenta previa, bleeding
    (management), 32
Marijuana, 49–50
  breastfeeding impact, 65
  fetus/neonate effects, 50
  pharmacology, 49–50
  pregnancy effects, 50
  usage, incidence, 49
MAS. *See* Meconium aspiration
    syndrome
Mask CPAP, 499–500
Mask of pregnancy, 3
Massage, benefits, 214
Mass conversion, 884
Maternal assessment, continuation,
    25
Maternal cardiac output, 23
Maternal cardiac output, decrease,
    23
Maternal complications, 24–25,
    178
Maternal Cushing syndrome, 650
Maternal diabetes, 121
Maternal disease
  classification, 544b
  impact, 543–544
Maternal drugs, withdrawal, 772
Maternal drug use
  care, continuity, 66–67
  documentation, 58
  follow-up, 66–67
  gender-specific treatment needs,
    67
  nursing considerations, 67
  problems, 65–67
  treatment/rehabilitation/
    recovery, 67
Maternal-fetal ABO
    incompatibilities, 675t
Maternal-fetal transfusion, 670
Maternal fever, 133

Maternal Graves disease, 647
  effects, 647
  treatment, effects, 648
Maternal HBsAg-negative
    treatment recommendations,
    80
Maternal HbsAg-positive treatment
    recommendations, 79
Maternal health problems, 351
Maternal heart rate, increase, 4
Maternal history, 545
  cardiovascular clinical signs, 701
  clinical manifestations, 700–701
  gastrointestinal clinical signs, 701
  internal organ manifestations,
    701
  metabolic disturbances, 701
  neurologic clinical signs, 700
  respiratory clinical signs, 700–701
  risk factors, identification, 699–
    700
  skin, signs, 701
  thermoregulatory instability, 700
Maternal illnesses, 82
Maternal-infant relationships, 65–
    66
Maternal infections, 11
  protozoan, impact, 792
Maternal Lifestyle Study, 46
Maternal medical history, 120
Maternal medications, adverse
    effects, 86
Maternal oxygen requirements,
    increase, 2
Maternal parenting outcomes
    evaluation, 354
  predictors, 354
Maternal physical stress, 24
Maternal physiologic changes, 1–6
Maternal-placental-fetal complex,
    status, 25
Maternal placental perfusion,
    cessation, 75
Maternal serum alpha-fetoprotein
    (MSAFP) testing, 27
Maternal serum screening, 121
Maternal vasoconstriction, impact,
    23
Maternal vasodilatation, impact, 23
Maternal vital signs, monitoring, 31
Maturational hypotonia, 215
Mature human milk, composition,
    195t
Mature milk, establishment, 18
Maturity
  classification, 127–132
  measurement, 127
  obtaining, 127
Maxilla, jaw (relationship), 141
MBC. *See* Minimal bactericidal
    concentration
MBD. *See* Metabolic bone disease
McCune-Albright syndrome, 647
MCH. *See* Mean corpuscular
    hemoglobin
MCHC. *See* Mean corpuscular
    hemoglobin concentration

McRoberts maneuver, usage, 34
M-CSF. *See* Monocyte colony-
forming stimulating factor
MCTs. *See* Medium-chain
triglycerides
MCV. *See* Mean corpuscular
volume
MDI. *See* Mental Development
Index
MDMA. *See* 3,4-Methylenedioxy-
methamphetamine
Mean 24-hour urine output,
increase, 4
Mean airway pressure (MAP), 495,
505
governance, 510
Mean arterial pressure (MAP),
persistence, 439
Mean corpuscular hemoglobin
concentration (MCHC), 669
Mean corpuscular hemoglobin
(MCH), 669
Mean corpuscular volume (MCV),
669
Mechanical dead space, definition,
495
Mechanical ventilation, 500–501
initiation, 503–505
parameters, 504–505
requirement, 502–505
usage, 437–438
Mechanoreceptors, 486
Meckel-Gruber syndrome, 590
Meconium
drug screening, 64
presence, 35
Meconium aspiration syndrome
(MAS), 468–470
appearance, 278f
clinical presentation/diagnosis,
469
complications, 469
definition, 468
delivery room management, 469
etiology, 468
incidence, 468
management/prevention, 469–
470
metabolic complication, 469
neurologic complication, 469
outcome, 470
pathophysiology, 468–469
pulmonary complications, 469
radiographic evaluation, 277–278
respiratory care, 469–470
Meconium aspirator, applicability,
303
Meconium ileus, 290, 607–609
definition, 607
diagnosis, 607
etiology, 607
free air, lateral film visibility,
290f
nonsurgical procedure, 607–608
perforation, lateral film visibility,
290f
postoperative care, 608–609

Meconium ileus *(Continued)*
postprocedural care, 608
postprocedural management,
608–609
pre-nonsurgical procedure, 607
prognosis, 607
radiologic studies, 607
surgical repair, 608
types, 607
Meconium peritonitis, radiographic
evaluation, 292
Meconium plug syndrome, 291, 609
definition, 609
diagnosis, 609
etiology, 609
incidence, 609
interventions, 609
pre-nonsurgical procedure, 609
prognosis, 609
Meconium-stained amniotic fluid
(MSAF), 468
Meconium-stained fluid, presence,
98, 100
Mediastinal air collection, 279
Mediastinum, anatomic/pathologic
x-ray changes, 273–274
Medical costs, increase, 384–385
Medical history, information, 6
Medical indications, case analysis
model component, 863
Medical management, change
(consideration), 267
Medical practice, nursing practice
(overlap), 872
Medical record
attorney usage, 874
court importance, 877
documentation, nurse
responsibility, 874
transfer system, establishment,
429
Medical therapy
implementation/adequacy,
absence, 265–266
interference, 266
Medication. *See* High-alert
medications; Off-label
medications
absorption, principles, 236–239
flowchart, 236f
absorption rate, skin thickness
(relationship), 238
absorptive response time,
variation, 238
action, mechanisms, 234–235
administration, 375–376
nursing implications, 250–251
categories, 243–246
chemical change, 241
concentration, alterations, 235
cross-checking, 250
definition, 233
desired effects, undesired effects
(contrast), 235
dispensing, 375
distribution, 239
principles, 239–241

Medication *(Continued)*
doses
checking, 250
clinical response, relationship,
235
dosing, documentation, 251
excretion, principles, 241–243
first-pass effect, 241
hepatic uptake, 241
improvement strategies, 377
intake/output measurements,
usage, 251
interactions, considerations, 267
levels, types, 234
metabolism
maturational changes, 241
principles, 241
movement, 240–241
blood flow, 240
ordering/delivery, stages, 374–
376
phase II metabolism, 241
phase I metabolism, 241
precautions, 251
prescribing, 374
reconciliation, 379
definition, 362b
response
factors, 235
time, 238
sensitivity, 235
serum level monitoring,
facilitation, 251
side effects, 235
solubility, 240–241
subtherapeutic effect, 235
teaching, 392
toxic effects, 235
transcribing, 375
Medication errors, 369, 374–377
identification
methods, addition, 372
reporting methods, 371–372
Medium-chain acetyl-CoA
dehydrogenase deficiency,
809–810
associated findings, 809
clinical findings, 809
diagnosis, 809
incidence/etiology, 809
treatment, 809–810
Medium-chain triglycerides
(MCTs), absorption, 87
ease, 189
Melasma, impact, 3
Membrane lung, development, 521
Membranes, artificial/spontaneous
rupture (assessment), 33
Membranous labyrinth, 846
Mendelian disorders, 783
Meningitis, 779–781
clinical presentation, 779–780
complication, 462
definition, 779
diagnostic evaluation, 780
neonatal infection, 706–707
outcome, 780–781

Meningitis *(Continued)*
  pathophysiology, 779
  patient care management, 780
  risk factors, 779
Menstrual cycle, opiates
    (interference), 51
Menstrual history, information, 8
Mental Development Index (MDI),
    48
Mesocardia, 285
Mesonephros, 724
Metabolic acidosis, 84, 104, 169–170
  causes/precipitating factors, 169
  clinical presentation/assessment,
    169–170
  complications, 170
  measurement, 517
  pathophysiology, 169
  patient care management, 170
  symptom, 179
Metabolic activity, types (division),
    241
Metabolic alkalosis, 163, 170
  causes/precipitating factors, 170
  complications, 170
  measurement, 517
  pathophysiology, 170
  patient care management, 170
Metabolic bone disease (MBD),
    166–167
  causes/precipitating factors,
    166
  clinical presentation/assessment,
    166
  diagnostic tests, 166–167
  pathophysiology, 166
  patient care management/
    prevention, 167
Metabolic changes, maternal
    physiologic changes, 6
Metabolic demands (decrease),
    supportive measures
    (usage), 438
Metabolic derangements, 580
  risk, increase, 192
Metabolic disorders, 837
  apnea cause, 488
  correction, 580
Metabolic disturbances, 582
Metabolic encephalopathies, 771
Metabolism. *See* Inborn errors of
    metabolism
  disorders, 807–811
  inborn errors, 174, 629
  rate, 72
Metabolites, presence, 254
Metanephros, 725
Metatarsus adductus, 150
Methadone
  absorption, 51
  breastfeeding impact, 65
  heroin, comparison, 52
  impact, 51
  obstetric complications, 52b
  synthetic opiate, 51
Methicillin-resistant *Staphylococcus
    aureus* (MRSA), 703

Methylxanthine, usage, 490–491,
    514
MIC. *See* Minimal inhibitory
    concentration
Microbiology tests, 254
Microcephaly, 755–756
  clinical presentation, 755
  definition, 755
  diagnostic evaluation, 755
  outcome, 756
  pathophysiology, 755
  patient care management, 755
  risk factors, 755
Microcytosis, 691
Microdeletions, FISH detection,
    542
Micrognathia, 478
Micropenis, 657
Microphthalmos, 839
Microscopic renal anatomy, 725
Microscopy tests, 254
Microstomia, 140
Microtia, 141
Midazolam (Versed), usage, 303–
    304
Middle cerebral flow velocity,
    increase, 122
Middle ear, 846
  lateral wall, 846
Midgut volvulus, 290–291
Midline catheter (MLC), insertion,
    310–311
MIH. *See* Müllerian-inhibiting
    hormone
Milia, 819
  photograph, 819f
Miliaria, 819–820
  types, 819–820
Miliaria crystallina, 819
Miliaria profunda, 820
Miliaria pustulosa, 820
Miliaria rubra, 820
Miliary tuberculosis, 194
Milk
  consumption, increase, 222
  expression, encouragement,
    198
  flow restriction, oral feeding
    facilitation, 222
  flow volume, 222
  intake, measurement methods,
    226
  secretion, initiation, 18
Milrinone, benefits, 584
Mineral retention, decrease, 194
Minimal bactericidal concentration
    (MBC), 243
Minimal inhibitory concentration
    (MIC), 243
Mirror image dextrocardia, 285
  appearance, 286f
Misidentification, reduction
    (improvement strategies),
    374
Mistaken entry, correction, 876
Mitochondrial disorders, 401
Mitral atresia, 286–287

Mivacurium (Mivacron), usage,
    304
Mixed apnea, 485
  definition, 485
Mixed gonadal dysgenesis, 658
Mixed hearing loss, 847
Mixed venous oxygen saturation
    (SvO_2), 526, 577
MLC. *See* Midline catheter
M-mode echocardiography, 552
Modified Allen's test, performing,
    318, 323
Modified biophysical profile, 10
Modified Finnegan Score, 54
  scoring tool, 54–55
Molecular cytogenics, 785
Molecules, concentration (changes),
    235
Momentary time-out, providing,
    212
Moment-to-moment care,
    formulation (assessment),
    211–212
Moment-to-moment caregiver
    adaptations, 212
Mongolian spots, 149, 788
Monoamine oxidase inhibitors
    (MAOIs), 54
Monocyte colony-forming
    stimulating factor (M-CSF),
    666–667
Monocytes, 669–670
  importance, 698
Moro reflex (startle reflex), 153
Morphine, usage, 303, 343
Mortality, etiology dependence,
    131
Mosaicism, 402
Mother-nurse interactions, 59–62
Mothers
  breast milk, providing
    (opportunity), 358
  hospital discharge, 358
  privacy/comfort, 226
Motilin, presence, 183
Motor assessment, 224
Motor efferents, 846
Motor functioning, infant abilities/
    sensitivities/thresholds, 209
Mottling, 134
MRI. *See* Magnetic resonance
    imaging
MRSA. *See* Methicillin-resistant
    Staphylococcus aureus
MSAF. *See* Meconium-stained
    amniotic fluid
MSAFP. *See* Maternal serum alpha-
    fetoprotein
MSUD. *See* Maple sugar urine
    disease
Mucocutaneous candidiasis, 712
Mucopolysaccharidosis, 140
Mucopurulent discharge, presence,
    837
Mucosal cysts, 140
Müllerian-inhibiting hormone
    (MIH), 655

Multicystic dysplastic kidney disease, 735–736
 clinical presentation, 736
 complications, 736
 definition, 735
 diagnostic studies, 736
 differential diagnosis, 736
 etiology, 736
 incidence, 736
 outcome, 736
 patient care management, 736
 physical examination, 736
Multidisciplinary team developmental care meetings, impact, 209
Multifactorial disorder, 841
Multifactorial genetic factor, 542
Multifocal clonic seizure, 772
Multigravida, quickening, 8
Multiinstitutional specialty-based reports, 371–372
Multiple gestation, 106
 definitions/characteristics, 106
 management, 106
 single gestation, contrast, 121
Murmur, 548–549. See also Physiologic murmurs
 absence, 548
 auscultation, 144–145
 evaluation, 548–549
 grading, 548
 presence, 106
 quality/pitch, 548
Muscle relaxants, usage, 467
Muscle tone
 examination, 753
 procession, 215
Mustard procedure, 568
Mydriatic eyedrops, 796
Myelomeningocele, 105, 758–760
 clinical presentation, 759
 definition, 758
 diagnostic evaluation, 759
 incidence, 759
 outcome, 760
 pathophysiology, 759
 patient care management, 759–760
 risk factors, 758–759
Myocardium, dependence, 84
Myoclonic seizure, 772
Myogenic mechanism, 726

N

Nails, changes (rarity), 3
Naloxone hydrochloride (Narcan) narcotic displacement, 103
Naloxone hydrochloride (Narcan), administration, 88
Narcotics, 50–52
 displacement, naloxone hydrochloride (impact), 103
 fetus/neonate effects, 51–52
 follow-up studies, results, 52
 pharmacology, 51
 pregnancy effects, 51
Narrative charting, usage, 874

Narrative notes, completion, 875
Narrow-bore cannula, usage, 507
Nasal breathing, preference, 92
Nasal cannula. See High-flow nasal cannula
 complications, 499
 usage, 499, 502
Nasal CPAP, 500
Nasal flaring retractions, 142
Nasal intubation, procedure, 201
Nasal periphery, vascularization, 840
Nasal prong CPAP, 502
Nasogastric (NG) tube feeding, 201
Nasolacrimal duct obstruction, 836–837
 clinical presentation, 836
 complications, 836
 congenital obstruction, 836
 nursing care, 836–837
 pathophysiology, 836
Nasolacrimal sac, hydrostatic pressure (increase), 837
Nasopharyngeal CPAP, 500, 502
Nasopharynx, communication, 846
National Association of Neonatal Nurses, 336
 guidelines, 371
National Guideline Clearinghouse (NGC), 370–371
National Institute for Nursing Research, 857–858
National Patient Safety Goals (The Joint Commission), 365t
National Quality Forum (NQF), 368–369
Natural opioids, 50
NDM. See Neonatal diabetes mellitus
Near-patient testing (NPT), 256
Near-term well newborns, risk designation, 626f
Necrotizing enterocolitis (NEC), 161, 198, 612–615
 appearance, 292f
 care, 614–615
 clinical presentation, 613–614
 considerations, 612–614
 definition, 612
 diagnosis, 613–614
 etiology, 612–613
 focal intestinal perforation, 613
 incidence, 613
 laboratory studies, 614
 medical management, 614
 physical examination, 613
 postoperative care, 615
 postrecovery phase, 187–188
 presence, 327
 prognosis, 614
 radiographic evaluation, 291–292
 radiologic examination, 614
 surgical management, 614–615
 surgical repair, 615
 x-ray findings, 291

Negligence. See Corporate negligence
 liability, 872
 standard of care, 872
Neisseria gonorrhoeae, 711–712, 835
 clinical presentation, 835
 complications, 835
 diagnostic findings, 835
 impact, 79
 incidence, 835
 infection, onset, 835
 nursing care, 835
 onset, 836
Neomycin, usage, 843
Neonatal abstinence, description, 54
Neonatal Abstinence Scoring System (Finnegan Score), 56
 illustration, 56t
Neonatal abstinence syndrome (NAS), 54. See also Iatrogenic NAS
 degree/severity, factors, 54
 nonpharmacologic treatment, 58
 pharmacologic treatment, 56–58
 presentation, variation, 54
 scoring methods, 54–56
Neonatal adrenocortical function, 650
Neonatal bile pigment metabolism, 628f
Neonatal calcium metabolism, 165
Neonatal conjunctivitis, 707
Neonatal death, history, 7
Neonatal delivery room resuscitation
 antepartum period, 93
 anticipation/preparation, 94–95
 complications, 107
 decision-making process, 97–103
 definitions, 91
 delivery room preparation, 94–95
 education/competency development, 94
 family support, 108
 intrapartum period, 93
 newly born period, 94
 non-delivery room preparation, 95
 personnel roles, 95
 risk factors, 93–94
 unusual situations, 103–107
Neonatal diabetes mellitus (NDM), 662
 pathophysiology, 180
 permanence, 178
Neonatal discharge checklist, 389f
Neonatal Drug Withdrawal Scoring System, 54
 scale, 55
Neonatal ECMO patient criteria, 522
Neonatal ECMO patient qualifying criteria, 523b
Neonatal endocrine disorders, 638
Neonatal GBS infections, occurrence, 11
Neonatal glucose homeostasis, 173

Neonatal hair/nails, drug
    screening, 64
Neonatal herpes simplex infection,
    826
Neonatal hyperglycemia, urinary
    loss (combination), 179
Neonatal hyperinsulinemia, 160
Neonatal hyperinsulinism,
    persistence, 174
Neonatal hypertension, 549–550
Neonatal hyperthyroidism,
    transience, 649
Neonatal immunodeficiencies, 698
Neonatal Infant Pain Scale, 340
    example, 340f
Neonatal infection, 460
    epidemiologic history, 706
    history, 706–708
    sites, 706–708
    types, 706–708
Neonatal Intensive Care Quality
    Improvement Collaborative
    (NIC/Q), 364
Neonatal intensive care unit
    (NICU)
    atmosphere, establishment, 220
    autonomy, impact, 861
    beneficence, principle, 861
    blood components, usage, 254–
        255
    challenges, evaluation, 208
    charting systems, 874–875
    comfort, 215
    design, change, 385
    developmental support, 208
    discharge, readiness criteria,
        386b
    ELBW admission, 436–437
    ELBW infant transfer, 435
    environment
        feeding method, 201
        human factors, 367
        language development/
            communication processing,
            relationship, 219
    ethical issues, 860
        examination, 860
    evacuation, 429
    flow sheets, usage, 874
    health care errors, 373–379
    health care workers, laboratory
        involvement, 252
    holistic nursing care, importance,
        434
    infants
        admission, 299
        discharge, 385
        discharge, parenting
            challenges, 386
        procedures, 334
    justice, questions, 861–862
    laboratory tests, 252–255
        list, 253t
        multidimensional
            characteristic, 255
    narrative charting, usage, 874
    noise, undesirable effects, 219

Neonatal intensive care unit
    (NICU) (Continued)
    nonpharmacologic pain relief, 215
    optimal pain management, 334–
        336
    painful procedures,
        pharmacologic/
        nonpharmacologic
        interventions, 334
    PIE charting, usage, 875
    Principle Approach, usage, 862
    problem-oriented charting,
        usage, 874–875
    procedures, pain, 333–334
    quiet times, scheduling, 219
    setting, infant development
        (barriers), 208–209
    sick newborn infant transfer, 87
    social components, absence, 208
    stress, coping, 212
    team, support, 864
    touch/handling, considerations,
        214
Neonatal intubation, laryngoscope
    hand position, 305f
Neonatal magnesium homeostasis,
    167
Neonatal morbidity, birth weight/
    gestational age (inclusion),
    132f
Neonatal mortality risk,
    determination, 130
Neonatal nurse practitioners
    (NNPs), 366–367, 873
    recognition, 873
    transport involvement, 420
Neonatal nurses
    challenges, 182
    practice parameters, 1
Neonatal nursing, exploration
    areas, 854
Neonatal Pain Agitation and
    Sedation Scale, 340
    example, 341f
Neonatal pancreatic function, 662
Neonatal period
    fluid losses, 157–158
    PN indications, 191
Neonatal pharmacology, study/
    clinical application, 233
Neonatal pneumonia, 461
Neonatal pneumonia, organisms
    (association), 460b
Neonatal population
    antimicrobial agent
        consideration, 244
    CNS medication considerations,
        247–248
    considerations, 246
    diuretics considerations, 248–249
    immunizations considerations,
        250
    pharmacodynamics, 244, 246
    pharmacokinetics, 244, 246
Neonatal procedural pain,
    prevention/treatment
    (guidelines), 334

Neonatal pustular melanosis,
    photograph, 822f
Neonatal research, 850
Neonatal resuscitation
    anticipation/preparation, 94–95
    complications, 107
    decision-making process, 97–103
    equipment, 95
        list, 96b
    ethics, 109
    family support, 108
    unusual situations, 103–107
Neonatal Resuscitation Program
    (NRP), 304
    skills, 435
Neonatal risk factors, 700
Neonatal sepsis, 694
Neonatal skull, views, 761f
Neonatal teaching needs, 392–393
Neonatal team, justification, 421
Neonatal thyroid physiology, 642–
    643
Neonatal transport
    incubator, thermal cover, 117f
    philosophy, 416
    process, 422–427
    program, crew/patient safety
        priority, 416
    referral call, 422–424
    supplies, 422
        list, 422b–423b
Neonatal transport team
    composition, 419–420
    medical director, involvement,
        421
    NICU evacuation assistance, 429
    NICU extension, 416
Neonatal triggers, 372
Neonatal Withdrawal Inventory, 54
    scale, 55
Neonates
    abdominal wall defect
        care, 597–599
        laboratory studies, 598
        postoperative care, 598–599
        repair, 598
    adrenal disorders, 650
    alcohol, effects, 44–45
    amphetamines
        effects, 49
        withdrawal, 49
    anatomy/physiology, 92–93
    arterial puncture technique, 324f
    breathing/crying, 97
    cocaine
        effects, 47
        withdrawal, 47
    contractility, 541
    definition, 91
    drug effects, 25–26
    early radiation effects, 272
    endocrine disorders, 640
    enzyme maturity, induction, 241
    epidermal layer, thinness, 92
    family unit member, 416
    first bath, 78
    fluid homeostasis, 156

Neonates *(Continued)*
  gastroschisis, care, 597–599
  glottis, anterior position, 92
  hyperbilirubinemia,
      management, 631t
  hyperthermia, iatrogenic
      characteristic, 118
  immature systems, 92
  infectious organisms,
      transmission, 698–699
  inhalants, effects, 53
  large head, body size
      (proportion), 92
  liability costs, 870
  marijuana, effects, 50
  MDMA, effects, 49
  medication administration,
      nursing implications, 250–
      251
  medication errors, 374–377
  muscle mass, decrease, 92
  muscle tone, appropriateness,
      97
  narcotics/opioids, effects, 51–52
  neck, shortness, 92
  nurses, duty, 870
  omphalocele, care, 597–599
  opioid-induced cardiorespiratory
      side effects, 343
  opioid therapy, monitoring, 343
  opioid withdrawal (reduction),
      drugs (usage), 57t
  pain management, special
      considerations, 343
  physical variations, 93
  physiologic/anatomic
      characteristics, 92–93
  preferential nasal breathing, 92
  radiographic examination, risks,
      272
  repetitive/unrelieved pain,
      consequences, 336
  respiratory support, 106–107
  resuscitation
      requirement, 91
      risk, 91
  risk factors, 93–94
  sedatives/hypnotics, effects,
      53
  standard of care, 866
  subcutaneous fat, decrease, 92
  surface area/body size ratio,
      92
  transient tachypnea, 277f
  transport, individualized
      developmental care
      techniques (usage), 426
  vasoconstriction, 93
  venous access, 93
      sites, usage, 309f
Neonatology consultation, 434
Nephron, 725
Nephropathy
  evidence, 27
  progression, 26
Nerve injury, impact, 261–262
Nesidioblastosis, 174

Neural tube defects (NTDs), 26–27,
      105, 149, 758
  acute clinical problems, 105
  etiology, 796–797
  impact, 160
  incidence, 796–797
  malformation disorders, 796–797
  management, 105
  risk, 796
  specific defects, 797
  types/characteristics, 105
Neural tube defects (NTDs),
      genetic screening, 9
Neurobehavioral subsystems, 210t–
      211t
  information, 211
Neurofibromatosis, 152
  indication, 823
  pigmented nevi, association, 822
  tumor formation, 790
Neurologic assessment, 752–753
  history/observation, 752
  physical examination, 752–753
Neurologic clinical signs, 700
Neurologic criteria, assessment
      technique, 124–126
Neurologic disorders, 753–766
Neurologic morbidities, increase,
      397
Neurologic recovery, assessment,
      531
Neurologic system
  anatomy, 748–751
  cerebral blood flow, 751–752
  embryologic development, 748–
      750
  glucose metabolism, 751
  neuronal migration, 749
  neuronal organization, 750
  neuronal proliferation, 749
  physiology, 751–752
Neuromotor deficits, 47
Neuromotor maturation, sequential
      patterns, 214–215
Neuromuscular blocking agents,
      usage, 304, 344
Neuromuscular disorders, 480
Neuroprotection, 107
Neurosensory morbidities,
      increase, 397
Neurotransmitters, amounts
      (decrease), 485
Neuro Ultrasounds (NUS), usage,
      444
Neutral thermal environment
      (NTE)
  establishment, 436
  maintenance, interventions,
      436
  providing, 114–118
  temperatures, 115t
Neutrophils, 669
  count, 701–702
  response, 698
  WBC representation, 702f
Nevus simplex/flammeus, 135
Nevus simplex (stork bite), 823

New Ballard Score, 123
  expansion, 125f
Newborn infants (newborns)
  abdomen, 146–147
      observation, 146
  abdominal wall defect,
      observation, 146
  abnormalities, radiographic
      evaluation, 270
  acrocyanosis, 133
  adventitious breath sounds, 143
  anocutaneous reflex (anal wink),
      153
  anterior fontanelle, 137
  anus, 147–149
  appearance, 133–134
  assessment, 25–26
      techniques, 133
  Babinski reflex, 153
  back, 149–150
  birth defect, evaluation, 408
  bladder, palpation, 146
  blood pressure, 145
  bowel sounds, auscultation, 146
  brachial plexus injury, 150
  bradycardia, 143
  breasts/nipples, inspection, 143
  breath sounds, auscultation, 143
  buttocks, 150
  café au lait spots, 135
  caphalohematoma, 138
  capillary refill/perfusion,
      assessment, 145
  caput succedaneum, 138
  cardiovascular system, 143–145
  care, 408–414
  chest, 142–143
  clavicles, 141–142
  clotting mechanisms,
      deficiencies, 671
  complete diagnosis, 408
  congenital defects, 134
  congenital spine defects, 149
  cornea, 139
  cranial nerves, 153–154
  craniotabes, 137
  defect, causation, 410
  delivery room examination, 133
  dental eruptions, 140
  diagnosis, 408–409
  dislocated/unstable hip,
      assessment, 151f
  disorders, examples, 411
  ears, 141
  ecchymosis, 135
  elbow flexion, 152
  epidermolysis bullosa, 136
  erythema toxicum, 135
  examinations, 410–411
      order, 133
      timing, 133
  extremities, 149–150
  eyes, 139–140
      movements, symmetry, 139–
      140
      relationship/location, 139–140
  face, 138–141

Newborn infants (newborns)
(*Continued*)
facial features, 140
facial skin, inspection, 141
females, inspection, 148–149
fontanelles, 136–138
frenulum, 140
frog-leg position, 152
gastroschisis, 146
genitalia, 147–149
hands/digits, observation, 150
harlequin sign, 134
head, 136–138
head circumference (HC)
    measurements, 136
head drop method, 153
hearing screening, examination,
    799
heart, 143–145
    rate, 143
    sounds, auscultation, 144
hemorrhagic disease, 678–679
hips, 150
history, 409
homeostasis, 724
hypothermia, thermoregulatory
    problem, 114–118
hypoxia, 84
intersex conditions, 149
intestinal obstruction, causes, 599t
iris, 139
jaundice, 134
jaw size, observation, 141
kidneys, palpation, 146
knots, presence, 146
labia/clitoris, 148
laboratory tests, 252
lanugo, 135
length conversion, 883
limb/digit amputation, 150
liver, enlargement, 146
lower extremities, 150
low thyroid states, 646t
lungs, 142–143
males, inspection, 147–148
mass conversion, 884
maturity rating, 123
metatarsus adductus, 150
molding, 136
Mongolian spots, 149
moro reflex (startle reflex), 153
mottling, 134
mouth
    region, 140
    relationship/location, 139–140
mucosal cysts, 140
murmur, auscultation, 144–145
neck, 141–142
neonatal teeth, 140
neurobehavioral effects, 43
neurofibromatosis, 152
neurologic examination, 150–154
nose, 140
    relationship/location, 139–140
NTDs, 149
obligate thumb flexion, 152
omphalocele, 146

Newborn infants (newborns)
(*Continued*)
pallor, 133
palmar grasp, 152
perioral region, 140
persistent neck extension, 152
petechiae, 135
physical examination, 132–154,
    410
plethora, 134
point of maximal intensity,
    location, 143–144
posterior fontanelle, 137
posture, assessment, 152
pulses, palpation, 145
pupils, 139
pustular melanosis, 135
rash, 135
red reflex, 139
reflexes, 152–153
respirations, depth/ease, 142
respiratory acidosis, 84
respiratory distress (assessment),
    Silverman-Andersen scale
    (usage), 511f
respiratory rate, 134
    pattern, 142
risk designation, 626f
rocker bottom feet, 150
rooting reflex, 152
rounded head, occurrence, 136
scalp, inspection, 138
scrotum/testes, 148
sensory function responses, 154
skin, 134–136
    assessment, 816–817
    care, 815–816
    differences, 814–815
    lesions, observation, 152
    variations, 817–820
skull, views, 137f
smoking, impact, 43
soft tissue, palpation, 138
spinal reflexes, 153
spine, 149–150
spontaneous movement,
    observation, 152
staphylococcal scalded skin
    syndrome, 136
stepping reflex, 153
strawberry hemangioma, 135–136
stridor, 134
Sturge-Weber syndrome, 152
subgaleal hemorrhage, 138
sucking reflex, 152
sutures, palpation, 136–138
swiping motions, 337
tachycardia, 143
talipes calcaneovalgus, 150
talipes equinovarus, 150
temperature conversion, 882
thermal stress, symptoms, 112b
thrush, 140
tongue, 140
tonic neck reflex, 152–153
truncal incurvation reflex (galant
    reflex), 153

Newborn infants (newborns)
(*Continued*)
tuberous sclerosis, 152
uncertainties, parental emotional
    support, 386
University of Colorado Medical
    Center classification, 131f
urine, observation, 148
vagina, 148
vascular nevi, 135
vernix caseosa, 135
webbing, 141
weight conversion, 884
wheezing, 134
x-ray views
    anteroposterior view, 271f
    cross-table lateral view, 271f
    lateral decubitus view, 271f
    usage, 271–272
Newborns' and Mothers' Health
    Protection Act (1996), 17
Newborn state system, information,
    211
Newly born, definition, 91
NG. *See* Nasogastric
Nicotine
    abuse, 42–43
    breastfeeding impact, 64
Nifedipine (Procardia), oral
    administration, 29
NIH. *See* Nonimmune hydrops
Nipples
    change, frequency, 222
    usage, 222
Nippling, contraindications, 81
Nissen fundoplication, 622f
Nitroglycerin 2%, usage, 310
Nitroprusside, impact, 468
Nitrous oxide (laughing gas/
    whippets), 53
N-methyl-D-aspartate, afferent fiber
    neurotransmitter
    stimulation, 335
NNPs. *See* Neonatal nurse
    practitioners
NNS. *See* Nonnutritive sucking
Nodule, 817
Nonchromosomal abnormalities,
    794–805
Nonemergency replacement
    transfusion, 677
Nonesterified fatty acids, release, 113
Nonimmune hydrops (NIH), 633–
    634
Noninvasive monitoring, 512–513,
    576–577
Nonmaleficence, 68
    action, intent, 861
    ethics principle, 861
Nonmultiples, number, 402
Nonnutritive sucking (NNS)
    increase. *See* Breast milk
        breast milk odor, impact, 223
    meta-analysis, 221
    provision, 202–203
    usage, 87
Nonoliguric hyperkalemia, 440

Nonopioid analgesics, usage, 344
Nonpathologic unconjugated hyperbilirubinemia, management, 630
Nonpharmacologic pain management, 217b
Nonreactive NST, 10
Nonreassuring fetal heart tracing, 122
Nonreassuring FHR, detection, 17
Nonreciprocal translocation, 402
Non-REM (NREM), EEG characteristics, 211
Non-salt losing, 810
Nonshivering thermogenesis, 112–113
Nonspecific cellular immunity, 697–698
Nonstreptococcal scarlatina, 827
Nonstress test (NST), 9–10. *See also* Serial NST
  indications, 10
  testing, 10
  usage, 27
Nontechnological improvement strategies definitions, 362b
Nonthyroidal illness (NTI) syndrome, 644
Nontracheal tubes, usage, 503
Nontraditional transport equipment, requirement, 429
Norepinephrine
  release, 113
  reuptake, cocaine inhibition, 46
Normoglycemia, ensuring, 108
Normothermia, maintenance, 114–118
Norwood procedure, 572–573
Nosocomial bloodstream infections, risk reduction, 441
Nosocomial infections, 377
Nostrils, patency, 140
NPT. *See* Near-patient testing
NREM. *See* Non-REM
NS flush solution, usage, 308
NST. *See* Nonstress test
NTE. *See* Neutral thermal environment
NTI. *See* Nonthyroidal illness
Nuchal cord, blood volume impact, 671
Nuchal translucency, screen reliability, 8
Nucleated RBCs, 668, 691
Numerical chromosomal abnormalities, 783
Numerical data, analysis, 853
Nursery
  infection control measures, 721
  thermoregulation considerations, 78–79
Nurses
  accountability, 870–871
  duty, breach, 869
  educational preparation, 851t
  float, refusal right, 872–873
  liability, 869–873

Nurses *(Continued)*
  malpractice, 869
  medical record documentation responsibility, 874
  patient/family signatures, obtaining, 878
  patient responsibility, 872
  practice, scope, 872
  preventive legal maintenance, practicing, 879–880
  research consumption, 813, 854–856
  research ethics advocates, 856–858
  research roles, 851t
  suit involvement, 877
Nurse-to-nurse communication, 108
Nursing
  care, 511–513
    quality, judgment, 866–867
  education, nursing process (foundation), 865–866
  knowledge, research/generation, 850–851
  malpractice cases, liability/damages (proof), 867–868
  notes, completeness, 874
  practice
    boundaries, limitation, 877–878
    ethical standards, 868
    medical practice, overlap, 872
  process, 865–866
    research process, similarities, 852t
    steps, 865–866
    usage. *See* Attorneys
  research
    findings, usage, 855–856
    standards, 851b
NUS. *See* Neuro Ultrasounds
Nutrition, feeding developmental framework, 221
Nutritional adequacy/toxicity, assessment, 203–204
Nutritional assessment/standards, 203–205
Nutritional intake, 203
Nutritive sucking, impact, 221–222
Nystatin (Mycostatin), usage, 826

O

Obligate thumb flexion (cortical thumb), 152
Obligation-based theory, 862
Obstetric analgesia, 35–39
  assessment/management, 36
  fetal/neonatal complications, 36
  IM/IV route, 35
  maternal complications, 36
  side effects/complications, 36
Obstetric anesthesia, 35–39
  allergic reaction, 38
  assessment/management, 36–37
  complications, 36
  fetal/neonatal complication, 36
  maternal complications, 36
  toxic reaction, 38

Obstetric history, 120
  writing, 6
Obstetrics, risk (consideration), 865
Obstruction, diagnosis (difficulty), 4
Obstructive apnea, 485
  definition, 485
Obstructive defects
  decreased pulmonary blood flow, inclusion, 562–567
  pulmonary venous congestion, inclusion, 560–562
Obstructive lesions, 85
Occipital frontal circumference (OFC), measurement, 752–753
Occlusive dressing, usage, 176
Occupational therapist (OT), resource, 215
Occurrence-basis policy, 879
Occurrences, documentation, 876
Ocular manifestations, 839
OFC. *See* Occipital frontal circumference
Office for Human Research Protections (OHRP), 858
Off-label medications, 376
OG. *See* Orogastric
Oligohydramnios syndrome, 733–735
Oliguria, 580
  persistence, 577
Omphalocele, 105, 146
  diagnosis, 596
  exomphalos, 595–596
  gastroschisis, comparison, 597t
  photograph, 595f
  prognosis, 596
One-way transports, 417
Open neural tube defects, 403
Ophthalmologic disorders
  birth history, 834
  complications, 839–840
  external assessment, 834
  family history, 834
  history, 834
  light/visual stimuli, reaction, 834
  pathologic conditions/management, 834–844
  patient assessment, 834
  pregnancy, impact, 834
Opiates
  analgesics, weaning, 531
  CNS depressants, 51
  interference, 51
  use, pregnancy incidence, 50–51
Opioids, 50–52
  fetus/neonate effects, 51–52
  follow-up studies, results, 52
  pharmacology, 51
  pregnancy effects, 51
  therapy, efficacy, 343
  tolerance/dependence, management, 343–344
  withdrawal (reduction), drugs (usage), 57t
Optic disc, 833

Optic nerve, 833
Oral breast/bottle feeding, 202
Oral endotracheal intubation
  advanced practice procedure,
    302–307
  equipment/supplies, 302–303
  indications, 302
  precautions, 302
Oral ETT, impact, 306
Oral feeding
  establishment, 531
  initiation, 202
  interventions, 224
  readiness, 202
Oral intubation, procedure, 201
Oral morphine, usage, 58
Oral-motor function, improvement,
  215
Orbital cellulitis, 836
Orchiopexy, 745
Order-writing policies, correctness,
  250
Organ injury, impact, 261–262
Organogenesis, gestation, 177
Orogastric (OG) tube
  feeding, 201
  passage, 83
  placement, 100
Oropharyngeal tissues, trauma/
  edema, 306
Oropharynx, suctioning, 304
Ostensible authority, 871
Osteogenesis imperfecta, 794–795
  associated findings, 795
  clinical presentation, 794–795
  clinical types, 794
  diagnosis, 795
  incidence/etiology, 794
  treatment, 795
Osteopenia. See Parenteral nutrition
  monitoring, 474
Ostium primum, closure, 537f
Ototoxic drugs, impact, 847
Out-of-state transport, 430
Output measurements, usage, 251
Over-the-counter medications,
  maternal use, 195
Ovotesticular DSD, 655–656, 658
Oxygenated blood, return, 523
Oxygenation
  assessment, 107–108
  determination, MAP (usage),
    510
Oxygen (O₂). See Blow-by oxygen
  analyzer, 513
  consumption, minimization, 438
  delivery
    continuation, 99
    devices, care, 502–503
  exposure, 438
  hood, 499
    usage, 502
  saturation
    monitor, usage, 303
    peripheral monitoring, 83
  supply, 88
  toxicity, 471

Oxygen (O₂) (Continued)
  transport, 495–497
    iron, importance, 185
  usage, precautions, 843
Oxytocin, secretion, 18

P

P. aeruginosa, 711
Packed red blood cells (PRBCs),
  688
  usage, 254
Pain
  behavioral expression, sedative
    suppression, 344
  behavioral responses, 337
  control, 584
  definition, 333
  Fentanyl, usage, 343
  IASP definition, 333
  long-term effects, 336
  NICU procedure, impact, 333–
    334
  nursing care, 340–344
  physiologic/behavioral
    measures, composite/
    multidimensional
    instruments (selection), 338
  physiologic measures, 337
  physiologic responses, 337
  responses, modification
    (contextual factors), 337–338
  standards of practice, 336
Pain assessment, 336–338
  fifth vital sign, 584
  golden rule, 336
  instruments, 338–340
  parents, role, 345
Pain management. See Extremely
  low birth weight infants;
  Nonpharmacologic pain
  management
  behavioral measures, 342
  goals, 342
  inadequacy, recognition, 336
  nonpharmacologic approaches,
    342
  nonpharmacologic methods, 35
  parents, role, 345
  pharmacologic approaches, 343–
    344
  preventive measures, 342
PAIS. See Partial AIS
Palivizumab (Synagis), usage, 474,
  715
Palliation, selection, 568
Palmar grasp, 152
Pancreas, disorders, 662–663
Pancreatic disorders, 662–663
  anatomy/physiology, 662
Pancreatic polypeptide, presence,
  183
Pancuronium (Pavulon), usage, 515
Papule, 817
Paracentesis, requirement, 104
Paralytic agents, usage, 515–516
Paramedics, transport involvement,
  421

Parental knowledge base,
  assessment, 386–387
Parental learning, barriers, 387
Parental needs, summary, 359
Parental skin-to-skin care,
  encouragement, 115
Parent Buddy Program,
  implementation, 220–221
Parenteral nutrition (PN), 190–194
  administration, 191
    complications, 192–194
  calcium intake, 192
  calories, 191
  central route, 191
  complications, prevention/
    minimization, 194
  fat intake, 192
  fluid intake, 191
  indications, 191
  intake, determination
    (guidelines), 191–192
  IV administration, guidelines,
    191–192
  nutrients, 191–192
  peripheral route, 191
  phosphorous intake, 192
  PN-induced osteopenia, 193–194
  preparations, compositions, 191–
    192
  protein intake, 192
  receiving, monitoring schedule,
    193t
Parent-infant bonding
  behaviors, concern, 359
  evaluation, 359
  positive attachment behaviors,
    359
Parent-infant interaction, feeding
  developmental framework,
    221
Parent-infant relationships,
  alteration, 383
Parenting behavior, nurturing, 358
Parents
  adaptation, determination, 350
  autopsy, options, 356
  care participation,
    encouragement, 353
  communication, adequacy, 863–
    864
  concerns/fears, sharing
    (encouragement), 353
  consent, absence, 878
  feeding, relationship, 224
  grief response
    assessment, 352
    determination, 350
  grieving process, parental
    understanding, 355
  guilt, feeling (acknowledgment),
    352
  infant body, disposition, 356
  infant death, responses, 355
  journal, keeping
    (encouragement), 352
  loss, 354–356
    pain, acknowledgment, 355

Parents *(Continued)*
  memorial/funeral service, 356
  NICU visit, information detail, 352
  perinatal loss
    information, providing, 356
  perinatal loss, interventions, 355–356
  power struggles, avoidance, 358
  relationship, maintenance, 353
  role, adaptation (facilitation), 352
  situation, understanding, 349–350
  social support network, determination, 353
  specific population, 349
  support group, encouragement, 353–354
  support systems, determination, 350
  treatment, refusal, 878
  visitors, reference (absence), 353
Parent teaching, 88–89
Parent-to-parent groups, usage, 89
Partial AIS (PAIS), 657
Partial exchange transfusions, 689
Partial placenta previa, bleeding (management), 32
Partial prothrombin time (PTT), usage, 671
Participant observation, 854
Passive immunization, 249
Patent airway, maintenance, 103, 300
Patent ductus arteriosus (PDA), 26–27, 160
  anatomy, 554
  clinical manifestations, 554–555
  clinical significance, 280
  commonness, 439
  complication, 530
  hemodynamics, 554
  illustration, 554f
  impact, 457, 553
  incidence, 553–554
  indomethacin management, 555–556
  management, 555–556
  manifestation, 439
  prognosis, 556
  radiographic evaluation, 286
Patent urachus, 740–741
  clinical presentation, 740
  complications, 741
  definition, 740
  diagnostic studies, 740
  differential diagnosis, 740
  etiology, 740
  incidence, 740
  patient care management, 741
  physical examination, 740
Paternal problems, 351
Pathogen, isolation, 704–705
Pathologic GER, 620
Pathologic unconjugated hyperbilirubinemia, 629–630
  management, 630–632

Patient care
  documentation, 428
  equipment, cleaning, 720
  practice, review, 267
Patient-focused testing (PFT), 256
Patients
  blood gas values, 526
  diagnosis, laboratory result (contribution), 263
  identification
    errors, bar coding (usage), 369–370
    system, establishment, 429
  misidentification, 373–374
    reduction, improvement strategies, 374
  nurse responsibility, 872
  nursing care, 502–505
  preferences, case analysis model component, 863
  signatures, obtaining, 878
  tracking system, establishment, 429
  triggers, 372
Patient safety
  establishment, strategic priority, 361–363
  priority, 347
  promotion, family empowerment, 364
Patient-triggered ventilation (PTV), 501–502
Pavlik harness, 802
  photograph, 802f
PBPs. *See* Potentially Better Practices
PCR. *See* Polymerase chain reaction
PDA. *See* Patent ductus arteriosus
PDAs. *See* Personal digital assistants
PDI. *See* Psychomotor Development Index
Peak medication level, 234
Pectin-based barriers, helpfulness, 816
Pediatric laryngoscope handle, 302
Pediatrix Medical Group, Inc., Growth Chart, 129
PEEP. *See* Positive end expiration pressure
Peer groups, loss, 351
Peer review, usage, 432
Pelvic examination, 8
Pelvic structures, enlargement, 327
Penetrance, definition, 400
Penis, cleaning, 325
Pentobarbital, usage, 543
Percutaneous central venous line, 296
Percutaneous medication administration, 238
Percutaneous umbilical blood sampling, 405–406
  indications, 406
  postsampling care, 406
  preparation, 406
  results, 406

Percutaneous umbilical blood sampling *(Continued)*
  risks, 406
  timing, 406
Perfusion, decrease, 628
Perihilar, definition, 271
Perihilar region, vascularity (presence), 284f
Perilymph, movement, 846
Perinatal asphyxia, 84, 161
  degree, 84
Perinatal factors, 108
Perinatal fetal distress, 82
Perinatal history, 120–123, 545
  review, 82
Perinatal loss
  information, providing. *See* Parents; Siblings
  interventions. *See* Parents
Perinatal mortality
  rate, increase, 178
  smoking, impact, 43
Perinatal nutrition, maternal physiologic changes, 1–2
Perinatal risk factors, 488
Perinatal stress, 174
Perinatal substance abuse, 41–42
  criminal model, harm-reduction model (contrast), 68
  drug screening, 63–64
    maternal characteristics, 63b
  epidemiologic evidence, 41
  ethical/legal considerations, 67–68
  legal implications, 68
  management recommendations, 58
  mother-nurse interactions, 59–62
  nursing interventions, 59–62
  prevalence, 41–42
  racial trends, 42
Perineum, inspection, 591
Periodic breathing, 142, 484
  definition, 484
Peripheral arterial line insertion, 319f
Peripheral cyanosis, central cyanosis (differentiation), 545
Peripheral glucose infusions, extravasations, 160
  equipment/supplies, 308
  precautions, 307–308
  procedure, 308–310
Peripheral intravenous line placement, 307–310
  complications, 310
  indications, 307
  multiple puncture technique, 310
  pharmacologic intervention, 310
Peripherally inserted central catheter (PICC)
  advanced practice procedure, 310–313
  catheter insertion kit, usage, 311–312
  complications, 313
  contraindications, 311

Peripherally inserted central
    catheter (PICC) *(Continued)*
  equipment/supplies, 311–312
  indications, 311
  precautions, 311
  procedure, 312–313
Peripherally inserted central
    catheter (PICC) removal, 314
  complications, 314
  equipment/supplies, 314
  indications, 314
  precautions, 314
  procedure, 314
Peripherally inserted midline
    catheter, advanced practice
    procedure, 310–313
Peripheral nervous system, acute
    pain (physiology), 335
Peripheral perfusion, decrease, 303
Peripheral pulses, 549
Peripheral vasoconstriction, 46
Peritoneal dialysis, 164
Peritoneal tap, 257
Periventricular-intraventricular
    hemorrhage, 768–771
  clinical presentation, 770
  definition, 768
  diagnostic evaluation, 770
  incidence, 769–770
  outcome, 771
  pathophysiology, 769
  patient care management, 770–771
  risk factors, 768–769
Periventricular leukomalacia (PVL),
    778
  clinical presentation, 778
  definition, 778
  diagnostic evaluation, 778
  incidence, 778
  outcome, 778
  pathophysiology, 778
Permanent neonatal diabetes, 179–
    180
  clinical presentation, 180
  complications, 180
  definition, 179
  incidence, 180
  management, 180
  outcomes, 180
  pathophysiology, 163
Permissive hypercapnia, 495
Permissive hypercarbia, 437
PERRL. *See* Pupils equal, round,
    and react to light
Persistent fetal shunts, 85
Persistent neck extension
    (opisthotonos), 152
Persistent neonatal
    hyperinsulinism, 174
Persistent pulmonary hypertension,
    complication, 462
Persistent pulmonary hypertension
    of the newborn (PPHN),
    463–468
  analgesics/sedatives, usage, 468
  cardiovascular abnormalities,
    465

Persistent pulmonary hypertension
    of the newborn (PPHN)
    (Continued)
  cardiovascular complications, 466
  clinical presentation, 465
  complications, 466
  definition, 463–464
  diagnosis, 465–466
  differential diagnosis, 466
  etiology, 464–465
  hematologic complications, 466
  iatrogenic complications, 466
  maladaptation, 464
  maldevelopment, 464
  management, 466–468
  metabolic abnormalities, 465
  metabolic complications, 466
  neurologic complications, 466
  outcome, 468
  pathophysiology, 464
  pulmonary complications, 466
  pulmonary vasodilators, usage,
    468
  renal complications, 466
  respiratory abnormalities, 465
  stimulation/handling, 467
  supportive care, 466
  underdevelopment, 464–465
  vasopressors, usage, 467–468
Personal digital assistants (PDAs),
    370
Personality, development, 349
Person-centered approach, 363
Petechiae, 135, 817, 835
  eruptions, 827
PFT. *See* Patient-focused testing
pH, 168
Pharmacodynamics, 234–235
  definition, 233
  neonatal population, 244, 246
Pharmacokinetics, 236–243
  definition, 233
  neonatal population, 244, 246
  usage, 490
Pharmacology
  definition, 233–234
  principles, 233–234
  terminology, 233–234
Pharmacotherapy, definition, 233
Pharynx, exposure, 304
Phase II medication metabolism,
    241
Phase I medication metabolism, 241
Phenobarbital, usage, 773
Phenotype, definition, 400
Phentolamine (Regitine), usage, 310
Phenylketonuria (PKU), 197, 807–
    808
  clinical findings, 808
  diagnosis, 808
  incidence/etiology, 807
  treatment, 808
Phenytoin (fetal hydantoin
    syndrome), 543
PHH. *See* Posthemorrhagic
    hydrocephalus
Phlebotomy, 321–322

Phosphatidylglycerol (PG), 10
  appearance, 454
Phosphatidylinositol concentration,
    454
Phosphorous, medications
    (negative effect), 204
Photoreceptors, 814
Phototherapy, hazard, 218–219
pH probe test, 593
Phrenic nerve injury, 280
Phrenic nerve paralysis, 765–766
  clinical presentation, 765
  diagnostic evaluation, 765
  outcome, 765–766
  pathophysiology, 765
  patient care management, 765
Physical assessment, 120
Physical environment, 367
Physical examination, 410
  criteria, 126
Physical therapist (PT), resource,
    215
Physicians, transport involvement,
    420
Physiologic dead space, definition,
    494
Physiologic murmurs, 548
Physiologic stress
  creation, 260
  impact, 260
  symptoms, 260
PICC. *See* Peripherally inserted
    central catheter
PIE. *See* Problem, intervention, and
    evaluation of problems;
    Pulmonary interstitial
    emphysema
Pierre Robin syndrome, 788
Pigmentary retinopathy, 839
Pigmentation, increase, 3
Pigmented nevi
  benign characteristic, 821
  neurofibromatosis, association,
    822
  tuberous sclerosis, association,
    822
Pigmented skin lesions, 821–823
Pigment specific lasers, usage, 822
Pinna
  development, 847
  lacerations, 835
PIP, 504, 508
Pituitary gland, 640–641
  anatomy/physiology, 640
  disorders, 640–641
  structures, 640
PIVKA. *See* Protein induced by
    vitamin K absence
PKU. *See* Phenylketonuria
Placenta
  anatomy/physiology, 72
  concept, 20
  location, ultrasonography
    (usage), 30
  nicotine, impact, 43
  perfusion, 75
Placental abnormality, 122

Placental circulation,
characteristics, 72–74
Placental complications, 25
Placental-fetal function tests, 25
Placental grading, usage (absence),
8
Placental infarction, 25
Placental insufficiency, 684
hypertensive/vascular disorder,
impact, 122
Placental membrane, thinning, 23
Placental transfusion, 670
Placental transport mechanisms,
20–24
Placental villi, edema
(development), 23
Placenta previa, 31–32, 43
assessment/management, 31–32
blood volume impact, 671
clinical presentation, 31
complications, 31
etiology/predisposing factors, 31
fetal/neonatal complications, 31
incidence, 31
maternal complications, 31
Planning, nursing process step, 865
Plantar creases, 126
Plaque, 817
Plasma
glucose, optimal range, 158
insulin levels, 180
protein concentrations, 240
usage, 254
Plasma blood glucose levels, 179
Plasma colloid osmotic pressure,
decrease, 24
Plasma thromboplastin component
(factor IX), 79
Platelets, 670
destruction, 682
production, impairment, 682
usage, 254
Pleural cavity exposure, 159
Plexiglas heat shields, usage
(avoidance), 117
Pluripotent stem cells, presence,
666
Plus disease, 841
PN. See Parenteral nutrition
Pneumomediastinum, 475–477
chest/abdominal x-ray
examination, 108
clinical presentation/diagnosis,
476
lateral view, 280f
management, 476
radiographic evaluation, 279
thymus lifted, appearance, 280f
Pneumonia, 460–462. See also
Congenital pneumonia;
Neonatal pneumonia
clinical presentation, 461
complications, 462
definition, 460
diagnostic evaluation, 461–462
differential diagnosis, 462
etiology, 460

Pneumonia (Continued)
incidence, 460
infection risk, 460
management, 462
neonatal infection, 707
organisms, association. See
Neonatal pneumonia
pathophysiology, 461
physical examination, 461
radiographic evaluation, 278
Pneumopericardium, 475–477
appearance, 280f
chest/abdominal x-ray
examination, 108
clinical presentation/diagnosis,
476
management, 477
radiographic evaluation, 279
Pneumoperitoneum
chest/abdominal x-ray
examination, 108
radiographic evaluation, 292
Pneumothorax, 475–477
chest/abdominal x-ray
examination, 108
clinical presentation/diagnosis,
476
management, 476
radiographic evaluation, 279
Poikilocytosis, 691
Poikilothermic response, 111
Point-of-care blood glucose
screening, 175
Point-of-care testing (POCT), 256
device, calibration, 266
Polycystic kidneys, 26–27
risk, increase, 43
Polycythemia, 26–27, 85, 684–685
clinical assessment, 685
clinical presentation, 684
complications, 685
diagnostic studies, 685
etiologic factors, 684
impact, 177
outcome, 685
partial exchange transfusion, 685
patient care management, 685
physical examination, 685
Polydactyly, 803–805
associated findings, 804
clinical findings, 804
diagnosis, 805
incidence/etiology, 803
photograph, 804f
treatment, 805
Polydrug abusers, 51
Polydrug use, commonness, 67
Polyethylene bag, usage, 116
Polygenic defects, definition, 402
Polyhydramnios
association, 10
presence, assessment, 33
Polymerase chain reaction (PCR),
406
detection, 703
Polymyxin B sulfate (Maxitrol),
usage, 843

Polyploidy, definition, 402
Polyuria, 180
Popliteal angle, 124–125
Port-wine stain, 823–824
confinement, 824
Positional hip abduction, 150
Positioning
deformities, prevention, 215
guidelines, 216b
usage, 214–215
Positive end expiration pressure
(PEEP), 469, 504. See also
Inadvertent PEEP
Positive Na balance, 162
Positive-pressure devices, 501
Positive-pressure ventilation (PPV),
99–101
Postamniocentesis care, 405
Post-CVS care, 405
Postdischarge, 395–397
Post-ECMO care, 531
Posterior fontanelles, 137
Posterior pole retinal vessels,
engorgement/tortuosity,
841
Posterior urethral valves, 738
Posthemorrhagic hydrocephalus
(PHH), 757–758
clinical presentation, 758
diagnostic evaluation, 758
etiology, 757
incidence, 757
outcome, 758
patient care management, 758
Postnatal circulation, 75
Postnatal growth curves, 205
Postnatal testing, 406
Postoperative cardiac management,
576–578
Postoperative disturbances, 578–
585
Postoperative pain management,
584
Postpartum blues, occurrence, 18
Postpartum care, terminology, 1
Postpartum depression
commonness, 386
occurrence, 18
Postpartum hemorrhage, 30
Postpartum period (early
discharge), parent teaching,
89
Postpartum thyroiditis, impact, 18
Postprandial hyperglycemia, 6
Postresuscitation care, 107–109
Postterm pregnancy, 1
Potassium (K), 163–165
function, 163
homeostasis, 163
intake, inadequacy, 163
laboratory assessment, 203–204
normalization, 164
regulation, 163
Potentially Better Practices (PBPs),
370–371
VON offering, 371
Potter facies, 734f

Potter syndrome (oligohydramnios syndrome), 26–27, 733–735
clinical assessment, 734
clinical presentation, 733–734
complications, 734
diagnostic studies, 734
differential diagnosis, 734
etiology, 733
incidence, 733
outcome, 735
patient care management, 735
physical examination, 734
Povidone-iodine (Betadine) absorption, impact, 238
PPHN. *See* Persistent pulmonary hypertension of the newborn
PPROM. *See* Preterm premature rupture of membranes
PPV. *See* Positive-pressure ventilation
Practice, scope, 872
increase, 872
permissibility, legal issue, 874
PRBCs. *See* Packed red blood cells
Preaccident planning, 429
Preauricular ear appendages, 141
Preauricular pits, 141
presence, 847
Preauricular sinuses, 141
Preconception counseling, 27
Preductal PaO₂, increase, 551
Preeclampsia, 24–26
assessment/management, 25–26
clinical presentation, 24
complications, 24–25
etiology/predisposing factors, 24
pathophysiologic events, 24
severity, 25
Pre-ECMO stabilization, 522
Preferential nasal breathing, 92
Pregnancy
alcohol
effects, 44
use, incidence, 44
blood pressure (BP), 24
cocaine
impact, 46–47
usage, incidence, 46
dating, placental grading (usage, absence), 8
history, 121–122
information, 6
inhalants, effects, 53
loss, history, 7
marijuana, effects, 50
mask, 3
methadone, impact, 51
narcotics/opioids, effects, 51
opiate use, incidence, 50–51
pharmacology, 43
sedatives/hypnotics, effects, 53
smoking
impact, 43
incidence, 42–43
Pregnancy-induced hypertension, 26

Pregnant addicts, medical complications, 51
Pregnant women
cigarette smokers, likelihood, 42
conditions/substances, 20
Preload, 541
changes, low cardiac output, 579
filling, 579
Premature, 106–107
definitions/characteristics, 106
infection control, 107
management, 106–107
neuroprotection, 107
Premature births, rate increase, 447
Premature human milk, composition, 195t
Premature Infant Pain Profile, 339–340
example, 339t
Premature infants, 187–190, 198–199
adipose tissue, minimum, 185
apnea, pathogenesis, 485–487
biphasic response. *See* Hypoxia
birth, crisis, 347–349
blood values, 668t
calcium, impact, 185
carbohydrate intake, 189–190
caregivers, usage, 358
commercial formulas, 194–199
commercially prepared human milk fortifiers/formulas, 199t
considerations, 187
crisis, discussion, 348–349
electrolytes, intake, 190
energy/caloric intake requirements, 188–189
energy intakes, 190
fat intake, 189–190
fluid requirements, 187–188
formulas, mixture, 199
functional development, 183
gastrointestinal (GI) function, postnatal development, 184
gastrointestinal (GI) tract anatomic/functional development, 182–183
anatomy/physiology, 182–185
functional development, 183
postnatal development, 183–184
growth charts, 205
human milk, 194–199
benefits, 198
importance, 198
IEM risk, 197
iron, role, 185
length board, 204
leukocyte values, 670t
magnesium, impact, 185
minerals
impact, 185
intake, 190
mother (human) milk, concentrations, 198
nutrient deficiencies, 184–185

Premature infants (*Continued*)
nutritional requirements, 186–190
list, 188t
phosphorous, impact, 185
pneumonia infection, risk, 460
poikilothermic response, 111
postnatal growth curves, 205
protein intake, 189–190
determination, 190
psychologic tasks, 348
trace elements
impact, 185
intake, 190
vitamins
impact, 185
intake, 190
Premature placental aging, 25
Premature rupture of membranes (PROM), 43
Prematurity
anemia, 675–676
apnea cause, 487
hypothyroxinemia, 643
treatment, 646–647
late metabolic acidosis, 169
problems, 397
Prematurity-related problems, 396b
Prenatal diagnosis, 402–406
advantages, 402–403
indications, 402–403
Prenatal drug exposure, caring strategies, 59t–62t
Prenatal high-risk factors, 21t–23t
Prenatal history, 409
Prenatal pulmonary hypertension, impact, 464
Prenatal records, review, 11
Prenatal screening tests, 7t
Prenatal teaching, providing, 89
Prenatal tests, 403–406
preparation, 403
results, 404
shortfalls, 403–404
Prescription medications, maternal use, 195
Presenting problem, history, 122
Pressure-cycled ventilator, 501
Pressure monitoring, 525
Pressure-support ventilator (PSV), 501
Pressure valves, cardiac catheterization, 576t
Preterm births, 25
costs, 383
percentage, 384t
rates, increase, 383
Preterm gestational age, 25
Preterm infants
breastfeeding, 224–226
day-night cycled lighting, 219
development, KC benefits, 214
endurance, 224
feeding facilitation techniques, 225b–226b
feeding modalities, alternative, 226–227

Preterm infants *(Continued)*
  fluid requirements,
      quantification, 158
  hypernatremic hyperosmolar
      dehydration, fluid
      management, 160
  intrauterine influence, 219
  NNS, receiving, 223
  oral feeding (facilitation), milk
      flow (restriction), 222
  problems, observation, 226
  skin
      care, 815–816
      differences, 814–815
  tears, secretion, 786
  transient hypothyroid states,
      643–644
Preterm labor, 28–29
  assessment/management, 28–29
  clinical presentation, 28
  complications, 28
  development, fetal factors, 28
  episodes, 29
  etiology/predisposing factors,
      28
  incidence, 28
      increase, 28
  medications, 29
  risk scoring systems, 28
Preterm neonates. *See* Late preterm
      neonate
  acute pain
      physiology, 334–336
      physiology, understanding,
          334–336
      supraspinal/integrative level,
          335–336
  evaporative heat loss, increase,
      114
Preterm newborn infants, tears
      (secretion), 836
Preterm pregnancy, terminology, 1
Preterm premature rupture of
      membranes (PPROM),
      122
Preterm skin, differences, 783
Preventive legal maintenance,
      nurse practice, 879–880
Prilocaine, usage, 344
Primary apnea, 484–485
  definition, 484
Primary health care practitioner,
      selection, 390–392
Primary hypothyroidism, 643. *See
      also* Atypical primary
      hypothyroidism
Primary myocardial disease, 550
Primary neurulation, 748
Primary subarachnoid hemorrhage,
      767
  clinical presentation, 767
  definition, 767
  diagnostic evaluation, 767
  incidence, 767
  outcome, 767
  pathophysiology, 767
Primigravida, quickening, 8

Principle Approach, 860
  assistance, 862
  usage. *See* Neonatal intensive
      care unit
Principle of double effect, 861
Principles of Biomedical Ethics,
      860
Probability sampling, 852
Problem, intervention, and
      evaluation of procedure
      (PIE) charting, usage, 875
Problem-oriented charting, usage,
      874–875
Proconvertin (factor VII), 79
Professional liability insurance,
      878–880
  carrying, 879
Professional organizations,
      standards, 868
Prolactin, secretion, 18
Prolapse. *See* Umbilical cord
      prolapse
      occurrence, 33
Prolapsed cord, examination, 35
Prometaphase banding, 406
Pronephros, 724
Proper technique, definition, 271
Prophylaxis treatment, 458
Propylthiouracil (PTU), TPO
      inhibition, 648
Prosencephalic development, 748–
      749
Prostaglandin E_1 (PGE$_1$), 561
Prostaglandins, 726
Protective reflexes, 486
Protein-bound calcium, 165
Protein induced by vitamin K
      absence (PIVKA), 678
Protein metabolism, errors, 807–
      808
Proteins
  ingestion, 183
  lymphatic drainage, 160
Proteinuria, renal perfusion
      (impact), 24
Prothrombin (factor II), 79
Prothrombin time (PT), 594–595
  usage, 671
Proton pump inhibitors, 622
Proximal airway pressures, 507
Proximal cause, 869
Prune belly syndrome
  management, 623–624
  surgical procedures, 624
PS. *See* Pulmonary stenosis
Pseudoglandular, term (usage),
      453
PSV. *See* Pressure-support
      ventilator
Psychologic morbidity, 532
Psychomotor Development Index
      (PDI), 48
Psychomotor retardation, 840
PTT. *See* Partial prothrombin time
PTU. *See* Propylthiouracil
PTV. *See* Patient-triggered
      ventilation

Puerperium (fourth trimester), 17–18
  emotional changes, 18
  immunizations, 18
Pulmonary adaptation, 75–77
Pulmonary air leaks, 107, 475–477
  clinical presentation/diagnosis,
      476
  definition, 475
  evaluation, 430
  incidence, 475
  management, 476–477
  outcome, 477
  pathophysiology, 475–476
  radiographic evaluation, 279
Pulmonary arteries, 74
  division, 538f
  hypertension, 497–499
  hypertensive crisis, 579
  pressure
      invasive monitoring, 577
      measurement, 552
  stenosis, detection, 552
Pulmonary atresia, 565–566
  anatomy, 565
  clinical manifestations, 565–566
  hemodynamics, 565
  illustration, 565f
  incidence, 565
  management, 566
  prognosis, 566
Pulmonary blood flow, 74
  decrease, 85
  increase, 85
      defects, 553–560
Pulmonary edema, 24, 160
  appearance, 282f
  diuretics, impact, 473–474
  radiographic evaluation, 280
  reduction, 197
Pulmonary hemorrhage, 300, 477–
      478
  clinical presentation, 478
  definition, 477
  etiology, 477–478
  management, 478
  outcome, 478
  pathophysiology, 477–478
Pulmonary hypertension, 132, 581
Pulmonary hypoplasia, 103–104,
      477
  definition, 477
  diagnosis, 477
  management, 477
  outcome, 477
  pathophysiology, 477
Pulmonary interstitial emphysema
      (PIE), 475–477
  appearance, 276f
  clinical presentation/diagnosis,
      476
  management, 477
  radiographic evaluation, 275
Pulmonary lymphatic system,
      impact, 463
Pulmonary parenchymal disease
  impact, 464
  radiographic evaluation, 275–278

Pulmonary stenosis (PS), 287, 564–565
  anatomy, 564
  clinical manifestations, 564–565
  hemodynamics, 564
  illustration, 564f
  incidence, 564
  management, 565
  prognosis, 565
Pulmonary valve atresia, 287
Pulmonary vascularity
  appearance, 284f
  increase, 285–287
  radiographic evaluation, 284–285
Pulmonary vascular resistance
  (PVR)
  decrease, 75, 464
  elevation, 463–464
  impact, 541
  increase, 579, 757
Pulmonary vasodilators, usage, 468
Pulmonary vasospasm, 581
Pulmonary venous congestion, 560–562
Pulmonary vessels
  abnormality, 464
  Po$_2$ increase response, 77
Pulsed-dye laser, success, 824
Pulse oximetry, 83, 513
  availability, 99
  noninvasive/inexpensive
    characteristic, 551
  usage, 513, 576
Pulse volume, gradation, 549
Puncture site
  determination, 323, 329
  examination, 329
Pupillary reflex, 815
Pupils, 833
  characteristics, 834
  dilation, 842
  rigidity, 841
Pupils equal, round, and react to
  light (PERRL), 139
Purpuric macules, eruption, 827
Pustular melanosis, 135
Pustular rash, appearance, 826
Pustule, 817
PVL. *See* Periventricular
  leukomalacia
PVR. *See* Pulmonary vascular
  resistance
Pyloric sphincter, relaxation, 2
Pyloric stenosis, 289, 602–603
  definition, 602
  diagnosis, 602–603
  etiology, 602
  incidence, 602
  medical repair, 603
  postoperative care, 603
  preoperative care, 603
  prognosis, 603
  surgical repair, 603

Q

Q-switched laser, usage, 822
Quad screen tests, 403–404

Qualitative research, 854
Quality
  improvement, attainment, 431–432
  indicators, 431
  management. *See* Total quality
    management
Quality assurance
  activities, 871
  protective shield, 871
  risk management, relationship,
    871
Quality of life, case analysis model
  component, 863
Quantitative research, 853–854

R

Rad, definition, 271
Radial artery catheterization
  advanced practice procedure,
    318–320
  complications, 320
  equipment/supplies, 318
  indications, 318
  precaution, 318
  procedure, 318–320
Radial artery puncture
  advanced practice procedure,
    322–324
  complications, 324
  equipment/supplies, 323
  indications, 322–323
  precautions, 323
  procedure, 323–324
Radiant energy, heat transfer, 114
Radiation, 114
Radio frequency identification
  (RFID), 370
Radiographic densities, 272
  differentiation, 272
Radiographic evaluation
  basic concepts, 270
  densities/shapes, comparison,
    270
  diagnostic imaging, 296–298
  terminology, 270–271
Radiographic examination, risks,
  272
Radiographs, imagery, 270
Radiologic studies, 593
Radiolucent, definition, 271
Radionuclide renal scans, usage,
  730
Radiopaque, definition, 271
Random medication level, 234
Rapid eye movement (REM), EEG
  characteristics, 211
Rastelli procedure, 568
RBCs. *See* Red blood cells
RDE. *See* Rule of double effect
Reactive hypoglycemia, 176
Reactive NST, 10
Read-backs, definition, 362b
Real-time echnocardiography, 552
Rebound tachycardia, fetal heart
  monitoring, 25
Receiving facility, arrival, 426

Receiving hospital, planning, 425–426
Receptor-medication complexes
  cell membrane permeability,
    change, 234
  gene expression regulation, 234
  second messenger molecule,
    intracellular concentration
    (increase), 234–235
  types, 234–235
Receptors, concept, 234
Recessive gene, definition, 400
Recessiveness, 400
Recombinant hematopoietic growth
  factors, 690
Rectal-genital GBS, screening, 11
Rectal medication administration,
  237
Red blood cells (RBCs), 668–669
  count, 668
    increase, 5
  function, 668
  indices, 669
    evaluation, 691
  metabolism, inherited disorders,
    627
  usage. *See* Packed red blood cells
Red tube (laboratory specimen
  tube), 257
Reference ranges. *See* Laboratory
  tests
Referral call, 422–424
  information, obtaining, 424
Referral hospital, stabilization, 424–425
Referring hospital, planning, 424
Reflex development, procession,
  215
Reflex stimulation, apnea cause,
  488
Reflux episodes, 620
Regional anesthetics
  assessment/management, 37–38
  complications, 37–38
  fetal/neonatal complications, 37
  management, 37–38
  maternal complications, 37
Registered nurses, transport
  involvement, 420
Regurgitation, minimization, 621–622
REM. *See* Rapid eye movement
Renal anatomy, 725
  gross anatomy, 725
Renal blood flow, 156, 726
  hormonal regulation, 726
  increase, 156
  medication excretion, 242
  regulation, 726
Renal cortical necrosis, 24
Renal disorders, 480
Renal excretion, improvement, 164
Renal failure, 161
  complication, 530
Renal function, monitoring, 251
Renal hemodynamics, 726
Renal losses, 157

Renal perfusion, decrease, 24
Renal physiology, 726–728
  acid-base balance, 728
  concentration, 728
  dilution mechanism, 728
  postnatal changes, 726–727
  tubular function, 727–728
Renal plasma flow, 726
  increase, 4
Renal system, urodynamic/
    hemodynamic changes
    (occurrence), 4
Renal tubular function, 156
Renal ultrasound, helpfulness, 730
Renal vein thrombosis, 178, 738–
    739
  diagnostic studies, 739
  outcome, 739
  patient care management, 739
  predisposing conditions, 738
  symptoms, clinical triad, 739
Renin-angiotensin-aldosterone
    system, 726
Reporting methods, 371
Repositioning, usage, 214
Research. See Neonatal research;
    Qualitative research;
    Quantitative research
  applications, 855b
  background, 852
  consumption, 817
  critique, 855b
  design
    bias control, levels, 853t
    types, 852
  ethics, nurse advocacy, 856–858
  evidence, levels, 856b
  findings
    application, 856
    usage, 855–856
  method, 852–853
  process, 851–853
    description, 850
    nursing process, similarities,
      852t
  question, 851
  sample, 852
  study, components, 851–853
  utilization, 856
  variables, 853
Research-based practice (Iowa
    Model), 857f
Residual anatomic lesions, 579
Resistance, definition, 243
RespiGam (RSV IGIV), usage, 474
Respiration
  evaluation, 98–99
  initiation, stimuli, 75
  physiologic changes, 78
  physiology, 455
Respiratory acidosis, 84, 104
  measurement, 517
Respiratory alkalosis,
    measurement, 517
Respiratory augmentation, 77
Respiratory changes, 3
Respiratory clinical signs, 700–701

Respiratory compromise,
    precipitation, 95
Respiratory disease, infant risk
    (identification), 130–132
Respiratory disorders, 455–475
  apnea cause, 487
Respiratory distress, 27, 453
  assessment, Silverman-Andersen
    scale (usage), 511f
  cardiovascular disorders, impact,
    480
  causes, 280, 478–480
  CNS disorders, impact, 480
  diaphragmatic disorders, impact,
    480
  hematologic disorders, impact,
    480
  lung development, 453–455
    anatomic events, 453–454
    antenatal steroids, role, 455
    biochemical events, 454–455
  renal disorders, impact, 480
  thoracic disorders, impact, 479–
    480
  upper airway disorders, impact,
    478–479
Respiratory distress syndrome
    (RDS), 122, 160, 455–459
  clinical presentation, 456–457
  complications, 457–458
  definition, 455
  diagnosis, 457
  differential diagnosis, 457
  etiology, 456
  incidence, 455–456
  management, 458–459
  mimicking, 457
  pathophysiology, 456
  prevention, 459
  radiographic evaluation, 275
  reticulogranular pattern,
    similarity, 278
  timing, treatment methods, 458–
    459
Respiratory losses, 158
Respiratory pattern, 546
Respiratory rate/pattern, changes,
    300
Respiratory situations, 103–104
Respiratory support. See Extremely
    low birth weight infants
  requirement, 502–505
Respiratory syncytial virus
    immune globulin (RSVIG),
    715
Respiratory syncytial virus (RSV),
    459, 714–715
  presentation, 714–715
  prevalence, 714
  prophylaxis, 715
    benefits, 474
  treatment, 715
Respiratory system
  maternal physiologic changes,
    2–3
  radiographic evaluation, 274–
    275

Respiratory therapists, transport
    involvement, 420
Respondeat superior, 870
Resuscitation. See Neonatal
    resuscitation
  bag, attachment, 306
  care. See Postresuscitation care
  complications, 107
  devices, 99
  documentation, 108
  equipment, availability, 435
  ethics, 109
  safety, 108
  therapies, controversy, 109
Retained fetal lung fluid, 277
  infant risk, 462–463
Retained lung fluid, 84
  syndromes, 462–463
Reticulogranular lung pattern,
    275f
Retina, 833
  avascular characteristic, 840
Retinal detachment, 25
Retinoic acid, usage, 543
Retinopathy
  progression, 26
  stages, 841–842
Retinopathy of prematurity (ROP),
    218, 840
  blinding complications, 844
  blood/fluid leakage, 841
  classification zones, 842
  complications, 844
  cryotherapy, 844
    nursing care, 844
  description, 841
  documentation, 842
  etiology, 841
  follow-up, 842
  incidence, 841
  laser photocoagulation, 843
  outcome, 844
  pathophysiology, 840–841
  physical examination, 842
  prevention, 843
  risk, 300
    factors, 841
  screening, 444
  sensory stimulation, 843
  treatment, 843–844
  vitreoretinal surgery, 844
  zones, 842f
Retrolental fibroplasia, 840
Reuptake, 53–54
RFID. See Radio frequency
    identification
Rh incompatibility, 175, 674–675
Rh-negative blood, usage, 102
RhoGAM, 674–675
Rib fractures, occurrence, 294
Right atrium blood, 74
Right lung, cystic adenomatoid
    malformation (appearance),
    283f
Right mainstem bronchus,
    endotracheal tube
    (placement), 295f

Right-sided cardiac pressures, invasive monitoring, 577
Right ventricle blood, 74
Right ventricular afterload, reduction, 580
Risk management, 871
  activities, protective shield, 871
  internal systematic process, 871
  quality assurance, relationship, 871
Ritodrine (Yutopar), IV administration, 29
Ritter disease, 827
Robin sequence, 103
Rocker bottom feet, 150
Roentgen, definition, 271
Role-model caregiving techniques, 358
Rooting reflex, 152
ROP. *See* Retinopathy of prematurity
Rotation, definition, 271
Routine care, 212–213
RSV. *See* Respiratory syncytial virus
RSVIG. *See* Respiratory syncytial virus immune globulin
Rubella virus, 713–714
Ruby laser, usage, 822
Rule of double effect (RDE), 861
Rush disease, 842

S

Sacral agenesis, 160
Sacrococcygeal teratoma, 149
Safe practices, NQF identification, 368–369
Safety briefings, definition, 362b
Safety discharge topics, selection, 379–380
Sail sign
  creation, 279
  demonstration, 280f
Salivary glands, medication excretion, 241
Salt losing, 810
Salt-wasting disease, 652
Sampling-induced anemia, minimization strategies, 262
Sampling-induced infection, minimization strategies, 261
Sampling-induced organ/nerve injury, minimization strategies, 262
Sampling-induced pain, minimization strategies, 260–261
Sampling-induced physiologic stress, minimization strategies, 260
Sampling-induced skin injury, minimization strategies, 261
SBAR. *See* Situation, background, assessment, and recommendation
Scalded skin syndrome, 827
Scalp lacerations, 820

Scaphoid abdomen, 131
Scarf sign, 125
School-age ECMO survivors, 532
Sclera, 782
Scoliosis, 149
Screening blood glucose test, 80
Screening tests, 403. *See also* Quad screen tests; Triple screen tests
Searching nystagmus, 837
Sebaceous glands, 813
  hyperplasia, 819
Secondary apnea, 485
  definition, 485
Secondary hypothyroidism, 643
Second heart sound, 547
Second messenger molecule, intracellular concentration (increase), 234–235
Second pain, association, 335
Second-stage management, 17
Second-trimester biochemical marker screening, 9
Second-trimester ultrasound, 9
Second victim, recognition (absence), 373
Secretory glands, changes, 3
Sedation, 584
Sedatives, 52–53, 246–247
  breastfeeding impact, 65
  fetus/neonate effects, 53
  impact, 344
  pharmacology, 52
  pregnancy effects, 53
  use, incidence, 52
Seizures, 771–774
  clinical presentation, 772
  definition, 771
  diagnostic evaluation, 772–773
  fosphenytoin, usage, 773–774
  incidence, 772
  Lorazepam, usage, 774
  outcome, 774
  pathophysiology, 772
  patient care management, 773–774
  phenobarbital, usage, 773
  phenytoin, usage, 773
  precautions, 25
  prevention, 25
  risk factors, 771–772
Selective serotonin reuptake inhibitors (SSRIs), 53–54
Self-insurance, implication, 879
Semicircular canals, 846
Semisynthetic opioids, 50
Senning procedures, 568
Sensorineural hearing loss, 839, 847
Sensory afferents, 798
Sensory cells, 846
Sensory-motor-oral stimulation, 202–203
Sensory stimulation, 794
Sepsis. *See* Neonatal sepsis
  diagnostic evaluation, 83
  ELBW deaths, 441
  impact, 311

Sepsis *(Continued)*
  infection, 194
  neonatal infection, 706
  variable nonspecific presentation, 700
Septic shock, indicators, 583
Septum primum, formation, 537f
Septum secundum, formation, 537f
Sequence, definition, 409
Serial NST, 25
Seronegative pregnant women, infant care (avoidance), 840
Serum bile acids, 595
Serum blood glucose levels, 179
Serum calcium
  levels, decrease, 5
  transportation, 165
Serum creatinine, 25
Serum glucose determination, 83
Serum glutamate-pyruvate transaminase (SGPT), 193
Serum glutamic-oxaloacetic transaminase (SGOT), increase, 193
Serum integrated biochemical marker screening, 8
Serum Na, acute drops, 162
Servocontrolled driving pressure, 507
Severe dehydration, management, 159
Sex chromosomes
  abnormalities, 792–794
  definition, 400
Sexual development, disorders, 655–662
Sexual differentiation, 655
Sexually transmitted diseases (STDs), presence, 47, 51
Sexually transmitted infections (STIs), 14t–15t
  maternal infection, 11
  presence, 47, 51
SGOT. *See* Serum glutamic-oxaloacetic transaminase
SGPT. *See* Serum glutamate-pyruvate transaminase
Shaken baby syndrome
  definition, 393b
  prevention, 392
Sharps program, 720
Shock, 581–584. *See also* Cardiogenic shock; Distributive shock; Hypovolemic shock
  blood volume
    inadequacy, 581
    indicators, 582–583
  cardiac function, indicators, 583
  cardiopulmonary status, changes, 582
  clinical indicators, 582–583
  coagulation defects, evidence, 582
  corticosteroids, usage, 584
  digitalis, consideration, 584

Shock (*Continued*)
Dobutamine (Dobutrex), usage, 584
dopamine, usage, 583–584
etiology, 581–582
indicators. *See* Septic shock
inotropic agents, usage, 583
Isoproterenol (Isuprel), usage, 583
management, 583–584
metabolic disturbances, 582
Milrinone, benefits, 584
nonspecific signs, 582
pathogenesis, 583
supportive care, 583
therapies, 583–584
treatment goals, 584
urinary output, decrease, 582
Short-acting barbiturates, replacement, 52
Short bowel syndrome, 615–617
care, 616–617
considerations, 615–616
definition, 615
diagnosis, 616
etiology, 615
incidence, 616
medical management, 616
prognosis, 616
surgical management, 616–617
Shoulder dystocia, 33–34, 123
assessment/management, 34
clinical presentation, 33
complications, 33–34
etiology/predisposing factors, 33
fetal/neonatal complications, 33–34
impact, 178
incidence, 33
maternal complications, 33
McRoberts, usage, 34
Wood corkscrew maneuver, usage, 34
Zavanelli maneuver, performing, 34
Shunt study, 465
SIADH. *See* Syndrome of inappropriate antidiuretic hormone
Siblings
infant death, information, 356
perinatal loss, information, 356
visitation, encouragement, 358
Sick infant
birth, crisis, 347–349
caregivers, usage, 358
crisis, discussion, 348–349
psychologic tasks, 348
Sickle cell anemia, ethnic predisposition, 7
Sick newborn infant
acute hypovolemic shock, 85
air leak, 84
anemia, 85
antibiotics, usage, 88
arterial blood gas determination, 83
blood glucose, examination, 87

Sick newborn infant (*Continued*)
cardiovascular problems, 85
clinical findings, 85
cardiovascular system, physical assessment, 82
chest x-ray examination, 83
clinical findings, 84
clinical presentation, 83–87
CNS, physical assessment, 82
complete blood cell count, 83
computed tomography, 83
congenital anomalies, 86–87
congenital heart disease, 85
delivery complications, 82
diagnostic tools, 83
echocardiography, 83
electrocardiography, 83
GI tract, physical assessment, 82
glucose
IV administration, 88
oral administration, 87–88
supply, 87–88
handling, excess (avoidance), 87
hematocrit determination, 83
hemodynamics, 85
hypoglycemia, 86
infection, 86
initial stabilization, 87–88
lumbar puncture, 83
magnetic resonance imaging, 83
maternal illnesses, 82
maternal medications, adverse effects, 86
metabolic problems, 86
morphologic features, 82
Naloxone hydrochloride (Narcan), administration, 88
neutral thermal environment, providing, 87
NICU transfer, 87
orogastric tube, passage, 83
oxygen
saturation, peripheral monitoring, 83
supply, 88
pathophysiologic sequelae, 84
physical assessment, 82
polycythemia, 85
problems, 83–87
pulmonary problems, 84–85
pulse oximetry, 83
recognition, 82–88
respiratory system, physical assessment, 82
sepsis, diagnostic evaluation, 83
serum glucose determination, 83
short-term observation, transition nursery, 87
skin, physical assessment, 82
substance abuse, medications/history, 82
transillumination, 83
ultrasonographic-biophysical profile, 82
ultrasonography, 83
urine sample collection, 83
volume expanders, supply, 88

Sick newborn infant (*Continued*)
white blood cells, differential examination, 83
whole-blood glucose screening test, 83
SIDS. *See* Sudden infant death syndrome
Silicone rubber, development, 521
Silverman-Andersen scale, 511f
Simple meconium ileus, 607
Simple virilizing, 651
SIMV. *See* Synchronized intermittent mandatory ventilation
Single-dimension echocardiography, 552
Single gene disorders, 783
Single gestation, multiple gestation (contrast), 121
Single-mutant-gene syndromes, 542
Single vessel, extension, 537–538
Sinusoidal FHR pattern, 30
Sirenomelia, 590
SIRS. *See* Systematic inflammatory response syndrome
Situation, background, assessment, and recommendation (SBAR), 366
Six Sigma, 374
Size classification, determination, 130
Skeletal changes, maternal physiologic changes, 5
Skeletal defects, 26–27
Skeletal system
anatomic/pathologic x-ray changes, 274
radiographic evaluation, 293–294
Skeleton articulation, 215
Skin
acidic surface, 814
anatomy, 813–815
appearance, factors, 816–817
bacteriostatic properties, decrease, 815
care. *See* Extremely low birth weight infants
chemical/bacterial function, 814
colonization, reduction, 816
disinfection, 784
emollient creams, benefit, 816
flap, closure, 598
fragility. *See* Very low birth weight
functions, 814
fungal infection, 826
gestational age, impact, 816
heat regulation, 814
injury
impact, 261
prevention, 176
integrity, infection/loss, 326
layers, 814f
anatomy, 813–814
lesions, 817–830. *See also* Pigmented skin lesions
description, 817

Skin *(Continued)*
  maternal physiologic changes, 3
  maturation, 814
  mechanical function, 814
  occlusive barriers, application, 118
  oxygenation status, 817
  permeability. *See* Immature skin increase, 816
  physical examination, 126
  physical protection, 814
  physiologic changes, 77–78
  physiology, 813–815
  structures, 814f
  tags, presence, 847
  temperature, 110
    monitoring, continuation, 111
  thermistors, attachment, 111
  variations, 817–820
  vascularity, degree, 157
Skinfold, definition, 271
Skin-to-skin holding, 213–214, 220
Skull
  deformities, risk (increase), 43
  views, 137f
Skull fractures, 27, 763–764
  clinical presentation, 764
  diagnostic evaluation, 764
  incidence, 764
  outcome, 764
  pathophysiology, 763
  patient care management, 764
  radiographic evaluation, 294
Sleep guidelines, 391b
Sleep states, 486–487
  EEG characteristics, 211
Sleep-wake behavior, touch (synchronization), 214
Sleep-wake behavioral organization, 221
Small bowel
  abnormalities, 290–291
  follow-through, 298
  motility, decrease, 2
Small-bowel atresia, 290
Small-for-gestational-age (SGA) infants
  hypoglycemia, incidence, 173
  outcomes, 161
Small left colon syndrome, 291
Smart infusion pumps, usage, 369
Smith-Lemli-Opitz syndrome, 657
Smoking
  breastfeeding impact, 64
  incidence, 42–43
  neurobehavioral effects, 43
Sniffing death, 53
Soap bubble appearance, 290
Social-cultural structure, 350–351
Social history, 120–121
Sodium bicarbonate, base buffer, 102
Sodium filtration, increase, 4
Sodium (Na), 161–163
  balance. *See* Positive Na balance
  fluid restriction, 162
  functions, 161–162

Sodium (Na) *(Continued)*
  homeostasis, 161–162
  laboratory assessment, 203
  monitoring, 162
  regulation, 162
Sodium polystyrene sulfonate (Kayexalate), impact, 165
Soft/loose bedding/objects, usage (avoidance), 216
Soft tissue
  dystocia, absence, 34
  palpation, 138
Somatostatin, 176
  presence, 183
So what question, answering, 263
SP-A (SP-D). *See* Hydrophilic surfactant proteins A/D
SP-B (SP-C). *See* Hydrophobic surfactant proteins B/C
Special-needs infants
  discharge, 385
  home readiness, 394b
  human milk/commercial formulas, 194–199
Special transport stabilization considerations, 426–427
Specimen. *See* Laboratory specimens
Speech delay, 219
Spherocytosis, 691
Sphingomyelin concentration, stability, 454
Spider angiomas, appearance, 3
Spina bifida, 26–27, 799–800
  associated findings, 799
  clinical presentation, 799
  diagnosis, 799
  incidence/etiology, 799
  treatment, 799–800
Spinal anesthesia, 37
Spinal cord, acute pain physiology, 335
Spinal immobilization. *See* Very low birth weight
Spironolactone (Aldactone), usage, 515
Spontaneous abortions, 43
  number, 6
Spontaneously breathing neonate, ventilation (control factors), 498b
Spontaneous movement, observation, 152
Sprintzen syndrome, 791–792
Square window, 124
SSIs. *See* Surgical site infections
SSRIs. *See* Selective serotonin reuptake inhibitors
Standard of care, 866–869. *See also* Negligence
  articulation, requirement, 867
  determination, 875
  ethical standards, 868–869
  expert witness testimony, 867–868
  federal regulations, 867

Standard of care *(Continued)*
  institutional policies/procedures/protocols, 867
  practice guidelines, 868–869
  state regulations, 867
Standard of professional organizations, 868
Stapedius muscles, 846
Staphylococcal scalded skin syndrome, 136
Staphylococcus aureus, 835
  coagulase-positive organism, 710
Startle reflex, 153
State subsystem functioning, infant abilities/sensitivities/thresholds, 209
Statistical significance, 853–854
Steady state, definition, 234
Stenosis, 290
Stepping reflex, 153
Sterile-water test feeding, 81
Steroids
  synthesis, 649
  usage, 473
Stimulants, 46–49
Stomach
  abnormalities, 289
  dilation, excess, 289
  positioning, correction (verification), 201
  radiographic evaluation, 289
  tone, loss, 2
  transpyloric tube feeding, bypass, 202
Stools
  blood, presence, 200
  examination, 593
  losses, 158
Stork bite, 823
Storytelling, definition, 362b
Stratum corneum, 813
  barrier effectiveness, 436
Strawberry hemangioma, 135–136, 824–825
  photograph, 825f
  size, increase, 825
  treatment, 825
Stress
  hormones, concentration, 75
  minimization, environmental modification, 227
Stretch marks, occurrence, 3
Striae gravidarum (stretch marks), occurrence, 3
Stroke volume, fixation, 541
Structural heart defects, impact, 574
Structural renal changes, 3–4
Stuart factor (factor X), 79
Sturge-Weber syndrome, 152, 824
  photograph, 824f
Subconjunctival hemorrhage, 784
Subcutaneous fat
  accumulation, 815
  insulation, 113
  necrosis, 820
    hypercalcemia, association, 820

Subcutaneous medication administration, 238
Subcutaneous microdialysis, 175
Subdural hemorrhage, 766–767
  clinical presentation, 767
  definition, 766
  diagnostic evaluation, 767
  incidence, 766
  outcome, 767
  pathophysiology, 766
  risk factors, 766
Subgaleal hemorrhage, 138, 763
  clinical presentation, 763
  diagnostic evaluation, 763
  incidence, 763
  outcome, 763
  pathophysiology, 763
  patient care management, 763
Subglottic stenosis, 306
Substances, radiodensities, 272
Substance use, medications/history, 82
Substance use disorders
  female characteristics, 66b
  psychologic profile, 66b
Subtle seizure, 772
Subtotal pancreatectomy, severity, 176
Subtotal retinal detachment, 793
Sucking pressure, 222
Sucking reflex, 152
Sucking rhythms, stability (increase), 223
Suck-swallow-breathe coordination, demonstration, 202
Suck-swallow-breathe sequence, coordination (increase), 221
Suck-swallow pattern, encouragement, 221
Suction catheter, determination, 301
Suctioning protocols, 503
Suction passes, number (limitation), 301
Sudden infant death syndrome (SIDS), 484
  incidence, 215–218
  increase, 43
  information, resource, 218
  reduction, 218
  strategies, 379
Superficial vesiculopustular lesions, rupture, 822
Superior vena cava (SVC)
  blood flow, 72–74
  unoxygenated blood return, 74
Supernumerary nipples, 143
Supine hypotension, maternal cardiac output (decrease), 23
Supplemental humidity, usage, 160
Supplemental oxygen
  initiation, 99
  maintenance, 438
Suprapubic pressure, application, 34
Surface absorptive properties, impact, 114
Surface-active phospholipids, presence, 454

Surface-area-to-weight ratio, increase, 113
Surfactant
  FDA approval, 458
  lipoprotein, 77
  medications, 513–516
  mixture, 454
  proteins, groups, 454
  replacement, 467
    therapy, 458–459
  secretion, 74
Surfactant/albumin ratio, measurement, 10–11
Surgical site infections (SSIs), 378
Surveillance plans, implementation (consideration), 267
Sutures
  illustration, 761f
  palpation, 136–138
Suxamethonium (succinylcholine) (Anectine), usage, 304
SVR. *See* Systemic vascular resistance
Sweat glands, 813
  medication excretion, 241
  presence, 815
Sympathetic nervous system, compensation, 337–338
Sympathomimetic amines, 245
Synchronized intermittent mandatory ventilation (SIMV), 473, 501–502
Syndrome, definition, 408, 783b
Syndrome of inappropriate antidiuretic hormone (SIADH), 161, 641
  management. *See* True SIADH
Synthetic opioids, 50
Syphilis, 719–720
  diagnosis, 719
  presentation, 719
  treatment, 720
Systematic inflammatory response syndrome (SIRS), 462
Systemic Candida infection, 826
Systemic corticosteroid therapy, usage, 825–826
Systemic hypotension, 104
Systemic opioids, analgesia induction, 343
Systemic vascular resistance (SVR), impact, 541
Systemic venous blood, right atrium entry, 75
Systemic venous return, inadequacy, 579
Systems approach, 363
Systolic murmurs, 548
  diagram, 144f
Systolic thrill, 561

T

Tachycardia, 30, 143
  cocaine, impact, 46
  hemodynamic management, 578
  mechanism, effectiveness, 541

Tachykinin receptors, afferent fiber neurotransmitter stimulation, 335
Tachyphylaxis, 235
Tachypnea, 142
Tactile sensations, 213–214
Talipes calcaneovalgus, 150, 806
  associated findings, 806
  clinical findings, 806
  diagnosis, 806
  incidence/etiology, 806
  treatment, 806
Talipes equinovarus, 150, 802–803
  associated anomalies, 803
  clinical presentation, 802–803
  diagnosis, 803
  incidence/etiology, 802
  treatment, 803
TALLman lettering, definition, 362b
TAPVR. *See* Total anomalous pulmonary venous return
TAR. *See* Thrombocytopenia with absent radii
Target cells, 691
Tay-Sachs, ethnic predisposition, 7
TBAs. *See* Thyroid-blocking antibodies
TBW. *See* Total body water
TCAs. *See* Tricylcic antidepressants
T-connector device, flushing, 308
TDM. *See* Therapeutic drug monitoring
Teamwork, methods (effectiveness), 366
Tears, secretion, 836
TEF. *See* Tracheoesophageal fistula
Temperature
  conversion, 882
  gradient, impact, 114
  infant physiologic response, 111
  monitoring, 78, 110
Temporal bone, petrous portion, 797
TENS. *See* Transcutaneous electrical nerve stimulation
Tensor tympani, 846
Teratogens, 543
  disorders, 783–784
  exposure, 7
Terbutaline (Brethine), subcutaneous administration, 29
Terminal air spaces, surface-active phospholipids (presence), 454
Term infants
  blood values, 668t
  carbohydrate, impact, 187
  commercially prepared formulas, 196t
  delivery failure, acknowledgment, 348
  energy/caloric intake requirements, 187
  fat, intake, 187
  fluid requirements, 186

Term infants *(Continued)*
  fluoride supplementation, 187
  formulas, commercial
    preparation, 195
  human milk/commercial
    formulas, 194–199
  iron supplementation,
    recommendation (absence),
    187
  leukocyte values, 670t
  milk, usage, 195
  minerals, intake, 187
  nutritional requirements, 186–190
    list, 186t
  protein, impact, 187
  tears, secretion, 836
  trace elements, intake, 187
  vitamins, impact, 187
Term neonate, hyperbilirubinemia
    (management), 631t
Term newborn infant, skin care, 815
Term pregnancy, terminology, 1
Term well newborns, risk
    designation, 626f
Tertiary hypothyroidism, 643
Testis-determining gene (SRY), 655
Tests, utilization. *See* Laboratory
    tests
Tetralogy of Fallot (TOF), 287, 562–
    564
  anatomy, 563
  clinical manifestations, 563
  hemodynamics, 563
  illustration, 563f
  incidence, 562
  management, 563–564
  prognosis, 564
TEWL. *See* Transepidermal water
    loss
TF. *See* Tissue factor
Thalidomide, usage, 543
Thanatophoric dwarf, appearance,
    295f
Theophylline
  caffeine, contrast, 491
  dosage, 490
  usage, 514
Therapeutic drug monitoring
    (TDM), definition, 234
Therapeutic interventions,
    laboratory data
    interpretation (importance),
    264–268
Therapeutic range, definition, 233
Therapeutic touch, tactile
    sensations, 213–214
Thermal afferents, 486
Thermal controlled environment,
    weaning, 118
Thermal cover. *See* Neonatal
    transport incubator
Thermal homeostasis, maintenance,
    302
Thermal instability, 110
  definition, 110
  infant risk, identification, 110–
    111, 130–132

Thermal receptor stimulation, 113
Thermal stability, 106
Thermal stress, symptoms, 112b
Thermal support, continuation, 98
Thermal window blinds, usage,
    116
Thermogenesis. *See* Nonshivering
    thermogenesis
Thermogenin, 113
Thermoregulation, 110. *See also*
    Extremely low birth weight
    infants
  heat loss/gain/production,
    balance, 111–113
  management strategies, 114–118
  physiology, 111–113
Thermoregulation considerations,
    78–79
Thermoregulatory instability, 700
Thermoregulatory problem, 114–
    118
Third heart sound, 547
Third-stage V time, 17
Thoracentesis, 256–257
  advanced practice procedure,
    307
  complications, 307
  equipment/supplies, 307
  indications, 307
  procedure, 307
  requirement, 104
Thoracic disorders, 479–480
Thoracic surgical problems,
    radiographic evaluation,
    281–284
3,4-Methylenedioxymetham-
    phetamine (MDMA), 48–49
  fetus, effects, 49
  incidence, 48
  neonate
    effects, 49
    withdrawal, 49
  nursing considerations, 49
  pharmacology, 49
  pregnancy effects, 49
Three-dimensional
    echocardiography, 552
Three-way transport, 418
Thrombocytopenia, 681–684
  clinical assessment, 683
  clinical presentation, 683
  complications, 683
  diagnostic studies, 683
  differential diagnosis, 683
  etiologic factors, 682–683
  impaired platelet production, 682
  infant management, 683–684
  neonatal conditions, 682
  outcome, 684
  physical examination, 683
  platelet destruction, 682
Thrombocytopenia with absent
    radii (TAR) syndrome, 682
Thrombopoietin (TPO), 666–667
Thrombosis, 27
  complication, 317
Thrush, 140, 826

Thymus
  anatomic/pathologic x-ray
    changes, 273
  radiographic evaluation, 274–275
Thyroid abnormalities, 643
Thyroid-binding globulin (TBG),
    641
  increase, 6
Thyroid-blocking antibodies
    (TBAs), production, 647
Thyroid dysgenesis, 643
Thyroid function testes, 645
Thyroid gland, 641–643
  anatomy, 641
  disorders, 641–649
  functions, 641
  metabolism, 641
  physiology, 641–642
  regulation, mechanisms, 642
Thyroid hormones
  physiologic effects, 642
  release (inhibition), lugol iodine
    (usage), 648
  transport, 641–642
Thyroid peroxidase (TPO), 641
  enzyme, defect, 643
  MMI inhibition, 648
  PTU inhibition, 648
Thyroid-stimulating hormone
    (TSH), release, 642
Thyroid-stimulating
    immunoglobulins (TSIs),
    production, 647
Thyrotoxicosis, manifestations, 648
Thyrotropin-releasing hormone
    (TRH), secretion, 642
Thyroxine (T$_4$), 641
  normalization, 646
  transplacental transfer, 6
Tidal volume (V$_T$), 504
  definition, 494
Time-cycled, pressure-limited,
    continuous-flow ventilator,
    501
Time Outs, definition, 362b
Tissue factor (TF), exposure, 671
Tissues
  infiltration, monitoring, 309
  radiodensities, 272
TLC. *See* Total lung capacity
T lymphocytes, migration, 697
Tobacco
  abuse, 42–43
  exposure, 121
TOF. *See* Tetralogy of Fallot
Tolerance, definition, 247
Tonic neck reflex, 152–153
Tonic seizure, 772
Topical medication administration,
    238
TORCH. *See* Toxoplasmosis others
    rubella cytomegalovirus
    infection and herpes simplex
Total anomalous pulmonary
    venous return (TAPVR),
    285–286, 570–571
  anatomy, 570–571

Total anomalous pulmonary
venous return (TAPVR)
(Continued)
clinical manifestations, 571
hemodynamics, 571
illustration, 570f
incidence, 570
management, 571
nonobstructed characteristic, 571
obstructed characteristic, 571
prognosis, 571
surgical treatment, 571
Total body water (TBW)
body compartment, 239
content, changes, 156
Total lung capacity (TLC),
definition, 494
Total pancreatectomy, severity, 176
Total parenteral nutrition (TPN), 310
management, 620
Total patient flow, 526
Total placenta previa, bleeding
(management), 32
Total quality management (TQM),
431–432
Total retinal detachment, 793
Total serum bilirubin (TSB)
level, elevation, 625–626
prediction, risk index, 627f
Touch
considerations, 214
usage, 213–214
Toxic epidermal necrolysis, 827
Toxicology screening, obtaining, 58
Toxic reaction, complication/
management, 38
Toxic substances, presence, 254
Toxoplasmosis, 719, 837, 840–844
clinical presentation, 840
etiology, 840
incidence, 840
nursing care, 840
outcome, 840
pathophysiology, 840
Toxoplasmosis others rubella
cytomegalovirus infection
and herpes simplex
(TORCH) infections, 12t–13t,
122
maternal infection, 11
T-Piece Resuscitator, 501
T-piece resuscitator, usage, 306
TPO. *See* Thrombopoietin; Thyroid
peroxidase
TQM. *See* Total quality
management
Trace, proteinuria, 4
Trachea
anatomic/pathologic x-ray
changes, 273
perforation, 306
radiographic evaluation, 275
Trachea, obstruction, 479
Tracheal aspirate specimens,
obtaining, 300
Tracheal suctioning/lavage,
requirement, 302

Tracheobronchial secretions,
clearance, 300
Tracheobronchial tree, immature
ciliary system, 460
Tracheoesophageal fistula (TEF),
26–27, 104, 479, 600–602
definition, 600
diagnosis, 601
esophageal fistula, absence, 289
etiology, 600
incidence, 600
postoperative care, 602
postoperative complications,
602
preoperative care, 601
prognosis, 601
surgical repair, 601
types, 600
Tracheostomy tube, usage, 503
Transcutaneous electrical nerve
stimulation (TENS), 35
Transepidermal water loss
(TEWL)
decrease, double-walled
incubators (usage), 440
estimation, 440–441
increase, 113, 157
occurrence, 157
prevention, 160
reduction, 160, 163
Transesophageal echo, 552
Transfusion therapies, 686–690
albumin, usage, 690
consent, recommendation, 686
cryoprecipitate, usage, 690
exchange transfusions, 689
FFP, usage, 689–690
fluid overload, 687
graft-*versus*-host disease, 687
granulocytes, usage, 690
infection, 687
informed consent, 687–689
partial exchange transfusions,
689
platelets, usage, 689
PRBCs, usage, 689
reactions, 687
risks, 687
volumes, 689–690
Transient bradycardia, fetal heart
monitoring, 25
Transient hypothyroidism, 646–647
outcome, 647
Transient hypothyroid states,
etiologies, 643
Transient neonatal diabetes, 179–
180
clinical presentation, 180
complications, 180
definition, 179
incidence, 180
management, 180
outcomes, 180
pathophysiology, 180
Transient neonatal pustular
melanosis, 822
Transient tachypnea, 277f

Transient tachypnea of the
newborn (TTN), 457, 462–463
clinical presentation, 462
definition, 462
diagnosis, 463
differential diagnosis, 463
etiology, 462
incidence, 462
management, 463
origination, 463
outcome, 463
pathophysiology, 462–463
radiographic evaluation, 277
supportive management, 463
Transillumination, 83
Transition
multidisciplinary approach, 387
parent teaching, 89
Transitional premature infant
formulas, 199
Transition nursery
assessment/observation, 77–78
clinical changes, 77
feeding guidelines, 81
infant transfer, 81
medications, 79–80
ongoing teaching, 81
routine care considerations, 77–
81
short-term observation, 87
Translocation. *See* Chromosome 21
definition, 402
Transmission-based precautions,
720–721
Transparency
model, incorporation, 863–864
process, 372–373
Transports. *See* Air transport;
Back/return transport;
Interfacility neonatal
transport; International
transport; Intrafacility
neonatal transport; One-way
transports; Out-of-state
transport; Three-way
transport; Two-way
transport
crew, hydration/nutrition (plan),
430
EMTs/paramedics, involvement,
421
equipment, 421–422
battery power, 422
selection, 424
neonatal nurse practitioners,
involvement, 420
personnel, 419–421
roles, 420
physicians, involvement, 420
programs, safety priority, 428
registered nurses, involvement,
420
respiratory therapists,
involvement, 420
stabilization considerations. *See*
Special transport
stabilization considerations

Transports (*Continued*)
  supplies, selection, 424
  team
    composition, considerations, 420–421
    expertise, 421
    family support, 425
    members, selection/ notification, 424
  types, 417–418
Transport vehicles
  communication equipment, 429
  considerations, 418–419
  dispatch, 424
  electrical outlets, type/ grounding (evaluation), 422
  lights/sirens (usage), written policy (establishment), 429
  selection, 418–419, 424
  survival/first-aid kit, location, 428
Transpyloric tube feeding, 202
Transthoracic echo, 552
Transvaginal/transabdominal sampling, 405
Trash disposal, 721
Trauma, 107
  impact, 820–821
Traumatic facial nerve palsy, 766
  clinical presentation, 766
  incidence, 766
  outcome, 766
  pathophysiology, 766
  patient care management, 766
TRH. *See* Thyrotropin-releasing hormone
Tricuspid atresia, 287, 566–567
  anatomy, 566–567
  clinical manifestations, 567
  hemodynamics, 567
  illustration, 566f
  incidence, 566
  management, 567
Tricylcic antidepressants (TCAs), 54
Triggering reflexes, avoidance, 489
Triggers, 372
Triiodothyronine (T$_3$), 641
  transplacental transfer, 6
Trimesters, terminology, 1
Trimethadione (fetal trimethoadione syndrome), 543
Triple screen tests, 403–404
Trisomies, 411–412
Trisomy 13, 413–414, 543, 790–791
  associated findings, 791
  care management, 414
  clinical presentation, 413–414, 790
  complications/outcome, 414
  diagnosis, 791
  etiology, 413, 790
  genetic ambiguity, relationship, 657
  genetic screening, 9
  history, 590

Trisomy 13 (*Continued*)
  incidence, 413, 790
  treatment, 791
Trisomy 18, 403, 413, 543, 788–790
  associated findings, 788
  care management, 413
  clinical presentation, 413, 788
  complications/outcome, 413
  diagnosis, 788–790
  etiology, 413, 788
  female neonates, 789f
  genetic screening, 9
  history, 590
  incidence, 413, 788
  precipitating factors, 413
  treatment, 790
Trisomy 21 (Down Syndrome), 403, 411–412, 543
  associated findings, 787
  chromosome abnormality, 786–788
  clinical presentation, 412, 786–787
  complications/outcome, 412
  diagnosis, 787
  frequency, 644
  history, 590
  incidence/etiology, 411–412, 786
  treatment, 788
Trophic feeding, 184
  minimum, 199–200
Trophic hormones, release, 640
Trophoblastic tissue, transabdominal/ transvaginal aspiration, 9
Trough medication level, 234
True SIADH, management, 162
Truncal incurvation reflex (Galant reflex), 153
Truncal septation, developmental abnormalities, 538–539
Truncus arteriosus, 286, 569–570
  anatomy, 569
  clinical manifestations, 569
  closure, 538f
  extension, 537–538
  hemodynamics, 569
  illustration, 569f
  incidence, 569
  management, 570
  prognosis, 570
  transformation, 540f
TSH. *See* Thyroid-stimulating hormone
TSIs. *See* Thyroid-stimulating immunoglobulins
TTN. *See* Transient tachypnea of the newborn
T-tube, illustration, 608f
Tuberculin (TB) syringe, usage, 307
Tuberous sclerosis, 152
  pigmented nevi, association, 822
Tubes/catheters, anatomic/ pathologic x-ray changes, 274
Tubular reabsorption, medication excretion, 242–243

Tubular secretion, medication excretion, 242
Tubuloglomerular feedback mechanism, 726
Tumor, 817
Turner syndrome, 792–793
  associated anomalies, 792
  clinical presentation, 792
  diagnosis, 792
  incidence/etiology, 792
  treatment, 792–793
22q11.2 deletion syndrome, 791–792
  associated findings, 791
  clinical presentation, 791
  diagnosis, 792
  incidence/etiology, 791
  treatment, 792
Twin-to-twin transfusion, 122
Twin-twin transfusion, 670
Two-dimensional echocardiography, 552
Two-way transport, 417–418
Tympanic membrane, 845–846
  thermometry, 110
Tyrosine, solubility (limitation), 192

U

UAC. *See* Umbilical artery catheterization
UACs. *See* Umbilical arterial catheters
uE3. *See* Unconjugated estriol
Ulcer, 817
Ultrasonographic-biophysical profile, 82
Ultrasonography, 404
  diagnostic capability, 404
  initial assessment, 404
  preparation, 404
  usage, 8
Ultrasound
  dating, reliability, 8
  diagnostic imaging, 296–297
Umbilical access, 93
Umbilical arterial catheters (UACs), presence, 200
Umbilical artery catheter, 294
  appearance, 296f
Umbilical artery catheterization (UAC), 315–317
Umbilical artery Doppler studies, 122
Umbilical blood sampling. *See* Percutaneous umbilical blood sampling
Umbilical catheters, usage (complications), 317–318
Umbilical cord
  care, 816
  clamping, 75
  compression, 24
  inspection, 146–147
Umbilical cord prolapse, 32–33
  assessment/management, 33
  clinical presentation, 32
  complications, 32–33
  etiology, 32

Umbilical cord prolapse *(Continued)*
fetal/neonatal complications, 32–33
incidence, 32
maternal complications, 32
predisposing factors, 32
Umbilical hernia, 132
Umbilical vein
catheterization, 317
oxygen flow, 72
Umbilical venous catheter, 294
Umbilical vessel catheterization
advance practice procedure, 314–318
catheter, malposition, 317
contraindications, 315
equipment/supplies, 315
indications, 314–315
insertion depth, calculation, 315–316
mechanical complications, 317
precautions, 315
procedure, 315
Umbilical vessel catheters, usage, 107
Umbilicus/umbilical cord, 591
Unbound substances, passive/facilitated diffusion, 20
Uncomplicated antepartum care, terminology, 1
Uncomplicated meconium ileus, surgical repair, 608
Unconjugated bilirubin, body compartment, 240
Unconjugated estriol (uE3), 403
Undescended testes, 132
Undescended testicles
(cryptorchidism), 744–745
clinical assessment, 744
clinical presentation, 744
complications, 745
diagnostic studies, 744
differential diagnosis, 745
disease states, 744
etiology, 744
incidence, 744
outcome, 745
patient care management, 745
physical examination, 744
University of Colorado Medical Center, newborn classification, 131f
Unplanned endotracheal extubations, 379
Unplanned extubations, 379
Upper airway disorders, 478–479
Upper-airway obstruction, 103
relief, 302
Upper extremities, numbness/tingling/weakness, 5
Upper-extremity pulses, 549
Upper GI series, 593
diagnostic imaging, 298
Upper respiratory tract, vascularity/vascular congestion (increase), 2

Urea cycle disorders, 197
Ureaplasma urealyticum colonization, 471
Ureteropelvic junction obstruction, 738
Urethra, stricture, 326
Urethral catheters, usage, 324–325
Urinary catheter tray, usage, 325
Urinary function, physiologic changes, 78
Urinary glucose, 179
Urinary meatus, position, 147–148
Urinary output, 576–577
decrease, 582
medication excretion, 243
Urinary system, maternal physiologic changes, 3–4
Urinary tract development, 725
Urinary tract infection (UTI), 739–740
clinical presentation, 739
diagnostic studies, 740
etiology, 739
incidence, 739
management, 740
neonatal infection, 707
outcome, 740
Urine
diagnostic evaluation, 704
dilution, 157
drug screen, 63t
drug screening, 64
osmolality, 158
output, 580
sample collection, 83
sampling, 256
Urodynamic changes, occurrence, 4
Uterine activity, measurement, 17
Uterine blood flow, maternal cardiac output, 23
Uterine contractions, impact, 75
Uterine involution, 17
Uterine relaxation, magnesium sulfate (IV administration), 29
Uteroplacental blood flow, 23–24
decrease, causes, 23–24
Uterus
blood flow, decrease, 23
enlargement, 30
size, determination, 8
Utilitarianism, 862
focus, 862
Uveal tract, 782

V

VA. *See* Venoarterial
Vaccine information statement (VIS), 249
Vaccines
contraindications, misconceptions, 250
documentation, requirements, 249

VACTERL. *See* Vertebral anomalies, anal atresia, cardiac abnormalities, tracheoesophageal fistula and/or esophageal atresia, renal agenesis and dysplasia, and limb defects
Vagina, hand examination, 33
Vaginal bleeding, 30
Vaginal CVS, 405
Vaginal secretions, fetal fibronectin test (performing), 29
Valproic acid, usage, 543
Vancomycin-resistant *S. aureus* (VRSA), 710
Varicella, 837
lesions, 194
Vascular abnormality, 122, 817
Vascular access sites, assessment, 820
Vascular anomalies, 825
Vascular disorders, 122
Vascular lesions, 823–826
Vascular markings, decrease, 285
Vascular nevi, 135
presence, 823
Vascular resistance, increase, 121
Vascular supply, development, 725
Vascular tunic. *See* Eyeball
Vasculogenesis, 840
Vasculopathy, progression, 26
Vasoconstriction
impact, 121
introduction, 464
Vasodilators, 245
Vasopressive agents, 245
Vasopressors, usage, 467–468
Vasoproliferation, 841
Vasoproliferative retinopathy, 840
Vasospasm, complication, 317
VATER. *See* Vertebral anomalies, anal atresia, tracheoesophageal fistula, and radial and renal dysplasia
VATERR. *See* Vertebral defects, imperforate Anus, TracheoEsophageal fistula and/or esophageal atresia, and Radial and Renal dysplasia
Vecuronium bromide (Norcuron), usage, 304
Vecuronium (Norcuron), usage, 516
Vegan mothers, infants (vitamin B_{12} supplementation), 187
VEGF, stimulation, 841
Velocardiofacial syndrome, 791–792
Venipuncture, 256, 261
complications, 322
contraindications, 321
equipment/supplies, 322
fundamental procedure, 321–322
indications, 321
precautions, 321–322
preference, 334
procedure, 322

Venoarterial (VA) bypass, institution, 526
Venoarterial (VA) perfusion, 522–523
  advantages, 523
  disadvantages, 523
  technique, 522–523
Venous access, 93
Venous cannula, size, 522
Venous catheterization, 314–315
Venous return
  decrease, 530
  servo-regulation, 525
Venovenous (VV) ECMO, oxygenation, 527
Venovenous (VV) perfusion, 523–524
  advantages, 523
  disadvantages, 524
  technique, 523
Ventilation. See Assist/control mode of ventilation; Assisted ventilation: Mechanical ventilation; Very low birth weight; Volume-targeted ventilation
  assessment, 107–108
  control, factors, 498b
  endotracheal tube, usage, 100–101
  weaning, 516–517
    process, nursing care, 517
Ventilation-perfusion ratio, 495
  impact. See Blood gas tension
Ventilation therapy
  bronchodilators, usage, 514
  corticosteroids, usage, 515
  diuretics, usage, 514–515
  iNO, usage, 516
  medications, usage, 513–516
  pain control/sedation, 516
  paralytic agents, usage, 515–516
Ventilator-associated pneumonia (VAP), 378
Ventilators
  breaths, present number, 501
  changes, effects, 506b
  circuits, prewarming, 116
  graphics, pattern change, 300
  manipulations, 458
  modes, 501–502
  selection, 504
  settings, reduction, 527
  waveforms, comparison, 505f
Ventilatory management, 522
Ventilatory support, maintenance, 438
Ventricles, blood volume, 541
  increase, 541
Ventricular contractility, 541
Ventricular septal defect (VSD), 26–27, 556–557
  anatomy, 556
  clinical manifestations, 557
  hemodynamics, 556–557
  incidence, 556
  management, 557

Ventricular septal defect (VSD) (Continued)
  prognosis, 557
  radiographic evaluation, 286
Ventricular septation, 537f
  result, 535
Vermont Oxford Network (VON), 364
  PBPs, offering, 371
Vernix caseosa, 135, 815
  absence, 131
  usage, 436
Vertebral anomalies, anal atresia, cardiac abnormalities, tracheoesophageal fistula and/or esophageal atresia, renal agenesis and dysplasia, and limb defects (VACTERL) association, 411, 590
  care management, 411
  clinical presentation, 411
  complications/outcome, 411
  etiology/precipitating factors, 411
  incidence, 411
Vertebral anomalies, anal atresia, tracheoesophageal fistula, and radial and renal dysplasia (VATER) association, 411
  care management, 411
  clinical presentation, 411
  complications/outcome, 411
  etiology/precipitating factors, 411
Vertebral defects, imperforate Anus, TracheoEsophageal fistula and/or esophageal atresia, and Radial and Renal dysplasia (VATERR), 590
Very low birth weight (VLBW), 106
  airway assist vehicles, 427
  hypothermia, 426–427
  infant, early discharge, 385
  inhaled nitric oxide, 427
  skin fragility, 427
  spinal immobilization, 427
  transport stabilization considerations, 426–427
  ventilation, 426
    devices, 427
Very low birth weight (VLBW) infants
  evaporative heat loss, 114
  feeding tolerance/intolerance, contraindications, 200–201
  fungal infections, risk, 826
  glucose renal threshold, 179
  management, considerations, 116–118
  protein requirements, 190
Vesicle, 817
  types, 828
Vesicoureteral reflux, 738
Vesicular rash, appearance, 826
Vesiculopustular lesions, rupture. See Superficial vesiculopustular lesions

Vestibular stimulation, recommendation, 214
Vestibule, 846
  sensory afferents, 846
Vestibulocochlear nerves, 846
Villi, edema (occurrence), 23
Viral infections, 713–719
  impact, 543–544
  transmission, mode, 713
  viral organisms, impact, 713–719
Virilized genitalia, management, 653–654
VIS. See Vaccine information statement
Visceromegaly, 177
Visual disturbances, 840
Visual impairments, 837
Visual system, animal models, 218–219
Vital capacity (VC), definition, 494
Vital signs
  assessment, 77
  changes, 300
  monitoring, 108
  parameters/clinical responses, assessment, 251
Vitamin A, pregnancy transfer, 185
Vitamin D
  deficiency, 194
  supplementation, AAP recommendation, 187
Vitamin E, pregnancy increase, 185
Vitamin K
  deficiency, 678
  pharmacologic antagonism, 679
Vitamin K1 (phytonadione)
  administration, 79
  deficiency, risk, 79
Vitamin K-dependent clotting factors, hepatic biosynthesis (promotion), 79
Vitreoretinal surgery, 844
Vitreous haze, 841
Vitreous humor, 833
VLBW. See Very low birth weight
Vocal cords
  identification, 305
  injury, 306
Voiding cystourethrogram (VCUG), 298
  usage, 730
Volume-cycled ventilator, 501
Volume expanders
  fluids, 102
  supply, 88
Volume support, 108
Volume-targeted ventilation, 502
von Willebrand disease, 685–686
VRSA. See Vancomycin-resistant S. aureus
VSD. See Ventricular septal defect
VV. See Venovenous

W

Wake County Hospital System v. National Casualty Co., 879
Ward stock, 377

Warfarin (Coumadin), usage, 543
Waste products, elimination, 72
Water, distribution, 156
Waterbeds, usage (avoidance), 216
Water bug, 711
WBCs. *See* White blood cells
Weak pulses, indication, 549
Weight conversion, 884
Weight gain, caloric intake (relationship), 580
Weight loss, 180
Wellbutrin, usage, 54
Wet lung disease, 277
Wheal, 817
White blood cells (WBCs), 669–670
  count, 670
    increase, 5
    interpretation difficulty, 701
  differential examination, 83
  types, 669–670
White pupil (leukocoria), 837
Whole blood, usage, 254
Whole-blood glucose screening test, 83
Witch's milk, 143

Withdrawal
  neonatal signs, 55t
  signs, evaluation, 58
Women, substance-use disorder
  characteristics, 65
    details, 66b
  psychologic profile, 65
    details, 66b
Wood corkscrew maneuver, usage, 34
Workforce, aging, 367

X

X-linked disorders, 401
X-linked dominant disorders, 401
  characteristics, 401
X-linked ichthyosis, 829
X-linked recessive disorders, 401, 657
  characteristics, 401
X-linked recessive inheritance, 685
X-linked situs inversus, 542
X-rays
  anatomic/pathologic changes, assessment, 273–274
  anteroposterior view, 271
    illustration, 271f

X-rays (*Continued*)
  beams, exit transmission, 297
  cross-table lateral view, 272
    illustration, 271f
  definition, 271
  delayed effects, 272
  early radiation effects, 272
  film, exposure assessment, 273
  film, interpretation, 272
  interpretation, 272–274
  labeling, 273
  lateral decubitus view, 272
    illustration, 271f
  personnel, risks, 272
  positioning, notation, 273
  views, usage. *See* Newborn infants

Y

Yellow tube (laboratory specimen tube), 258
Younger pregnant women, cigarette smoking (likelihood), 42

Z

Zavanelli maneuver, usage, 34